THERAPYED'S

National Physical Therapy Examination Review & Study Guide

SUSAN B. O'SULLIVAN, PT, EDD
Professor Emerita
Department of Physical Therapy
School of Health and Environment
University of Massachusetts Lowell
Lowell, Massachusetts

RAYMOND P. SIEGELMAN, PT, DPT, MS
President
TherapyEd
Evanston, Illinois

TherapyEd
Evanston, Illinois
United States of America

Library of Congress Control Number: 96-78846

ISBN: 978-0-9843393-4-1

The authors and contributors have made a faithful attempt to include relevant summaries of current physical therapy practice and other information at the time of publication. It is recognized that recommended practices, drug therapies, equipment, devices, governmental regulations, administrative procedures and other protocols and factors may change or be open to other interpretations. Therapists should take responsibility for updating their knowledge of technological advances, new information or conclusions available through publications, research, new regulations or guidelines.

The publisher disclaims any liability or loss incurred as a result of direct or indirect use of this book. Use of this book does not guarantee successful passage of the National Physical Therapy Examination.

Copies of this book and software may be obtained from:
TherapyEd
500 Davis Street, Suite 512
Evanston, IL 60201
Telephone (888) 369-0743
FAX (847) 328-5049
www.TherapyEd.com

Preface

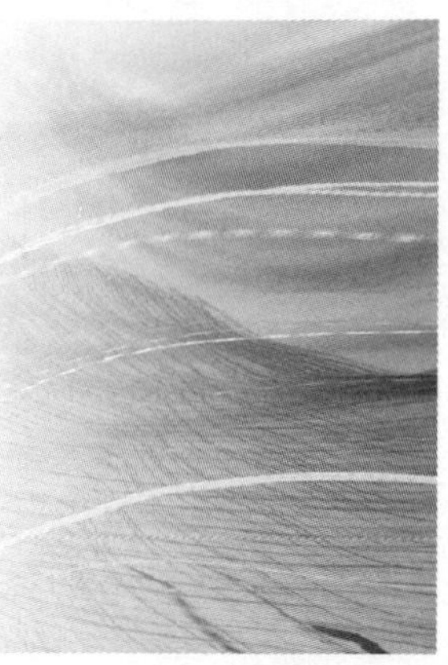

One of the final hurdles for physical therapists to become licensed to practice in the United States is successful completion of the National Physical Therapy Examination (NPTE). This exam often requires candidates to combine basic physical therapy knowledge with clinical experience in order to interpret, evaluate, or solve problems that may occur in clinical situations. In order to protect the public, licensing boards use NPTE results as the main resource to determine whether a candidate has demonstrated minimal standards necessary for safe and effective practice.

Since 1988, TherapyEd has offered Examination Preparatory Courses for physical therapists, physical therapist assistants, occupational therapists and occupational therapy assistants. The physical therapist and physical therapist assistant courses help exam candidates assess their strengths and weaknesses vis-à-vis NPTE expectations and help shape and focus their preparation. Building on the years of experience of both the organization and the authors and contributors, the *National Physical Therapy Examination Review & Study Guide* provides a comprehensive content review, practice tests, critical reasoning rationales, strategies for study, and review and licensure information. Practice tests help familiarize therapists with the format and type of questions to expect on the national exam.

The authors recognize that the Review & Study Guide is an ongoing project that is updated every year. We encourage and appreciate the feedback we have received from our many readers over the years. It is our hope that all exam candidates who use this book receive good news about their results and go on to reap the rewards of patient care and contribute to the development of physical therapy in the United States and throughout the world.

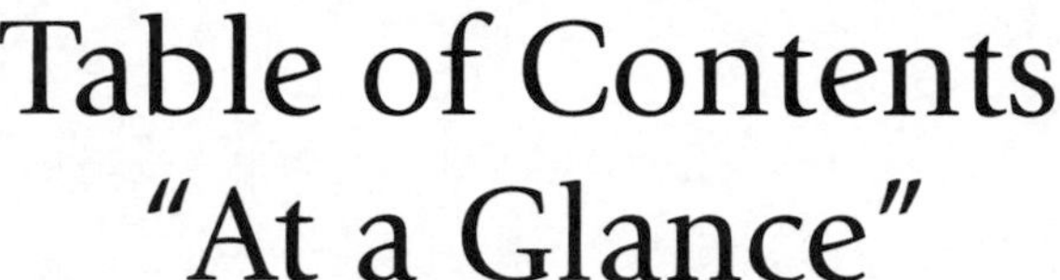

Table of Contents "At a Glance"

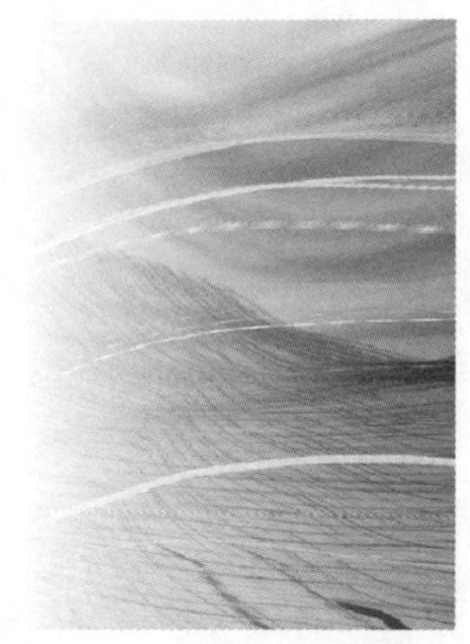

Table of Contents

Contributors

Thomas Bianco, PT, MSPT
President
Sensible Ergonomic Solutions
Wilbraham, Massachusetts

Suzanne Robben Brown, PT, MPH
Associate Professor and Director
School of Physical Therapy
Touro University Nevada
Henderson, Nevada

John Carlos, Jr., PT, PhD
Professor
Department of Physical Therapy and Associate Director
Behavioral Sciences Coordinator
Andrews University
Berrien Springs, Michigan

Sean Collins, PT, ScD, CCS
Associate Professor and Chair
Department of Physical Therapy
School of Health and Environment
University of Massachusetts, Lowell
Lowell, Massachusetts

Gerard J. Dybel, PT, ScD, GCS
Associate Professor
Department of Physical Therapy
School of Health and Environment
University of Massachusetts, Lowell
Lowell, Massachusetts

William Farina, PT, DPT, MBA, FACHE
Vice President for Rehabilitation Services
Radius Management Services
Framingham, Massachusetts

Rita P. Fleming-Castaldy, PhD, OTL, FAOTA
Associate Professor
Occupational Therapy Program
University of Scranton
Scranton, Pennsylvania

Kari Inda, OTR, PhD
Professional Entry Program Director
Professor
Occupational Therapy Department
Mount Mary College
Milwaukee, Wisconsin

Linda Kahn-D'Angelo, PT, ScD
Professor
Department of Physical Therapy
School of Health and Environment
University of Massachusetts, Lowell
Lowell, Massachusetts

L. Vincent Lepak III, PT, DPT, MPH, CWS
Assistant Professor
Division of Rehabilitation Sciences
University of Oklahoma Health Sciences Center
Tulsa, Oklahoma

Elizabeth Oakley, PT, DHSc, MSPT
Associate Professor
Department of Physical Therapy
Andrews University
Berrien Springs, Michigan

Robert Rowe, PT, DMT, MHS, FAAOMPT
Residency/Fellowship Program Manager
Brooks Health Systems
Jacksonville, Florida

Julie Ann Starr, DPT, MS, CCS
Clinical Associate Professor
Physical Therapy Program
Department of Rehabilitation Sciences
Sargent College of Health and Rehabilitation Sciences
Boston University
Boston, Massachusetts

Acknowledgements

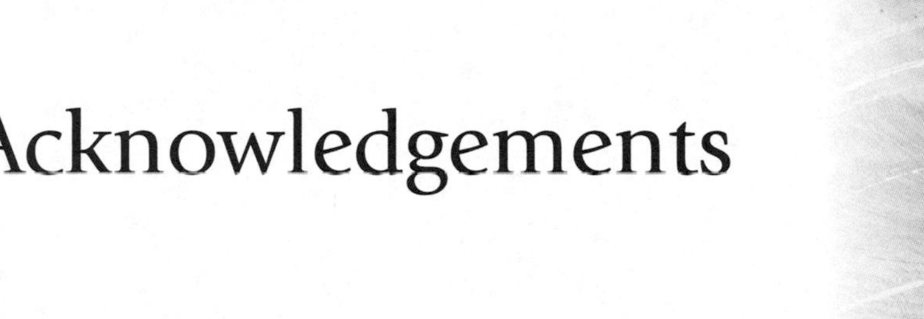

Al Beringer
Publishing Services
Cherry Hill, New Jersey

Harjeet Singh
Head: US Operations
Spearhead Group
Bear, Delaware

Surinder Sharma
Accounts Manager
Spearhead Group
Bear, Delaware

Kathleen McCullough
Copyeditor
Philadelphia, Pennsylvania

Ruth Ann Cassidy
President and Creative Director
Zographix, Inc.
Roseville, California

Laura Girardeau
Copyeditor
Pullman, Washington

Shannon Gleason
Copyeditor
Pullman, Washington

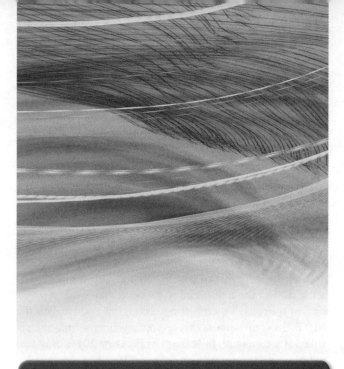

Introduction

RAYMOND P. SIEGELMAN

Purpose of This Book and Software

The *National Physical Therapy Examination Review & Study Guide* is designed to help physical therapist candidates prepare for the National Physical Therapy Examination (NPTE). Each chapter is presented in an easy-to-read outline format. Specific chapters focus on musculoskeletal, neuromuscular, cardiovascular, pulmonary, integumentary, psychological, and other aspects of physical therapy practice. Relevant anatomy, kinesiology, and pathophysiology of different diagnostic categories are briefly reviewed. Important medical, pharmacological, and surgical interventions are also identified. Each chapter reviews the elements of physical therapy practice, including: examination, evaluation of data, determination of an appropriate diagnosis, prognosis, plan of care, interventions, and reevaluation of interventions selected. Additional chapters focus on the professional roles assumed by the physical therapist: consultant, administrator, educator, and researcher. Chapters on pediatrics, geriatrics, therapeutic exercise, research and evidence-based practice, physical agents, and functional devices are also included.

It is vital for candidates to master the elements of physical therapy practice in order to apply the information to clinical situations. This book was developed to help you organize and focus your review efficiently and effectively. However, you may elect to pursue a more in-depth review of topics, terms, or procedures by referring to our recommended references.

The practice-exam software will help you assess your understanding of particular content areas and your ability to apply this knowledge to real-world situations. The practice exam format simulates the actual NPTE format, with a question counter and running clock on the top of the screen to help you keep track of your progress. The software also allows you to go back to questions you would like to review. When you are finished, the computer program will analyze your results and provide feedback to help you focus on areas for additional study.

At the back of the text are the question explanations along with critical reasoning rationales to help you understand how the answers were derived. Reading and interpreting these practice questions will also help prepare you for the various forms of multiple-choice questions you may encounter on the actual NPTE.

It is important to note that although the practice tests are designed to help you diagnose the strengths and weaknesses of your academic and clinical preparation, they should not be used to measure minimal entry-level competency or predict your score on the NPTE.

What Is the Procedure for Obtaining a License?

Licensure of healthcare practitioners protects the public from unsafe practices. In the U.S. and its territories, all physical therapists require a license to practice. Licensure is a function of state or territorial governments, not the federal government. It should be noted that physical therapist employees of the federal government are exempt from state regulation. However, a valid license in at least one state or jurisdiction is usually required by federal employers, such as the military or Public Health Service.

All jurisdictions require candidates to complete the NPTE successfully to obtain a license, but because the U.S. is made up of numerous states and governing entities, each state may have different requirements for you to become eligible to take the NPTE. Different states may also have different practice restrictions after you have passed the NPTE. These requirements can even differ within the same state, according to whether you graduated from a program accredited by the Commission on Accreditation in Physical Therapy Education (CAPTE). The CAPTE no longer accredits baccalaureate degree programs. In the

United States, all candidates must have graduated from an entry-level masters or doctoral program or an equivalent international program. Each state has sovereignty over physical therapy licensure and regulation. Contact the individual licensing board in your jurisdiction to obtain applications and information about requirements and procedures.

Jurisprudence Examination

Some states require candidates to pass a separate examination concerning the rules, regulations, and laws governing physical therapy practice in that state. Licensed therapists who wish to obtain another license when moving to another state may have to pass a jurisprudence examination if it is required by that state. The Federation of State Boards of Physical Therapy (FSBPT) administers some, but not all, jurisprudence exams.

Fees

All states require a fee to apply for and renew a license. There are separate fees to sit for the NPTE. Fees vary widely and can change yearly.

Special Accommodation

1. Candidates with documented current disabilities can apply to their jurisdiction for special accommodation during the NPTE.
2. Medical or health conditions that may require a snack, water, medications, visual aids, a reader, extra time, wheelchair placement and so on may be considered. Pregnancy without complications is not considered a disability by the ADA.
3. English as a second language is not considered a disability. No dictionaries or extra time will be granted.
4. Test anxiety and technophobia are not considered disabilities.
5. All accommodations must be approved at least 15 days before the exam date.
6. If special accommodation is denied, the jurisdiction may have an appeal process.

Other Requirements and Issues

Tests of English Language Proficiency. Various tests of spoken, written, or comprehended English may be required if English is not your first language. Standards and requirements differ from state to state. Personal interviews may also be required.

AIDS Awareness Training. Some states require AIDS awareness training for licensure.

Fingerprinting, FBI Check, Vaccination, Malpractice Insurance. One or more of these may be required by some jurisdictions.

Credentials Evaluation. Currently, most states require physical therapists educated outside of the United States who graduated from programs not accredited by CAPTE to submit transcripts and other credentials to approved agencies for evaluation. Credentials often include course content, credit hours, grades earned, and degrees granted. This process is required to establish eligibility to take the NPTE.

Supervised Practice Period. Some states may require therapists educated outside of the United States to undergo a period of supervised practice after successfully completing the NPTE. Permanent license is not granted until this supervised practice period is successfully completed.

Temporary License. Some states grant a temporary license to candidates eligible to take the NPTE. This temporary license allows the individual to practice under the supervision of a licensed therapist before taking and passing the NPTE. In some states, this temporary license may be revoked if a candidate fails the NPTE. As of 2011, only two states extend this temporary license if the candidate applies to retake the examination. In some states, if a temporary license is not offered, a physical therapist may *not* practice in that state until all requirements for licensure have been satisfied. In other states without a temporary license provision, applicants who have filed to take the exam may be allowed to practice under supervision of a licensed therapist. Therefore, it is prudent for you to keep current on the rules and regulations of the state(s) in which you wish to practice.

Transfer of Scores to Other Jurisdictions. All jurisdictions use the criterion referenced grading method, which standardizes exam scoring and allows transfer of passing scores. The Federation of State Boards of Physical Therapy (FSBPT) is responsible for score transfer (http://www.fsbpt.net/ptorg). For a fee, you may transfer your scores online or download the Score Transfer Request Form and mail the completed form to the FSBPT. If you maintain a license, you should not have to retake the NPTE if you move to a different state. However, if you are unlicensed, let your license lapse, or never took the examination, you will have to take the NPTE when seeking a license in that jurisdiction.

Retaking the Examination. Candidates may take the NPTE exam up to three times per 12-month period, which is the limit set by the FSBPT. A candidate never takes the same form of an exam he or she had previously taken. Some states allow only three opportunities to take the NPTE in total. If you fail, the state may impose a stipulation that you show evidence of remedial work or study before retaking the NPTE. The state licensure board has an obligation to protect the public from practitioners who do not demonstrate competency.

License Renewal. After 1, 2, or 3 years, a license must be renewed for a physical therapist to continue practicing. Renewal notices are sent out by the state or territory in which the therapist is practicing. Sometimes, renewal simply involves paying the fee and returning the form. However, some states require verification of continuing education units. If you fail to notify the state of a change of address and do not receive a renewal notice, fail to respond to renewal in a timely manner, or do not meet other requirements, your license could lapse. It is illegal to practice without a valid license. The state may require a number of conditions be met to reinstate a lapsed license. One condition might include retaking the NPTE even if you had previously passed the exam. *Inform the board of any change of address. Do not let your license lapse!*

Continuing Education or Active Practice. Many states require the physical therapist to acquire a specific number of continuing education units (CEUs) to renew a license. Documentation, approval, and reporting of CEUs vary from state to state. Some states require evidence of continuing active practice to renew. The FSBPT and the American Physical Therapy Association (APTA) are exploring alternative means to ascertain continued competency.

Endorsement. With a valid license in one state or jurisdiction, a physical therapist may apply to another state for a "license by endorsement." All criteria established by the new state must be met. This can include taking a jurisprudence exam for that state, attending interviews, providing letters of recommendation, taking English competency exams, attending AIDS awareness training, and accruing CEUs. Contact the licensure board in the state where licensure by endorsement is sought to get information and applications. Start the process early; it can take months.

How Is the NPTE Developed?

The FSBPT is the organization that develops and owns the NPTE. The exam is based on a survey of practice conducted periodically by the FSBPT, from which the "blueprint" for the exam is developed. Numerous clinicians, educators, and others contribute questions to the NPTE. Questions are designed to test knowledge and problem-solving skills that reflect current clinical practice and entry-level competency (defined as the first 6 months of practice). Various content experts and clinicians review the questions (item-reviewers). Finally, the FSBPT committees and psychometricians fine-tune the questions and construct the final exam blueprint. The APTA or the individual state licensing boards do not develop, oversee, or administer the NPTE.

Each examination adheres closely to the blueprint to fairly and comprehensively assess a candidate's competency to practice. The blueprint imparts a degree of stability, consistency, and continuity between different forms of the exam. However, each exam is a unique document with its own mix of questions. Questions are referenced to physical therapy textbooks in common use (a list of textbooks is available on fsbpt.org), and are not derived from a specific textbook or point of view. Terminology is consistent with that used in the *Guide to Physical Therapist Practice* and other commonly used texts.

NPTE Security Agreement

Each candidate who takes the NPTE must accept the NPTE Security Agreement. In part, this agreement states that it is illegal and unethical to recall (memorize) and share NPTE questions or solicit questions from candidates who have taken the exam. The FSBPT will continue to prosecute individuals who violate the security agreement.

What Areas Does the Exam Cover?

The exam places great emphasis on evaluation, plan of care, and interventions for a variety of patient/client problems. The exam also covers topics that are peripheral to direct patient care, often including professional roles in research, evidence-based practice, education, ethical decision-making, communication, administration, and other supporting activities. The exam is very comprehensive. Ensure that your preparation reflects the composition of the current exam. Naturally, not every item or sub-item listed here is covered in each examination. The NPTE currently consists of 250 questions, but only 200 questions count for your score. The additional 50 questions are used by the FSBPT to check their validity for future use. The content outline is based on the 200 questions that are scored.

The following information has been adapted from the NPTE Content Outline Federation of State Boards of Physical Therapy (effective March 2008, Copyright 2007). The use of category and domain designations is specific to the practice exams, and is used for the purposes of reporting your results.

Category A

Clinical Applications of Foundational Sciences (Pediatric and Adult): 29 Total Questions, or 14.5% of the NPTE

- Anatomy and Physiology of Systems
- Pharmacology as Related to Specific Systems
- Effects of Activity and Exercise
- Physiological Response to Environmental Factors and Aquatic Therapy
- Motor Learning and Control
- Cognition, Affect, Arousal, and Memory (neuromuscular questions only)
- Joint Structure and Function (musculoskeletal questions only)
- Normal Interrelationships among Multiple Systems (multiple system involvement questions only)

Category A: Number of Questions by System

Domain I.
Cardiac, Vascular, Lymphatic, and Pulmonary — 5 questions
Domain II.
Musculoskeletal — 6 questions
Domain III.
Neuromuscular — 6 questions
Domain IV.
Integumentary — 3 questions
Domain V.
Metabolic/Endocrine — 2 questions
Gastrointestinal — 1 question
Genitourinary — 1 question
Multiple System Involvement — 5 questions

Category B

Examination of the Patient/Client (Pediatric and Adult): 26 Total Questions, or 13% of the NPTE

- Tests and Measures and Their Application
- Information Collected During Systems Review and History
- Kinesiology/Kinematics (musculoskeletal and neuromuscular only)
- Movement Analysis (including gait deviations, prosthetic/orthotic gait deviations, thoracic excursion [pulmonary only], friction, pressure, shear, and scar ([integumentary only])
- Physiological Response to Tests and Measures

Category B: Number of Questions by System

Domain I.
Cardiac, Vascular, Lymphatic, and Pulmonary — 4 questions
Domain II.
Musculoskeletal — 9 questions
Domain III.
Neuromuscular — 9 questions
Domain IV.
Integumentary — 3 questions
Domain V.
Metabolic/Endocrine — 1 question
Gastrointestinal — 0 questions
Genitourinary — 0 questions
Multiple System Involvement — 0 questions

Category C

Foundations for Evaluation, Differential Diagnosis, and Prognosis (Pediatric and Adult): 47 Total Questions, or 23.5% of the NPTE

- Interpretation of Knowledge (regarding conditions, diseases, and pathologies to ensure safe, appropriate, and effective patient/client management decisions)
- Differential Diagnosis
- Diagnostic Imaging
- Medical/Surgical Management
- Impact of Comorbidities or Coexisting Conditions Affecting Multiple Systems
- Psychiatric or Psychological Conditions (multiple system involvement only)
- Conditions or Pathologies Affecting Connective Tissue (musculoskeletal only)

Category C: Number of Questions by System

Domain I.
Cardiac, Vascular, Lymphatic, and Pulmonary — 7 questions
Domain II.
Musculoskeletal — 10 questions
Domain III.
Neuromuscular — 9 questions
Domain IV.
Integumentary — 3 questions
Domain V.
Metabolic/Endocrine — 3 questions
Gastrointestinal — 2 questions
Genitourinary — 2 questions
Multiple System Involvement — 11 questions

Category D

Interventions (Pediatric and Adult): 37 Total Questions, or 18.55% of the NPTE

- Selection, Types, Sequencing, and Application of Appropriate Interventions
- Physiological Response to Interventions
- Complications or Secondary Effects of Interventions
- Motor Control and Motor Learning (neuromuscular system only)
- Wound Management Techniques (including topical agents, debridement, and dressings [integumentary only])
- Genitourinary Interventions (including biofeedback, bladder programs, and pelvic floor retraining)

Category D: Number of Questions by System

Domain I.
Cardiac, Vascular, Lymphatic, and Pulmonary — 7 questions
Domain II.
Musculoskeletal — 11 questions
Domain III.
Neuromuscular — 10 questions
Domain IV.
Integumentary — 5 questions
Domain V.
Metabolic/Endocrine — 2 questions
Gastrointestinal — 1 question

Genitourinary	1 question
Multiple System Involvement	0 questions

Category E

Equipment, Devices, and Modalities (Pediatric and Adult): 22 Total Questions, or 11% of the NPTE

- Selection and Application of Devices and Equipment for Patient Management
- Assistive, Supportive, Protective, and Adaptive Devices
- Prosthetics
- Orthotics
- Bariatric Equipment and Devices
- Gravity-Assisted Devices (e.g., body weight support locomotor training)
- Principles of and Justification for Therapeutic Modalities
- Indications, Precautions, and Contraindications for Modality Use
- Physical Agents (including sound, light, hydrotherapy, thermotherapy, cryotherapy, and athermal agents)
- Mechanical Modalities (such as compression, traction, and motion devices [CPM])
- Electrical Stimulation (including TENS, NMES, HVPC, and FES)

Category E: Number of Questions by Category

Equipment and Devices	10 questions
Modalities	12 questions

Category F

Teaching and Learning; Research and Evidence-Based Practice; Safety, Protection, and Emergencies; Healthcare Roles: 39 Questions, or 19.5% of the NPTE

- Teaching and Learning Theories, Strategies, and Techniques (including motor learning and cognitive models of education, for patient/client management)
- Effective Communication with Patients/Clients
- Health Behavior Change Models (such as positive reinforcement)
- Qualitative and Quantitative Interpretation of Research Design
- Common Statistical Methods of Measurement (including reliability and validity)
- Outcome Measures
- Types of Data Collection (such as surveys and observation)
- Evidence Hierarchy (including randomized control studies, cohort studies, and case studies)
- Injury Prevention and Patient/Client Safety (including fall risk, environmental factors, restraints, and equipment-related issues)
- Infection Control (including standard/universal precautions)
- Use of Proper Body Mechanics
- Emergency First Aid and CPR
- Response to Emergency Situations and Disasters
- Patient/Client Rights (including HIPAA, IDEA, ADA, DNR, and advance directives)
- Reporting Neglect or Abuse
- Legal Issues (relating to OSHA, sexual harassment, or other human resource problems)
- Standards of Documentation
- Risk Guidelines (including accident reporting and policies and procedures)
- Roles and Responsibilities (of support staff, students, and other healthcare practitioners)

Category F: Number of Questions by Category

Teaching, Learning, and Communication:	11 questions
Research and Evidence-Based practice:	13 questions
Safety, Protection, Emergencies, and Healthcare Roles:	15 questions

What Is the Procedure for Taking the Exam?

To start the process of preparing for the exam, contact the licensing agency in the state or jurisdiction in which you wish to apply for a license. Return the completed application to the appropriate agency. If you are eligible, the FSBPT will send you an "Authorization to Test" letter. Once you are eligible, you should receive information about how to contact Prometric to establish your test location. You may contact the FSBPT Examination Services by phone at (703) 739-9420 to check on the status of your application or inquire about other general information. Note that you are *not* required to take the exam in the state where you seek a license. You may take the NPTE in any Prometric Center in the United States. (See Box A for an outline of these steps).

Determine the exam site for your exam. If it is necessary to travel the day before and seek lodging, make arrangements in advance. Plan to arrive at the exam site early. You *must* arrive at least 30 minutes *before* your scheduled examination. Bring a map or use GPS (you can also get directions at www.2test.com), know the traffic patterns (including rush hour times), and bring money to cover possible parking fees.

Test Dates

Prior to 2011, a system of open-ended, continuous computer-based testing existed for taking the NPTE. Security breaches and item sharing among candidates compromised exam questions, possibly endangering the public and

Box A ➤ PROCEDURE FOR REGISTERING FOR THE EXAM

1. Contact the appropriate board or agency in the jurisdiction (state, district, territory) where you seek a license once you are eligible to take the exam.
2. Complete the application materials. If you are a new graduate or soon-to-be a new graduate, your academic program must certify your eligibility. *Do this as soon as possible.*
3. Register for the exam at the FSBPT website (*http://www.fsbpt.org*) as soon as you can. The registration deadline is *30 days prior to the exam date you wish to take.* There is a fee.
4. If the jurisdiction approves your eligibility, they must notify the Federation no later than 15 days prior to the scheduled exam. If the jurisdiction does not notify the Federation in time, you will not get an "Authorization to Test" letter for the exam date you requested.
5. If you receive an "Authorization to Test" letter, you will be instructed to contact Prometric to schedule the site where you wish to take the NPTE.
6. You do not have to take the exam in the jurisdiction where you seek a license. You may take it at any Prometric Center in another jurisdiction. Contact Prometric at *www.prometric.com. Do this as soon as possible after receiving the ATT letter. Some sites may fill up rapidly, and you may have to choose alternative sites that involve travel or overnight stays.*

eroding confidence in the testing procedure. Therefore, the Federation of State Boards of Physical Therapy (FSBPT) implemented fixed-date testing for all candidates. The number of fixed dates is limited, and all questions will be new on each form of the exam.

Fixed NPTE dates for 2012

January 30th (Monday)
March 29th (Thursday)
July 2nd (Monday)
July 31st (Tuesday)
October 23rd (Tuesday)

Candidates with documented disabilities may receive special accommodation during the exam. Special seating, extra time, a reader, and other considerations are possible. Any special accommodation must be approved in advance by the licensing board.

Prometric personnel will orient you regarding exam procedures. A tutorial before the exam should familiarize you with keyboard commands and other functions. We urge you to take the tutorial and ask for clarification of any detail before the start of the exam. If you are dissatisfied with the lighting, seating, ability to read the computer screen, noise levels, or other factors, request a change to another computer

Box B ➤ TEST CENTER PROCEDURES

1. Check in at least 30 minutes prior to the exam. When you arrive at the exam site, visit the restroom before you check in. The whole examination procedure can last up to 6 hours. You may use the restroom during breaks.
2. Remember to bring proper identification and your "Authorization to Test" letter, since you will not be allowed to take the exam without either of them. Two forms of identification are required. One must be a government-issued photo ID such as a passport and driver's license. Another can be an ID preprinted with your name and signature, such as a credit card. Social Security cards are not accepted. IDs will be scanned. *Your first and last names on the IDs must be the same as the names on the "Authorization to Test" letter. If there is any problem with the IDs, you will not be allowed to take the exam. All fees will be forfeited, and you will have to reschedule for the next fixed date.* Photocopies of identification are not acceptable.
3. You will be fingerprinted and photographed. All testing sessions are videotaped. If you leave the testing room for any reason (e.g, visit the restroom), you will be fingerprinted again.
4. You may request a dry erase board to make notes. You may not bring in your own scratch paper. The boards will be collected when you leave the testing center.
5. Personal items such as eyeglasses/contacts and medications are allowed. Some comfort items such as tissues or mints may be allowed.
6. Earplugs are not permitted. Prometric will supply sound dampening headphones upon request. Keep in mind that background noise may be distracting.
7. A locker will be provided for personal items. The locker cannot be accessed during the exam.
8. Wear multi-layer clothing to stay comfortable in various room temperatures. Jackets with pockets, "hoodie" sweatshirts, hats or scarves are not permitted. If you remove a sweater or outer shirt, you must wrap it around your waist. These items cannot be placed on the back of a chair or elsewhere in the testing room. If you must wear a head covering for health or religious reasons, you must receive approval before the testing date. Prometric personnel cannot grant approval on site.
9. No electronic devices of any kind (such as cell phones, MP3 players, digital watches) are allowed in the testing room. They must be put in the locker.
10. Eat a good meal before taking the exam. Food or drink is officially not allowed at the computer cubicle during the examination. At some centers, water may be available in the reception area, or you may keep your own drink there.
11. You may not talk or read aloud during the exam.

cubicle *before* the exam starts. Contact Prometric personnel immediately if there is any computer malfunction.

Test-Taking Strategies

The exam is divided into sections of 50 questions each. The sections are balanced in terms of the content covered on the exam blueprint. Once you have completed a section and you take a break, you may not go back to any questions in that section. However, before you complete any section, you may review marked questions and change answers, if you wish. The computer screen shows a running clock of your remaining time to complete the exam. There will be a scheduled break of 15 minutes when the clock is stopped. During other breaks, the clock will run. You may also choose not to take a break. If you complete the exam before the allocated time, you may leave early.

During the exam, you may electronically mark questions you have skipped or wish to review at a later time. We do not recommend skipping questions. Answer each question to the best of your ability. Use educated guesses if you must. Guessing is not penalized. If time permits, use the computer review commands to return to previously marked items. Answers may be changed if necessary. If in doubt, stick with your original choice. Return to the marked questions before you exit each section. Once you exit a section of the exam, you cannot return to that section.

Time management is crucial. There are 250 items to answer in a 5-hour period not counting breaks. This amounts to a time allotment of just over one minute per question. You must complete an average of 50 questions per hour to finish all of the examination questions. When you have completed the first 50 questions, check the running clock on the computer screen. Have you completed them in an hour or less? If not, you must increase your pace or you may not get to answer all of the questions. Check again at questions #100 and #150. Some people prefer to check the computer clock at the end of each hour and note the number of questions answered. Either way, pace yourself properly.

Also keep in mind that during the third hour of the examination, reading skills tend to deteriorate and it may take longer to process each question. If English is your second language, you should think in English when answering questions. Otherwise, it may be very difficult to finish the examination on time, and this could also cause interpretation errors.

What should you do if there are only two minutes left and you have not answered all of the questions? Do not leave anything blank. Quickly choose answers for each question, even if you have not had a chance to read them all. Since there is no penalty for entering incorrect answers, you may be lucky and get a few correct! Over the years, many candidates have been unsuccessful on the NPTE because of failure to budget their time properly.

Once the exam has begun, communicate only with Prometric personnel. An innocent remark to a nearby test-taker or glancing at another computer screen might be mistaken for an attempt to cheat. Candidates attempting to cheat can face serious consequences. Trying to obtain a physical therapy license by fraudulent means is a crime. Don't even think about doing it.

How Is the NPTE Graded, and How Are Scores Reported?

The FSBPT employs criterion-referenced performance standards. Using this system, a test score is interpreted in terms of an individual's mastery of a specified content domain. A passing criterion or standard is established by the FSBPT for each examination. A candidate must reach or exceed the designated cut score of competency to pass the exam. The cut score represents the minimal acceptable level of exam performance consistent with safe and effective practice expected of physical therapists. A panel of physical therapy content experts establishes the passing score after screening questions for performance characteristics and bias. The examinee's performance is not compared with the performance of others who took the same test. Each form of the NPTE has its own criterion-referenced passing grade, and these may vary from exam to exam. Grading on a curve, using a fixed percentage, and using the number of questions answered correctly are methods that are not used to determine passing scores.

Reporting of grades to candidates can be confusing. Scaled scores, rather than the absolute number of questions answered correctly (raw score), are reported to candidates. The scaled scoring range is from 200–800, with 600 always reflecting the cut score. For example, if the passing raw score is determined to be 149 out of 200 questions for an exam, this would equal a scaled score of 600. If a candidate achieved a score of 600 or better, the state licensing board would notify the candidate of his or her success and issue a license provided that all other conditions were satisfied.

Some states still convert the passing scaled score to another system based on the number 70 or 75. Your score can be reported as being above or below the number 70 or 75. This does not mean that you scored above or below 70% or 75% or correctly or incorrectly answered 70 or 75 questions. It is merely an arbitrary numbering system used to denote a pass/fail line.

Planning Your Exam Review

After you have completed your entry-level physical therapy education, you bring all of your academic and clinical experiences to the table in preparation for the NPTE. Four to six weeks of structured independent review should be adequate. More time might be necessary for candidates who are not native English speakers or for candidates who were not educated through an APTA accredited program.

Candidates with learning disabilities might require more preparation time because the processing of information may be slower. Most candidates probably do not need to take a lengthy refresher/remedial course. However, a Licensure Examination Preparatory course, such as the type offered since 1988 by TherapyEd, can be quite helpful. Extensive student feedback has indicated that this type of preparation course, when used in combination with this text, is an effective tool to provide information about current exam expectations and trends. The course manual and additional means of self-assessment provide even more focus and direction for exam preparation.

Please show respect for the examination process. Procrastination, skimpy review, and lack of understanding about the nature of the NPTE could lead to disappointing results. The expenses incurred to retake the examination, along with the potential loss of income because of failure to obtain a license, are significant. If you are unsuccessful, your self-esteem may take a mighty blow.

Discipline. About a month or two before your scheduled exam, establish a routine and spend 6 days per week reviewing material. Set up realistic and potentially achievable short-term goals as to what you wish to accomplish each day. Take one day off per week to pursue interests other than physical therapy. Give yourself a break! When you are reviewing, however, allot 2 to 3 hours of uninterrupted study time each day. Study in a quiet and well-lit space. Do not study when you are tired or ill. If you work during the week, weekends may give you more flexibility and time for review.

If you break your routine, add compensatory time. Answer the computer-based sample questions as a means of diagnosing strengths and weaknesses. Trying to memorize hundreds of sample questions and rationales is not a satisfactory means of preparation. Practice questions serve as templates for a multitude of item possibilities and primarily serve as diagnostic tools. You must review basic physical therapy knowledge and be able to apply that knowledge to a variety of problems, settings, circumstances, and situations. Some individuals may benefit from small group study sessions.

Although the review is for the purpose of passing the NPTE, we have received feedback through the years that this retrospective overview of one's physical therapy education has helped to sharpen and focus many aspects of clinical practice as well.

Analysis of Strengths and Weaknesses

A "shotgun" approach to exam preparation is not the best way to use your time. Try to form a composite picture of your physical therapy education and experiences.

Academic Program. Even accredited physical therapist programs can vary widely in terms of the quantity and quality of the content covered. Many programs are superb. Others may have problems with curricula or faculty. There could be a lack of emphasis on content that might be important for the NPTE. Be sure to request a copy of your school's report on performance of previous classes on the exam according to the exam blueprint. Some information is available at the FSBPT website.

Consider which content areas were presented in a comprehensive manner and which areas left something to be desired. Were there any gaps in your basic preparation that may be emphasized on the NPTE? Will this require you to spend more time gathering or reviewing information in these areas? Were academic standards poorly enforced, were grades inflated, or were some marginal students given social promotions to help enhance their self-esteem or the status of the program? Your study plan should compensate for weaknesses in your academic program, since the NPTE conforms to a standard outside the academic setting.

Classroom Performance. Generally, strong classroom performers with good English skills should fare well on the NPTE *as long as they take the time to prepare properly*. Students who performed marginally in their program, whose basic physical therapy education program lacked rigor, or whose English skills are not well developed are often disappointed when they receive NPTE results.

Clinical Experiences/Affiliations. If the range of clinical experiences was limited in terms of settings, patient populations, types of treatments, or degree of responsibility, exam candidates may have difficulty answering questions that require the application of clinical knowledge or judgment. For example, an exam candidate with no clinical exposure in such areas as prosthetics, cardiac rehabilitation, or wound or burn care may have difficulty in reaching conclusions requiring systems review, evaluation, outcome projection, or interventions in these areas. Many NPTE questions require an amalgam of clinical experience and academic knowledge to solve problems. Selected use of the *Guide to Physical Therapist Practice* may prove helpful in areas of deficient clinical preparation. Specific practice patterns, examinations, goals, interventions, and outcomes may be delineated.

Analysis of Sample Question Results. At appropriate times, you should attempt to answer the practice questions in the simulated exams in the accompanying software. The computer scoring will assist you in identifying content areas, domains, and critical reasoning categories in which your performance was good and those areas that need more work. This analysis can serve as a basis for structuring further study and review. After taking the exams, be sure to read the rationale and critical reasoning strategies for the practice exam questions in the *Review & Study Guide*.

Based on your personal analysis, write down areas of weakness and try to rank order them in terms of which areas might require the most remedial work. Set priorities based on the Content Outline, *Guide to Physical Therapist Practice,* 2nd edition, and expectations of the examination. Keep in mind that the NPTE emphasis is primarily on entry-level knowledge and judgment.

Levels of Question Difficulty

The NPTE attempts to ascertain how a candidate deals with a variety of different situations to determine how the applicant would function in the role of a physical therapist in a clinical setting. Most of the questions require problem solving at the upper levels of cognitive functioning (see Box C: Levels of NPTE Exam Questions).

Methods of Reading Multiple-Choice Questions

Carefully read the stem of each question. What is the focus of the question? Think about the information using your knowledge as well as your judgment. Then read each choice carefully. Begin the process by eliminating one option at a time. Every time you are able to rationalize eliminating an incorrect option, the odds of answering the question correctly increase dramatically. Be careful; sometimes options have some correct information that does not apply to the question asked. If the stem of the question is long or involved, you might wish to read the options first. This may help you focus better on the relevance of the information presented.

As the exam progresses, your reading skills may tend to deteriorate. You may have to rest your eyes for a minute or stand up and walk away from the computer screen for a short time. If your mind is no longer processing information properly, you may answer questions incorrectly that you normally would get right. Stop and rest for a few moments until you can refocus on the question. You might have to take a longer break after you complete a section.

Strategies for Answering Multiple-Choice Questions

1. Look for opposites in the list of options. These are the extremes of a concept, such as positive/negative, inversion/eversion, hypoglycemia/hyperglycemia, or spasticity/flaccidity. Examine opposites first. If you cannot eliminate both of them immediately, there is a good chance that one is the correct answer. If you can eliminate both opposites right away, the chances drop to 50/50 for selecting the correct response from the remaining two choices.
2. Identify choices that are so similar that it is difficult to choose between them. These may be choices that say the same thing in slightly different ways. If you cannot discriminate between them, it is possible that both are incorrect. For example, if one option in a question is "the primary muscle of inspiration," and another choice in the same question is "the diaphragm," they both say the same thing and need to be eliminated. Sometimes a choice that is unique but not far-fetched merits greater consideration than others.
3. Identify clues in the stem that may be helpful in focusing your thoughts. For example, a question presents a recently discharged patient who can transfer independently, but cannot ambulate independently for more than 20 feet. Your judgment should lead you to conclude that the patient is probably homebound. A response requiring outpatient management, use of a therapeutic pool, or elaborate therapeutic exercise equipment might be inappropriate.
4. Look for key words or phrases in the stem. If you see **best, most important, first,** or **primary,** you will need to set priorities. All of the choices could correctly answer the question; however, you must go through a process of rank ordering and elimination to reach the best option. Try to eliminate any obvious, unrealistic choices first, and work backwards toward what you consider to be the top priority.
5. Look for overlapping facts in the options. If you ascertain that a fact or statement in one option is incorrect, and you see the same fact or statement in another option, both choices can be eliminated. For example, given a patient problem, two options in the question are (1) pallor and diaphoresis and (2) tachycardia and diaphoresis. If you determine that diaphoresis is never a sign of the problem with choice (1), then you must automatically eliminate choice (2) as well.
6. Identify options that are crucial for the survival or safety of the patient. These always receive a high priority. You should give less credibility to responses that provide false reassurance to the patient, are overly optimistic, or do not address the patient's or family's feelings. Also give less credibility to responses in which the therapist gives away decision-making capability or responsibility to other health care workers. Consider abdicating responsibility if there is a medical situation outside of the scope of practice for physical therapists, or if the therapist does not possess the skills to treat a particular type of patient problem.
7. Look for negative words or phrases in the stem. Phrases and words such as **least important, not,** and other negatives denote that you must search for an answer that is false, unacceptable, low priority, or contraindicated. Negative words are often in bold type. If you consider each choice as either *true* or *false* relative to the scenario presented, you should end up with three *trues* and one *false*, and therefore be able to answer the question. The

Box C ➤ LEVELS OF NPTE EXAM QUESTIONS

QUESTION LEVEL AND DESCRIPTION

1. Knowledge
   Recall of basic information such as characteristics of diagnoses, spinal cord level functionality, wheelchair measurements, shapes of joints and so on.

   Relevance to the NPTE
   A solid knowledge foundation of all information related to entry-level PT practice is required to answer various scenarios proposed on NPTE questions.
   It is HIGHLY UNLIKELY that any NPTE questions are solely at this level. Ready recall of this information is needed in order to help solve advanced-level questions.

   NPTE Exam Preparation Strategy
   A strong commitment to studying is needed to remember all the relevant information acquired during PT entry-level education. This is a short-term goal of about 2 months. Fortunately, this Review & Study Guide (and the Course Manual, if you took a TherapyEd prep course) provides extensive information in an outline format to make your review easier.

2. Comprehension
   Understanding of basic information to determine significance, consequences or implications. For example, the impact of a tenodesis grasp on function or the possible consequences of using aquatic therapy for a group of patients with multiple sclerosis.

   Relevance to the NPTE
   The NPTE is not a matching test. Therefore, you must do more than recall information to succeed on the exam; you must have a firm grasp of content to understand the nuances and meaning of the questions. This may be the "who, what, where, when and how" of the question.

   NPTE Exam Preparation Strategy
   When reviewing foundational knowledge, think about why this information might be important. Studying with a peer/study group and explaining to the group the relevance, significance, consequences and implications of the study material may help you master it. Having a family member or friend quiz you on basic information may help you determine your ability to "think on your feet." Don't enter the test without strong comprehension abilities in all major areas of PT practice.

3. Application
   Use of information and application of rules, procedures or theories to new situations. For example, how to apply ergonomic principles to modify a work station for someone with bilateral carpal tunnel syndrome.

   Relevance to the NPTE
   The NPTE requires one to integrate knowledge and comprehension as well as competencies developed during clinical experiences in order to best answer a practice scenario. Many NPTE questions should be at this level, since a main goal of the exam is to assess the candidate's ability to respond competently to different situations.

   NPTE Exam Preparation Strategy
   If your knowledge and comprehension are solid in all major domains of the exam as put forth in this Review & Study Guide, take one of the computer-based practice exams that accompany this text. The challenging questions follow the format of the NPTE. Use your results to determine areas of academic, clinical and reasoning strengths and weaknesses.

4. Analysis
   Recognition of interrelationships between principles and interpretation or evaluation of data presented. For example, the most beneficial focus for discharge planning sessions for a parent and an adolescent with acquired traumatic brain injury.

   Relevance to the NPTE
   The NPTE assumes that test-takers have mastery and comprehension of entry-level knowledge and can apply it competently in diverse situations. Therefore, expect to analyze and respond to ambiguous situations. Direct "textbook answers" may not apply, which causes problems for some concrete thinkers. Many items are at this level, since the main objective of the exam is to determine competency in complex practice or ethical situations. In other words, practice your ability to think "outside of the box" to solve problems in real-world situations.

   NPTE Exam Preparation Strategy
   Use the analyses of the practice exams to reflect on your reasoning and judgment. Critically review the explanations for each question that you struggled with. Use peer or study groups to help determine gaps in analyses of exam questions. Ascertain what actions to take regarding deficiencies in critical reasoning skills to adequately prepare for the complexities of the NPTE.

   Modified and adapted with permission from the National Occupational Therapy Certification Examination Review & Study Guide, 5th edition by Rita Fleming-Castaldy

Box D ➤ GENERAL STRATEGIES FOR ANSWERING NPTE ITEMS

- Read the exam item carefully but quickly before selecting a response.
- Read the exam item for key words that set a priority.
- Use knowledge of medical terminology to decipher unknown words using prefixes, suffixes and root words.
- Employ *relevant* clinical experience. Do not call on unusual or atypical cases.
- Apply clinical reasoning skills to determine the relevance of the information in the question (diagnosis, setting, intervention, theoretical principles).
- Check the answer to see if it is theoretically, diagnostically and developmentally consistent with the item scenario.
- Choose patient/client-centered actions that focus on the emotional well-being of the person, if they are relevant to the question.
- Eliminate choices that contain contraindications (unless asked for a contraindication) and unsafe options.
- Use both your academic knowledge and clinical judgment to support your answer.
- Work rapidly but accurately. Time management is an important criterion for success.
- The NPTE is a five-hour exam. Fight fatigue and eye strain.
- Exam boredom can be a factor, especially after you have answered 200 questions, with 50 more to go. Losing interest in reading and answering questions can cost you points.

false choice would be the correct answer if you categorized everything appropriately. These types of negative questions are becoming less common on the NPTE.

8. Don't look for a particular pattern of answers that would cause you to alter a choice you believe to be correct. For instance, do not eliminate a correct choice because you chose the same letter or number choice as a response in the item immediately preceding the one you are currently answering. Questions are selected and randomly placed in the exam. Don't look for or think about answer patterns.
9. Don't overanalyze a question. Read the question at face value. Don't go outside of the gist of the information in the stem of the question to reach a conclusion. Sufficient information should be available. Adding your own hypothetical conditions to the situation presented could lead you in the wrong direction.
10. Some questions may present graphic or visual representations with an accompanying question. These may include x-rays; wounds; ECG readouts; therapists performing various tests, measures, or interventions; or depictions of patients with impairments such as scoliosis or amputations. A useful strategy for these types of questions is to look at the choices first. With the choices in mind, look at the graphic representation next, and finally look at the question. Looking at the choices first may help you focus on the aspect of the graphic representation that may be most relevant to answer the question.

Final Review

A review consisting of *just* answering or memorizing sample questions is often unsatisfactory, since the sample questions in the accompanying computer software are not actual NPTE questions. These questions are meant to be used for diagnostic or learning purposes. Although some questions on the NPTE may seem similar to the practice questions, the NPTE questions may have entirely different answers. You most likely will also encounter some questions on the actual NPTE that have a different focus than the practice exam questions.

Your final review should refocus on the areas that are emphasized on the NPTE and that you have identified as areas of personal weakness. You may wish to retake the practice exams, if time permits.

Box E ➤ STRATEGY REVIEW FOR ANSWERING MULTIPLE-CHOICE ITEMS

- Identify the question theme. What is the question really asking?
- Avoid reading "into" the question. Don't make up a story. Read the question, and nothing but the question.
- Identify choices that are equally plausible. If two choices say basically the same thing, eliminate them both.
- Carefully consider opposites. If you cannot eliminate both right away, one may be the correct answer.
- More than one choice may correctly answer the question. Choose the one that is MOST correct.
- In most cases, select positive, active choices rather than passive, negative ones.
- When changing an answer, make sure you have a good reason to eliminate your original choice, and an even better reason to make a new choice. Don't let second-guessing talk you out of the correct answer.

The Day Before the Exam

The day before the examination, make sure you have gathered all necessary documents, materials, medications, eyeglasses, and personal items you may need. It will heighten your anxiety to look for these things on the day of the exam. Do not use medications such as antihistamines or muscle relaxants, drink alcohol, or use other substances that may affect your alertness. Do not "cram" or stay up late the night before, reviewing material. Do not go to a party the night before the exam. (After it's over, OK)! Try to get a good night's sleep. On the day of the test, eat a meal before the exam. You may not have the opportunity to eat again for many hours. Finally, allow extra time to arrive at the test site in case travel is delayed.

Expect to be a little nervous. Prometric personnel are trained to put you at ease and explain what will happen. However, if you are unrealistic in your expectations at the testing site, Prometric personnel may react negatively to your demands. This will not put you in the proper frame of mind to take the NPTE. Also, if you are overly anxious, your ability to process questions and recall information could be impaired. Anxiety can also lead you to dwell more on the consequences of the exam rather than the questions presented. Practice relaxation strategies you find helpful. If you have disciplined yourself to review material thoroughly, you should feel confident, and there is more likelihood of a positive outcome.

The Role of Critical Reasoning in Your Performance

Critical reasoning is an important part of NPTE preparation. At this moment, you have achieved a certain level of critical reasoning skill that has helped you succeed in academic and clinical arenas. Critical reasoning skills are the foundation for how we reason the situations we encounter in everyday life. We often do not acknowledge how important this implicit skill is for exam success.

It is important to define critical reasoning and why you should spend time focusing your attention on this process. Critical reasoning is a decision-making process by which one uses one's knowledge, skills, experience, and logic to draw conclusions about everyday situations. When this process is used judiciously, it is undertaken with purpose, clarity, accuracy, and thoroughness. It is the foundation by which individuals draw conclusions about their world and what one determines to be true.

How does this relate to the NPTE, and why should you be concerned about it? The NPTE provides opportunities for you to demonstrate how well you can reason out challenging clinical, ethical, administrative, or other circumstances with the 250 questions you will need to answer for the exam. Each question will require you to draw on your knowledge, skills, and experiences to arrive at a correct conclusion. The way you arrive at a correct conclusion is primarily by using critical reasoning.

Some individuals erroneously believe that the NPTE only tests your ability to recall facts that are readily found in books. Although factual knowledge is important and provides a foundation for the exam, the NPTE also tests your ability to reason out challenging circumstances correctly and to make prudent decisions about the situations described in each question. The exam often moves beyond simple recall of knowledge and facts to contextualized clinical information. This means that you will be given clinical scenarios in which you will need to draw conclusions about a patient's symptoms, diagnosis, response to therapy, and expected outcomes. You must draw on your knowledge to take your reasoning to the next level application of information.

One should be aware of critical reasoning processes and skills. (See Table 1). The following section helps you become aware of the different skills involved in the process of critical reasoning, and how NPTE success is, in part, tied to these processes.

Sub-skills of Critical Reasoning

There are five sub-skills of critical reasoning that underlie the foundation for good critical reasoning skill. They are based on expert consensus of many critical thinking experts and reported by Peter and Noreen Facione (1990a, 1990b, 2006), who describe the skills used in reasoning out challenging circumstances. These skills include **inductive reasoning, deductive reasoning, analysis, inference,** and **evaluation**.

Inductive Reasoning

Inductive reasoning is the process of reasoning in which the assumptions of an argument are believed to endorse the conclusion, but do not guarantee it. It starts with reasoning in specific situations and then moves to more generalized situations. It may start with observations about a specific situation and then require one to draw conclusions about larger circumstances.

For example, if we observe a patient who experienced a stroke demonstrating dysarthria, we might conclude that all patients with stroke have dysarthria. We know that this is, in fact, not true. Inductive reasoning skill was used to draw this conclusion because we took observations from a specific situation and applied them to a larger, more global assumption. Recognizing that inductive reasoning can be flawed is an important part of successful exam performance. Inductive reasoning is an important skill clinically, because it helps us examine all possible options in a clinical situation and determine the most reasonable action. It is used in diagnostic thinking, where we form assumptions about what to expect from a diagnosis as it evolves over time.

Deductive Reasoning

Deductive reasoning is the process of reasoning whereby one draws conclusions based on facts, laws, rules, or accepted principles. It is the reverse thinking process of inductive reasoning, whereby the individual starts with larger circumstances and theories and applies them to specific situations.

For example, if we read the *Physical Therapy Guide for Professional Conduct,* which states that fraudulent billing for therapy services is unethical, we could reasonably conclude that when we witness therapist A in a clinic billing for services for patient B that did not occur, therapist A is acting unethically. Here the circumstance started with a global principle and was applied to a specific circumstance.

However, deductive reasoning also has its flaws. Sometimes individuals make erroneous assumptions about the premises of a theory and then apply this error in thinking to the specific circumstance. If we start with a premise that all patients enjoy physical therapy, then patients B, C, and D all will enjoy physical therapy. Can we say this for sure? Of course not! This is a type of flawed premise that leads to a faulty conclusion. We must be sure that our deductive reasoning begins with sound theory and known principles.

Deductive reasoning is important to physical therapists because it helps them apply rules and laws, without necessitating independent judgment for the situation. This is especially beneficial when applying protocols for treatment approaches (e.g., functional electrical stimulation, assuming one is following a published protocol) or research guidelines, (e.g., how to carry out correlational analysis of an array of data).

Analysis

Analytical reasoning or analysis is defined as the process of interpreting the meaning of information as well as relationships within the information presented, and then making assumptions or judgments about that information. Information presented in the form of graphs, charts, tables, and pictures encourages analytical reasoning skills, because one must interpret the information and determine what it means. Other times, information is presented in such a manner that one must make a "mental chart" of the information.

Popular questions that test one's analytical reasoning contain descriptors assigned to a group, with the key features of the group given in part. This leaves the test-taker to make assumptions about what is true about the whole group based on the information provided. Questions of this nature tend to place groups of people into categories, and the test-taker must determine the characteristics are of each group, based on limited information. These questions tend to frustrate people. Nonetheless, analytical reasoning is a necessary evil!

In physical therapy practice, analytical reasoning is important because it helps one to interpret an ECG strip or determine the diagnosis when analyzing the x-ray of a patient with a "Scotty dog" fracture in the spine (What is the significance?). Often, questions of this nature provide a host of symptoms, and the test-taker must determine the diagnosis (categorization of information). We also use analytical reasoning to give definitions to symptoms we are reading about (How can we describe this symptom?). Overall, analytical reasoning helps us to examine ideas and concepts and the relationships between them.

Inference

Inference or inferential reasoning is the process of drawing conclusions or making logical judgments based on concepts, assumptions, and evidence, rather than direct observations. Questions that ask you to determine what is best, most important, or most likely to occur, in addition to what something is *not*, often test your inferential reasoning ability. Questions of this nature also ask you to determine what is believed to be true, even though you cannot be 100% sure.

Inferential reasoning skills are used in clinical situations when a physical therapist must determine what symptoms to expect from a diagnosis or what is the likely functional result from a disease process or disorder. Because we cannot be 100% sure about the nature of a disease and all its possible symptoms, we must infer this information based on our knowledge and experiences. This is an important skill for a physical therapist to possess.

Pitfalls to inferential reasoning commonly occur when we fail to consider all the information presented or use faulty logic to determine what may occur in certain situations. An example of this might be a physical therapist who determines that it is most appropriate for a patient with T12 paraplegia to focus on strengthening upper trapezius and levator scapulae muscles in preparation for ambulation with crutches, rather than triceps and lower trapezius muscles. Here, the therapist did not consider the nature of the task at hand (ambulation with crutches) or tie the muscle functions with the use of crutches for ambulation. Hasty decisions can lead to suboptimal treatment planning with patients.

Evaluation

Evaluation and evaluative reasoning is a process by which one weighs the merits of an argument for its validity and the inherent value of the argument itself. Here, the individual determines if an argument "holds water," if there is value to be found in the argument itself, and what value one can assign to it.

Individuals make value judgments all the time. We are often unaware of the thought processes involved. Every day, we evaluate ideas that are presented to us, sometimes in the form of a news story or a discussion with a friend. We tend to judge the merits and value of the information we receive. However, a good evaluative thinker listens with a skeptical ear, determining how truthful the information is and how much value one should assign to that information. Accepting information at face value can be a pitfall because we are not considering the possibility that there is more information to be heard that may complete the story.

There are also times where we may have to make difficult decisions in areas that have no clear-cut answers. In physical therapy practice, we may be faced with dilemmas that pose a challenge for the correct course of action. Pay close attention to questions with the picture of the cogwheels next to them because they will help you to identify questions that pose difficult clinical and ethical situations and require evaluative reasoning.

An example of such a dilemma is a situation in which a therapist is working with a patient who becomes short of breath. The therapist must determine whether to immediately notify the physician, document the symptoms, or continue with the treatment session as planned. It is also helpful to know whether shortness of breath is an expected symptom, given the patient's medical history and past response to treatment. This information helps the therapist guide his or her thinking about a correct course of action. Nonetheless, these types of situations are not clear-cut, and require the therapist to evaluate the circumstances, weigh the information presented, and determine a correct course of action, given his or her knowledge and experience.

Pitfalls in evaluative reasoning involve assigning great value to information that has little value to the situation, not assigning enough value to highly valuable information, and not using principles and guidelines that are put into place to

TABLE 1 ➤ CRITICAL REASONING SELF-ASSESSMENT QUESTIONS

OBSERVED EXAM DIFFICULTY	REASONING CHALLENGE	NPTE EXAM PREPARATION STRATEGY
Do You: - Have difficulty with taking specific information and applying it to larger populations? - Selecting incorrect answers because you don't know how to generalize your knowledge?	Inductive	When studying a specific content area, think about how to apply the information you are reviewing to a diversity of situations. Use a reflective "what if" stance to think about how this information may be generalized to a broader context. This can be a fun and effective study group activity.
Do you: - Prefer to follow your instincts rather than the guidelines that a protocol may provide? - Select incorrect answers because you are unfamiliar with established practice standards or major theoretical approaches?	Deductive	When studying, be sure to master all major concepts, laws, rules, and accepted principles that guide PT practice. Carefully review all frames of reference, practice guidelines, and intervention protocols and procedures. Review the APTA Code of Ethics and Guidelines for Professional Conduct.
Do You: - Tend to misinterpret information provided and make poor judgments and apply inadequately conceived assumptions about it? - Select incorrect answers because you misjudged the effects of a clinical condition on functional performance?	Analytical	Obtain knowledge of all major clinical conditions, their symptoms, diagnostic testing and criteria, anticipated sequelae, and expected outcomes. This information is extensively reviewed in this text to help you make accurate judgments and correct assumptions about the potential impact of a clinical condition on functional performance. Review potential adverse effects (red flags in this text) and common errors associated with training.
Do You: - Have difficulty with thinking about how clinical conditions and practice situations may evolve over time? - Assume information is valid when it is not true? - Select incorrect answers because you have difficulty deciding the best course of action in a practice scenario?	Inferential	When studying clinical conditions, think about how the presentation of these conditions may sometimes vary from textbook descriptions. Use the knowledge and experience you acquired during your clinical education experiences to assess the trustworthiness of your assumptions. Study guidelines and models developed from evidence-based practice to develop a solid foundation on how to decide the best course of action.
Do you: - Feel anxious when you have questions that are ambiguous and you cannot find answers to them in a textbook? - Rely on protocols and guidelines more that gut instinct? - Select incorrect answers because you become overwhelmed by questions that present ethical dilemmas?	Evaluative	When reviewing specific content, think about the practice ambiguities and ethical dilemmas you observed during your clinical education experiences related to these areas. Review the APTA Code of Ethics and Guidelines for Professional Conduct and practice applying this information to determine a correct course of action using practice examples and case studies.

This table was adapted with permission from Dr. Kari Inda, from a table published in Fleming-Castaldy, R: *National Occupational Therapy Certification Exam – Review & Study Guide*, 5th ed. Evanston IL, TherapyEd, 2009, p. x.

help guide one's thinking (such as the Code of Ethics and *Guide to Professional Conduct*).

Summary of Reasoning Skills

You are encouraged to pay particular attention to the five types of critical reasoning listed with each practice question in the simulated examination section. The following five symbols have been assigned to help you key into areas that may be weaknesses:

 = inductive reasoning

 = deductive reasoning

 = analysis

 = inference

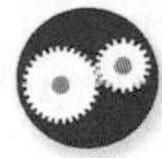 = evaluation

As you complete the simulated examination items, pay attention to any patterns that emerge. Are you particularly weak in a certain area of reasoning? Often, individuals are stronger in certain areas of reasoning than others. Our skill in reasoning ability comes from not only our knowledge, but also our day-to-day experiences. If you notice that you have a weakness in a certain area of reasoning, do not despair. Being aware of the issue is a good first step. The next section will help you to determine your next course of action.

Improving Your Critical Reasoning Skills

Critical reasoning is not learned or improved in a quick lesson or by simply reading basic definitions. It requires practice with items that test these skill areas and provide feedback on your performance. The good news is that you already have this information contained in this study guide! Each practice question in the book has an accompanying rationale for the correct and incorrect choices. Additionally, each question has an explanation about the sub-skill of critical reasoning and the knowledge or skill required to arrive at a correct conclusion. Paying attention to these areas will help you to build your knowledge and experiences with critical reasoning skills and prepare you for the NPTE and all its challenges.

After you receive the results of your CD practice test, refer back to your incorrect responses. This may help you uncover a pattern in the types of questions you are answering incorrectly, as related to a sub-skill of critical reasoning. Do you notice that you have difficulty with certain types of questions, such as ones that encourage evaluative or inferential reasoning? This will help you to identify a potential area for improvement and an area to help base study strategies. Once you have identified a weakness in critical reasoning, take some time to reflect on why this is so. Refer back to Table 1.

Other Courses of Action. This study guide was designed to help you to identify potential weak areas and prepare you to succeed on the NPTE. More detailed information about critical reasoning is beyond the scope and focus of this book. However, if you would like additional information about critical reasoning and practice with questions that test critical thinking and reasoning skills, the following resources may help you practice honing these skill areas:

- **Insight Assessment, Inc.** http://www.insight-assessment.com/. Offers periodic free mini-tests with rationales for correct and incorrect answers. Also offers resources that discuss the various types of reasoning.
- **Coping.org.** http://www.coping.org/write/percept/critical.htm. Offers information about the various types of reasoning and challenges with the reasoning process.
- Nosich, G. M. (2001). *Learning to Think Things Through: A Guide to Critical Thinking in the Curriculum,* 2nd ed. Prentice Hall. A handy guide written to help students engage in critical thinking.
- **Richard Bowles.** http://richardbowles.tripod.com/gmat/critreas/critreas.htm. Richard Bowles offers a practice critical reasoning test to improve critical reasoning skills on his personal website.
- **San Jose State University.** http://www.sjsu.edu/depts/itl/7/part2/indded.html. Offers free practice tests for inductive and deductive reasoning and explanations of the difference between the two types of reasoning.

Reasoning References

Facione, P. (2006). *Critical Thinking: What It Is and Why It Counts.* Millbrae, CA: The California Academic Press.

Facione, P. (1990a). Critical Thinking: A Statement of Expert Consensus for Purposes of Educational Assessment and Instruction: Research Findings and Recommendations. Newark, DE: The American Psychological Association. ERIC Document Reproduction Service. No. ED 315423.

Facione, P. (1990b). Critical Thinking: A Statement of Expert Consensus for Purposes of Educational Assessment and Instruction ("Executive Summary: The Delphi Report"). Millbrae, CA: The California Academic Press.

Facione, N. C., & Facione, P. A. (2006). *The Health Sciences Reasoning Test HSRT: Test Manual 2006 Edition.* Millbrae, CA: The California Academic Press.

Retaking the Examination

Remember, most candidates are successful the first time! If you receive bad news about your NPTE results, life goes on, but gets a bit more complicated. You might lose your temporary license if your state or jurisdiction has granted you one. If applicable, your visa to work as a physical therapist in the United States may be revoked. In two states you may retain a temporary license if you reapply to take the NPTE. If you are working as a physical therapist, you could lose your job, or you might continue to work, albeit with a different title, responsibilities, or salary until you pass the examination. If you have accepted a future position and fail to get a license, your employer might opt not to save the position for you. Undoubtedly, you will experience various emotions, which could include frustration, anger, depression, low self-esteem, and embarrassment.

What can be done? You can go online and download the Performance Feedback Request Form from the FSBPT. This report compares your test performance in various categories with other candidates who sat for the same examination. It gives the number of questions in a category, your percentage score, and the average percentage score of other test takers in that category. The current cost is $90 plus a $3 credit card fee. No personal checks are accepted. Due to examination security rules, you will not be able access or revisit your actual examination. You may contact http://www.fsbpt.org, or call (703) 739-9420.

Our advice is not to dwell on past failures. Carefully evaluate your performance. Think about areas on the previous exam with which you had some difficulty. Were there any gaps in your academic or clinical knowledge? Did you find it difficult to make decisions and answer questions requiring clinical judgment or analysis? Were your English language skills inadequate?

Focus on the next exam. Reinstitute a program of disciplined study. Consider taking a preparation course if you had not previously attended one. We have found that candidates who retake the exam without adjusting their behaviors or correcting deficiencies wind up with the same disappointing results. There is no magic potion that helps you pass the exam. It is your responsibility to demonstrate competency to practice. Take a positive and determined outlook. Approach the next examination with self-confidence.

Useful Web Links and E-Mail Addresses

http://www.fsbpt.org: information on licensure, the NPTE, and the role of the FSBPT, as well as addresses and links to state physical therapy boards.

http://www.fsbpt.net/pt: covers transfer of exam scores and other related information.

http://www.2test.com: provides locations of Prometric Testing Centers.

http://www.apta.org: information on the profession, policies regarding the role of the physical therapist, and resources in selected areas of practice.

http://www.TherapyEd.com: information on examination preparatory courses as well as materials for physical and occupational therapists and assistants.

chapter 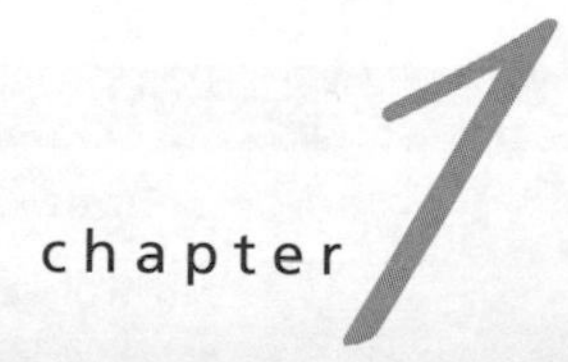

Musculoskeletal Physical Therapy

ROBERT ROWE

Anatomy and Biomechanics of the Musculoskeletal System

General Principles of Biomechanics

1. **Levers.** Rotations of a rigid surface about an axis. There are three types of levers.
   a. First class lever occurs when two forces are applied on either side of an axis.
      (1) The effort force attempts to cause movement.
      (2) The resistance is the force that opposes movement.
      (3) Example in human body is the contraction of triceps at elbow joint.
   b. Second class lever occurs when two forces are applied on one side of the axis.
      (1) Resistance lies between the effort force and axis of rotation.
      (2) Few examples in human body (toe raises).
   c. Third class lever occurs when two forces are applied on one side of the axis.
      (1) The effort force lies closer to the axis than the resistance force.
      (2) Most muscles in the human body are third class levers (elbow flexion).
2. **Selected kinematics.**
   a. Arthrokinematics is defined as the movement between joint surfaces.
   b. Three motions describe the movement of one joint surface on another.
      (1) Roll consists of one joint surface rolling on another, such as a tire rolling on the road (e.g., movement between the femoral and tibial articular surfaces of knee).
      (2) Glide consists of a pure translatory motion of one surface gliding on another as when a braked wheel skids (e.g., movement of the joint surface of the proximal phalanx at head of the metacarpal bone of the hand).
      (3) Spin consists of a rotation of the movable component of the joint (e.g., movement between joint surfaces of radial head with humerus).
      (4) Combinations of all three motions can occur at joints (e.g., between joint surfaces of humerus and scapula of shoulder).
   c. Osteokinematics: movement between two bones.
   d. Convex-concave rule describes relationship between arthrokinematics and osteokinematics.
      (1) When a convex surface is moving on a fixed concave surface, the convex surface moves opposite to the direction of the shaft of the bony lever.
      (2) When a concave surface moves on a fixed convex surface, the concave articulating surface moves in the same direction as the bony lever. (Table 1-1).
      (3) In the spine, the convex rule applies at the atlanto-occipital joint. Below the second vertebra, concave rule applies.
3. **Capsular positions.**
   a. Resting or loose-packed position (Table 1-2).
      (1) Joint position where capsule and other soft tissues are in most relaxed position.
      (2) Minimal joint surface contact.
      (3) May perform joint play and mobilization techniques in this joint position.

Table 1-1 ➤ CONCAVE-CONVEX RULE APPLICATION

JOINT	FUNCTION	DISTAL MOVING PART	SHAPE
Fingers	Flexion/extension	Distal phalanx	Concave
Metacarpal-phalangeal	Abduction/adduction	Proximal phalanx	Concave
Wrist	Flexion/extension	Capitate, scaphoid,	
		Lunate, triquetrum	Convex
		Trapezoid	Concave
Radio-ulnar			
Distal	Pronation/supination	Radius	Concave
Proximal	Pronation/supination	Radius	Convex
Humeroradial	Flexion/extension	Radius	Concave
Humeroulnar	Flexion/extension	Ulna	Concave
Glenohumeral	All movements	Humerus	Convex
Sternoclavicular	Elevation/depression	Clavicle	Convex
	Protraction/retraction	Clavicle	Concave
Acromioclavicular	All movements	Scapula	Concave
Toes	Flexion/extension	Distal phalanx	Concave
Metatarsal-phalangeal	Abduction/adduction	Proximal phalanx	Concave
Ankle/Foot			
Subtalar	All movements	Navicular, cuneiform	Concave
	Inversion/eversion	Cuboid, calcaneus	Convex
Talocrural	Dorsal/plantar flexion	Talus	Convex
Tibio-fibular	All movements	Fibular head	Concave
Knee	All movements	Tibia	Concave
Hip	All movements	Femur	Convex
TMJ	All movements	Mandible	Convex

From: Kaltenborn, FM. Manual Mobilization of the Extremity Joints, 4th ed., 1989 FM Kaltenborn, Oslo, with permission.

b. Close-packed position. (Table 1-3).
   (1) Joint position where capsule and other soft tissues are maximally tensed.
   (2) Maximal contact between joint surfaces.
   (3) Joint play and mobilization cannot be properly performed in this position.

c. Selected capsular patterns. (Table 1-4).

d. End feels.
   (1) Normal physiological end-feel.
      (a) Soft: occurs with soft tissue approximation.
      (b) Firm: capsular and ligamentous stretching.
      (c) Hard: when bone and/or cartilage meet.
   (2) Pathological end-feel.
      (a) Boggy: edema, joint swelling.
      (b) Firm with decreased elasticity: fibrosis of soft tissues.
      (c) Rubbery: muscle spasm.
      (d) Empty: loose, then very hard; associated with muscle guarding or patient avoiding painful part of range.
      (e) Hypermobility: end-feel at a later time than opposite side.

e. Grading of accessory joint movement.
   (1) Accessory joint movement or joint play is graded to assess arthrokinematic motion of the joint and/or when it is impractical or impossible to measure joint motion with a goniometer (Table 1-5).
   (2) Although interrater reliability is poor, intrarater reliability is acceptable.
   (3) Data gleaned provides clinician with more specific data on source of patient's problem.

4. Muscle substitutions.

a. Occur when muscles have become shortened/lengthened, weakened, lost endurance, developed impaired coordination, or paralyzed.

b. Stronger muscles compensate for loss of motion.

c. Common muscle substitutions:
   (1) Use of scapular stabilizers to initiate shoulder motion when shoulder abductors are weakened.
   (2) Use of lateral trunk muscles, or tensor fascia latae (TFL) when hip abductors are weak.
   (3) Use of passive finger flexion by contraction of wrist extensors when finger flexors are weak (tenodesis).
   (4) Use of long head of biceps, coracobrachialis, and anterior deltoid when pectoralis major is weak.
   (5) Use of lower back extensors, adductor magnus, and quadratus lumborum when hip extensors are weak.

Table 1-2 ➤ JOINT LOOSE-PACKED POSITIONS

JOINT(S)	POSITION
Vertebral	Midway between flexion and extension
Temporomandibular	Jaw slightly open (freeway space)
Sternoclavicular	Arm resting by side
Acromioclavicular	Arm resting by side
Glenohumeral	55–70° abduction; 30° horizontal adduction; neutral rotation
Elbow	
Humeroulnar	70° flexion and 10° supination
Humeroradial	Full extension and supination
Forearm	
Proximal radioulnar	70° flexion and 35° supination
Distal radioulnar	10° supination
Radio/ulnocarpal	Neutral with slight ulnar deviation
Hand	
Midcarpal	Neutral with slight flexion and ulnar deviation
Carpometacarpal (2 through 5)	Midway between flexion/extension, mid flexion, and mid extension
Trapeziometacarpal	Midway betweeen flexion/extension and between abduction/adduction
Metacarpophalangeal (MCP)	First MCP joint: slight flexion MCP joints 2–5: slight flexion with ulnar deviation
Interphalangeal (IP)	Proximal IP joints: 10° flexion Distal IP joints: 30° flexion
Hip	30° flexion, 30° abduction, and slight lateral rotation
Knee	25° flexion
Ankle/Foot	
Talocrural	Mid inversion/eversion and 10° plantar flexion
Subtalar and mid-tarsal	Midway between extremes of range of motion with 10° plantar flexion
Tarsometatarsal	Midway between supination and pronation
Toes	
Metatarsophalangeal	Neutral (extension 10°)
Interphalangeal	Slight flexion

From: Hertling, DH; Kessler, RM. Management of Common Musculoskeletal Disorders; Physical Therapy Principles and Methods, 3rd ed., Philadelphia, Lippincott, 1996, with permission.

Table 1-3 ➤ JOINT CLOSE-PACKED POSITIONS

JOINT(S)	POSITION
Vertebral	Maximal extension
Temporomandibular	Maximal retrusion (mouth closed with teeth clenched) or maximal anterior position (mouth maximally opened)
Sternoclavicular	Arm maximally elevated
Acromioclavicular	Arm abducted 90°
Glenohumeral	Maximum abduction and external rotation
Elbow	
Humeroulnar	Full extension and supination
Humeroradial	90° flexion and 5° supination
Forearm	
Proximal radioulnar	5° supination and full extension
Distal radioulnar	5° supination
Radiocarpal	Full extension with radial deviation
Hand	
Midcarpal	Full extension
Carpometacarpal	Full opposition
Trapeziometacarpal	Full oppostition
Metacarpophalangeal (MCP)	First MCP joint: full extension MCP joints 2–5: full flexion
Interphalangeal	Full extension
Hip	Ligamentous: full extension, abduction, and internal rotation Bony: 90° flexion, slight abduction, and slight external rotation
Knee	Full extension and external rotation
Ankle/Foot	
Talocrural	Full dorsiflexion
Subtalar	Full inversion
Mid-tarsal	Full supination
Tarsometatarsal	Full supination
Toes	
Metatarsophalangeal	Full extension
Interphalangeal	Full extension

From: Hertling, DH; Kessler, RM. Management of Common Musculoskeletal Disorders; Physical Therapy Principles and Methods, 3rd ed., Philadelphia, Lippincott, 1996, with permission.

(6) Use of lower abdominal, lower obliques, hip adductors and latissimus dorsi when hip flexors are weak.

Functional Anatomy and Biomechanics

1. **Shoulder region.**
   a. Osteology (humerus, scapula, and clavicle).
      (1) Humerus.
         (a) Proximal end of humerus is approximately half a spheroid.
         (b) Articular surface is covered by hyaline cartilage.
         (c) Head is retroverted 20°–30°.
         (d) Longitudinal axis of head is 135° from axis of neck.
      (2) Scapula.
         (a) Large, flat triangular bone that sits over 2nd to 7th ribs.
         (b) Costal surface and a dorsal surface.
         (c) Three angles—medial, superior, and lateral.
         (d) Lateral angle bears glenoid fossa, which faces anteriorly, laterally, and superiorly.
            - Pear-shape of fossa allows for freer range of motion (ROM) in abduction and flexion.
            - Concave shape receives convex humeral head.
            - Orientation of the glenoid fossa places true abduction at 30° anterior to frontal plane.

Table 1-4 ➤ CAPSULAR PATTERNS

JOINT(S)	PROPORTIONAL LIMITATIONS
Temporomandibular	Limitation of mouth opening
Upper cervical spine (occiput - C2)	
Occipitoatlantal joint	Forward bending more limited than backward bending
Atlantoaxial joint	Restriction with rotation
Lower cervical spine (C3 - T2)	Limitation of all motions except flexion (sidebending = rotation > backward bending)
Sternoclavicular	Full elevation limited; pain at extreme range of motion
Acromioclavicular	Full elevation limited; pain at extreme range of motion
Glenohumeral	Greater limitation of external rotation, followed by abduction and internal rotation
Humeroulnar	Loss of flexion > extension
Humeroradial	Loss of flexion > extension
Forearm	Equally restricted in pronation and supination in presence of elbow restriction
Proximal radioulnar	Limitation: pronation = supination
Distal radioulnar	Limitation: pronation = supination
Wrist	Limitation: flexion = extension
Midcarpal	Limitation: equal all directions
Trapeziometacarpal	Limitation: abduction > extension
Carpometacarpals II - V	Equally restricted all directions
Upper extremity digits	Limitation: flexion > extension
Thoracic spine	Limitation of sidebending and rotation > loss of extension > flexion
Lumbar spine	Marked and equal limitation of sidebending and rotation; loss of extension > flexion
Sacroiliac, symphysis pubis, sacrococcygeal	Pain when joints are stressed
Hip	Limited flexion/internal rotation; some limitation of abduction; no or little limitation of adduction and external rotation
Tibiofemoral (knee)	Flexion grossly limited; slight limitation of extension
Tibiofibular	Pain when joint is stressed
Talocrural (ankle)	Loss of plantarflexion > dorsiflexion
Talocalcaneal (subtalar)	Increasing limitations of varus; joint fixed in valgus (inversion > eversion)
Midtarsal	Supination > pronation (limited dorsiflexion, plantar flexion, adduction, and medial rotation)
First metatarsophalangeal	Marked limitation of extension; slight limitation of flexion
Metatarsophalangeal (II - V)	Variable; tend toward flexion restrictions
Interphalangeal	Tend toward extension restrictions

From: Hertling, DH; Kessler, RM. Management of Common Musculoskeletal Disorders; Physical Therapy Principles and Methods, 3 ed., Philadelphia, Lippincott, 1996, with permission.

Table 1-5 ➤ MANUAL GRADING OF ACCESSORY JOINT MOTION

GRADE	JOINT STATUS
0	Ankylosed
1	Considerable hypomobility
2	Slight hypomobility
3	Normal
4	Slight hypermobility
5	Considerable hypermobility
6	Unstable

From: Grieve, GP. Mobilization of the Spine; A Primary Handbook of Clinical Method, ed 5., Churchill Livingstone, NY, 1991 with permission.

(3) Clavicle.
  (a) Extends laterally and links manubrium to acromion.
  (b) Connects shoulder complex to axial skeleton.

b. Arthrology (glenohumeral, sternoclavicular, acromioclavicular, and scapulothoracic).
  (1) Glenohumeral joint.
    (a) Convex humeral head articulates with concave glenoid fossa.
    (b) Glenoid fossa very shallow.
  (2) Sternoclavicular joint.
    (a) Convex (superior/inferior) and concave (anterior/posterior) articulates with reciprocal shape of sternum.
    (b) Both articulations covered with fibrocartilage.
  (3) Acromioclavicular joint.
    (a) A plane joint with relatively flat surfaces.
  (4) Scapulothoracic joint.
    (a) A "clinical" articulation.

c. Muscles (depressors, elevators, protractors, retractors, internal rotators, external rotators, flexors, abductors, adductors, and extensors) (Table 1-6).

d. Noncontractile structures (acromioclavicular, trapezoid, conoid, and sternoclavicular ligament, subacromial bursa, shoulder capsule, glenoid labrum and associated nerves and vessels).
  (1) Capsule.
    (a) Attaches medially to glenoid margin, glenoid labrum, coracoid process.
    (b) Attaches laterally to humeral anatomical neck and descends approximately 1 cm on the shaft.
    (c) Supported by tendons of supraspinatus, infraspinatus, teres minor, subscapularis and long head of triceps below.
    (d) Inferiorly capsule is least supported and most lax.
  (2) Ligaments.
    (a) Coracohumeral ligament.
      - Base of coracoid process to greater and lesser tubercle of humerus.

Table 1-6 ➤ SHOULDER GIRDLE AND UPPER EXTREMITY MUSCULAR & NEUROLOGICAL SCREENING

ACTION TO BE TESTED	MUSCLES	MYOTOMES	REFLEXES	CORD SEGMENT	NERVES
Neck flexion Neck extension Neck rotation Neck lateral bending	Sternoclei-domastoid, trapezius, Other deep neck muscles			C1-C4	Cervical spinal accessory
Shoulder shrug, scapular upward rotation	Upper trapezius	C4		C1-C4	Spinal accessory
Shoulder horiz. adduction	Pect. major/minor			C5-C8 T1	Medial/lateral pectoral
Scapular downward rotation	Pectoralis minor			C8-T1	Medial pectoral
Shoulder protraction, scapular upward rotation	Serratus anterior			C5-C7	Long thoracic
Scapular elevation, downward rotation	Levator scapula			C5	Dorsal scapular
Scapular adduction, elevation, downward rotation	Rhomboids			C4-C5	Dorsal scapular
Shoulder abduction	Supraspinatus			C4-C6	Suprascapular
Shoulder lateral rotation	Infraspinatus			C4-C6	Suprascapular
Shoulder medial rotation, adduction	Latissimus dorsi, teres major and subscapularis			C5-C8	Subscapular thoracodorsal
Shoulder abduction, flexion, extension	Deltoid	C5		C5-C6	Axillary
Shoulder lateral rotation	Teres minor			C4-C5	Axillary
Elbow flexion, forearm supination	Biceps brachii	C6	C5	C5-C6	Musculocutaneous
Shoulder flexion, adduction	Coracobrachialis			C6-C7	Musculocutaneous
Elbow flexion	Brachialis			C5-C6	Musculocutaneous
4th & 5th digit DIP flexion	Flexor digitorum profundus (ulnar part)			C7-T1	Ulnar
Wrist ulnar flexion	Flexor carpi ulnaris	C7		C7-T1	Ulnar
Thumb adduction	Adductor pollicis			C8-T1	Ulnar
5th digit abduction	Abductor digiti quinti			C8-T1	Ulnar
5th digit opposition	Opponens digiti quinti			C7-T1	Ulnar
5th digit MCP flexion	Flexor digiti quinti brevis			C7-T1	Ulnar
2nd–5th digit MCP flexion, adduction, abduction	Interossei	T1		C8-T1	Ulnar
Forearm pronation	Pronator teres, pronator quadratus			C6-C7	Median
Wrist radial flexion	Flexor carpi radialis			C6-C7	Median
Wrist flexion	Palmaris longus			C7-T1	Median
2nd–5th digit PIP flexion	Flexor digitorum sublimis			C7-T1	Median
Thumb IP flexion	Flexor pollicis longus			C7-T1	Median
2nd–3rd digit DIP flexion	Flexor digitorum profundus (radial part)			C7-T1	Median
Thumb abduction	Abductor pollicis brevis			C6-T1	Median
Thumb MCP flexion	Flexor pollicis brevis			C6-T1	Median/ulnar
Thumb opposition	Opponens pollicis			C8-T1	Median
2nd–5th digit MCP flexion, IP extension	Lumbricals			C8-T1	Median/ulnar
Elbow flexion	Brachioradialis		C6	C5-C6	Radial
Elbow extension	Triceps brachii, anconeus		C7	C6-C8	Radial

(Continued on following page)

Table 1-6 ➤ continued

ACTION TO BE TESTED	MUSCLES	MYOTOMES	REFLEXES	CORD SEGMENT	NERVES
Wrist radial extension	Extensor carpi radialis			C6-C8	Radial
2nd–5th digit MCP, IP extension	Extensor digitorum communis extensor digiti quinti proprius			C6-C8	Radial
Wrist ulnar extension	Extensor carpi ulnaris			C6-C8	Radial
Forearm supination	Supinator			C5-C6	Radial
Thumb MCP abduction	Abductor pollicis longus	C8		C7-C8	Radial
Thumb extension	Extensor pollicis longus/ brevis			C6-C8	Radial
2nd digit extension	Extensor indicis proprius			C6-C8	Radial

Adapted from Chusid, JG. Correlative Neuroanatomy and Functional Neurology, Lange Medical Publications, Los Altos, CA, 1970; and Kendall, FP; McCreary, EK, and Provance, PG. Muscles Testing and Function: 4th ed., Baltimore, Williams & Wilkins, 1993.

- Primary function to reinforce biceps tendon, reinforce superior capsule, and prevents caudal dislocation of humerus. Taut with external rotation.

(b) Coracoacromial ligament.
- Strong triangular ligament runs from coracoid to acromion.
- Not a "true" ligament; connects two points of same bone.

(c) Glenohumeral ligaments.
- Three bands (superior, middle, and inferior) located on anterior glenohumeral joint.
- Reinforce anterior glenohumeral capsule.

(d) Transverse humeral ligament.
- Broad band passing over top of bicipital groove.
- Acts as a retinaculum for long biceps tendon.

(3) Labrum.
(a) Glenoid labrum is a fibrocartilaginous ring that deepens glenoid fossa.
(b) Attached to capsule superiorly and inferiorly as well as to the long head of the biceps tendon superiorly.
(c) Internal surface covered with articular cartilage which is thicker peripherally and thinner centrally.
(d) Aids in lubrication like meniscus of knee and serves to protect the bone.

(4) Bursae.
(a) Multiple bursae found within this region.
(b) Primary bursa involved with pathology is subacromial bursa between deltoid and capsule. Also runs under acromion and coracoacromial ligament and between the supraspinatus tendon.

e. Shoulder biomechanics.
(1) Glenohumeral joint arthrokinematics/osteokinematics.
(a) Occurs in opposite directions. With elevation of humerus, head of humerus moves in an inferior direction because of convex moving on concave.
(b) Rolling-gliding occurs during elevation of the humerus, so that the instantaneous centers of rotation varies considerably during the complete range.
(c) At approximately 75° of elevation, external rotation (conjunct rotation) occurs, preventing compression of greater tubercle against the acromion.

(2) Scapulothoracic and glenohumeral rhythm (scapulohumeral rhythm) is the ratio of movement of the glenohumeral with the scapulothoracic joint.
(a) With 180° of abduction, there is a 2:1 ratio of movement between the two joints.
(b) First 30°–60° of elevation occurs mainly in the glenohumeral joint.
(c) 120° of movement occurs at glenohumeral joint.
(d) 60° of movement occurs at scapulothoracic joint.

(3) Requirements of full elevation.
(a) Scapular stabilization.
(b) Inferior glide of humerus.
(c) External rotation of humerus.
(d) Rotation of the clavicle at sternoclavicular joint.
(e) Scapular abduction and lateral rotation of acromioclavicular joint.
(f) Straightening of thoracic kyphosis.

2. Elbow region.

a. Osteology and arthrology (ulnohumeral, radiohumeral, superior and inferior radioulnar).
(1) Humeroulnar joint.
(a) Distal end humerus (trochlea) articulates with proximal end of ulna.

(b) Trochlea and trochlear notch face anteriorly at a 45° angle, allowing space between ulna and humerus during flexion.

(2) Humeroradial joint.

(a) Distal end humerus (capitulum) articulates with concave oval facet of proximal radius.

(3) Proximal radioulnar joint.

(a) Radial head is ovoid and cone-shaped.

(b) Medial radius articulates with radial notch (of ulna).

(4) Distal radioulnar joint.

(a) Convex ulna articulates with concave radius (opposite to proximal articulation of these two bones).

b. Muscles (flexors, extensors, supinators, and pronators) (see Table 1-6).

c. Noncontractile structures (medial collateral ligament, radial collateral ligament, annular ligament, elbow capsule, associated bursae, nerves, and vessels).

(1) Capsule.

(a) Encloses entire elbow joint complex. It is thin, both anteriorly and posteriorly. Continuous medially with ulnar collateral ligament, and laterally with radial collateral ligament.

(2) Ligaments.

(a) Ulnar collateral.

- Ligament is triangular shaped consisting of three parts.
- Reinforces humeroulnar joint medially.

(b) Radial collateral.

- Ligament is fan shaped, and runs from lateral epicondyle of humerus to annular ligament.
- Reinforces humeroradial joint laterally and is stronger (histologically) than ulnar collateral ligament.

(c) Annular.

- An osteofibrous ring attached to medial ulna and encircles radial head.
- Cone-shaped, and inner surface is lined with fibrocartilage.
- Protects radial head, especially in semi-flexion, where it is very unstable. Taut in extremes of pronation and supination.

(d) Quadrate.

- Extends from radial notch (ulna) to the neck of radius.
- Reinforces inferior joint capsule, maintains radial head in opposition to ulna, limits amount of spin in supination and pronation.

(e) Distal radioulnar.

- Anterior radioulnar ligament: primarily strengthens capsule.
- Posterior radioulnar ligament: primarily strengthens capsule.

(3) Bursa.

(a) Olecranon bursa located on posterior aspect of elbow over olecranon process.

(4) Blood supply.

(a) Elbow joint receives blood supply from brachial artery, anterior ulnar recurrent artery, posterior ulnar recurrent artery, radial recurrent artery, and middle collateral branch of the deep brachial artery.

(5) Elbow joint stability.

(a) Elbow joint complex possesses significant inherent stability.

(b) Main contributor to bony stability is articulation between the trochlea (humerus) and trochlear fossa (ulna).

(c) Medial collateral ligament provides strong resistance to valgus forces.

(d) Resistance of lateral collateral ligament to varus forces minimal, due to its attachment to another soft tissue structure (annular ligament).

(e) Functionally, this relationship is beneficial, since functional activities place tensile forces medially and compressive forces laterally. Therefore, the lateral ligament does not have to be as strong as the medial ligament.

d. Elbow biomechanics.

(1) Conjunct rotations.

(a) Ulna pronates slightly with extension. Ulna supinates slightly with flexion.

(b) Proximal ulna glides medially during extension and laterally during flexion.

(c) Flexion/extension of elbow is accompanied by a screw-home mechanism with conjunct rotation of ulna. Ulna externally rotates (or supinates) during elbow flexion and internally rotates (or pronates) during elbow extension.

3. Wrist and hand region.

a. Osteology (radius, ulna, carpals, metacarpals, and phalanges).

(1) Radius is biconcave relative to carpals.

(2) Ulna is convex at its distal end relative to the triquetrum.

(3) Proximal aspect of proximal row is biconvex. Distal aspect of proximal row is concave at lunate/capitate and triquetrum/hamate articulations. Scaphoid is convex anterior/posterior and concave medial/lateral relative to trapezium/trapezoid. Capitate is convex, and articulates with concavities of scaphoid, hamate and trapezoid.

(4) Metacarpal heads are biconvex, and bases are generally flat relative to distal row of carpals.

(5) Phalanges' proximal ends are mostly biconcave, with a ridge running down the center, dividing it into two surfaces. Distal end is pulley-shaped, and mostly biconvex, with a groove running through the center.

b. Arthrology (radiocarpal, midcarpal, carpometacarpal, metacarpophalangeal [MCP], and interphalangeal [IP]).
   (1) Radiocarpal joint.
      (a) Convex scaphoid and lunate articulate with concave radius.
   (2) Midcarpal joint.
      (a) Articulation between four proximal and four distal carpal bones is known as midcarpal joint.
      (b) Functional rather then anatomical joint.
      (c) Can be divided into middle pillar (lunate and triquetrum with capitate and hamate) and lateral pillar (scaphoid with trapezoid and trapezium).
   (3) Carpometacarpal (CMC) joint.
      (a) First CMC (thumb) is a saddle articulation with trapezium being convex in medial/lateral direction and concave in anterior/posterior direction.
      (b) First metacarpal is opposite in shape to trapezium.
      (c) 2nd–5th CMC are essentially flat between bases of metacarpals and distal row of carpals.
   (4) Metacarpalphalangeal (MCP) joints consist of convex metacarpals with concave proximal phalanges.
   (5) Proximal interphalangeal (PIP) joints consist of convex distal aspects proximal phalanges with concave proximal aspect of middle phalanges. Same orientation exists at distal interphalangeal (DIP) joints.

c. Muscles (wrist flexors, wrist extensors, radial deviators, ulnar deviators, extrinsic finger flexors, extrinsic finger extensors, and intrinsic finger muscles) (see Table 1-6).

d. Noncontractile structures (volar carpal, radiocarpal, collateral, and palmar ligaments; extensor hood; associated capsules; volar plate; nerves; and vessels).
   (1) Ligaments.
      (a) Fingers.
         - Collateral: run from lateral condyle to distal phalanx and lateral volar plate. All fibers tighten with flexion and volar fibers tighten with extension.
         - Accessory: run from condylar head to volar plate.
         - Transverse: present at MCP joints. Provide stability linking MCP joints and providing reinforcement to anterior capsule.
      (b) Wrist.
         - Radial collateral: limits ulnar deviation.
         - Ulnar collateral: limits radial deviation.
         - Palmar ulnocarpal: limits extension and supination.
         - Palmar radiocarpal: limits extension and supination.
         - Dorsal radiocarpal: limits flexion, pronation, and possibly radial deviation.
         - Radiate: stabilizes hand for any impact through knuckles.
   (2) Extensor hood.
      (a) Fibrous mechanism on the dorsum of each finger that is a fibrous expansion of the extensor digitorum tendon.
      (b) Its purpose is to assist with extension of the PIP and DIP joints.
   (3) Capsule.
      (a) Fingers.
         - MCP, PIP, and DIP joints all have fibrous capsules that are strong but lax and supported by ligaments.
      (b) Wrist.
         - Radiocarpal joint shares fibrous capsule (which is thicker palmarly and dorsally) with midcarpal joint, but usually has its own synovial membrane.
   (4) Volar plate.
      (a) Present on palmar aspect of the MCP, PIP, and DIP joints. Thickening of capsule. Functions to increase articular surface during extension and protect joint volarly. Volar plate more mobile at MCP than at IPs.
   (5) Nerves.
      (a) Ulnar innervates hypothenar region (palmarly and dorsally), 5th digit, and medial half of 4th digit.
      (b) Median nerve innervates remainder of palmer surface not innervated by ulnar nerve and dorsal portions of 2nd, 3rd, and lateral half of 4th digit from DIP joint to tip of finger.
      (c) Radial nerve innervates remainder of dorsum of hand not innervated by ulnar or median nerves.
   (6) Blood supply from ulna and radial arteries. Merge to form palmar arch and then send digital branches that run up medial and lateral aspects of each digit.

e. Hand and wrist biomechanics.
   (1) Hand.
      (a) PIPs and DIPs.
         - During flexion digits rotate radially to enhance grasp and opposition.
      (b) MCPs.
         - During flexion digits rotate radially to enhance grasp and opposition.
      (c) First CMC.
         - Due to position of trapezium (anteriorly and medially rotated relative to other carpals) plane of flexion/extension is perpendicular to other digits.
         - During flexion/extension it is concave moving on convex.

- During abduction/adduction, it is convex moving on concave.
- During flexion and abduction, the first metacarpal rotates ulnarly.
- During extension and adduction, the first metacarpal rotates radially.

(2) Wrist.

(a) Flexion.

- Proximal aspect of scaphoid/lunate glide dorsally relative to radius.

(b) Extension.

- Proximal aspect of scaphoid/lunate glide ventrally relative to radius.

(c) Radial deviation.

- Proximal row glides ulnarly. Proximal surface of scaphoid rotates palmarly.

(d) Ulnar deviation.

- Proximal row glides radially as a unit.

4. Hip region.

a. Osteology (femur and acetabulum of pelvis).

(1) Femur.

(a) Head is two thirds of a sphere with a depression at its center called the fovea capitis femoris.

(b) Head is oriented superiorly, anteriorly, and medially.

(c) Articular cartilage covers entire head, except for fovea capitis.

(d) Angle of inclination normally 115°– 125°.

- Coxa valga is angle > 125°.
- Coxa vara is angle < 115°.

(e) Femoral neck angles anteriorly 10°–15° from frontal plane to form anterior antetorsion angle.

- Anteversion: considered excessive if anterior antetorsion angle > 25°–30°.
- Retroversion: considered excessive if anterior antetorsion angle < 10°.

(2) Acetabulum.

(a) Acetabulum faces laterally, inferiorly, and anteriorly.

(b) Made of union between ischium, ilium, and pubis bones.

(c) Acetabular fossa: center of acetabulum, which is nonarticulating and filled with fat pad for shock absorption.

(d) Acetabulum is not completely covered with cartilage. Lined with a horseshoe-shaped articular cartilage with interruption inferiorly forming acetabular notch.

b. Arthrology (coxofemoral).

(1) Synovial joint.

(2) Convex femoral head articulates with concave acetabulum.

(3) Very stable joint due to bony anatomy as well as strength of ligaments and capsule.

c. Muscles (flexors, extensors, adductors, abductors, internal rotators [IRs], and external rotators [ERs]) (Table 1-7).

d. Noncontractile structures (capsule, labrum, bursae, iliofemoral ligament, ischiofemoral ligament, pubofemoral ligament, and associated nerves and vessels).

(1) Capsule is strong, dense, and encloses the entire joint.

(2) Labrum.

(a) Triangular shaped, made up of a fibrocartilaginous ring, thickest superiorly.

(b) Attaches to bony rim of acetabulum, bridging acetabular notch.

(c) Serves to deepen acetabulum.

(d) Inner surface is lined with articular cartilage, and outer surface connects to joint capsule.

(3) Ligaments.

(a) Iliofemoral ligament ("Y" or ligament of Bigelow).

- Two bands, both starting from anterior inferior iliac spine (AIIS). Medial running to distal intertrochanteric line. Lateral running to proximal aspect of intertrochanteric line.
- Very strong.
- Both bands taut with extension and external rotation. Lateral band taut with abduction.

(b) Pubofemoral ligament.

- Runs from iliopectineal eminence, superior rami of pubis, obturator crest, and obturator membrane, laterally blending with capsule; inserts into same point as medial iliofemoral ligament.
- Taut with extension, external rotation, and abduction.

(c) Ischiofemoral ligament.

- Runs from ischium and posterior acetabulum, superiorly and laterally, blending with zona articularis, and attaching to greater trochanter.
- Taut with medial rotation, abduction, and extension.

(d) Zona orbicularis.

- Runs in a circular pattern around femoral neck.
- Has no bony attachments, but helps to hold head of femur in acetabulum.

(e) Inguinal ligament.

- 12–14 cm long, running from ASIS medially and inferiorly, attaching to pubic tubercle.
- Forms tunnel for muscles, arteries, veins, and nerves.

(4) Bursae.

(a) Subtendinous iliac, located between hip and os pubis.

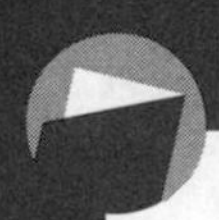

Table 1-7 ➤ PELVIC GIRDLE AND LOWER EXTREMITY MUSCULAR & NEUROLOGICAL SCREENING

ACTION TO BE TESTED	MUSCLES	MYOTOMES	REFLEXES	CORD SEGMENT	NERVES
Hip flexion	Iliopsoas	L2		L1-L3	Femoral
Hip flexion, abduction, lat. rotation	Sartorius	L2		L2-L3	Femoral
Knee extension	Quadriceps femoris	L3	L4	L2-L4	Femoral
Hip adduction	Pectineus, adductor longus			L2-L3	Obturator
Hip adduction	Adductor brevis			L2-L4	Obturator
Hip adduction	gracilis			L2-L4	Obturator
Hip abduction, flexion, medial rotation	Gluteus medius, minimus	L5		L4-S1	Sup. gluteal
Hip flexion, abduction, medial rotation	Tensor fascia lata			L4-L5	Sup. gluteal
Hip lateral rotation	Piriformis			L5-S1	Sup. gluteal
Hip extension, lateral rot.	Gluteus maximus			L4-S2	Inf. gluteal
Hip lateral rotation	Obturator internus			L5-S1	Sacral plexus
Hip lateral rotation	Gemelli, quadratus femoris			L4-S1	Sacral plexus
Hip extension, knee flexion, leg lateral rotation	Biceps femoris			L5-S2	Sciatic
Hip extension, knee flexion,	Semitendinosus		L5	L5-S2	Sciatic
Leg medial rotation	Semimembranosus			L5-S2	Sciatic
Ankle dorsiflexion	Tibialis anterior	L4		L4-L5	Deep peroneal
2nd–5th digit MTP extension	Extensor digitorum longus			L4-S1	Deep peroneal
Great toe MTP extension	Extensor hallucis longus	L5		L4-S1	Deep peroneal
Foot eversion	Peroneus longus/ brevis	S1		L5-S1	Sup. peroneal
Leg medial rotation	Popliteus			L4-S1	Tibial
Foot inversion	Tibialis posterior	S1	S1	L5-S2	Tibial
Ankle plantar flexion	Gastrocnemius/ soleus		S1	L5-S2	Tibial
2nd–5th digit DIP flexion	Flexor digitorum longus			L5-S2	Tibial
Great toe IP flexion	Flexor hallucis longus			L5-S2	Tibial
2nd–5th digit PIP flexion	Flexor digitorum brevis			L5-S1	Medial plantar
Great toe MTP flexion	Flexor hallucis brevis			L5-S2	Medial plantar
Toe adduction/abduction	Dorsal/plantar interossei			S1-S2	Lateral plantar
Pelvic floor control	Perineals and sphincters			S2-S4	Pudendal

Adapted from Chusid, JG. Correlative Neuroanatomy and Functional Neurology, Lange Medical Publications, Los Altos, CA, 1970; and Kendall, FP; McCreary, EK, and Provance, PG. Muscles Testing and Function: 4th ed., Baltimore, Williams & Wilkins, 1993.

(b) Iliopectineal between tendons of psoas major, iliacus, and capsule. Lies close to femoral nerve.

(c) Ischiofemoral between ischial tuberosity and gluteus maximus muscle. May cause pain in sciatic distribution.

(d) Deep trochanteric between gluteus maximus and posterior lateral greater trochanter. May cause pain with hip flexion and internal rotation due to compression of gluteus maximus.

(e) Superficial trochanteric located over greater trochanter.

(5) Innervation of hip joint comes from femoral, obturator, sciatic, and superior gluteal nerves.

(6) Blood supply.

(a) Medial and lateral femoral circumflex supplies proximal femur.
(b) Femoral head is supplied by a small branch off obturator artery.
(c) Acetabulum is supplied by branches from superior and inferior gluteal arteries.

(7) Hip biomechanics.
(a) Coxofemoral joint arthrokinematics/osteokinematics occur in opposite directions due to relationship of convex femoral head moving within concave acetabulum.

5. Knee region.

a. Osteology (femur, tibia, fibula, and patella).

(1) Femur.
(a) Femoral condyles are convex in anterior/posterior and medial/lateral planes. Both femoral condyles are spiral, but lateral one has a longer surface area and medial one descends further inferiorly.

(2) Tibia.
(a) Medial tibial condyle is biconcave, has a larger surface area and is more stable, and therefore less mobile.
(b) Lateral tibial condyle is convex anterior/posterior and concave medial/lateral. Smaller surface area, more circular, and less stable, therefore more mobile.
(c) Both tibial surfaces are raised where they border intercondylar area.

(3) Patella.
(a) A vertical ridge divides patella into a larger and smaller medial part. Patella can further be divided by two faint horizontal ridges which divide it into its facets.

b. Arthrology (tibiofemoral, patellofemoral, and proximal tibiofibular).

(1) Proximal tibiofibular joint.
(a) Oval tibial facet is flat or slightly convex. Fibular head has an oval, slightly concave to flat surface.

(2) Tibiofemoral joint.
(a) Synovial hinge joint with two degrees of freedom. Minimal bony stability thus relies on capsule, ligaments, and muscles.

(3) Patellofemoral joint.
(a) Patella articular surface is adapted to patellar surface of femur. An oblique groove running inferiorly and laterally is the guiding mechanism on femur for patellar tracking. Patellar surface of femur is concave transversely and convex sagittally, creating its saddle (sellar) shape.

c. Muscles (flexors, tibial rotators, and extensors) (see Table 1-7).

d. Noncontractile structures (medial collateral ligament, lateral collateral ligament, anterior cruciate ligament, posterior cruciate ligament, menisci, capsule, bursae and associated nerves and vessels).

(1) Capsule.
(a) Tibiofemoral capsule is a fibrous sleeve attached to distal femur and proximal tibia. Inner wall is covered by a synovium. Shaped as a cylinder with a posterior invagination, which posteriorly divides cavity into medial and lateral halves. Anterior surface has a window cut out for patella.
(b) Proximal tibiofibular joint has a fibrous capsule, which is continuous with knee joint capsule 10% of time.

(2) Ligaments.
(a) Tibiofemoral and patellofemoral joints (knee joint proper).

- Medial collateral ligament (MCL): runs from medial aspect of medial femoral condyle to upper end of tibia. Posterior fibers blend with capsule. Runs oblique anteriorly and inferiorly. Taut in extension and slackened in flexion. Prevents external rotation and provides stability against valgus forces. Runs in same direction as ACL.
- Lateral collateral ligament (LCL): runs from lateral femoral condyle to head of fibula. Free of any capsular attachment. Runs oblique inferiorly and posteriorly in same direction as PCL. Taut in extension and slackened in flexion. Prevents external rotation and provides stability against varus forces.
- Anterior cruciate ligament (ACL): attached to anterior intercondylar fossa of tibia and to femur at medial aspect of lateral condyle. Runs oblique superiorly and laterally. Extracapsular, but more correctly a thickening of the capsule. Checks forward gliding of tibia on femur and limits internal rotation of tibia during flexion as it twists around posterior cruciate ligament.
- Posterior cruciate ligament (PCL): attaches to posterior intercondylar fossa of tibia and on lateral surface of femoral medial condyle. Runs oblique medially and anteriorly-superiorly. Checks posterior displacement of tibia on femur.
- Meniscofemoral ligament: runs with PCL. Attaches below posterior horn of lateral meniscus. Has common insertion into lateral aspect of medial condyle. Occasionally a similar ligament exists medially.
- Oblique popliteal ligament: inserts into expansion from tendon of semimembranosus. It partially blends with capsule. Forms floor of popliteal fossa and is in contact with popliteal anterior artery. Strengthens posteromedial capsule.

- Arcuate popliteal ligament: Y-shaped and commonly described as having two bands (medial and lateral). Stem attaches to fibular head. Medial band attaches to posterior border of intercondylar area of tibia. Lateral band extends to lateral epicondyle of femur. Strengthens posterolateral capsule.
- Transverse ligament connects lateral and medial meniscus anteriorly.
- Meniscopatellar ligament: runs from inferolateral edges of patella to lateral borders of each meniscus. Pulls menisci forward with extension.
- Alar fold: runs from lateral borders of patella to medial and lateral aspects of femoral condyles. Keeps patella in contact with femur.

(b) Infrapatellar fold: formed by attachments of patella fat pad and tendons via a fibroadipose band lying in intercondylar notch. Acts as stop gap as it is compressed by patella tendon in full flexion.

(c) Proximal tibiofibular joint ligaments.
- Anterior tibiofibular ligament: located on anterior aspect of joint. Reinforces capsule anteriorly.
- Posterior tibiofibular ligament: located on posterior aspect of joint. Reinforces capsule posteriorly.

(3) Menisci.

(a) Medial meniscus.
- Medial meniscus is large, C-shaped and fairly stable. Laterally, it is firmly attached to MCL and fibrous capsule. Other structures that attach to the medial meniscus are semimembranosus muscle and medial meniscopatellar ligament.

(b) Lateral meniscus.
- Smaller than medial meniscus and more circular. Structures that attach to lateral meniscus include popliteus muscle, lateral meniscopatellar ligament, and meniscofemoral ligament. Lateral meniscus is separated from LCL and lateral capsule by popliteus muscle tendon.

(c) Function of menisci.
- Deepens fossa of tibia.
- Increase congruency of tibia and femur.
- Provides stability to tibiofemoral joint.
- Provides shock absorption and lubrication to knee.
- Reduces friction during movement.
- Improves weight distribution.

(d) Movement of menisci.
- Menisci follow tibia with flexion/extension and femoral condyles with internal/external rotation.
- Medial meniscus moves a total of 6 mm while lateral moves 12 mm. With isolated tibial rotation, the menisci move opposite; e.g., with tibial IR, the medial meniscus moves anteriorly and the lateral meniscus moves posteriorly.
- Meniscal motion is also influenced by soft tissue structures. Medial meniscus is pulled posteriorly (flexion) by semimembranosus muscle and ACL. Pulled anteriorly (extension) by medial meniscopatellar ligament. Held firm by attachment to MCL and fibrous capsule.
- Lateral meniscus pulled posteriorly (flexion) by popliteus muscle and anteriorly (extension) by lateral meniscopatellar ligament and meniscofemoral ligament.

(4) Bursae.

(a) Prepatellar, between skin and anterior distal patella.

(b) Superficial infrapatellar, anterior to ligamentum patella.

(c) Deep infrapatellar, between posterior ligamentum patella and anterior tibial tuberosity.

(d) Suprapatellar, between patella and tibia femoral joint.

(e) Popliteal, posterior knee often connected to synovial cavity.

(f) Semimembranosus, between muscle and femoral condyle.

(g) Gastrocnemius, one for each head. Medial bursa usually communicates with semimembranosus bursa.

(h) Pes anserine bursa, between pes anserine and MCL.

(5) Blood supply comes from descending branch from lateral circumflex femoral branch of the deep femoral artery. Genicular branches of popliteal artery and recurrent branches of anterior tibial artery.

(6) Articular innervation is provided by obturator, femoral, tibial, and common fibular nerves.

e. Biomechanics knee joint proper.

(1) Arthrokinematics/osteokinematics.

(a) Movements of femoral condyles during flexion and extension.
- Condyles roll and glide simultaneously (only way that posterior dislocation of femoral condyle can be avoided). Initially, movement is pure rolling and ends in pure gliding. For medial condyle, pure rolling occurs during first 10°–15° of flexion. For lateral condyle, rolling continues until 20° of flexion.
- During flexion, femoral condyles roll posteriorly; ACL becomes taut causing condyles to glide anteriorly.

- During extension, femoral condyles roll anteriorly; PCL becomes taut, causing condyles to glide posteriorly.

(b) During walking, normal range of knee flexion is approximately 15°. We are essentially using pure rolling of femur on tibia.

(2) Conjunct rotations.

(a) During flexion at 10°–15°, ACL tightens, causing femur to glide anteriorly, then 5° further, rolling occurs on lateral condyle, causing a conjunct medial rotation of tibia.

(b) During extension, PCL causes femur to glide posteriorly, while condyles roll anteriorly 10°–15°. Then a further 5° of rolling occurs anteriorly on lateral side, causing a medial femoral rotation or a lateral rotation of tibia as a conjunct rotation with extension.

(c) "Screw home" mechanism describes the 5° of tibial external rotation, which occurs during terminal knee extension.

- Occurs as closed-chain internal femoral rotation during weight-bearing to provide increased stability of knee joint during weight-bearing activities. Can also occur as open-chain external tibial rotation.
- Lateral or external rotation of tibia occurs as knee moves toward terminal extension, due to anatomical relationship of surfaces of tibia and femur.
- Unlocking occurs through action of popliteus. Open-chain unlocking occurs primarily with popliteal action.

(d) Causes for screw home mechanism.

- Lateral femoral condyle glides more freely on lateral convex (anterior-posterior) facet of tibia. Causes greater tibial motion in posteror direction on lateral side.
- Medial femoral condyle has a longer articular surface than lateral condyle. During femoral rolling, more motion occurs on lateral side (20°) than on medial side (10°–15°).
- Medial meniscus is attached to MCL which tightens during extension. Medial meniscus stops gliding, while lateral meniscus continues to glide forward. Creates internal rotation of femur, which is same as external rotation of tibia.
- Twisted cruciate ligaments create external rotation force on tibia, while preventing an internal rotation.
- Lateral angle of pull of quadriceps muscle creates external rotation of tibia.

f. Biomechanics proximal tibiofibular joint.

(1) Dorsiflexion of talocrural joint.

(a) Fibular head glides superiorly and posteriorly. Fibular shaft rotates externally.

(2) Plantar flexion of talocrural joint.

(a) Fibular head glides inferiorly and anteriorly. Fibular shaft rotates internally.

6. Foot and ankle region.

a. Osteology and arthrology (talocrural, subtalar, talocalcaneonavicular, calcaneocuboid, transverse tarsal, tarsometatarsal, metatarsophalangeal, and interphalangeal).

(1) Talocrural joint.

(a) Ankle mortise formed by three components including (1) distal end of tibia and its medial malleolus; (2) with lateral malleolus of fibula and inferior transverse tibiofibular ligament; (3) and trochlear surface of talus.

(b) Three articulations involved in the talocrural joint: (1) tibiofibular, (2) tibiotalar, (3) fibulotalar.

(c) Transversely (medial/lateral), trochlear surface is gently concave. Trochlear surface is wedge shaped, wider anteriorly than posteriorly.

(d) Laterally, talus is triangular shaped and concave in superior/inferior direction, and convex in anterior/posterior direction. Articulates with reciprocally curved fibula. Medial part of trochlear surface is comparatively flat, and articulates with distal end of tibia, which is also flat.

(2) Subtalar joint.

(a) Two separate articulations; anterior and posterior talocalcaneal.

- Posterior talocalcaneal articulation (subtalar joint proper): posterior superior articulation is convex in anterior/posterior direction, and concave in medial/lateral direction. This articulates with reciprocally curved posterior part of inferior surface of talus.
- Anterior talocalcaneal articulation consists of obliquely oriented surfaces of biconvex inferior surface of neck and head of talus, resting on the biconcave anterior surface of calcaneus. Anterior talocalcaneal articulation, when described functionally, also includes posterior surface of navicular bone, which articulates with head of talus. Joint is properly referred to as talocalcaneonavicular joint.

(3) Talonavicular joint.

(a) Biconvex head of talus articulates with biconcavity, formed by posterior navicular surfaces and upper edge of plantar calcaneonavicular ligament.

(4) Calcaneocuboid joint.

(a) Anterior calcaneus is concave medial/lateral and convex superior/inferior. Posterior cuboid

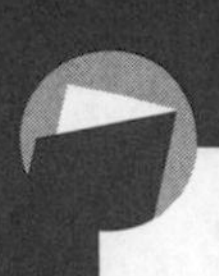

is concave superior/inferior and convex medial/lateral. Bony prominence on inferior/medial surface of cuboid articulates with inferior surface of calcaneus, making saddle shape deeper. Cuboid is key to lateral arch.

(5) Tarsometatarsal joints.
  (a) Proximally, three cuneiforms medially and cuboid laterally. Distally bases of five metatarsals. First metatarsal (MT) is largest and strongest, second MT is longest. Third MT articulates primarily with the third cuneiform. Fourth and fifth MT articulate with cuboid.

(6) Cuneonavicular joint.
  (a) Biconvex anterior surface of navicular has three facets to articulate with concave posterior surfaces of three cuneiform bones.

(7) Metatarsalphalangeal joint.
  (a) Metatarsal heads are convex and proximal phalanges are concave.

(8) Interphalangeal joints.
  (a) Same as fingers of hand.

b. Muscles (ankle plantarflexors, ankle dorsiflexors, everters, inverters, and intrinsics) (see Table 1-7).

c. Noncontractile structures (deltoid ligament, anterior talofibular, posterior talofibular, calcaneofibular, calcaneonavicular [spring ligament], interosseous, bifurcate ligament, plantar aponeurosis, long plantar ligament, and short plantar ligament, capsule, bursae, fascia, nerves, and vessels).

(1) Capsule.
  (a) Talocrural joint.
    - Fibrous capsule lined with synovial membrane strengthened by collateral, anterior, and posterior ligaments. Thin anteriorly and posteriorly and thickened laterally.
  (b) Subtalar joint.
    - Posterior articulation has an independent capsule with synovial membrane. Anterior articulation has capsule with synovial membrane that includes talonavicular joint.
  (c) Talonavicular joint.
    - Fibrous capsule with synovial lining is shared with anterior subtalar joint.
  (d) Calcaneocuboid.
    - Independent fibrous capsule with synovial membrane independent from other tarsal articulations.
  (e) Tarsometatarsal (three capsular cavities).
    - 1st MT with medial cuneiform.
    - 2nd and 3rd cuneiform capsule is continuous with intercuneiform and cuneonavicular joint cavity.
    - 3rd cuneiform with base of 4th MT capsule encloses 4th MT with cuboid and 3rd cuneiform.
  (f) Cuneonavicular.
    - Continuous with those of intercuneiform and cuneocuboid joints, as is its synovial cavity. Capsule is connected to second and third cuneometatarsal joints between 2nd and 4th metatarsal bones.
  (g) Metatarsalphalangeal joint.
    - Fibrous capsule present for each articulation.
  (h) Interphalangeal joints.
    - Fibrous capsule present for each articulation.

(2) Ligaments.
  (a) Talocrural joint.
    - Medial collateral ligament (deep fibers): anterior talotibial ligament and posterior talotibial ligament.
    - Medial collateral ligament (superficial fibers): deltoid ligament.
    - Lateral collateral ligament: anterior talofibular ligament, calcaneofibular ligament, posterior talofibular ligament.
  (b) Subtalar joint.
    - Interosseous talocalcaneal ligament: two fibrous bands taut with eversion.
    - Lateral talocalcaneal ligament.
    - Posterior talocalcaneal ligament.
    - Medial talocalcaneal ligament.
  (c) Talonavicular joint.
    - Plantar calcaneonavicular ligament (spring ligament).
    - Dorsal talonavicular ligament.
  (d) Calcaneocuboid joint.
    - Medial band of the bifurcate ligament (lateral calcaneonavicular ligament).
    - Medial calcaneocuboid (lateral band of the bifurcated ligament).
    - Long plantar ligament (superficial plantar calcaneocuboid).
    - Plantar calcaneocuboid (short plantar).
  (e) Tarsometatarsal joint.
    - Medially, dorsal ligament runs from medial cuneiform to base of 2nd MT.
    - Laterally, dorsal ligaments with straight fibers from middle cuneiform to second MT, lateral cuneiform to third MT, cruciate fibers from lateral cuneiform to 2nd MT, and middle cuneiform to 3rd MT.
  (f) Cuneonavicular joint.
    - 3 dorsal cuneonavicular ligaments, one attached to each cuneiform.
    - Plantar ligaments have similar attachments and receive slips from tendons of posterior tibialis muscle.
  (g) Metatarsalphalangeal joint.
    - Plantar ligaments and collateral ligaments present.

(h) Interphalangeal joints.
- Plantar ligaments and collateral ligaments present.

(3) Plantar fascia.
(a) Also known as plantar aponeurosis.
(b) A broad, dense band of longitudinally arranged collagen fibers that can be divided into three components, running from medial calcaneus to phalanges.
(c) Fascia tightens with dorsiflexion of MTP joints as occurs during push off. Known as "windlass effect." Tightening of this fascia causes supination of calcaneus and inversion of subtalar joint, creating a rigid lever for push off.

(4) Bursa.
(a) Posterior calcaneal bursa.
(b) Retrocalcaneal bursa.

(5) Blood supply comes from malleolar rami of anterior tibial and fibular arteries.

(6) Articular innervation comes from deep fibular and tibial nerves.

d. Ankle and foot biomechanics.
(1) Talocrural joint.
(a) Conjunct rotations.
- Talus rotates medially 30° from dorsiflexion to plantar flexion. Also slight side-to-side gliding, rotation, and abduction/adduction are permitted when foot is plantar flexed.

(b) Arthrokinematics/osteokinematics.
- Open chain: Δuring plantar flexion talus describes anterior glide on mortise with slight medial rotation or adduction. Dorsiflexion occurs as reciprocally opposite motion.
- Closed chain: Δuring plantar flexion tibia glides posteriorly on talus with slight lateral rotation. Dorsiflexion occurs as a reciprocally opposite motion.

(2) Subtalar joint.
(a) Joint axes.
- Oblique axis extends from posterior, plantar, and lateral to anterior, dorsal, and medial. Joint is oriented obliquely, with the average at 42° from the horizontal and 16° from midline of foot.
- Variances in joint axis are fairly common.
- With a high inclination of axis, movement at subtalar joint is increased in transverse plane and decreased in frontal plane.
- With a low inclination of axis joint will be more frontal plane dominant, leading to greater calcaneal pronation/supination.

(b) Conjunct rotation.
- Calcaneus can move in many directions, due to its multiple articulations. Like a ship in the waves—rotation around a vertical axis, tilts medially and laterally, glides anteriorly and posteriorly.

(c) Arthrokinematics/osteokinematics.
- Occurs in same direction when mobilizing calcaneus on a fixed talus. Subtalar joint represents the purest triplanar movement.
- Open chain: Δuring inversion, calcaneus moves into adduction, supination, and plantar flexion on fixed talus. Eversion occurs as a reciprocally opposite motion.
- Closed chain: Δuring inversion, supination of calcaneus (talus guides laterally) with abduction and dorsiflexion of talus. Produces external rotation of tibia. Eversion occurs as a reciprocally opposite motion. Produces internal rotation of tibia.

(3) Talonavicular joint.
(a) Arthrokinematics/osteokinematics.
- Arthokinematics and osteokinematics occur in same direction when mobilizing navicular on a fixed talus. Rotational movements of midtarsal joint allow forefoot to twist on rearfoot. Talus and navicular rotate in opposite directions.
- Open chain: Δuring inversion, navicular plantarflexes, adducts, and externally rotates on talus. Eversion occurs as a reciprocally opposite motion.
- Closed chain: Δuring inversion, navicular plantarflexes (talus glides dorsally on navicular), adducts (talus abducts), and internally rotates. Eversion occurs as a reciprocally opposite motion.

(4) MTPs and PIPs same as fingers.

7. Spine.

a. General function of the vertebral column.
(1) Support for head and internal organs.
(2) Stable attachment for all soft tissues, extremities, rib cage, and pelvis.
(3) Protection of internal organs and spinal cord.
(4) Attenuates forces from above and below.

b. Components of the vertebral column.
(1) Consists of 24 freely movable and 9 fused bones.
(2) Divided into five distinct regions (cervical, thoracic, lumbar, sacral, and coccygeal).

c. Osteology.
(1) Typical vertebra (vertebral body, pedicles, lamina which includes superior and inferior articular processes or facets, transverse processes, and the spinous process).
(2) Regional variations.
(a) Cervical: two atypical (atlas and axis) which allow for increase active range of motion (AROM) in rotation without compressing the spinal cord), uncinate processes, and transverse foramen.

- Vertebral body is rectangular shaped.
- Uncinate joints (joints of von Luschka) found at C_3-C_7 limit lateral cervical motion.

(b) Thoracic: demifacets for articulation with the ribs. Vertebral body is heart shaped. Prominent spinous processes are angled following "Rules of 3."

- Rules of 3: spinous process of T_{1-3} even with transverse process of same level vertebra; T_{4-6} spinous processes are found one half level below transverse processes of same level; T_{7-9} spinous processes are one full level below transverse process of same level; T_{10} is full level below; T_{11} is one half level below; and T_{12} is level.

(c) Lumbar: vertebra larger than other regions and body is kidney shaped. Very prominent spinous processes.

(d) Sacrum is wedge shaped, both anteriorly/posteriorly and inferiorly/superiorly. Made of five fused vertebrae.

(e) Ilium is made up of three fused bones (ischium, ilium, and pubis). Shape varies widely among people, with significant difference in shape between men and women.

d. Arthrology.

(1) Atypical joints.

(a) Atlanto-occipital joint: synovial articulation between occiput and C_1. Also known as "yes" joint, since much of head nodding motion comes from this articulation.

(b) Atlanto-axial joint: nonsynovial articulation between dens of C_2 and anterior arch of C_1. Known as "no" joint, since much of head rotation comes from this articulation.

(c) Costotransverse and costovertebral: articulations between rib and transverse process and vertebral body respectively.

(2) Apophyseal or facet joints which guide movement of spine. Synovial/diarthrodial joints with capsule and synovial membrane. Composed of superior and inferior articulatory processes of adjacent vertebrae. In lumbar region, facet surfaces may be flat or curved. In cervical and thoracic regions, surfaces are generally flat.

(3) Intervertebral joints between intervertebral disc and adjacent superior and inferior vertebral bodies. Allow movement between vertebral bodies and transmit loads from one vertebral segment to another.

(4) Sacroiliac (SI) joint: composed of auricular-shaped joint surfaces of sacrum and ilium. Diarthrosis/synarthrosis (syndesmosis) combination. Ilial articulation is primarily convex and covered with a thin layer of fibrocartilage. Sacral articulation is primarily concave and covered with hyaline cartilage. SI joints attenuate forces from trunk and lower extremities.

e. Fibroadipose meniscoid.

(1) Structure composed of dense connective tissue and adipose tissue.

(2) Found at superior and inferior aspects of facet joints.

(3) Protects cartilage of facet surface during extremes in motion.

f. Muscles (see Table 1-6).

g. Intervertebral disc/endplate.

(1) Annulus fibrosis/fibrosus.

(a) Concentric layers or lamellae composed of collagen (type II) and fibrocartilage. 65% water.

Table 1-8 ➤ TRUNK AND RIBCAGE MUSCULAR & NEUROLOGICAL SCREENING

ACTION TO BE TESTED	MUSCLES	CORD SEGMENT	NERVES
Inspiration	Diaphragm Levator costarum, external intercostals, anterior Internal intercostals	C3-C5 T1-T12	Phrenic Intercostal
Forced expiration	Internal obliques,transverse abdominis, external obliques, posterior internal intercostals, rectus abdominis	T7-L1 T7-T12 T1-T12 T7-T12	Intercostal Intercostal Intercostal Intercostal
Spine extension	Erector spinae, transversospinalis, interspinales, rotatores intertransversarii	T1-T12, L1-L5, S1-S3	
Spine flexion	Rectus abdominis/external obliques, internal obliques, psoas minor	T7-T12 T7-L1 L1	Intercostal Intercostal Lumbar plexus
Spine lateral flexion (hip hiking in reverse)	Quadratus lumborum	T12-L3	Lumbar plexus
Spine rotation	Rotators, internal/external obliques, intertransversarii, transversospinalis	as above	

Adapted from Chusid, JG. Correlative Neuroanatomy and Functional Neurology, Lange Medical Publications, Los Altos, CA, 1970; and Kendall, FP; McCreary, EK, and Provance, PG. Muscles Testing and Function: 4th ed., Baltimore, Williams & Wilkins, 1993.

(b) Outer one third of annulus is innervated by branches from sinovertebral nerve.
(c) Functions to sustain compressive, torsional, shearing, and distraction loads.

(2) Nucleus pulposis/pulposus.
(a) Gel with imbibing capabilities composed of water and proteoglycans with a minimal amount of collagen (type I). 70%–90% water.
(b) Avascular and aneural structure.
(c) Makes up 20%–33% height of vertebral column.
(d) Functions to sustain compressive, torsional, shearing, and distraction loads.

(3) Vertebral endplate.
(a) Structure continuous with annulus and nucleus. Sits inside ring apophysis of vertebral body.
(b) Composed of proteoglycans, collagen, and water as well as both fibrocartilage (on side closest to disc) and hyaline cartilage (on side closest to vertebral body).
(c) Functions to provide passive diffusion of nutrients.

h. Other noncontractile soft tissues.

(1) Ligaments.
(a) Alar ligament.
(b) Tectorial membrane.
(c) Anterior longitudinal ligament.
(d) Posterior longitudinal ligament.
(e) Ligamentum flavum.
(f) Interspinous ligament.
(g) Supraspinous ligament.
(h) Transforaminal ligaments.
(i) Costotransverse ligament (superior, posterior, and lateral).
(j) Iliolumbar ligament.
(k) Posterior sacroiliac ligaments (short, transverse, and long).
(l) Anterior sacroiliac ligament.
(m) Sacrotuberous ligament.
(n) Posterior interosseous ligament (sacroiliac joint [SIJ]).

(2) Capsules.
(a) Facet joint: assist ligaments in providing limitation of motion and stability of spine. Strongest in the thoracolumbar and cervicothoracic regions.
(b) Sacroiliac joints: synovial capsule present in surrounding joint, which is very prominent anteriorly; posteriorly, it is lost within posterior interosseous ligament.

(3) Thoracolumbar fascia.
(a) Provides stability of vertebral column when a force is applied.
(b) Acts as a corset when tension is created by contraction of abdominals, gluteals, and lumbar muscles.

i. Nerves.

(1) Dorsal roots transmit sensory fibers to spinal cord and ventral roots; mainly transmit motor fibers from spinal cord to spinal nerve.

(2) Spinal nerves are connected centrally to spinal cord by a dorsal and ventral root, which join to become the spinal nerve in the intervertebral foramen. Spinal nerve divides into dorsal and ventral rami.
(a) Dorsal rami innervate structures on posterior trunk.
(b) Ventral rami.
- Cervical ventral rami form cervical and brachial plexuses.
- Thoracic ventral rami innervate anterior structures of trunk within thoracic region.
- Lumbar ventral rami form lumbar and lumbosacral plexuses.

(3) Spinal nerves in various sections of spine.
(a) Cervical: spinal nerves come out at the level above its associated vertebra.
(b) Thoracic/lumbar: spinal nerves come out at level below its associated vertebra.

(4) Spinal cord terminates approximately at level of L_{1-2} disc.

j. Spinal biomechanics.

(1) Arthrokinematics.
(a) Flexion: upper facets glide anteroproximally and tilt forward.
(b) Extension: upper facets move downward, slightly posterior, and tilt backward.
(c) Side bending: when side bending right, upper facet moves down and slightly anterior. Left facet moves upward and slightly posterior. Both facets move to the left.
(d) Rotation.
(e) Cervical: right rotation causes facets on right to glide down and back, causing approximation of facet joints on right.
(f) Lumbar/thoracic: very little, but clinically important because this motion causes separation and approximation of the facet joints; e.g., if L_3 rotates right, there is separation at right L_{3-4} joint and approximation at left L_{3-4} joint.

(2) Coupled motions.
(a) Cervical.
- Side bending and rotation occur in same direction from C_{2-7}, regardless of whether spine is in neutral/extension or flexion. When occiput side bends, C_1 rotates in opposite direction.

(b) Lumbar/thoracic.
- Neutral/extension: lumbar segments will side bend and rotate in opposite directions; e.g., side bend right results in segment rotating left.

- Flexion: lumbar segments will side bend and rotate in the same direction.
- This coupling described above is a very basic interpretation. In reality, there are significant variations in coupling motions between individuals. Coupling motion may depend on whether a side bend or rotation is done first. Direction of spinal segmental coupling should always be checked with each patient prior to performing a manual technique.

(3) Lumbopelvic rhythm.
(a) During flexion, spine (primarily lumbar spine) goes through 60°–70° of motion and then pelvis will rotate anteriorly to allow more movement, eventually followed by flexion of hips.
(b) During extension (coming from flexed position) hips extend, pelvis rotates posteriorly, and then spine begins to extend.

(4) Sacroiliac joint osteokinematics.
(a) Motion limited, but during gait movements takes place in multiple planes.
(b) Nutation and counternutation: coupling movement that occurs between sacrum and ilium during gait.

- Nutation: describes a movement that involves flexion of sacrum and posterior rotation of ilium.
- Counternutation: describes a movement that involves extension of sacrum and anterior rotation of ilium.

8. Temporomandibular joint (TMJ).
a. Functional anatomy. A bilateral articulation between mandible and cranium (craniomandibular joint).
b. Arthrology.
(1) Synovial joint with articular surfaces covered by dense fibrous connective tissue rather than hyaline cartilage.
(2) Articular disc composed of dense fibrous connective tissue without blood vessels or nerves in pressure bearing areas.
(3) Discal ligaments function to restrict movement in sagittal plane.
(4) Superior retrodiscal lamina (superior stratum) composed of elastic connective tissue; counteracts forward pull of superior lateral pterygoid muscle on articular disc.
(5) Retrodiscal pad consists of loose neurovascular connective tissue.
c. Joint movement.
(1) Combination of hinge axis rotation in disc condyle complex and sliding movement of the upper joint.
(2) Functional range of opening is 40 mm, with 25 mm of rotation and 15 mm of translatory glide.

Physical Therapy Examination

Patient/Client History (or Interview), Systems Review, and Tests and Measures

1. Patient/client history.
a. Gather information to develop a hypothetical diagnosis, which dictates flow of examination. Delineate any precautions and/or contraindications when performing components of examination (Table 1-9).
b. Components of history.
(1) Demographics: age, gender, diagnosis and referral (if appropriate), hand dominance, etc.
(2) Social and family history.
(3) Current condition(s)/chief complaint.
(4) General health status.
(5) Social health.
(6) Employment/work.
(7) Growth and development.
(8) Living environment.
(9) Functional status and activity level.
(10) Medical/surgical history, including previous treatment and review of systems.

2. Systems review.
a. Components of system review. (See Table 1-10).
(1) Musculoskeletal.
(2) Neuromuscular.
(3) Cardiopulmonary.
(4) Integumentary systems.
b. Determine if identified condition(s) are comorbidity(ies) and/or complicating factor(s).
c. Determine if a referral to an additional healthcare provider is appropriate, and if so, make the referral.

3. Tests and measures.
a. Gather specific data regarding patient/client. Choosing specific components as well as order of exam will be dictated by history.
b. Components that may be a part of tests and measures include:

Table 1-9 ➤ QUESTIONS RELATED TO SPECIFIC AREAS OF DYSFUNCTION

AREA OF DYSFUNCTION	RELATED QUESTIONS
Shoulder	Do you have pain raising your arm up, and if so, what part of the range does that occur? Have you ever dislocated your shoulder? Do you have pain sleeping on your shoulder at night?
Elbow	Have you recently changed your activities? Have you recently changed the type of tools you use at work or the instruments you use for recreational activities?
Hand	Have you been doing more or different work with your hands than the usual, such as typing, sewing, gardening, etc?
Cervical	Do you have dizziness when looking overhead? Any previous motor vehicle accidents with resulting neck injury? How many pillows do you use at night?
TMJ	Do you have any popping or clicking in the TMJ? Do you have pain trying to eat specific foods? Does your jaw ever get stuck open or closed?
Thoracic	Do you have pain with breathing? Have you had a recent upper respiratory infection?
Lumbar	Have you had any changes in your ability to urinate or have a bowel movement? Do you have any symptoms such as pain, tingling, burning, etc. in either of your legs?
Sacroiliac	Did you fall onto your buttocks? Did you step off a curb and experience pain? Do you have pain with walking and/or sustained postures?
Hip	Do you have pain in your groin? Do you have stiffness in the morning that feels better with movement?
Knee	Does your knee "pop"? Does your knee ever give way and/or lock? Did your knee swell as soon as you were injured or did the swelling come later?
Ankle/Foot	Have you ever sprained your ankle and if yes, how many times? Do you have pain in your foot when you first try to step out of bed in the morning?

Table 1-10 ➤ SUMMARY OF SYMPTOMS OBSERVED IN COMMON AND UNCOMMON DYSFUNCTIONS

DYSFUNCTION	SYMPTOMS OBSERVED
DJD/ Osteoarthritis	Pain and stiffness upon rising Pain eases through the morning (4 to 5 hours) Pain increases with repetitive bending activities Constant awareness of discomfort with episodes of exacerbation Describes pain as more soreness and nagging
Facet Joint Dysfunction	Stiff upon rising. Pain eases within an hour Loss of motion accompanied by pain Patient will describe pain as sharp with certain movements Movement in painfree range usually reduces symptoms Stationary positions increase symptoms
Discal, with nerve root compromise	No pain in reclined or semireclined position Pain increases with increasing weightbearing activities Describes pain as shooting, burning, or stabbing Patient may describe altered strength or ability to perform ADLs
Spinal Stenosis	Pain is related to position Flexed positions decrease pain, and extended positions increase pain Describes symptoms as a numbness, tightness, or cramping

Table 1-10 ➤ continued

DYSFUNCTION	SYMPTOMS OBSERVED
	Walking for any distance brings on symptoms Pain may persist for hours after assuming a resting position
Vascular Claudication	Pain is consistent in all spinal positions Pain is brought on by physical exertion Pain is relieved promptly with rest (1 to 5 minutes) Pain is described as a numbness Patient usually has decreased or absent pulses
Neoplastic Disease	Patient will describe pain as gnawing, intense, or penetrating Pain is not resolved by changes in position, time of day, or activity level Pain will wake the patient

(1) Anthropometric characteristics.
(2) Postural alignment and position (Table 1-11, Figure 1-1).
  (a) Dynamic.
  (b) Static.
(3) Range of motion (see Tables 1-12 and 1-13).
  (a) AROM.
  (b) Passive range of motion (PROM).
  (c) Flexibility testing.

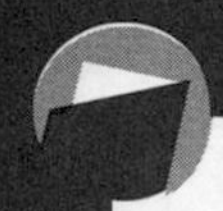

Table 1-11 ➤ EFFECTS OF FORWARD HEAD POSTURE ON THE SPINE, TMJ AND ASSOCIATED SOFT TISSUE STRUCTURES

STRUCTURE	POSTURE CHANGES
1. Cranium	Extended on upper cervical spine
2. Mandible	Elevated and retruded
3. TMJ	Posterior close-packed position
4. Maxillomandibular relationship	Increased freeway space with significant posterior intercuspation
5. Hyoid	Elevated (suprahyoids shorten, infrahyoids lengthen)
6. Tongue	Drops to the floor of mouth
7. Upper cervical spine	Extended (can compress neurovascular structures)
8. Middle and lower cervical spine	Lordosis decreased (flexed positioning)
9. First and second ribs	Elevated
10. Scalenes, Suboccipital, Sternocleidomastoids, Longus colli, Upper trapezius, Levator scapulae	Shorten
11. Pectoralis major and minor	Shorten, creating rounded shoulder position
12. Scapular stabilizers Rectus capitis anterior	Stretched
13. Longus capitis	Stretched suboccipital region, shorten C2-C6

Adapted from Darnell, M. A proposed chronology of events for forward head posture. Journal of Craniomandibular Practice, 1983, 1(4): 50–54.

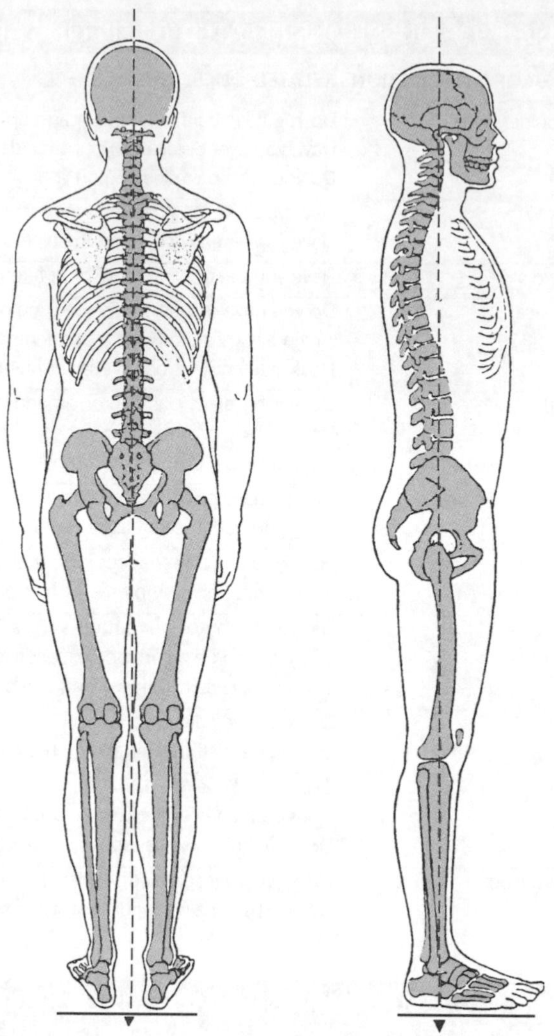

Figure 1-1 • Vertical line of gravity.
(Adapted from Kendall, FP, McCreary, EK, Provance, PG. Muscle Testing and function, 4th ed. Baltimore, Williams & Wilkins, 1993).

(4) Muscle performance: resisted tests, manual muscle testing, muscle tension (Table 1-14).
(5) Motor function.
(6) Cranial and peripheral nerve integrity (see Tables 1-7, 1-8, 1-9, Figure 1-2).
(7) Reflex integrity.
(8) Sensory integrity.
(9) Joint integrity and mobility.
(10) Pain.
(11) Assistive and adaptive devices.
(12) Orthotic, protective, and supportive devices.
(13) Ergonomics and body mechanics.
(14) Self-care and home management.
(15) Gait, locomotion, and balance.
(16) Work, community, and leisure integration or reintegration.
(17) Special tests (see specifics for each joint/region).

4. Diagnostic testing.

a. Diagnostic tests are utilized for correlation with history and tests and measures to determine patient's primary physical therapy diagnosis as well as identify any medical conditions that may be a contributing factor or comorbidity.

b. If further diagnostic tests are warranted and/or beneficial, make appropriate referral or recommendation.

c. Most common types of diagnostic testing for musculoskeletal dysfunctions include imaging, laboratory tests, and electrodiagnostic testing.

d. Imaging.

(1) Plain film radiograph (x-rays).

(a) X-rays are used to demonstrate bony tissues. Beams pass through the tissues resulting in varying shades of gray on film depending on density of tissue it passed through. The more dense the structure (bone), the more white the structure will appear on the film.

(b) Readily available, relatively inexpensive, and shows bony anatomy very well.

(c) Negative is patient exposure to radiation.

(d) Requires two different projections, since structures may be superimposed on each

Table 1-12 ➤ EXTREMITY RANGE OF MOTION

JOINT	FLEXION/ EXTENSION	ABDUCTION/ ADDUCTION	EXTERNAL/ INTERNAL ROTATION	HORIZONTAL ADDUCTION	SUPINATION/ PRONATION	RADIAL/ ULNAR DEVIATION	PLANTARFLEXION/ DORSIFLEXION
Shoulder	160–180/ 50–60	170–180/ 50–75	80–90/ 60–100	130/45			
Elbow	140–150/ 0–10				90/80–90		
Wrist	80–90/ 70–90					15/30–45	
MCP	85–90/ 30–45						
PIP	100–115/0						
DIP	80–90/20						
1st CMC	45–50	60–70/30					
1st MCP	50–55/0						
1st IP	85–90/0–5						
Hip	110–120/ 10–15	30–50/30	40–60/30–40				
Knee	135/0–15		30–40/20–30				
Ankle					45–60/15–30		50/20
2nd–5th MTP	40/40						
1st MTP	45/70						
1st IP	90/0						
2nd–5th PIP	35/0						
2nd–5th DIP	60/30						

other, making it difficult to identify pathology with one view. Typical views are anterior-posterior and lateral, although other views may be used.

(e) Used for viewing dysfunction and/or disease of bones. Does not demonstrate soft tissues well or at all.

(2) Computed tomography (CT scan).

(a) Uses plain film x-ray slices that are enhanced by a computer to improve resolution. It is multiplanar so can image in any plane; therefore, tissue can be viewed from multiple directions.

(b) Typically used to assess complex fractures as well as facet dysfunction, disc disease, or stenosis of the spinal canal or intervertebral foramen. CT demonstrates better quality and better visualization of bony structures than plain films. CT also demonstrates soft tissue structures, although not as well as MRI.

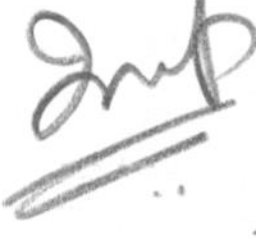

(c) Fairly expensive, and patient is exposed to radiation.

(3) Discography.

(a) Radiopaque dye is injected into the disc to identify abnormalities within the disc (annulus or nucleus). The needle is inserted into the disc with the assistance of radiography (fluoroscopy).

(b) Not commonly used. Requires a high level of skill and proper equipment to perform. Fairly specific technique to identify internal disc disruptions of the nucleus and/or annulus.

(c) Expensive, may be painful, and since it is invasive, there is a risk of infection.

(4) Magnetic resonance imaging (MRI).

(a) Uses magnetic fields rather than radiation.

(b) Offers excellent visualization of tissue anatomy. Utilizes two types of images known as T1 and T2. T1 demonstrates fat within the

Table 1-13 ➤ SPINE RANGE OF MOTION

REGION	FLEXION/ EXTENSION	SIDEBENDING	ROTATION	OPENING	PROTRUSION/ RETRUSION	LATERAL DEVIATION
Cervical	80–90/70	20–45	70–90			
Thoracic	20–45/25–45	20–40	35–50			
Lumbar	40–60/20–35	15–20	3–18			
TMJ				35–50 mm	3–6 mm/3–4 mm	10–15 mm

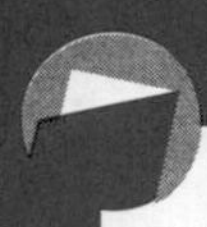

Table 1-14 ➤ MUSCLE GRADING

Normal	N	5/5	Lift or hold against gravity with maximal resistance
Good +	G +	4+/5	Good grades include lifting or holding against gravity with moderate to minimal resistance
Good	G	4/5	
Good –	G –	4–/5	
Fair +	F +	3+/5	Fair grades include lifting or holding against gravity without resistance
Fair	F	3/5	
Fair	F –	3–/5	Some assistance may be required to complete the motion in the minus category
Poor +	P +	2+/5	Poor grades include movement with gravity eliminated
Poor	P	2/5	
Poor –	P –	2–/5	Some assistance may be required to complete the motion in the minus category
Trace	T	1/5	Muscle contraction can be seen or felt No movement is produced
Zero	0	0/5	No contraction is seen or felt

Adapted from Kendall, FP, McCreary, EK, Provance, PG, Muscles Testing and Function: 4th ed., Baltimore, Williams & Wilkins, 1993.

tissues and is typically used to assess bony anatomy, while T2 suppresses fat and demonstrates tissues with high water content. T2 is used to assess soft tissue structures.

(c) Fairly expensive, and patients with claustrophobia do not tolerate this test well. Quality of open MRI is inferior to closed. May not be able to use with patients who have metallic implants.

(5) Arthrography.

(a) Invasive technique that injects water-soluble dye into area, and is observed with a radiograph. Dye is observed as it surrounds tissues, demonstrating the anatomy where fluid moves within joint.

(b) Typically used to identify abnormalities within joints such as tendon ruptures.

(c) Expensive, and carries risks since it is invasive.

(6) Bone scans (osteoscintigraphy).

(a) Chemicals laced with radioactive tracers are injected.

(b) Isotope settles in areas where there is a high metabolic activity of bone.

(c) Radiograph is taken to demonstrate any "hot spots" of increased metabolic activity.

(d) Patients with dysfunctions, such as rheumatoid arthritis, possible stress fractures, bone cancer, infection within bone, often receive a bone scan, since these dysfunctions increase metabolic activity of bone in the affected regions.

(7) Diagnostic ultrasound.

(a) Utilizes transmission of high-frequency sound waves, similar to therapeutic ultrasound.

(b) Limited by contrast resolution, small viewing field, how deep it penetrates, and poor penetration of bone. Interpretation of data is subjective, so results depend on skill of operator.

(c) Provides real-time dynamic images, and can assess soft tissue dysfunctions.

(d) No known harmful effects at this time.

(8) Myelography.

(a) Invasive technique using water-soluble dye. Dye is visualized as it passes through vertebral canal to observe anatomy within region.

(b) Seldom used due to side effects versus MRI or CT scan, which provide as good, if not better, information. Very expensive, since it often involves a hospital stay overnight.

(c) Traditionally used for diagnostic assessment of the discs and stenosis. May still be beneficial to identify stenosis.

e. Laboratory tests.

(1) Laboratory tests are typically used to screen patients, assist with making a diagnosis, or for monitoring.

(2) Since many patients with musculoskeletal dysfunction present with other medical pathology, it is important to monitor clinical laboratory findings.

(3) Multiple tests available that fall into the following categories.

(a) Blood tests.

(b) Serum chemistries.

(c) Immunological tests.

(d) Pulmonary function tests.

(e) Arterial blood gases.

(f) Fluid analysis.

f. Electrodiagnostic testing. (Also refer to Chapter 2: Neuromuscular Physical Therapy.)

(1) Electroneuromyography (ENMG) and nerve conduction velocity (NCV) tests are commonly used to assess and/or monitor musculoskeletal conditions.

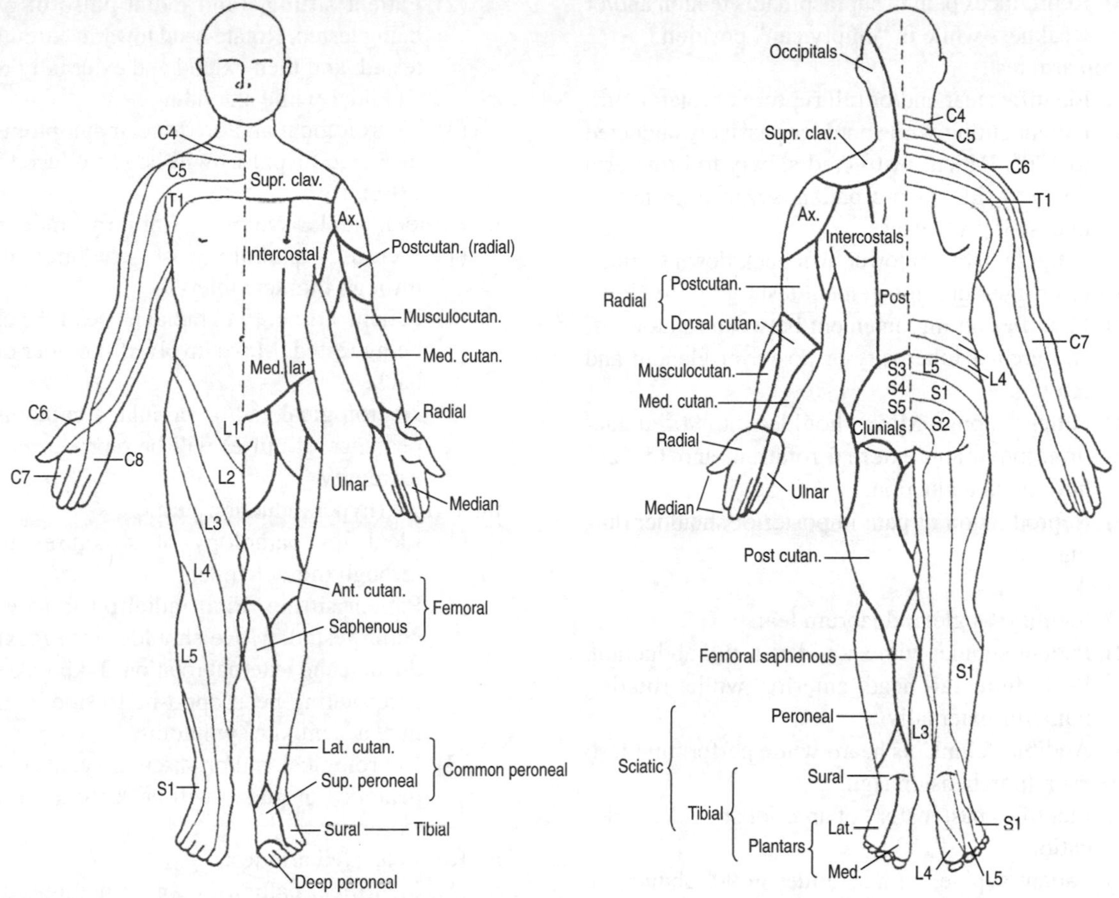

Figure 1-2 • Segmental and peripheral nerve distribution.
(From Hertling, DH, Kessler, RM. Management of Common Musculoskeletal Disorders: Physical Therapy Principles and Methods. 3rd ed. Philadelphia, Lippincott, 1996, with permission).

Special Tests of the Upper Extremity

1. **Shoulder special tests.**
   a. Yergason's test.
      (1) Tests for integrity of transverse ligament; may also identify bicipital tendonitis.
      (2) Patient sitting with shoulder in neutral stabilized against trunk, elbow at 90°, and forearm pronated. Resist supination of forearm and external rotation of shoulder.
      (3) Tendon of biceps long head will "pop out" of groove. May also reproduce pain in long head of biceps tendon.
   b. Speed's test (Biceps straight arm).
      (1) Identifies bicipital tendonitis or tendonosis.
      (2) Patient sitting or standing with upper limb in full extension and forearm supinated. Resist shoulder flexion. May also place shoulder in 90° flexion and push upper limb into extension, causing an eccentric contraction of the biceps.
      (3) Reproduces symptoms (pain) in long head of biceps tendon.
   c. Neer's impingement test.
      (1) For impingement of soft tissue structures of shoulder complex (long head of biceps and supraspinatus tendon).
      (2) Patient sitting, and shoulder is passively internally rotated, then fully abducted.
      (3) Reproduces symptoms of pain within shoulder region.
   d. Supraspinatus (empty can) test.
      (1) Identifies tear and/or impingement of supraspinatus tendon or possible suprascapular nerve neuropathy.
      (2) Patient sitting, with shoulder at 90° and no rotation. Resist shoulder abduction. Then place shoulder in "empty can" position, which is internal rotation and 30° forward (horizontal adduction) and resist abduction. Differentiate whether pain is present between two positions.

(3) Reproduces pain in supraspinatus tendon and/or weakness while in "empty can" position.

e. Drop arm test.
   (1) Identifies tear and/or full rupture of rotator cuff.
   (2) Patient sitting with shoulder passively abducted to 120°. Patient instructed slowly to bring arm down to side. Guard patient's arm from falling in case it gives way.
   (3) Patient unable to lower arm back down to side.

f. Posterior internal impingement test.
   (1) Identifies an impingement between rotator cuff and greater tuberosity or posterior glenoid and labrum.
   (2) Patient supine. Move shoulder into 90° abduction, maximum external rotation, and 15°–20° horizontal adduction.
   (3) Reproduction of pain in posterior shoulder during test.

g. Clunk test.
   (1) Identifies a glenoid labrum tear.
   (2) Patient supine, with shoulder in full abduction. Push humeral head anterior while rotating humerus externally.
   (3) Audible "clunk" is heard while performing test.

h. Anterior apprehension sign.
   (1) Identifies past history of anterior shoulder dislocation.
   (2) Patient supine, with shoulder in 90° abduction. Slowly take shoulder into external rotation.
   (3) Patient does not allow and/or does not like shoulder to move in direction to simulate anterior dislocation.

i. Posterior apprehension sign.
   (1) Identifies past history of posterior shoulder dislocation.
   (2) Patient supine with shoulder abducted 90° (in plane of scapula) with scapula stabilized by table. Place a posterior force through shoulder via force on patient's elbow while simultaneously moving shoulder into medial rotation and horizontal adduction.
   (3) Patient does not allow and/or does not like shoulder to move in direction to simulate posterior dislocation.

j. Acromioclavicular (AC) shear test.
   (1) Identifies dysfunction of AC joint (such as arthritis, separation).
   (2) Patient sitting with arm resting at side. Examiner clasps hands and places heel of one hand on spine of scapula and heel of other hand on clavicle. Squeeze hands together, causing compression of AC joint.
   (3) Reproduces pain in AC joint.

k. Adson's test.
   (1) Identifies pathology of structures that pass through thoracic inlet.
   (2) Patient sitting. Find radial pulse of extremity being tested. Rotate head toward extremity being tested, and then extend and externally rotate the shoulder while extending head.
   (3) Neurological and/or vascular symptoms (disappearance of pulse) will be reproduced in upper extremity.

l. Costoclavicular syndrome (military brace) test.
   (1) Identifies pathology of structures that pass through thoracic inlet.
   (2) Patient sitting. Find radial pulse of the extremity being tested. Move involved shoulder down and back.
   (3) Neurological and/or vascular symptoms (disappearance of pulse) will be reproduced in upper extremity.

m. Wright (hyperabduction) test.
   (1) Identifies pathology of structures that pass through thoracic inlet.
   (2) Patient sitting. Find radial pulse of extremity being tested. Move shoulder into maximal abduction and external rotation. Taking deep breath and rotating head opposite to side being tested may accentuate symptoms.
   (3) Neurological and/or vascular symptoms (disappearance of pulse) will be reproduced in upper extremity.

n. Roos elevated arm test.
   (1) Identifies pathology of structures that pass through thoracic inlet.
   (2) Patient standing, with shoulders fully externally rotated, 90° abducted, and slightly horizontally abducted. Elbows flexed to 90° and patient opens/closes hands for 3 minutes slowly.
   (3) Neurological and/or vascular symptoms (disappearance of pulse) will be reproduced in upper extremity.

o. Upper limb tension tests (Table 1-15).
   (1) Evaluation of peripheral nerve compression.
   (2) Neurological symptoms will be reproduced in upper extremity.

2. Elbow special tests.

a. Ligament instability tests (medial and lateral stability).
   (1) Identifies ligament laxity or restriction.
   (2) Patient sitting or supine. Entire upper limb is supported and stabilized and elbow placed in 20°–0° of flexion. Valgus force placed through elbow tests ulnar collateral ligament. Varus force placed through elbow tests radial collateral ligament.
   (3) Primary finding is laxity, but pain may be noted as well.

b. Lateral epicondylitis ("tennis elbow") test.
   (1) Identifies lateral epicondylitis.
   (2) Patient sitting with elbow in 90° flexion and supported/stabilized. Resist wrist extension,

Table 1-15 ➤ UPPER LIMB TENSION TESTS SHOWING ORDER OF JOINT POSITIONING AND NERVE BIAS

	ULTT1	ULTT2	ULTT3	ULTT4
Shoulder	Depression and abduction (110°)	Depression and abduction (10°)	Depression and abduction (10°)	Depression and abduction (10° to 90°) hand to ear
Elbow	Extension	Extension	Extension	Flexion
Forearm	Supination	Supination	Pronation	Supination
Wrist	Extension	Extension	Flexion and ulnar deviation	Extension and radial deviation
Fingers and thumb	Extension	Extension	Flexion	Extension
Shoulder	—	Lateral rotation	Medial rotation	Lateral rotation
Cervical spine	Contralateral side flexion	Contralateral side flexion	Contralateral side flexion	Contralateral side flexion
Nerve bias	Median nerve, anterior interosseous nerve, C5, C6, C7	Median nerve musculocutaneous nerve, axillary nerve	Radial nerve	Ulnar nerve, C8 and T1 nerve roots

From: Magee, D: Orthopedic Physical Assessment, 4th ed., Philadelphia, Saunders, 2002, with permission.

wrist radial deviation, and forearm pronation with fingers fully flexed (fist) simultaneously.
- (3) Reproduces pain at lateral epicondyle.

c. Medial epicondylitis ("golfer's elbow") test.
- (1) Identifies medial epicondylitis.
- (2) Patient sitting with elbow in 90° flexion and supported/stabilized. Passively supinate forearm, extend elbow, and extend wrist.
- (3) Reproduces pain at medial epicondyle.

d. Tinel's sign.
- (1) Identifies dysfunction of ulnar nerve at olecranon.
- (2) Tap region where the ulnar nerve passes through cubital tunnel.
- (3) Reproduces a tingling sensation in ulnar distribution.

e. Pronator teres syndrome test.
- (1) Identifies a median nerve entrapment within pronator teres.
- (2) Patient sitting with elbow in 90° flexion and supported/stabilized. Resist forearm pronation and elbow extension simultaneously.
- (3) Reproduces a tingling or paresthesia within median nerve distribution.

3. Wrist and hand special tests.

a. Finkelstein's test.
- (1) Identifies deQuervain's tenosynovitis (paratendonitis of the abductor pollicis longus and/or extensor pollicis brevis).
- (2) Patient makes fist with thumb within confines of fingers. Passively move wrist into ulnar deviation.
- (3) Reproduces pain in wrist. Often painful with no pathology, so compare to uninvolved side.

b. Bunnel-Littler test.
- (1) Identifies tightness in structures surrounding the MCP joints.
- (2) MCP joint is stabilized in slight extension while PIP joint is flexed. Then MCP joint is flexed and PIP joint is flexed.
- (3) Differentiates between a tight capsule and tight intrinsic muscles. If flexion is limited in both cases, capsule is tight. If more PIP flexion with MCP flexion, then intrinsic muscles are tight.

c. Tight retinacular test.
- (1) Identifies tightness around proximal interphalangeal joint.
- (2) PIP is stabilized in neutral while DIP is flexed. Then PIP is flexed and DIP is flexed.
- (3) Differentiates between a tight capsule and tight retinacular ligaments. If flexion is limited in both cases capsule is tight. If more DIP flexion with PIP flexion then retinacular ligaments are tight.

d. Ligamentous instability tests (medial and lateral stability).
- (1) Identifies ligament laxity or restriction.
- (2) Fingers are supported and stabilized. Valgus and varus forces applied to PIP joints all digits. Repeated at DIP joints.
- (3) Primary finding is laxity, but pain may be noted as well.

e. Froment's sign.
- (1) Identifies ulnar nerve dysfunction.
- (2) Patient grasps paper between 1st and 2nd digits of hand. Pull paper out and look for IP flexion of thumb, which is compensation due to weakness of adductor pollicis.
- (3) Patient unable to perform test without compensating may indicate ulnar nerve dysfunction.

f. Tinel's sign.
- (1) Identifies carpal tunnel compression of median nerve.
- (2) Tap region where median nerve passes through carpal tunnel.

(3) Reproduces tingling and/or paresthesia into hand following median nerve distribution.

g. Phalen's test.
(1) Identifies carpal tunnel compression of median nerve.
(2) Patient maximally flexes both wrists holding them against each other for 1 minute.
(3) Reproduces tingling and/or paresthesia into hand following median nerve distribution.

h. Two point discrimination test.
(1) Identifies level of sensory innervation within hand which correlates with functional ability to perform certain tasks involving grasp.
(2) Patient sitting with hand stabilized. Using a caliper, two-point discriminator, or paper clip apply device to palmar aspect of fingers to assess patients ability to distinguish between two points of testing device. Record smallest difference that patient can sense two separate points.
(3) Normal amount that can be discriminated is generally less than 6 mm.

i. Allen's test.
(1) Identifies vascular compromise.
(2) Identify radial and ulnar arteries at wrist. Have patient open/close fingers quickly several times and then make a closed fist. Using your thumb, occlude the ulnar artery and have patient open hand. Observe palm of hand and then release the compression on artery and observe for vascular filling. Perform same procedure with radial artery.
(3) Positive finding will present by abnormal filling of blood within hand during test. Under normal circumstances, there is a change in color from white to normal appearance on palm of hand.

Special Tests of the Lower Extremity

1. Hip special tests.

a. Patrick's (FABER) test.
(1) Identifies dysfunction of hip, such as mobility restriction.
(2) Patient lies supine. Passively flex, abduct, and externally rotate test leg so that foot is resting just above knee on opposite leg. Slowly lower testing leg down toward table surface.
(3) Positive test when involved knee is unable to assume relaxed position and/or reproduction of painful symptoms.

b. Grind (Scouring) test.
(1) Identifies degenerative joint disease (DJD) of hip joint.
(2) Patient supine with hip in 90° flexion and knee maximally flexed. Place compressive load into femur via knee joint, therefore loading hip joint.
(3) May reproduce pain within hip joint.

c. Trendelenburg's sign.
(1) Identifies weakness of gluteus medius or unstable hip.
(2) Patient standing, and asked to stand on one leg (flex opposite knee). Observe pelvis of stance leg.
(3) Positive when ipsilateral pelvis drops when lower limb support is removed while standing.

d. Thomas' test.
(1) Identifies tightness of hip flexors.
(2) Patient supine with one hip and knee maximally flexed to chest and held there. Opposite limb is kept straight on table. Observe whether hip flexion occurs on straight leg as opposite limb is flexed.
(3) Weakness of test is that it does not differentiate between tightness in iliacus versus psoas major.
(4) Positive if straight limb's hip flexes and/or patient is unable to remain flat on table when opposite limb is flexed.

e. Ober's test.
(1) Identifies tightness of tensor fascia latae and/or iliotibial band.
(2) Patient lying on side, with lower limb flexed at hip and knee. Passively extend and abduct testing hip with knee flexed to 90°. Slowly lower uppermost limb and observe if it reaches table.
(3) Positive if uppermost limb is unable to come to rest on table.

f. Ely's test.
(1) Identifies tightness of rectus femoris.
(2) Patient prone, with knee of testing limb flexed. Observe hip of testing limb.
(3) Positive if hip of testing limb flexes.

g. 90-90 Hamstring test.
(1) Identifies tightness of hamstrings.
(2) Patient supine, with hip and knee of testing limb is supported in 90° flexion. Passively extend knee of testing limb until a barrier is encountered.
(3) Positive if knee is unable to reach 10° from neutral position (lacking 10° of extension).

h. Piriformis test.
(1) Identifies piriformis syndrome.
(2) Patient supine, with foot of test leg passively placed lateral to opposite limb's knee. Testing hip is adducted. Observe position of testing knee relative to opposite knee.
(3) Positive if testing knee is unable to pass over resting knee, and/or reproduction of pain in buttock, and/or along sciatic nerve distribution.

i. Leg length test.
(1) Identifies true leg length discrepancy.
(2) Patient supine, with pelvis balanced/aligned with lower limbs and trunk. Measure distance from ASIS to lateral malleolus on each limb several times for consistency and compare results.

(3) A difference in lengths between two limbs identifies, a true leg length discrepancy. This test will determine if the limb discrepancy is true or functional. True discrepancy is caused by an anatomical difference in bone lengths (either tibia or femur). Functional discrepancies are not anatomical in origin, and are the result of compensation due to abnormal position or posture, such as pronation of a foot or pelvic obliquity.

j. Craig's test.
 (1) Identifies abnormal femoral antetorsion angle.
 (2) Patient prone with knee flexed to 90°. Palpate greater trochanter and slowly move hip through internal/external rotation. When greater trochanter feels most lateral, stop and measure the angle of leg relative to a line perpendicular with table surface.
 (3) Based on findings, patient may have an anteverted or retroverted hip. Normal angle is between 8° and 15° hip internal rotation. Less than 8° indicates a retroverted hip, and greater than 15° indicates an anteverted hip.

2. Knee special tests.

a. Collateral ligament instability tests (medial and lateral stability).
 (1) Identifies ligament laxity or restriction.
 (2) Patient is supine. Entire lower limb is supported and stabilized and knee placed in 20°–30° of flexion. Valgus force placed through knee tests medial collateral ligament. Varus force placed through knee tests lateral collateral ligament.
 (3) Primary finding is laxity, but pain may be noted as well.

b. Lachman's stress test.
 (1) Indicates integrity of anterior cruciate ligament.
 (2) Patient supine, with testing knee flexed 20°–30°. Stabilize femur and passively try to glide tibia anterior.
 (3) Positive finding is excessive anterior glide of tibia.

c. Pivot shift (anterolateral rotary instability).
 (1) Indicates anterior cruciate ligament integrity.
 (2) Patient supine, with testing knee in extension, hip flexed and abducted 30° with slight internal rotation. Hold knee with one hand and foot with other hand. Place valgus force through knee and flex knee.
 (3) Positive finding is ligament laxity as indicated by tibia relocating during the test. As knee is flexed, the tibia clunks backward at approximately 30°–40°. The tibia at beginning of test was subluxed, and then was reduced by pull of iliotibial band as knee was flexed.

d. Posterior sag test.
 (1) Indicates integrity of posterior cruciate ligament.
 (2) Patient supine with testing hip flexed to 45° and knee flexed to 90°. Observe to see if tibia "sags" posteriorly in this position.
 (3) Positive finding is sag of tibia relative to femur.

e. Posterior drawer test.
 (1) Indicates integrity of posterior cruciate ligament.
 (2) Patient supine and testing hip flexed to 45° and knee flexed to 90°. Passively glide tibia posteriorly following the joint plane.
 (3) Positive finding is excessive posterior glide.

f. Reverse Lachman.
 (1) Indicates integrity of posterior cruciate ligament.
 (2) Patient prone with knees flexed to 30°. Stabilize femur and passively try to glide tibia posterior.
 (3) Positive finding is ligament laxity.

g. McMurray's test.
 (1) Identifies meniscal tears.
 (2) Patient supine, with testing knee in maximal flexion. Passively internally rotate and extend the knee. This tests lateral meniscus. Test medial meniscus with same procedure, except rotate tibia into lateral rotation.
 (3) Positive finding is reproduction of click and/or pain in knee joint.

h. Apley test.
 (1) Helps differentiate between meniscal tears and ligamentous lesions.
 (2) Patient prone, with testing knee flexed to 90°. Stabilize patient's thigh to table with your knee. Passively distract the knee joint, then slowly rotate tibia internally and externally. Next, apply a compressive load to knee joint and again slowly rotate tibia internally and externally.
 (3) Pain or decreased motion during compression indicates a meniscal dysfunction. If pain or decreased motion occurs during the distraction, then it is most likely a ligamentous dysfunction.

Table 1-16 ➤ POSITIONS/ACTIVITIES THAT PRECIPITATE SI DYSFUNCTION

TYPE OF DYSFUNCTION	ACTIVITIES THAT PRECIPITATE DYSFUNCTION
Anterior Torsion of Innominate	Squatting/lifting/lowering Pregnancy Hip at 90° with axial loading Golfing/batting/tennis
Posterior Torsion of Innominate	Vertical thrust onto extended LE Sprint starting position Fall onto ischial tuberosity Unilateral standing
Sacral Dysfunction	Long-term postural abnormalities Fall onto sacrum/coccyx Carrying a load during ambulation Trauma during childbirth Loss of balance during ambulation Sitting combined with rotation and lifting

i. Hughston's plica test.
   (1) Identifies dysfunction of the plica.
   (2) Patient is supine and testing knee is flexed with tibia internally rotated. Passively glide the patella medially, while palpating the medial femoral condyle. Feel for popping as you passively flex and extend the knee.
   (3) Positive finding is pain and/or "popping" noted during the test.

j. Patellar apprehension test.
   (1) Indicates past history of patella dislocation.
   (2) Patient supine, with patella passively glided laterally.
   (3) Patient does not allow and/or does not like patella to move in lateral direction to simulate subluxation/dislocation.

k. Clarke's sign.
   (1) Indicates patellofemoral dysfunction.
   (2) Patient supine, with knee in extension resting on table. Push posterior on superior pole of patella, then ask patient to perform an active contraction of the quadriceps muscle.
   (3) Pain is produced in knee as a result of the test.

l. Ballotable patella (Patellar tap test).
   (1) Indicates infrapatellar effusion.
   (2) Patient supine, with knee in extension resting on table. Apply a soft tap over the central patella.
   (3) Positive finding is perception of the patella floating ("dancing patella" sign).

m. Fluctuation test.
   (1) Indicates knee joint effusion.
   (2) Patient supine, with knee in extension resting on table. Place one hand over suprapatellar pouch and other over anterior aspect of knee joint. Alternate pushing down with one hand at a time.
   (3) Positive finding is fluctuation (movement) of fluid noted during the test.

n. Q-angle measurement.
   (1) Measurement of angle between the quadriceps muscle and the patellar tendon.
   (2) Normal is 13° for men and 18° for women.
   (3) Angles < or > normal may be indicative of knee dysfunction and/or biomechanical dysfunctions within the lower limb.

o. Noble compression test.
   (1) Identifies whether distal iliotibial (IT) band friction syndrome is present.
   (2) Patient supine, with hip flexed to 45° and knee flexed to 90°. Apply pressure to lateral femoral epicondyle then extend knee.
   (3) Reproduces same pain over lateral femoral condyle. Patient will complain of pain over lateral femoral epicondyle at approximately 30° flexion.

p. Tinel's sign.
   (1) Identifies dysfunction of common fibular nerve posterior to fibula head.
   (2) Tap region where common fibular nerve passes through posterior to fibula head.
   (3) Reproduces tingling and/or paresthesia into leg following common fibular nerve distribution.

3. Ankle and foot special tests.

a. Neutral subtalar positioning.
   (1) Examination identifies abnormal rearfoot to forefoot positioning.
   (2) Patient prone, with foot over edge of table. Palpate dorsal aspect of talus on both sides with one hand, and grasp lateral forefoot with other hand. Gently dorsiflex foot until resistance is felt, then gently move foot through arc of supination and pronation.
   (3) Neutral position is point at which you feel foot fall off easier to one side or other. At this point, compare rearfoot to forefoot and rearfoot to leg.

b. Anterior drawer test.
   (1) Identifies ligamentous instability (particularly anterior talofibular ligament).
   (2) Patient supine, with heel just off edge of table in 20° plantar flexion. Stabilize lower leg and grasp foot. Pull talus anterior.
   (3) Positive finding if talus has excessive anterior glide and/or pain is noted.

c. Talar tilt.
   (1) Identifies ligamentous instability (particularly calcaneofibular ligament).
   (2) Patient sidelying, with knee slightly flexed and ankle in neutral. Move foot into adduction testing calcaneofibular ligament and into abduction testing deltoid ligament.
   (3) Positive finding if excessive adduction or abduction occurs and/or pain is noted.

d. Thompson's test.
   (1) Evaluates integrity of the Achilles' tendon.
   (2) Patient prone, with foot off edge of table. Squeeze calf muscles.
   (3) No movement of foot while squeezing calf indicates positive finding.

e. Tinel's sign.
   (1) Identifies dysfunction of posterior tibial nerve posterior to the medial malleolus or deep fibular nerve anterior to talocrural joint.
   (2) Patient supine, with foot supported on the table. Tap over region of posterior tibial nerve as it passes posterior to medial malleolus. Tap over region of deep fibular nerve as it passes under dorsal retinaculum (anterior to ankle joint).
   (3) Reproduces tingling and/or paresthesia into the respective nerve distributions.

f. Morton's test.
   (1) Identifies stress fracture or neuroma in forefoot.
   (2) Patient supine, with foot supported on table. Grasp around metatarsal heads and squeeze.
   (3) Positive finding is pain in forefoot.

Special Tests of the Spine, Pelvis, and Temporomandibular Joint

1. Cervical special tests.

a. Vertebral artery test.
   (1) Assesses the integrity of the vertebrobasilar vascular system.
   (2) Patient supine, with head supported on table and follow the progression.
      (a) Extend head and neck for 30 seconds. If no change in symptoms, progress to next step.
      (b) Extend head and neck with rotation left, then right, for 30 seconds. If no change in symptoms, progress to next step.
      (c) With head being cradled off table, extend head and neck for 30 seconds. If no change in symptoms, progress to next step.
      (d) With head being cradled off table, extend head and neck with rotation left for 30 seconds. Repeat same procedure with rotation to the right.
   (3) Patient should be continuously monitored for any change in symptoms during entire test. Caution should be used with this test, since there is an inherent danger in test itself; therefore, progressive flow should be followed.
   (4) Performing mobilization/manipulation within cervical region without performing this test beforehand would be considered by most to be a breach in standard of care.
   (5) Positive findings are, e.g., dizziness, visual disturbances, disorientation, blurred speech, nausea/vomiting.

b. Hautant's test.
   (1) Differentiates vascular versus vestibular causes of dizziness/vertigo.
   (2) Two steps to this test.
      (a) Patient sitting, with shoulders at 90° and palms up. Have patient close eyes and remain in this position for 30 seconds. If arms lose their position, there may be a vestibular condition.
      (b) Patient sitting, with shoulders at 90° and palms up. Have patient close eyes, and cue patient into head and neck extension with rotation right, then left, remaining in each position for 30 seconds. If arms lose their position, the condition may be vascular in nature.
   (3) Position/movement of arms determines positive finding.

c. Transverse ligament stress test.
   (1) Tests integrity of transverse ligament.
   (2) Patient supine, with head supported on table. Glide C1 anterior. Should be firm end feel.
   (3) Positive findings: soft end feel, dizziness, nystagmus, lump sensation in throat, nausea.

d. Anterior shear test.
   (1) Assesses integrity of upper cervical spine ligaments and capsules.
   (2) Patient supine, with head supported on table. Glide C2-7 anterior. Should be firm end feel.
   (3) Laxity of ligaments is positive finding, as well as dizziness, nystagmus, a lump sensation in the throat, nausea.

e. Foraminal compression (Spurling's) test.
   (1) Identifies dysfunction (typically compression) of cervical nerve root.
   (2) Patient sitting, with head side bent toward uninvolved side. Apply pressure through head straight down. Repeat with head side bent toward involved side.
   (3) Positive finding is pain and/or paresthesia in dermatomal pattern for involved nerve root.

f. Maximum cervical compression test.
   (1) Identifies compression of neural structures at intervertebral foramen and/or facet dysfunction.
   (2) Patient sitting. Passively move head into side bending and rotation towards nonpainful side, followed by extension. Repeat this toward painful side.
   (3) Be careful since this is very similar to vertebral artery test.
   (4) Positive finding is pain and/or paresthesia in dermatomal pattern for involved nerve root, or localized pain in neck if facet dysfunction.

g. Distraction test.
   (1) Indicates compression of neural structures at the intervertebral foramen or facet joint dysfunction.
   (2) Patient sitting with head passively distracted.
   (3) Positive finding is a decrease in symptoms in neck (facet condition) or a decrease in upper limb pain (neurological condition).

h. Shoulder abduction test.
   (1) Indicates compression of neural structures within intervertebral foramen.
   (2) Patient sitting, and asked to place one hand on top of their head. Repeat with opposite hand.
   (3) Positive finding is a decrease in symptoms into upper limb.

i. Lhermitte's sign.
   (1) Identifies dysfunction of spinal cord and/or an upper motor neuron lesion.
   (2) Patient in long sitting on table. Passively flex patient's head and one hip, while keeping knee in extension. Repeat with other hip.
   (3) Positive finding is pain down the spine and into the upper or lower limbs.

j. Romberg's test.
   (1) Identifies upper motor neuron lesion.
   (2) Patient standing, and closes eyes for 30 seconds.
   (3) Excessive swaying during test indicates positive finding.

k. Thoracic outlet syndrome (TOS) tests (see shoulder special tests).
l. Upper limb tension tests (see shoulder special tests).

2. Thoracic special tests.
a. Rib springing.
(1) Evaluates rib mobility.
(2) Patient prone. Begin at upper ribs applying a posterior/anterior force through each rib progressively working through entire rib cage. Following prone test, position patient side lying and repeat. Be careful with springing the 11th and 12th ribs, since they have no anterior attachments and therefore are less stable.
(3) Positive finding is pain, excessive motion of rib, or restriction of rib.
b. Thoracic springing.
(1) Evaluates intervertebral joint mobility in thoracic spine.
(2) Patient prone. Apply posterior/anterior glides/springs to transverse processes of thoracic vertebra. Remember that the spinous process and transverse process of the same vertebra may not be at the same level in the thoracic region.
(3) Positive finding is pain, excessive movement, and/or restricted movement.
c. Slump test.
(1) Identifies dysfunction of neurological structures supplying the lower limb.
(2) Patient sitting on edge of table with knees flexed. Patient slump sits, while maintaining neutral position of head and neck. The following progression is then followed.
(a) Passively flex patient's head and neck. If no reproduction of symptoms, move on to next step.
(b) Passively extend one of patient's knees. If no reproduction of symptoms, move on to next step.
(c) Passively dorsiflex ankle of limb with extended knee.
(d) Repeat flow with opposite leg.
(3) Positive finding is reproduction of pathological neurological symptoms.

3. Lumbar special tests.
a. Slump test (see thoracic special tests).
b. Lasegue's (straight leg raising) test.
(1) Identifies dysfunction of neurological structures that supply lower limb.
(2) Patient supine, with legs resting on table. Passively flex hip of one leg with knee extended until patient complains of shooting pain into lower limb. Slowly lower limb until pain subsides, then passively dorsiflex foot.
(3) Positive finding is reproduction of pathological neurological symptoms when foot is dorsiflexed.
c. Femoral nerve traction test.
(1) Identifies compression of femoral nerve anywhere along its course.
(2) Patient lies on nonpainful side with trunk in neutral, head flexed slightly, and lower limb's hip and knee flexed. Passively extend hip while knee of painful limb is in extension. If no reproduction of symptoms, flex knee of painful leg.
(3) Positive finding is neurological pain in anterior thigh.
d. Valsalva's maneuver.
(1) Identifies a space-occupying lesion.
(2) Patient sitting. Instruct patient to take a deep breath and hold while they "baear down" as if having a bowel movement.
(3) Positive finding is increased low back pain or neurological symptoms into lower extremity.
e. Babinski's test.
(1) Identifies upper motor neuron lesion.
(2) Patient supine or sitting. Glide bottom end of a standard reflex hammer along plantar surface of patient's foot.
(3) Positive finding is extension of big toe and splaying (abduction) of other toes.
f. Quadrant test.
(1) Identifies compression of neural structures at the intervertebral foramen and facet dysfunction.
(2) Patient standing.
(a) Intervertebral foramen: cue patient into side bending left, rotation left, and extension to maximally close intervertebral foramen on the left. Repeat on other side.
(b) Facet dysfunction: cue patient into side bending left, rotation right, and extension to maximally compress facet joint on left. Repeat on other side.
(3) Positive finding is pain and/or paresthesia in the dermatomal pattern for the involved nerve root, or localized pain if facet dysfunction.
g. Stork standing test.
(1) Identifies spondylolisthesis.
(2) Patient standing on one leg. Cue patient into trunk extension. Repeat with opposite leg on ground.
(3) Positive finding is pain in low back with ipsilateral leg on ground.
h. McKenzie's side glide test.
(1) Differentiates between scoliotic curvature versus neurological dysfunction causing abnormal curvature (lateral shift) of trunk.
(2) Test is performed if "lateral shift" of trunk is noted. Patient standing. Stand on side of patient so that upper trunk is shifted toward you. Place your shoulders into patient's upper trunk and wrap your arms around patient's pelvis. Stabilize upper trunk and pull pelvis, to bring pelvis and trunk into proper alignment.

(3) Positive test is reproduction of neurological symptoms as alignment of trunk is corrected.

i. Bicycle (van Gelderen's) test.
(1) Differentiates between intermittent claudication and spinal stenosis.
(2) Patient seated on stationary bicycle. Patient rides bike while sitting erect. Time how long they can ride at a set pace/speed. After a sufficient rest period, have patient ride bike at same speed while in a slumped position.
(3) Determination is based on length of time patient can ride bike in sitting upright versus sitting slumped. If pain is related to spinal stenosis, patient should be able to ride bike longer while slumped.

4. Sacroiliac joint (SIJ) special tests.

a. Gillet's test.
(1) Assessing posterior movement of the ilium relative to the sacrum.
(2) Patient standing. Place thumb of your hand under PSIS of limb to be tested and place your other thumb on center of sacrum at same level as thumb under PSIS. Ask patient to flex hip and knee of limb being tested as if bringing their knee to chest. Assess movement of PSIS via comparison of positions of your thumbs. Make sure your eyes are level with your thumbs. PSIS should move in an inferior direction.
(3) Positive finding is no identified movement of PSIS as compared to sacrum.

b. Ipsilateral anterior rotation test.
(1) Assessing anterior movement of ilium relative to sacrum.
(2) Place your thumb under PSIS of limb to be tested, and place your other thumb on center of sacrum, at same level as thumb under PSIS. Ask patient to extend hip of limb being tested. Assess movement of PSIS via comparison of positions of your thumbs. Make sure your eyes are level with your thumbs. PSIS should move in a superior direction.
(3) Positive finding is no identified movement of PSIS compared to sacrum.

c. Gaenslen's test.
(1) Identifies sacroiliac joint dysfunction.
(2) Patient side lying at edge of table while holding bottom leg in maximal hip and knee flexion (knee to chest). Standing behind patient, passively extend hip of uppermost limb. This places stress on SIJ associated with uppermost limb.
(3) Positive finding is pain in SIJ.

d. Long sitting (supine to sit) test.
(1) Identifies dysfunction of SIJ that may be cause of functional leg length discrepancy.
(2) Patient supine with correct alignment of trunk, pelvis, and lower limbs. Stand at edge of table near patient's feet, palpating the medial malleoli to assess symmetry (one longer than other). Have patient come into long sitting position, and once again assess their leg length, making a comparison between supine and long sitting.
(3) Abnormal finding is reversal in limb lengths between supine and long sitting.

e. Goldthwait's test.
(1) Differentiates between dysfunction in lumbar spine versus SIJ.
(2) Patient supine with your fingers in between spinous processes of lumbar spine. With your other hand, passively perform a straight leg raise.
(3) If pain presents prior to palpation of movement in lumbar segments, dysfunction is related to SIJ.

5. TMJ special tests.

a. TMJ compression.
(1) Evaluates for pain with compression of the retrodiscal tissues.
(2) Patient sitting or supine. Support/stabilize patient's head with one hand. With other hand, push mandible superior, causing a compressive load to the TMJ.
(3) Positive finding is pain in TMJ.

Assessment of Normal Gait Pattern

1. Divided into two phases of gait (stance phase and swing phase).

a. Stance phase is subdivided into initial contact, foot flat, midstance, heel off, and preswing.
(1) Initial contact: heel strikes the ground and the limb prepares to absorb the ground reaction forces.
(2) Foot flat: as the limb is being loaded, the individual makes a subconscious decision regarding the ability to tolerate the loading, and may compensate as necessary.
(3) Midstance: the foot fully flattens and the trunk is aligned over the stance leg.
(4) Heel-off: the weight distribution shifts from the entire foot to the forefoot.
(5) Preswing: as the toe takes on the final contact of the stance phase, the force is accelerated to provide momentum for propulsion.

b. Swing phase is subdivided into initial swing, midswing, and terminal swing.
(1) Initial swing: the foot loses contact with the ground and accelerates forward.
(2) Midswing: the limb transitions from acceleration to deceleration.
(3) Terminal swing: the limb decelerates and prepares for heel strike.

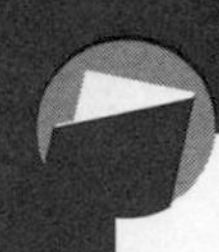

Table 1-17 ➤ SUMMARY OF JOINT MOTIONS AT THE HIP, KNEE, TIBIA, FOOT, AND ANKLE DURING THE STANCE PHASE OF GAIT

HIP

PHASE	KINEMATIC MOTION	KINETIC MOTION: EXTERNAL FORCES	KINETIC MOTION: INTERNAL FORCES
Heel strike	20° to 40° of hip flexion moving toward extension Slight adduction and lateral rotation	Reaction force in front of joint; flexion moment moving toward extension; forward pelvic rotation	Gluteus maximus and hamstrings working eccentrically to resist flexion moment Erector spinae working eccentrically to resist forward bend
Foot flat	Hip moving into extension, adduction, medial rotation	Flexion moment	Gluteus maximus and hamstrings contracting concentrically to bring hip into extension
Midstance	Moving through neutral position Pelvis rotating posteriorly	Reaction force posterior to hip joint; extension moment	Iliopsoas activity continuing
Toe-off	Moving toward 10° extension, abduction, lateral rotation	Decrease of extension moment	Adductor magnus working eccentrically to control or stabilize pelvis Iliopsoas activity continuing

KNEE AND TIBIA

PHASE	KINEMATIC MOTION: KNEE	KINEMATIC MOTION: TIBIA	KINETIC MOTION: EXTERNAL FORCES	KINETIC MOTION: INTERNAL FORCES
Heel Strike	In full extension before heel contact; flexing as heel strikes floor	Slight lateral rotation	Rapidly increasing reaction forces behind knee joint, causing flexion moment	Quadriceps femoris contracting eccentrically to control rapid knee flexion and to prevent buckling
Foot flat	In 20° flexion moving toward extension	Medial rotation	Flexion moment	After foot is flat, quadriceps femoris activity, becoming concentric to bring femur over tibia
Midstance	In 15° flexion moving toward extension	Lateral rotation	Reaction forces moving anterior to joint extension moment	Gastrocnemius beginning to work concentrically to start knee flexion
Toe-off	Moving from near full extension to 40° flexion	Lateral rotation	Reaction forces moving posterior to joint as knee flexes, flexion moment	Quadriceps femoris contracting eccentrically

FOOT AND ANKLE

PHASE	KINEMATIC MOTION: FOOT	KINEMATIC MOTION: ANKLE	KINETIC MOTION: EXTERNAL FORCES	KINETIC MOTION: INTERNAL FORCES
Heel Strike	Supination (rigid) at heel contact	Moving into plantar flexion	Reaction forces behind joint axis; plantar flexion moment at heel strike	Dorsiflexors (tibialis anterior, extensor digitorum longus, and extensor hallucis longus) contracting eccentrically to slow plantar flexion
Foot flat	Pronation, adapting to support surface	Plantar flexion to dorsiflexion over a fixed foot	Maximum plantar flexion moment; reaction forces beginning to shift anterior, producing a dorsiflexion moment	Plantar flexor muscles (gastrocsoleus and peroneal muscles), activated to control dorsiflexion of the tibia and fibula over a fixed foot, contracting eccentrically
Midstance	Neutral	3° of dorsiflexion	Slight dorsiflexion moment	Plantar flexor muscles (gastrocsoleus and peroneal muscles), activated to control dorsiflexion of the tibia and fibula over a fixed foot, contracting eccentrically
Heel-off	Supination as foot becomes rigid for push-off	15° dorsiflexion toward plantar flexion	Maximal dorsiflexion moment	Plantar flexor muscles beginning to contract concentrically to prepare for push-off
Toe-off	Supination	20° plantar flexion	Dorsiflexion moment	Plantar flexor muscles at peak activity but becoming inactive as foot leaves ground

Modified from Giallonardo, LM. Gait. In Myers, RS (ed): Saunders Manual of Physical Therapy Practice. Philadelphia, Saunders, 1995, pp 1108–1109.

Table 1-18 ➤ SUMMARY OF JOINT MOTION AND FORCES DURING SWING PHASE: ACCELERATION TO MIDSWING AND MIDSWING TO DECELERATION

	ACCELERATION TO MIDSWING		MIDSWING TO DECELERATION	
JOINT	KINEMATIC MOTION	KINETIC MOTION	KINEMATIC MOTION	KINETIC MOTION
Hip	Slight flexion (0° to 15°) moving at 30° flexion and lateral rotation to neutral	Hip flexors working concentrically to bring limb through; contralateral gluteus medius concentrically contracting to maintain pelvis position	Continued flexion at about 30° to 40°	Gluteus maximus contracting eccentrically to slow hip flexion
Knee	30° to 60° knee flexion and lateral rotation of tibia moving toward neutral	Hamstrings concentrically contracting	Moving to near full extension and slight lateral tibial rotation	Quadriceps femoris contracting concentrically and hamstrings contracting eccentrically
Ankle and foot	20° dorsiflexion and slight pronation	Dorsiflexors contracting concentrically	Ankle in neutral; foot in slight supination	Dorsiflexors contracting isometrically

From: Giallonardo, LM. Gait. In Myers, RS (ed): Saunders Manual of Physical Therapy Practice. Philadelphia, Saunders, 1995, p 1110.

Table 1-19 ➤ TYPICAL COUPLING PATTERNS THROUGHOUT THE LOWER KINEMATIC CHAIN

Lumbar Spine	1. Lumbar spine flexion is coupled with ilial posterior rotation. 2. Lumbar spine extension is coupled with ilial anterior rotation.
Pelvis	1. During unilateral ilial posterior rotation, the ilium simultaneously moves in the direction of an outflare, causing external rotation of the acetabulum (i.e., the hip joint), leading to hip external rotation.
Femur	1. External rotation of the femur causes external rotation of the tibia.
Tibia	1. Tibial external rotation is coupled with an upward glide of the talus and supination of the foot.
Fibula	1. Supination of the foot is coupled with cranial and anterior glide of the fibula head.

Table 1-20 ➤ LOWER KINEMATIC CHAIN COMPENSATIONS*,**

REGION	TRUE LEG LENGTH DISCREPANCY ON THE RIGHT
Lumbar Spine	Side bent right. Rotated left.
Pelvis	Right ilium rotated posteriorly.
Femur	Right femur adducted and in external rotation at hip joint. Right femur in relative extension at hip joint.
Tibia	External rotation of right tibia.
Fibula	Fibular head glides cranially and anteriorly.
Ankle/Foot	Supination of right foot. Talus rotated externally and glides upwardly.

*Describes the potential functional compensational movements that may be seen in a patient with a leg length discrepancy.

**Individuals may not demonstrate some or any of the compensations for the related conditions listed above. The functional compensations described above are commonly seen, but must be assessed for each patient to determine if they are truly present.

Musculoskeletal Conditions

Arthritic Conditions

1. **Degenerative joint disease (DJD; degenerative osteoarthritis/osteoarthrosis [OA]).** (See Table 1-10).
   a. A degenerative process of varied etiology which includes mechanical changes, diseases, and/or joint trauma.
   b. Characterized by degeneration of articular cartilage, with hypertrophy of subchondral bone and joint capsule of weight bearing joints.
   c. Many different medications are used to control pain, including corticosteroids and nonsteroidal anti-inflammatory drugs (NSAIDs). Glucocorticoids injected into joints that are inflamed and not responsive to NSAIDs. For mild pain without inflammation, acetaminophen may be used.

d. Diagnostic tests utilized: plain film imaging demonstrates characteristic findings of OA (diminished joint space, decreased height of articular cartilage, presence of osteophytes) and lab tests help to rule out other disorders such as rheumatoid arthritis (RA).
e. Clinical examination assists in confirming diagnosis.
f. Physical therapy goals, outcomes, and interventions.
   (1) Joint protection strategies.
   (2) Maintain/improve joint mechanics and connective tissue functions.
   (3) Implementation of aerobic capacity/endurance conditioning or reconditioning, such as aquatic programs.

2. Rheumatoid conditions.

a. Ankylosing spondylitis (Marie-Strümpell, Bechterew's, rheumatoid spondylitis).
   (1) Progressive inflammatory disorder of unknown etiology that initially affects axial skeleton.
   (2) Initial onset (usually mid and low back pain for 3 months or greater) before fourth decade of life.
   (3) First symptoms include mid and low back pain, morning stiffness, and sacroiliitis.
   (4) Results in kyphotic deformity of the cervical and thoracic spine and a decrease in lumbar lordosis.
   (5) Degeneration of peripheral and costovertebral joints may be observed in advanced stages.
   (6) Affects men three times more often than women.
   (7) Medications: NSAIDs such as aspirin are used to reduce inflammation and pain. Corticosteroid therapy or medications to suppress immune system may be used to control various symptoms. Cytotoxic drugs (drugs that block cell growth) may be used in people who do not respond well to corticosteroids or who are dependent on high doses of corticosteroids. Tumor necrosis factor (TNF) inhibitors have been shown to improve some symptoms of ankylosing spondylitis.
   (8) Diagnostic tests utilized: HLA-B27 antigen may be helpful, but not diagnostic by itself.
   (9) Clinical examination will assist in confirming diagnosis.
   (10) Physical therapy goals, outcomes, and interventions.
      (a) Implementation of flexibility exercises for trunk to maintain/improve normal joint motion and length of muscles in all directions, especially extension.
      (b) Implementation of aerobic capacity/endurance conditioning or reconditioning such as aquatic programs.
      (c) Implementation of relaxation activities to maintain/improve respiratory function.
         • Breathing strategies to maintain/improve vital capacity.

b. Gout.
   (1) Genetic disorder of purine metabolism, characterized by elevated serum uric acid (hyperuricemia). Uric acid changes into crystals and deposits into peripheral joints and other tissues (e.g., kidneys).
   (2) Most frequently observed at knee and great toe of foot.
   (3) Medications: NSAIDS (specifically indomethacin), COX-2 inhibitors (cardiac side effects may limit use), colchicine, corticosteroids, adrenocorticotropic hormone (ACTH), allopurinol, probenecid, and sulfinpyrazone.
   (4) Diagnostic tests utilized: lab tests identify monosodium urate crystals in synovial fluid and/or connective tissue samples.
   (5) Clinical examination assists in confirming diagnosis.
   (6) Physical therapy goals, outcomes, and interventions.
      (a) Patient/client education for injury prevention and reduction of involved joint(s).
      (b) Early identification of condition, with fast implementation of intervention, is very important.

c. Psoriatic arthritis.
   (1) Chronic, erosive inflammatory disorder of unknown etiology, associated with psoriasis.

Table 1-21 ➤ PREFERRED PRACTICE PATTERNS MUSCULOSKELETAL

Pattern A:	Primary Prevention/Risk Reduction for Skeletal Demineralization
Pattern B:	Impaired Posture
Pattern C:	Impaired Muscle Performance
Pattern D:	Impaired Joint Mobility, Motor Function, Muscle Performance, and Range of Motion Associated with Connective Tissue Dysfunction
Pattern E:	Impaired Joint Mobility, Motor Function, Muscle Performance, and Range of Motion Associated with Localized Inflammation
Pattern F:	Impaired Joint Mobility, Motor Function, Muscle Performance, Range of Motion, and Reflex Integrity Associated with Spinal Disorders
Pattern G:	Impaired Joint Mobility, Muscle Performance, and Range of Motion Associated with Fracture
Pattern H:	Impaired Joint Mobility, Motor Function, Muscle Performance, and Range of Motion Associated with Joint Arthroplasty
Pattern I:	Impaired Joint Mobility, Motor Function, Muscle Performance, and Range of Motion Associated with Bony or Soft Tissue Surgery
Pattern J:	Impaired Motor Function, Muscle Performance, Range of Motion, Gait, Locomotion, and Balance Associated with Amputation

From: Guide for Physical Therapist Practice, 2nd ed., Phys Ther 81:9, 2001.

Table 1-22 ➤ DIFFERENTIAL DIAGNOSIS OF CERVICAL FACET SYNDROME, CERVICAL NERVE ROOT LESION, AND THORACIC OUTLET SYNDROME

SIGNS AND SYMPTOMS	FACET SYNDROME	CERVICAL NERVE ROOT	THORACIC OUTLET SYNDROME
Pain referral	Possible	Yes	Possible
Pain on hyperextension and rotation	Yes (often without increased referral of symptoms)	Yes, with increased symptoms	No
Spine stiffness	Yes	Possible	Possible
Paresthesia	No	Yes	Possible
Reflexes	Not affected	May be affected	May be affected
Muscle spasm	Yes	Yes	Yes
Tension tests	May or may not be positive	Positive	May be positive
Pallor and coolness	No	No	Possible
Muscle weakness	No	Possible	Not early (later smaller muscles)
Muscle fatigue and cramps	No	No	Possible

From: Magee, D. Orthopedic Physical Assessment, 3rd ed., Philadelphia, Saunders 1997, p 148, with permission.

(2) Erosive degeneration usually occurs in joints of digits as well as axial skeleton.
(3) Both sexes are affected equally.
(4) Medications: acetaminophen for pain, NSAIDs, corticosteroids, disease-modifying antirheumatic drugs (DMARDs) can slow the progression of psoriatic arthritis, and biological response modifiers (BRMs) such as Enbrel (etanercept) are a newly developed class of medicines.
(5) Diagnostic tests utilized: lab tests are not useful except to rule out rheumatoid arthritis.
(6) Clinical examination assists in confirming diagnosis.
(7) Physical therapy goals, outcomes, and interventions.
   (a) Joint protection strategies.
   (b) Maintain/improve joint mechanics and connective tissue functions.
   (c) Implementation of aerobic capacity/endurance conditioning or reconditioning, such as aquatic programs.

d. Rheumatoid arthritis (RA).
   (1) Chronic systemic disorder of unknown etiology, usually involving a symmetrical pattern of dysfunction in synovial tissues and articular cartilage of joints of hands, wrists, elbows, shoulders, knees, ankles, and feet.

Table 1-23 ➤ DIFFERENTIAL DIAGNOSIS OF CERVICAL SPONDYLOSIS AND TEMPOROMANDIBULAR JOINT (TMJ) DYSFUNCTION

	CERVICAL SPONDYLOSIS	TMJ DYSFUNCTION
History	Insidious onset May complain of referred pain into arm or head Stiff neck	Insidious onset May be related to biting something hard Pain may be referred to neck or head
Observation	Muscle guarding of neck muscles	Minimal or no muscle guarding
Active movements	Cervical spine movement limited TMJ movements normal	Cervical movements may be limited if they compress or stress TMJ TMJ movements may or may not be painful, but range of motion is altered
Passive movements	Restricted May have altered end feel: muscle spasm or bone-to-bone	Restricted
Resisted isometric movements	Relatively normal Myotomes may be affected	Normal
Special tests	Spurling's test may be positive Distraction test may be positive	None
Reflexes and cutaneous distribution	Deep tendon reflexes may be hyporeflexic See history for referred pain	No effect See history for referred pain

From: Magee, D. Orthopedic Physical Assessment, 3rd ed., Philadelphia, Saunders 1997, p 173, with permission.

Table 1-24 ➤ DIFFERENTIAL DIAGNOSIS OF ANKYLOSING SPONDYLITIS AND THORACIC SPINAL STENOSIS

	ANKYLOSING SPONDYLITIS	THORACIC SPINAL STENOSIS
History	Morning stiffness Male predominance Sharp pain → ache Bilateral sacroiliac pain may refer to posterior thigh	Intermittent aching pain Pain may refer to both legs with walking (neurogenic intermittent claudication)
Active movements	Restricted	May be normal
Passive movements	Restricted	May be normal
Resisted isometric movements	Normal	Normal
Special tests	None (Scober's test)	Bicycle test of van Gelderen may be positive Stoop test may be positive
Reflexes	Normal	May be affected in long-standing cases
Sensory deficit	None	Usually temporary
Diagnostic imaging	Plain films are diagnostic	Computed tomography scans are diagnostic

From: Magee, D. Orthopedic Physical Assessment, 3rd ed., Philadelphia, Saunders 1997, p 359, with permission.

(2) Metacarpophalangeal (MCP) and proximal interphalangeal (PIP) joints are usually affected, with characteristic pannus formation (inflammatory granulation tissue that covers joint surface), ulnar drift, and volar subluxation of MCP joints; ulnar drift observed at PIPs in severe forms. Distal interphalangeal (DIP) joints are usually spared. Other deformities include swan-neck and boutonniere deformities and Bouchard's nodes (excessive bone formation on dorsal aspect of PIP joints).

(3) Women have two to three times greater incidence than men.

(4) Juvenile rheumatoid arthritis (JRA) onset prior to age 16, with complete remission in 75% of children.

(5) Pharmacological management varies with disease progression, and may include gold compounds and antirheumatic drugs (DMARDs) (e.g., hydroxychloroquine and methotrexate) early. Nonsteroidal anti-inflammatory drugs (e.g., ibuprofen), immunosuppressive agents (e.g., cyclosporine, azathioprine, and mycophenolate), or corticosteroids are commonly prescribed for long-term management.

Table 1-25 ➤ DIFFERENTIAL DIAGNOSIS OF LUMBAR STRAIN AND POSTEROLATERAL LUMBAR DISC HERNIATION AT L5-S1

	LUMBAR STRAIN	LUMBAR DISC (L5-S1)
History	Mechanism of injury: flexion, side flexion and/or rotation under load or without control	Quick movement into flexion, rotation, side flexion, or extension (may or may not be load)
Pain	In lumbar spine, may be referred into buttocks May increase with extension (muscle contraction) or flexion (stretch)	In lumbar spine with referral into posterior foot (radicular pain) Increases with extension
Observation	Scoliosis may be present Muscle spasm	Scoliosis may be present Muscle guarding
Active movements	Pain especially on stretch (flexion, side flexion, and rotation) Pain on unguarded movement Limited range of motion	Pain especially on extension and flexion Side flexion and rotation may be affected Limited range of motion
Resisted isometric movements	Pain on muscle contraction (often minimal pain) Myotomes normal	Minimal pain unless large protrusion L5-S1 myotomes may be affected
Special tests	Neurological tests negative	Straight leg raising and slump test often positive
Sensation	Normal	L5-S1 dermatomes may be affected
Reflexes	Normal	L5-S1 reflexes may be affected
Joint play	Muscle guarding	Muscle guarding

From: Magee, D. Orthopedic Physical Assessment, 3rd ed., Philadelphia, Saunders 1997, p 428, with permission.

(6) Diagnostic tests: plain film imaging demonstrating symmetrical involvement within joints as well as laboratory testing. Positive test findings include increased white blood cell count and erythrocyte sedimentation rate. Hemoglobin and hematocrit tests will show anemia, and rheumatoid factor will be elevated.
(7) Clinical examination assists in confirming diagnosis.
(8) Physical therapy goals, outcomes, and interventions.
(a) Joint protection strategies.
(b) Maintain/improve joint mechanics and connective tissue functions.
(c) Implementation of aerobic capacity and endurance conditioning or reconditioning, such as aquatic programs.

Skeletal and Soft Tissue Conditions

1. Osteoporosis.
a. A metabolic disease that depletes bone mineral density/mass, predisposing individual to fracture.
b. Affects women 10 times more frequently than men.
c. Common sites of fracture include thoracic and lumbar spine, femoral neck, proximal humerus, proximal tibia, pelvis, and distal radius.
d. Primary or postmenopausal osteoporosis is directly related to a decrease in estrogen production.
e. Senile osteoporosis occurs due to a decrease in bone cell activity secondary to genetics or acquired abnormalities.
f. Medications: calcium, vitamin D, estrogen, calcitonin, and biophosphonates.
g. Diagnostic tests utilized: CT scan to assess bony density. Single and dual photon absorptiometry are also used, but very expensive.
h. Clinical examination will assist in confirming diagnosis.
i. Physical therapy goals, outcomes, and interventions.
(1) Joint/bone protection strategies.
(2) Maintain/improve joint mechanics and connective tissue functions.
(3) Implementation of aerobic capacity/endurance conditioning or reconditioning, such as aquatic programs.

2. Osteomalacia.
a. Characterized by decalcification of bones due to vitamin D deficiency.
b. Symptoms include: severe pain, fractures, weakness, and deformities.
c. Medications: calcium, vitamin D, and vitamin D injection in the form of calciferol (vitamin D_2).
d. Diagnostic tests: plain films, lab tests (urinalysis and blood work), bone scan, and bone biopsy if warranted.
e. Clinical examination assists in confirming diagnosis.
f. Physical therapy goals, outcomes, and interventions.
(1) Joint/bone protection strategies.
(2) Maintain/improve joint mechanics and connective tissue functions.
(3) Implementation of aerobic capacity/endurance conditioning or reconditioning, such as aquatic programs.

3. Osteomyelitis.
a. An inflammatory response within bone caused by an infection.
b. Usually caused by *Staphylococcus aureus*, but could be another organism.
c. More common in children and immunosuppressed adults than healthy adults; more common in males than females.
d. Medical treatment consists of antibiotics. Proper nutrition is important as well. Surgery may be indicated if infection spreads to joints.
e. Diagnostic tests utilized: lab tests for infection and possibly a bone biopsy.
f. Clinical examination will assist in confirming diagnosis.
g. Physical therapy goals, outcomes, and interventions.
(1) Joint/bone protection strategies and cast care.
(2) Maintain/improve joint mechanics and connective tissue functions.

4. Arthrogryposis multiplex congenita.
a. Congenital deformity of skeleton and soft tissues, characterized by limitation in joint motion and a "sausage-like" appearance of limbs.
b. Intelligence develops normally.
c. Ongoing communication with family and school is important in therapeutic management.
d. Diagnostic tests utilized: plain films.
e. Clinical examination assists in confirming diagnosis.
f. Physical therapy goals, outcomes, and interventions.
(1) Joint/bone protection strategies.
(2) Maintain/improve joint mechanics and connective tissue functions.
(3) Implementation of aerobic capacity/endurance conditioning or reconditioning such as aquatic programs.
(4) Application of and patient education regarding adaptive devices, assistive devices, orthotic devices, and supportive devices.
(5) Implementation of flexibility exercises to maintain/improve normal joint motion and length of muscles.

5. Osteogenesis imperfecta.
a. Inherited disorder transmitted by an autosomal dominant gene.

b. Characterized by abnormal collagen synthesis, leading to an imbalance between bone deposition and reabsorption.
c. Cortical and cancellous bones become very thin, leading to fractures and deformity of weight-bearing bones.
d. Medications: calcium, vitamin D, estrogen, calcitonin, and biophosphonates.
e. Diagnostic tests utilized: bone scan and plain films will show old fractures and deformities. Serological testing is also indicated.
f. Clinical examination assists in confirming diagnosis.
g. Physical therapy goals, outcomes, and interventions.
   (1) Joint/bone protection strategies.
   (2) Maintain/improve joint mechanics and connective tissue functions.
   (3) Implement of aerobic capacity/endurance conditioning or reconditioning, such as aquatic programs.

6. Osteochondritis dissecans.
a. A separation of articular cartilage from underlying bone (osteochondral fracture), usually involving medial femoral condyle near intercondylar notch; observed less frequently at femoral head and talar dome. Also affects the humeral capitellum.
b. Surgical intervention is indicated if fracture is displaced.
c. Diagnostic tests utilized: plain film or CT scan imaging to identify defect.
d. Clinical examination assists in confirming diagnosis.
e. Physical therapy goals, outcomes, and interventions.
   (1) Joint/bone protection strategies.
   (2) Implementation of flexibility exercises to maintain/improve normal joint motion and length of muscles.
   (3) Implementation of aerobic capacity/endurance conditioning or reconditioning, such as aquatic programs.
   (4) Implementation of strength, power, and endurance exercises.

7. Myofascial pain syndrome.
a. Characterized by clinical entity known as a "trigger point," which is a focal point of irritability found within a muscle. Trigger point can be identified as a taut, palpable band within the muscle.
b. Trigger points may be active or latent. Active trigger points are tender to palpation and have a characteristic referral pattern of pain when provoked. Latent trigger points are palpable taut bands that are not tender to palpation, but can be converted into an active trigger point.
c. Onset is hypothesized to sudden overload, overstretching, and/or repetitive/sustained muscle activities.
d. Medical intervention may include dry needling and/or injection of analgesic, possibly combined with a corticosteroid.
e. Diagnosis is made by clinical assessment, with no diagnostic tests available.
f. Clinical examination will assist in confirming diagnosis.
g. Physical therapy goals, outcomes, and interventions.
   (1) Implementation of flexibility exercises to maintain/improve normal joint motion and length of muscles.
   (2) Implementation of manual therapy for maintenance of normal joint mechanics.
      (a) Soft tissue/massage techniques and joint oscillations to reduce pain and/or muscle guarding.
      (b) Biomechanical faults caused by joint restrictions should be corrected with joint mobilization to the specific restrictions identified during the examination.
      (c) Use of "spray and stretch" technique.
      (d) Cryotherapy, thermotherapy, hydrotherapy, sound agents, and transcutaneous electrical nerve stimulation (TENS) for symptomatic relief of pain.
      (e) Desensitization of trigger point with manual pressure.
   (3) Implementation of strength, power, and endurance exercises.
      (a) Active assistive, active, and resistive exercises.
      (b) Task specific performance training.

8. Tendonitis.
a. An inflammation of tendon as result of microtrauma from overuse, direct blows, and/or excessive tensile forces.
b. Medications: acetaminophen, NSAIDs, and/or steroid injection.
c. Diagnostic tests utilized: possibly MRI.
d. Clinical examination assists in confirming diagnosis. Specific special tests assist with making diagnosis within each region/joint.
e. Physical therapy goals, outcomes, and interventions.
   (1) Implementation of flexibility exercises to maintain/improve normal joint motion and length of muscles.
   (2) Implementation of manual therapy for maintenance of normal joint mechanics.
      (a) Soft tissue/massage techniques and joint oscillations to reduce pain and/or muscle guarding.
      (b) Biomechanical faults caused by joint restrictions should be corrected with joint mobilization to the specific restrictions identified during the examination.

(3) Implementation of aerobic capacity/endurance conditioning or reconditioning.
(4) Application of thermal agents for pain reduction, edema reduction, and muscle performance.
(a) Cryotherapy, thermotherapy, hydrotherapy, and sound agents.
(5) Patient/client education and training/retraining for instrumental activities of daily living (IADL).
(a) Household chores, yard work, shopping, caring for dependents, and home maintenance.

9. Tendonosis.

a. Common chronic tendon dysfunction whose cause and pathogenesis are poorly understood. Often referred to as chronic tendonitis; however, there is no inflammatory response noted.
b. Common in many tendons throughout body (supraspinatus, common extensor tendon of elbow, patella, Achilles').
c. Histological characteristics include hypercellularity, hypervascularity, no indication of inflammatory infiltrates, and poor organization and loosening of collagen fibrils.
d. Medications: acetaminophen, NSAIDs, and/or steroid injection.
e. Diagnostic tests utilized: possibly MRI.
f. Clinical examination assists in confirming diagnosis. Specific special tests are available to assist with making diagnosis within each region/joint.
g. Physical therapy goals, outcomes, and interventions.
(1) Implementation of flexibility exercises to maintain/improve normal joint motion and length of muscles.
(2) Implementation of manual therapy for maintenance of normal joint mechanics.
(a) Soft tissue/massage techniques and joint oscillations to reduce pain and/or muscle guarding.
(b) Biomechanical faults caused by joint restrictions should be corrected with joint mobilization to the specific restrictions identified during the examination.
(3) Implementation of aerobic capacity/endurance conditioning or reconditioning.
(4) Application of thermal agents for pain reduction, edema reduction, and muscle performance.
(a) Cryotherapy, thermotherapy, hydrotherapy, and sound agents.
(5) Patient/client education and training/retraining for instrumental activities of daily living (IADL).
(a) Household chores, yard work, shopping, caring for dependents, and home maintenance.

10. Bursitis.

a. Inflammation of bursa secondary to overuse, trauma, gout, or infection.
b. Signs and symptoms of bursitis.
(1) Pain with rest.
(2) PROM and AROM are limited due to pain, but not in a capsular pattern.
c. Medications: acetaminophen, NSAIDs, and/or steroid injection.
d. Clinical examination assists in confirming diagnosis.
e. Physical therapy goals, outcomes, and interventions.
(1) Implementation of flexibility exercises to maintain/improve normal joint motion and length of muscles.
(2) Implementation of manual therapy for maintenance of normal joint mechanics.
(a) Soft tissue/massage techniques and joint oscillations to reduce pain and/or muscle guarding.
(b) Biomechanical faults caused by joint restrictions should be corrected with joint mobilization to the specific restrictions identified during the examination.
(3) Implementation of aerobic capacity/endurance conditioning or reconditioning.
(4) Application of thermal agents for pain reduction, edema reduction, and muscle performance.
(a) Cryotherapy, thermotherapy, hydrotherapy, and sound agents.
(5) Patient/client education and training/retraining for instrumental activities of daily living (IADL).
(a) Household chores, yard work, shopping, caring for dependents, and home maintenance.

11. Muscle strains.

a. Inflammatory response within a muscle following a traumatic event that caused microtearing of the musculotendinous fibers.
b. Pain and tenderness within that muscle.
c. Seen within muscles throughout the body.
d. Medications: acetaminophen and/or NSAIDs.
e. Diagnostic tests utilized: MRI if necessary.
f. Clinical examination will assist in confirming diagnosis.
g. Physical therapy goals, outcomes, and interventions.
(1) Implementation of flexibility exercises to maintain/improve normal joint motion and length of muscles.
(2) Implementation of manual therapy for maintenance of normal joint mechanics.
(a) Soft tissue/massage techniques and joint oscillations to reduce pain and/or muscle guarding.
(b) Biomechanical faults caused by joint restrictions should be corrected with joint mobilization to the specific restrictions identified during the examination.
(3) Implementation of aerobic capacity/endurance conditioning or reconditioning.
(4) Application of thermal agents for pain reduction, edema reduction, and muscle performance.

(a) Cryotherapy, thermotherapy, hydrotherapy, and sound agents.

(5) Patient/client education and training/retraining for instrumental activities of daily living (IADL).

(a) Household chores, yard work, shopping, caring for dependents, and home maintenance.

12. Myositis ossificans.

a. Painful condition of abnormal calcification within a muscle belly.

b. Usually precipitated by direct trauma which results in hematoma and calcification of the muscle.

c. Can also be induced by early mobilization and stretching, with aggressive physical therapy following trauma to muscle.

d. Most frequent locations are quadriceps, brachialis, and biceps brachii muscles.

e. Medications: acetaminophen and/or NSAIDs.

f. Surgical care is warranted only in patients with nonhereditary myositis ossificans, and only after maturation of the lesion (6–24 months). Surgery is indicated when lesions mechanically interfere with joint movement or impinge on nerves.

g. Diagnostic tests utilized: imaging (plain films, CT scan, and/or MRI).

h. Clinical examination assists in confirming diagnosis.

i. Physical therapy goals, outcomes, and interventions.

(1) Implementation of flexibility exercises to maintain/improve normal joint motion and length of muscles. Avoid being overly aggressive with muscle flexibility exercises, which may worsen condition.

(2) Implementation of manual therapy for maintenance of normal joint mechanics.

(a) Soft tissue/massage techniques and joint oscillations to reduce pain and/or muscle guarding. Avoid aggressive soft tissue/massage techniques, which may worsen condition.

(b) Biomechanical faults caused by joint restrictions should be corrected with joint mobilization to the specific restrictions identified during the examination.

(3) Implementation of aerobic capacity/endurance conditioning or reconditioning, such as aquatic programs.

13. Complex regional pain syndrome (CRPS).

a. Formerly referred to as reflex sympathetic dystrophy (RSD).

b. Etiology largely unknown, but thought to be related to trauma. Can affect upper and lower extremities, trunk, head, and neck.

c. Results in dysfunction of sympathetic nervous system to include pain, circulation, and vasomotor disturbances.

d. Two types of CRPS.

(1) CRPS I is frequently triggered by tissue injury; term describes all patients with the above symptoms, but with no underlying nerve injury.

(2) Patients with CRPS II experience same symptoms but their cases are clearly associated with a nerve injury.

e. Medical intervention may include sympathetic nerve block, surgical sympathectomy, spinal cord stimulation, intrathecal drug pumps.

f. Medications: multiple forms including topical analgesic drugs that act locally on painful nerves, skin, and muscles; antiseizure drugs; antidepressants, corticosteroids, and opioids.

g. Long-term changes include muscle wasting, trophic skin changes, decreased bone density, decreased proprioception, loss of muscle strength from disuse, and joint contractures.

h. Diagnostic tests utilized: none.

i. Clinical examination will assist in confirming diagnosis.

j. Physical therapy goals, outcomes, and interventions.

(1) Patient/client education for injury prevention and reduction.

(2) Desensitization activities that focus on return to work/school/home activities.

(3) Implementation of flexibility exercises to maintain/improve normal joint motion and length of muscles.

(4) Electrical stimulation (TENS) for pain relief.

14. Paget's disease (osteitis deformans).

a. Etiology is largely unknown, but thought to be linked to a type of viral infection along with environmental factors.

b. Considered to be a metabolic bone disease involving abnormal osteoclastic and osteoblastic activity.

c. Results in spinal stenosis, facet arthropathy, and possible spinal fracture.

d. Primary medical intervention is drug therapy, such as acetaminophen for pain control. Drugs such as calcitonin and etidronate disodium may be beneficial, since they limit osteoclast activity.

e. Diagnostic tests utilized: plain film imaging identifies bony changes. Lab tests look for increased levels of serum alkaline phosphatase and urinary hydroxyproline.

f. Clinical examination assists in confirming diagnosis.

g. Physical therapy goals, outcomes, and interventions.

(1) Joint/bone protection strategies should be taught to patient.

(2) Maintain/improve joint mechanics and connective tissue functions.

(3) Implementation of aerobic capacity/endurance conditioning or reconditioning, such as aquatic programs.

15. Idiopathic scoliosis.

a. Two types: structural and nonstructural, both of unknown etiology.
b. Structural scoliosis is an irreversible lateral curvature of spine with a rotational component.
c. Nonstructural scoliosis is a reversible lateral curvature of spine without a rotational component, and straightening as individual flexes spine.
d. Intervention for structural scoliosis includes bracing and possible surgery, with placement of Harrington rod instrumentation. For less than 25°, do conservative physical therapy (see below); between 25°–45°, use spinal orthoses; and surgery is performed for curves greater than 45°.
e. Diagnostic tests utilized: plain film imaging using full-length Cobb's method. CT scan and/or MRI may be used to rule out associated conditions.
f. Clinical examination assists in confirming diagnosis.
g. Physical therapy goals, outcomes, and interventions.
   (1) Implementation of flexibility exercises to maintain/improve normal joint motion and length of muscles throughout trunk and pelvis.
   (2) Implementation of strength, power, and endurance exercises.
   (3) Electrical stimulation to improve muscle performance.
   (4) Application and patient education regarding spinal orthoses.

16. Torticollis.

a. Spasm and/or tightness of sternocleidomastoid (SCM) muscle, with varied etiology.
b. Dysfunction observed is sidebending towards and rotation away from the affected SCM.
c. Medications: acetaminophen, muscle relaxants, and/or NSAIDs.
d. Diagnostic tests utilized: none.
e. Physical therapy goals, outcomes, and interventions.
   (1) Implementation of flexibility exercises to maintain/improve normal joint motion and length of muscles.
   (2) Implementation of manual therapy for maintenance of normal joint mechanics.
      (a) Soft tissue/massage techniques and joint oscillations to reduce pain and/or muscle guarding.
      (b) Biomechanical faults caused by joint restrictions should be corrected with joint mobilization to the specific restrictions identified during the examination.

Upper Extremity Disorders

1. Shoulder conditions.

a. Glenohumeral subluxation and dislocation.
   (1) Most dislocations (95%) occur in anterior-inferior direction.
   (2) Anterior-inferior dislocation occurs when abducted upper extremity is forcefully, externally rotated, causing tearing of inferior glenohumeral ligament, anterior capsule and occasionally glenoid labrum.
   (3) Posterior dislocations are rare, and occur with multidirectional laxity of glenohumeral joint.
   (4) Posterior dislocation occurs with horizontal adduction and internal rotation of glenohumeral joint.
   (5) Complications may include compression fracture of posterior humeral head (Hill-Sachs lesion), tearing of superior glenoid labrum from anterior to posterior (SLAP lesion), an avulsion of anteroinferior capsule and ligaments associated with glenoid rim (Bankart's lesion), and bruising of axillary nerve.
   (6) Following surgical repair for dislocation/chronic subluxation, patients should avoid apprehension position (flexion to 90° or greater, horizontal abduction to 90° or greater, and external rotation to 80°).
   (7) Diagnostic tests utilized: plain film imaging, CT scan, and/or MRI.
   (8) Diagnosis made by clinical examination. Apprehension tests will be positive.
   (9) Medications.
      (a) Acetaminophen for pain.
      (b) NSAIDs for pain and/or inflammation.
   (10) Physical therapy goals, outcomes, and interventions.
      (a) Physical therapy intervention is varied, depending on specific patient problems and whether surgery is performed.
      (b) Biomechanical faults caused by joint restrictions should be corrected with joint mobilization to the specific restrictions identified during the examination.
      (c) Restoration of normal shoulder mechanics via strengthening/endurance/coordination exercises that focus on regaining dynamic scapulothoracic, glenohumeral stabilization and muscular reeducation.

b. Instability.
   (1) Divided into two categories: traumatic (common in young throwing athletes) and atraumatic (individuals with congenitally loose connective tissue around the shoulder).
   (2) Characterized by popping/clicking and repeated dislocation/subluxation of the glenohumeral joint.
   (3) Unstable injuries require surgery to reattach the labrum to the glenoid. Bankart's lesions require surgery.
   (4) Diagnosis made by clinical examination by comparing results of patient history with the AROM,

PROM, resistive tests, and palpation. MRI arthrograms are very effective in identifying labral tears.

(5) Medications.
  (a) Acetaminophen for pain.
  (b) NSAIDS for pain and/or inflammation.

(6) Physical therapy goals, outcomes, and interventions.
  (a) Physical therapy intervention emphasizes return of function without pain.
  (b) Functional training and restoration of muscle imbalances using exercise to normalize strength, endurance, coordination, and flexibility.
  (c) Biomechanical faults caused by joint restrictions should be corrected with joint mobilization to the specific restrictions identified during the examination.
  (d) For patients requiring surgery, the shoulder is usually kept in a sling for 3 or 4 weeks. After 6 weeks, more sports-specific training can be done, although full fitness may take 3 or 4 months.

c. Labral tears.

(1) Glenoid labrum injuries are classified as either superior (toward the top of the glenoid socket) or inferior (toward the bottom of the glenoid socket). A superior injury is known as a SLAP lesion (superior labrum, anterior [front] to posterior [back]) and is a tear of the rim above the middle of the socket that may also involve the biceps tendon. A tear of the rim below the middle of the glenoid socket is called a Bankart lesion, and also involves the inferior glenohumeral ligament. Tears of the glenoid labrum may often occur with other shoulder injuries, such as a dislocated shoulder.

(2) Characterized by the following signs and symptoms.
  (a) Shoulder pain which cannot be localized to a specific point.
  (b) Pain is made worse by overhead activities or when the arm is held behind the back.
  (c) Weakness.
  (d) Instability in the shoulder.
  (e) Pain on resisted flexion of the biceps (bending the elbow against resistance).
  (f) Tenderness over the front of the shoulder.

Biceps load test

(3) Unstable injuries require surgery to reattach the labrum to the glenoid. Bankart's lesions require surgery.

(4) Diagnosis made by clinical examination, through comparing results of AROM, PROM, resistive tests, and palpation. MRI arthrograms are very effective in identifying labral tears. The "gold" standard for identifying a labral tear is through arthroscopic surgery of the shoulder.

(5) Medications.
  (a) Acetaminophen for pain.
  (b) NSAIDS for pain and/or inflammation.

(6) Physical therapy goals, outcomes, and interventions.
  (a) Physical therapy intervention emphasizes return of function without pain.
  (b) Functional training and restoration of muscle imbalances using exercise to normalize strength, endurance, coordination, and flexibility.
  (c) Any underlying causes which contributed to the injury such as shoulder instability should be addressed.
  (d) Biomechanical faults caused by joint restrictions should be corrected with joint mobilization to the specific restrictions identified during the examination.
  (e) Following surgery, the shoulder is usually kept in a sling for 3 or 4 weeks. After 6 weeks, more sports-specific training can be done, although full fitness may take 3 or 4 months.

d. Thoracic outlet syndrome (TOS).

(1) Compression of neurovascular bundle (brachial plexus, subclavian artery and vein, vagus and phrenic nerves, and the sympathetic trunk) in thoracic outlet between bony and soft tissue structures.

(2) Compression occurs when size or shape of thoracic outlet is altered.

(3) Common areas of compression are:
  (a) Superior thoracic outlet.
  (b) Scalene triangle.
  (c) Between clavicle and 1st rib.
  (d) Between pectoralis minor and thoracic wall.

(4) Surgery may be performed to remove a cervical rib or a release of anterior and/or middle scalene muscle.

(5) Diagnostic tests utilized: plain film imaging to identify abnormal bony anatomy and MRI to identify abnormal soft tissue anatomy. Electrodiagnostic test to assess nerve dysfunction.

(6) Clinical examination including the following special tests will be useful to make diagnosis.
  (a) Adson's test.
  (b) Roos' test.
  (c) Wright's test.
  (d) Costoclavicular test.

(7) Medications.
  (a) Acetaminophen for pain.
  (b) NSAIDs for pain and/or inflammation.

(8) Physical therapy goals, outcomes, and interventions.
  (a) Physical therapy intervention varies, depending on the exact cause.
  (b) Includes postural reeducation.

(c) Functional training and restoration of muscle imbalances using exercise to normalize strength, endurance, coordination, and flexibility.
(d) Biomechanical faults caused by joint restrictions should be corrected with joint mobilization to the specific restrictions identified during the examination.
(e) Manipulations (typically 1st rib articulation) to diminish pain and soft tissue guarding.

e. Acromioclavicular and sternoclavicular joint disorders.
(1) Mechanism of injury is a fall onto shoulder, with upper extremity adducted, or a collision with another individual during a sporting event.
(2) Traditionally, degree of injury is graded from first to third degree. Rockwood classification scale uses grades from I to IV, with grades IV–VI as variations of the traditional grade III.
(3) Upper extremity is positioned in neutral with use of sling in acute phase. Avoid shoulder elevation during the acute phase of healing.
(4) Diagnostic tests utilized: plain film imaging.
(5) Clinical examination including the following special tests will be useful to make diagnosis.
(a) Shear test.
(6) Surgical repair is rare, due to tendency of acromioclavicular joint degeneration following the repair.
(7) Medications.
(a) Acetaminophen for pain.
(b) NSAIDs for pain and/or inflammation.
(8) Physical therapy goals, outcomes, and interventions.
(a) Emphasize return of function without pain.
(b) Functional training and restoration of muscle imbalances using exercise to normalize strength, endurance, coordination, and flexibility.
(c) Manual therapy techniques to AC and SC joints and surrounding connective tissues, such as soft tissue/massage, joint oscillations, and mobilizations to normalize soft tissue and joint biomechanics.

f. Subacromial/subdeltoid bursitis.
(1) Subacromial and subdeltoid bursae (which may be continuous) have a close relationship to rotator cuff tendons, making them susceptible to overuse.
(2) They can also become impinged beneath the acromial arch.
(3) Diagnosis made by clinical examination. Differentiate from contractile condition by comparing results of AROM, PROM, and resistive tests.
(4) Medications.
(a) Acetaminophen for pain.
(b) NSAIDs for pain and/or inflammation.
(5) Physical therapy goals, outcomes, and interventions.
(a) Refer to intervention for general bursitis/tendonitis/tendonosis.

g. Rotator cuff tendonitis.
(1) Tendons of rotator cuff are susceptible to tendonitis, due to relatively poor blood supply near insertion of muscles.
(2) Results from mechanical impingement of the distal attachment of the rotator cuff on the anterior acromion and/or coracoacromial ligament with repetitive overhead activities.
(3) Diagnostic tests utilized: MRI may be used, but sometimes not sensitive enough for accurate assessment.
(4) Clinical examination including the following special tests will be useful to make diagnosis.
(a) Supraspinatus test.
(b) Neer's impingement test.
(5) Medications.
(a) Acetaminophen for pain.
(b) NSAIDs for pain and/or inflammation.
(6) Physical therapy goals, outcomes, and interventions.
(a) Refer to intervention for general bursitis/tendonitis/tendonosis.

h. Impingement syndrome.
(1) Characterized by soft tissue inflammation of the shoulder from impingement against the acromion with repetitive overhead AROM.
(2) Diagnostic tests utilized: arthrogram or MRI.
(3) Clinical examination including the following special tests will be useful to make diagnosis.
(a) Neer's impingement test.
(b) Supraspinatus test.
(c) Drop arm test.
(4) Surgical repair of shoulder impingement. The patient should avoid shoulder elevation greater than 90°.
(5) Medications.
(a) Acetaminophen for pain.
(b) NSAIDs for pain and/or inflammation.
(6) Physical therapy goals, outcomes, and interventions.
(a) Restoration of posture.
(b) Correction of muscle imbalances and biomechanical faults using strengthening, endurance, coordination, and flexibility exercises to gain restoration of normal function.
(c) Biomechanical faults caused by joint restrictions should be corrected with joint mobilization to the specific restrictions identified during the examination.

i. Internal (posterior) impingement.
(1) Characterized by an irritation between the rotator cuff and greater tuberosity or posterior glenoid and labrum.

(2) Often seen in athletes performing overhead activities. Pain commonly noted in posterior shoulder.
(3) Diagnostic tests utilized: None.
(4) Clinical examination including posterior internal impingement test helps to identify this condition.
(5) Medications.
 (a) Acetaminophen for pain.
 (b) NSAIDs for pain and/or inflammation.
(6) Physical therapy goals, outcomes, and interventions.
 (a) Correction of muscle imbalances and biomechanical faults using strengthening, endurance, coordination, and flexibility exercises to gain restoration of normal function.
 (b) Biomechanical faults caused by joint restrictions should be corrected with joint mobilization to the specific restrictions identified during the examination.

j. Bicipital tendonitis.
 (1) Most commonly an inflammation of the long head of the biceps.
 (2) Results from mechanical impingement of the proximal tendon, between the anterior acromion and the bicipital groove of the humerus.
 (3) Diagnostic tests utilized: MRI may be used, but sometimes not sensitive enough for accurate assessment.
 (4) Clinical examination including the following special tests will be useful to make diagnosis.
  (a) Speed's test.
 (5) Medications.
  (a) Acetaminophen for pain.
  (b) NSAIDs for pain and/or inflammation.
 (6) Physical therapy goals, outcomes, and interventions.
  (a) Refer to intervention for general bursitis/tendonitis/tendonosis.

k. Proximal humeral fractures.
 (1) Humeral neck fractures frequently occur with a fall onto an outstretched upper extremity among older osteoporotic women. Generally does not require immobilization or surgical repair, since it is a fairly stable fracture.
 (2) Greater tuberosity fractures are more common in middle-aged and elder adults. Usually related to a fall onto the shoulder, and does not require immobilization for healing.
 (3) Diagnostic tests utilized: plain film imaging.
 (4) Medications.
  (a) Acetaminophen for pain.
  (b) NSAIDs for pain and/or inflammation.
 (5) Physical therapy goals, outcomes, and interventions.
  (a) Physical therapy intervention emphasizes return of function without pain.
  (b) Functional training and restoration of muscle imbalances using exercise to normalize strength, endurance, coordination, and flexibility.
  (c) Biomechanical faults caused by joint restrictions should be corrected with joint mobilization to the specific restrictions identified during the examination.
  (d) Early PROM is important in preventing capsular adhesions.

l. Adhesive capsulitis (frozen shoulder).
 (1) Characterized by a restriction in shoulder motion as a result of inflammation and fibrosis of the shoulder capsule, usually due to disuse following injury or repetitive microtrauma.
 (2) Restriction follows a capsular pattern of limitation:
  (a) Greatest limitation in external rotation, followed by abduction and flexion, and least restricted in internal rotation.
 (3) Commonly seen in association with diabetes mellitus.
 (4) Diagnosis made by clinical examination by comparing results of AROM, PROM, resistive tests, and palpation.
 (5) Medications.
  (a) Acetaminophen for pain.
  (b) NSAIDs for pain and/or inflammation.
 (6) Physical therapy goals, outcomes, and interventions.
  (a) Physical therapy intervention emphasizes return of function without pain.
  (b) Functional training and restoration of muscle imbalances using exercise to normalize strength, endurance, coordination, and flexibility.
  (c) Biomechanical faults caused by joint restrictions should be corrected with joint mobilization to the specific restrictions identified during the examination.

2. Elbow conditions.

a. Elbow contractures.
 (1) Loss of motion in capsular pattern (loss of flexion greater than extension).
 (2) Loss of motion in noncapsular pattern as the result of a loose body in the joint, ligamentous sprain, and/or complex regional pain syndrome.
 (3) Diagnosis made by clinical examination by comparing results of AROM, PROM, resistive tests, and palpation.
 (4) Medications.
  (a) Acetaminophen for pain.
  (b) NSAIDs for pain and/or inflammation.
 (5) Physical therapy goals, outcomes, and interventions.
  (a) Biomechanical faults caused by joint restrictions should be corrected with joint

Table 1-26 ➤ DIFFERENTIAL DIAGNOSIS OF ROTATOR CUFF DEGENERATION, FROZEN SHOULDER, ATRAUMATIC INSTABILITY, AND CERVICAL SPONDYLOSIS

	ROTATOR CUFF LESIONS	FROZEN SHOULDER	ATRAUMATIC INSTABILITY	CERVICAL SPONDYLOSIS
History	Age 30–50 years Pain and weakness after eccentric load	Age 45+(insidious type) Insidious onset or after trauma or surgery Functional restriction of lateral rotation, abduction, and medial rotation Normal bone and soft-tissue outlines	Age 10–35 years Pain and instability with activity No history of trauma	Age 50+ years Acute or chronic
Observation	Normal bone and soft tissue outlines Protective shoulder hike may be seen	Normal bone and soft-tissue outlines	Normal bone and soft-tissue outlines	Minimal or no cervical spine movement Torticollis may be present
Active movement	Weakness of abduction or rotation, or both Crepitus may be present	Restricted ROM Shoulder hiking	Full or excessive ROM	Limited ROM with pain
Passive movement	Pain if impingement occurs	Limited ROM, especially in lateral, rotation, abduction, and medial rotation (capsular pattern)	Normal or excessive ROM	Limited ROM (symptoms may be exacerbated)
Resisted isometric movement	Pain and weakness on abduction and lateral rotation	Normal, when arm by side	Normal	Normal, except if nerve root compressed Myotome may be affected
Special tests	Drop-arm test positive Empty can test positive	None	Load and shift test positive Apprehension test positive Relocation test positive Augmentation tests positive	Spurling's test positive Distraction test positive ULTT positive Shoulder abduction test positive
Sensory function and reflexes	Not affected	Not affected	Anterior or posterior pain	Dermatomes affected Reflexes affected
Palpation	Tender over rotator cuff	Not painful unless Capsule is stretched	Negative	Tender over appropriate vertebra or facet
Diagnostic imaging	Radiography: upward displacement of humeral head; acromial spurring MRI diagnostic	Radiography: negative Arthrography: decreased capsular size		Radiography: narrowing osteophytes

MRI = magnetic resonance imaging; ROM = range of motion; ULTT = upper limb tension test.

mobilization to the specific restrictions identified during the examination.

(b) Soft tissue/massage techniques, modalities, flexibility exercises, and functional exercises, including strengthening, endurance, and coordination.

(c) Splinting may be an effective adjunct to physical therapy management in regaining loss of motion for capsular restrictions.

b. Lateral epicondylitis ("tennis elbow").

(1) Most often a chronic inflammation of the extensor carpi radialis brevis tendon (ECRB) at its proximal attachment to the lateral epicondyle of the humerus.

(2) Onset is gradual, usually the result of sports activities or occupations that require repetitive wrist extension or strong grip with the wrist extended, resulting in overloading the ECRB.

(3) Must rule out involvement or relationship to cervical spine condition.

(4) Clinical examination including lateral epicondylitis test helps to identify this condition.

(5) Medications.

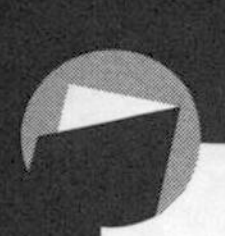

Table 1-27 ➤ DIFFERENTIAL DIAGNOSIS OF SHOULDER PATHOLOGY

PATHOLOGY	SYMPTOMS
External primary impingement (stage I)	Intermittent mild pain with overhead activities Over age 35
External primary impingement (stage II)	Mild to moderate pain with overhead activities or strenuous activities
External primary impingement (stage III)	Pain at rest or with activities Night pain may occur Scapular or rotator cuff weakness is noted
Rotator cuff tears (full thickness)	Classic night pain Weakness noted predominantly in abduction and lateral rotators Loss of motion
Adhesive capsulitis (idiopathic frozen shoulder)	Inability to perform activities of daily living owing to loss of motion Loss of motion may be perceived as weakness
Anterior instability (with or without external secondary impingement)	Apprehension to mechanical shifting limits activities Slipping, popping, or sliding may present as suitable instability Apprehension usually associated with horizontal abduction and lateral rotation Anterior or posterior pain may be present Weak scapular stabilizers
Posterior instability	Slipping or popping of the humerus out the back This may be associated with forward flexion and medial rotation while the shoulder is under a compressive load
Multidirectional instability	Looseness of shoulder in all directions This may be most pronounced while carrying luggage or turning over while asleep
Pain may or may not be present	

Modified from Maughon, TS, Andrews, JR: The subjective evaluation of the shoulder in the athlete. In Andrews, JR, Wilk, KE (eds): The Athlete's Shoulder. New York, Churchill-Livingstone, 1994, p 36.

(a) Acetaminophen for pain.
(b) NSAIDs for pain and/or inflammation.

(6) Physical therapy goals, outcomes, and interventions.
(a) Correction of muscle imbalances and biomechanical faults using strengthening, endurance, coordination, and flexibility exercises to gain restoration of normal function.
(b) Biomechanical faults caused by joint restrictions should be corrected with joint mobilization to the specific restrictions identified during the examination.
(c) Education regarding prevention.
(d) Cryotherapy, thermotherapy, hydrotherapy, sound agents, and TENS for symptomatic relief of pain.
(e) Counterforce bracing is frequently used to reduce forces along the ECRB.

c. Medial epicondylitis (golfer's elbow).
(1) Usually an inflammation of the pronator teres and flexor carpi radialis tendons at their attachment to the medial epicondyle of the humerus.
(2) Occurs with overuse in sports, such as baseball pitching, driving golf swings, swimming, or occupations that require a strong hand grip and excessive pronation of the forearm.
(3) Diagnostic tests utilized: none.
(4) Clinical examination including medial epicondylitis test helps to identify this condition.
(5) Physical therapy goals, outcomes, and interventions.
(a) Intervention is similar to lateral epicondylitis.

d. Distal humeral fractures.
(1) Complications can include loss of motion, myositis ossificans, malalignment, neurovascular compromise, ligamentous injury, and CRPS.
(2) Supracondylar fractures must be examined quickly for neurovascular status, due to high number of neurological (typically radial nerve involvement) and vascular structures that pass through this region (may lead to Volkmann's ischemia). In youth, it is important to assess growth plate as well. These fractures have a high incidence of malunion.
(3) Lateral epicondyle fractures are fairly common in young people, and typically require an open reduction internal fixation (ORIF) to ensure absolute alignment.
(4) Diagnostic tests utilized: plain film imaging.
(5) Medications.
(a) Acetaminophen for pain.
(b) NSAIDs for pain and/or inflammation.
(6) Physical therapy goals, outcomes, and interventions.
(a) Physical therapy intervention includes pain reduction and limiting the inflammatory response following trauma and/or surgery.
(b) Improving flexibility of shortened structures, strengthening, and training to restore functional use of UE.

e. Osteochondrosis of humeral capitellum.
(1) Osteochondritis dissecans affects central and/or lateral aspect of capitellum or radial head. An osteochondral bone fragment becomes detached from articular surface, forming a loose body in joint. Caused by repetitive compressive forces between radial head and humeral capitellum.

Occurs in adolescents between 12 and 15 years of age.

(2) Panner's disease is a localized avascular necrosis of capitellum leading to loss of subchondral bone, with fissuring and softening of articular surfaces of radiocapitellar joint. Etiology is unknown, but occurs in children age 10 or younger.

(3) Diagnostic tests utilized: plain film imaging.

(4) Medications.

(a) Acetaminophen for pain.

(b) NSAIDs for pain and/or inflammation.

(5) Physical therapy goals, outcomes, and interventions.

(a) Physical therapy intervention includes rest with avoidance of any throwing or upper extremity-loading activities (e.g., gymnastics).

(b) When patient is pain-free, initiate flexibility and strengthening/endurance/coordination exercises.

(c) During late phases of rehabilitation, a program to slowly increase load on joint is initiated. If symptoms persist, surgical intervention is necessary.

(d) After surgery, initial focus of rehabilitation is to minimize pain and swelling using modalities. Flexibility exercises are begun immediately following surgery.

(e) Thereafter, a progressive strengthening program is initiated.

(f) Biomechanical faults caused by joint restrictions should be corrected with joint mobilization to the specific restrictions identified during the examination.

f. Ulnar collateral ligament injuries.

(1) Occurs as result of repetitive valgus stresses to medial elbow with overhead throwing.

(2) Clinical signs include pain along medial elbow at distal insertion of ligament. In some cases, paresthesias are reported in ulnar nerve distribution with positive Tinel's sign.

(3) Diagnostic tests utilized: MRI.

(4) Clinical examination including medial ligament instability test helps to identify this condition.

(5) Medications.

(a) Acetaminophen for pain.

(b) NSAIDs for pain and/or inflammation.

(6) Physical therapy goals, outcomes, and interventions.

(a) Initial intervention includes rest and pain management.

(b) After resolution of pain and inflammation, strengthening exercises that focus on elbow flexors are initiated. Taping can also be used for protection during return to activities.

g. Nerve entrapments.

(1) Ulnar nerve entrapment.

Table 1-28 ➤ SIGNS AND SYMPTOMS OF POSSIBLE PERIPHERAL NERVE INVOLVEMENT

Nerve	Signs and symptoms
Spinal accessory nerve	Inability to abduct arm beyond 90° Pain in shoulder on abduction
Long thoracic nerve	Pain on flexing fully extended arm Inability to flex fully extended arm Winging starts at 90° forward flexion
Suprascapular nerve	Increased pain on forward shoulder flexion Shoulder weakness (partial loss of humeral control) Pain increases with scapular abduction Pain increases with cervical rotation to opposite side
Axillary (circumflex) nerve	Inability to abduct arm with neutral rotation
Musculocutaneous nervel	Weak elbow flexion with forearm supinated

(a) Various causes including direct trauma at the cubital tun, nel, traction due to laxity at medial aspect of elbow, compression due to a thickened retinaculum or hypertrophy of flexor carpi ulnaris muscle, recurrent subluxation or dislocation and DJD that affects the cubital tunnel.

(b) Clinical findings include medial elbow pain, paresthesias in ulnar distribution, and a positive Tinel's sign.

(2) Median nerve entrapment.

(a) Occurs within pronator teres muscle and under superficial head of flexor digitorum superficialis with repetitive gripping activities required in occupations (e.g., electricians) and with leisure time activities (e.g., tennis).

(b) Clinical signs include an aching pain with weakness of forearm muscles and positive Tinel's sign, with paresthesias in median nerve distribution.

(3) Radial nerve entrapment.

(a) Entrapment of distal branches (posterior interosseous nerve) occurs within radial tunnel (radial tunnel syndrome) as result of overhead activities and throwing.

(b) Clinical signs, include lateral elbow pain that can be confused with lateral epicondylitis, pain over supinator muscle, and paresthesias in a radial nerve distribution. Tinel's sign may be positive.

(4) Diagnostic tests utilized: electrodiagnostic tests.

(5) Clinical examination helps to identify this condition.

(6) Medications.

(a) Acetaminophen for pain.

(b) NSAIDs for pain and/or inflammation.

(c) Neurontin for neuropathic pain.

(7) Physical therapy goals, outcomes, and interventions.

(a) Early intervention includes rest, avoiding exacerbating activities, use of NSAIDs, modalities and soft tissue/massage techniques to reduce inflammation and pain.
(b) Protective padding and night splints to maintain slackened position of involved nerves.
(c) With reduction in pain and paresthesias, rehabilitation program should focus on strengthening/endurance/coordination exercise of involved muscles to achieve muscle balance between agonists and antagonists, normal flexibility of shortened structures, and normalization of strength/endurance/coordination.
(d) Intervention should also include functional training, patient education, and self-management techniques.

h. Elbow dislocations.
(1) Posterior dislocations account for most dislocations occurring at elbow.
(a) Posterior dislocations are defined by position of olecranon relative to the humerus.
(b) Posterolateral dislocations are most common, and occur as the result of elbow hyperextension from a fall on the outstretched upper extremity.
(c) Posterior dislocations frequently cause avulsion fractures of medial epicondyle secondary to traction pull of medial collateral ligament.
(2) Anterior and radial head dislocations account for only 1%–2% of all elbow dislocations.
(3) With a complete dislocation, ulnar collateral ligament will rupture, with possible rupture of anterior capsule, lateral collateral ligament, brachialis muscle, and/or wrist flexor and extensor muscles.
(4) Clinical signs include rapid swelling, severe pain at the elbow, and a deformity with olecranon pushed posteriorly.
(5) Diagnostic tests utilized: plain film imaging.
(6) Medications.
(a) Acetaminophen for pain.
(b) NSAIDs for pain and/or inflammation.
(7) Physical therapy goals, outcomes, and interventions.
(a) Initial intervention includes reduction of the dislocation.
(b) If elbow is stable, there is an initial phase of immobilization, followed by rehabilitation focusing on regaining flexibility within limits of stability and strengthening.
(c) If elbow is not stable, surgery is indicated.

3. Wrist and hand conditions.

a. Carpal tunnel syndrome (repetitive stress syndrome).
(1) Compression of the median nerve at the carpal tunnel of the wrist due to inflammation of the flexor tendons and/or median nerve.
(2) Commonly occurs as result of repetitive wrist motions or gripping, with pregnancy, diabetes, and rheumatoid arthritis.
(3) Must rule out potential of cervical spine dysfunction, thoracic outlet syndrome, or peripheral nerve entrapment that mimics this condition.
(4) Diagnostic tests utilized: electrodiagnostic testing.
(5) Common clinical findings include exacerbation of burning, tingling, pins and needles, and numbness into median nerve distribution at night, and a positive Tinel's sign and/or Phalen's test. Long-term compression causes atrophy and weakness of thenar muscles and lateral two lumbricals.
(6) Medications.
(a) Acetaminophen for pain.
(b) NSAIDs for pain and/or inflammation.
(7) Physical therapy goals, outcomes, and interventions.
(a) Biomechanical faults caused by joint restrictions should be corrected with joint mobilization to the specific restrictions identified during the examination.
(b) Soft tissue/massage techniques, modalities, flexibility exercises, and functional exercises including strengthening, endurance, and coordination.

b. DeQuervain's tenosynovitis.
(1) Inflammation of extensor pollicis brevis and abductor pollicis longus tendons at first dorsal compartment.
(2) Results from repetitive microtrauma or as a complication of swelling during pregnancy.
(3) Diagnostic tests utilized: MRI, but usually not necessary to make diagnosis.
(4) Clinical signs include: pain at anatomical snuffbox, swelling, decreased grip and pinch strength, positive Finkelstein's test (which places tendons on a stretch).
(5) Medications.
(a) Acetaminophen for pain.
(b) NSAIDs for pain and/or inflammation.
(6) Physical therapy goals, outcomes, and interventions.
(a) Biomechanical faults caused by joint restrictions should be corrected with joint mobilization to the specific restrictions identified during the examination.
(b) Soft tissue/massage techniques, modalities, flexibility exercises, and functional exercises including strengthening, endurance, and coordination.

c. Colles' fracture.
(1) Most common wrist fracture, resulting from a fall onto an outstretched upper extremity (UE). These fractures are immobilized between 5 and

8 weeks. Complication of median nerve compression can occur with excessive edema.
- (2) Characteristic "dinner fork" deformity of wrist and hand results from dorsal or posterior displacement of distal fragment of radius, with a radial shift of wrist and hand.
- (3) Diagnostic tests utilized: plain film imaging.
- (4) Complications may include loss of motion, decreased grip strength, CRPS, and carpal tunnel syndrome.
- (5) Medications.
  - (a) Acetaminophen for pain.
  - (b) NSAIDs for pain and/or inflammation.
- (6) Physical therapy goals, outcomes, and interventions.
  - (a) Early physical therapy intervention that focuses on normalizing flexibility is paramount to functional recovery of wrist and hand.
  - (b) Biomechanical faults caused by joint restrictions should be corrected with joint mobilization to the specific restrictions identified during the examination.
  - (c) Soft tissue/massage techniques, modalities, flexibility exercises, and functional exercises including strengthening, endurance, and coordination.

d. Smith's fracture.
- (1) Similar to Colles' fracture, except distal fragment of radius dislocates in a volar direction, causing a characteristic "garden spade deformity."
- (2) Diagnostic tests utilized: plain film imaging.
- (3) Medications.
  - (a) Acetaminophen for pain.
  - (b) NSAIDs for pain and/or inflammation.
- (4) Physical therapy goals, outcomes, and interventions.
  - (a) Intervention is similar to Colles' fracture.

e. Scaphoid fracture.
- (1) Results from a fall onto outstretched UE in a younger person. Most commonly fractured carpal.
- (2) Diagnostic tests utilized: plain film imaging.
- (3) Complications include a high incidence of avascular necrosis of the proximal fragment of the scaphoid secondary to poor vascular supply. Carpals are immobilized between 4 and 8 weeks.
- (4) Medications.
  - (a) Acetaminophen for pain.
  - (b) NSAIDs for pain and/or inflammation.
- (5) Physical therapy goals, outcomes, and interventions.
  - (a) Early intervention includes maintenance of flexibility of distal and proximal joints while UE is casted. Later intervention emphasizes strengthening, stretching, and joint and soft tissue mobilizations to regain full functional use of wrist and hand.

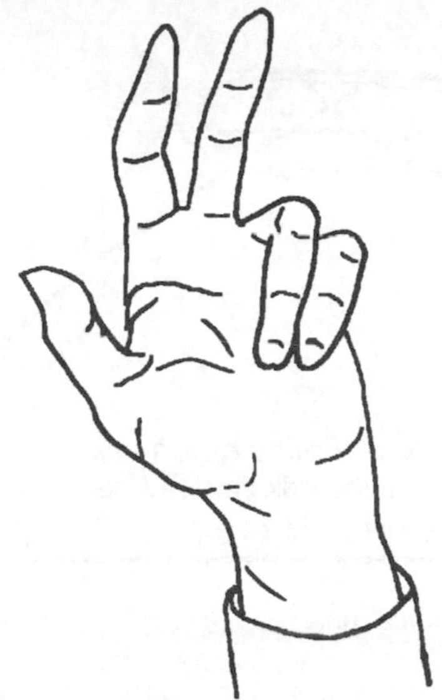

Figure 1-3 • Dupuytren's contracture.
(Adapted from Magee, DJ. Orthopedic Physical Assessment. 2nd ed. Philadelphia, Saunders, 1992).

f. Dupuytren's contracture (Figure 1-3).
- (1) Observed as banding on palm and digit flexion contractures, resulting from contracture of palmar fascia which adheres to skin.
- (2) Affects men more often than women.
- (3) Contracture usually affects the metacarpophalangeal (MCP) and proximal interphalangeal (PIP) joints of fourth and fifth digits in nondiabetic individuals and affects third and fourth digits most often in individuals with diabetes.
- (4) Medications.
  - (a) Acetaminophen for pain.
  - (b) NSAIDs for pain and/or inflammation.
- (5) Physical therapy goals, outcomes, and interventions.
  - (a) Physical therapy intervention includes flexibility exercise to prevent further contracture and splint fabrication/application.
  - (b) Once contracture is under control, promote restoration of normal hand function through functional exercises.
  - (c) Physical therapy intervention following surgery includes wound management, edema control, and progression of functional exercise.

g. Boutonnière deformity (Figure 1-4).
- (1) Results from rupture of central tendinous slip of extensor hood.
- (2) Observed deformity is extension of MCP and distal interphalangeal (DIP) with flexion of PIP.
- (3) Commonly occurs following trauma, or in rheumatoid arthritis with degeneration of the central extensor tendon.

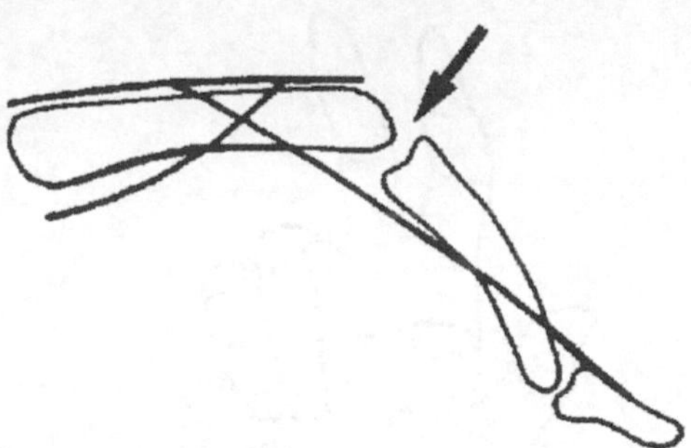

Figure 1-4 • Boutonnière deformity.
(From Magee, DJ. Orthopedic Physical Assessment. 2nd ed. Philadelphia, Saunders, 1992).

(4) Medications.
(a) Acetaminophen for pain.
(b) NSAIDs for pain and/or inflammation.
(5) Physical therapy goals, outcomes, and interventions.
(a) Physical therapy intervention includes edema management, flexibility exercises of involved and uninvolved joints, splinting or taping, and functional strengthening/endurance/coordination exercises.

h. Swan neck deformity (Figure 1-5).
(1) Results from contracture of intrinsic muscles with dorsal subluxation of lateral extensor tendons.
(2) Observed deformity is flexion of MCP and DIP with extension of PIP.
(3) Commonly occurs following trauma, or with rheumatoid arthritis following degeneration of lateral extensor tendons.
(4) Diagnostic tests utilized: plain film imaging, but may not be necessary.
(5) Medications.
(a) Acetaminophen for pain.
(b) NSAIDs for pain and/or inflammation.
(6) Physical therapy goals, outcomes, and interventions.
(a) Physical therapy intervention includes edema management, flexibility exercises of involved and uninvolved joints, splinting or taping, and functional strengthening/endurance/coordination exercises.

i. Ape hand deformity (Figure 1-6).
(1) Observed as thenar muscle wasting, with first digit moving dorsally until it is in line with second digit.
(2) Results from median nerve dysfunction.
(3) Diagnostic tests utilized: electrodiagnostic testing.
(4) Medications.
(a) Acetaminophen for pain.
(b) NSAIDs for pain and/or inflammation.
(5) Physical therapy goals, outcomes, and interventions.
(a) Physical therapy intervention includes edema management, flexibility exercises of involved and uninvolved joints, splinting or taping, and functional strengthening/endurance/coordination exercises.

j. Mallet finger (Figure 1-7).
(1) Rupture or avulsion of extensor tendon at its insertion into distal phalanx of digit.
(2) Observed deformity is flexion of DIP joint.
(3) Usually occurs from trauma, forcing distal phalanx into a flexed position.
(4) Diagnostic tests utilized: possibly MRI.
(5) Medications.
(a) Acetaminophen for pain.
(b) NSAIDs for pain and/or inflammation.
(6) Physical therapy goals, outcomes, and interventions.
(a) Physical therapy intervention includes edema management, flexibility exercises of involved and uninvolved joints, splinting or taping, and functional strengthening/endurance/coordination exercises.

k. Gamekeeper's thumb.
(1) A sprain/rupture of ulnar collateral ligament of MCP joint of first digit.
(2) Results in medial instability of thumb.
(3) Frequently occurs during a fall while skiing, when increasing forces are placed on thumb through ski pole. Immobilized for 6 weeks.

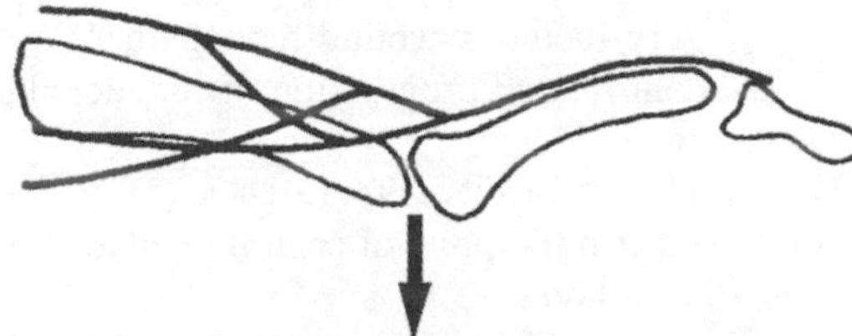

Figure 1-5 • "Swan neck" deformity.
(From Magee, DJ. Orthopedic Physical Assessment. 2nd ed. Philadelphia, Saunders, 1992).

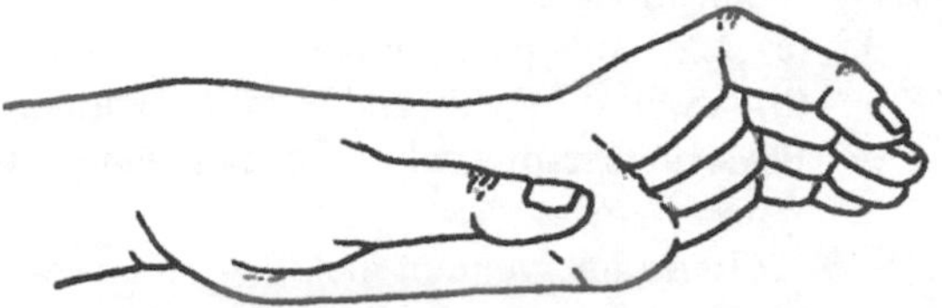

Figure 1-6 • "Ape hand" deformity.
(From Magee, DJ. Orthopedic Physical Assessment. 2nd ed. Philadelphia, Saunders, 1992).

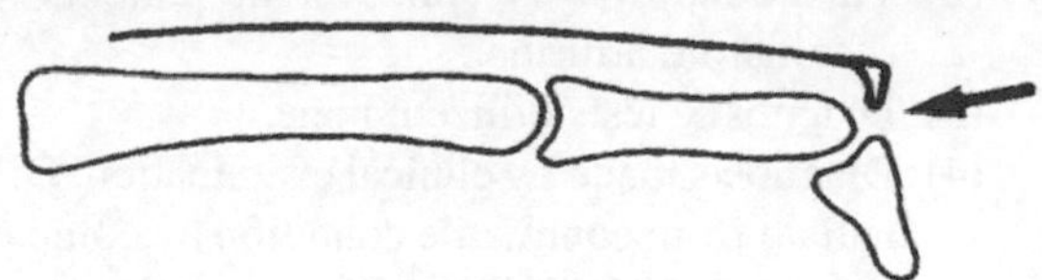

Figure 1-7 • Mallet finger.
(From Magee, DJ. Orthopedic Physical Assessment. 2nd ed. Philadelphia, Saunders, 1992).

(4) Diagnostic tests utilized: possibly MRI.
(5) Medications.
(a) Acetaminophen for pain.
(b) NSAIDs for pain and/or inflammation.
(6) Physical therapy goals, outcomes, and interventions.
(a) Physical therapy intervention includes edema management, flexibility exercises of involved and uninvolved joints, splinting or taping, and functional strengthening/endurance/coordination exercises.

l. Boxer's fracture.
(1) Fracture of neck of 5th metacarpal.
(2) Frequently sustained during a fight, or from punching a wall in anger or frustration.
(3) Casted for 2–4 weeks.
(4) Diagnostic tests utilized: plain film imaging.
(5) Medications.
(a) Acetaminophen for pain.
(b) NSAIDs for pain and/or inflammation.
(6) Physical therapy goals, outcomes, and interventions.
(a) Physical therapy intervention includes edema management, flexibility exercise initially at uninvolved joints, followed by involved joints after sufficient healing has occurred.
(b) Initiation of functional strengthening/endurance/coordination occurs when flexibility is restored.

Lower Extremity Conditions

1. Hip conditions.

a. Avascular necrosis (AVN) of the hip (osteonecrosis).
(1) Multiple etiologies resulting in an impaired blood supply to the femoral head.
(2) Hip ROM is decreased in flexion, internal rotation, and abduction.
(3) Diagnostic tests utilized: plain film imaging, bone scans, CT, and/or MRI may be utilized.
(4) Symptoms include pain in the groin and/or thigh, and tenderness with palpation at the hip joint.
(5) Coxalgic gait.
(6) Medications.
(a) Acetaminophen for pain.
(b) NSAIDs for pain and/or inflammation.
(c) Corticosteroids contraindicated since they may be causative factor. Patient taking steroids for some other condition should have dose decreased.
(7) Physical therapy goals, outcomes, and interventions.
(a) Joint/bone protection strategies.
(b) Maintain/improve joint mechanics and connective tissue functions.
(c) Implementation of aerobic capacity/endurance conditioning or reconditioning such as aquatic programs.
(d) Postsurgical intervention includes regaining functional flexibility, improving strength/endurance/coordination, and gait training.

b. Legg-Calvé-Perthe's disease (osteochondrosis).
(1) Age of onset between 2 and 13 years; average age of onset is at 6 years.
(2) Males have a four times greater incidence than females.
(3) Characteristic psoatic limp due to weakness of psoas major; affected lower extremity (LE) moves in external rotation, flexion, and adduction.
(4) Gradual onset of "aching" pain at hip, thigh, and knee.
(5) AROM limited in abduction and extension.
(6) Diagnostic tests utilized: MRI is imaging technique of choice. Positive bony crescent sign (collapse of subchondral bone at femoral neck/head).
(7) Medications.
(a) Acetaminophen for pain.
(b) NSAIDs for pain and/or inflammation.
(8) Physical therapy goals, outcomes, and interventions.
(a) Joint/bone protection strategies.
(b) Maintain/improve joint mechanics and connective tissue functions.
(c) Implementation of aerobic capacity/endurance conditioning or reconditioning such as aquatic programs.
(d) Postsurgical intervention includes regaining functional flexibility, improving strength/endurance/coordination, and gait training.

c. Slipped capital femoral epiphysis.
(1) Most common hip disorder observed in adolescents, and is of unknown etiology.
(2) Onset in males: 10–17 years of age, with the average age of onset at 13 years.
(3) Onset in females: 8–15 years of age, with the average age of onset at 11 years.
(4) Males have two times the incidence of females.

(5) AROM is restricted in abduction, flexion, and internal rotation.
(6) Patient describes pain as vague at knee, thigh, and hip.
(7) With chronic conditions, patient may demonstrate a Trendelenburg gait.
(8) Diagnostic tests utilized: plain film imaging show a positive displacement of upper femoral epiphysis.
(9) Medications.
(a) Acetaminophen for pain.
(b) NSAIDs for pain and/or inflammation.
(10) Physical therapy goals, outcomes, and interventions.
(a) Joint/bone protection strategies.
(b) Maintain/improve joint mechanics and connective tissue functions.
(c) Implementation of aerobic capacity/endurance conditioning or reconditioning such as aquatic programs.
(d) Postsurgical intervention includes regaining functional flexibility, improving strength/endurance/coordination, and gait training.

d. Femoral anteversion.
(1) Excessive femoral anteversion (25°–30° or greater) leads to squinting patellae and toeing in.
(2) With an angle less than 0° (retroversion), femoral neck is rotated backward in relation to femoral condyles.
(3) Diagnostic tests utilized: plain film imaging.
(4) Clinical examination including Craig's test helps to identify this condition.
(5) Physical therapy goals, outcomes, and interventions.
(a) Maintain/improve joint mechanics and connective tissue functions.

e. Coxa vara and coxa valga.
(1) Angle of femoral neck with shaft of femur is < 115°; coxa vara results.
(2) Angle of femoral neck with shaft of femur is > 125°; coxa valga results.
(3) Coxa vara usually results from a defect in ossification of head of femur. Coxa vara and coxa valga may result from necrosis of femoral head occurring with septic arthritis.
(4) Diagnostic tests utilized: plain film imaging.
(5) Physical therapy goals, outcomes, and interventions.
(a) Maintain/improve joint mechanics and connective tissue functions.

f. Trochanteric bursitis.
(1) An inflammation of deep trochanteric bursa from a direct blow, irritation by iliotibial band (ITB), and biomechanical/gait abnormalities causing repetitive microtrauma.
(2) This condition is common in patients with rheumatoid arthritis.
(3) Diagnostic tests utilized: none.
(4) Diagnosis made by clinical examination. Differentiate from contractile condition by comparing results of AROM, PROM, and resistive tests.
(5) Medications.
(a) Acetaminophen for pain.
(b) NSAIDs for pain and/or inflammation.
(6) Physical therapy goals, outcomes, and interventions.
(a) Refer to intervention for general bursitis/tendonitis/tendonosis.

g. Iliotibial band tightness/friction disorder.
(1) Etiology: tight iliotibial band, abnormal gait patterns.
(2) Results in inflammation of trochanteric bursa.
(3) Noble compression test is positive when friction is introduced over the lateral femoral condyle during knee extension. Ober's test will also demonstrate tightness in ITB.
(4) Medications.
(a) Acetaminophen for pain.
(b) NSAIDs for pain and/or inflammation.
(5) Physical therapy goals, outcomes, and interventions.
(a) Reduction of pain and inflammation utilizing modalities, soft tissue techniques, and manual therapy techniques such as soft tissue/massage and joint oscillations.
(b) Correction of muscle imbalances and biomechanical faults using strengthening, endurance, coordination, and flexibility (IT band, hamstrings, quadriceps, and hip flexors) exercises to gain restoration of normal function.
(c) Biomechanical faults caused by joint restrictions should be corrected with joint mobilization to the specific restrictions identified during the examination.
(d) Gait training and patient education regarding the selection of running shoes and running surfaces. Orthoses may be fabricated.

h. Piriformis syndrome.
(1) Piriformis muscle is an external rotator of hip and can become overworked with excessive pronation of foot, causing abnormal femoral internal rotation. Considered a tonic muscle which is active with motion of sacroiliac joint, particularly sacrum.
(2) Tightness or spasm of piriformis muscle can result in compression of sciatic nerve and/or sacroiliac dysfunction.
(3) Diagnostic tests utilized: possibly electrodiagnostic tests for sciatic nerve.
(4) Signs and symptoms include:
(a) Restriction in internal rotation.

(b) Pain with palpation of piriformis muscle.
(c) Referral of pain to posterior thigh.
(d) Weakness in external rotation, positive piriformis test.
(e) Uneven sacral base.

(5) Perform lower extremity biomechanical examination to determine if abnormal biomechanics are the cause. Must rule out involvement of lumbar spine and/or sacroiliac joint.

(6) Medications.
(a) Acetaminophen for pain.
(b) NSAIDs for pain and/or inflammation.
(c) Neurontin for neuropathic pain.

(7) Physical therapy goals, outcomes, and interventions.
(a) Reduction of pain utilizing modalities and manual therapy techniques, such as soft tissue/massage to piriformis muscle.
(b) Joint oscillations to hip or pelvis to inhibit pain.
(c) Correction of muscle imbalances and biomechanical faults using strengthening, endurance, coordination, and flexibility exercises to gain restoration of normal function.
(d) Restore muscle balance and patient education regarding protection of the sacroiliac joint (e.g., instruction not to step off a curb onto the dysfunctional lower extremity).
(e) Correction of biomechanical faults may include orthoses or orthotic devices for feet.

2. Knee conditions.

a. Ligament sprains.

(1) Four major ligaments may be involved (anterior cruciate, posterior cruciate, medial collateral, and lateral collateral).

(2) Injury to the ligaments may result in a single plane or rotary instability.
(a) ACL laxity may result in single plane anterior instability.
(b) PCL laxity may result in single plane posterior instability.
(c) ACL and MCL laxity may result in anteromedial rotary instability.
(d) ACL and LCL laxity may result in anterolateral rotary instability.
(e) PCL and MCL laxity may result in posteromedial rotary instability.
(f) PCL and LCL laxity may result in posterolateral rotary instability.

(3) Classification of injury.
(a) First degree, resulting in little or no instability.
(b) Second degree, resulting in minimal to moderate instability.
(c) Third degree, resulting in extreme instability.

(4) "Unhappy triad" includes injury to the medial collateral ligament, anterior cruciate ligament, and the medial meniscus, resulting from a combination of valgum, flexion, and external rotation forces applied to knee when the foot is planted.

(5) Diagnostic tests utilized: MRI. Difficult to visualize complete ACL on MRI, so often read incorrectly as partially torn even if normal.

(6) Refer to knee special tests that help to identify ligamentous instabilities of knee joint.

(7) Reconstruction frequently involves a combination of intra-articular and extra-articular procedures.

(8) Medications.
(a) Acetaminophen for pain.
(b) NSAIDs for pain and/or inflammation.

(9) Physical therapy goals, outcomes, and interventions.
(a) Physical therapy intervention is varied depending on whether the patient undergoes a surgical procedure, as well as type of surgery performed.
(b) Reduction of pain and inflammation utilizing modalities, soft tissue techniques, and manual therapy techniques such as oscillations.
(c) Postoperatively, continuous passive motion (CPM) devices may be used to maintain promote flexibility of the joint.
(d) Correction of muscle imbalances and biomechanical faults using strengthening, endurance, coordination, and flexibility exercises to gain restoration of normal function.
(e) Biomechanical faults caused by joint restrictions should be corrected with joint mobilization to the specific restrictions identified during the examination.
(f) Progression to functional training based on patient's occupation and/or recreational goals.

b. Meniscal injuries.

(1) Result from a combination of forces to include tibiofemoral joint flexion, compression, and rotation which places abnormal shear stresses on the meniscus.

(2) Symptoms include lateral and/or medial joint pain, effusion, joint popping, knee giving way during walking, limitation in flexibility of knee joint, and joint locking.

(3) Diagnostic tests utilized: MRI typically done, but not always sensitive enough to confirm tear.

(4) Clinical examination including the following special tests will be useful to make diagnosis.
(a) McMurray's test.
(b) Apley's test.

(5) Medications.
(a) Acetaminophen for pain.
(b) NSAIDs for pain and/or inflammation.

(6) Physical therapy goals, outcomes, and interventions.

(a) Reduction of pain and inflammation utilizing modalities, soft tissue/massage techniques to surrounding muscles, and manual therapy techniques, such as joint oscillations to inhibit pain.
(b) Correction of muscle imbalances and biomechanical faults using strengthening, endurance, coordination, and flexibility exercises to gain restoration of normal function.
(c) Biomechanical faults caused by joint restrictions should be corrected with joint mobilization to the specific restrictions identified during the examination.
(d) Progression to functional training based on patient's occupation and/or recreational goals.

c. Patellofemoral conditions.
(1) Abnormal patella positions.
(a) Patella alta.
- Malalignment in which patella tracks superiorly in femoral intercondylar notch.
- May result in chronic patellar subluxation.
- Positive camel back sign (two bumps over anterior knee region instead of typical one). Two bumps, since patella rides high within femoral condyles, creating a superior bump with tibial tuberosity forming second bump inferiorly).

(b) Patella baja.
- Malalignment in which patella tracks inferiorly in femoral intercondylar notch.
- Results in restricted knee extension with abnormal cartilaginous wearing, resulting in DJD.

(c) Lateral patellar tracking.
- Could result if there is an increase in "Q angle" with a tendency for lateral subluxation or dislocation.

(d) Diagnostic tests utilized: plain film imaging including "sunrise" view.
(e) Physical therapy goals, outcomes, and interventions.
- Regaining functional strength of structures surrounding knee, particularly vastus medialis oblique (VMO) muscle, regain normal flexibility of ITB and hamstrings, orthoses (if appropriate), and patellar bracing/taping.

(2) Patellofemoral pain syndrome (PFPS).
(a) Common dysfunction that may occur on its own or in conjunction with other entities. May have been caused by trauma or by congenital/developmental dysfunction.
(b) May be interrelated with chondromalacia patellae and/or patella tendonitis.
(c) Common result is an abnormal patellofemoral tracking leading to abnormal patellofemoral stress.
(d) Occasionally, surgery is indicated.
(e) Diagnostic tests utilized: possibly MRI to rule out other dysfunctions.
(f) Medications.
- Acetaminophen for pain.
- NSAIDs for pain and/or inflammation.

(g) Physical therapy goals, outcomes, and interventions.
- Patellofemoral (McConnell) taping is helpful to inhibit pain during rehabilitation.
- Patella mobilization indicated with restrictions of patella glides (e.g., if patella is in a lateral glide position and has decreased medial glide, perform a medial glide joint mobilization to the patella).
- Correction of muscle imbalances and biomechanical faults using strengthening, endurance, coordination, and flexibility exercises to gain restoration of normal function.

(3) Patellar tendonitis.
(a) May be related to overload and/or jumping related activities/sports.
(b) May also be interrelated to patellofemoral dysfunction.
(c) Diagnosis made by clinical examination.
(d) Medications.
- Acetaminophen for pain.
- NSAIDs for pain and/or inflammation.
- Corticosteroid injection or by mouth.

(e) Physical therapy goals, outcomes, and interventions.
- Refer to intervention for general bursitis/tendonitis/tendonosis.

d. Pes anserine bursitis.
(1) Typically caused by overuse or a contusion.
(2) Must be differentiated from tendonitis.
(3) Diagnosis made by clinical examination. Differentiate from contractile condition by comparing results of AROM, PROM, and resistive tests.
(4) Medications.
(a) Acetaminophen for pain.
(b) NSAIDs for pain and/or inflammation.
(c) Corticosteroid injection or by mouth.
(5) Physical therapy goals, outcomes, and interventions.
(a) Refer to intervention for general bursitis/tendonitis/tendonosis.

e. Osgood-Schlatter (jumper's knee).
(1) Mechanical dysfunction resulting in traction apophysitis of the tibial tubercle at the patellar tendon insertion.
(2) Diagnostic tests utilized: plain film findings demonstrate irregularities of the epiphyseal line.
(3) Occasionally surgery is indicated.
(4) Diagnosis made by clinical examination.

(5) Medications.
(a) Acetaminophen for pain.
(b) NSAIDs for pain and/or inflammation.
(6) Physical therapy goals, outcomes, and interventions.
(a) Modify activities to prevent excessive stress to irritated site.

f. Genu varum and valgum.
(1) Normal tibiofemoral shaft angle is 6° of valgum.
(2) Genu varum is an excessive medial tibial torsion, commonly referred to as "bowlegs."
(3) Genu varum results in excessive medial patellar positioning and the pigeon-toed orientation of the feet.
(4) Genu valgum is an excessive lateral tibial torsion commonly referred to as "knock-knees."
(5) Genu valgum results in excessive lateral patellar positioning.
(6) Diagnostic tests utilized: plain film imaging.
(7) Diagnosis made by clinical examination.
(8) Physical therapy goals, outcomes, and interventions.
(a) Intervention includes decreased loading of knee while maintaining strength and endurance.

g. Fractures involving knee joint.
(1) Femoral condyle.
(a) Medial femoral most often involved due to its anatomical design.
(b) Numerous etiological factors include trauma, shearing, impacting, and avulsion forces.
(c) Common mechanism of injury is a fall, with knee subjected to a shearing force.
(2) Tibial plateau.
(a) Common mechanism of injury is a combination of valgum and compression forces to knee when knee is in a flexed position.
(b) Often occurs in conjunction with a medial collateral ligamentous injury.
(3) Epiphyseal plate.
(a) Mechanism of injury is frequently a weight-bearing torsional stress.
(b) Presents more frequently in adolescents where an ACL injury would occur in an adult.
(4) Patella.
(a) Most common mechanism of injury is a direct blow to patella due to a fall.
(5) Diagnostic tests utilized: plain film imaging most likely, unless complex fracture, which would benefit from CT.
(6) Medications.
(a) Acetaminophen for pain.
(b) NSAIDs for pain and/or inflammation.
(7) Physical therapy goals, outcomes, and interventions.
(a) Physical therapy intervention emphasizes return of function without pain.
(b) Early flexibility is important in preventing capsular adhesions.

3. Conditions of the lower leg.

a. Anterior compartment syndrome (ACS).
(1) Increased compartmental pressure resulting in a local ischemic condition.
(2) Multiple etiologies; direct trauma, fracture, overuse, and/or muscle hypertrophy.
(3) Symptoms of chronic or exertional compartment syndrome are produced by exercise or exertion and described as a deep, cramping feeling.
(4) Symptoms of acute ACS are produced by sudden trauma causing swelling within the compartment.
(5) Diagnosis made by clinical examination.
(6) Acute ACS is considered a medical emergency and requires immediate surgical intervention with fasciotomy.

b. Anterior tibial periostitis (shin splints).
(1) Musculotendinous overuse condition.
(2) Three common etiologies include:
(a) Abnormal biomechanical alignment.
(b) Poor conditioning.
(c) Improper training methods.
(3) Muscles involved include anterior tibialis and extensor hallucis longus.
(4) Pain elicited with palpation of lateral tibia and anterior compartment.
(5) Diagnosis made by clinical examination.
(6) Medications.
(a) Acetaminophen for pain.
(b) NSAIDS for pain and/or inflammation.
(7) Physical therapy goals, outcomes, and interventions.
(a) Correction of muscle imbalances and biomechanical faults using strengthening, endurance, and coordination exercises.
(b) Flexibility exercises for anterior compartment muscles, as well as the triceps surae, to gain restoration of normal function.

c. Medial tibial stress syndrome.
(1) Overuse injury of the posterior tibialis and/or the medial soleus, resulting in periosteal inflammation at the muscular attachments.
(2) Etiology is thought to be excessive pronation.
(3) Pain elicited with palpation of the distal posteromedial border of the tibia.
(4) Diagnosis made by clinical examination.
(5) Medications.
(a) Acetaminophen for pain.
(b) NSAIDs for pain and/or inflammation.
(6) Physical therapy goals, outcomes, and interventions.
(a) Correction of muscle imbalances and biomechanical faults using strengthening, endurance, and coordination exercises.

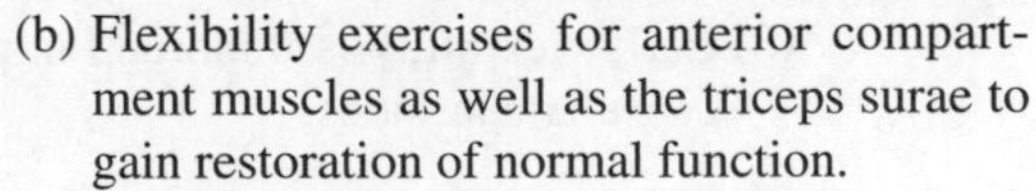

(b) Flexibility exercises for anterior compartment muscles as well as the triceps surae to gain restoration of normal function.

d. Stress fractures.
(1) Overuse injury resulting most often in microfracture of the tibia or fibula.
(2) 49% of all stress fractures involve the tibia, and 10% involve the fibula.
(3) Three common etiologies: abnormal biomechanical alignment, poor conditioning, and improper training methods.
(4) Diagnostic tests utilized: plain film imaging and bone scan.
(5) Medications.
(a) Acetaminophen for pain.
(b) NSAIDs for pain and/or inflammation.
(6) Physical therapy goals, outcomes, and interventions.
(a) Correction of muscle imbalances and biomechanical faults using strengthening, endurance, and coordination exercises.
(b) Flexibility exercises for anterior compartment muscles as well as the triceps surae to gain restoration of normal function.

4. Foot and ankle conditions.

a. Ligament sprains.
(1) 95% of all ankle sprains involve lateral ligaments.
(2) With lateral sprains, foot is plantar flexed and inverted at time of injury.
(3) The most common grading system is as follows:
(a) Grade I: no loss of function, with minimal tearing of the anterior talofibular ligament.
(b) Grade II: some loss of function, with partial disruption of the anterior talofibular and calcaneofibular ligaments.
(c) Grade III: complete loss of function, with complete tearing of the anterior talofibular and calcaneofibular ligaments, with partial tear of the posterior talofibular ligament.
(4) Diagnostic tests utilized: MRI if necessary.
(5) Instability is evaluated using anterior drawer and talar tilt special tests.
(6) Medications.
(a) Acetaminophen for pain.
(b) NSAIDs for pain and/or inflammation.
(7) Physical therapy goals, outcomes, and interventions.
(a) Physical therapy intervention is varied, depending on whether the patient undergoes a surgical procedure as well as type of surgery that is performed.
(b) Reduction of pain and inflammation utilizing modalities, soft tissue techniques, and manual therapy techniques, such as oscillations.
(c) Correction of muscle imbalances and biomechanical faults using strengthening, endurance, coordination, and flexibility exercises to gain restoration of normal function.
(d) Biomechanical faults caused by joint restrictions should be corrected with joint mobilization to the specific restrictions identified during the examination.
(e) Progression to functional training based on patient's occupation and/or recreational goals.

b. Achilles tendonitis/tendonosis.
(1) Differentiate whether an inflammatory tendonitis or a chronic tendonosis.
(2) Clinical examination including Thompson's test helps to identify this condition.
(3) Medications.
(a) Acetaminophen for pain.
(b) NSAIDs for pain and/or inflammation.
(c) Corticosteroid injection or by mouth.
(4) Physical therapy goals, outcomes, and interventions.
(a) Refer to intervention for general bursitis/tendonitis/tendonosis.

c. Fractures of foot and ankle.
(1) Unimalleolar involves the medial or lateral malleolus.
(2) Bimalleolar involves the medial and lateral malleoli.
(3) Trimalleolar involves the medial and lateral malleoli, and the posterior tubercle of the distal tibia.
(4) Diagnostic tests utilized: plain film imaging.
(a) Growth plate fractures are a concern, since bone growth can be affected. Types III and IV fractures, according the the Salter Harris classification, are of most concern and can have a high complication rate. (See Table 1-29).
(5) Medications.
(a) Acetaminophen for pain.
(b) NSAIDs for pain and/or inflammation.
(6) Physical therapy goals, outcomes, and interventions.
(a) Physical therapy intervention emphasizes return of function without pain.
(b) Functional training and restoration of muscle imbalances using exercise to normalize strength, endurance, coordination, and flexibility.
(c) Early PROM is important in preventing capsular adhesions.

d. Tarsal tunnel syndrome.
(1) Entrapment of the posterior tibial nerve or one of its branches within the tarsal tunnel.
(2) Over/excessive pronation, overuse problems resulting in tendonitis of the long flexor and posterior tibialis tendon, and trauma may compromise space in the tarsal tunnel.

Table 1-29 ➤ SALTER-HARRIS FRACTURE CLASSIFICATION

TYPE	ANATOMICAL DEFORMITY	COMMON CAUSE	GENERAL PROGNOSIS	MEDICAL MANAGEMENT
I	Entire epiphysis	Caused by shearing, torsion, or avulsion forces.	Good, with very few complications to growth of the bone.	Relocated if necessary, and immobilized with cast.
II	Entire epiphysis and portion of the metaphysis	Usually caused by a shear or avulsion with angular force. Most common type.	May cause decreased bone growth, but typically minimal, so limited negative impact on long term function.	Relocated and immobilized with cast.
III	Portion of the epiphysis.	Typically occurs when the growth plate is partially fused. Rare, but most commonly occurs to the distal tibia in adolescents.	This type of fracture may lead to long term problems secondary to the fracture, crossing the physis and extending into the articular surface of the bone. Even with this potential, the prognosis is typically favorable, since these fractures rarely result in significant deformity.	Relocated and immobilized. Occasionally requires surgical intervention (i.e. ORIF). A specific fracture known as the Tillaux fracture (a type III fracture of the distal tibia) has a particularly poor prognosis.
IV	Portion of the epiphysis and portion of the metaphysis.	Similar to Type III. Most commonly seen in the distal humerus.	Since this fracture interferes with the cartilage growth, it may lead to premature focal fusion of the involved bone causing deformity of the joint.	Generally, surgery (i.e. ORIF) is necessary to restore alignment. Prognosis is correlated to quality of alignment achieved.
V	Nothing "broken off," compression injury of the epiphyseal plate.	This is caused by a compression or crush injury of the epiphyseal plate, with no associated epiphyseal or metaphyseal fracture.	Type V fractures are associated with growth disturbances at the physis, and generally will have a poor functional prognosis.	These are usually found "after the fact," so no immediate intervention is provided. If it is identified acutely, patient is placed on non-weight-bearing protocols.

(3) Symptoms include; pain, numbness and paresthesias along the medial ankle to the plantar surface of the foot.
(4) Diagnostic tests utilized: electrodiagnostic tests.
(5) Positive Tinel's sign at the tarsal tunnel.
(6) Medications.
 (a) Acetaminophen for pain.
 (b) NSAIDs for pain and/or inflammation.
 (c) Neurontin for neuropathic pain.
(7) Physical therapy goals, outcomes, and interventions.
 (a) Intervention includes the use of orthoses to maintain neutral alignment of the foot.

e. Flexor hallucis tendonopathy.
(1) Identified as a tendonitis in the acute stage, or can present as a chronic tendonosis. Commonly seen in ballet performers.
(2) Medications.
 (a) Acetaminophen for pain.
 (b) NSAIDs for pain and/or inflammation.
 (c) Corticosteroid injection or by mouth.
(3) Physical therapy goals, outcomes, and interventions.
 (a) Refer to intervention for general bursitis/tendonitis/tendonosis.

f. Pes cavus (hollow foot).
(1) Numerous etiologies to include genetic predisposition, neurological disorders resulting in muscle imbalances, and contracture of soft tissues.
(2) Deformity observed includes an increased height of longitudinal arches, dropping of anterior arch, metatarsal heads lower than hindfoot, plantar flexion and splaying of forefoot, and claw toes.
(3) Function is limited due to altered arthrokinematics, reducing ability to absorb forces through foot.
(4) Diagnosis made by clinical examination including thorough biomechanical lower quarter exam.
(5) Physical therapy goals, outcomes, and interventions.
 (a) Intervention includes patient education emphasizing limitation of high impact sports (i.e., long-distance running and ballet), use of proper footwear and fitting for orthoses.

g. Pes planus (flat foot).
(1) Etiologies include genetic predisposition, muscle weakness, ligamentous laxity, paralysis, excessive pronation, trauma or disease (e.g., rheumatoid arthritis).

(2) Normal in infant and toddler feet.
(3) Deformity observed may include a reduction in height of medial longitudinal arch.
(4) Decreased ability of foot to provide a rigid lever for push-off during gait, due to altered arthrokinematics.
(5) Diagnosis made by clinical examination, including thorough biomechanical lower quarter exam.
(6) Physical therapy goals, outcomes, and interventions.
(a) Intervention emphasizes patient education, use of proper footwear, and orthotic fitting.

h. Talipes equinovarus (clubfoot).
(1) Two types: postural and talipes equinovarus.
(2) Etiology.
(a) Postural type results from intrauterine malposition.
(b) Talipes equinovarus type is an abnormal development of the head and neck of the talus, due to heredity or neuromuscular disorders; e.g., myelomeningocele.
(3) Deformity observed.
(a) Plantar flexed, adducted, and inverted foot (postural).
(b) Talipes equinovarus has three components: plantar flexion at talocrural joint; inversion at subtalar, talocalcaneal, talonavicular, and calcaneocuboid joints; and supination at midtarsal joints.
(4) Diagnosis made by clinical examination including thorough biomechanical lower quarter exam.
(5) Physical therapy goals, outcomes, and interventions.
(a) Manipulation followed by casting or splinting for postural condition.
(b) Talipes equinovarus requires surgical intervention to correct deformity followed by casting or splinting.

i. Equinus.
(1) Etiology can include congenital bone deformity, neurological disorders such as cerebral palsy, contracture of gastrocnemius and/or soleus muscles, trauma, or inflammatory disease.
(2) Deformity observed: plantar flexed foot.
(3) Compensation secondary to limited dorsiflexion includes subtalar or midtarsal pronation.
(4) Diagnosis made by clinical examination, including thorough biomechanical lower quarter exam.
(5) Physical therapy goals, outcomes, and interventions.
(a) Physical therapy intervention includes flexibility exercises of shortened structures within foot, joint mobilization to joint restrictions identified in examination, strengthening to intrinsic and extrinsic foot muscles, and orthotic management.

j. Hallux valgus.
(1) Etiology is varied to include biomechanical malalignment (excessive pronation), ligamentous laxity, heredity, weak muscles, and footwear that is too tight.
(2) Deformity observed: a medial deviation of head of first metatarsal from midline of body; metatarsal and base of proximal first phalanx move medially, while distal phalanx then moves laterally.
(3) Normal metatarsophalangeal angle is 8°–20°.
(4) Diagnosis made by clinical examination, including thorough biomechanical lower quarter exam.
(5) Physical therapy goals, outcomes, and interventions.
(a) Early orthotic fitting and patient education.
(b) Later management requires surgery, followed by flexibility exercises to restore normal function, strengthening exercises, and possible joint mobilization to identified restrictions.

k. Metatarsalgia.
(1) Etiologies.
(a) Mechanical: tight triceps surae group and/or Achilles' tendon, collapse of transverse arch, short first ray, pronation of forefoot.
(b) Structural changes in transverse arch, possibly leading to vascular and/or neural compromise in tissues of forefoot.
(c) Changes in footwear.
(2) Complaint frequently heard is pain at first and second metatarsal heads after long periods of weight bearing.
(3) Diagnosis made by clinical examination including thorough biomechanical lower quarter exam.
(4) Medications.
(a) Acetaminophen for pain.
(b) NSAIDs for pain and/or inflammation.
(c) Neurontin for neuropathic pain.
(5) Physical therapy goals, outcomes, and interventions.
(a) Intervention includes correction of biomechanical abnormality (improving flexibility of triceps surae), modalities to decrease pain.
(b) Prescription and/or creation of orthoses.
(c) Patient education regarding selection of footwear.

l. Metatarsus adductus.
(1) Etiology: congenital, muscle imbalance, or neuromuscular diseases such as polio.
(2) Two types: rigid and flexible.
(3) Deformity observed.
(a) Rigid form results in a medial subluxation of tarsometatarsal joints. Hindfoot is slightly in valgus with navicular lateral to head of talus.
(b) Flexible form is observed as adduction of all five metatarsals at the tarsometatarsal joints.

(4) Diagnosis is made by clinical examination, including thorough biomechanical lower quarter exam.
(5) Physical therapy goals, outcomes, and interventions.
(a) Intervention includes strengthening and regaining proper alignment of foot (i.e., through use of orthoses).

m. Charcot-Marie-Tooth disease.
(1) Peroneal muscular atrophy that affects motor and sensory nerves.
(2) May begin in childhood or adulthood.
(3) Initially affects muscles in lower leg and foot, but eventually progresses to muscles of hands and forearm.
(4) Slowly progressive disorder with varying degrees of involvement, depending on degree of genetic dominance.
(5) Diagnostic tests utilized: electrodiagnostic tests.
(6) Diagnosis made by clinical examination including thorough biomechanical lower quarter exam.
(7) Medications.
(a) Acetaminophen for pain.
(b) NSAIDs for pain and/or inflammation.
(c) Neurontin for neuropathic pain.
(8) Physical therapy goals, outcomes, and interventions.
(a) No specific treatment to prevent, since it is an inherited disorder.
(b) Physical therapy intervention centers on preventing contractures/skin breakdown and maximizing patient's functional capacity to perform activities.
(c) Patient education and training regarding braces and ambulatory assistive devices.

n. Plantar fasciitis.
(1) Etiology is usually mechanical.
(a) Chronic irritation of plantar fascia from excessive pronation.
(b) Limited ROM of first MTP and talocrural joint.
(c) Tight triceps surae.
(d) Acute injury from excessive loading of foot
(e) Rigid cavus foot.
(2) Results in microtears at attachment of plantar fascia.
(3) Diagnostic tests utilized: none.
(4) Diagnosis made by clinical examination including thorough biomechanical lower quarter exam. Differentiated from tarsal tunnel syndrome by a negative Tinel sign.
(5) Medications.
(a) Acetaminophen for pain.
(b) NSAIDs for pain and/or inflammation.
(c) Corticosteroid injection or by mouth.
(6) Physical therapy goals, outcomes, and interventions.
(a) Physical therapy intervention includes regaining proper mechanical alignment.
(b) Modalities to reduce pain and inflammation.
(c) Flexibility of the plantar fascia for the pes cavus foot.
(d) Careful flexibility exercises for triceps surae.
(e) Joint mobilization to identified restrictions.
(f) Night splints.
(g) Strengthening of invertors of foot.
(h) Patient education regarding selection of footwear, and orthotic fitting.

o. Forefoot/rearfoot deformities.
(1) Rearfoot varus (subtalar varus, calcaneal varus).
(a) Etiology: abnormal mechanical alignment of tibia, shortened rearfoot soft tissues, or malunion of calcaneus.
(b) Deformity observed: rigid inversion of calcaneus when subtalar joint is in neutral position.
(c) Diagnosis made by clinical examination including thorough biomechanical lower quarter exam.
(d) Physical therapy goals, outcomes, and interventions.
- Regaining proper mechanical alignment.
- Improving flexibility of shortened soft tissues.
- Orthotic fitting and patient education regarding selection of footwear.

(2) Rearfoot valgus.
(a) Etiology: abnormal mechanical alignment of the knee (genu valgum), or tibial valgus.
(b) Deformity observed: eversion of calcaneus with a neutral subtalar joint.
(c) Due to increased mobility of hindfoot, fewer musculoskeletal problems develop from this deformity than with rearfoot varus.
(d) Diagnosis made by clinical examination, including thorough biomechanical lower quarter exam.
(e) Physical therapy goals, outcomes, and interventions.
- Regaining proper mechanical alignment.
- Improving flexibility of shortened soft tissues.
- Orthotic fitting and patient education regarding selection of footwear.

(3) Forefoot varus.
(a) Etiology: congenital abnormal deviation of head and neck of talus.
(b) Deformity observed: inversion of forefoot when subtalar joint is in neutral.
(c) Diagnosis made by clinical examination, including thorough biomechanical lower quarter exam.
(d) Physical therapy goals, outcomes, and interventions.

- Regaining proper mechanical alignment.
- Improving flexibility of shortened soft tissues.
- Orthotic fitting and patient education regarding selection of footwear.

(4) Forefoot valgus.
(a) Etiology: congenital abnormal development of head and neck of talus.
(b) Deformity observed: eversion of forefoot when the subtalar joint is in neutral.
(c) Diagnosis made by clinical examination, including thorough biomechanical lower quarter exam.
(d) Physical therapy goals, outcomes, and interventions.
- Regaining proper mechanical alignment.
- Improving flexibility of shortened soft tissues.
- Orthotic fitting and patient education regarding selection of footwear.

Spinal Conditions

1. Muscle strain.

a. May be related to sudden trauma, chronic or sustained overload, or abnormal muscle biomechanics secondary to faulty function (abnormal joint or muscle biomechanics).
b. Commonly will resolve without intervention, but if trauma is too great or if related to chronic etiology, patient will benefit from intervention.
c. Diagnosis made by clinical examination through comparing results of flexibility (AROM/PROM), resistive tests, and palpation.
d. Medications.
(1) Acetaminophen for pain.
(2) NSAIDs for pain and/or inflammation.
(3) Corticosteroid injection or by mouth.
(4) Muscle relaxants; e.g., as Flexeril (cyclobenzaprine) or Valium (diazepam).
(5) Trigger point injections.
e. Physical therapy goals, outcomes, and interventions.
(1) Biomechanical faults caused by joint restrictions should be corrected with joint mobilization.
(2) Patient education regarding the elimination of harmful positions and postural reeducation.
(3) Spinal manipulation for pain inhibition is generally indicated for this condition.

2. Spondylolysis/spondylolisthesis.

a. Etiology: thought to be congenitally defective pars interarticularis.
b. Spondylolysis is a fracture of the pars interarticularis with positive "Scotty dog" sign on oblique radiographic view of spine.
c. Spondylolisthesis is the actual anterior or posterior slippage of one vertebra on another, following bilateral fracture of pars interarticularis.
d. Spondylolisthesis can be graded according to amount of slippage from 1 (25% slippage) to 4 (100% slippage).
e. Diagnostic tests utilized: plain film (oblique to see fracture and lateral views to see slippage).
f. Clinical examination, including stork test, helps identify this condition.
g. Medications.
(1) Acetaminophen for pain.
(2) NSAIDs for pain and/or inflammation.
(3) Corticosteroid injection or by mouth.
(4) Muscle relaxants.
(5) Trigger point injections.
h. Physical therapy goals, outcomes, and interventions.
(1) Biomechanical faults caused by joint restrictions should be corrected with joint mobilization to the specific restrictions identified during the examination.
(2) Exercise should focus on dynamic stabilization of trunk, with particular emphasis on abdominals.
(3) Avoid extension and/or other positions that add stress to defect (i.e., extension, ipsilateral sidebending, and contralateral rotation).
(4) Patient education regarding the elimination of positions of extension and postural reeducation.
(5) Braces such as Boston brace and TLSO (thoracolumbrosacral orthosis) have traditionally been used, but frequency is decreasing.
(6) Spinal manipulation may be contraindicated for this condition, particularly at the level of defect.

3. Spinal or intervertebral stenosis.

a. Etiology: congenital narrow spinal canal or intervertebral foramen, coupled with hypertrophy of the spinal lamina and ligamentum flavum or facets, as the result of age-related degenerative processes or disease.
b. Results in vascular and/or neural compromise.
c. Signs and symptoms (see Table 1-10).
(1) Bilateral pain and paresthesia in back, buttocks, thighs, calves, and feet.
(2) Pain decreases in spinal flexion, increases in extension.
(3) Pain increases with walking.
(4) Pain relieved with prolonged rest.
d. Diagnostic tests utilized: imaging including plain films, MRI, and/or CT scan. Occasionally, myelography is helpful.
e. Clinical examination, including bicycle (van Gelderen's test), helps identify this condition and differentiate it from intermittent claudication.

f. Medications.
   (1) Acetaminophen for pain.
   (2) NSAIDs for pain and/or inflammation.
   (3) Corticosteroid injection or by mouth.
   (4) Muscle relaxants.
   (5) Trigger point injections.
g. Physical therapy goals, outcomes, and interventions.
   (1) Biomechanical faults caused by joint restrictions should be corrected with joint mobilization to the specific restrictions identified during the examination.
   (2) Perform flexion-based exercise, and exercises that promotes dynamic stability throughout the trunk and pelvis.
   (3) Avoid extension and/or other positions that narrow the spinal canal or intervertebral foramen (i.e., extension, ipsilateral side bending, and ipsilateral rotation).
   (4) Manual and/or mechanical traction.
      (a) Traction.
         - Cervical spine positioned at 15° of flexion to provide the optimum intervertebral foraminal opening.
         - Contraindications include joint hypermobility, pregnancy, rheumatoid arthritis, Down's syndrome, or any other systemic disease which affects ligamentous integrity.

4. Disc conditions.

a. Internal disc disruption.
   (1) Internal structure of disc annulus is disrupted; however, external structures remain normal. Most common in lumbar region.
   (2) Symptoms include constant deep, achy pain, and increased pain with movement. No objective neurological findings, although patient may have referred pain in lower extremity.
   (3) Regular CT or myelogram will not demonstrate any abnormal findings. Can be diagnosed by CT discogram or an MRI.
   (4) Clinical examination helps to identify this condition.
   (5) Medications.
      (a) Acetaminophen for pain.
      (b) NSAIDs for pain and/or inflammation.
      (c) Muscle relaxants.
      (d) Trigger point injections.
      (e) Corticosteroid injection or by mouth.
   (6) Physical therapy goals, outcomes, and interventions.
      (a) Biomechanical faults caused by joint restrictions should be corrected with joint mobilization to the specific restrictions identified during the examination.
      (b) Spinal manipulation may be contraindicated for this condition.
      (c) Patient education regarding proper body mechanics, positions to avoid, limiting repetitive bending and twisting movements, limiting upper extremity overhead and sitting activities, and carrying heavy loads.
b. Posterolateral bulge/herniation.
   (1) Most commonly observed disc disorder of lumbar spine due to three structural deficiencies:
      (a) Posterior disc is narrower in height than anterior disc.
      (b) Posterior longitudinal ligament is not as strong and only centrally located in lumbar spine.
      (c) Posterior lamellae of annulus are thinner.
   (2) Etiology: overstretching and/or tearing of annular rings, vertebral endplate and/or ligamentous structures, from high compressive forces or repetitive microtrauma.
   (3) Results in loss of strength, radicular pain, paresthesia and inability to perform activities of daily living (see Table 1-25).
   (4) Diagnostic tests utilized: MRI.
   (5) Clinical examination helps to identify this condition.
   (6) Medications.
      (a) Acetaminophen for pain.
      (b) NSAIDs for pain and/or inflammation.
      (c) Muscle relaxants.
      (d) Trigger point injections.
      (e) Corticosteroid injection or by mouth.
   (7) Physical therapy goals, outcomes, and interventions.
      (a) Exercise program to promote dynamic stability throughout trunk and pelvis and to provide optimal stimulus for regeneration of disc.
      (b) Positional gapping for 10 minutes to increase space within region of space occupying lesion. If left posterolateral lumbar is herniation present:
         - Have patient sidelying on right side, with pillow under right trunk (accentuating trunk side bending right).
         - Flex both hips and knees.
         - Rotate trunk to left (or pelvis to right).
         - Patient can be taught to perform this at home.
      (c) Spinal manipulation may be contraindicated for this condition, particularly at the level of the herniation.
      (d) Patient education regarding proper body mechanics, positions to avoid, limiting repetitive bending and twisting movements, limiting upper extremity overhead and sitting activities, and carrying heavy loads.
      (e) Manual and/or mechanical traction.
         - Traction: cervical spine positioned at 15° degrees of flexion to provide the optimum intervertebral foraminal opening.

- Contraindications include joint hypermobility, pregnancy, rheumatoid arthritis, Down's syndrome, or any other systemic disease which affects ligamentous integrity.
- Efficacy of traction for intervention of disc conditions is currently under scrutiny.

c. Central posterior bulge/herniation.
  (1) More commonly observed in the cervical spine but can also be seen in the lumbar spine.
  (2) Etiology: overstretching and/or tearing of annular rings, vertebral endplate, and/or ligamentous structures (posterior longitudinal ligament) from high compressive forces and/or long-term postural malalignment.
  (3) Results in loss of strength, radicular pain, paresthesia, inability to perform activities of daily living, and possible compression of the spinal cord. Patient exhibits central nervous system symptoms, e.g., hyperreflexia, and a positive Babinski reflex (see Table 1-8).
  (4) Diagnostic tests utilized: MRI.
  (5) Clinical examination helps to identify this condition.
  (6) Medications.
    (a) Acetaminophen for pain.
    (b) NSAIDs for pain and/or inflammation.
    (c) Muscle relaxants.
    (d) Trigger point injections.
    (e) Corticosteroid injection or by mouth.
  (7) Physical therapy goals, outcomes, and interventions.
    - Refer to posterolateral intervention above.

d. Anterior bulge/herniation is very rare due to structural integrity of anterior intervertebral disc.

5. Facet joint conditions.

a. Degenerative joint disease (DJD).
  (1) Etiology: Part of normal aging process due to weight-bearing properties of facets and intervertebral joints.
  (2) Results in bone hypertrophy, capsular fibrosis, hypermobility or hypomobility of joint, and proliferation of synovium.
  (3) Symptoms include reduction in mobility of the spine, pain, and possible impingement of associated nerve root, resulting in loss of strength and paresthesias (see Table 1-8).
  (4) Diagnostic tests utilized: plain film imaging.
  (5) Clinical examination including lumbar quadrant test helps to identify this condition.
  (6) Medications.
    (a) Acetaminophen for pain.
    (b) NSAIDs for pain and/or inflammation.
    (c) Muscle relaxants.
    (d) Trigger point injections.
    (e) Corticosteroid injection or by mouth.
  (7) Physical therapy goals, outcomes, and interventions.
    (a) Exercise program to promote dynamic stability throughout trunk and pelvis and to provide optimal stimulus for regeneration of facet cartilage and/or capsule.
    (b) Biomechanical faults caused by joint restrictions should be corrected with joint mobilization to the specific restrictions identified during the examination.
    (c) Spinal manipulation may be useful.

b. Facet entrapment (acute locked back).
  (1) Caused by abnormal movement of fibroadipose meniscoid in facet during extension (from flexion). Meniscoid does not properly reenter joint cavity and bunches up, becoming a space-occupying lesion, which distends capsule and causes pain.
  (2) Flexion is most comfortable for patient, and extension increases pain.
  (3) Clinical examination, including lumbar quadrant test, helps to identify this condition.
  (4) Medications.
    (a) Acetaminophen for pain.
    (b) NSAIDs for pain and/or inflammation.
    (c) Muscle relaxants.
    (d) Trigger point injections.
    (e) Corticosteroid injection or by mouth.
  (5) Physical therapy goals, outcomes, and interventions.
    (a) Positional facet joint gapping and/or manipulation are appropriate treatments.

6. Acceleration/deceleration injuries of cervical spine.

a. Formerly known as "whiplash."

b. Occurs when excess shear and tensile forces are exerted on cervical structures.

c. Structures injured may include facets/articular processes, facet joint capsules, ligaments, disc, anterior/posterior muscles, fracture to odontoid process and spinous processes, TMJ, sympathetic chain ganglia, spinal and cranial nerves.

d. Signs and symptoms.
  (1) Early include headaches, neck pain, limited flexibility, reversal of lower cervical lordosis and decrease in upper cervical kyphosis, vertigo, change in vision and hearing, irritability to noise and light, dysesthesias of face and bilateral upper extremities, nausea, difficulty swallowing, and emotional lability.
  (2) Late include chronic head and neck pain, limitation in flexibility, TMJ dysfunction, limited tolerance to ADLs, disequilibrium, anxiety, and depression.

e. Common clinical findings include postural changes, excessive muscle guarding with soft tissue fibrosis, segmental hypermobility, and gradual development of restricted segmental motion, cranial and caudal to the injury (segmental hypomobility).

f. Diagnostic tests utilized: plain film imaging, CT, and/or MRI.
g. Clinical examination helps to identify this condition.
h. Medications.
   (1) Acetaminophen for pain.
   (2) NSAIDs for pain and/or inflammation.
   (3) Muscle relaxants.
   (4) Trigger point injections.
   (5) Corticosteroid injection or by mouth.
i. Physical therapy goals, outcomes, and interventions.
   (1) Spinal manipulation is generally indicated.
   (2) Correction of muscle imbalances and biomechanical faults using strengthening, endurance, coordination, and flexibility exercises to gain restoration of normal function.
   (3) Biomechanical faults caused by joint restrictions should be corrected with joint mobilization to the specific restrictions identified during the examination.
   (4) Progression to functional training based on patient's occupation and/or recreational goals.
   (5) Patient education regarding the elimination of harmful positions and postural reeducation.
   (6) Manual and/or mechanical traction.
      (a) Traction.
         • Cervical spine positioned at 15° of flexion to provide the optimum intervertebral foraminal opening.
         • Contraindications include joint hypermobility, pregnancy, rheumatoid arthritis, Down's syndrome, or any other systemic disease which affects ligamentous integrity.

7. Hypermobile spinal segments.

a. An abnormal increase in ROM at a joint due to insufficient soft tissue control (i.e., ligamentous, discal, muscle, or a combination of all three).
b. Diagnostic tests utilized: plain film imaging, particularly dynamic flexion/extension views.
c. Clinical examination helps to identify this condition.
d. Medications.
   (1) Acetaminophen for pain.
   (2) NSAIDs for pain and/or inflammation.
   (3) Muscle relaxants.
   (4) Trigger point injections.
   (5) Sclerosing injections.
   (6) Corticosteroid injection or by mouth.
e. Physical therapy goals, outcomes, and interventions.
   (1) Pain reduction modalities to reduce irritability of structures.
   (2) Passive ROM within a normal range of movement.
   (3) Passive stabilization with corsets, splints, casts, tape, and collars.
   (4) Increase strength/endurance/coordination, especially in the multifidus, abdominals, extensors, and gluteals, which control posture.
   (5) Regain muscle balance.
   (6) Patient education regarding postural reeducation, limiting excessive overloading, limiting sustained activities, and limiting end range postures.

8. Sacroiliac joint (SIJ) conditions.

a. Cause and specific pathology is unknown. Since this is a joint, it may become inflamed, develop degenerative changes, or develop abnormal movement patterns.
b. Anatomically and functionally, SIJ is closely related to lumbar spine, so a thorough examination of both regions is indicated if a patient presents with pain in either.
c. Diagnostic tests utilized: plain film imaging and possibly MRI. Occasionally, double-blind injections may be used to assist in making the diagnosis (1st injection is provocative in nature, and 2nd injection is analgesic). If increased "same" pain with 1st injection and decreased pain following 2nd injection, joint is determined to be pathological.
d. Clinical examination, including the following special tests, will be useful to make diagnosis.
   (1) Gillet's test.
   (2) Ipsilateral anterior rotation test.
   (3) Gaenslen's test.
   (4) Long-sitting (supine to sit) test.
   (5) Goldthwait's test.
e. Medications.
   (1) Acetaminophen for pain.
   (2) NSAIDs for pain and/or inflammation.
   (3) Muscle relaxants.
   (4) Trigger point injections.
   (5) Corticosteroid injection or by mouth.
f. Physical therapy goals, outcomes, and interventions.
   (1) Spinal manipulation such as SIJ gapping is generally indicated to inhibit pain, reduce muscle guarding, and restore normal joint motion.
   (2) Correction of muscle imbalances throughout pelvis using strengthening, endurance, coordination, and flexibility exercises to gain restoration of normal function.
   (3) Biomechanical faults caused by joint restrictions should be corrected with joint mobilization to the specific restrictions identified during the examination.
   (4) Patient education regarding the elimination of harmful positions and postural reeducation.
   (5) Sacroiliac belts may be useful in some patients.

9. Repetitive/cumulative trauma to back.

a. Disorders of the nerves, soft tissues, and bones precipitated or aggravated by repeated exertions or movements of the back, occurring most often in the workplace.
b. Repetitive trauma disorders account for 48% of all reported occupational diseases.

c. Diagnosis is difficult, with up to 85% of back pain nondiagnosed.
d. Typically causes one of the conditions previously listed above: muscle, disc, and/or joint impairment.
e. Vocational factors which contribute to back pain include physically heavy static work postures, lifting, frequent bending and twisting, repetitive work and vibration.
f. Chronic disability may be reduced by enrollment in a work-conditioning program, including patient education, aerobic exercises, general strengthening, and functional stability exercises that promote endurance for work-related activities.
g. Clinical examination helps to identify this condition.
h. Intervention should focus on prevention, consisting of education. If this phenomenon leads to a condition listed above, follow the specific intervention associated with that condition.

10. Other conditions affecting the spine. (See Table 1-10).

a. Bone tumors.
  (1) May be primary or metastatic.
    (a) Primary tumors include multiple myeloma (the most common primary bone tumor), Ewing's sarcoma, malignant lymphoma, chondrosarcoma, osteosarcoma, and chondromas.
    (b) Metastatic bone cancer has primary sites in lung, prostate, breast, kidney, and thyroid.
    (c) Patient history should always include questions about a prior episode of cancer.
    (d) Signs and symptoms include pain which is unvarying and progressive, is not relieved with rest or analgesics, and is more pronounced at night (see Table 1-8).
    (e) Diagnostic tests utilized: plain film imaging, CT, and/or MRI as well as laboratory tests.
b. Visceral tumors.
  (1) Esophageal cancer symptomatology may include pain radiating to the back, pain with swallowing, dysphagia, and weight loss.
  (2) Pancreatic cancer symptomatology includes a deep, gnawing pain that may radiate from the chest to the back.
  (3) Diagnostic tests utilized: plain film imaging, CT, and/or MRI as well as laboratory tests.
c. Gastrointestinal conditions.
  (1) Acute pancreatitis may manifest itself as midepigastric pain radiating through to the back.
  (2) Cholecystitis may present with abrupt, severe abdominal pain and right upper quadrant tenderness, nausea, vomiting, and fever.
  (3) Diagnostic tests utilized: plain film imaging, CT, and/or MRI as well as laboratory tests.
d. Cardiovascular and pulmonary conditions.
  (1) Heart and lung disorders can refer pain to chest, back, neck, jaw, and upper extremity.
  (2) Abdominal aortic aneurysm (AAA) usually appears as nonspecific lumbar pain.
  (3) Diagnostic tests utilized: plain film imaging, CT, and/or MRI, as well as laboratory tests.
  (4) Will be identified as pain during examination of abdominal region.
e. Urological and gynecological conditions.
  (1) Kidney, bladder, ovary, and uterus disorders can refer pain to the trunk, pelvis, and thighs.
  (2) Diagnostic tests utilized: plain film imaging, CT, and/or MRI as well as laboratory tests.
f. (See Figure 1-8).

11. Temporomandibular joint conditions.

a. Common signs and symptoms include joint noise (i.e., clicking, popping, and/or crepitation), joint locking, limited flexibility of jaw, lateral deviation of mandible during depression or elevation of mandible, decreased strength/endurance of muscles of mastication, tinnitus, headaches, forward head posture, and pain with movement of mandible.
b. Cervical spine must be thoroughly examined due to close biomechanical and functional relationships between TMJ and the cervical region. Many patients with TMJ have a component of cervical dysfunction.
c. Dysfunctions fall into three diagnostic categories.
  (1) DJD, such as OA or RA in TMJ. (Refer to OA and RA for causes, characteristic findings, diagnostic methods, medical and physical therapy intervention).
  (2) Myofascial pain is most common form of temporomandibular dysfunction (TMD), which is discomfort or pain in muscles controlling jaw function, as well as neck and shoulder muscles. (Refer to myofascial pain syndrome for causes, characteristic findings, diagnostic methods, medical and physical therapy intervention.)
  (3) Internal derangement of joint, meaning a dislocated jaw, displaced articular disc, or injury to condyle.
    (a) Loss of functional mobility may result from increased activity in muscles of mastication due to stress and anxiety.
    (b) Causes.
      - Trauma: leading to joint edema, capsulitis, hypomobility/hypermobility, or abnormal function of ligaments, capsule, and/or muscles.
      - Congenital anatomical anomalies: change in shape of palate.
      - Abnormal function, such as repeatedly chewing ice or hard candy, paranormal breathing (mouth breather), forward head posture.
    (c) Diagnostic tests utilized: plain film imaging and/or MRI if necessary.

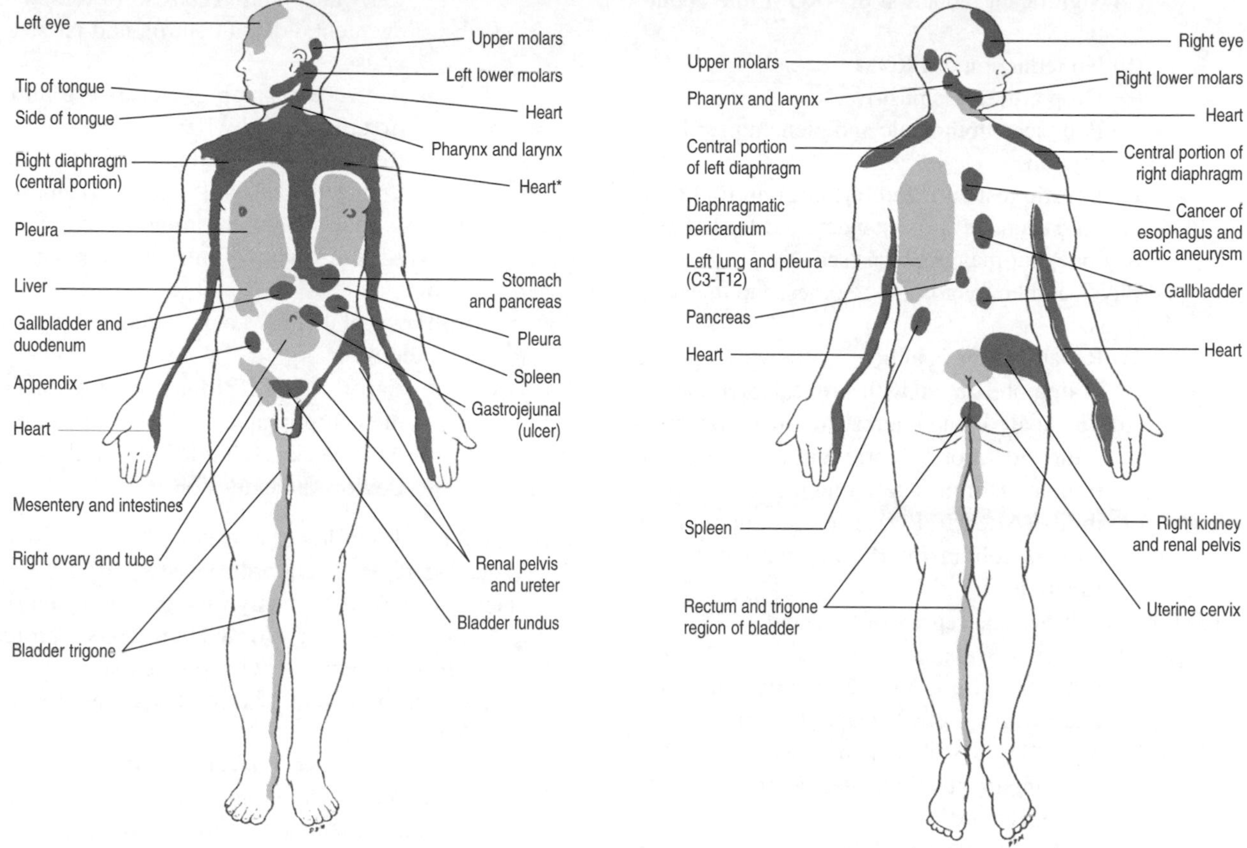

Figure 1-8 • Pain referred from viscera.
(From Rothstein, J et al. The Rehabiltation Specialists' Handbook. 2nd ed. Philadelphia, Davis, 1998, pp 484–485).

(d) Clinical examination helps to identify this condition.

(e) Medications.
- Acetaminophen for pain.
- NSAIDs for pain and/or inflammation.
- Muscle relaxants.
- Trigger point injections.
- Corticosteroid injection or by mouth.

(f) Physical therapy goals, outcomes, and interventions.
- Postural reeducation regarding regaining the normal anterior-posterior curves and left-right symmetry of the spine.
- Modalities for reduction of pain and inflammation.
- Biofeedback to minimize effects of stress and/or anxiety.
- Joint mobilization if restriction in TMJ is present. Primary glide is inferior, which gaps joint, stretches the capsule, and allows relocation of anteriorly displaced disc.
- Flexibility and muscle-strengthening exercises (e.g., Rocobado's jaw opening while maintaining the tongue in contact with the palate and isometric mandibular exercises).
- Patient education (e.g., foods to avoid, maintaining proper postural alignment).
- Night splints may be prescribed by the dentist to maintain resting jaw position.
- Educate patient regarding resting position of tongue on hard palate.
- It is critical to normalize the cervical spine posture before the patient receives any permanent dental procedures and/or appliances.

Orthopaedic Surgical Repairs

1. Surgical repairs of upper extremity.

a. Rotator cuff tears.

(1) Usually degenerative and occur over time, with impingement of supraspinatus tendon between greater tuberosity and acromion.

(2) Signs and symptoms include:

(a) Significant reduction of AROM into abduction.
(b) No reduction of PROM.
(c) Drop arm test is positive.
(d) Poor scapulothoracic and glenohumeral rhythm.

(3) Diagnostic tests utilized: arthrogram traditionally had been the "gold standard" test. MRI may be done, but may not be as sensitive.

(4) Physical therapy goals, outcomes, and interventions.
(a) Rehabilitation is initiated, following a period of immobilization with surgical intervention.
(b) Physical therapy intervention emphasizes return of normal strength/endurance/coordination of muscles, joint mechanics, flexibility (AROM/PROM), and scapulothoracic and glenohumeral rhythm with overhead function.

b. Tendon injuries and repairs of the hand.

(1) Flexor tendon repairs.
(a) First 3–4 weeks, distal extremity is immobilized with a protective splint, with wrist and digits flexed. Rubber band traction is applied to maintain interphalangeal joints in 30°–50° of passive flexion.
(b) Physical therapy goals, outcomes, and interventions.
- Patient can perform resisted extension and passive flexion within constraints of splint. AROM to tolerance is initiated at 4 weeks.
- Goal is to manage all soft tissues through wound-healing phases by providing collagen remodeling, which preserves free tendon gliding.
- Early intervention consists of wound management, edema control, and passive exercises.
- Active extension exercises are initiated first followed by flexion.
- Resistive and functional exercises are introduced when full AROM is achieved.

(2) Extensor tendon repairs.
(a) Distal repairs are immobilized such that the distal interphalangeal joints are in neutral for 6–8 weeks.
(b) Physical therapy goals, outcomes, and interventions.
- AROM is initiated at 6 weeks, with proximal interphalangeal joints in neutral.
- Goal is to manage all soft tissues through wound-healing phases by providing collagen remodeling, which preserves free tendon gliding.
- Early intervention consists of wound management, edema control, and passive exercises.
- Active extension exercises are initiated first, followed by flexion.
- Resistive and functional exercises are introduced when full AROM is achieved.

(c) Proximal repairs are immobilized, with the wrist and digital joints in extension for 4 weeks.
(d) Physical therapy goals, outcomes, and interventions.
- Early AROM/PROM in flexion with metacarpophalangeal joint in extension. At 6 weeks, full AROM is initiated into flexion and extension.

2. Surgical repairs of lower extremity.

a. Total hip replacement/arthroplasty (THR).

(1) This information may vary, depending on surgical procedure and/or MD preference/protocol. Must be familiar with postoperative protocol for each patient relative to procedure and/or MD.

(2) Cemented versus noncemented.
(a) Cemented hips can tolerate full weight bearing immediately following surgery.
(b) Cement may crack with aging, causing a loosening of prosthesis. Noncemented technique is more stressful on bones during the surgical procedure.
(c) Noncemented procedures are typically used with younger and/or more active individuals. Cemented technique may be better for individuals with fragile bones, or for those who will benefit from immediate ability to weight bear; e.g., those with dementia or significant debilitation.

(3) Bed positioning with a wedge to prevent adduction.

(4) Patient should avoid the position of hip flexion > 90° with adduction and internal rotation. Partial weight bearing to tolerance is initiated on the second postsurgery day, using crutches or a walker with typical surgical procedures.

(5) Physical therapy goals, outcomes, and interventions.
(a) Physical therapy interventions focus on bed mobility, transitional movements, ambulation, and return to premorbid activities of daily living.

b. Open reduction internal fixation (ORIF) following femoral fracture.

(1) Patient will typically be non–weight bearing for 1–2 weeks, using crutches or a walker.

Thereafter, the patient will be partial weight-bearing as tolerated.

(2) Physical therapy goals, outcomes, and interventions.

(a) Physical therapy interventions focus on bed mobility, transitional movements, ambulation, and return to premorbid activities of daily living.

Important to note that guidelines/precautions can vary significantly.

c. Total knee replacements/arthroplasty (TKR).

(1) TKR surgery is typically performed as a result of severe DJD of the knee joint, which has led to pain and impaired function.

(2) Physical therapy goals, outcomes, and interventions.

(a) Goals of early rehabilitation (1–3 weeks) include muscle reeducation, soft tissue mobilization, lymphedema reduction, initiation of PROM (e.g., a continuous passive motion [CPM] machine is used in the hospital following surgery), AROM, and reduction of postsurgical swelling.

(b) Goals of the second phase of rehabilitation include regaining endurance, coordination, and strength of the muscles surrounding the knee. Functional activities include progressive ambulation stair climbing, as well as transitional training based on healing and the type of prosthesis used.

(c) Goals and outcomes of the last phase of rehabilitation include returning the patient to premorbid activities of daily living. Functional and endurance training and proprioceptive exercises are introduced during this phase.

(d) The weight-bearing status of patients with a cemented prosthesis is at the level of the patient's tolerance. Patients with cementless prostheses are progressed according to the time frame for fracture healing. Weight bearing at 1–7 weeks is 25%, 50% by week 8, 75% by week 10, and 100% without an assistive device by week 12.

(e) Avoidance of forceful mobilization and PROM into flexion > 90° is important, because of the mechanical restraints of the prosthesis.

(f) Biomechanical faults caused by joint restrictions should be corrected with joint mobilization to the specific restrictions identified during the examination.

Table 1-30 ➤ TOTAL HIP GUIDELINES/PRECAUTIONS

ACTIVITY	CEMENTED	CEMENTLESS	
Internal rotation of hip Joint	Do not perform for 3-6 months.	Do not perform for 3-6 months.	
Adduction of hip joint	Do not perform for 3-6 months.	Do not perform for 3-6 months.	
Flexion of hip joint beyond 90°	Do not perform for 3-6 months.	Do not perform for 3-6 months.	
Ambulation	Partial weight-bearing (PWB) for approximately 3 weeks. Begin ambulation with cane at week 4 post-op. Begin transition to full weight-bearing at week 5.	Varies from weight-bearing as tolerated (WBAT) to touch-down weight bearing (TDWB), based on the surgeons philosophy and the surgical approach.	
		WBAT	TDWB
		Partial weight-bearing (PWB) for approximately 3 weeks.	Progress to 1/3 weight-bearing at week 6.
		Begin ambulation with cane at week 4 post-op.	Progress to 2/3 weight-bearing at week 8.
		Begin transition to full weight-bearing at week 6.	Progress to full weight-bearing at week 10 with walker.
			Begin transition to cane at week 12.
			Progress to no assistive device when safe, and no Trendelenberg gait.
Isometric exercise	Immediately post-op as tolerated by the patient.	Immediately post-op as tolerated by the patient.	
Active exercise	Initiation is variable between weeks 1 through 4, depending on surgeon's guidelines.	Initiation is variable between weeks 1 through 4, depending on the surgeon's guidelines.	

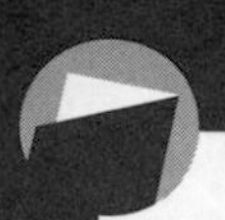

Table 1-31 ➤ TOTAL KNEE ARTHROPLASTY (TKA) GUIDELINES/PRECAUTIONS

ACTIVITY	CEMENTED	CEMENTLESS	
Range of motion	0°-90° within 2 weeks 0°-120° within 3-4 weeks	0°-90° within 2 weeks 0°-120° within 3-4 weeks	
Ambulation	Weight-bearing as tolerated with walker immediately post-op. Ambulation with cane at week 3. Transition to full weight-bearing at week 4.	Varies from weight bearing as tolerated (WBAT) to touch-down weight bearing (TDWB) based on surgeon's philosophy and surgical approach.	
		WBAT	TDWB
		Weight-bearing as tolerated with walker immediately post-op. Ambulation with cane at week 5-6. Transition to full weight-bearing at week 6.	Touch down weight bearing with walker immediately post-op. Weight-bearing as tolerated with walker at week 6. Ambulation with cane at week 8-10. Transition to full weight-bearing at week 10.
Isometric and active exercise	Immediately post-op	Immediately post-op	
Resisted exercise	Begin at week 2-3	Begin at week 2-3.	

Important to note that guidelines/precautions can vary significantly.

d. Ligamentous repairs of knee.
   (1) Six phases of rehabilitation are followed with ACL and PCL reconstructive surgery.
   (2) Anterior cruciate ligament reconstruction.
      (a) Immediately following surgery, a continuous passive motion unit (CPM) is utilized, with PROM from 0°–70° of flexion.
      (b) Motion is increased to 0°–120° by the 6th week.
      (c) Reconstruction is usually protected with a hinged brace set at 20°–70° of flexion initially.
      (d) Patient is non–weight bearing for approximately one week.
      (e) Weight-bearing progresses as tolerated to full weight-bearing.
      (f) Patient is weaned from brace between the 2nd and 4th weeks.
   (3) Posterior cruciate ligament reconstruction.
      (a) Generally similar to ACL repair, except patient is often initially in hinged brace at 0° during ambulation.
   (4) Physical therapy goals, outcomes, and interventions following ACL and PCL surgical repairs.
      (a) Six phases of rehabilitation are as follows: (1) preoperative, (2) maximum protection, (3) controlled motion, (4) moderate protection, (5) minimum protection, and (6) return to activity.
      (b) Specific interventions.
         - Soft tissue/massage techniques to quadriceps and hamstring muscles to reduce muscle guarding.
         - Joint oscillations to inhibit joint pain and muscle guarding.
         - Correction of muscle imbalances and biomechanical faults using strengthening, endurance, coordination, and flexibility exercises to gain restoration of normal function.
         - Biomechanical faults caused by joint restrictions should be corrected with joint mobilization to the specific restrictions identified during the examination.
         - Progression to functional training based on patient's occupation and/or recreational goals.

e. Lateral retinacular release.
   (1) Typically performed as a result of patellofemoral pain syndrome (PFPS). Purpose of procedure is to restore normal tracking of the patella during contraction of the quadriceps muscle.
   (2) Physical therapy goals, outcomes, and interventions.
      (a) Intervention should emphasize closed kinetic chain exercises to strengthen quadriceps, muscles and regain dynamic balance of all structures (contractile and non-contractile) surrounding knee.

(b) Normalize the flexibility of the hamstrings, triceps surae, and ITB will help restore mechanical alignment.
(c) Mobilization of patella is important to maintain nutrition and decrease the likelihood of adhesions.

f. Meniscal arthroscopy.
   (1) Partial meniscectomy.
      (a) Partial weight-bearing as tolerated when full knee extension is obtained.
      (b) Physical therapy goals, outcomes, and interventions.
         - Initial goals focus on edema/effusion control.
         - AROM is urged after surgical day 1.
         - Isotonic and isokinetic strengthening by day 3.
         - Jogging on the ball of the foot or toes is recommended to decrease the loading of the knee joint.
   (2) Repairs.
      (a) Patient will be non–weight bearing for 3–6 weeks.
      (b) Rehabilitation of the joint begins within 7–10 days of procedure.
      (c) Physical therapy goals, outcomes, and interventions.
         - Soft tissue/massage techniques to quadriceps and hamstring muscles to reduce muscle guarding.
         - Joint oscillations to inhibit joint pain and muscle guarding.
         - Correction of muscle imbalances and biomechanical faults using strengthening, endurance, coordination, and flexibility exercises to gain restoration of normal function.
         - Biomechanical faults caused by joint restrictions should be corrected with joint mobilization to the specific restrictions identified during the examination.
         - Progression to functional training, based on patient's occupation and/or recreational goals.

3. Surgical repairs of spine.

a. Rehabilitation varies according to the type of surgery performed.
b. A back protection program and early mobilization exercises should be initiated prior to surgery.
c. Patients should avoid prolonged sitting, heavy lifting, and long car trips for approximately 3 months.
d. Repetitive bending with twisting should always be avoided.
e. With microdiscectomies, rehabilitation time is decreased because the fibers of the annulus fibrosus are not damaged.
f. With laminectomy/discectomy, early movement and activation of paraspinal musculature (especially multifidus) is necessary.
g. Multilevel vertebra fusion:
   (1) Typically requires 6 weeks of trunk immobility with bracing.
   (2) Once brace is removed and movement is allowed, important to regain as much normal/functional movement as possible, while restoring functional activation of muscles.
   (3) With combined anterior/posterior surgical approach, bracing is seldom used.
h. With Harrington rod placement for idiopathic scoliosis, rehabilitation goals focus on early mobilization in bed and effective coughing.
   (1) The patient can begin ambulation between the 4th and 7th postoperative days.
   (2) The patient should avoid heavy lifting and excessive twisting and bending.
i. Physical therapy goals, outcomes, and interventions following surgical interventions.
   (1) Soft tissue/massage techniques to paraspinal muscles to reduce muscle guarding.
   (2) Joint oscillations to inhibit joint pain and muscle guarding.
   (3) Correction of muscle imbalances using strengthening, endurance, coordination, and flexibility exercises to gain restoration of normal function. Make sure that multifidus function is restored.
   (4) Must develop dynamic stabilization for muscles of trunk and pelvis during all functional activities.
   (5) Biomechanical faults caused by joint restrictions should be corrected with joint mobilization to the specific restrictions identified during the examination.
   (6) Progression to functional training based on patient's occupation and/or recreational goals.

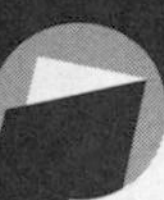

Interventions for Patients/Clients with Musculoskeletal Conditions

Interventions for Patients/Clients with Acute Conditions

1. **Acute phase.**
   a. Immobilization with limited (1–2 days) bed rest. Use of braces, slings, corsets, cervical collars, assistive devices, and taping.
   b. Control inflammatory response (rest, ice, compression, elevation [RICE]).
      (1) Physical agents: ice and electric stimulation.
      (2) Compression and elevation to reduce and prevent effusion and swelling.
      (3) NSAIDs.
      (4) Rest/relaxation to reduce pain.
      (5) Soft tissue/massage techniques.
   c. Assisted movement of injured tissues.
   d. Joint oscillations (grades I and II) for pain relief.
   e. Therapeutic exercise.
      (1) Dose of 40%–60% of one repetition maximum (i.e., high repetition with low resistance) to stimulate regeneration of tissue and revascularization.
      (2) Exercise should be nontraumatic, meaning no pain and/or increased edema as a result of the exercise.
   f. Educate patient/client on joint protection strategies.

2. **Subacute phase.**
   a. Avoidance of continued irritation and repetitive trauma.
      (1) Modify activities at home/work/recreational.
      (2) Modify use of equipment or type of equipment at home/work/recreational.
      (3) Correct biomechanical faults, such as leg length discrepancy, abnormal foot biomechanics, abnormal throwing motion.
   b. Joint mobilization.
   c. Continued therapeutic exercise, including flexibility/endurance/coordination exercise.
   d. Postural reeducation.
   e. Biomechanical education.

3. **Functional restoration phase.**
   a. Maintain or return to optimum level of patient function.
   b. Normalize flexibility of joints and related soft tissues.
   c. Restore loading capacity of connective tissues to normal strength.
   d. Functional strengthening exercises.
   e. Functional stabilization of the involved joint/region.

Interventions for Patients/Clients with a Chronic Condition

1. **Determine possible causative factors.**
   a. Abnormal remodeling of injured tissues.
   b. Chronic low-grade inflammation due to repetitive stresses of tissues.

2. **Reduce stresses to tissues.**
   a. Identify/eliminate the magnitude of loading.
   b. Identify/eliminate direction of forces.
   c. Identify and eliminate any biomechanical barriers that are preventing healing; e.g., leg length discrepancy.
   d. Patient education regarding protection of joints and associated soft tissues.

3. **Regain structural integrity.**
   a. Improving flexibility.
   b. Postural reeducation.
   c. Increasing tissue's capacity to tolerate loading.
   d. Functional strengthening, endurance, and coordination exercises.

4. **Resume optimal patient function and prevention of reoccurrence.**
   a. Patient education regarding causative factors in dysfunction.
   b. Work conditioning.

Specific Interventions

1. **Soft tissue/myofascial techniques.**
   a. Aid in reduction of metabolites from muscle, reactivating a muscle which has not been functioning secondary to guarding and ischemia, revascularization of muscle, and also decrease guarding in a muscle.
   b. Autonomic: stimulation of skin and superficial fascia to facilitate a decrease in muscle tension.
   c. Mechanical: movement of skin, fascia, and muscle causes histological and mechanical changes to occur in soft tissues to produce improved mobility and function (e.g., acupressure and osteopathic mechanical stretching techniques).
   d. Goals: decrease pain, edema, and muscle spasm, increase metabolism and cutaneous temperature, stretch tight muscles and other soft tissues, improve circulation, strengthen weak muscles, and mobilize joint restrictions.

e. Indications: patients with soft tissue and joint restriction that result in pain and limits ADLs.
f. Contraindications.
   (1) Absolute: soft tissue breakdown, infection, cellulitis, inflammation, and/or neoplasm.
   (2) Relative: hypermobility, and sensitivity.
g. Traditional massage techniques, such as effleurage and petrissage.
h. Functional massage.
   (1) Three techniques used to assist in reactivation of a debilitated muscle and/or to increase vascularity to a muscle.
      (a) Soft tissue without motion.
         - Traditional technique; however, hands do not slide over skin; instead, they stay in contact with skin while hands and skin move together over the muscle.
         - Direction of force is parallel to muscle fibers, and total stroke time should be 5–7 seconds.
      (b) Soft tissue with passive pumping.
         - Place muscle in shortened position and with one hand place tension on muscle parallel to muscle fibers.
         - Other hand passively lengthens muscle and simultaneously gradually releases tension of hand in contact with muscle.
      (c) Soft tissue with active pumping.
         - Place muscle in lengthened position m and with one hand place, tension on muscle perpendicular to muscle fibers.
         - Other hand, guides limb as patient actively shortens muscle. As muscle shortens, gradually release tension of hand in contact with muscle.
i. Transverse friction massage.
   (1) Used to initiate an acute inflammatory response for a tissue that is in metabolic stasis, such as a tendonosis.
   (2) Involved tendon is briskly massaged in a transverse fashion (perpendicular to the direction of the fibers).
   (3) Performed for 5–10 minutes and tends to be very uncomfortable for the patient.
j. Movement approaches require the patient to actively participate in treatment. Examples include:
   (1) Feldenkrais.
      (a) Facilitates development of normal movement patterns.
      (b) The practitioner uses skillful, supportive, gentle hands to create a sense of safety, maintain supportive contact, while introducing new movement possibilities in small, easily available increments.
   (2) Muscle energy techniques.
      (a) Include voluntary contraction in a precisely controlled direction, at varying levels of intensity, against an applied counterforce from the clinician.
      (b) Purpose is to gain motion that is limited by restrictions of the neuromuscular system.
      (c) Modification of proprioceptive neuromuscular facilitation (PNF) technique.
   (3) PNF hold-relax-contract technique.
      (a) Antagonist of the shortened muscle is contracted to achieve reciprocal inhibition and increased range.
      (b) Refer to Chapter 2 (Neuromuscular Physical Therapy) for details.

2. Articulatory techniques.
a. Joint oscillation.
   (1) Inhibit pain and/or muscle guarding.
   (2) Lubricate joint surfaces.
   (3) Provide nutrition to the joint structures.
   (4) Maitland suggests that grades III and IV oscillations are beneficial to stretch tight connective tissues.
   (5) Grades of movement as described by Maitland (Figure 1-9).
      (a) Five grades of joint play in neutral.
         - Grade I oscillations are small amplitude at the beginning of the range of joint play.
         - Grade II oscillations are large amplitude at the midrange of joint play.
         - Grade III oscillations are large amplitude at the end range of joint play.
         - Grade IV oscillations are small amplitude at the end range of joint play.
         - Grade V is a manipulation of high velocity and low amplitude to the anatomical endpoint of a joint. Technically, this is not an oscillation, since it is a single movement rather than a repetitive movement.
      (b) Indications for use of oscillation grades, per Maitland.

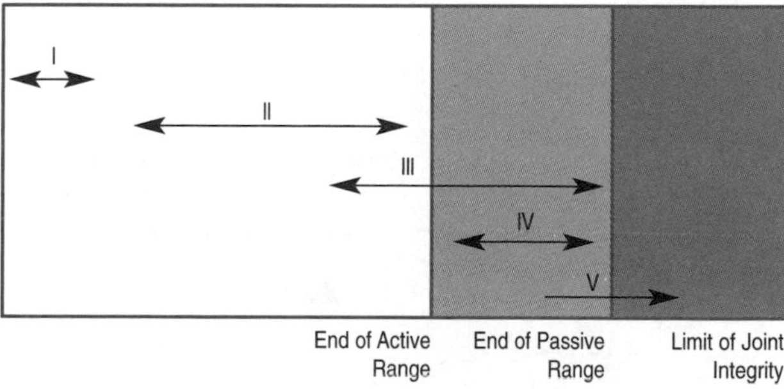

Figure 1-9 • Grades of movement.
(Adapted from Grieve, GP. Mobilization of the Spine. A Primary Handbook of Clinical Method. 5th ed. Churchill Livingstone, New York, 1991).

- Grades I and II are used to improve joint lubrication/nutrition, as well as decrease pain and muscle guarding.
- Grades III and IV are used to stretch tight muscles, capsules, and ligaments.
- Grade V is used to regain normal joint mechanics, as well as decrease pain and muscle guarding.

(6) Contraindications.

(a) Absolute: joint ankylosis, malignancy involving bone, diseases that affect the integrity of ligaments (RA and Down's syndrome), arterial insufficiency, and active inflammatory and/or infective process.

(b) Relative: arthrosis (DJD), metabolic bone disease (osteoporosis, Paget's disease, and tuberculosis), hypermobility, total joint replacement, pregnancy, spondylolisthesis, use of steroids, and radicular symptoms.

b. Joint mobilization.

(1) To stretch/lengthen/deform collagen and normalize the arthrokinematic glide of joint structures.

(2) Grades of translatoric glide, as described by Kaltenborn (Figure 1-10).

(a) Grade I.

- "Loosening" translatoric glide.
- Movement is a very small amplitude traction force.
- Used to relieve pain and/or decompress a joint during joint glides, performed within examination or intervention.

(b) Grade II.

- "Tightening" translatoric glide.
- Movement takes up slack in tissues surrounding joint.
- Used to alleviate pain, assess joint play, and/or reduce muscle guarding.

(c) Grade III.

- "Stretching" translatoric glide.
- Movement stretches the tissues crossing joint.
- Used to assess end feel, or to increase movement (stretch tissue).

(3) Traction: manual, mechanical, and self or auto-traction.

(a) Vertebral bodies separating.

(b) Distraction and gliding of facet joints.

(c) Tensing of the ligamentous structures of the spinal segment.

(d) Intervertebral foramen widening.

(e) Spinal muscles stretching.

(4) Contraindications.

(a) Absolute: joint ankylosis, malignancy involving bone, diseases that affect the integrity of ligaments (RA and Down's syndrome), arterial insufficiency, and active inflammatory and/or infective process.

(b) Relative: arthrosis (DJD), metabolic bone disease (osteoporosis, Paget's disease, and tuberculosis), hypermobility, total joint replacement, pregnancy, spondylolisthesis, use of steroids, and radicular symptoms.

c. Manipulation.

(1) Inhibit pain and/or muscle guarding.

(2) Improve translatoric glide in cases of joint dysfunction due to restriction.

(3) Health-care practitioners who commonly perform manipulative thrusts include physical therapists, osteopaths, chiropractors, and medical doctors.

(4) Types of manipulations.

(a) Generalized.

- Fairly forceful, long lever techniques intended to include as many vertebral segments as possible.
- More commonly performed by chiropractic practitioners.

(b) Specific.

- Aimed at having an effect on either a specific segment or only a few vertebral segments.
- Uses minimal force with short lever arms.
- Often includes "locking" techniques based on biomechanics to ensure that a specific vertebral segment receives the manipulative thrust.
- More commonly performed by physical therapists.

(c) Mid-range.

- Very gentle, short lever arm techniques.
- Barrier is created in mid-range by specific positioning of patient as well as creating tautness in surrounding soft tissues.
- More commonly performed by osteopathic practitioners.

(5) Contraindications.

(a) Absolute: joint ankylosis, malignancy involving bone, diseases that affect the

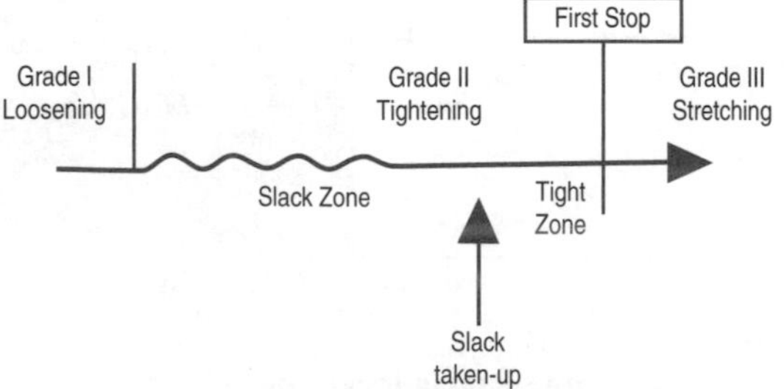

Figure 1-10 • Manual mobilization of the joints. (From Kaltenborn, F. Manual Mobilization of the Joints: Volume II The Spine. 4th ed. Minneapolis,OPTP, 2003, with permission).

integrity of ligaments (RA and Down syndrome), arterial insufficiency, and active inflammatory and/or infective process.
(b) Relative: arthrosis (DJD), metabolic bone disease (osteoporosis, Paget's disease, and tuberculosis), hypermobility, total joint replacement, pregnancy, spondylolisthesis, use of steroids, and radicular symptoms.

3. Neural tissue mobilization.
a. Movement of neural structures to regain normal mobility.
b. Tension tests for upper and lower extremities (i.e., dural stretch test).
(1) Movement of soft tissues that may be restricting neural structures (e.g., cross friction massage for adhesions of the radial nerve to the humerus at a fracture site).
(2) Indications: used for patients who have some type of restriction in neural mobility, anywhere along the course of the nerve.
(3) Postural reeducation: to open up the intervertebral foramen, and decrease tension to tissues.
(4) Contraindications: extreme pain and/or increase in abnormal neurological signs.

4. Therapeutic exercise for musculoskeletal conditions.
a. Therapeutic exercise is indicated to:
(1) Decrease muscle guarding.
(2) Decrease pain.
(3) Increase vascularity of tissue.
(4) Promote regeneration and/or speed up recovery of connective tissues, such as cartilage, tendons, ligaments, capsules, intervertebral discs.
(5) Mobilize restricted tissue to increase flexibility.
(6) Increase endurance of muscle.
(7) Increase coordination of muscle.
(8) Increase strength of muscle.
(9) Sensitize muscles to minimize joints going into excessive range, in cases of hypermobility.
(10) Develop dynamic stability and functional movement patterns, allowing for optimal function within the environment.
b. Home exercise program for patients/clients with musculoskeletal conditions.
(1) Patient's home program will consist of exercises to reinforce clinical program.
(2) Necessary to perform enough repetitions for desired physiological effect on appropriate tissues, as well as to develop coordination and endurance in order to promote dynamic stability within functional patterns.
c. See Chapter 9, Therapeutic Exercise Foundations.

Manual Therapy Approaches in Rehabilitation

1. All approaches provide: a philosophical basis, subjective evaluation, objective examination, a diagnosis, and a plan of care.

2. Approaches can be divided into two categories.
a. Physician generated.
(1) Mennell believed the joint is the dysfunctional unit.
(2) Osteopaths suggest that any component of the somatic system is responsible for dysfunction.
(3) Cyriax contends that dysfunction is due to interplay between contractile and noncontractile tissues.
b. Physical therapist generated.
(1) McKenzie feels that postural factors precipitate discal dysfunction. Treatment emphasizes the use of extension exercises.
(2) Maitland proposes that the subjective evaluation should be integrated with objective measures to determine the dysfunctional area.
(3) Kaltenborn believes that abnormal joint mobility and soft tissue changes account for dysfunction.
c. Chiropractic generated.
(1) Focus is to restore normal joint function through soft tissue and joint manipulation. Chiropractors believe that restoration of normal biomechanical function affects other systems of the body as well, thus improving the state of health in many ways.

Table 1-32 ➤ HAMSTRING VERSUS PATELLA TENDON GRAFT FOR ACL RECONSTRUCTION

PROS/CONS	HAMSTRING GRAFTS	PATELLA TENDON GRAFTS
Pros	1. Typically fewer symptoms. postoperatively	1. Better at maintaining graft tension postoperatively
	2. Greater return to preinjury level of activity.	2. Typically less expensive.
	3. Typically allows earlier rehabilitation.	3. Faster healing time.
Cons	1. Typically more expensive.	1. Increased potential for anterior knee pain and later patellofemoral osteoarthrosis.
	2. Believed to be more technically difficult procedure.	2. Increased potential for knee extension deficit.
	3. Rehabilitation can be more difficult (i.e., slower).	3. Potential delay in rehabilitation secondary to more atrophy of quadriceps.

CHAPTER 1

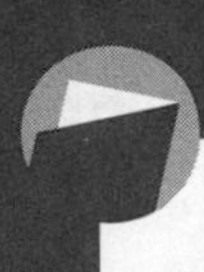

Relevant Pharmacology

1. **Nonsteroidal anti-inflammatory drugs (NSAIDs).**
   a. Most commonly prescribed medication for pain relief for musculoskeletal dysfunction.
   b. Examples include: ibuprofen (Motrin), naproxen sodium (Aleve), salsalate (Discalced), and indomethacin (Indocin).
   c. Provide analgesic, anti-inflammatory, and antipyretic capabilities.
   d. Adverse side effects could include gastrointestinal irritation, fluid retention, renal or liver problems, and prolonged bleeding.
   e. COX-2 inhibitors have decreased gastrointestinal irritation, but rofecoxib (Vioxx) was withdrawn for the market secondary to its relationship with heart-related conditions. Other COX-2 inhibitors such as colecoxib (Celebrex) and valdecoxib (Bextra) are being evaluated for their safety and possible association with heart-related conditions.

2. **Muscle relaxants.**
   a. Commonly prescribed for skeletal muscle spasm.
   b. Examples include: cyclobenzaprine HCl (Flexeril), methocarbamol (Robaxin), and carisoprodol (Soma).
   c. Act on the central nervous system to reduce skeletal muscle tone by depressing the internuncial neurons of the brain stem and spinal cord.
   d. Adverse side effects could include drowsiness, lethargy, ataxia, and decreased alertness.

3. **Nonnarcotic analgesics.**
   a. Prescribed when NSAIDs are contraindicated.
   b. Examples include: acetaminophen (Tylenol).
   c. Act on the central nervous system to alter response to pain, and have antipyretic capabilities.
   d. Adverse side effects are negligible when taken in recommended doses. Excessive amounts of acetaminophen may lead to liver disease or acute liver shutdown.

Psychosocial Considerations

1. **Malingering** (symptom magnification syndrome).
   a. Defined as a behavioral response where displays of symptoms control the life of the patient, leading to functional disability.
   b. There may be psychological advantages to illness.
      (1) The patient may feel protected from the threatening world.
      (2) Uncertainty or fear about the future.
      (3) Social gain.
      (4) Reduces stressors.
   c. Therapist needs to recognize symptoms and respond to the patient.
      (1) Tests to evaluate malingering back pain may include the Hoover and Burn's tests and Waddell's signs.
         (a) Hoover test involves the therapist's evaluation of the amount of pressure the patient's heels place on the therapist's hands when the patient is asked to raise one lower extremity while in a supine position.
         (b) Burn's test requires the patient to kneel and bend over a chair to touch the floor.
         (c) Waddell's signs evaluate tenderness, simulation tests, distraction tests, regional disturbances, and overreaction. Waddell's scores can be predictive of functional outcome.
      (2) Functional capacity evaluations are used to evaluate psychosocial as well as physical components of disability.
      (3) Emphasize regaining functional outcomes, not pain reduction.

2. **Secondary gain.**
   a. Usually some type of financial gain for staying ill.
      (1) Workers compensation.
      (2) Larger settlement for injury claims.
   b. Frequently seen in clinics that manage industrial injuries.
   c. May not want to return to work for various reasons associated with the work environment; e.g., stress, disliking coworkers.

Radiology

This section and Appendix F prepared by:

L. Vincent Lepak III

Professionals

1. **Radiologists:** physicians that train and subspecialize in different types of imaging.
2. **Radiographers:** the technicians trained to perform specific types of imaging.
3. **Physical therapists:** receive basic training in the interpretation of these studies and the type of studies indicated for their clients.
   a. This knowledge better informs the therapists when developing a diagnosis, prognosis, and plan of care.

Diagnostic Exams and Procedures

1. **Radiography (x-rays).**
   a. Noninvasive test used to identify and screen for lung or heart disease, fractures, dislocations, bone growth, foreign objects, etc.
   b. X-ray photons pass through the body and are captured on plain film or digitally. The radiodensity of the anatomical structure determines whether the object is seen as white, black, gray-black, or gray.
      (1) A structure that is radiodense (bone) will absorb more x-rays and leave the film white, while a less radiodense structure (air) will not absorb as much X-radiation, allowing penetration to the film and turning it black.
      (2) The radiograph (x-ray) is a 2-D (dimensional) view of a 3-D object, causing structures to be superimposed. At least two views (often three) are required so the diagnostician does not neglect an abnormality that is viewable in another plane (sagittal, frontal, or transverse).
   c. Use the ABCs to interpret the musculoskeletal radiograph: **A**lignment - size contour, alignment with adjacent bones; **B**one density - density and texture; **C**artilage spaces - joint space width, presence of subchondral bone, epiphyseal plates.
   d. Advantages: quick, easy, portable, and relatively inexpensive.
   e. Disadvantages: ionizing radiation, poor at visualizing soft tissues and small fractures.
2. **Magnetic resonance imaging (MRI).**
   a. Noninvasive test that provides sectional imaging of anatomy that is especially helpful for visualizing soft tissues. These images can be configured into detailed 3-D models.
   b. MRI uses radio waves and magnetic fields to provide detailed imaging of the body that is often not visible to other types of imaging. The two basic types of an MRI are T1 and T2.
      (1) T1: fat is brighter, and is helpful in defining anatomy.
      (2) T2: fluid appears brighter, and the fat is suppressed, which is helpful for various joint pathologies.
   c. Functional MRIs are used to detect metabolic changes in the brain.
   d. Advantages: high-quality imaging of almost any structure of the body (e.g., organs, bone, soft tissues). Does not rely on ionizing radiation. Contrasts can be used to increase details.
   e. Disadvantages: expensive, time-consuming, must remain perfectly still to avoid artifacts, may not be able to distinguish between edema and cancer tissue, may cause implanted metal device to malfunction, claustrophobic environment, and relatively non-portable.
3. **Computed Tomography (CT) or CAT scan.**
   a. Noninvasive test that provides sectional imaging of bone and most soft tissues. Especially useful for the chest and abdomen, with better anatomical resolution than an x-ray. Able to measure bone density (predict fractures) and identify tumors.
   b. A special radiography device with advanced computer analysis that configures images from x-rays at various angles to show high-quality cross-sectional and 3-D imaging of body tissues (e.g., bone, lungs, vessels, brain, tendons) and organs.
   c. Advantages: fast; provides high-quality imaging of bone, soft tissue, and blood vessels all at the same time. Contrasts can be used to increase details.
   d. Disadvantages: large amounts of ionizing radiation; not as good at soft tissue structures as MRI. Not portable, expensive, may result in a claustrophobic reaction, and has bariatric limits.
4. **Bone scan or bone scintigraphy.**
   a. Helps to diagnose fractures not detected by x-ray, and areas of damage to bone caused by cancer, trauma, infection, or other conditions.
   b. Uses gamma ray emission to detect newly forming bone. A radionuclide is injected intravenously, and the distribution (uptake) is recorded on radiographic film. Increased areas of uptake equal increased metabolic activity, and show up on the film as black. This test has poor specificity and good sensitivity.

c. Advantages: noninvasive, small amounts of radiation, and improved detection of abnormal bone metabolism.

d. Disadvantages: slow (about 1 hour for whole body), ionizing radiation, potential adverse reaction from contrast.

5. **Angiography.**
   a. A common procedure that helps the medical team evaluate and diagnose a client's condition. Also provides valuable information for prognosis and treatment intervention.
   b. A catheter and a contrast material are often used in conjunction with x-rays, CT-scan, or MRI. The primary purpose of this procedure is to examine blood vessels throughout the body. Also may be used to guide intervention, e.g., stent placement.

6. **Bone density scan:** or dual-energy x-ray absorptiometry (DEXA) or bone densitometry.
   a. Measures bone mineral density. Used to delineate osteopenia from osteoporosis.
   b. An enhanced x-ray technique; gold standard for measuring bone mineral density.

7. **Ultrasound.**
   a. Helps diagnose partial tendon tears, soft-tissue masses (e.g., tumors, hematomas), pockets of fluid, muscle development or activation.
   b. Sound waves capture real-time images of various body structures and blood flowing through the vessels.

8. **Positron emission tomography or PET scan.**
   a. Used to detect non-perfusing areas of the heart or to evaluate the brain in cases of undetermined dementia, stroke, seizures, memory disorders, or suspected tumors.
   b. Captures positrons emitted from radioactive substance.

Table 1-33 ➤ TISSUE APPEARANCE ACCORDING TO IMAGING STUDY

	RADIOGRAPH	CT	T1 MRI	T2 MRI
Air	Black	Black	Black	Black
Fat	Poorly visualized or absent	Black	White	Gray
Bone cortex	White	White	Black	Black
Bone marrow	White	Gray	White	Gray

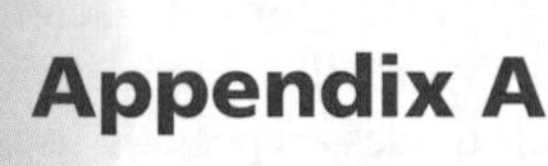

Appendix A

Clinical Practice Guidelines: Grades of Evidence

GRADES OF RECOMMENDATION BASED ON		STRENGTH OF EVIDENCE
A	Strong evidence	A preponderance of Level I and/or Level II studies support the recommendation. This must include at least one Level I study
B	Moderate evidence	A single, high-quality, randomized controlled trial or a preponderance of Level II studies support the recommendation
C	Weak evidence	A single Level II study or a preponderance of Level III and IV studies, including statements of consensus by content experts support the recommendation
D	Conflicting evidence	Higher-quality studies conducted on this topic disagree on conclusions. The recommendation is based on these conflicting studies
E	Theoretical/foundational evidence	A preponderance of evidence from animal or cadaver studies, from conceptual models/principles, or from basic sciences/bench research support this conclusion
F	Expert opinion	Best practice based on the clinical experience of the guidelines development team

Knee Pain and Mobility Impairments: Meniscal and Articular Cartilage Lesions Clinical Practice Guidelines Linked to the International Classification of Functioning, Disability, and Health from the Orthopaedic Section of the APTA, Summary of Recommendations page A30 from JOSPT June 2010, Number 6, Vol 40.

Appendix B

Clinical Practice Guidelines: Meniscal and Articular Cartilage Lesions

1. Clinical Course. (C).
Knee pain and mobility impairments associated with meniscal and articular cartilage tears can be the result of a contact or noncontact incident. This can result in damage to one or more structures. Clinicians should assess for impairments in range of motion, motor control, strength, and endurance of the limb associated with the identified meniscal or articular cartilage pathology or following meniscal or chondral surgery.

2. Risk Factors: Meniscus. (C).
Clinicians should consider age and greater time from injury as predisposing factors for having a meniscal injury. Patients who participated in high-level sports or had increased knee laxity after an ACL injury are more likely to have late meniscal surgery.

3. Risk Factors: Articular Cartilage. (C).
Clinicians should consider the patients' age and presence of a meniscal tear for the odds of having a chondral lesion subsequent to an ACL injury. Greater patient age and longer time from initial ACL injury are predictive factors of the severity of chondral lesions. Time from initial ACL injury is significantly associated with the number of chondral lesions.

4. Diagnosis/Classification. (C).
Knee pain, mobility impairments, and effusion are useful clinical findings for classifying a patient with knee pain and mobility disorders into the following International Statistical Classification of Diseases and Related Health Problems (ICD) categories: tear of the meniscus and tear of the articular cartilage.

5. Differential Diagnosis. (C).
Clinicians should consider diagnostic classifications associated with serious pathological conditions or psychosocial factors when the patient's reported activity limitations or impairments of body function and structure are not consistent with those presented in the diagnosis/classification section of this guideline, or, when the patient's symptoms are not resolving with interventions aimed at normalization of the patient's impairments of body function.

6. Examination - Outcome Measures. (C).
Clinicians should use a validated, patient-reported outcome measure, a general health questionnaire, and a validated activity scale for patients with knee pain and mobility impairments. These tools are useful for identifying a patient's baseline status relative to pain, function, and disability and for monitoring changes in the patient's status throughout the course of treatment.

7. Examination - Activity Limitation Measures. (C).
Clinicians should utilize easily reproducible physical performance measures, such as single-limb hop tests, 6-minute walk test, or timed up-and-go test, to assess activity limitation and participation restrictions associated with their patient's knee pain or mobility impairments and to assess the changes in the patient's level of function over the episode of care.

8. Interventions - Progressive Knee Motion. (C).
Clinicians may utilize early progressive knee motion following knee meniscal and articular cartilage surgery.

9. Interventions - Progressive Weight Bearing. (D).
There are conflicting opinions regarding the best use of progressive weight-bearing for patients with meniscal repairs or chondral lesions.

10. Interventions - Progressive Return to Activity - Meniscus. (C).
Clinicians may utilize early progressive return to activity following knee meniscal repair surgery.

11. Interventions - Progressive Return to Activity - Articular Cartilage. (E).
Clinicians may need to delay return to activity, depending on the type of articular cartilage surgery.

12. Interventions - Supervised Rehabilitation. (D).
There are conflicting opinions regarding the best use of clinic-based programs for patients following arthroscopic meniscectomy to increase quadriceps strength and functional performance.

13. Interventions - Therapeutic Exercises. (B).
Clinicians should consider strength training and functional exercise to increase quadriceps and hamstrings strength, quadriceps endurance, and functional performance following meniscectomy.

14. Interventions - Neuromuscular Electrical Stimulation. (B).
Neuromuscular electrical stimulation can be used with patients following meniscal or chondral injuries to increase quadriceps muscle strength.

Knee Pain and Mobility Impairments: Meniscal and Articular Cartilage Lesions Clinical Practice Guidelines Linked to the International Classification of Functioning, Disability, and Health from the Orthopaedic Section of the APTA, Summary of Recommendations page A30 from JOSPT June 2010, Number 6, Vol 40.

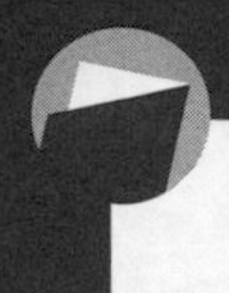

Appendix C

Clinical Practice Guidelines: Hip Pain and Mobility Deficits/Hip Osteoarthritis

1. **Pathoanatomical Features.** (B).
Clinicians should assess for impairments in mobility of the hip joint and strength of the surrounding muscles, especially the hip abductor muscles, when a patient presents with hip pain.

2. **Risk Factors.** (A).
Clinicians should consider age, hip developmental disorders, and previous hip joint injury as risk factors for hip osteoarthritis.

3. **Diagnosis/Classification.** (A).
Moderate lateral or anterior hip pain during weight bearing, in adults over the age of 50 years, with morning stiffness less than 1 hour, with limited hip internal rotation and hip flexion by more than 15° when comparing the painful to the nonpainful side are useful clinical findings to classify a patient with hip pain into the International Statistical Classification of Diseases and Related Health Problems (ICD).

4. **Differential Diagnosis.** (E).
Clinicians should consider diagnostic classifications other than osteoarthritis of the hip when the patient's history, reported activity limitations, or impairments of body function and structure are not consistent with those presented in the diagnosis/classification section of this guideline, or when the patient's symptoms do not diminish with interventions aimed at normalization of the patient's impairments of body function.

5. **Examination - Outcome Measures.** (A).
Clinicians should use validated functional outcome measures, such as the Western Ontario and McMaster Universities Osteoarthritis Index, the Lower Extremity Functional Scale, and the Harris Hip Score before and after interventions intended to alleviate the impairments of body function and structure, activity limitations, and participation restrictions associated with hip osteoarthritis.

6. **Examination - Activity Limitation and Participation Restriction Measures.** (A).
Clinicians should utilize easily reproducible physical performance measures, such as the 6-minute walk, self-paced walk, stair measure, and timed up-and-go tests to assess activity limitation and participation restrictions associated with their patient's hip pain, and to assess changes in the patient's level of function over the episode of care.

7. **Interventions - Patient Education.** (B).
Clinicians should consider the use of patient education to teach activity modification, exercise, weight reduction when overweight, and methods of unloading the arthritic joints.

8. **Interventions - Functional, Gait, and Balance Training.** (C).
Functional, gait, and balance training, including the use of assistive devices such as canes, crutches, and walkers, can be used in patients with hip osteoarthritis to improve function associated with weight-bearing activities.

9. **Interventions - Manual Therapy.** (B).
Clinicians should consider the use of manual therapy procedures to provide short-term pain relief and improve hip mobility and function in patients with mild hip osteoarthritis.

10. **Interventions - Flexibility, Strengthening, and Endurance Exercises.** (B).
Clinicians should consider the use of flexibility, strengthening, and endurance exercises in patients with hip osteoarthritis.

Hip Pain and Mobility Deficits – Hip Osteoarthritis: Clinical Practice Guidelines Linked to the International Classification of Functioning, Disability, and Health from the Orthopaedic Section of the APTA, Summary of Recommendations page A18 from JOSPT April 2009, Number 4, Vol 39.

Appendix D

Clinical Practice Guidelines: Neck Pain

1. Pathoanatomical Features. (E).
Although the cause of neck pain may be associated with degenerative processes or pathology identified during diagnostic imaging, the tissue causing a patient's neck pain is most often unknown. Thus, clinicians should assess for impaired function of muscle, connective, and nerve tissues associated with the identified pathological tissues when a patient presents with neck pain.

2. Risk Factors. (B).
Clinicians should consider age greater than 40, coexisting low back pain, a long history of neck pain, cycling as a regular activity, loss of strength in the hands, worrisome attitude, poor quality of life, and less vitality as predisposing factors for the development of chronic neck pain.

3. Diagnosis/Classification. (B).
Neck pain, without symptoms or signs of serious medical or psychological conditions, associated with (1) motion limitations in the cervical and upper thoracic regions, (2) headaches, and (3) referred or radiating pain into an upper extremity are useful clinical findings for classifying a patient into one of the following international Statistical Classification of Diseases and Related Health Problems (ICD) categories: cervicalgia, pain in thoracic spine, headaches, cervicocranial syndrome, sprain and strain of cervical spine, spondylosis with radiculopathy, and cervical disc disorder with radiculopathy; and the associated International Classification of Functioning, Disability, and Health (ICF) impairment-based category neck pain.

The following physical examination measures may be useful in classifying a patient in the ICF impairment-based category of neck pain with mobility impairments and the associated ICD categories of cervicalgia or pain in thoracic spine.

- Cervical active range of motion
- Cervical and thoracic segmental mobility

The following physical examination measures may be useful in classifying a patient in the ICF impairment-based category of neck pain with headaches and the associated ICD categories of headaches or cervicocranial syndrome.

- Cervical active range of motion
- Cervical segmental mobility
- Cranial cervical flexion test

The following physical examination measures may be useful in classifying a patient in the ICF impairment-based category of neck pain with movement coordination impairments, and the associated ICD category of sprain and strain of cervical spine.

- Cranial cervical flexion test
- Deep neck flexor endurance

The following physical examination measures may be useful in classifying a patient in the ICF impairment-based category of neck pain with radiating pain, and the associated ICD categories of spondylosis with radiculopathy or cervical disc disorder with radiculopathy.

- Upper limb tension test
- Spurling's test
- Distraction test

4. Differential Diagnosis. (B).
Clinicians should consider diagnostic classifications associated with serious pathological conditions or psychosocial factors when the patient's reported activity limitations or impairments of body function and structure are not consistent with those presented in the diagnosis/classification section of this guideline, or, when the patient's symptoms are not resolving with interventions aimed at normalization of the patient's impairments of body function.

5. Examination – Outcome Measures. (A).
Clinicians should use validated self-report questionnaires, such as the Neck Disability Index and the Patient-Specific Functional Scale for patients with neck pain. These tools are useful for identifying a patient's baseline status relative to pain, function, and disability, as well as for monitoring a change in patient's status throughout the course of treatment.

6. Examination – Activity Limitation Measures. (F).
Clinicians should utilize easily reproducible activity limitation and participation restriction measures associated with their patient's neck pain to assess changes in the patient's level of function over the episode of care.

7. Interventions – Cervical Mobilization/Manipulation. (A).
Clinicians should consider utilizing cervical manipulation and mobilization procedures, thrust and non-thrust, to reduce neck pain and headache. Combining cervical manipulation and mobilization with exercise is more effective for reducing neck pain, headache, and disability than manipulation and mobilization alone.

8. Interventions – Thoracic Mobilization/ Manipulation. (C).
Thoracic spine thrust manipulation can be used for patients with primary complaints of neck pain. Thoracic spine thrust manipulation can also be used for reducing

pain and disability in patients with neck and neck-related arm pain.

9. Interventions – Stretching Exercises. (C).
Flexibility exercises can be used for patients with neck symptoms. Examination and targeted flexibility exercises for the following muscles are suggested by the authors: anterior/medial/posterior scalenes, upper trapezius, levator scapulae, pectoralis minor, and pectoralis major.

10. Interventions – Coordination, Strengthening, and Endurance Exercises. (A).
Clinicians should consider the use of coordination, strengthening, and endurance exercises to reduce neck pain and headache.

11. Interventions – Centralization Procedures and Exercises. (C).
Specific repeated movements or procedures to promote centralization are not more beneficial in reducing disability than other forms of interventions.

12. Interventions – Upper Quarter and Nerve Mobilization Procedures. (B).
Clinicians should consider the use of upper quarter and nerve mobilization procedures to reduce pain and disability in patients with neck and arm pain.

13. Interventions – Traction. (B).
Clinicians should consider the use of mechanical intermittent cervical traction, combined with other interventions such as manual therapy and strengthening exercises, for reducing pain and disability in patients with neck and neck-related arm pain.

14. Interventions – Patient Education and Counseling. (A).
To improve the recovery in patients with whiplash-associated disorder, clinicians should (1) educate the patient that early return to normal, non-provocative pre-accident activities is important, and (2) provide reassurance to the patient that good prognosis and full recovery commonly occurs.

Neck Pain: Clinical Practice Guidelines Linked to the International Classification of Functioning, Disability, and Health from the Orthopaedic Section of the APTA, Summary of Recommendations pages A28-A29 from JOSPT September 2008, Number 9, Vol 38.

Appendix E

Clinical Practice Guidelines: Heel Pain/Plantar Fasciitis

1. Pathoanatomical Features. (F).
Clinicians should assess for impairments in muscles, tendons, and nerves, as well as the plantar fascia, when a patient presents with heel pain.

2. Risk Factors. (B).
Clinicians should consider limited ankle dorsiflexion range of motion and a high body mass index in nonathletic populations as factors predisposing patients to the development of heel pain/plantar fasciitis.

3. Diagnosis/Classification. (B).
Functional limitations associated with pain in the plantar medical heel region, most noticeable with initial steps after a period of inactivity, but also worse following prolonged weight bearing, and often precipitated by a recent increase in weight-bearing activity, are useful in classifying a patient into the ICD category of plantar fasciitis and the associated ICF impairment-based category of heel pain.

The following physical examination measures may be useful in classifying a patient with heel pain:

- Symptom reproduction with palpatory provocation of the proximal plantar fascia insertion
- Active and passive talocrural joint dorsiflexion range of motion
- Tarsal tunnel syndrome test
- Windlass test
- Longitudinal arch angle

4. Differential Diagnosis. (F).
Clinicians should consider diagnostic classifications other than heel pain/plantar fasciitis when the patient's reported functional limitations or physical impairments are not consistent with those presented in the diagnosis/classification section of this guideline, or, the patient's symptoms are not resolving with interventions aimed at normalization of the patient's physical impairments.

5. Examination: Outcome Measures. (A).
Clinicians should use validated self-report questionnaires, such as the Foot Function Index (FFI), Foot Health Status Questionnaire (FHSQ), or the Foot and Ankle Ability Measure (FAAM), before and after interventions intended to alleviate the physical impairments, functional limitations, and activity restrictions associated with heel pain/plantar fasciitis. Physical therapists should consider measuring change

over time using the FAAM, as it has been validated in a physical therapy practice setting.

6. Examination: Functional Limitation Measures. (F).
Clinicians should utilize easily reproducible functional limitations and activity restrictions measures associated with the patient's heel pain/plantar fasciitis to assess changes in the patient's level of function over the episode of care.

7. Interventions: Modalities. (B).
Dexamethasone 0.4% or acetic acid 5% delivered via iontophoresis can be used to provide short-term (2 to 4 weeks) pain relief and improved function.

8. Interventions: Manual Therapy. (E).
There is minimal evidence to support the use of manual therapy and nerve mobilization procedures short-term (1 to 3 months) for pain and function improvement. Suggested manual therapy procedures include: talocrural joint posterior glide, subtalar joint lateral glide, anterior and posterior glides of the first tarsometatarsal joint, subtalar joint distraction manipulation, soft tissue mobilization near potential nerve entrapment sites, and passive neural mobilization procedures.

9. Interventions: Stretching. (B).
Calf muscle and/or plantar fascia-specific stretching can be used to provide short-term (2 to 4 months) pain relief and improvement in calf muscle flexibility. The dosage for calf stretching can be either 2 or 3 times a day, utilizing either a sustained (3 minutes) or intermittent (20 seconds) stretching time, since both dosages have been shown to have the same effect.

10. Interventions: Taping. (C).
Calcaneal or low-Dye taping can be used to provide short-term (7 to 10 days) pain relief. Studies indicate that taping does improve function.

11. Interventions: Orthotic Devices. (A).
Prefabricated or custom foot orthoses can be used to provide short-term (3 months) reduction in pain and improvement in function. There appear to be no differences in the amount of pain reduction or improvement in function created by custom foot orthoses compared to prefabricated orthoses. There is currently no evidence to support the use of prefabricated or custom foot orthoses for long-term (1 year) pain management or function improvement.

12. Interventions–Night Splints. (B).
Night splints should be considered as an intervention for patients with symptoms greater than 6 months in duration. The desired length of time for wearing the night splint is 1 to 3 months. The type of night splint used (ie, posterior, anterior, sock-type) does not appear to affect the outcome.

Heel Pain – Plantar Fasciitis: Clinical Practice Guidelines Linked to the International Classification of Functioning, Disability, and Health from the Orthopaedic Section of the APTA, Summary of Recommendations page A16 from JOSPT April 2008, Number 4, Vol 38.

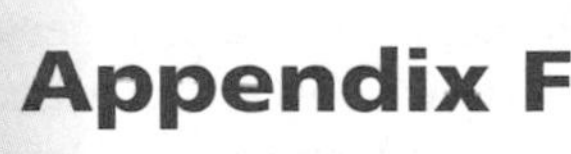

Appendix F

Clinical Practice Guidelines: Knee Ligament Sprains

1. Risk Factors. (B).
Clinicians should consider the shoe-surface interaction, increased body mass index, narrow femoral notch width, increased joint laxity, preovulatory phase of the menstrual cycle in females, combined loading pattern, and strong quardiceps predisposing activation during eccentric contractions as predisposing factors for the risk of sustaining a non-contact anterior cruciate ligament (ACL) injury.

2. Diagnosis/Classification. (A).
Passive knee instability, joint pain, joint effusion, and movement coordination impairments are useful clinical findings for classifying a patient with knee instability into the following International Statistical Classification of Diseases and Related Health Problems (ICD) categories: Sprain and strain involving collateral ligament of knee, Sprain and strain involving cruciate ligament of knee, Injury to multiple structures of knee; and the associated International Classification of Functioning, Disability, and Health (ICF) impairment-based category of knee instability.

3. Differential Diagnosis. (B).
Clinicians should consider diagnostic classifications associated with serious pathological conditions or psychosocial factors when the patient's reported activity limitations or impairments of body function and structure are not consistent with those presented in the diagnosis/classification section of this guideline or when the patient's symptoms are not resolving with interventions aimed at normalization of the patient's impairments of body function.

4. Examination: Outcome Measures. (A).
Clinicians should use a validated patient-reported outcome

measure with a general health questionnaire, along with a validated activity scale for patients with knee stability and movement coordination impairments. These tools are useful for identifying a patient's baseline status relative to pain, function, and disability and for monitoring changes in the patient's status throughout the course of treatment.

5. **Examination: Activity Limitation Measures.** (C).
Clinicians should utilize easily reproducible physical performance measures, such as single-limb hop tests, to assess activity limitation and participation restriction associated with their patient's knee stability and movement coordination impairments, to assess the changes in the patient's level of function over the episode of care, and to classify and screen knee stability and movement coordination.

6. **Interventions: Continuous Passive Motion.** (C).
Clinicians can consider using passive motion in the immediate postoperative period to decrease postoperative pain.

7. **Intervention: Early Weight Bearing.** (C).
Early weight-bearing can be used for patients following ACL reconstruction without incurring detrimental effects on stability or function.

8. **Interventions: Knee Bracing.** (C).
The use of functional knee bracing appears to be more beneficial than not using a brace in patients with ACL deficiency.

(B).
The use of immediate postoperative knee bracing appears to be no more beneficial then not using a brace in patients following ACL reconstruction.

(D).
Conflicting evidence exists for the use of functional knee bracing in patients following ACL reconstruction.

Knee bracing can be used for patients with acute PCL injuries, severe MCL injuries, or PLC injuries.

9. **Interventions: Immediate Vs. Delayed Mobilization.** (B).
Clinicians should consider the use of immediate mobilization following ACL reconstruction to increase range of motion, reduce pain, and limit adverse change to soft tissue structures.

10. **Interventions: Cryotherapy.** (C).
Clinicians should consider the use of cryotherapy to reduce postoperative knee pain immediately post-ACL reconstruction.

11. **Interventions: Supervised Rehabilitation.** (B).
Clinicians should consider the use of exercises as part of the in-clinic program, supplemented by a prescribed home-based program supervised by a physical therapist in patients with knee stability and movement coordination impairments.

12. **Intervention: Therapeutic Exercises.** (A).
Clinicians should consider the use of non-weight-bearing (open chain) exercises in conjunction with weight-bearing (closed-chain) exercises in patients with knee stability and movement coordination impairments.

13. **Interventions: Neuromuscular Electrical Stimulation.** (B).
Neuromuscular electrical stimulation can be used with patients following ACL reconstruction to increase quadriceps muscle strength.

14. **Interventions: Neuromuscular Reeducation.** (B).
Clinician should consider the use of neuromuscular training as a supplementary program to strength training in patients with knee stability and movement coordination impairments.

15. **Interventions: "Accelerated" Rehabilitation.** (B).
Rehabilitation that emphasizes early restoration of knee extension and early weight-bearing activity appears safe a for patients with ACL reconstruction. No evidence exists to determine the efficacy and/or safety of early return to sports.

16. **Interventions: Eccentric Strengthening.** (B).
Clinicians should consider the use of an eccentric exercise ergometer in patients following ACL reconstruction to increase muscle strength and functional performance. Clinicians should consider the use of eccentric squat program in patients with PCL injury to increase muscle strength and functional performance.

Clinical Practice Guidelines Linked to the International Classification of Functioning, Disability, and Health, American Physical Therapy Association (2010). Summary of Recommendations, JOSPT 4 (40): A31–32.

Appendix G

Selected Medical Images for Physical Therapists

1. Region: Head and Neck

Lateral Radiographic View of Cervical Spine:

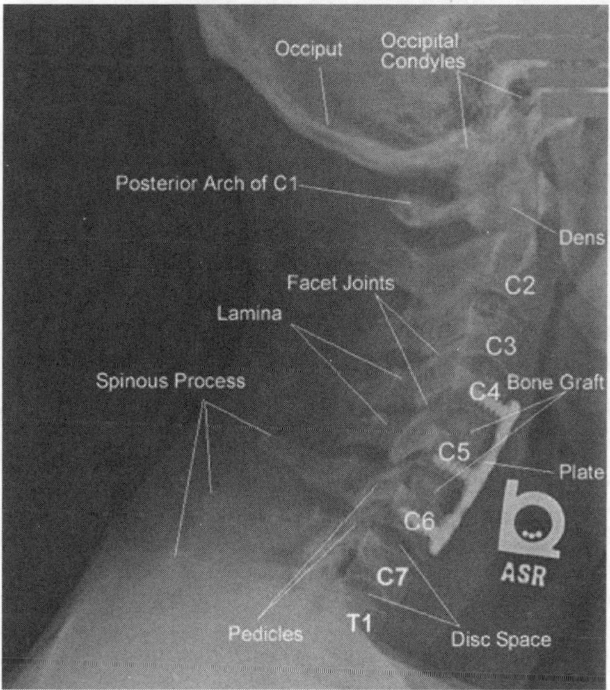

Reference: http://www.neckpainexplained.com/degenerative-disc-disese.htm

MRI of Circle Willis and Other Cerebral Arteries:

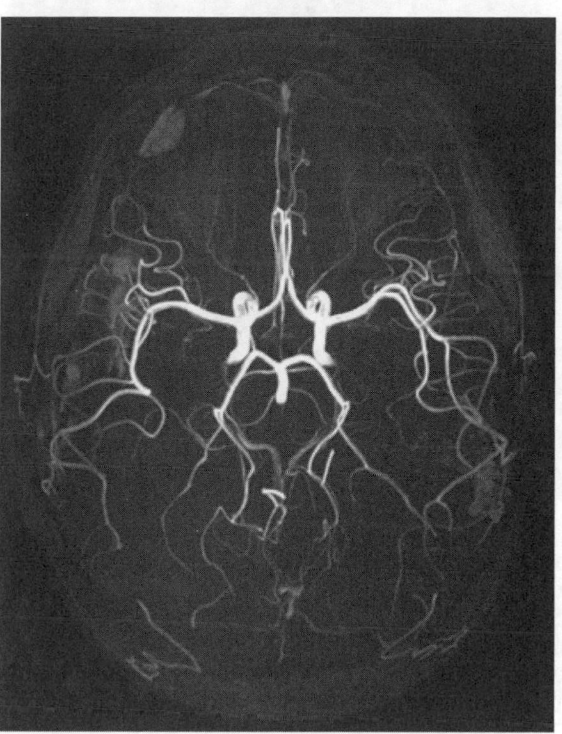

From: http://wsunews.wsu.edu/Content/Publications/MRI1.jpg

Axial T2 MRI:

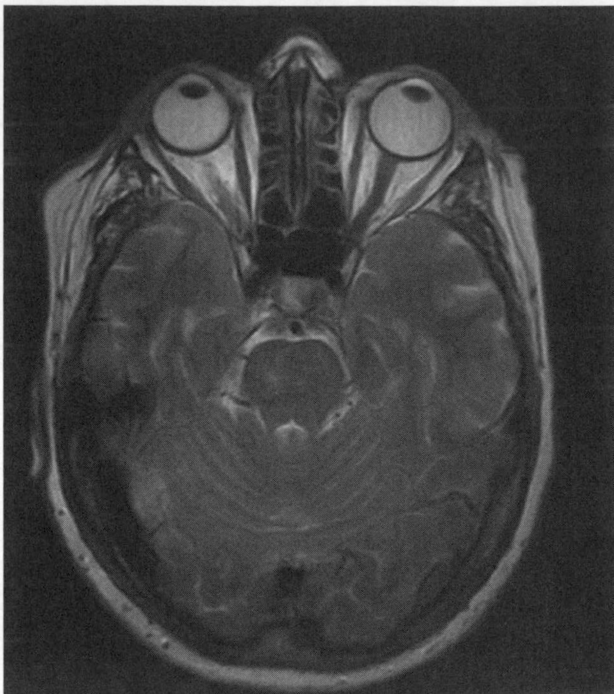

A student studying for NPTE.:☺ This view shows the eyeballs with optic nerves, chiasm, and tracts. The temporal, occipital, and cerebellar tissues are also visible.

➤

Source: http://wsunews.wsu.edu/pages/publications.asp?Action5Detail&PublicationID510646

Axial CT of Hemorrhagic Stroke (arrows indicate bleeding):

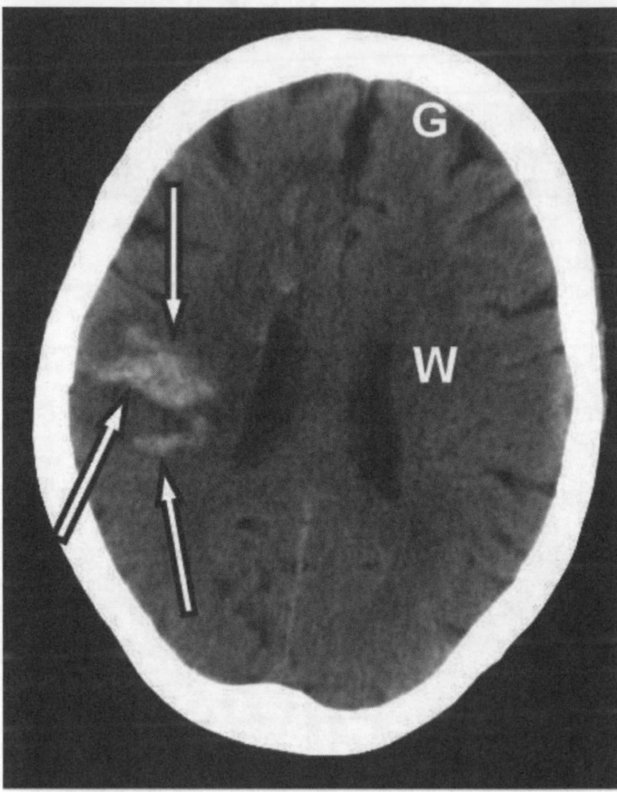

The blood is white, with slightly darker than normal areas surrounding this, due to local brain swelling (edema). G = normal brain gray matter; W = normal brain white matter (darker on CT scans than gray matter).

From: http://www.radiologyinfo.org/en/photocat/gallery3. cfm?image=CTHemStroke.jpg

Axial CT of Epidural Hematoma:

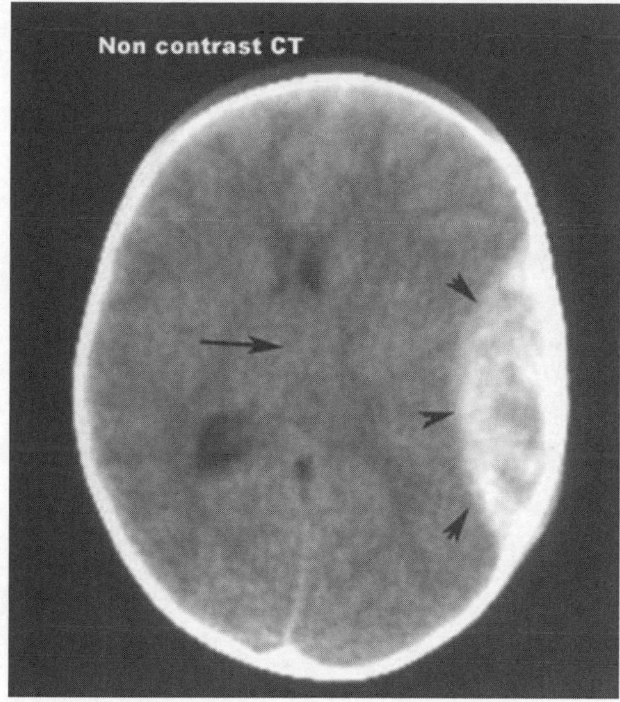

Arrowheads point to the collection of blood between the skull and dura. The arrow demonstrates a shift of midline to the right.

➤

From: http://www.meddean.luc.edu/lumen/MedEd/Radio/curriculum/Neurology/IC_hemorrhage2.htm

2. Region: Thorax and Spine

Posterior-Anterior (PA) Radiographic View of Normal Thoracic Radiograph of a Female:

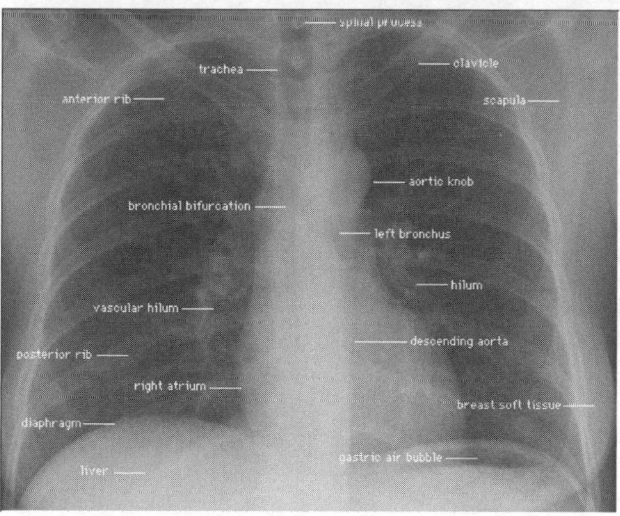

From: http://www.med.yale.edu/intmed/cardio/imaging/cases/normal_female_1/index.html

PA Radiographic View: Demonstrates Signs of Congestive Heart Failure:

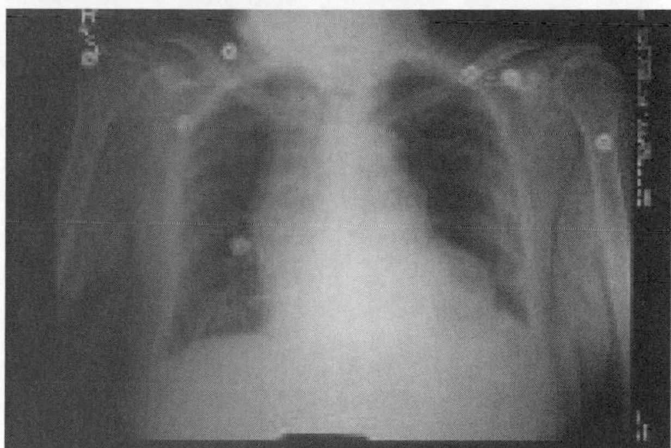

The size of the heart and edema at the lung bases are indications of congestive heart failure.

➤

From: http://emedicine.medscape.com/article/354666-imaging

Coronal T1 MRI Thoracic View of Normal Female:

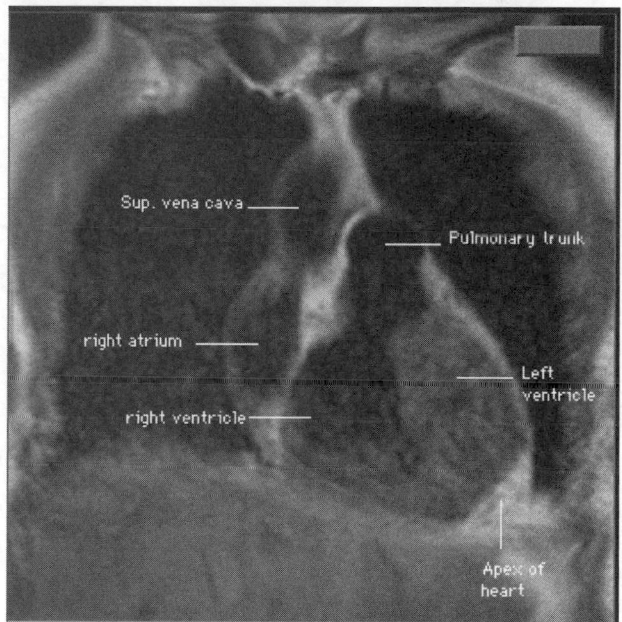

Lateral Radiographic View of Normal Lumbar Spine:

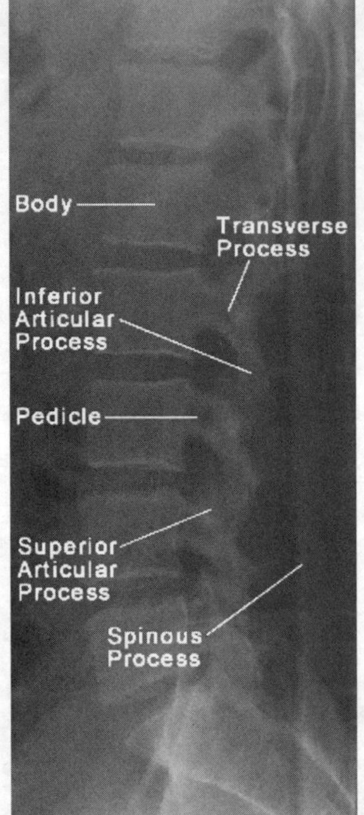

Oblique Radiographic View Demonstrates Fracture Through the Pars Interarticularis (arrows):

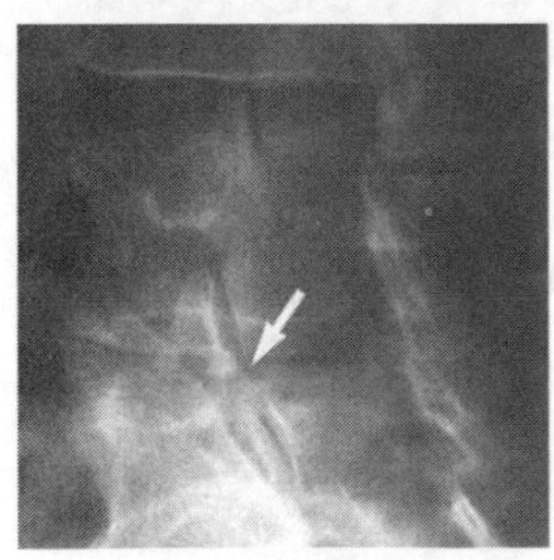

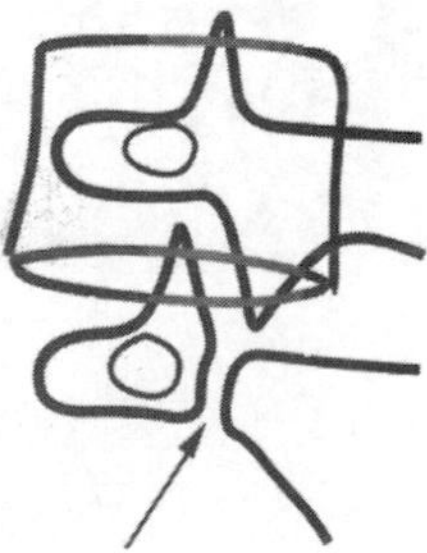

Sagittal View of T2 and T1 with Contrast MRIs of Lumbar Disc Annular Tear:

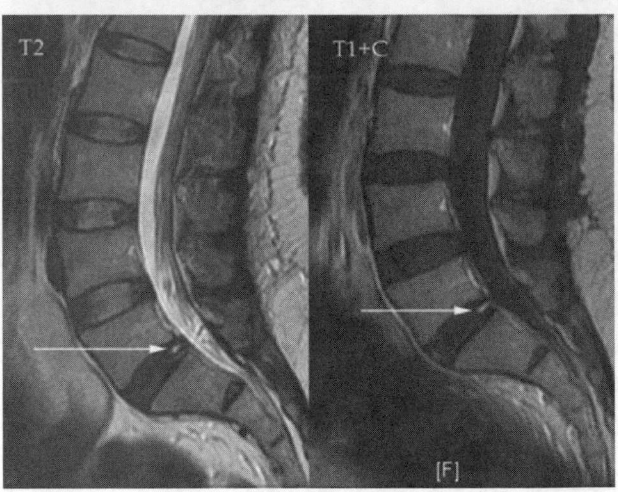

3. Region: Upper Extremity

Anterior-Posterior (AP) Radiographic View of Right Shoulder in External Rotation:

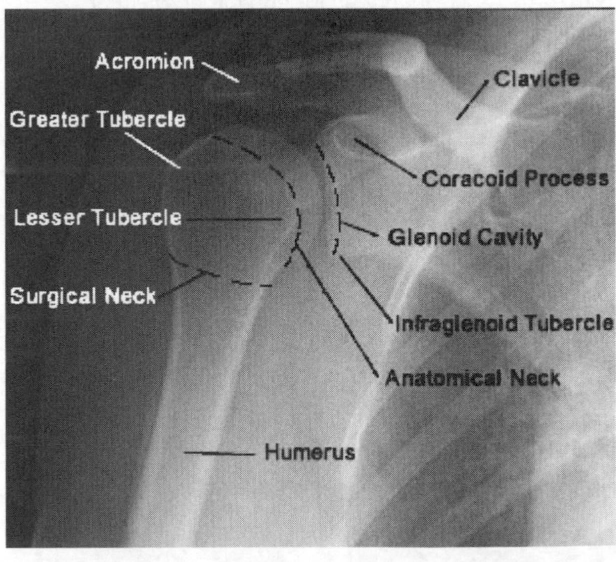

AP Radiographic Stress View of Type II Separation:

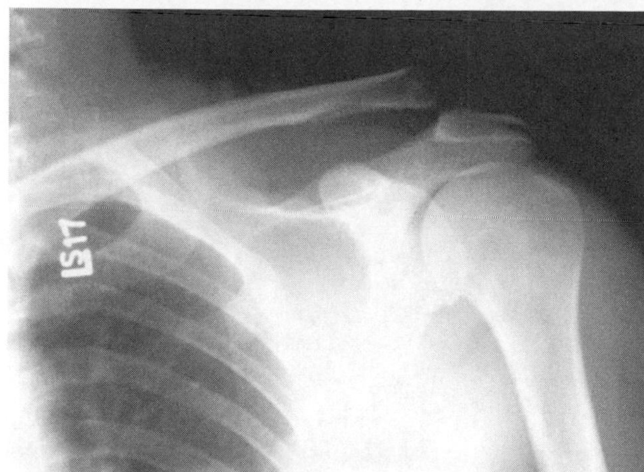

Coronal T1 (Figure 1-normal) and T2 (Figure 2-torn supraspinatus) MRIs of Left Shoulder:

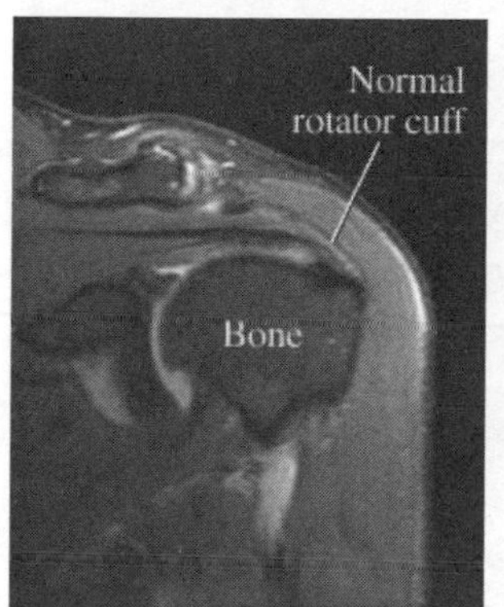

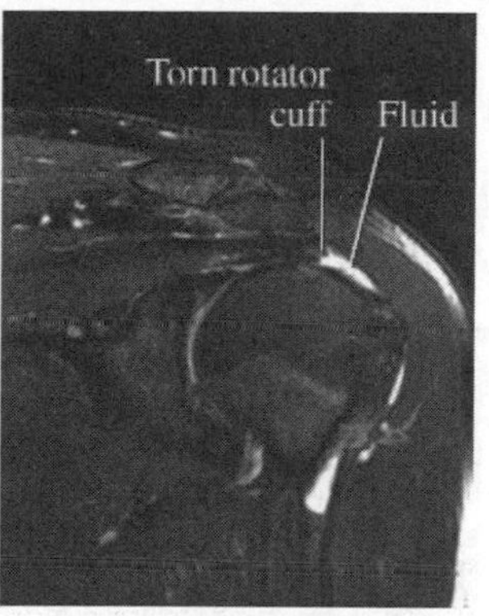

Lateral and AP Radiographic Views of Normal Elbow:

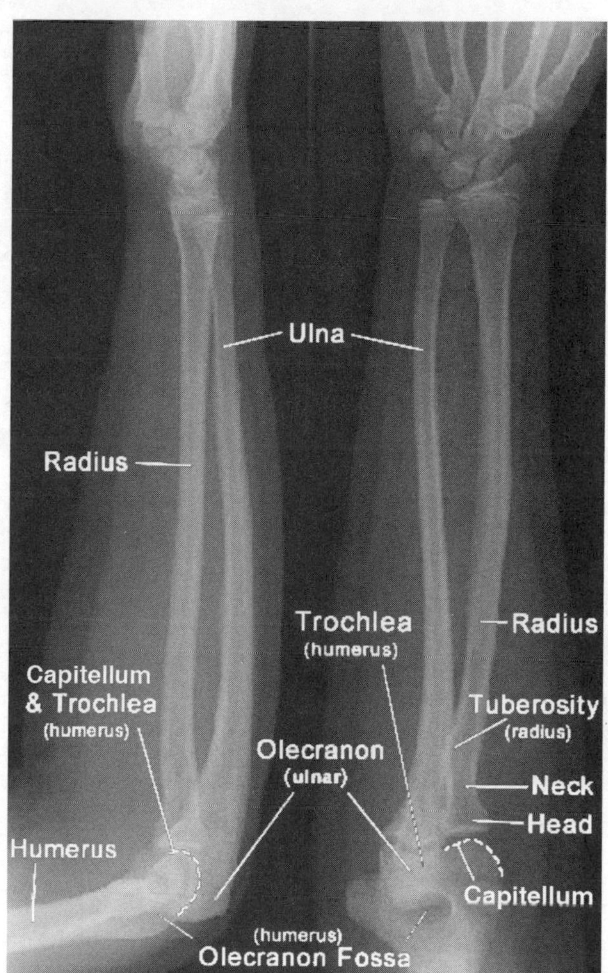

AP Radiographic View of Wrist:

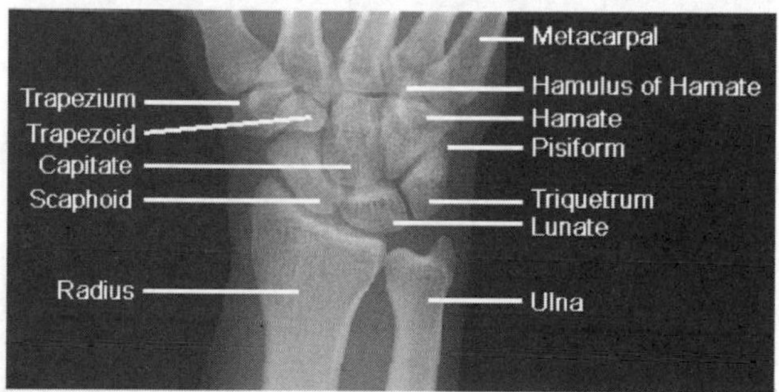

Mnemonic for remembering carpals: Some Lovers Try Positions That They Can't Handle.
Scaphoid, Lunate, Triquetrum, Pisiform, Trapezium, Trapezoid, Capitate, Hamate

➤

From: http://www.med-ed.virginia.edu/courses/rad/

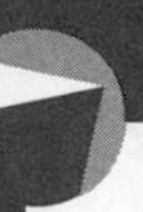

Radiographic View of Boxer's Fracture of Fifth Metacarpal (white pointer):

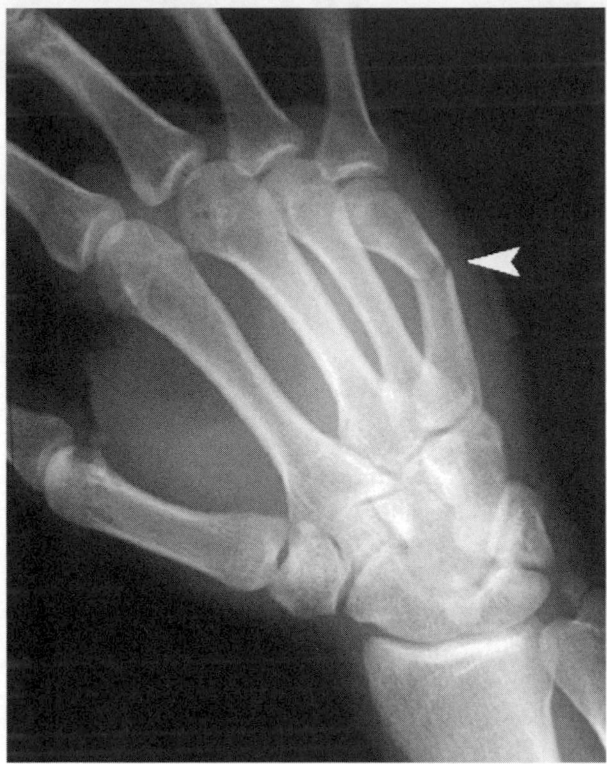

Radiograph Demonstrates Ulnar Deviation of the Metacarpophalangeal Joints due to Rheumatoid Arthritis:

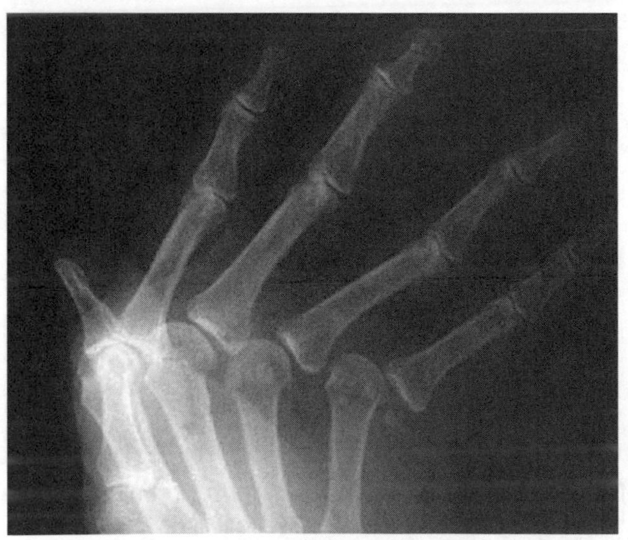

4. Region: Lower Extremity

AP Radiographic View of Normal Pelvis:

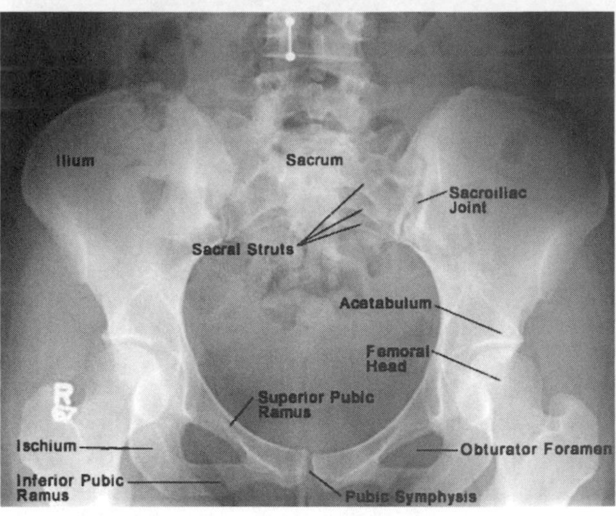

AP Radiographic View of Right Acetabular Fracture (arrow)

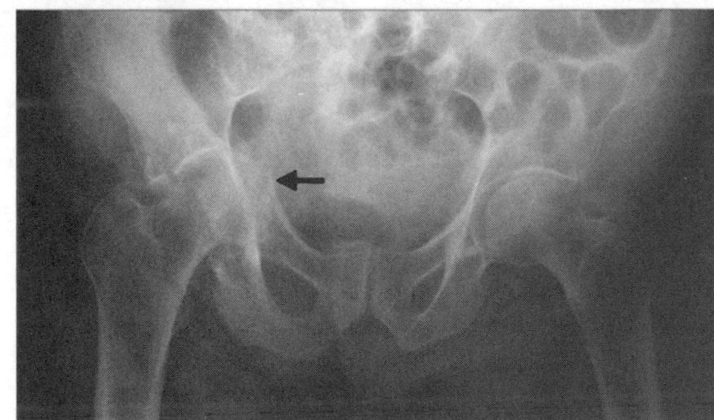

Axial CT Scan of Right Acetabular Fracture (arrows):

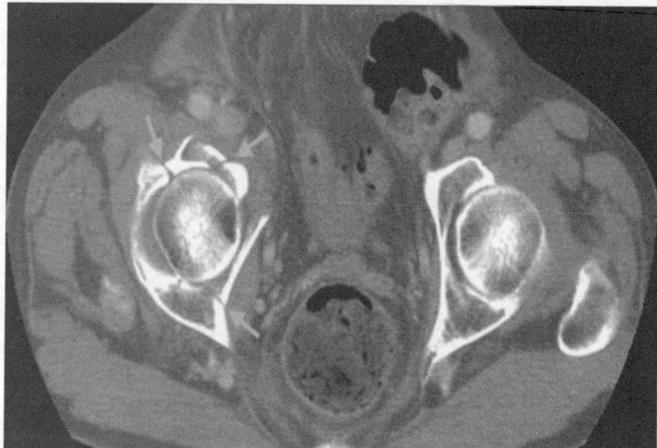

Reference: *J Orthop Sports Phys Ther 2009;39(9):703*

AP Radiographic View of Normal Child's Leg:

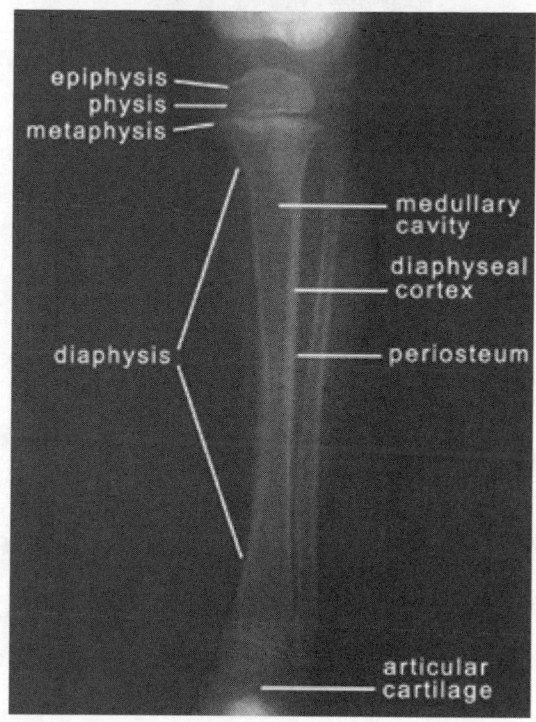

The epiphyseal gaps would be absent or sclerosed in a radiograph of an adult.

➤

Image from: http://www.med-ed.virginia.edu/courses/rad/ext/index.html

MRI Figure 1 Normal:

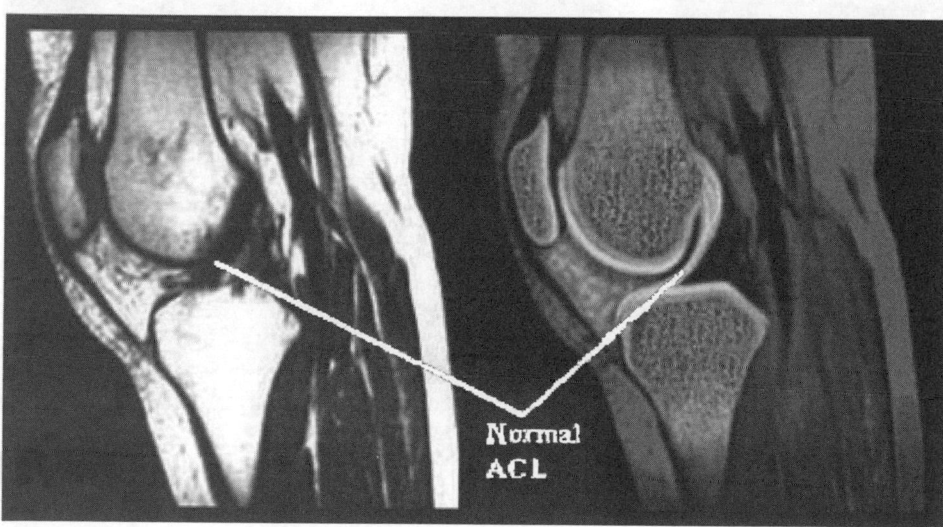

Coronal MRI of Tibial Stress Fracture (arrow):

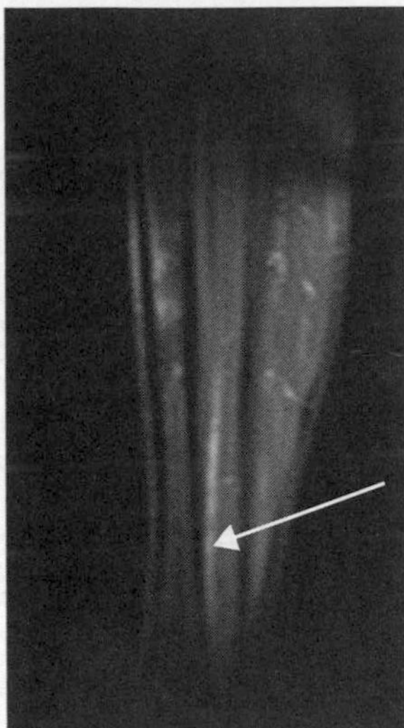

This fat suppressed MRI of right tibia demonstrates a high signal consistent with edema associated with a stress fracture.

➤
Image from: http://www.eurorad.org/

Lateral Radiographic View of Normal Ankle:

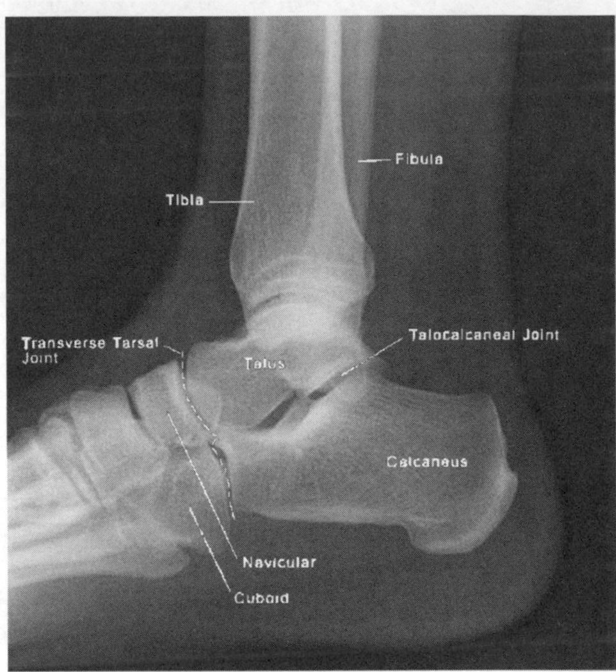

Axial MRI of Tibial Stress Fracture (arrow):

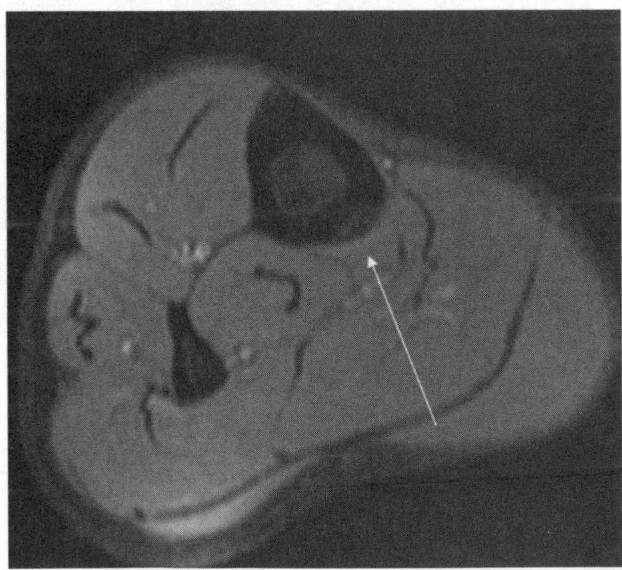

This fat suppressed MRI of right tibia demonstrates a transversal line (arrow) transgressing the tibial cortex associated with a stress fracture.

➤
Image from: http://www.eurorad.org/

Lateral Radiographic View of Heel Spur:

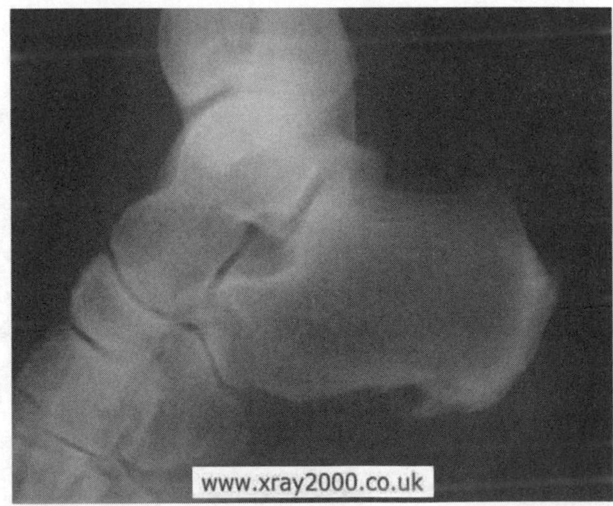

PA Radiographic View of Talocrural Demonstrates Fibular Fracture and Widening of Ankle Mortise:

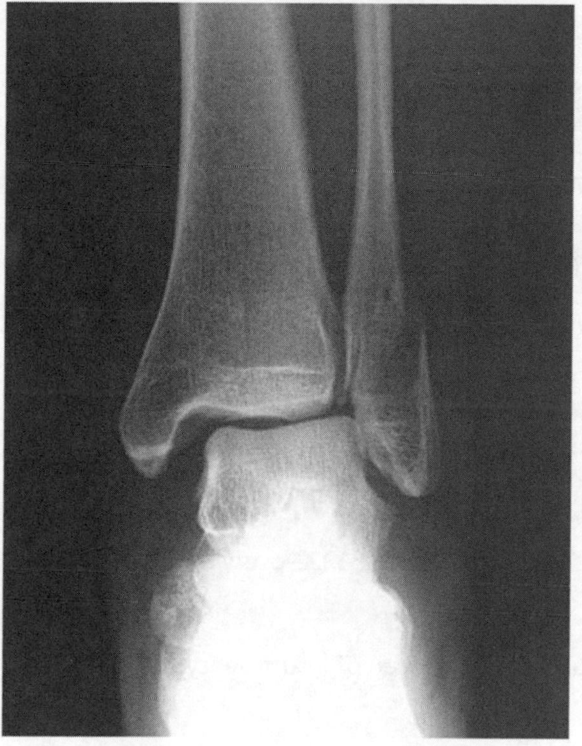

AP Radiographic View of Medial Malleolus Fracture (arrow):

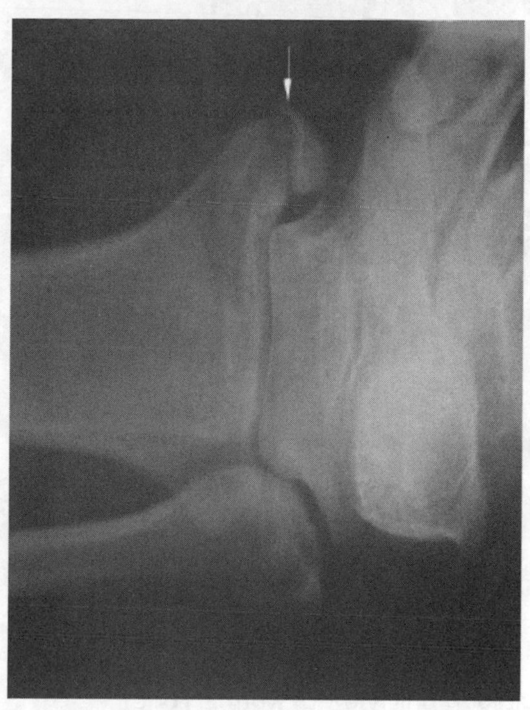

T1 MRI (Figure 1 - Normal) and T2 MRI (Figure 2 - Torn) of Achilles Tendon:

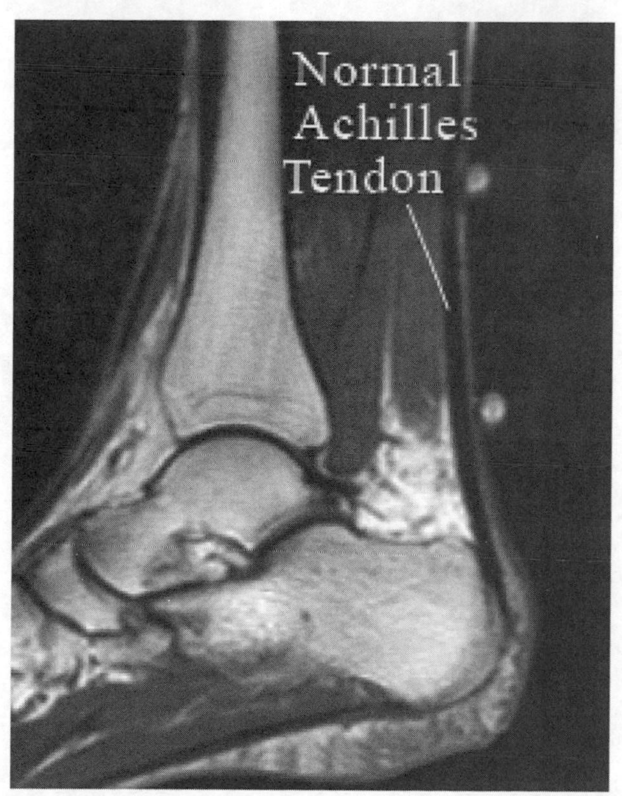

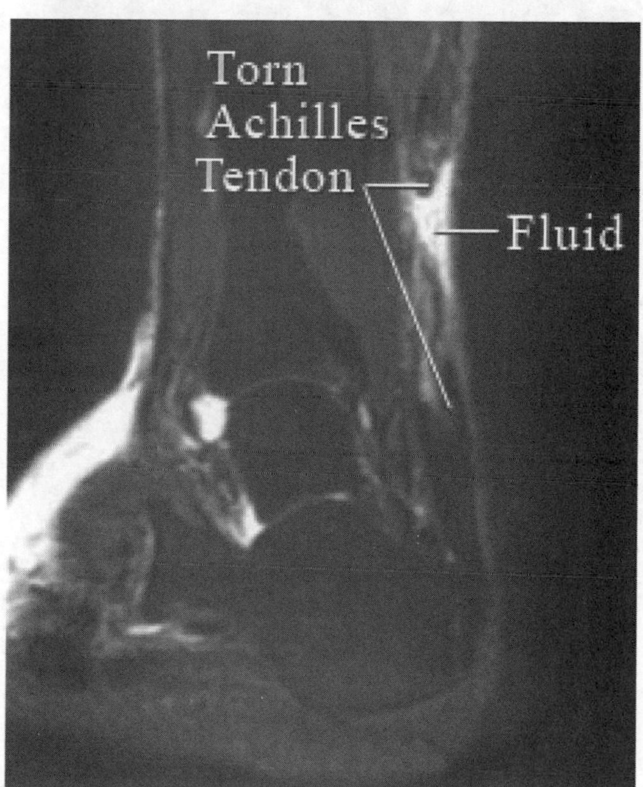

Coronal T1 MRI (Left) and Axial T2 MRI (Right) of Posterior Tibial Tendonitis (arrows):

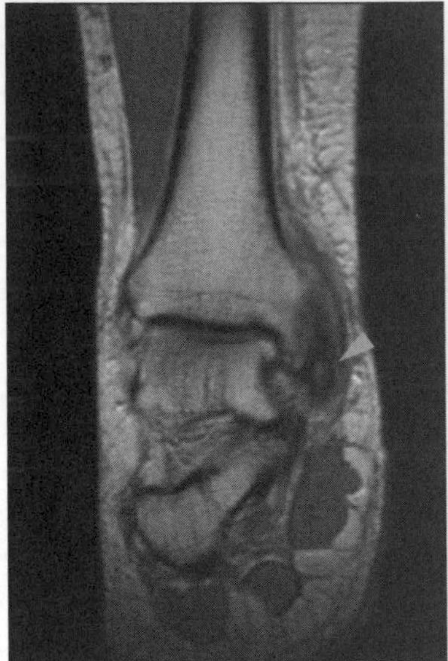

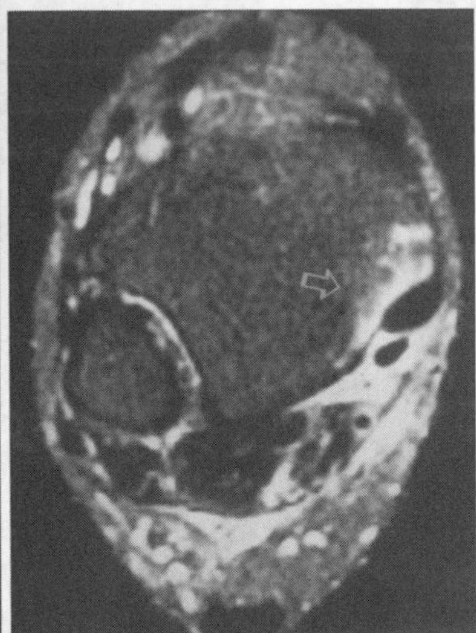

Posterior Tibial Tendonitis MRIs from: http://emedicine.medscape.com/article/386322-overview

AP Radiographic View of Normal Foot:

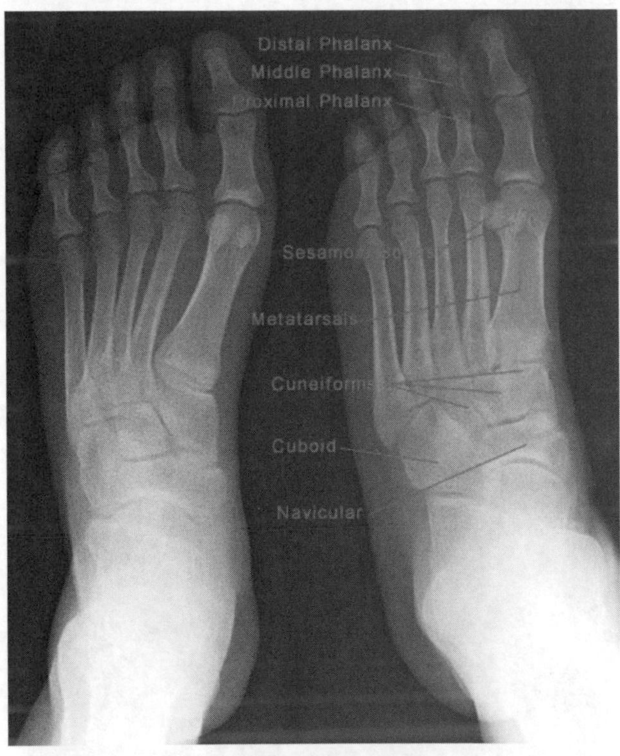

Full Body Bone Scan of Insufficiency Rib Fractures:

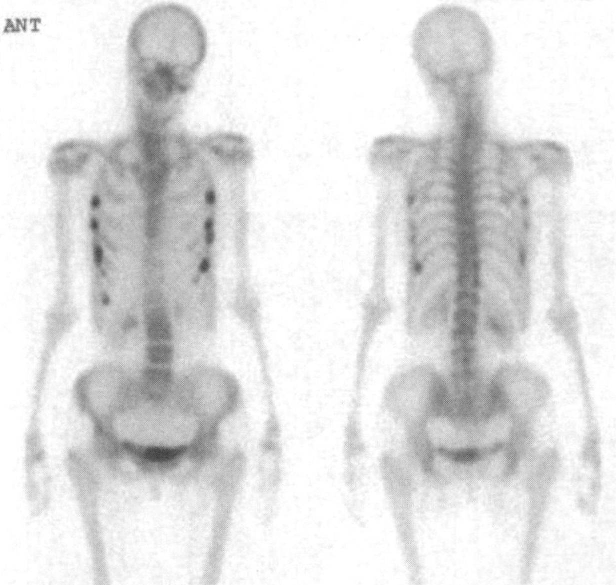

85 year-old female diagnosed with insufficiency fractures of the ribs following several falls at home. No metastases.

➤

From: http://www.ruh.nhs.uk/archive/nm_training/bone/Bone%20Case%209.htm

Acknowledgments

The authors wish to acknowledge the contributions of Connie J. Seymour, PT, PhD, OCS to previous editions of this chapter.

The authors also wish to acknowledge L. Vincent Lepak III for the creation of Appendix G.

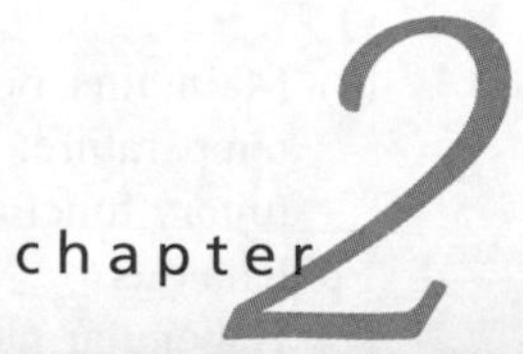

chapter 2

Neuromuscular Physical Therapy

SUSAN B. O'SULLIVAN

Anatomy and Physiology of the Nervous System

Brain

1. **Cerebral hemispheres (telencephalon).**
   a. Convolutions of gray matter composed of gyri (crests) and sulci (fissures).
      (1) Lateral central fissure (fissure of Sylvius) separates temporal lobe from frontal and parietal lobes.
      (2) Longitudinal cerebral fissure separates the two hemispheres.
      (3) Central sulcus separates the frontal lobe from the parietal lobe.
   b. Paired hemispheres, consisting of six lobes on each side: frontal, parietal, temporal, occipital, insular, limbic.
      (1) Frontal lobe.
         (a) Precentral gyrus: primary motor cortex for voluntary muscle activation.
         (b) Prefrontal cortex: controls emotions and judgments.
         (c) Broca's area: controls motor aspects of speech.
      (2) Parietal lobe.
         (a) Postcentral gyrus: primary sensory cortex for integration of sensation.
         (b) Receives fibers conveying touch, proprioceptive, pain, and temperature sensations from opposite side of body.
      (3) Temporal lobe.
         (a) Primary auditory cortex: receives/processes auditory stimuli.
         (b) Associative auditory cortex: processes auditory stimuli.
         (c) Wernicke's area: language comprehension.
      (4) Occipital lobe.
         (a) Primary visual cortex: receives/processes visual stimuli.
         (b) Visual association cortex: processes visual stimuli.
      (5) Insula.
         (a) Deep within lateral sulcus, associated with visceral functions.
      (6) Limbic system.
         (a) Consists of the limbic lobe (cingulate, parahippocampal, and subcallosal gyri), hippocampal formation, amygdaloid nucleus, hypothalamus, and anterior nucleus of thalamus.
         (b) Phylogenetically oldest part of the brain, concerned with instincts and emotions contributing to preservation of the individual.
         (c) Basic functions include feeding, aggression, emotions, and endocrine aspects of sexual response.
   c. White matter: myelinated nerve fibers located centrally.

(1) Transverse (commissural) fibers: interconnect the two hemispheres, including the corpus callosum (the largest), anterior commissure, and hippocampal commissure.
(2) Projection fibers: connect cerebral hemispheres with other portions of the brain and spinal cord.
(3) Association fibers: connect different portions of the cerebral hemispheres, allowing cortex to function as an integrated whole.

d. Basal ganglia.
(1) Masses of gray matter deep within the cerebral hemispheres, including the corpus striatum (caudate nucleus and lenticular nuclei) amygdaloid nucleus, and claustrum. The lenticular nuclei are further subdivided into the putamen and the globus pallidus.
(2) Forms an associated motor system (extrapyramidal system) with other nuclei in the subthalamus and the midbrain.
(3) Circuits of the basal ganglia (BG).
(a) Oculomotor circuit (caudate loop): originates in frontal and supplementary motor eye fields; projects to caudate; functions with saccadic eye movements.
(b) Skeletomotor circuit (putamen loop): originates in precentral motor and postcentral somatosensory areas; projects to putamen; functions to scale amplitude and velocity of movements; reinforces selected pattern, suppresses conflicting patterns; preparatory for movement (i.e., motor set, anticipatory movement).
(c) Limbic circuit: originates in prefrontal and limbic areas of cortex; to BG; to prefrontal cortex; functions to organize behaviors (executive functions, problem solving, motivation) and for procedural learning.

2. Diencephalon.

a. Thalamus.
(1) Sensory nuclei: integrate and relay sensory information from body, face, retina, cochlea, and taste receptors to cerebral cortex and subcortical regions; smell (olfaction) is the exception.
(2) Motor nuclei: relay motor information from cerebellum and globus pallidus to precentral motor cortex.
(3) Other nuclei: assist in integration of visceral and somatic functions.

b. Subthalamus: involved in control of several functional pathways for sensory, motor, and reticular function.

c. Hypothalamus.
(1) Integrates and controls the functions of the autonomic nervous system and the neuroendocrine system.
(2) Maintains body homeostasis: regulates body temperature, eating, water balance, anterior pituitary function/sexual behavior, and emotion.

d. Epithalamus.
(1) Habenular nuclei: integrate olfactory, visceral, and somatic afferent pathways.
(2) Pineal gland: secretes hormones that influence the pituitary gland and several other organs; influences circadian rhythm.

3. Brainstem.

a. Midbrain (mesencephalon).
(1) Connects pons to cerebrum; superior peduncle connects midbrain to cerebellum.
(2) Contains cerebral peduncles (two lateral halves), each divided into an anterior part or basis (crus cerebri and substantia nigra) and a posterior part (tegmentum).
(3) Tegmentum contains all ascending tracts and some descending tracts; the red nucleus receives fibers from the cerebellum, is the origin for the rubrospinal tract, important for coordination; contains cranial nerve nuclei: oculomotor and trochlear.
(4) Substantia nigra is a large motor nucleus connecting with the basal ganglia and cortex; it is important in motor control and muscle tone.
(5) Superior colliculus is an important relay station for vision and visual reflexes; the inferior colliculus is an important relay station for hearing and auditory reflexes.
(6) Periaqueductal gray contains endorphin-producing cells (important for the suppression of pain) and descending autonomic tracts.

b. Pons.
(1) Connects the medulla oblongata to the midbrain, allowing passage of important ascending and descending tracts.
(2) Anterior basal part acts as a bridge to cerebellum (middle cerebellar peduncle).
(3) Midline raphe nuclei project widely and are important for modulating pain and controlling arousal.
(4) Tegmentum contains several important cranial nerve nuclei: abducens, trigeminal, facial, vestibulocochlear.

c. Medulla oblongata.
(1) Connects spinal cord with pons.
(2) Contains relay nuclei of dorsal columns (gracilis and cuneatus); fibers cross to give rise to medial lemniscus.
(3) Inferior cerebellar peduncle relays dorsal spinocerebellar tract to cerebellum.
(4) Corticospinal tracts cross (decussate) in pyramids.
(5) Medial longitudinal fasciculus arises from vestibular nuclei and extends throughout brainstem

and upper cervical spinal cord; important for control of head movements and gaze stabilization (vestibulo-ocular reflex).

(6) Olivary nuclear complex connects cerebellum to brainstem and is important for voluntary movement control.

(7) Contains several important cranial nerve nuclei: hypoglossal, dorsal nucleus of vagus, and vestibulocochlear.

(8) Contains important centers for vital functions: cardiac, respiratory, and vasomotor centers.

4. Cerebellum.

a. Located behind dorsal pons and medulla in posterior fossa.

b. Structure.

(1) Joined to brainstem by three pairs of peduncles: superior, middle, and inferior.

(2) Comprises two hemispheres and midline vermis; cerebellar cortex, underlying white matter, and four paired deep nuclei.

(3) Archicerebellum (flocculonodular lobe) connects with vestibular system and is concerned with equilibrium and regulation of muscle tone; helps coordinate vestibulo-ocular reflex.

(4) Paleocerebellum (rostral cerebellum, anterior lobe; also known as spinocerebellum) receives input from proprioceptive pathways and is concerned with modifying muscle tone and synergistic actions of muscles; it is important in maintenance of posture and voluntary movement control.

(5) Neocerebellum (cerebellar hemisphere, posterior lobe; also known as pontocerebellum); receives input from corticopontocerebellar tracts and olivocerebellar fibers; it is concerned with the smooth coordination of voluntary movements; ensures accurate force, direction, and extent of movement. Important for motor learning, sequencing of movements, and visually triggered movements. May have a role in assisting cognitive function and mental imagery.

Spinal Cord

1. General structure.

a. Cylindrical mass of nerve tissue extending from the foramen magnum in the skull continuous with the medulla to the lower border of the first lumbar vertebra in the conus medullaris.

b. Divided into 30 segments: 8 cervical, 12 thoracic, 5 lumbar, 5 sacral, and a few coccygeal segments.

2. Central gray matter. Two anterior (ventral) and two posterior (dorsal) horns united by gray commissure with central canal.

a. Anterior horns contain cell bodies that give rise to efferent (motor) neurons: alpha motor neurons to effect muscles and gamma motor neurons to muscle spindles.

b. Posterior horns contain afferent (sensory) neurons with cell bodies located in the dorsal root ganglia.

c. Two enlargements (cervical and lumbosacral) for origins of nerves of upper and lower extremities.

d. Lateral horn is found in thoracic and upper lumbar segments for preganglionic fibers of the autonomical nervous system.

3. White matter. Anterior (ventral), lateral, and posterior (dorsal) white columns or funiculi.

a. Ascending fiber systems (sensory pathways).

(1) Dorsal columns/medial lemniscal system: convey sensations of proprioception, vibration, and tactile discrimination; divided into fasciculus cuneatus (upper extremity tracts, laterally located) and fasciculus gracilis (lower extremity tracts, medially located); neurons ascend to medulla where fibers cross (lemniscal decussation) to form medial lemniscus; ascend to thalamus and then to somatosensory cortex.

(2) Spinothalamic tracts: convey sensations of pain and temperature (lateral spinothalamic tract), and crude touch (anterior spinothalamic tract); tracts ascend one or two ipsilateral spinal cord segments (Lissauer's tract), synapse and cross in spinal cord to opposite side and ascend in ventrolateral spinothalamic system.

(3) Spinocerebellar tracts: convey proprioception information from muscle spindles, Golgi tendon organs, and touch and pressure receptors to cerebellum for control of voluntary movements; dorsal spinocerebellar tract ascends to ipsilateral inferior cerebellar peduncle, and ventrospinocerebellar tract ascends to contralateral and ipsilateral superior cerebellar peduncle.

(4) Spinoreticular tracts: convey deep and chronic pain to reticular formation of brainstem via diffuse, polysynaptic pathways.

b. Descending fiber systems (motor pathways).

(1) Corticospinal tracts: arise from primary motor cortex, descend in brainstem, cross in medulla (pyramidal decussation), via lateral corticospinal tract to ventral gray matter (anterior horn cells); 10% of fibers do not cross and travel in anterior corticospinal tract to cervical and upper thoracic segments; important for voluntary motor control.

(2) Vestibulospinal tracts: arise from vestibular nucleus and descend to spinal cord in lateral (uncrossed) and medial (crossed and uncrossed) vestibulospinal tracts; important for control of muscle tone, antigravity muscles, and postural reflexes.

(3) Rubrospinal tracts: arise in contralateral red nucleus and descend in lateral white columns to spinal gray; assist in motor function.
(4) Reticulospinal system: arises in the reticular formation of the brainstem and descends (crossed and uncrossed) in ventral and lateral columns, terminates both on dorsal gray (modifies transmission of sensation, especially pain) and on ventral gray (influences gamma motor neurons and spinal reflexes).
(5) Tectospinal tract: arises from superior colliculus (midbrain) and descends to ventral gray; assists in head-turning responses to visual stimuli.

4. Autonomic nervous system (ANS).
a. Concerned with innervations of involuntary structures: smooth muscle, heart, glands; helps maintain homeostasis (constant internal body environment).
b. Two divisions: sympathetic and parasympathetic; both have afferent and efferent nerve fibers; preganglionic and postganglionic fibers.
(1) Sympathetic (thoracolumbar division, T1-L2): prepares body for fight or flight, emergency responses; increases heart rate and blood pressure, constricts peripheral blood vessels, and redistributes blood; inhibits peristalsis.
(2) Parasympathetic (craniosacral division, CN III, VII, IX, X; pelvic nerves): conserves and restores homeostasis; slows heart rate and reduces blood pressure; increases peristalsis and glandular activity.
c. Autonomic plexuses: cardiac, pulmonary, celiac (solar), hypogastric, pelvic.
d. Modulated by brain centers.
(1) Descending autonomic system: arises from control centers in hypothalamus and lower brainstem (cardiac, respiratory, vasomotor) and projects to preganglionic ANS segments in thoracolumbar (sympathetic) and craniosacral (parasympathetic) segments.
(2) Cranial nerves: visceral afferent sensations via glossopharyngeal and vagus nerves; efferent outflow via oculomotor, facial, glossopharyngeal, and vagus nerves.

CNS Support Structures

1. Bony structure.
a. Skull (cranium): rigid bony chamber that contains the brain and facial skeleton, with an opening (foramen magnum) at its base.

2. Meninges. Three membranes that envelop the brain.
a. Dura mater: outer, tough, fibrous membrane attached to inner surface of cranium; forms falx and tentorium.
b. Arachnoid: delicate, vascular membrane.
c. Subarachnoid space: formed by arachnoid and pia mater, contains cerebrospinal fluid (CSF) and cisterns, major arteries.
d. Pia mater: thin, vascular membrane that covers the brain surface; forms tela choroidea of ventricles.

3. Ventricles.
a. Four cavities or ventricles that are filled with CSF and communicate with each other and with the spinal cord canal.
b. Lateral ventricles: large, irregularly shaped with anterior (frontal), posterior (occipital), and inferior (temporal) horns; communicates with third ventricle through foramen of Monro.
c. Third ventricle: located posterior and deep between the two thalami; cerebral aqueduct communicates third ventricle with fourth ventricle.
d. Fourth ventricle: pyramid-shaped cavity located in pons and medulla; foramina (openings) of Luschka and Magendie communicate fourth ventricle with subarachnoid space.

4. CSF.
a. Provides mechanical support (cushions brain), controls brain excitability by regulating ionic composition, aids in exchange of nutrients and waste products.
b. Produced in choroid plexuses in ventricles.
c. Normal pressure: 70–200 mm H_2O.
d. Appearance: clear, colorless.

5. Blood-brain barrier.
a. Selective restriction of blood-borne substances from entering the CNS.
b. Associated with capillary endothelial cells.

6. Blood supply.
a. Brain is 2% of body weight with a circulation of 18% of total blood volume.
b. Carotid system: internal carotid arteries arise off of common carotids and branch to form anterior and middle cerebral arteries; supplies a large area of brain and many deep structures.
c. Vertebrobasilar system: vertebral arteries arise off of subclavian arteries and unite to form the basilar artery; this vessel bifurcates into two posterior cerebral arteries; supplies the brainstem, cerebellum, occipital lobe, and parts of thalamus.
d. Circle of Willis: formed by anterior communicating artery, connecting the two anterior cerebral arteries and the posterior communicating artery, connecting each posterior and middle cerebral artery.
e. Venous drainage: includes cerebral veins and dural venous sinuses.
f. See Neurological Dysfunction, Cerebrovascular Accident for a discussion of specific stroke syndromes (characteristic signs and symptoms associated with occlusion of specific cerebral vessels).

Neurons

1. Structure.

a. Neurons vary in size and complexity.
   (1) Cell bodies (genetic center) with dendrites (receptive surface area to receive information via synapses).
   (2) Axons conduct impulses away from the cell body (one-way conduction).
   (3) Synapses allow communication between neurons; chemical neurotransmitters are released (chemical synapses) or electrical signals pass directly from cell to cell (electrical synapses).

b. Neuron groupings and types.
   (1) Nuclei are compact groups of nerve cell bodies; in the peripheral nervous system, these groups are called ganglia.
   (2) Projection neurons carry impulses to other parts of the CNS.
   (3) Interneurons are short relay neurons.
   (4) Axon bundles are called tracts or fasciculi; in the spinal cord, collections of tracts are called columns or funiculi.

c. Neuroglia: support cells that do not transmit signals; important for myelin and neuron production; maintenance of K^+ levels and reuptake of neurotransmitters after neural transmission at synapses.

2. Function. Neuronal signaling.

a. Resting membrane potential: positive on outside, negative on inside (about –70 mV).

b. Action potential: increased permeability of Na^+ and influx into cell with outflow of K^+ results in polarity changes (inside to about +35 mV) and depolarization; generation of an action potential is all-or-none.

c. Conduction velocity is proportional to axon diameter; the largest myelinated fibers conduct the fastest.

d. Repolarization results from activation of K^+ channels.

e. Myelinated axons: many axons are covered with myelin with small gaps (nodes of Ranvier) where myelin is absent; the action potential jumps from one node to the next, termed *saltatory conduction*; myelin functions to increase speed of conduction and conserve energy.

f. Nerve fiber types.
   (1) A fibers: large, myelinated, fast-conducting.
      (a) Alpha: proprioception, somatic motor.
      (b) Beta: touch, pressure.
      (c) Gamma: motor to muscle spindles.
      (d) Delta: pain, temperature, touch.
   (2) B fibers: small, myelinated, conduct less rapidly; preganglionic autonomic.
   (3) C fibers: smallest, unmyelinated, slowest conducting.
      (a) Dorsal root: pain, reflex responses.
      (b) Sympathetic: postganglionic sympathetics.

Peripheral Nervous System

1. Peripheral nerves (lower motor neurons, LMNs).

a. Motor (efferent) fibers originate from motor nuclei (cranial nerves) or anterior horn cells (spinal nerves).

b. Sensory (afferent) fibers originate in cells outside of brainstem or spinal cord with sensory ganglia (cranial nerves) or dorsal root ganglia (spinal nerves).

c. Autonomic nervous system fibers: sympathetic fibers at thoracolumbar spinal segments and parasympathetic fibers at craniosacral segments.

2. Cranial nerves (CN).

a. Twelve pairs of cranial nerves; all nerves are distributed to the head and neck, except CN X, which is distributed to the thorax and abdomen (Table 2-1).

b. CN I, II, and VIII are pure sensory, carry special senses of smell, vision, hearing, and equilibrium.

c. CN III, IV, and VI are pure motor, controlling eye movements and pupillary constriction.

d. CN XI and XII are pure motor, innervating sternocleidomastoid, trapezius, and tongue.

e. CN V, VII, IX, and X are mixed motor and sensory; involved in chewing (V), facial expression (VII), swallowing (IX, X), vocal sounds (X); sensations from head (V, VII, IX), alimentary tract, heart, vessels, and lungs (IX, X), and taste (VII, IX, X).

f. CN III, VII, IX, and X carry parasympathetic fibers of ANS; involved in control of smooth muscles of inner eye (III); salivatory and lacrimal glands (VII); parotid gland (IX); muscles of heart, lung, and bowel (X).

3. Spinal nerves.

a. 31 pairs of spinal nerves; spinal nerves are divided into groups (8 cervical, 12 thoracic, 5 lumbar, 5 sacral, and 1 coccygeal) and correspond to vertebral segments; each has a ventral root and a dorsal root.

b. Ventral (anterior) root: efferent (motor) fibers to voluntary muscles (alpha motor neurons, gamma motor neurons), and to viscera, glands, and smooth muscles (preganglionic ANS fibers).

c. Dorsal (posterior) root: afferent (sensory) fibers from sensory receptors from skin, joints, and muscles; each dorsal root possesses a dorsal root ganglion (cell bodies of sensory neurons); there is no dorsal root for C1.

d. The term *dermatome* refers to a specific segmental skin area innervated by sensory spinal axons; the term *myotome* refers to the skeletal muscles innervated by motor axons in a given spinal root. A motor unit consists of the alpha motor neurons and the muscle fibers it innervates.

e. Nerve roots exit from the vertebral column through the intervertebral foramina.

Table 2-1 ➤ EXAMINATION OF CRANIAL NERVE INTEGRITY

NERVE	FUNCTION	TEST	POSSIBLE ABNORMAL FINDINGS
I Olfactory	Smell	Test sense of smell on each side: use common, nonirritating odors; close off other nostril	Anosmia (inability to detect smells), seen with frontal lobe lesions
II Optic	Vision	Test visual acuity	Blindness, myopia (impaired far vision); presbyopia (impaired near vision)
		Central: Snellen eye chart; test each eye separately by covering other eye; test at distance of 20 feet	
		Visual fields: test peripheral vision by confrontation	Visual field defects: (homonymous hemianopsia)
II, III Optic and Oculomotor	Pupillary reflexes	Test pupillary reactions (constriction) by shining light in eye; if abnormal, test near reaction	Absence of pupillary constriction
		Examine pupillary size/shape	Anisocoria (unequal pupils); Horner's syndrome, CN III paralysis
III, IV, VI Oculomotor, Trochlear, and Abducens	Extraocular movements	Test extraocular movements in each of six directions	Strabismus (eye deviates from normal conjugate position). Impaired eye movements
	CN III: turns eye up, down, in	Observe position of eye	Strabismus: eye pulled outward by CN VI; eye cannot look upward, downward, inward movements
	Elevates eyelid	Test pursuit eye movement	May see ptosis, pupillary dilation
	CN IV: turns adducted eye down	Test pursuit eye movement	Eye cannot look down when eye is adducted
	CN VI: turns eye out	Observe position of eye	Esotropia (eye pulled inward)
		Test pursuit eye movement	Eye cannot look out
V Trigeminal	Sensory: face	Test pain, light touch sensations: forehead, cheeks, jaw (eyes closed)	Loss of facial sensations, numbness with CN V lesion
	Sensory: cornea	Test corneal reflex: touch lightly with wisp of cotton	Loss of corneal reflex ipsilaterally (blinking in response to corneal touch)
	Motor: temporal and masseter muscles	Palpate muscles; have patient clench teeth, hold against resistance	Weakness, wasting of muscles of mastication
			Deviation of jaw when opened to ipsilateral side
VII Facial	Facial expression	Test motor function facial muscles: raise eyebrows, frown, show teeth, smile, close eyes tightly, puff out both cheeks	Paralysis ipsilateral facial muscles: inability to close eye, droop in corner of mouth, difficulty with speech articulation; PNI CN VII Bell's palsy; CNS facial paralysis stroke
VIII Vestibulocochlear (Acoustic)	Vestibular function	Test balance: vestibulospinal function	Vertigo, dysequilibrium
	Test eye-head coordination: vestibular ocular reflex (VOR)	Gaze instability with head rotations	Nystagmus (constant, involuntary cyclical movement of the eyeball)
	Cochlear function	Test auditory acuity	Deafness, impaired hearing, tinnitus
		Test for lateralization (Weber's test): place vibrating tuning fork on top of head, mid position; check if sound heard in one ear, or equally in both	Unilateral conductive loss: sound lateralized to impaired ear
			Sensorineural loss: sound heard in good ear
		Compare air and bone conduction (Rinne's test): place vibrating tuning fork on mastoid bone, then close to ear canal; sound heard longer through air than bone	Conductive loss: sound heard through bone is equal to or longer than air
			Sensorineural loss: sound heard longer through air
IX/X Glossopharyngeal and Vagus	Phonation	Listen to voice quality	Dysphonia: hoarseness denotes vocal cord paralysis; nasal quality denotes palatal weakness
	Swallowing	Examine for difficulty in swallowing	Dysphagia

Table 2-1 ➤ EXAMINATION OF CRANIAL NERVE INTEGRITY (continued)

NERVE	FUNCTION	TEST	POSSIBLE ABNORMAL FINDINGS
IX/X Glossopharyngeal and Vagus	Palatal, pharynx control	Have patient say "ah"; observe motion of soft palate (elevates) and position of uvula (remains midline)	Paralysis: palate fails to elevate (lesion of CN X); Asymmetrical elevation: unilateral paralysis
	Gag reflex	Stimulate back of throat lightly on each side	Absent reflex: lesion of CN IX; possibly CN X
XI Spinal Accessory	Muscle function	Examine bulk, strength	Atrophy, fasciculations, weakness (PNI):
	Trapezius muscle		Inability to shrug ipsilateral shoulder; shoulder droops
	Sternoclei-domastoid	Shrug both shoulders upward against resistance	Inability to turn head to opposite side
		Turn head to each side against resistance	
XII Hypoglossal	Tongue movements	Listen to patient's articulation	Dysarthria (lesions of CN X or CN XII)
		Examine resting position of tongue	Atrophy or fasciculations of tongue
		Examine tongue movements (move side-to-side, protrude)	Impaired movements, deviation to weak side on protrusion

(1) In the cervical spine, numbered roots exit horizontally above the corresponding vertebral body, with C8 exiting below C7 and above T1.

(2) In the thoracic, lumbar, and sacral segments, the roots exit below the corresponding vertebral body.

(3) Spinal cord ends at the level of L1; in the lumbosacral region, the nerve roots descend almost vertically below the cord to form the cauda equina (horse's tail).

f. After emerging from the intervertebral foramen, each spinal nerve divides into a large anterior ramus (supplying the muscles and skin of the anterolateral body wall and limbs) and a small posterior ramus (supplying the muscles and skin of the back); each ramus contains motor and sensory fibers.

g. The anterior rami join at the root of the limbs to form nerve plexuses. The cervical and brachial plexuses are at the root of the upper limbs; the lumbar and sacral plexuses are at the root of the lower limbs.

(1) The cervical plexus arises from C1 through C4 nerve roots. The brachial plexus arises from C5 through T1 nerve roots that split into anterior and posterior divisions, redistributing fibers into three cords (lateral, posterior, and medial) and finally into the peripheral nerves that supply the upper extremity.

(2) The lumbar plexus arises from T12 through L4 nerve roots. The sacral plexus arises from L4 through S3 nerve roots. Nerve fibers from both are redistributed into the peripheral nerves that supply the lower extremity.

(3) Refer to Tables 1-6 and 1-7 for specific cord segments, nerves, and muscles innervated.

Spinal Level Reflexes

Involuntary responses to stimuli; basic, specific, and predictable; dependent on intact neural pathway (reflex arc); reflexes may be monosynaptic or polysynaptic (involving interneurons); provides basis for unconscious motor function and basic defense mechanisms.

1. **Stretch (myotatic) reflexes.**
   a. Stimulus: muscle stretch.
   b. Reflex arc: afferent Ia fiber from muscle spindle to alpha motor neurons projecting back to muscle of origin (monosynaptic).
   c. Functions for maintenance of muscle tone, support agonist muscle contraction, and to provide feedback about muscle length.
   d. Clinically, sensitivity of the stretch reflex and intactness of spinal cord segment are tested by applying stretch to the deep tendons.
   e. Reciprocal inhibition: via an inhibitory interneuron, the same stretch stimulus inhibits the antagonist muscle.
   f. Reciprocal innervation: describes the effects of a stretch stimulus on agonist (autogenic facilitation), antagonist (reciprocal inhibition), and synergistic muscles (facilitation).

2. **Inverse stretch (myotatic) reflex.**
   a. Stimulus: muscle contraction.
   b. Reflex arc: afferent Ib fiber from Golgi tendon organ via inhibitory interneuron to muscle of origin (polysynaptic).
   c. Functions to provide agonist inhibition, diminution of force of agonist contraction, stretch-protection reflex.

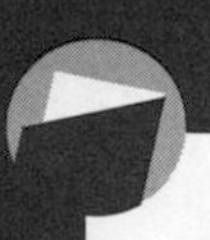

3. Gamma reflex loop.
   a. Stretch reflex forms part of this loop.
   b. Allows muscle tension to come under control of descending pathways (reticulospinal, vestibulospinal, and others).
   c. Descending pathways excite gamma motor neurons, causing contraction of muscle spindle, and in turn increased stretch sensitivity and increased rate of firing from spindle afferents; impulses are then conveyed to alpha motor neurons.

4. Flexor (withdrawal) reflex.
   a. Stimulus: cutaneous sensory stimuli.
   b. Reflex arc: cutaneous receptors via interneurons to largely flexor muscles; multisegmental response involving groups of muscles (polysynaptic).
   c. Functions as a protective withdrawal mechanism to remove body part from harmful stimuli.

5. Crossed extension reflex.
   a. Stimulus: noxious stimuli and reciprocal action of antagonists; flexors of one side are excited, causing extensors on same side to be inhibited; opposite responses occur in opposite limb.
   b. Reflex arc: cutaneous and muscle receptors diverging to many spinal cord motor neurons on same and opposite side (polysynaptic).
   c. Function: coordinates reciprocal limb activities such as gait.

Neurological Examination: History, Systems Review, Tests, and Measures

Patient Interview

1. **Presenting symptoms.** Onset, progression, nature of symptoms, patient's insight into medical condition.

2. **Past medical history.** Other diagnoses, surgeries, health factors.

3. **Social history.** Current living situation, family/social support, education level, employment, lifestyle, risk factors.

Examine Level of Consciousness

1. Determine orientation to person, place, and time (oriented × 3).

2. Determine response to stimuli.
   a. Purposeful, nonpurposeful, no response.
   b. Verbal, tactile, simple commands.
   c. Painful stimuli: pinch, pinprick.

3. Determine level of consciousness (arousal).
   a. Alertness: alert patient responds appropriately; can open eyes, look at examiner, respond fully and appropriately to stimuli.
   b. Lethargy: patient appears drowsy; can open eyes and look at examiner, respond to questions, but falls asleep easily.
   c. Obtundation: patient can open eyes, look at examiner, but responds slowly and is confused; demonstrates decreased alertness and interest in environment.
   d. Stupor: patient can be aroused from sleep only with painful stimuli; verbal responses are slow or absent; patient returns to unresponsive state when stimuli are removed; demonstrates minimal awareness of self and environment.
   e. Coma: patient cannot be aroused, eyes remain closed; no response to external stimuli or environment.

4. Glasgow Coma Scale (GCS) (Teasdale and Jennette, 1974).
   a. Relates consciousness to three elements of response: eye opening, motor response, and verbal response.
   b. Scoring range from 3–15: severe brain injury (scores of 1–8); moderate brain injury (scores of 9–12); minor brain injury (scores of 13–15).
   c. Coma: a state defined by no eye opening, even to pain; failure to obey commands; and inability to speak with recognizable words.
   d. Unresponsive vigilance (vegetative) state: a state characterized by the return of sleep/wake cycles, normalization of vegetative functions (respiration, heart rate, blood pressure, digestion), and lack of cognitive responsiveness (can be aroused but is unaware).

Examine Cognitive Function

1. Memory.
   a. Immediate recall: name three items previously presented after a brief interval (i.e., 5 minutes).
   b. Recent memory (short-term): recall of recent events (i.e., What did you have for breakfast?)
   c. Remote memory (long-term): recall of past events (i.e., Where were you born? Where did you grow up?)

2. **Attention.**
   a. Length of attention span: digit span retention test (i.e., recall of up to seven numbers in order presented).
   b. Ability to attend to task without redirection (sustained attention); determine time on task, frequency of redirection.
   c. Ability to shift attention from one task to another (divided attention); assess ability of dual task control; assess also for perseveration (mental inertia): getting stuck on a task.
   d. Ability to stay on task in presence of detractors (focused attention); assess impact of environmental versus internal detractors.
   e. Ability to follow commands: one- or two-step, multilevel commands.

3. **Emotional responses/behaviors.**
   a. Safety, judgment: impulsivity and lack of inhibition.
   b. Affect, mood: irritability, agitation, depression, and withdrawal.
   c. Frustration tolerance.
   d. Self-centeredness (egocentricity).
   e. Insight into disability.
   f. Ability to follow rules of social conduct.
   g. Ability to tolerate criticism.

4. **Higher level cognitive abilities.**
   a. Judgment, problem solving.
   b. Abstract reasoning.
   c. Fund of general knowledge: current events, ability to learn new information, generalize learning to new situations.
   d. Calculation: serial 7 test (count backward from 100 by 7s).
   e. Sequencing: ability to order components of cognitive or functional task; assess if cueing is necessary, frequency of cues.

5. **Mini-mental status examination (MMSE)** (Folstein, Flostein, and McHugh, 1975).
   a. Brief screening test for cognitive dysfunction.
   b. Includes screening items for orientation, registration, attention and calculation, recall, and language.
   c. Maximum score is 30; 21–24 indicates mild cognitive impairment, 16–20 indicates moderate impairment, and 15 or less indicates severe impairment.

6. **Cognitive scale: Rancho Los Amigos Levels of Cognitive Function (LOCF)** (Hagen et al., 1979).
   a. Assesses cognitive recovery from traumatic brain injury (TBI).
   b. Includes eight levels of behavior: No Response (I), decreased response levels (II and III), confused levels (IV, V, and VI), appropriate (automatic, purposeful) levels (VII and VIII).
   c. Delineates emerging behaviors; patients may plateau at any level.

Examine Speech and Communication

1. **Expressive function.**
   a. Examine fluency of speech, speech production.
   b. Nonfluent aphasia (Broca's motor aphasia, expressive aphasia).
      (1) A central language disorder in which speech is typically awkward, restricted, interrupted, and produced with effort.
      (2) The result of a lesion involving the third frontal convolution of the left hemisphere (Broca's area).
   c. Verbal apraxia: impairment of volitional articulatory control secondary to a cortical, dominant hemisphere lesion.
   d. Dysarthria: impairment of speech production in the CNS/PNS mechanisms that control respiration, articulation, phonation, and movements of jaw and tongue.

2. **Receptive function.**
   a. Examine comprehension.
   b. Fluent aphasia (Wernicke's aphasia, receptive aphasia).
      (1) A central language disorder in which spontaneous speech is preserved and flows smoothly, while auditory comprehension is impaired.
   c. The result of a lesion in the posterior first temporal gyrus of the left hemisphere (Wernicke's area).

3. **Global aphasia.**
   a. Severe aphasia.
   b. Examine for marked impairments in comprehension and production of language.

4. **Nonverbal communication.**
   a. Examine ability to read and write.
   b. Use of gestures, symbols, and pictographs.

Examine Cranial Nerves

See Table 2-1, Examination of Cranial Nerve Intergrity.

Examine Vital Signs

1. **Determine heart rate (HR), blood pressure (BP).**
   a. Examine for any irregularities in pulse: bounding, thready (fine, barely perceptible).
   b. Examine for decrease or increase in BP: hypertension ≥140 mm Hg systolic blood pressure (SBP), ≥90 mm Hg diastolic blood pressure (DBP).
   c. Examine for changes in response to activity: normally, HR increases in direct proportion to intensity of exercise; SBP increases, while DBP remains the same or decreases moderately (a widening of pulse pressure).
   d. With increasing intracranial pressures, examine for changes in HR and BP that occur late.

CHAPTER 2

2. **Examine respiratory rate (RR), depth, rhythm, and characteristics of inspiratory and expiratory phases.**
   a. Cheyne-Stokes respiration: a period of apnea lasting 10–60 seconds followed by gradually increasing depth and frequency of respirations; accompanies depression of frontal lobe and diencephalic dysfunction.
   b. Hyperventilation: increased rate and depth of respirations; accompanies dysfunction of lower midbrain and pons.
   c. Apneustic breathing: abnormal respiration marked by prolonged inspiration; accompanies damage to upper pons.
3. **Examine temperature.**
   a. Elevation may indicate infection, damage to hypothalamus or brainstem.

Examine for CNS Infection or Meningeal Irritation

1. **Signs are global, not focal.**
2. **Neck mobility.**
   a. Patient is positioned in supine, flex neck to chest.
   b. Positive sign: neck pain in the neck, with limitation and guarding of head flexion due to spasm of posterior neck muscles; can result from meningeal inflammation, arthritis, or neck injury.
3. **Kernig's sign.**
   a. Patient is positioned in supine; flex hip and knee fully to chest, and then extend knee.
   b. Positive sign: causes pain and increased resistance to extending the knee due to spasm of hamstring; when bilateral, suggests meningeal irritation.
4. **Brudzinski's sign.**
   a. Patient is positioned in supine; flex neck to chest.
   b. Positive sign: causes flexion of hips and knees (drawing up); suggests meningeal irritation.
5. **Irritability.**
   a. Examine for photophobia, disorientation, restlessness.
6. **Slowed mental function.**
   a. Examine for persistent headache, increased in head-down position.
   b. May progress to delirium, lethargy, and coma.
7. **Altered vital signs.**
   a. Examine for increased HR and RR, fever; fluctuating BP.
8. **Generalized weakness.**

Examine for Increased Intracranial Pressure Secondary to Cerebral Edema and Brain Herniation

1. **Altered level of consciousness.**
   a. Progresses from restlessness and confusion to decreasing level of consciousness, unresponsiveness, and coma.
2. **Altered vital signs.**
   a. Examine for increased BP; widening pulse pressure and slowing of pulse; irregular respirations including periods of apnea, Cheyne-Stokes respirations; elevated temperature.
3. **Headache.**
4. **Vomiting.**
   a. Secondary to irritation of vagal nuclei, CN X.
5. **Pupillary changes (CN III signs).**
   a. Examine for ipsilateral dilation of pupil (unequal pupils), slowed reaction to light progressing to fixed, dilated pupils (a poor prognostic sign).
6. **Papilledema at entrance to eye.**
7. **Progressive impairment of motor function.**
   a. Examine for weakness, hemiplegia, positive Babinski's response, decorticate or decerebrate rigidity.
8. **Seizure activity.**

Examine Autonomic Nervous System Function (Table 2-2)

Table 2-2 ➤ AUTONOMIC NERVOUS SYSTEM FUNCTIONS

SYMPATHETIC NERVOUS SYSTEM	PARASYMPATHETIC NERVOUS SYSTEM
Activated in stressful situations, producing an arousal reaction (fight or flight)	Results in conservation and restoration of body energy and homeostasis (system balance)
Effects are widespread	Effects are localized and short-acting
Dilates pupils (mydriasis)	Constricts pupils
Increases heart rate and force of contraction	Decreases force of contraction
Breaks down glycogen into glucose Increases blood sugar level Increases blood flow in skeletal muscles Constricts blood flow to skin and abdomen	
Increases blood pressure and peripheral vascular resistance	Decreases blood pressure
Dilates bronchi for maximum respiratory flow	Constricts bronchi
Constricts bronchial arteries	Dilates bronchial arteries
Stimulates cortex and medulla; produces hyperalertness	
Decreases peristalsis, intestinal motility	Increases peristalsis, intestinal motility
Increases sweating	
Reduces glandular secretions	Increases glandular secretions

Examine Sensory Function

1. **Subjective.**
   a. Ask patient to describe (map out areas) where sensation does not feel normal; provide sensory clues.

2. **Topographical organization.**
   a. Use sensory dermatome chart.

3. **Testing considerations.**
   a. Document key sensory systems: test superficial and proprioceptive sensations first, then combined (cortical) sensations.
   b. Ensure that patient comprehends instructions and can communicate responses.
   c. Occlude vision: consider barrier method (use a piece of paper to block vision) versus blindfolding the patient.
   d. Apply stimulus in random, unpredictable order; avoid summation.
   e. To assess responses, always pose a choice (e.g., hot or cold).
   f. Examine for objective manifestations: withdrawal, wincing, blinking.
   g. Consider skin condition (calluses, scars) for areas of desensitivity.
   h. Look for signs of repetitive trauma, skin lesions.

4. **Evaluation and documentation.**
   a. Determine if the patient can readily distinguish one sensation from another.
   b. Determine the sensory threshold, the lightest stimulus perceived.
   c. Determine the degree and location of deficits (dermatome mapping).
   d. Determine the patient's subjective feelings, level of awareness of sensory losses.
   e. Determine functional impact of sensory losses.

Examine Perceptual Function

1. **Testing considerations.**
   a. Suspect perceptual dysfunction if patient has difficulty with functional mobility skills or activities of daily living for reasons that cannot be accounted for by specific sensory, motor, or comprehension deficits.
   b. Rule out specific sensory and motor loss, language impairment, hearing loss, or visual disturbance as cause of loss of function.
   c. Rule out psychological/emotional and cognitive factors.

2. **Test for homonymous hemianopsia.**
   a. Loss of half of visual field in each eye, contralateral to the side of a cerebral hemisphere lesion.
   b. Slowly bring two fingers from behind head into the patient's visual field while asking the patient to gaze straight ahead; the patient indicates when and where the fingers first appear.

3. **Examine for body scheme/body image disorders.**
   a. Body scheme disorder (somatognosia): have patient identify body parts or their relationship to each other.
   b. Visual spatial neglect (unilateral neglect): determine whether patient ignores one side of the body and stimuli coming from that side.

Table 2-3 ➤ EXAMINATION OF SENSORY INTEGRITY

Test Superficial Sensations	
Pain	Test sharp/dull sensation in response to sharp/dull stimuli with paper clip
Temperature	Test hot/cold sensation in response to hot/cold stimuli with test tubes filled with hot or cold water
Touch	Test touch/nontouch in response to slight touch stimulus (cotton ball) or no touch
Test Proprioceptive (deep) Sensations	
Joint position sense:	Test ability to perceive joint position at rest in response to your positioning the patient's limb (up or down, in or out)
Kinesthesia (movement sense)	Test ability to perceive movement in response to your moving the patient's limb; patient can duplicate movement with opposite limb or give a verbal report
Vibration sense (pallesthesia)	Test proprioceptive pathways by applying vibrating tuning fork or pressure only (sham vibration) on bony areas
Test Combined (Cortical) Sensations	Use a sample of two or three from this group
Stereognosis	Test ability to identify familiar objects placed in the by manipulation and touch
Tactile localization	Test ability to identify location of a touch stimulus on the body by verbal report or pointing
Two-point discrimination	Test ability to recognize one or two blunt points applied to the skin simultaneously; determine minimal distance on skin where two points can still be distinguished in millimeters using an aesthesiometer (the two tips must be applied simultaneously)
Barognosis	Test ability to identify similar size/shaped objects placed in the hand with different gradations of weight
Graphesthesia	Test ability to identify numbers, letters, or symbols traced on skin, typically the hand
Bilateral simultaneous stimulation	Test ability to identify simultaneous touch on the two sides/segments of the body

c. Right/left discrimination disorder: have patient identify right and left sides of his or her own body and your body.
d. Anosognosia: severe denial, neglect, or lack of awareness of severity of condition; determine whether patient shows severe impairments in neglect and body scheme.

4. Examine for spatial relations syndrome.
a. Figure-ground discrimination: have patient pick out an object from an array of objects (e.g., brake from rest of wheelchair).
b. Form constancy: have patient pick out an object from an array of similarly shaped but different-sized objects (e.g., large block from group of blocks).
c. Spatial relations: have patient duplicate a pattern of two or three blocks.
d. Position in space: have patient demonstrate different limb positions (e.g., put your arm overhead; put your foot underneath the chair).
e. Topographical disorientation: determine whether patient can navigate a familiar route on his or her own (e.g., travel from room to physical therapy clinic).
f. Depth and distance imperceptions: determine whether patient can judge depth and distance (e.g., navigate stairs, sit down into chair accurately).
g. Vertical disorientation: determine whether patient can accurately identify when something is upright (e.g., hold a cane, ask patient when it is vertical; ask patient to determine if own body is vertical).

5. Examine for agnosia.
a. The inability to recognize familiar objects with one sensory modality, while retaining the ability to recognize the same object with other sensory modalities.
b. The subject doesn't recognize an object (clock) by sight, but can recognize it by sound (ticking).

6. Examine for apraxia.
a. The inability to perform voluntary, learned movements in the absence of loss of sensation, strength, coordination, attention, or comprehension; represents a breakdown in the conceptual system, motor production system or both.
b. Ideomotor apraxia: patient cannot perform the task on command, but can do the task when left on own.
c. Ideational apraxia: patient cannot perform the task at all, either on command or on own.

Examine Motor Function

1. Examine muscle bulk, firmness.
a. Determine whether there is atrophy.
(1) Determine if atrophy is due to denervation, disuse, or primary atrophy.

Table 2-4 ➤ DIFFERENTIAL DIAGNOSIS: COMPARISON OF MAJOR TYPES OF CENTRAL NERVOUS SYSTEM DISORDERS

LOCATION OF LESION	CEREBRAL CORTEX CORTICOSPINAL TRACTS	BASAL GANGLIA: SUBCORTICAL GRAY	CEREBELLUM	SPINAL CORD
Disorder	Stroke	Parkinsonism	Cerebellar lesion: tumor, stroke	SCI: trauma, complete incomplete
Sensation	Impaired or absent, depending on lesion location; contralateral sensory loss	Not affected	Not affected	Impaired or absent below
Tone	Hypertonia/spasticity; clasp-knife phenomena present; spasticity is velocity-dependent; with cerebral shock, may see initial flaccidity	Leadpipe rigidity: uniform increased resistance to movement; cogwheel rigidity: rachet-like resistance to movement; rigidity is not velocity-dependent	Normal or may be decreased	Hypertonia/spasticity below the level of the lesion; initial flaccidity: spinal shock
Reflexes	Increased hyperreflexia	Normal or may be decreased	Normal or may be decreased	Increased hyperreflexia
Strength	Contralateral weakness or paralysis: hemiplegia	Slowness of movement	Normal or weak: asthenia	Impaired or absent below the level of the lesion: paraplegia or tetraplegia
Bulk	Normal: acute; disuse atrophy: chronic	Normal or disuse atrophy	Normal	Disuse atrophy
Involuntary Movements	Spasms	Resting tremor	None	Spasms
Voluntary Movements	Dyssynergic: abnormal timing, coactivation, activation, fatigability	Bradykinesia/akinesia slowness, lack of spontaneous and automatic movements	Ataxia: intention tremor dysdiadochokinesia, dysmetria, dyssynergia nystagmus	Intact: above level of lesion
Postural	Impaired or absent, depends on lesion location	Impaired: stooped	Impaired: truncal ataxia, dysequilibrium	Impaired below level of lesion
Gait	Impaired: gait deficits due to abnormal synergies, spasticity, timing deficits	Impaired: shuffling, festinating gait	Impaired: ataxic gait deficits, wide-based, unsteady	Impaired or absent: depends on level of lesion

Table 2-5 ➤ DIFFERENTIAL DIAGNOSIS: COMPARISON OF UPPER MOTOR NEURON (UMN) AND LOWER MOTOR NEURON (LMN) SYNDROMES

	UMN LESION	LMN LESION
Location of Lesion	Central nervous system	Peripheral nervous system
Structures Involved	Cortex, brainstem, corticospinal tracts, spinal cord	SC: anterior horn cell, spinal roots, peripheral nerves. CN: cranial nerves
Disorders	Stroke, traumatic brain injury, spinal cord injury	Polio, Guillain-Barré, PNI, peripheral neuropathy, radiculopathy
Tone	Increased: hypertonia Velocity-dependent	Decreased or absent: hypotonia, flaccidity Not velocity dependent
Reflexes	Increased: hyperreflexia, clonus Exaggerated cutaneous and autonomic reflexes: + Babinski response	Decreased or absent: hyporeflexia Cutaneous reflexes decreased or absent
Involuntary Movements	Muscle spasms: flexor or extensor	With denervation: fasciculations
Strength	Weakness or paralysis: ipsilateral (stroke) or bilateral (SCI) Corticospinal: contralateral if above decussation in medulla; Ipsilateral if below Distribution: never focal	Limited distribution: segmental or focal pattern, Root-innervated pattern
Muscle Bulk	Variable, disuse atrophy	Neurogenic atrophy; rapid, focal, severe wasting
Voluntary Movements	Impaired or absent: dyssynergic patterns, obligatory synergies	Weak or absent if nerve interrupted

(2) The presence of persistent fasciculations suggests neurogenic injury.
(3) Examine by inspection, palpation, and girth measurement.

b. Check muscle firmness, tenderness, and reactivity.

2. Examine muscle tone.

a. Use passive range of motion (PROM) to assess muscle stretch reflexes and responsiveness to passive elongation.

b. Flaccidity (absent tone), hypotonia (decreased tone).
(1) Seen in segmental/LMN lesions: nerve roots and peripheral nerve injury.
(2) Seen initially after suprasegmental/upper motor neuron (UMN) lesions (i.e., brief period of spinal shock in spinal cord injuries, cerebral shock in stroke). There is decreased or no resistance to PROM.

c. Spasticity (spastic hypertonia).
(1) Seen in suprasegmental/UMN lesions.
(2) There is increased resistance to PROM; determine whether increasing the speed increases the resistance (spasticity is velocity-dependent) (Table 2-6).
(3) Examine for additional signs of spastic hypertonia.
(a) Clasp-knife response: marked resistance to PROM suddenly gives way.
(b) Clonus: maintained stretch stimulus produces a cyclical, spasmodic contraction; common in plantar flexors, also seen in wrist flexors and jaw.
(c) Hyperactive cutaneous reflexes, positive Babinski's response: dorsiflexion of great toe with fanning of other toes in response to stroking up the lateral side of the sole of the foot; indicative of corticospinal (pyramidal) tract disruption.
(d) Hyperreflexia: increased deep tendon reflexes (DTRs).
(e) Some degree of muscle weakness is usually present.
(4) Modified Ashworth Scale: six grades are used for grading spasticity.
0—No increase in muscle tone.
1—Slight increase in muscle tone, minimal resistance at end of ROM.
1+—Slight increase in muscle tone, minimal resistance through less than half of ROM.
2—More marked increase in muscle tone, through most of ROM, affected part easily moved.
3—Considerable increase in muscle tone, passive movement difficult.
4—Affected part rigid in flexion or extension.

d. Rigidity: increased resistance to PROM that is independent of the velocity of movement.
(1) Rigidity seen in basal ganglia/nigrostriatal disorders: increased resistance to passive movement in agonist and antagonist muscle.
(2) Rigidity can be leadpipe (uniform throughout the range) or cogwheel (interrupted by a series of jerks).
(3) Associated with Parkinson's disease, resting tremor, bradykinesia; strength and reflexes are not affected.

e. Decerebrate rigidity/posturing.
(1) Seen in comatose patients with brainstem lesions between the superior colliculus and the vestibular nucleus.

Table 2-6 ➤ TYPICAL PATTERNS OF SPASTICITY IN UPPER MOTOR NEURON SYNDROME

UPPER LIMBS	ACTIONS	MUSCLES AFFECTED
Scapula	Retraction, downward rotation	Rhomboids
Shoulder	Adduction and internal rotation, depression	Pectoralis major, latissimus dorsi, teres major, subscapularis
Elbow	Flexion	Biceps, Brachialis, Brachioradialis
Forearm	Pronation	Pronator teres, Pronator quadratus
Wrist	Flexion, adduction	F. carpi radialis
Hand	Finger flexion, clenched fist Thumb adducted in palm	F. dig. profundus/sublimis, Add. pollicis brevis, F. pollicis brevis
LOWER LIMBS		
Pelvis	Retraction (hip hiking)	Quadratus lumborum
Hip	Adduction (scissoring) Internal rotation Extension	Add. longus/brevis Add. magnus, gracilis Gluteus maximus
Knee	Extension	Quadriceps
Foot & ankle	Plantarflexion Inversion Equinovarus Toes claw (MP ext., PIP flex, DIP ext.) Toes curl (PIP, DIP flex)	Gastrocsoleus Tibialis posterior Long toe flexors Ext. hallucis longus Peroneus longus
Hip & knee (prolonged sitting posture)	Flexion Sacral sitting	Iliopsoas Rectus femoris, pectineus Hamstrings
Trunk	Lateral flexion with concavity rotation	Rotators Internal/external obliques
COG forward (prolonged sitting posture)	Excessive forward flexion Forward head	Rectus abdominis, external obliques Psoas minor

The form and intensity of spasticity may vary greatly, depending upon the CNS lesion site and extent of damage. The degree of spasticity can fluctuate within each individual (i.e., due to body position, level of excitation, sensory stimulation, and voluntary effort). Spasticity predominates in antigravity muscles (i.e., the flexors of the upper extremity and the extensors of the lower extremity). If left untreated, spasticity can result in movement deficiencies, subsequent contractures, degenerative joint changes, and deformity.
Adapted from Mayer NH, Esquenazi A, Childers MK. Common patterns of clinical motor dysfunction. Muscle and Nerve 6:S21, 1997.

(2) Results in increased tone and sustained posturing of all limbs; trunk/ neck in rigid extension.

f. Decorticate rigidity/posturing
   (1) Seen in comatose patients with lesions above the superior colliculus.
   (2) Results in increased tone and sustained posturing of upper limbs in flexion and the lower limbs in extension.

g. Opisthotonos.
   (1) Prolonged, severe spasm of muscles, causing the head, back, and heels to arch backwards; arms and hands are held rigidly flexed.
   (2) Seen in severe meningitis, tetanus, epilepsy, and strychnine poisoning.

h. Use active ROM, active movement control to assess tone in automatic postural adjustments.
   (1) Check stiffness of limbs and trunk in maintaining posture against gravity.
   (2) Examine for abnormal movements: are movements restricted, are they performed with great effort, are there limitations in voluntary movements?

i. Evaluation and documentation.
   (1) Determine which body parts and joints have abnormal tone.
   (2) Determine if asymmetries exist, upper extremities versus lower extremities, axial (trunk) versus appendicular (limbs), distal versus proximal.
   (3) Describe the character of the resistance (e.g., velocity-dependent versus uniform, clasp-knife, leadpipe, cogwheel).
   (4) Describe the effects of tone on active movement, upright posture.

3. Examine reflexes. (See Table 2-7).

a. Categories of reflexes
   (1) Deep Tendon Reflexes: normally occurring reflexes in response to stretch of muscle.

Table 2-7 ➤ EXAMINATION OF REFLEXES

Deep Tendon Reflexes (DTRs)	Tap directly on tendon: stretch stimulus produces contraction of agonist muscle with corresponding quick movement Reflexes commonly tested: jaw reflex, trigeminal CN V; biceps, C5-C6; triceps, C7-C8; brachioradialis, C5-C6; hamstrings, L5-S3; quadriceps (knee jerk, patellar), L2-4; Achilles (ankle jerk), S1-2 Scoring: 0 absent reflex; 1+ decreased response; 2+ normal response; 3+ exaggerated; 4+ hyperactive DTRs: may be abnormal in CNS lesions (hyporeflexia, hyperreflexia) or PNS lesions (hyporeflexia)
Superficial Cutaneous Reflexes	
Plantar Reflex (S1-2, tibial nerve):	Stroking of the lateral sole of foot from calcaneus to base of fifth metatarsal and medially across metatarsal heads plantar flexion of toes produces plantar flexion of the toes Occurs in neurologically intact individual
Positive Babinski Response	Stroking of the lateral sole of foot from calcaneus to base of fifth metatarsal and medially across metatarsal heads produces dorsiflexion of the great toe and fanning (abduction) of the four lesser toes Seen in patients with corticospinal lesions
Abdominal Reflexes (T6-L1)	Lateral to medial scratching of skin (toward umbilicus) in each of four quadrants produces deviation of the umbilicus toward the stimulus Occurs in neurologically intact individual Loss of abdominal reflexes is a sign of corticospinal lesions
Cremasteric Reflex (L1-L2)	Stroking of skin of the proximal and medial thigh produces elevation of the testicle (neurologically intact individuals) Absent in spinal cord injury and corticospinal lesions
Primitive/spinal Reflexes	Present developmentally in normal infants (see Chapter 7) and in some patients with brain injury
Flexor Withdrawal	Noxious stimulus (pinprick) to sole of foot produces toe extension, dorsiflexion of the foot and flexion of entire LE
Crossed Extension	Noxious stimulus to ball of foot produces rigid extension of that LE with flexion of the opposite LE
Traction	Stretch stimulus from grasping the forearm and pulling produces total flexion response of the UE
Grasp	Maintained pressure to palm of hand (palmar grasp) or ball of foot (plantar grasp) produces maintained flexion of fingers or toes
Tonic/Brainstem Reflexes	Present developmentally in normal infants (see Chapter 7) and in some patients with brain injury
Asymmetrical Tonic Neck (ATNR)	Rotation of the head to one side produces flexion of the skull limbs and extension of the jaw limbs
Symmetrical Tonic Neck (STNR)	Flexion of the head produces flexion of the UEs with extension of the LEs Extension of the head produces extension of the UEs and flexion of the LEs
Positive Supporting	Contact to the ball of the foot in the standing position produces rigid extension (co-contraction) of the LEs
Associated Reactions	Strong voluntary movement in one body segment produces involuntary movement in another resting extremity

LE = lower extremity; UE = upper extremity

(2) Superficial cutaneous reflexes: normally occurring reflexes in response to noxious stimulus (light scratch) applied to skin.
(3) Primitive spinal reflexes.
(4) Midbrain/cortical reactions.

b. Reflex Scoring Scale (Capute) for primitive/spinal and tonic/brainstem reflexes:
0 absent.
1+ Tone change; no visible movement of extremities.
2+ Visible movement of extremities.
3+ Exaggerated, full movement of extremities.
4+ Obligatory and sustained movement, lasting for >30 seconds.

4. Examine muscle performance. Strength, power, and endurance.

a. Determine/document: relative strength/peak power, ability to initiate/accelerate contraction, control torque output at varying speeds.

b. Methods: patient's self-report, manual muscle test (MMT), dynamometry, muscle performance tests, physical capacity tests, technology-assisted analyses, timed activity tests.

c. Observe muscle strength, power, and endurance during functional activities (e.g., basic and instrumental activities of daily living, functional mobility skills).

d. Decreased strength: paresis (weakness) or paralysis (loss of voluntary motion).
(1) Cerebrovascular accident: hemiparesis or hemiplegia.
(2) Spinal cord injury: paraplegia or tetraplegia (quadriplegia).
(3) Traumatic brain injury: any level or degree possible.

e. Clinical issues with strength testing (standard MMT): patients with CNS, UMN lesions.
(1) Passive restraint: soft tissue changes restrict ability to move (e.g., contractures).

(2) Active restraint: spastic muscles restrict ability to move.
(3) Abnormal synergistic activity, inappropriate coactivation of muscles.
(4) Recruitment problems: abnormal type II fiber recruitment.
(5) Abnormal reflex activity: restricts ability to move.
(6) Isokinetic dynamometry: patients with UMN syndrome (i.e., stroke) typically demonstrate decreased torque development with increased problems at higher speeds, decreased limb excursion, extended time to peak torque development, extended time peak torque held, increased time intervals between reciprocal contractions, and changes on "supposedly normal" extremities.

f. Clinical issues with strength testing: patients with PNS, LMN lesions.
(1) With myopathies: see proximal weakness of extremities.
(2) With neuropathies: see distal weakness of extremities.
(3) Some conditions produce decremental strength losses (e.g., myasthenia gravis).

5. Examine for fatigue.

a. Fatigue is the failure to generate the required or expected force during sustained or repeated contractions.
(1) Fatigue is protective: guards against overwork and injury.
(2) Fatigue is task-dependent.
(3) Sources of fatigue.
(a) CNS/central fatigue: seen in multiple sclerosis, amyotrophic lateral sclerosis, chronic fatigue syndrome.
(b) Neural/myoneural junction: seen in multiple sclerosis, postpolio syndrome, Guillain-Barré syndrome, myasthenia gravis.
(c) Muscle contractile failure: metabolic changes at the level of the muscle (e.g., depleted Ca^{2+} stores) seen in muscular dystrophy.

b. Determine/document.
(1) Source of fatigue.
(2) Frequency and severity of fatigue episodes.
(3) Threshold for fatigue: level of exercise that cannot be sustained indefinitely.
(a) Onset is typically gradual, not abrupt.
(b) Dependent on the intensity and duration of activity attempted.
(4) Factors that influence fatigue: health status, environmental temperature, stress.
(5) Level of functional performance: independence, modified dependence, dependence, level of assistance, assistive devices.
(6) Episodes of exhaustion: limit of endurance beyond which no further performance is possible.
(7) Overwork weakness or injury: prolonged decrease in absolute strength and endurance due to excessive activity of partially denervated muscle. Common in postpolio syndrome, Duchenne's muscular dystrophy.
(8) Test and measures.
(a) Modified Fatigue Impact Scale (MFIS): subjective scale that includes three subscales assessing the impact of fatigue on physical, cognitive, and psychosocial function.
(b) Isokinetic dynamometry, electromyography (EMG): can observe decrements in force production.

6. Examine voluntary movement control.

a. Determine/document.
(1) Quality (synergistic organization) of muscle activation patterns.
(2) Are movements appropriate and timely in response to stimulus or command?
(3) Able to vary easily type of contraction pattern (i.e., isometric, concentric, eccentric)?
(4) Are movements symmetrical?
(5) Adequate control of multiple body segments, postural stabilization?
(6) Assess for presence of abnormal synergy patterns: muscle synergistic patterns that are highly stereotyped and obligatory; commonly seen in UMN dysfunction (e.g., cerebrovascular accident, TBI) (Table 2-8).

7. Examine for presence of involuntary movements.

a. Extrapyramidal disorders, basal ganglia dysfunction.
(1) Tics: spasmodic contractions of specific muscles, commonly involving face, head, neck, or shoulder muscles.

Table 2-8 ➤ ABNORMAL SYNERGY PATTERNS OF THE EXTREMITIES SEEN IN PATIENTS FOLLOWING STROKE

UPPER EXTREMITY
Flexion synergy components: scapular retraction/elevation, shoulder abduction, external rotation, elbow flexion*, forearm supination, wrist and finger flexion* Extension synergy components: scapular protraction, shoulder adduction*, and internal rotation, elbow extension, forearm pronation, wrist and finger flexion.
LOWER EXTREMITY
Flexion synergy components: hip flexion, abduction, external-rotation, knee flexion, ankle dorsiflexion and inversion. Extension synergy components: hip extension, adduction*, internal rotation, knee extension*, ankle plantarflexion* and inversion. The form and intensity of abnormal synergy patterns may vary greatly, depending upon the CNS lesion site, extent of damage, and stage of recovery. Synergies can fluctuate due to body position (presence of reflexes), degree of spasticity, level of excitation, sensory stimulation, and voluntary effort.

*Generally the strongest components are starred.

(2) Chorea: relatively quick twitches or "dancing" movements.
(3) Athetosis: slow, irregular, twisting, sinuous movements, occurring especially in upper extremities.
(4) Tremor: continuous quivering movements; rhythmic, oscillatory movement observed at rest (resting tremor).
(5) Myoclonus: single, quick jerk.

b. Cerebellar disorders: intention tremor occurring when voluntary movement is attempted.
c. Cortical disorders: epileptic seizures, tonic/ clonic convulsive movements.
d. Determine/document.
(1) Are movements extraneous and spontaneous, apparently unintended?
(2) Part of body involved, orientation in space.
(3) Frequency, amplitude, pattern.
(4) Effect of triggering stimuli or changes in environment.
(5) Methods: patient's self-report, observation/ functional assessment, videotaped analysis.

8. Examine coordination.

a. Gross motor coordination: body posture, balance, and extremity movements involving large muscle groups.
(1) Upper extremity tests: unilateral (finger to nose); rapid alternating movements (RAM), supination/pronation; bilateral symmetrical movements (clapping, RAM), bilateral asymmetrical movements (alternate touch knee/shoulder), bilateral unrelated movements (knee pat/elbow extension).
(2) Lower extremity tests: unilateral (heel to shin, foot tapping); bilateral symmetrical (foot tapping, alternate knee flexion/extension); bilateral asymmetrical (alternate knee flexion/extension); bilateral unrelated movements (knee flexion/extension and hip abduction/adduction).
(3) Postural/trunk tests: whole body movements.

b. Fine motor coordination: extremity movements concerned with use of small muscle groups.
(1) Thumb/finger opposition (unilateral, bilateral).
(2) Manual/finger dexterity: grasp and release.
(3) Standardized tests and measures: Jebsen-Taylor Hand Function Test, Minnesota Rate of Manipulation Test, Purdue Pegboard.

c. Evaluation and documentation.
(1) Speed/rate control: does increasing the speed of performance affect quality of motor performance?
(2) Control: Are movements precise? Are continuous and appropriate motor adjustments made if speed and direction are changed? Can movement and distance be judged following a moving target? Does occluding vision alter performance?
(3) Steadiness: Is there consistency over time? Can a position be maintained without swaying, tremors, or extra movements? Does patient fatigue rapidly?
(4) Response orientation: Does correct movement occur in response to a specific stimulus?
(5) Reaction time: Does movement occur in a reasonable amount of time?
(6) Descriptive comments/terms.
(a) Dyssynergia: impaired ability to associate muscles together for complex movement.
(b) Dysmetria: impaired ability to judge the distance or range of movement.
(c) Dysdiadochokinesia: impaired ability to perform rapid alternating movements.
(7) Scoring: 0 (unable), 1 (severe impairment), 2 (moderate impairment), 3 (minimal impairment), 4 (normal performance).
(8) Methods.
(a) Patient's self-report.
(b) Observation/functional assessment.
(c) Timed tests.
(d) Videotaped analysis.

9. Examine balance.

a. The control of relative positions of body parts by skeletal muscles, with respect to gravity and to each other.
b. Sensory elements of balance.
(1) Visual system: check visual acuity, depth perception, visual field defects.
(2) Somatosensory: check proprioception, cutaneous sensation (touch, pressure), lower extremities and trunk, especially feet and ankles.
(3) Vestibular: check motor responses to positional and movement testing.
(a) Move or position the body; observe automatic adjustments that restore normal alignment of the head position (face vertical, mouth horizontal) (righting reactions).
(b) Alter the body's center of mass (COM) or base of support (BOS) or both; observe automatic postural adjustments that serve to maintain body posture and balance (keep COM within the BOS).
(c) Alter the body's COM outside of the BOS; observe the automatic adjustments of the arms (protective reaching) or legs (protective stepping) or both to extend and support the body weight in anticipation of a fall.
(d) Testing considerations: can use a displacing manual force against the COM (a perturbation or push) or displace the BOS using a movable surface (platform, gymnastic ball, equilibrium board).
(4) Test of sensory interaction/organization: Clinical Test for Sensory Interaction in Balance (CTSIB) (also know as the Sensory Organization Test, Shumway-Cook and Horak, 1986).

(a) Equipment: computerized moving platform (e.g., NeuroComBasic and Balance Master Systems); stopwatch.

(b) Examines six different sensory conditions, progressing in difficulty.

Condition 1: eyes open, stable surface (EOSS).

Condition 2: eyes closed, stable surface (ECSS).

Condition 3: visual conflict (sway-referenced vision using a moving surround screen or dome using force-platform surround screen), stable support.

Condition 4: eyes open, moving surface (EOMS), using moving platform.

Condition 5: eyes closed, moving surface (ECMS).

Condition 6: visual conflict, moving surface.

(c) Evaluation and documentation.

- Record time that standing posture is maintained (30 seconds); record changes in the amount and direction of postural sway, on a scale of 1 (minimal sway) to 4 (fall).
- Patients dependent on vision become unstable in conditions 2, 3, 5, and 6.
- Patients dependent on surface/somatosensory inputs become unstable in conditions 4, 5, and 6.
- Patients with vestibular loss become unstable in conditions 5 and 6.
- Patients with sensory selection problems become unstable in conditions 3–6.

(d) Modified Clinical Test of Sensory Interaction on Balance (mCTSIB)

- Patients stand for 30 seconds in each of four conditions: EOSS, ECSS, EOFS (foam surface), ECFS.

c. Musculoskeletal elements and limits of stability (LOS).

(1) Determine musculoskeletal strength and range of motion (ROM), lower extremities, and trunk.

(2) Determine LOS: ability to move their COM over the BOS during self-initiated movements; can document with force plate analysis.

(3) Determine center of alignment: location of COM within the center of the BOS; center of pressure documented using force plate analysis.

(4) Determine availability of postural synergies (strategies) used to preserve balance.

(a) Ankle strategy: ankle muscles (dorsiflexors and plantar flexors) maintain balance by shifting COM forward or back using a long axis of motion (lower extremity is relatively fixed).

(b) Hip strategy: hip and lower trunk muscles maintain balance by shifting COM using hip motions (flexion or extension).

(c) Stepping strategy: rapid steps are taken to realign COM within BOS.

(5) Check static balance: ability to maintain a position and response to perturbation.

(a) Sitting: holding a steady position, arm support, no arm support.

(b) Standing: double-limb and single-limb support.

(c) Romberg's test: standing with feet in normal stance position, first with eyes open, then with eyes closed; used to detect posterior column (sensory) ataxia.

(d) Sharpened or tandem Romberg: have patient stand in a tandem heel-to-toe position, first with eyes open, then eyes closed; increases sensitivity of Romberg's test.

(6) Check dynamic balance: response to dynamic movement challenges.

(a) Functional movement tasks: standing up and sitting down, walking, turning.

(b) Navigation through obstacle course, dual tasks Walks While Talking test, walk, carry items.

(c) BOS challenges: sitting on Swiss ball, balance/wobble board or dyna disc; standing on balance/wobble board, dense foam, and foam rollers.

(d) See Table 2–9 for functional balance grades.

d. Standardized tests and measures. (See Table 2–10 and Chapter 12, Appendix E).

10. Examine gait and locomotion.

a. Gait is the manner in which a person walks, characterized by rhythm, cadence, step, stride, and speed (Guide to Physical Therapist Practice).

Table 2-9 ➤ FUNCTIONAL BALANCE GRADES

Grade	Description
Normal	Accepts maximal challenge Patient is able to maintain steady balance without hand-hold support (static). Accepts maximal challenge and can shift weight easily at full range in all directions (dynamic).
Good	Accepts moderate challenge Patient is able to maintain balance without hand-hold support, limited postural sway (static). Accepts moderate challenge; able to maintain balance while picking object off floor (dynamic).
Fair	Accepts minimal challenge Patient is able to maintain balance with hand-hold support; may required occasional minimal assistance (static). Accepts minimal challenge; able to maintain balance while turning head/trunk (dynamic).
Poor	Patient requires hand-hold support and moderate to maximal assistance to maintain position (static). Unable to accept challenge or move without loss of balance (dynamic).

From: O'Sullivan S, Schmitz,T. Physical Rehabilitation: Assessment and Treatment. Philadelphia, FA Davis, 2007, pp 476–477, with permission.

(1) Kinematic gait analysis analyzes gait characteristics and deviations (see chapter 11).

b. Locomotion is the ability to move from one place to another (Guide to Physical Therapist Practice). (Table 2-10).

(1) Timed walking test: patient is asked to walk first at preferred speed and then at maximal speed over a set distance; e.g., 10-m or 50-foot walk test. Velocity, cadence (steps/min), and stride length are calculated.

(2) Six minute walk test (6MWT): test examines ability to walk at self-selected speed for a set time interval (also 12 MWT or 2MWT). Total distance walked is measured and overall exercise tolerance is determined.

Table 2-10 ➤ FUNCTIONAL BALANCE AND LOCOMOTION TESTS

TEST	DESCRIPTION	REFERENCE VALUES
Performance-Oriented Mobility Assessment, (POMA,Tinetti)	Examines balance (balance subtest, nine items including sitting, sit-to-stand, standing, standing feet together, turn 360 degrees, sternal nudge, stand on one leg, tandem stand, reaching up, bending over, stand-to-sit, timed rising) and walking (gait subtest, eight items including gait initiation, path, turning timed walk, step over obstacles)	Maximum score is 28; patients who score <19 are at high risk for falls; patients who score 19–24 are at moderate risk
Berg Balance Scale	Examines functional balance (14 items) including sitting unsupported, sit-to-stand, stand-to-sit, transfers; in standing: EO to EC, feet together, forward reach, pick object off floor, head turns, turning 360 degrees, stepping up, tandem stand, stand on one leg	Maximum score is 56; patients who score <45 are at high risk for falls; with scores 54–46, a 1-point drop is associated with a 6–8% increase in fall risk
Timed Up and Go (TUG)	Examines functional balance during rise from a chair, walk 3 m, turn, and return to chair. Performance on the GUG is timed	Normal intact adults can perform the test in ≤10 seconds; 11–20 seconds is considered normal for frail elderly or disabled patients; patients who take >20 seconds are at increased risk for falls; patients who take >30 seconds are at high risk
Functional Reach (FR)	Examines maximal distance a person can reach forward beyond arm's length while maintaining a fixed position in standing (single item test)	Forward reach norms: above average >12.2 inches, below average <5.6 inches; a forward reach of < 10 is indicative of increased fall risk
Multidirectional Reach Test (MDRT)	Examines maximal distance a person can reach forward, backward, and lateral to right and left	Backward: above average >7.6 inches, below average <1.6 inches; lateral: above average >9.4 inches, below average <3.8 inches
Short Physical Performance Battery (SPPB)	Includes repeated chair stands (sit-to-stand rises), semitandem, tandem, and side-by-side stands as well as a timed 8 ft (2.44 meter) walk	Tests are scored in terms of time to complete: 5 sit-to-stands, 10 sec in each of the standing conditions and 8 ft walk. An ordinal score is given for each section. Summary ordinal score: 0 (worst performance) to 12 (best performance).
Dynamic Gait Index (DGI)	Examines dynamic gait (eight items) including changes in gait speed, head turns, pivot turns, obstacles, and stairs	Normal intact adults received a score of 21 ± 3; patients with history of falls received a mean score of 11 ± 4
Balance Efficacy Scale (BES)	Examines level of self-confidence when performing functional tasks encountered in daily life; 18 questions are scored from 0–100% confidence; activities include getting out of chair, walking up and down flight of 10 stairs, getting out of bed, getting into and out of tub or shower, removing items from cupboard, walking on uneven ground, standing on one leg	Total score is divided by 18 to yield mean BES score; scores <50 indicate low confidence
Walkie-Talkie Test (Stops Walking When Talking, SWWT)	Test examines ability to talk while walking, a measure of dual task control	Test is positive if the person must stop walking in order to respond to a question
Functional Gait Assessment (FGA)	A 10-item gait assessment is based the Dynamic Gait Index. It includes additional items on walking (ambulating backward, with narrow base of support, with eyes closed)	Total posible score is 30
Modified Emory Functional Ambulation Profile Scale (mEFAP)	A timed measure of walking using 5 environmental challenges (floor, carpet, up and go, obstacles, stairs)	Recorded time is multiplied by a a factor related to use of assistive device: no assistance = × 1; AFO = × 2; single point cane = ×3; hemiwalker or quad cane = × 4; AFO + single-point cane = × 5; AFO + hemiwalker (or quad cane) = × 6

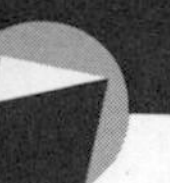

Review Medical Record for Diagnostic Procedures and Results

1. **Radiological procedures.** Skull x-rays.
   a. Delineates lesions of bone.
   b. Tomograms (tomography) are layered x-ray exposures, either vertical or horizontal.

2. **Ventriculography.** X-rays of skull after injection of air into lateral ventricles.
   a. Delineates ventricles, helps localize tumors.
   b. Useful with increased intracranial pressures.

3. **Myelography.** X-rays of spine after injection of air or dye into spinal subarachnoid space.
   a. Delineates abnormalities impinging on subarachnoid space.
   b. Complications: dye may result in meningeal irritation.

4. **Cerebral angiography.** X-rays of skull after injection of dye into carotid or vertebral arteries or both.
   a. Useful in showing areas of increased and decreased vascularity.
   b. Detects displacement of vessels by masses, occlusions, malformations, and aneurysms.
   c. Provides information about dynamics of circulation time.
   d. Complications: invasive technique; may cause meningeal irritation, hemorrhage, vasospasm, or anaphylactic reaction to dye.

5. **Computed tomography (CT).** Neuroimaging technique in which narrow x-ray beams are transmitted through tissues of varying densities and precisely measured; allows cross-sections (slices) of the brain to be visualized with three-dimensional localization.
   a. Contrast agents (intravenous iodinated agents) can be used to increase diagnostic sensitivity, to detect brain abnormalities (e.g., tumor, calcifications).
   b. Useful for showing presence of abnormal changes in tissue density: areas of hyperemia (hemorrhage) appear denser, edematous tissue less dense.

6. **Magnetic resonance imaging (MRI).** Neuroimaging technique in which nuclear particles (protons and neutrons) are depicted in a strong external magnetic field; no radiation is used.
   a. Useful for superior structural imaging of soft tissues and for flow of blood within medium and larger arteries and veins; bone is poorly imaged.
   b. Allows three-dimensional localization with high spatial resolution.
   c. Primary method of examination of tumors, demyelination, and vascular abnormalities.
   d. Contraindications: metal implants, pacemakers.

7. **Positron emission tomography (PET).** Neuroimaging technique in which radioisotopes are inhaled or injected, and emissions are measured with a gamma-ray detector system.
   a. Allows physiological mapping; a major clinical research tool for imaging cerebral blood flow, brain metabolism.
   b. Lacks detailed resolution of CT or MRI.

8. **Electroencephalography (EEG).** Ongoing electrical activity of brain is recorded, appearing as periodic waves.
   a. Provides useful information about structural disease of the brain, especially when seizures are present or likely.
   b. Can assist in localization of intracranial lesions in the brain.

9. **Evoked potentials/evoked responses.** External visual, auditory, or somatosensory stimuli are used to evoke potentials in brain; visual evoked potential (VEP), brainstem auditory evoked potential (BAEP), somatosensory evoked potential (SEP).
   a. Potentials are recorded from surface electrodes and processed by computer.
   b. Delineates conduction times along these sensory pathways.
   c. Detects lesions if responses are delayed or absent.

10. **Echoencephalogram (ultrasound/Doppler techniques).** Reflected ultrasonic waves are recorded and analyzed.
    a. Useful for imaging lumen of carotid artery and analyzing flow, detection of plaques in carotid arteries.
    b. Measures position and shifts of midline structures (e.g., tumors or hematomas).

11. **Lumbar puncture (LP).** Insertion of spinal needle below level of L1-2.
    a. Purposes.
       (1) Withdraw CSF for chemical analysis and cytological examination: measurement of protein, glucose, immunoglobulin content, cell count.
       (2) Measure intracranial pressures and spinal fluid dynamics.
       (3) Injection of contrast medium for radiological examination.
       (4) Injection of therapeutic agents (e.g., treatment of cancer, meningitis).
    b. Complications: severe headache caused by CSF leakage (relieved by lying down); more severe complications include infection, epidural hematoma, uncal herniation.
    c. Normal CSF: clear and colorless.
       (1) Manometric pressure CSF: 70–200 mm H_2O (average 125 mm H_2O).
       (2) Normal protein: 20–40 mg/dL.
    d. Pathological CSF findings.
       (1) Red blood cells (RBCs) indicate hemorrhage or traumatic tap; elevated white blood cells (WBCs) indicate significant inflammation and infection.

(2) Elevated proteins may indicate tumors or inflammation.

12. Neuromuscular diagnostic procedures.

a. Electromyography (EMG): detects electrical activity arising from muscles, both resting states and active contraction.

(1) Useful in diagnosing LMN disease or primary muscle disease, defects in transmission at neuromuscular junction.

(2) Insertional activity (burst of action potentials when EMG needle is inserted into normal muscle) is increased in denervated muscle and many muscle diseases.

(3) Number of motor unit potentials (MUPs) is decreased in LMN injury (denervated muscles); overall configurations remain normal.

(4) Alterations in MUP configurations (increased in size and duration, polyphasic shape) occur with reinnervation of previously denervated muscles.

(5) Spontaneous, ongoing EMG activity.

(a) Fibrillation (spontaneous independent contractions of individual muscle fibers) evident with denervation for 1–3 weeks after losing nerve.

(b) Fasciculations (spontaneous contractions of all or most of the fibers in a motor unit; muscle twitches that can be observed or palpated) are present with LMN disorders and denervation.

(c) Complete LMN lesions show only fibrillation potentials; partial LMN lesions show fibrillation and fasciculation potentials.

b. Nerve conduction velocity (NCV): conduction velocities are obtained by stimulating peripheral nerves through the skin and recording muscle and sensory nerve action potentials.

(1) Distance between two points (conduction distance) is divided by the difference between the corresponding latencies (conduction time), expressed as meters/second (m/s).

(2) Decreased conduction velocities are seen in peripheral neuropathies characterized by demyelination (e.g., Guillain-Barré syndrome, chronic demyelinating polyneuropathy, Charcot-Marie-Tooth disease).

(3) Slowed conduction velocities seen with focal compression of peripheral nerve.

Neurological Dysfunction

Table 2-11 ➤ NEUROMUSCULAR PREFERRED PRACTICE PATTERNS

Pattern A:	Primary Prevention/Risk Reduction for Loss of Balance and Falling
Pattern B:	Impaired Neuromotor Development
Pattern C:	Impaired Motor Function and Sensory Integrity Associated with Nonprogressive Disorders of the Central Nervous System—Congenital Origin or Acquired in Infancy or Childhood
Pattern D:	Impaired Motor Function and Sensory Integrity Associated with Nonprogressive Disorders of the Central Nervous System — Acquired in Adolescence or Adulthood
Pattern E:	Impaired Motor Function and Sensory Integrity Associated with Progressive Disorders of the Central Nervous System
Pattern F:	Impaired Peripheral Nerve Intergrity and Muscle Performance Associated with Peripheral Nerve Injury
Pattern G:	Impaired Motor Function and Sensory Integrity Associated with Acute or Chronic Polyneuropathies
Pattern H:	Impaired Motor Function, Peripheral Nerve Integrity, and Sensory Integrity Associated with Nonprogressive Disorders of the Spinal Cord
Pattern I:	Impaired Arousal, Range of Motion, and Motor Control Associated with Coma, Near Coma or Vegetative State

From: APTA Guide for Physical Therapist Practice, 2nd ed, 2001.

Infectious Diseases

1. Examine for signs of CNS infection, meningeal irritation.

2. Examine for signs of increased intracranial pressure.

3. Meningitis. Inflammation of the membranes of the spinal cord or brain.

a. Etiology: can be bacterial (*Escherichia coli, Haemophilus influenzae, Streptococcus pneumoniae,* other streptococci) or viral; patients with bacterial meningitis are usually sicker with more rapid time course.

b. Treat infective organism (bacterial meningitis) with antibacterial therapy (antibiotic, antipyretic); maintain fluid and electrolyte balance.

c. Provide supportive symptomatic therapy, including bed positioning, PROM, skin care to prevent complications of immobility; safety measures if confusion is present.

4. Encephalitis. Severe infection and inflammation of the brain.

a. Etiology: arboviruses, or a sequela in influenza (Reye's syndrome, eastern equine encephalitis,

measles), chronic and recurrent sinusitis, otitis, or other infections; bacterial encephalitis, prion-caused disease (kuru, "mad cow" disease).
   b. Treat infective organism (bacterial encephalitis).
   c. Provide supportive symptomatic therapy.

5. **Brain abscess.** Infectious process in which there is a collection of pyogenic material in the brain parenchyma.
   a. Signs and symptoms: headaches, fever, brainstem compression, focal signs CN II and VI.
   b. Can be an extension of an infection (e.g., meningitis, otitis media, sinusitis, post-TBI); typically frontal or temporal lobes or cerebellum.
   c. Treat infective organism, surgical intervention.
   d. Provide supportive symptomatic therapy.

6. **Acquired immunodeficiency syndrome (AIDS).**
   a. Viral syndrome characterized by acquired and severe depression of cell-mediated immunity.
   b. Symptoms: wide ranging; one third of patients exhibit CNS or PNS deficits.
      (1) AIDS dementia complex (ADC): symptoms range from confusion and memory loss to disorientation.
      (2) Motor deficits: ataxia, weakness, tremor, loss of fine motor coordination.
      (3) Peripheral neuropathy: hypersensitivity, pain, sensory loss.
   c. Treat with anti-HIV drugs (see Chapter 6).
   d. Provide palliative and supportive therapy.

Cerebrovascular Accident (Stroke)

1. **Sudden, focal neurological deficit resulting from ischemic or hemorrhagic lesions in the brain.** (See Table 2-12).

2. **Etiological categories.**
   a. Cerebral thrombosis: formation or development of a blood clot or thrombus within the cerebral arteries or their branches.
   b. Cerebral embolism: traveling bits of matter (thrombi, tissue, fat, air, bacteria) that produce occlusion and infarction in the cerebral arteries.
   c. Cerebral hemorrhage: abnormal bleeding as a result of rupture of a blood vessel (extradural, subdural, subarachnoid, intracerebral).

3. **Risk factors.**
   a. Atherosclerosis.
   b. Hypertension.
   c. Cardiac disease (rheumatic valvular disease, endocarditis, arrhythmias, cardiac surgery).
   d. Diabetes, metabolic syndrome.
   e. Transient ischemic attacks: brief warning episodes of dysfunction (<24 hours); a precursor of major stroke in more than one third of patients.

4. **Pathophysiology.**
   a. Cerebral anoxia: lack of oxygen supply to the brain (irreversible anoxic damage to the brain begins after 4–6 minutes).
   b. Cerebral infarction: irreversible cellular damage.
   c. Cerebral edema: accumulation of fluids within brain; causes further dysfunction; elevates intracranial pressures, can result in herniation and death.

5. **Neurovascular clinical syndromes.** Characteristic signs and symptoms associated with occlusion of specific cerebral vessels.
   a. Internal carotid artery (ICA) syndrome: ICA arises off the common carotid artery and ICA, gives off an ophthalmic branch, and terminates in the anterior cerebral artery (ACA) and middle cerebral artery (MCA); occlusions commonly produce signs and symptoms of MCA involvement with reduced levels of consciousness; ACA may also be affected; lesions involving MCA and ACA distributions may produce massive edema, brain herniation, and death.
      (1) ACA syndrome: ACA supplies anterior two thirds of the medial cerebral cortex; occlusions produce contralateral sensory loss and hemiparesis, with leg more involved than arm. Occlusions proximal to anterior communicating artery produce minimal deficits due to collateral circulation (Circle of Willis).
      (2) MCA syndrome: MCA supplies lateral cerebral cortex, basal ganglia, and large portions of the internal capsule; occlusions produce contralateral sensory loss and hemiparesis, with arm more involved than leg; may also produce motor speech dysfunction (Broca's area); perceptual dysfunction (parietal sensory association cortex); homonymous hemianopsia (optic radiation, internal capsule); loss of conjugate gaze to the opposite side (frontal eye fields); sensory ataxia (parietal lobe).
   b. Vertebrobasilar artery syndrome: two vertebral arteries arise off the subclavian arteries and supply the ventral surface of the medulla and the posterior inferior aspect of the cerebellum before joining to form the basilar artery at the junction of the pons and the medulla; the basilar artery supplies the ventral portion of the pons and terminates in the posterior cerebral artery (PCA). Numerous syndromes may occur.
      (1) Medial medullary syndrome (vertebral artery occlusion or branch of lower basilar artery): produces ipsilateral paralysis of tongue, contralateral paralysis of arm and leg with impaired sensation.
      (2) Lateral medullary (Wallenberg's) syndrome (vertebral, posterior inferior cerebellar, or basilar artery occlusion): produces ipsilateral cerebellar symptoms (ataxia, vertigo, nausea and vomiting, nystagmus), Horner's syndrome (miosis, ptosis, decreased sweating); dysphagia, impaired speech,

diminished gag reflex; sensory loss of ipsilateral arm, trunk, or leg; contralateral loss of pain and temperature of half of body, sometimes face.

(3) Basilar artery syndrome: produces brainstem signs and symptoms and PCA signs and symptoms; locked-in syndrome (basilar artery occlusion at the level of the pons): occlusions produce quadriplegia and bulbar paralysis; anarthria with preserved consciousness—the patient is unable to move or speak, but has full cognitive function; often fatal. Sensation may be intact.

(4) Medial inferior pontine syndrome (occlusion of paramedian branch of basilar artery): produces (1) ipsilateral signs and symptoms—cerebellar (nystagmus, ataxia), paralysis of conjugate gaze (to the side of the lesion), diplopia—and (2) contralateral signs and symptoms—hemiparesis, impaired sensation.

(5) Lateral inferior pontine syndrome (occlusion of anterior inferior cerebellar artery): produces (1) ipsilateral signs and symptoms—cerebellar (nystagmus, vertigo, nausea, vomiting, ataxia), facial paralysis, paralysis of conjugate gaze to the side of the lesion, deafness, tinnitus, impaired facial sensation—and (2) contralateral signs and symptoms—impairment of pain and temperature of half of body.

(6) PCA syndrome: PCA and posterior communicating arteries supply the midbrain, temporal lobe, diencephalon, and posterior third of cortex; occlusions may produce contralateral homonymous hemianopsia, contralateral sensory loss, thalamic syndrome, involuntary movements (choreoathetosis, intention tremor, hemiballismus), transient contralateral hemiparesis, Weber's syndrome (oculomotor nerve palsy with contralateral hemiplegia), and visual symptoms (paralysis of vertical eye movements, miosis, ptosis, decreased pupillary light reflex); occlusions proximal to posterior communicating artery produce minimal deficits owing to collateral circulation (same as for ACA).

6. Sequential recovery stages.

a. Stage 1: initial flaccidity, no voluntary movement.
b. Stage 2: emergence of spasticity, hyperreflexia, synergies (mass patterns of movement).
c. Stage 3: voluntary movement possible, but only in synergies; spasticity strong.
d. Stage 4: voluntary control in isolated joint movements emerging, corresponding decline of spasticity and synergies.
e. Stage 5: increasing voluntary control out-of-synergy; coordination deficits present.
f. Stage 6: control and coordination near normal.

7. Examine.

a. Generalized signs of increased intracranial pressure.
b. Level of consciousness, cognitive function.
c. Speech and communication.
   (1) Examine for aphasia with lesions of parieto-occipital cortex of dominant hemisphere (typically left hemisphere).
   (2) Examine for perceptual deficits with lesions of parietal lobe of nondominant hemisphere (typically right hemisphere).
d. Behaviors.
   (1) Patients with lesions of the left hemisphere (right hemiplegia) are slow, cautious, hesitant, and insecure.
   (2) Patients with lesions of the right hemisphere (left hemiplegia) are impulsive, quick, indifferent; often exhibit poor judgment and safety, overestimating their abilities, while underestimating their problems.
e. Sensory deficits (Figure 2–1).
   (1) Superficial, proprioceptive, and combined sensations of contralateral extremities, trunk, and face.
   (2) Hearing, vision; examine for homonymous hemianopsia.
   (3) Cranial nerve function with brainstem, vertebrobasilar strokes (pseudobulbar palsy).
f. Motor function (Figure 2–2).
   (1) Presence of abnormal tone and primitive reflexes.
   (2) Spasticity (see Table 2–6).

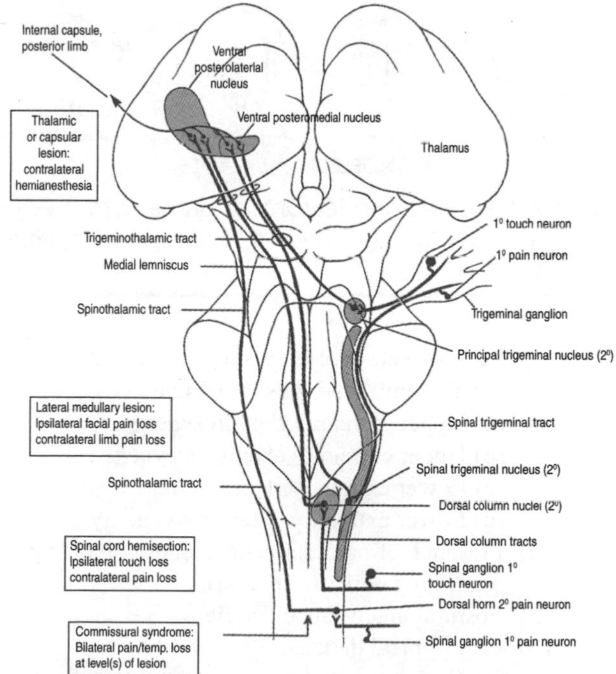

Figure 2-1 • Schematic synopsis of somatosensory pathways and their clinical syndromes.
From: Young P, Youp P. Basic Clinical Neuroanatomy. Baltimore, Williams & Wilkins, 1997, p 147, with permission.

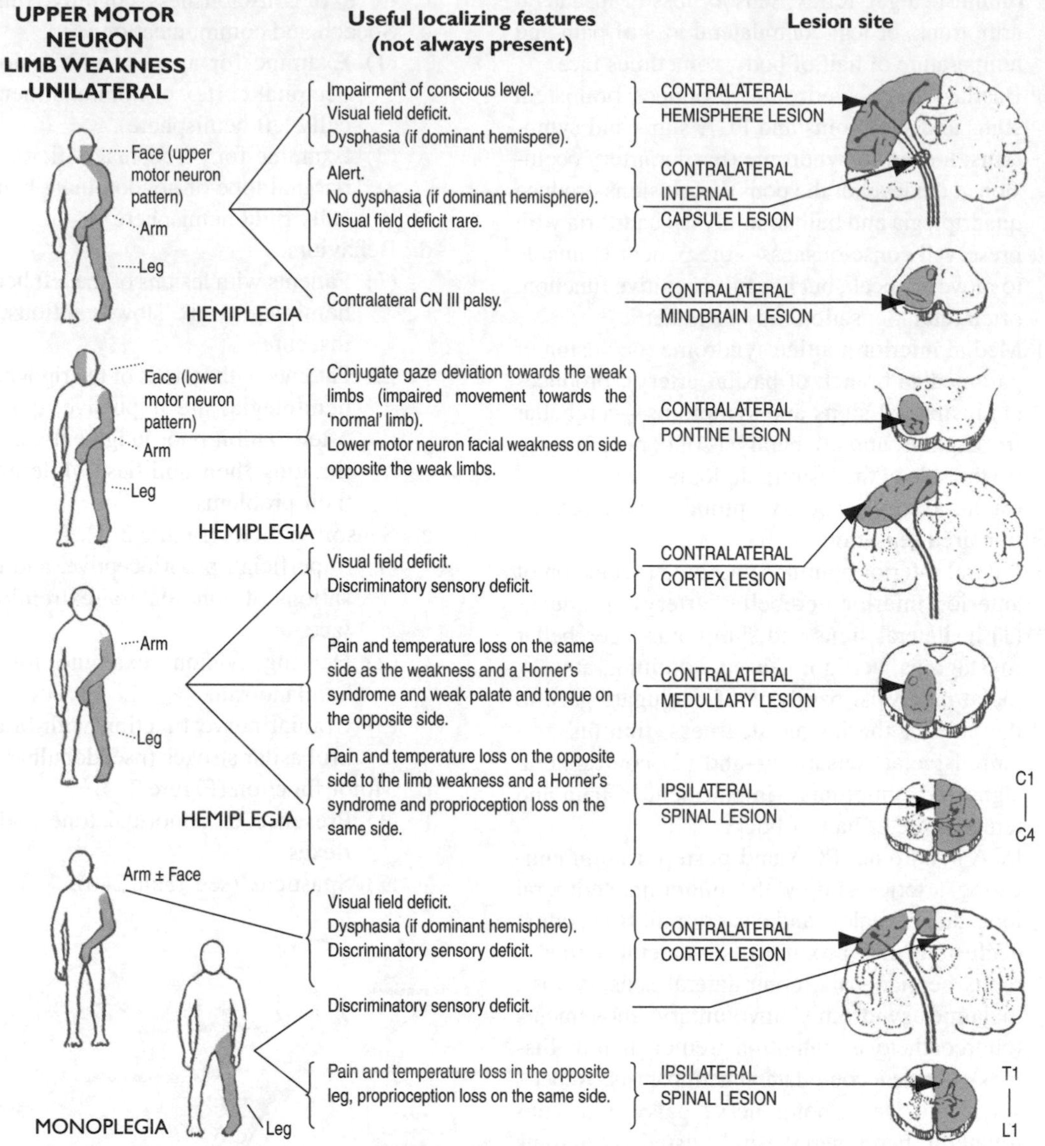

UPPER MOTOR NEURON LIMB WEAKNESS -UNILATERAL | **Useful localizing features (not always present)** | **Lesion site**

HEMIPLEGIA (Face (upper motor neuron pattern), Arm, Leg)
- Impairment of conscious level. Visual field deficit. Dysphasia (if dominant hemispere). — CONTRALATERAL HEMISPHERE LESION
- Alert. No dysphasia (if dominant hemisphere). Visual field deficit rare. — CONTRALATERAL INTERNAL CAPSULE LESION
- Contralateral CN III palsy. — CONTRALATERAL MINDBRAIN LESION

HEMIPLEGIA (Face (lower motor neuron pattern), Arm, Leg)
- Conjugate gaze deviation towards the weak limbs (impaired movement towards the 'normal' limb). Lower motor neuron facial weakness on side opposite the weak limbs. — CONTRALATERAL PONTINE LESION

HEMIPLEGIA (Arm, Leg)
- Visual field deficit. Discriminatory sensory deficit. — CONTRALATERAL CORTEX LESION
- Pain and temperature loss on the same side as the weakness and a Horner's syndrome and weak palate and tongue on the opposite side. — CONTRALATERAL MEDULLARY LESION
- Pain and temperature loss on the opposite side to the limb weakness and a Horner's syndrome and proprioception loss on the same side. — IPSILATERAL SPINAL LESION (C1–C4)

MONOPLEGIA (Arm ± Face; Leg)
- Visual field deficit. Dysphasia (if dominant hemisphere). Discriminatory sensory deficit. — CONTRALATERAL CORTEX LESION
- Discriminatory sensory deficit. — CONTRALATERAL CORTEX LESION
- Pain and temperature loss in the opposite leg, proprioception loss on the same side. — IPSILATERAL SPINAL LESION (T1–L1)

Figure 2-2 • Localizing features of damage to specific areas of the brain and spinal cord.
From: Lindsay KW, Bone I, Callander R. Neurology and Neurosurgery Illustrated. New York, Chuchill Livingstone, 1986, p 181, with permission.

(3) Loss of selective movements, presence of abnormal limb synergies (see Table 2–8).
   (a) Upper extremity flexion synergy.
   (b) Upper extremity extension synergy.
   (c) Lower extremity flexion synergy.
   (d) Lower extremity extension synergy.

(4) Presence of paresis, incoordination, motor programming deficits (apraxia).

(5) Postural and balance deficits.

(6) Gait: typical deficits.
   (a) Hip: poor hip position (retracted, flexed); Trendelenburg's limp (weak abductors); scissoring (spastic adductors); insufficient pelvic rotation during swing.
   (b) Weak hip flexors during swing may yield circumducted gait, external rotation with adduction, backward leaning of trunk, or exaggerated flexion synergy.
   (c) Knee: weak knee extensors (knee flexes during stance) may result in compensatory locking of knee in hyperextension; spastic quadriceps may also yield a hyperextended knee.
   (d) Ankle: footdrop; equinus gait (heel does not touch down); varus foot (weight is borne on lateral side of foot); or equinovarus position.
   (e) Unequal step lengths: leg does not advance through the end of stance into toe-off.
   (f) Decreased cadence, uneven timing.
   (g) Function: functional mobility skills (FMS), activities of daily living (ADLs).

(h) Standardized tests and measures for examination of patients with stroke. (See also Chapter 14, Appendix E)
(1) Fugl-Meyer Assessment of Physical Performance (FMA) (1980): provides objective criteria for scoring of movements (0, cannot perform, to 2, fully performed). Includes subtests for upper extremity function, lower extremity function, balance, sensation, ROM, and pain.
(2) NIH Stroke Scale provides measurements of acute cerebral infarction (1989).
(3) Postural Assessment Scale for Stroke Patients (PASS) provides a standardized assessment of postural control and balance in patients recovering from stroke (Benaim et al., 1999).
(4) Stroke Impact Scale provides a brief assessment of physical and social functioning after stroke (Duncan, Wallace, Lai et al., 1999).
(5) Functional Independence Measure (FIM) is a widely used instrument that provides measurement of 18 items of physical (functional mobility and basic ADL), psychological, and social functioning (Guide for the Uniform Data Set for Medical Rehabilitation [Adult FIM] version 4.0 [1993] State University of New York at Buffalo).
(6) Functional Assessment Measure (FAM). In addition to FIM items, the FAM includes additional functional areas including community access, instrumental ADL, safety, employability and adjustment (Functional Assessment Measure. J of Rehabil. Outcomes Measurement 1997;1(3):63–65).

8. Physical therapy goals, outcomes, and interventions.

a. Monitor changes associated with recovery and inactivity.
(1) Prevent or minimize indirect impairments/secondary complications.
(a) Maintain ROM and prevent deformity through optimal positioning, PROM, and mobilization.
(b) Maintain skin integrity.
(c) Avoid traction injuries to arm, development of painful shoulder.
(2) Teach sensory compensation strategies for sensory and perceptual losses.

b. Promote awareness, active movement, and use of hemiplegic side (remediation-facilitation approach).
(1) Promote normalization of tone through tone-reducing activities and techniques.
(2) Promote selective movement control (out-of-synergy movements) of involved extremities; emphasize functional patterns of movement.

c. Improve postural control, symmetry, and balance.

d. Task-specific training.
(1) Promote active problem-solving independence.
(2) Focus on goal-directed tasks, functional mobility skills (e.g., rolling, supine-to-sit, sitting, sit-to-stand, transfers, wheelchair mobility, and ambulation).
(3) Focus on adapting movements to specific environmental demands.
(4) Organize feedback inputs (knowledge of results, knowledge of performance) and practice schedules to facilitate learning.

e. Promote independence in ADL/self-care; compensatory training as appropriate.

f. Improve respiratory and oromotor function; promote functional cardiorespiratory endurance.
(1) Improve chest expansion, diaphragmatic breathing pattern.
(2) Oromotor training.
(3) Exercise conditioning: cycle ergometry, walking.

g. Isokinetic training: useful to improve timing deficits, velocity control of movement.

h. Treadmill training using body weight–supported treadmill training (BWS) (see section IV.C).

i. EMG—biofeedback training: useful to decrease firing in spastic muscles, increase firing in paretic muscles, and improve motor control.
(1) Functional electrical stimulation (FES): useful to stimulate muscle action, reduce spasticity, and substitute for an orthosis.

j. Constraint-induced movement therapy.

9. Guidelines to promote learning with hemispheric differences.

a. Patients with left hemisphere lesions (right hemiplegia).
(1) Develop an appropriate communication base: words, gestures, pantomime; assess level of understanding.
(2) Give frequent feedback and support.
(3) Do not underestimate ability to learn.

b. Patients with right hemisphere lesions (left hemiplegia).
(1) Use verbal cues; demonstrations or gestures may confuse patients with visuospatial deficits.
(2) Give frequent feedback: focus on slowing down and controlling movement.
(3) Focus on safety.
(4) Avoid environmental (spatial) clutter.
(5) Do not overestimate ability to learn.

Trauma

1. Traumatic brain injury (TBI).

a. Etiology: mechanism of injury is contact forces to skull and rotational acceleration forces, causing varying degrees of injury to the brain.

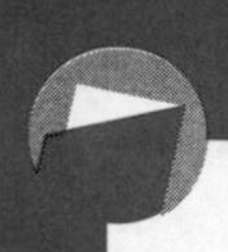

b. Pathophysiology (Table 2–12).
  (1) Primary brain damage.
    (a) Diffuse axonal injury: disruption and tearing of axons and small blood vessels from shear-strain of angular acceleration; results in neuronal death and petechial hemorrhages.
    (b) Focal injury: contusions, lacerations, mass effect from hemorrhage and edema (hematoma).
    (c) Coup-contracoup injury: injury at point of impact and opposite point of impact.
    (d) Closed or open injury (with fracture of the skull).
  (2) Secondary brain damage.
    (a) Hypoxic-ischemic injury: results from systemic problems (respiratory or cardiovascular) that compromise cerebral circulation.
    (b) Swelling/edema: can result in mass effect, with increased intracranial pressures, brain herniation (uncal, central, or tonsillar), and death.
    (c) Electrolyte imbalance and mass release of damaging neurotransmitters.
  (3) Concussion: loss of consciousness, either temporary or permanent, resulting from injury or blow to head, with impaired functioning of the brainstem reticular activating system (RAS); may see changes in HR, RR, BP.
    (a) Mild concussion syndrome: momentary loss of consciousness or confusion after TBI; may see retrograde amnesia (loss of memory that goes back in time before the injury occurred).
    (b) Classic concussion: moderate in severity, with loss of consciousness that is transient and mostly reversible in 24 hours; may see retrograde and posttraumatic amnesia (loss of memory for events after the traumatic event).
    (c) Severe concussion: loss of consciousness for >24 hours; associated with diffuse axonal injury and coma.

Table 2-12 ➤ SIGNS ASSOCIATED WITH LOCALIZED LESIONS OF THE CORTEX

LOBE	STRUCTURE	FUNCTION	DESTRUCTIVE LESION
Frontal	Area 4	Discrete volitional movements	Contralateral paralysis and paresis (most pronounced in distal parts of limbs and lower part of face)
	Area 8	Conjugate eye movements	Transitory paralysis of conjugate eye movements to opposite side
	Broca Speech (areas 44 and 45)	Language production	Nonfluent aphasia
	Prefrontal Cortex:		
	Dorsolateral	Motivation, problem solving, judgment	Bilateral lesions: Impaired ability to concentrate, easily distracted, loss of initiative, apathy, cannot make decisions
	Orbitofrontal	Emotions, behavior	Unstable emotions; unpredictable and frequent unacceptable behavior
	Orbital Gyri (posterolateral part)	Olfaction	Inability to discriminate odors
Parietal	Areas 3, 1, 2	Somesthetic sensations	Loss of contralateral stimulus location and intensity; severe impairment of two-point and limb position senses
	Area 43	Taste	Impairment of taste in contralateral side of tongue
	Superior and Inferior Parietal Lobules	Processing of somatic and visual information, especially related to use of hands	Tactile and visual agnosia, visual disorientation, neglect of contralateral self and surroundings
Temporal	Area 41	Hearing	Subtle decrease in hearing and ability to localize sounds, both contralaterally
	Wernicke Speech (area 22) Middle Inferior, and Occipito-temporal Gyri (dominant side)	Language understanding and formulation; storage of auditorially presented information	Fluent aphasia Impairment of learning and memory
	Temporal Cortex (nondominant side)	Storage of visually presented information	Impairment of learning and memory
	Parahippocampal Region	Recent memory	Bilateral lesions: Profound memory loss of recent events and no new learning
Occipital	Area 17	Vision	Contralateral homonymous hemianopsia
	Parastriate and Peristriate (areas 18 and 19)	Visual association	Bilateral lesions: Color agnosia and loss of spatial relationships (cannot draw floor plan of home, map of route to work or church, etc.)

From: Gilroy J. Basic Clinical Neurology, Elmsford, NY, 2nd ed, Pergamon Press, 1990, pp 228–229, with permission.

c. Standardized tests and measures for examination of patients with traumatic brain injury.
   (1) Glasgow Coma Scale (GCS): allows classification into mild (score 13–15), moderate (score 9–12), or severe (score ≤8) head injury (coma) (Jennett and Teasdale, 1974).
   (2) Rancho Los Amigos Levels of Cognitive Functioning (LOCF): delineates eight general cognitive and behavioral levels (Rancho Professional Staff Association, 1979).
   (3) Rappaport's Disability Rating Scale (DRS): classifies levels of disability using a wide range of functional behaviors (Rappaport et al., 1982).
   (4) Glasgow Outcome Scale (GOS): expands original scale; includes major disability categories for outcome assessment (Jennett and Bond, 1975).
   (5) High Level Mobility Assessment Tool (HI-MATP) provides measurement of high level functional mobility skills (Williams et al., 2005).
   (6) Functional Independence Measure/Functional Assessment Measure (FIM/FAM): see previous discussion.

d. Recovery stages from diffuse axonal injury (Alexander).
   (1) Coma: a state of unconsciousness in which there is neither arousal nor awareness; eyes remain closed, no sleep/wake cycles.
   (2) Unresponsive vigilance/vegetative state: marked by the return of sleep/wake cycles and normalization of vegetative functions (respiration, digestion, BP control); persistent vegetative state is determined if patient remains in vegetative state ≥1 year after TBI.
   (3) Mute responsiveness/minimally responsive: state in which patient is not vegetative and does show signs, even if intermittent, of fluctuating awareness.
   (4) Confusional state: mainly a disturbance of attention mechanisms; all cognitive operations are affected, patient is unable to form new memories; may demonstrate either hypoarousal or hyperarousal.
   (5) Emerging independence: confusion is clearing and some memory is possible; significant cognitive problems and limited insight remain; frequently uninhibited social behaviors.
   (6) Intellectual/social competence: increasing independence, although cognitive difficulties (problem solving, reasoning) persist along with behavioral and social problems (enhancement of premorbid traits, mood swings).
   (7) Patient can plateau at any stage or regress under conditions of stress or repetitive brain injury.

e. Examine.
   (1) For generalized signs of increased intracranial pressure.
   (2) Level of consciousness (GCS), cognitive function (LOCF), examine for disorders of learning, attention, memory, and complex information processing.
   (3) Cranial nerve function.
   (4) For changes in behavior: examine for inappropriate physical, verbal, sexual behaviors; poor judgment; irritability, low frustration tolerance, and aggression; impulsivity and safety issues; depressed mood; restricted affect.
   (5) Speech and communication.
   (6) Sensory deficits.
   (7) Motor function: examine for paresis, apraxia (dyspraxia), reflexive behaviors, balance deficits, ataxia, and incoordination (cerebellar damage is common).
   (8) Functional mobility skills (FMS), ADLs.
   (9) Level of general deconditioning; after prolonged hospitalization (comatose, vegetative, decreased response levels), patients experience severe deconditioning and effects of prolonged immobilization (disuse atrophy, contractures and deformity, skin breakdown).

f. Physical therapy goals, outcomes, and interventions.
   (1) Monitor changes associated with recovery and inactivity.
   (2) Management based on decreased response levels (LOCF I–III).
      (a) Maintain ROM, prevent contracture development: PROM, positioning, splinting, and serial casting.
      (b) Maintain skin integrity; prevent development of decubitus ulcers through frequent position changes.
      (c) Maintain respiratory status, prevent complications: postural drainage, percussion, vibration, suctioning to keep airway clear.
      (d) Provide sensory stimulation for arousal and to elicit movement: environmental and direct stimulation (auditory, visual, olfactory, gustatory, tactile stimuli).
      (e) Promote early return of FMS: upright positioning for improved arousal, proper body alignment.
   (3) Management based on mid-level recovery (LOCF IV–VI).
      (a) Provide structure, prevent overstimulation for confused, agitated patient: closed, reduced stimulus environment, daily schedules, and memory logs; relaxation techniques.
      (b) Provide consistency: use team-determined behavioral modification techniques, give clear feedback, written contracts.
      (c) Engage the patient in task-specific training; limit activities to familiar, well-liked ones; offer options; break down complex tasks into component parts.

(d) Provide verbal or physical assistance.
(e) Control rate of instruction; provide frequent orientation to time, place, your name, and task.
(f) Emphasize safety, behavioral management techniques.
(g) Model calm, focused behavior.

(4) Management based on high-level recovery (LOCF VII–VIII).
(a) Allow for increasing independence: wean patient from structure (closed to open environments); involve patient in decision making.
(b) Assist patient in behavioral, cognitive, emotional reintegration: provide honest feedback, prepare for community reentry.
(c) Promote independence in functional tasks: FMS, ADLs, in real-life environments.
(d) Improve postural control, symmetry, and balance.
(e) Encourage active lifestyle, improved cardiovascular endurance.

(5) Provide emotional support, encourage socialization, behavioral control, and motivation.
(a) Reorient and reassure.
(b) Provide patient and family education.

2. Spinal cord injury (SCI).

a. Etiology: partial or complete disruption of spinal cord resulting in paralysis, sensory loss, altered autonomic and reflex activities.
(1) Traumatic causes: motor vehicle accident (most common cause of SCI), jumps and falls, diving, gunshot wounds.
(2) Mechanisms of injury: flexion (most common lumbar injury), flexion-rotation (most common cervical injury), compression, hyperextension.
(3) Spinal areas of greatest frequency of injury: C5, C7, T12, and L1.
(4) Nontraumatic causes: disc prolapse, vascular insult, infections.

b. Pathophysiology.
(1) Primary injury, interruption of blood supply.
(2) Secondary sequelae: ischemia, edema, demyelination, and necrosis of axons, progressing to scar tissue formation.

c. Classification.
(1) Level of injury: UMN injury.
(a) Lesion level indicates most distal uninvolved nerve root segment with normal function; muscles must have a grade of at least 3+/5 or fair + function.
(b) Tetraplegia (quadriplegia): injury occurs between C1 and C8, involves all four extremities and trunk.
(c) Paraplegia: injury occurs between T1 and T12-L1, involves both lower extremities and trunk (varying levels).

(2) Degree of injury.
(a) Complete: no sensory or motor function below level of lesion.
(b) Incomplete: preservation of sensory or motor function below level of injury; spotty sensation, some muscle function (<3+/5 grades).
(c) American Spinal Injury Association (ASIA) Impairment Scale.
A = Complete, no motor or sensory function is preserved in the sacral segments S4-5.
B = Incomplete: sensory but not motor function is preserved below the neurological level and includes the sacral segments S4-5.
C = Incomplete: motor function is preserved below the neurological level, and most key muscles below the neurological level have a muscle grade of less than 3.
D = Incomplete: motor function is preserved below the neurological level, and most key muscles below the neurological level have a muscle grade of 3 or more.
E = Normal: motor and sensory function is normal.

(3) Syndromes (Figure 2–3).
(a) Anterior cord syndrome: damage is mainly in anterior cord, resulting in loss of motor function, pain and temperature with preservation of light touch, proprioception, and position sense.
(b) Brown-Séquard syndrome: hemisection of spinal cord, resulting in ipsilateral weakness and loss of position and vibration sense below the level of lesion, with contralateral loss of pain and temperature a few segments below the level of lesion.
(c) Central cord syndrome: loss of more centrally located cervical tracts/arm function, with preservation of more peripherally located lumbar and sacral tracts/leg function; early loss of pain and temperature.
(d) Cauda equina: injury below L1 results in injury to lumbar and sacral roots of peripheral nerves (LMN) with sensory loss and paralysis and some capacity for regeneration; LMN, autonomous or nonreflex bladder.
(e) Sacral sparing: sparing of tracts to sacral segments, with preservation of perianal sensation, rectal sphincter tone, or active toe flexion.

d. Examine.
(1) Vital signs.
(2) Respiratory function: action of diaphragm, respiratory muscles, intercostals; chest expansion, breathing pattern, cough, vital capacity; respiratory insufficiency or failure occurs in lesions above C4 (phrenic nerve, C3-5 innervates diaphragm).

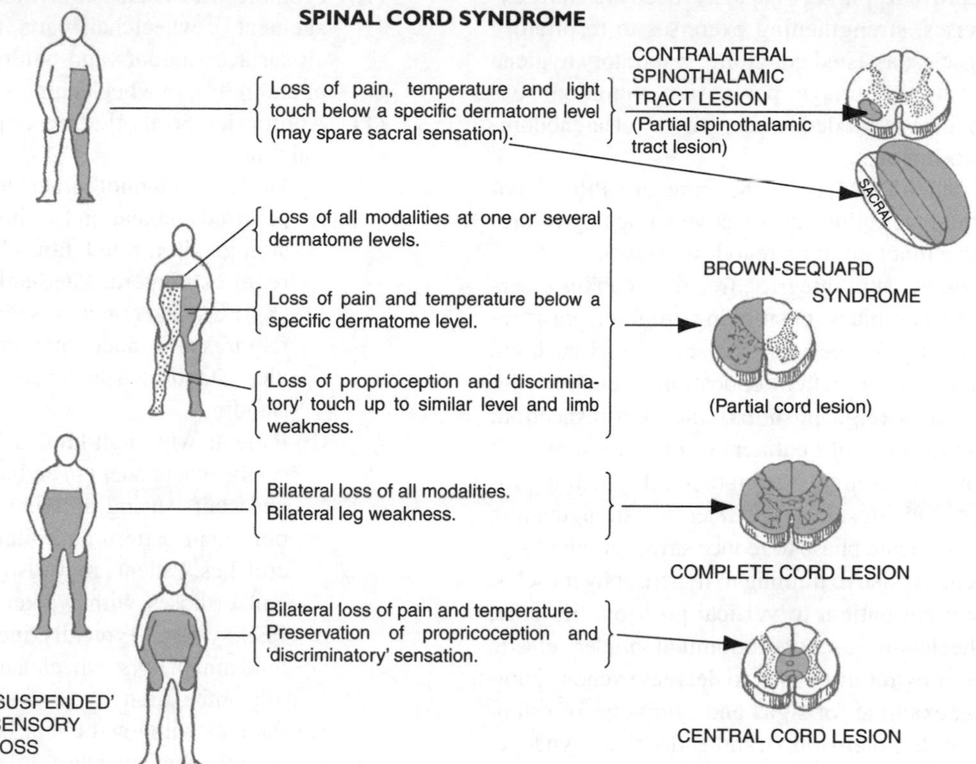
SPINAL CORD SYNDROME
Loss of pain, temperature and light touch below a specific dermatome level (may spare sacral sensation).
CONTRALATERAL SPINOTHALAMIC TRACT LESION
(Partial spinothalamic tract lesion)
SACRAL
Loss of all modalities at one or several dermatome levels.
Loss of pain and temperature below a specific dermatome level.
Loss of proprioception and 'discriminatory' touch up to similar level and limb weakness.
BROWN-SEQUARD SYNDROME
(Partial cord lesion)
Bilateral loss of all modalities.
Bilateral leg weakness.
COMPLETE CORD LESION
Bilateral loss of pain and temperature.
Preservation of proprioception and 'discriminatory' sensation.
'SUSPENDED' SENSORY LOSS
CENTRAL CORD LESION

Figure 2-3 • Spinal cord syndromes.
From: Lindsay KW, Bone I, Callander R. Neurology and Neurosurgery Illustrated. New York, Chuchill Livingstone, 1986, p 188, with permission.

(3) Skin condition, integrity: check areas of high pressure.
(4) Muscle tone and DTRs.
(5) Sensation/spinal cord level of injury: check to see if sensory level corresponds to motor level of innervation (may differ in incomplete lesions).
(6) Muscle strength (MMT)/spinal cord level of injury: lowest segmental level of innervation includes muscle strength present at a fair + grade (3+/5); use caution when doing MMT in acute phase with spinal immobilization.
(7) Functional status: full functional assessment possible only when patient is cleared for activity and active rehabilitation.

e. Standardized tests and measures for examination of patients with spinal cord injury.
(1) FIM/FAM. See previous discussion.
(2) Wheelchair skills test provides for measurement of functional and wheelchair management skills for the patient who uses the wheelchair for primary mobility (Kirby et al., 2004; http://www.wheelchairskills program.ca/eng/overview.htm).

f. Physical therapy goals, outcomes, and interventions.
(1) Monitor changes associated with recovery and inactivity.
(a) Spinal shock: transient period of reflex depression and flaccidity; may last several hours or up to 24 weeks.
(b) Spasticity/spasms: determine location and degree of tone. Examine for nociceptive stimuli that may trigger increased tone (e.g., blocked catheter, tight clothing or straps, body position, environmental temperature, infection, decubitus ulcers).
(c) Autonomic dysreflexia (hyperreflexia): an emergency situation in which a noxious stimulus precipitates a pathological autonomic reflex with symptoms of paroxysmal hypertension, bradycardia, headache, diaphoresis (sweating), flushing, diplopia, or convulsions; examine for irritating stimuli; treat as a medical emergency, elevate head, check and empty catheter first.
(d) Heterotopic bone formation (ectopic bone): abnormal bone growth in soft tissues; examine for early changes—soft tissue swelling, pain, erythema, generally near large joint; late changes—calcification, initial signs of ankylosis.
(e) Deep venous thrombosis: check lower extremities for edema and tenderness.

(2) Improve respiratory capacity: deep breathing exercises, strengthening exercises to respiratory muscles; assisted coughing, respiratory hygiene (postural drainage, percussion, vibration, suctioning) as needed to keep airway clear; abdominal support.
(3) Maintain ROM, prevent contracture: PROM, positioning, splinting; selective stretching to preserve function (e.g., tenodesis grasp).
(4) Maintain skin integrity, free of decubitus ulcers and other injury: positioning program, pressure-relieving devices (e.g., cushions, gel cushion, ankle boots), patient education: pressure relief activities (e.g., pushups) and skin inspection; provide prompt treatment of pressure sores.
(5) Improve strength: strengthen all remaining innervated muscles; use selective strengthening during acute phase to reduce stress on spinal segments; resistive training to hypertrophy muscles.
(6) Reorient patient to vertical position: tilt table, wheelchair; use of abdominal binder, elastic lower extremity wraps to decrease venous pooling; examine for signs and symptoms of orthostatic hypotension (lightheadedness, syncope, mental or visual blurring, sense of weakness).
(7) Promote early return of FMS and ADLs: emphasis on independent rolling and bed mobility, assumption of sitting, transfers, sit-to-stand, and ambulation as indicated (see section on transfer training in Chapter 11).
(8) Improve sitting tolerance, postural control, symmetry, and balance; standing balance as indicated.
(9) Appropriate wheelchair prescription.
   (a) Patients with high cervical lesions (C1-4): require electric wheelchair with tilt-in space seating or reclining seat back; microswitch or puff-and-sip controls; portable respirator may be attached.
   (b) Patients with cervical lesions, shoulder function, elbow flexion (C5): can use a manual chair with propulsion aids (e.g., projections); independent for short distances on smooth, flat surfaces; may choose electric wheelchair for distances and energy conservation.
   (c) Patients with cervical lesions, radial wrist extensors (C6): manual wheelchair with friction surface hand rims; independent.
   (d) Patients with cervical lesions, triceps (C7): same as for C6, but with increased propulsion.
   (e) Patients with hand function (C8-T1 and below): manual wheelchair, standard hand rims.
   (f) Significant changes in lighter, more durable, sports-oriented chairs.
(10) Promote wheelchair skills/independence: management of wheelchair parts, turns, propulsion all surfaces indoors and outdoors, safe fall out of and return to wheelchair.
(11) Appropriate orthotic prescription/ambulation training.
   (a) Patients with midthoracic lesions (T6-9): supervised ambulation for short distances (physiological, limited household ambulator); requires bilateral knee-ankle-foot orthoses (KAFOs) and crutches, swing-to gait pattern; requires assistance; may prefer standing devices/standing wheelchairs for physiological standing.
   (b) Patients with high lumbar lesions (T12-L3): can be independent in ambulation all surfaces and stairs; using a swing-through or four-point gait pattern and bilateral KAFOs and crutches. Patients may also use reciprocating gait orthoses with walker with or without FES system. Typically independent household ambulators; wheelchair use for community ambulation.
   (c) Patients with low lumbar lesions (L4-5); can be independent with bilateral AFOs and crutches or canes. Typically independent community ambulators; may still use wheelchair for activities with high-endurance requirements.
   (d) High rate of rejection of orthoses/ambulation in favor of wheelchair mobility and energy conservation.
(12) Improve cardiovascular endurance.
   (a) Methods: arm crank ergometry; functional electrical stimulation–leg cycle ergometry; hybrid: arm crank ergometry and functional electrical stimulation–leg cycle ergometry; wheelchair propulsion.
   (b) Precautions: individuals with tetraplegia and high-lesion paraplegia experience blunted tachycardia, lack of pressor response, and very low VO_2 peak, substantially higher variability of most responses.
   (c) Trunk stabilization and skin protection important.
   (d) Vascular support may be needed (elastic stockings, abdominal binder).
   (e) Absolute contraindications to exercise testing and training of individuals with SCI (from American College of Sports Medicine, ACSM).
      - Autonomic dysreflexia
      - Severe or infected skin on weight-bearing surfaces
      - Symptomatic hypotension
      - Urinary tract infection
      - Uncontrolled spasticity or pain

- Unstable fracture
- Uncontrolled hot and humid environments
- Insufficient ROM to perform exercise task

(13) Treadmill training using BWS (see section IV.C).
(a) Indications: incomplete cervical/thoracic injuries (ASIA levels B, C, and D).
(b) Promotes spinal cord learning/activation of spinal locomotor pools.
(c) Uses body harness to support weight; variable levels of loading from 40%, decreasing to 10% of full loading.
(d) Early training: therapists assist with foot placement.
(e) High frequency (4 days/week); moderate duration (30 minutes); typically for 8–12 weeks.

(14) Promote maximum mobility in home and community environment; assist patient in community reintegration; ordering of proper equipment, home modification.

f. Provide psychological and emotional support, encourage socialization and motivation.
(1) Reorient and reassure.
(2) Promote independent problem solving, self-direction.
(3) Provide patient and family education. Focus on strategies to prevent skin breakdown, and maintain ROM, strength, and function.

Degenerative Disorders

1. Multiple sclerosis (MS). A chronic, progressive, demyelinating disease of the CNS affecting mostly young adults.

a. Etiology: unknown; most likely viral, autoimmune (active immune responses detected in CSF).

b. Characteristics.
(1) Demyelinating lesions (plaques) impair neural transmission, cause nerves to fatigue rapidly.
(2) Variable symptoms: lesions scattered throughout CNS, common in pyramidal tract, dorsal columns, and periventricular areas of cerebrum, cerebellar peduncles.
(3) Variable course with fluctuating periods: exacerbations (worsening of symptoms) and remissions, progressing to permanent dysfunction; lesions are scattered "in time and place."
(4) Precipitating or exacerbating factors: infections, trauma, pregnancy, stress.
(5) Transient worsening of symptoms: adverse reactions to heat, hyperventilation, dehydration, fatigue.
(6) Variable course: four main types identified—benign, exacerbating-remitting, remitting-progressive, progressive.
(7) Categories of MS.
(a) Relapsing-remitting MS: characterized by relapses with either full recovery or some remaining neurological signs/symptoms and residual deficit on recovery; periods between relapses characterized by lack of disease progression.
(b) Primary-progressive MS: characterized by disease progression from onset, without plateaus or remissions or with occasional plateaus and temporary minor improvements.
(c) Secondary-progressive MS: characterized by initial relapsing-remitting course, followed by progression at a variable rate that may also include occasional relapses and minor remissions.
(d) Progressive-relapsing MS: characterized by progressive disease from onset but without clear, acute relapses that may or may not have some recovery or remission; commonly seen in individuals who develop the disease after 40 years of age.

c. Diagnostic tests: LP/CSF, elevated gamma globulin, CT or MRI, myelogram, EEG.

d. Examine.
(1) History: symptoms, disease progression, functional deficits.
(2) Cognitive/behavioral status: mild-to-moderate cognitive impairment common; also euphoria, emotional dysregulation.
(3) Communication: dysarthria and scanning speech common; dysphasia.
(4) ROM, deformity: associated with disuse and inactivity.
(5) Sensation: sensory symptoms common; e.g., paresthesias, hyperpathia (hypersensitivity to sensory stimuli), dysesthesias (abnormal sensations), trigeminal neuralgia, Lhermitte's sign (electric shock-like sensation throughout the body produced by flexing the neck).
(6) Vision: diplopia or blurred vision common; also optic neuritis, scotoma (blind spot), nystagmus.
(7) Skin integrity and condition.
(8) Muscle tone, DTRs: spasticity and hyperreflexia are common (pyramidal tract lesions).
(9) Muscle strength and control: paresis is common; if spasticity is severe, MMT may be invalid.
(10) Coordination: ataxia is common; intention tremors, dysmetria, dysdiadochokinesia.
(11) Balance: vestibular involvement common, with vertigo, dizziness, unsteadiness, paroxysmal or sudden onset of symptoms.
(12) Gait: ataxic gait is common.
(13) Fatigue patterns: early afternoon fatigue and exhaustion common with high energy periods in early morning, and some recovery in early evening.

(14) Respiratory status.
(15) Functional status: FMS, ADLs.

e. Standardized tests and measures for examination of patients with MS.
   (1) Expanded Disability Status Scale (EDSS) (Kurtzke, 1955).
   (2) Minimum Record of Disability (MRD) (International Federation of MS Societies, 1985).
   (3) Modified Fatigue Impact Scale (Fisk et al., 1994).

f. Medical management.
   (1) Immunosuppressant drugs: treat acute flare-ups and shorten duration of episode; adrenocorticotropic hormone (ACTH) and steroids (e.g., prednisone, dexamethasone, betamethasone, methylprednisolone).
   (2) Interferon drugs: slow progression of disease, decrease symptoms (e.g., Avonex, Betaseron, Copaxone).
   (3) Symptomatic management of spasticity: drugs (e.g., baclofen, diazepam [Valium], dantrolene [Dantrium]), baclofen pump, phenol block surgery.
   (4) Symptomatic management of urinary problems: anticholinergic drugs.

g. Physical therapy goals, outcomes, and interventions.
   (1) Monitor changes associated with disease progression; revise rehabilitation plan accordingly; develop/supervise maintenance program.
      (a) Examine for signs of urinary tract infection, respiratory infection (common causes of death).
   (2) Rehabilitation goals.
      (a) Restorative: intensive, time-limited rehabilitation services designed to improve/ stabilize patient status after a relapse.
      (b) Functional maintenance: services designed to manage effects of progressive disease and prevent/minimize indirect impairments associated with disuse and inactivity.
   (3) Maintain ROM, prevent contracture.
   (4) Maintain skin integrity, free of decubitus ulcers and other injury.
   (5) Improve respiratory function.
   (6) Improve sensory awareness, sensory compensation to prevent injury; consider eye patching with diplopia.
   (7) Improve strength.
   (8) Improve motor control, coordination: teach tone reduction techniques, compensatory strategies, safety.
   (9) Improve postural control, symmetry, and balance; teach compensatory strategies and safety, provide assistive devices for gait.
   (10) Promote independence in functional mobility skills and ADLs; supervise family/home health aides in assisting patient.
   (11) Promote maximum mobility in home and community; provide appropriate mobility aids and adaptive equipment (wheelchair use common); anticipate changes, rate of disease progression.
   (12) Teach energy conservation techniques, activity pacing.
   (13) Avoid precipitating exacerbations: schedule therapy sessions during optimal times for function; minimize fatigue, establish schedule of rest and moderate exercise; avoid stressors, overheating.

h. Provide psychological and emotional support.
   (1) Emphasize realistic expectations; focus on remaining abilities.
   (2) Provide patient, family, and caregiver education.
   (3) Teach problem-solving skills, emphasize coping skills.

2. Parkinson's disease. A chronic, progressive disease of the CNS with degeneration of dopaminergic substantia nigra neurons and nigrostriatal pathways.

a. Etiology: several different causes identified: infectious/postencephalitic, atherosclerosis, idiopathic, toxic, drug induced.
   (1) Deficiency of dopamine within the basal ganglia corpus striatum with degeneration of substantia nigra.
   (2) Loss of inhibitory dopamine results in excessive excitatory output from cholinergic system (acetylcholine) of basal ganglia.

b. Characteristics.
   (1) Classic symptoms: rigidity (leadpipe or cogwheel), bradykinesia (hypokinesia), resting tremor (resting), impaired postural reflexes.
   (2) Slowly progressive with emergence of secondary impairments and permanent dysfunction.
   (3) Stages (Hoehn and Yahr classification).
      I. Minimal or absent disability, unilateral symptoms.
      II. Minimal bilateral or midline involvement, no balance involvement.
      III. Impaired balance, some restrictions in activity.
      IV. All symptoms present and severe; stands and walks only with assistance.
      V. Confinement to bed or wheelchair.

c. Examine.
   (1) History: symptoms, disease progression, functional deficits.
   (2) Cognitive/behavioral status: intellectual impairment/dementia occurs in advanced stages; examine for memory deficits, bradyphrenia (slowing of thought processes), and depression.
   (3) Communication: dysarthria, hypophonia (decreased volume) are common; mutism in advanced stages; mask-like face with infrequent blinking and expression, writing becomes progressively smaller.
   (4) Oromotor control, nutritional status: dysphagia is common, problems in chewing and swallowing.

(5) Respiratory status: breathing patterns, vital capacity; decreased chest expansion common.
(6) ROM, deformity associated with disuse and inactivity: contractures common in flexors, adductors; persistent posturing in kyphosis with forward head; many patients osteoporotic with high risk of fracture.
(7) Sensation/perceptual function: examine for aching and stiffness, abnormal sensations (cramp-like sensations, poorly localized), problems in spatial organization, perception of vertical, extreme restlessness (akathisia).
(8) Vision: examine for blurring, cogwheeling eye pursuit, eye irritation from decreased blinking, decreased pupillary reflexes.
(9) Skin integrity and condition, circulatory changes: edema may occur in lower extremities; increased sweating (ANS dysfunction); decubitus ulcers in late stages.
(10) Muscle tone: examine for rigidity, including location, distribution, and symmetry between two sides of body, type (cogwheel or leadpipe).
(11) Muscle strength: weakness is associated with disuse and atrophy; assess torque output at varying speeds (isokinetics).
(12) Motor function: examine for bradykinesia (slowed movement) or akinesia (absent movement), ability to initiate movement (number of freezing episodes, precipitating factors); assess reaction time versus movement time, overall poverty of movement.
(13) For involuntary movements: examine for presence, location of tremor, precipitating factors; resting tremor common, especially pill-rolling of hands; tremors during movement may occur in advanced stages; postural tremors.
(14) Balance: impaired postural reactions are common (worse with severe rigidity of trunk, lack of trunk rotation); examine for ability to maintain static and dynamic balance, reactive adjustments and anticipatory adjustments.
(15) Gait: characterized by poverty of movements, with generalized lack of extension; festination common (an abnormal, involuntary increase in the speed of walking, often with forward acceleration, but may occur with backward progression).
(16) Functional status.
(17) Overall level of endurance: fatigue and inability to sustain performance is common, affected by stress, high effort; cardiovascular deconditioning occurs with long-standing disease.
(18) Patients on levodopa: examine for fluctuations in symptoms related to dosing (end-of-dose deterioration, on-off phenomenon, dyskinesia); common with disease progression and long-term use of levodopa (e.g., 2–3 years).

d. Standardized tests and measures for examination of patients with Parkinson's disease.
  (1) Unified Rating Scale for Parkinsonism documents the overall effects of the disease on an individual (UPDRS) (1987).
  (2) The Parkinson's Disease Questionnaire (PDQ-39) is a quality of life questionnaire hat focuses on the subjective report of the impact of Parkinson's disease on daily life (Petro et al., 1995).
e. Medical management.
  (1) Sinemet (levodopa/carbidopa) or sustained-release Sinemet: provides dopamine (crosses blood-brain barrier) and decreases effects of disease; effect is prolonged with low-protein diet. Numerous adverse effects including nausea and vomiting, orthostatic hypotension, cardiac arrhythmias, involuntary movements (dyskinesias), and psychoses and abnormal behaviors (hallucinations are common). In on-off phenomenon, patients experience sudden changes from normal function to immobility to severe dyskinetic movements.
  (2) Dopamine agonist drugs: enhance the effects of Sinemet therapy (bromocriptine, pergolide mesylate).
  (3) Anticholinergic drugs: for control of tremor.
  (4) Amantadine: enhances dopamine release.
  (5) Selegiline (deprenyl): monoamine oxidase inhibitor increases dopamine; used during early disease to slow progression.
  (6) Surgery: thalamotomy, pallidotomy, deep brain stimulation in thalamus or subthalamic nucleus, cell transplant.
f. Physical therapy goals, outcomes, and interventions.
  (1) Monitor changes associated with disease progression and pharmacological interventions; revise rehabilitation plan accordingly; develop/supervise maintenance program.
  (2) Prevent or minimize secondary impairments associated with disuse and inactivity (see section on MS).
  (3) Teach compensatory strategies to initiate movement (unlock freezing episodes); repetitive auditory stimulation.
  (4) Improve strength: emphasis on improving overall mobility, rotational patterns (consider proprioceptive neuromuscular facilitation patterns, rhythmic initiation technique).
  (5) Teach relaxation skills.
  (6) Improve postural control, symmetry, and balance; teach compensatory strategies, safety.
  (7) Promote independence in FMS and ADLs; supervise family/home health aides in assisting patient.
  (8) Promote maximum mobility and safety in home and community, improve gait: provide

appropriate aids and adaptive equipment; anticipate changes, progression of disease.
(9) Improve cardiovascular endurance.
(10) Teach energy conservation techniques, activity pacing.
(11) Provide psychological and emotional support (see section on MS).

3. **Myasthenia gravis.** A neuromuscular junction disorder characterized by progressive muscular weakness and fatigability on exertion.
a. Etiology: autoimmune antibody–mediated attack on acetylcholine receptors at neuromuscular junction.
b. Characteristics.
(1) Muscular strength worse with continuing contraction, improved with rest.
(2) Classified into four types: ocular myasthenia (confined to extraocular muscles), mild generalized myasthenia, severe generalized myasthenia, and crisis.
(3) Generalized myasthenia: usually involves bulbar (extraocular, facial, and muscles of mastication) and proximal limb-girdle muscles.
(4) Course varies: may progress from mild to severe, typically within 18 months.
(5) Myasthenic crisis: myasthenia gravis with respiratory failure; treat as medical emergency.
c. Examine.
(1) Cranial nerves: examine for diplopia and ptosis; progressive dysarthria or nasal speech; difficulties in chewing and swallowing; difficulties in facial expression, drooping facial muscles.
(2) Respiratory function: breathing difficulties, hoarse voice.
(3) Muscle strength: proximal more involved than distal. Fatigability is characteristic of this disease; repeated muscle use results in rapid weakness.
(4) Functional mobility skills: common difficulties with climbing stairs, rising from chair or lifting (similar to myopathies).
(5) EMG and repetitive nerve stimulation studies conclusive: show abnormal responses to repetitive nerve stimulation (failure of transmission, decreased EMG-recorded responses).
d. Medical interventions.
(1) Acetylcholinesterase inhibitors: pyridostigmine.
(2) Corticosteroids: prednisone, methylprednisolone.
(3) Immunosuppressants: azathioprine, intravenous immunoglobulin (IVIG).
(4) Alternative treatments: plasmapheresis (removal of blood with filtering and separation of cellular elements from plasma); thymectomy.
e. Physical therapy goals, outcomes, and interventions.
(1) Monitor changes in patient's condition for complications: vital signs, respiration, swallowing.
(2) Promote independence in FMS and ADLs.
(3) Teach energy conservation techniques; activity pacing: promote optimal activity with rest as indicated.
(4) Provide psychological and emotional support.

Epilepsy

1. **Abnormal and excessive neuronal discharges resulting from disturbances of CNS.**

2. **Characteristics.**
a. Etiology: brain tumor; trauma; stroke; progressive neurological disease; hereditary disorders, congenital anomalies; febrile states; idiopathic.
b. Symptoms.
(1) Altered consciousness.
(2) Altered motor activity (convulsion): characterized by involuntary contractions of muscles; tonic activity (stiffening and rigidity of muscles); clonic activity (rhythmic jerking of extremities).
(3) Sensory phenomena: patient experiences somatosensory, visual, auditory, olfactory, gustatory, and vertiginous sensations.
(4) Autonomic phenomena: associated with sudden attack of anxiety, tachycardia, sweating, piloerection, abnormal sensation rising up in upper abdomen and chest.
(5) Cognitive phenomena: sudden failure of comprehension, inability to communicate, intrusion of thought, illusions, hallucinations, affective disturbances (intense feelings of fear, anger, and hate).
c. Primary, generalized seizures: bilateral and symmetrical, without local onset.
(1) Tonic-clonic (grand mal): dramatic loss of consciousness, with a cry, fall, and tonic-clonic convulsions of all extremities; often with tongue biting and arrested breathing, urinary and fecal incontinence; after 2–5 minutes, contractions subside, and consciousness is gradually regained; patient is confused, drowsy, and amnesiac about the event; full recovery may take several hours; some attacks are preceded by a brief aura.
(2) Absence seizures (petit mal): brief, almost imperceptible lapse of consciousness followed by immediate and full return to consciousness; posture is maintained, with no convulsive muscle contractions; may occur as often as a hundred times a day.
d. Partial seizures.
(1) Simple partial seizures: focal, begin locally, limited to a portion of the body, usually have an identifiable structural cause.
(a) Focal motor: clonic activity involving a specific area of the body.

(b) Focal motor with march (Jacksonian): an orderly spread or march of clonic movements from initial muscles to involve adjacent muscles, with spread to the entire side.

(c) Temporal lobe seizure: characterized by episodic changes in behavior, with complex hallucinations; automatisms (e.g., lip smacking, chewing, pulling on clothing); altered cognitive and emotional function (e.g., sexual arousal, depression, violent behaviors); preceded by an aura.

(2) Complex partial seizures: simple partial seizures followed by impairment of consciousness.

e. Status epilepticus: prolonged seizure or a series of seizures (lasting >30 minutes) with very little recovery between attacks; may be life threatening; medical emergency (generalized status epilepticus).

3. Examine/determine.

a. Time of onset, duration, type of seizure, sequence of events.

b. Patient activity at onset, presence of aura.

c. Sensory elements, motor activity: type, degree, and location of involvement.

d. Presence of tongue biting, incontinence, respiratory distress.

e. Behavioral elements, changes in mood and perception.

f. Patient responses after the seizure.

4. Medical interventions.

a. Antiepileptic medications: phenytoin (Dilantin), carbamazepine (Tegretol), phenobarbital.

b. Surgical intervention: lobe resection, hemispherectomy.

5. Physical therapy goals, outcomes, and interventions.

a. Protect patient from injury during seizure: remain with patient, remove potentially harmful nearby objects, loosen restrictive clothing, and do not restrain limbs.

b. Establish airway, prevent aspiration: turn head to side or sidelying position; check to see if airway is open, wait for tonic-clonic activity to subside before initiating artificial ventilation, if needed.

c. Promote regular routines for physical activity and emotional health.

Cerebellar Disorders

1. Diseases/lesions of the cerebellum.

a. Hereditary ataxia, Friedreich's ataxia.

b. Neoplastic or metastatic tumors.

c. Infection.

d. Vascular: stroke.

e. Developmental: ataxic cerebral palsy, Arnold-Chiari syndrome.

f. Trauma: TBI.

g. Drugs, heavy metals.

h. Chronic alcoholism.

2. Lesions/impairments of the cerebellum. Cerebellar lesions tend to produce ipsilateral signs and symptoms.

a. Lesions of the archicerebellum.

(1) Central vestibular symptoms: ocular dysmetria, poor eye pursuit, dysfunctional vestibular ocular reflex (VOR), impaired eye-hand coordination.

(2) Gait and trunk ataxia: poor postural control and orientation, wide-based gait.

(3) Little change in tone or dyssynergia of extremity movements.

b. Lesions of the paleocerebellum.

(1) Hypotonia.

(2) Truncal ataxia: dysequilibrium, static postural tremor, increased sway, wide BOS and high guard arm position. Posture worse with eyes closed, narrow BOS (Romberg, sharpened Romberg).

(3) Ataxic gait: unsteady, increased falls, uneven/decreased step length, increased step width.

c. Lesions of the neocerebellum produce ataxic limb movements.

(1) Intention tremor: irregular, oscillatory voluntary movements.

(2) Dysdiadochokinesia: impaired rapid alternating movements (RAM).

(3) Dysmetria: hypermetria (overshooting), errors or force, direction, amplitude, rebound phenomenon (Holmes).

(4) Dyssynergia: abnormal timing (errors of velocity, onset and stop), movement decomposition of agonist/antagonist interactions. Impairments of multijoint coordination, movement sequences, complex motor tasks.

(5) Errors in timing related to perceptual tasks.

d. Additional impairments.

(1) Asthenia: generalized weakness (F to G muscle grades).

(2) Hypotonia: especially in acute cerebellar lesions, difficulty with postural control of proximal (axial) muscles.

(3) Motor learning impairments: decreased anticipatory control, feedback and learning delays.

(4) Cognition: deficits in information procession, attention deficits.

(5) Emotional dysregulation: changes in emotional behaviors.

3. Examine.

a. Muscle strength, tone.

b. Range of motion.

c. Coordination: determine abnormalities of coordinated movement.

d. Balance: determine abnormalities of postural control and balance.
e. Gait: determine abnormalities of gait (ataxic gait).
f. Motor function: determine abnormalities of motor learning.
g. Functional status.
h. Endurance and fatigue level: fatigue is common with dysmetric patients.

4. **Standardized.** Tests and measures for examination of patients with disorders of balance. See discussion standardized tests and measures for the examination of balance (previous section); see also Table 2–7.

5. **Physical therapy goals, outcomes, and interventions.**
   a. Goals.
      (1) Improve accuracy of limb movements.
      (2) Improve postural stability and dynamic postural control.
      (3) Improve functional mobility and safety: transfers and gait.
      (4) Stabilize VOR/vision.
   b. Eye-head coordination exercise: slow head movements with visual fixation; active eye and head movements.
   c. Stability exercises: use of weight-bearing postures, carefully graded resistance and approximation to promote steady holding. Use of theraband, weights (ankle and wrist cuffs), weighted waist belts and walkers to decrease ataxic movements.
   d. Dynamic stability exercises: promote small range control, smooth reversals of movements, movement transitions, using carefully graded resistance.
   e. Balance training: compensatory training/ safety important. Standing balance and gait activities.
   f. Therapeutic pool: water provides graded resistance, decreases ataxic movements and postural instability.
   g. Coordination exercises: PNF patterns, Frenkel's exercises, ball gymnastics to promote balance.
   h. Stationary bike: assists timing of reciprocal movements.
   i. Motor learning strategies: low-stimulus environment (closed environment) ideal; focus on practice and repetition; distributed practice (endurance may be low).
   j. Biofeedback: augmented feedback to enhance stability and postural control (i.e., balance training platform).
   k. Energy conservation techniques, assistive devices as needed.

Vestibular Disorders

1. **Characteristics.**
   a. Dizziness: sensation of lightheadedness, giddiness, faintness; increased risk of falls.
   b. Vertigo: sensation of moving around in space or having objects move around a person; tends to come in attacks; if severe, accompanied by nausea and vomiting.
   c. Visual changes.
      (1) Nystagmus: involuntary, cyclical movement of the eyeball; e.g., horizontal, rotary.
      (2) Blurred vision: gaze instability secondary to vestibular ocular reflex (VOR) dysfunction.
   d. Dysequilibrium or postural instability: vestibular spinal reflex (VSR) dysfunction; ataxia, gait disturbances; increased risk of falls.
   e. Anxiety, fear, depression.
   f. Indirect impairments: physical deconditioning, decreased cervical ROM.

2. **Etiology: unilateral vestibular disorders (UVD).**
   a. Trauma: vestibular symptoms seen in 30%–65% of patients with TBI.
   b. Vestibular neuronitis, labyrinthitis: an acute infection with prolonged attack of symptoms, persisting for several days or several weeks; caused by viral or bacterial infection.
   c. Ménière's disease: recurrent and usually progressive vestibular disease; episodic attacks may last from minutes to several hours with severe symptoms; usually associated with tinnitus, deafness, sensation of pressure/fullness within ear; etiology unknown, edema of membranous labyrinth is a consistent finding.
   d. Benign paroxysmal positional vertigo (BPPV): brief attacks of vertigo and nystagmus that occur with certain head positions (lying down, turning over in bed, tilting head back); may be related to degenerative processes, mechanical impairment of peripheral vestibular system.
   e. Tumor: acoustic neuroma, gliomas/brainstem or cerebellar medulloblastoma.

3. **Etiology: bilateral vestibular disorders (BVD).**
   a. Toxicity: ototoxic drugs.
   b. Bilateral infection: neuritis, meningitis.
   c. Vestibular neuropathy, otosclerosis (Paget's disease).

4. **Examine.**
   a. History: determine type, nature, duration of symptoms, triggering stimuli/activity.
   b. Subjective assessment: Dizziness Handicap Inventory (DHI).
   c. VOR function: examine for nystagmus, blurred vision with head and total body movements.
   d. Sensory function.
      (1) Examine for intact vision, proprioception, especially of feet/ankles. Important for compensatory postural adjustments with vestibular losses.
      (2) Examine for sensory interaction in balance (CTSIB).
   e. VSR function: examine posture and balance; examine for instability in sitting, standing, during functional activities and gait.

f. Hallpike Dix test.
   (1) Patient sits on table; clinician turns patient's head horizonatally 45° and quickly moves patient down to supine position, with neck extended 30° beyond horizontal.
   (2) Check for symptoms (vertigo and nystagmus).
   (3) Return patient to sitting and test other side.
   (4) Positive for benign paroxysmal positional vertigo (BPPV) on side that produces symptoms.
g. ROM: special attention to cervical ROM.
h. Vertebral artery compression: can produce vestibular symptoms (i.e., in supine position, extend, laterally flex, and rotate head, hold for 30 seconds; each side tested separately).
i. Functional status: determine current level of activity.
j. Standardized tests and measures for examination of patients with vestibular disorders.
   (1) See discussion of standardized tests and measures for examination of patients with balance disorders (previous section); see also Table 2–7.
   (2) DHI measures a patient's self-perceived handicap as a result of vestibular disorders. It includes 25 questions grouped into functional, emotional, and physical components (Jacobson and Newman, 1990).

5. **Medical interventions.** Vestibular suppressant medications; prolonged use may delay recovery; severe cases may require ablative surgery.

6. **Physical therapy goals, outcomes, and interventions.**
   a. Bed rest: brief, useful during initial stages only; prolonged bed rest may delay recovery.
   b. Implement safety measures: teach sensory substitution, compensatory strategies; provide ambulatory aids as indicated; e.g., cane, walker.
   c. Provide active exercises to promote vestibular adaptation (recalibration of system).
      (1) Habituation training: repetition of movements and positions that provoke dizziness and vertigo.
      (2) Encourage movement; engage VOR and VSR as much as possible.
         (a) Eye and head exercises; e.g., eye movements up and down, side to side; head movements up and down, side to side progressing slow to fast.
         (b) Exercises to improve postural stability: sitting and standing, static and dynamic activities; e.g., bending forward, turning, Swiss ball exercises.
      (3) Emphasize functional mobility skills: walking, turning, stairs, community activities, activities with spatial and timing constraints.
      (4) Relaxation training: to decrease anxiety levels.
      (5) Begin conservatively, avoid excessive exacerbation of symptoms.
   d. Recovery is better, generally faster in unilateral than bilateral vestibular dysfunction.
   e. Provide psychological support and reassurance.

Cranial and Peripheral Nerve Disorders

1. **Peripheral nerve disease/injury.**
   a. Etiology: wide range of etiological factors (more than 100 distinct diseases).
   b. Basic pathological processes.
      (1) Wallerian degeneration: transection (neurotmesis) results in degeneration of the axon and myelin sheath distal to the site of axonal interruption.
         (a) Chromatolysis and repair processes occurs in nerve cell body.
         (b) Endoneurium (sheath) does not degenerate but forms a tube directing regeneration.
      (2) Segmental demyelination: axons are preserved (no wallerian degeneration); remyelination restores function (e.g., Guillain-Barré syndrome).
      (3) Axonal degeneration: degeneration of axon cylinder and myelin, progressing from distal to proximal, "dying back" of nerves (e.g., peripheral neuropathy).
   c. Terminology.
      (1) Neuropathy (peripheral neuropathy): any disease of nerves characterized by deteriorating neural function; e.g., diabetic neuropathy, alcoholic neuropathy.
         (a) Polyneuropathy: bilateral symmetrical involvement of peripheral nerves, usually legs more than arms, distal segments earlier and more involved than proximal.
         (b) Mononeuropathy: involvement of a single nerve.
      (2) Radiculopathy: involvement of nerve roots.
      (3) Traumatic nerve injury.
         (a) Neurapraxia (Class 1): injury to nerve that causes a transient loss of function (conduction block ischemia); nerve dysfunction may be rapidly reversed or persist a few weeks; e.g., compression.
         (b) Axonotmesis (Class 2): injury to nerve interrupting the axon and causing loss of function and wallerian degeneration distal to the lesion; with no disruption of the endoneurium, regeneration is possible; e.g., crush injury.
         (c) Neurotmesis (Class 3): cutting of the nerve with severance of all structures and complete loss of function; reinnervation typically fails without surgical intervention because of aberrant regeneration (failure of regenerating axon to find its terminal end).
   d. Clinical symptoms LMN syndrome (see Table 2–3).
      (1) Weakness/paresis of denervated muscle, hyporeflexia and hypotonia, (rapid) atrophy, fatigue.

(2) Sensory loss: corresponds to motor weakness; proprioceptive losses may yield sensory ataxia; insensitivity may yield limb trauma.

(3) Autonomic dysfunction: vasodilation and loss of vasomotor tone (dryness, warm skin, edema, orthostatic hypotension).

(4) Hyperexcitability of remaining nerve fibers.

(a) Sensory dysesthesias: hyperalgesia, pins and needles, numbness, tingling, burning.

(b) Motor: fasciculations, spasms.

(5) Muscle pain (myalgia) with inflammatory myopathies (e.g., postpolio syndrome).

e. Diagnostic tests.

(1) Nerve conduction studies (NCV): conduction times (motor, sensory) are slowed or complete conduction block may be evident.

(2) EMG (motor nerve function): examine for signs of widespread denervation atrophy (spontaneous fibrillation potentials); evidence of reinnervation (low-amplitude, short-duration, polyphasic motor unit potentials).

2. Trigeminal neuralgia (tic douloureux). Neuralgia of the trigeminal nerve (CNV).

a. Etiology: results from degeneration (etiology unknown) or compression (tortuous basilar artery or cerebellopontine tumor); occurs in older population (mean age ~50); abrupt onset.

b. Characteristics: brief paroxysms of neurogenic pain (stabbing and/or shooting pain); reoccurring frequently.

(1) Occurs along the distribution of the trigeminal nerve, mandibular and maxillary divisions (involvement of ophthalmic division is rare); restricted to one side of the face.

(2) There is autonomic instability: exacerbated by stress, cold; relieved by relaxation.

c. Examine/determine.

(1) Pain: location, intensity.

(2) Trigger points: light touch to face, lips, or gums will cause pain.

(3) Triggering stimuli: extremes of heat or cold, chewing, talking, brushing teeth, movement of air across the face.

(4) Motor function: control is normal.

d. Medical: medications (anticonvulsants, vitamin B_{12}); alcohol injections, surgery (sectioning of nerve, permanent anesthesia).

e. Transcutaneous nerve stimulation (TENS) can be effective for pain relief.

3. Bell's palsy (facial paralysis). LMN lesion involving CN VII (facial nerve), resulting in unilateral facial paralysis.

a. Etiology: acute inflammatory process of unknown etiology (immune or viral disease) resulting in compression of the nerve within the temporal bone.

b. Characteristics.

(1) Muscles of facial expression on one side are weakened or paralyzed.

(2) Loss of control of salivation or lacrimation.

(3) Onset is acute, with maximum severity in a few hours or days; commonly preceded by a day or two of pain behind the ear; most recover fully in several weeks or months.

(4) Sensation is normal.

c. Examine/determine.

(1) Drooping of corner of mouth, eyelids that don't close.

(2) Function of muscles of facial expression: have patient wrinkle forehead, raise eyebrows, frown, smile, close eyes tightly, puff cheeks.

(3) Taste of the anterior two thirds of tongue.

d. Medications: corticosteroids (prednisone); analgesics.

e. Physical therapy goals, outcomes, and interventions.

(1) Protect cornea (artificial tears or temporary patching) until recovery allows for eyelid closure.

(2) Electrical stimulation to maintain tone, support function of facial muscles.

(3) Provide active facial muscle exercises.

(4) May require face sling to prevent overstretching of facial muscles.

(5) Provide functional retraining: foods that can be easily eaten, chewing with opposite side.

(6) Provide emotional support and reassurance.

4. Bulbar palsy (bulbar paralysis). Refers to weakness or paralysis of the muscles innervated by the motor nuclei of the lower brainstem, affecting the muscles of the face, tongue, larynx, and pharynx.

a. Etiology: the result of tumors, vascular or degenerative diseases of lower cranial nerve motor nuclei, (e.g., amyotrophic lateral sclerosis).

b. Examine/determine.

(1) Glossopharyngeal and vagal paralysis: phonation, articulation, palatal action, gag reflex, swallowing.

(2) Changes in voice quality: dysphonia (hoarseness or nasal quality).

(3) Bilateral involvement: severe airway restriction with dyspnea, difficulty with coughing.

(4) Possible complications: aspiration pneumonia.

c. Pseudobulbar palsy: bilateral dysfunction of corticobulbar innervation of brainstem nuclei; a central or UMN lesion analogous to corticospinal lesions disrupting function of anterior horn cells.

(1) Produces similar symptoms as bulbar palsy.

(2) Examine for hyperactive reflexes: increased jaw jerk, and snout reflex (tapping on lips produces pouting of lips).

d. Medical/surgical treatment of underlying cause.

e. Physical therapy goals, outcomes, and interventions.

(1) Suctioning, oral care.
(2) Maintenance of respiratory function, open airway.
(3) Elevate head of bed.
(4) Dietary changes: soft foods, liquids.

5. **Guillain-Barré syndrome (GBS, acute ascending, symmetrical polyneuropathy).** Polyneuritis with progressive muscular weakness that develops rapidly.
 a. Etiology: unknown; associated with an autoimmune attack, usually occurs after recovery from an infectious illness (respiratory or gastrointestinal).
 b. Characteristics.
  (1) Involves acute demyelination of both cranial and peripheral nerves (LMN disease).
  (2) Sensory loss, paresthesias (tingling, burning), pain; sensory loss is typically less than motor loss.
  (3) Motor paresis or paralysis: relative symmetrical distribution of weakness; progresses from lower extremities to upper (ascending pattern) and from distal to proximal; may produce full tetraplegia with respiratory failure.
  (4) Dysarthria, dysphagia, diplopia, and facial weakness may develop in severe cases.
  (5) Progression evolves over a few days or weeks; recovery usually slow (6 months to 2 years) and usually complete (85% of cases); some mild weakness may persist; 3% mortality.
  (6) Complications.
   (a) Respiratory impairment and failure.
   (b) Autonomic instability: tachycardia, arrhythmias, BP fluctuations.
   (c) Pain: myalgia.
   (d) Risk of pneumonia.
   (e) Prolonged hospitalizations and immobility: deep venous thrombosis, skin breakdown, contracture.
   (f) Relapse: if treatment is inadequate.
 c. Examine.
  (1) Cardiac and respiratory status, vital signs.
  (2) Cranial nerve function (VII, IX, X, XI, XII).
  (3) Motor strength (serial MMTs indicated).
  (4) Reflexes: decreased or absent tendon reflexes.
  (5) Sensation: changes can include paresthesias, anesthesias, hyperesthesias, pain (muscle aching, burning); may have stocking and glove distribution (anesthesia of distal extremities in a pattern as if the patient were wearing long gloves and stockings).
  (6) Functional status.
 d. Medical.
  (1) Good nursing care.
  (2) Plasmapheresis.
  (3) IVIG.
  (4) Analgesics for relief of pain.
 e. Physical therapy goals, outcomes, and interventions.
  (1) Maintain respiratory function: may require endotracheal intubation, tracheotomy and ventilation; pulmonary physical therapy.
  (2) Prevent indirect impairments: PROM within pain tolerance, positioning and skin care.
  (3) Prevent injury to denervated muscles: monitor recovery; splinting, positioning.
  (4) Provide muscle reeducation, moderate exercise program (active assistance and active exercise progressing to resistive), functional training as recovery progresses.
  (5) Teach energy conservation techniques and activity pacing: avoid overuse and fatigue which may prolong recovery.
  (6) Improve cardiovascular fitness following prolonged bed rest and deconditioning.
  (7) Provide emotional support and reassurance to patient and family.

6. **Amyotrophic lateral sclerosis (ALS, "Lou Gehrig's disease").** A degenerative disease affecting both upper and LMNs (degeneration of anterior horn cells and descending corticobulbar and corticospinal tracts).
 a. Etiology: unknown (viral/autoimmune, toxic); 5%–10% genetic (autosomal dominant).
 b. Characteristics.
  (1) Progressive disease, often leading to death, typically in 2–5 years; highly variable symptoms.
   (a) Bulbar onset (progressive bulbar palsy).
   (b) Spinal cord onset (progressive muscular atrophy).
  (2) Muscular weakness that spreads over time: early onset involves limbs progressing to whole body; atrophy, cramping, muscle fasciculations, or twitching (LMN signs).
  (3) Spasticity, hyperreflexia (UMN signs).
  (4) Dysarthria, dysphagia, dysphonia secondary to pseudobulbar palsy and progressive bulbar palsy.
  (5) Usually absence of sensory changes; small number (20%) may show sensory deficits.
  (6) Autonomic dysfunction in about one third of patients.
  (7) Pain due to spasticity, cramping, postural stress syndrome, joint hypomobility, or instability.
  (8) Respiratory impairments: weakness > paralysis, nocturnal difficulty, exertional dyspnea, accessory muscle use; paradoxical breathing, ventilator dependent; poor cough, clearance of secretions.
  (9) Typical sparing of bowel and bladder function.
  (10) Cognition is normal, similar to locked-in syndrome (CVA).
  (11) Depression common.
 c. Stages of ALS.
  (1) Stage I: early disease, mild focal weakness, asymmetrical distribution; symptoms of hand cramping and fasciculations.

(2) Stage II: moderate weakness in groups of muscles, some wasting (atrophy) of muscles; modified independence with assistive devices.
(3) Stage III: severe weakness of specific muscles, increasing fatigue; mild to moderate functional limitations, ambulatory.
(4) Stage IV: severe weakness and wasting of LEs, mild weakness of UEs; moderate assistance and assistive devices required; wheelchair user.
(5) Stage V: progressive weakness with deterioration of mobility and endurance, increased fatigue, moderate to severe weakness of whole limbs and trunk; spasticity, hyperreflexia; loss of head control; maximal assist.
(6) Stage VI: bedridden, dependent ADLs, FMS; progressive respiratory distress.

d. Examine.
(1) History: varied pattern of onset.
(2) Vital signs, respiratory function.
(3) Cranial nerve function: especially lower cranial nerves (VII, IX, X, XI, XII).
(4) Motor function.
(a) Examine for atrophy, widespread weakness; a symmetrical distribution, muscle cramping, and muscle twitching.
(b) Examine for spasticity, hyperreflexia.
(c) Coordination tests: manual skills.
(5) Sensory function.
(6) Gait: timed walk (10-m walk test).
(7) Functional status: monitor closely for overwork fatigue, persistent weakness following exercise or activity; e.g., keep activity log.
(8) ALS Functional Rating Scale (ALSFRS): assesses disease progression and function across 10 functional categories; scored 0 (loss of function) to 4 (normal function); 40 maximal score.

e. Medical management: there is no effective treatment for this disease.
(1) Riluzole, a glutamate antagonist, may slow progression, prolong survival, especially with bulbar-onset disease.
(2) Symptomatic relief: i.e., spasticity, pain, respiratory failure.

f. Physical therapy goals, outcomes, and interventions.
(1) Maintain respiratory function: may require airway clearance techniques, cough facilitation, breathing exercises, chest stretching, suctioning, incentive spirometry, long-term mechanical ventilation.
(2) Provide for nutritional needs: assist in management of dysphagia; may require nasogastric tube or percutaneous gastrostomy in later stages.
(3) Prevent indirect impairments: maintain activity levels as long as possible, PROM, positioning, skin care.
(4) Provide moderate exercise program.
(a) Prevent further deconditioning and disuse atrophy while avoiding overwork damage in weakened, denervated muscle; e.g., mild resistive exercises if muscles are in good to normal ranges; active exercises or functional activities as weakness progresses.
(b) Mild aerobic activities: e.g., swimming, walking, stationary bike (submaximal levels).
(c) Exercise precautions: monitor fatigue levels closely; avoid overwork injury (avoid exercise if less than one third of motor units are functioning); limited positions with decreased pulmonary function.
(d) As disease progresses, replace resistance exercises with functional training activities.
(5) Teach energy conservation activity, pacing techniques; e.g., balance activity with rest.
(6) Maintain maximal functional independence: provide appropriate assistive devices, orthotic support, wheelchair, environmental adaptations; anticipate needs.
(7) Symptomatic treatment of pain, spasms, spasticity.
(8) Teach patient, family, caregivers all care, ADLs; assist in utilization of community resources.
(9) Provide psychological support and reassurance, maximum comfort; loss of control is an important issue.

7. **Postpolio syndrome (PPS), progressive postpolio muscular atrophy (PPPMA).** New, slowly progressive muscle weakness occurring in individuals with a confirmed history of acute poliomyelitis; follows a stable period of functioning.

a. Etiology: unknown; possible hyperfunctioning of motor neurons, long-term overuse at high levels resulting in new denervation.

b. Characteristics:
(1) New weakness and atrophy, asymmetrical in distribution. Occurs in both initially weak and uninvolved muscles.
(2) Abnormal fatigue: may not be related to activity levels, doesn't recover easily with usual rest periods.
(3) Pain: myalgia, cramping pain, joint pain with repetitive injury, hypersensitivities.
(4) Decreased function with reduced endurance for routine activities.
(5) Slow progression, either steady or stepwise.
(6) Environmental cold intolerance.
(7) Difficulty in concentration, memory, attention; damage to reticular formation, hypothalamus, dopaminergic neurons (brain fatigue generator model).
(8) Sleep disturbances.
(9) Decreased functional mobility, aerobic capacity, labile exercise blood pressures.
(10) Slow progression, can be steady or stepwise.

c. Examine.
   (1) History: confirm original acute polio illness; document onset of present symptoms, presentation, course, chronology.
   (2) Motor function: strength, atrophy, muscle fatigue, muscle twitching and cramps.
      (a) Identify problem musculature, weakness found in both new muscles and muscles previously affected by polio.
      (b) Identify functional contractions (fair grades or above).
      (c) Look for spotty involvement, asymmetrical paralysis.
   (3) ROM and deformity.
   (4) Pain.
      (a) Muscle pain: check tenderness to touch.
      (b) Skeletal, soft tissue pain: chronic overuse, poor alignment.
   (5) Sensory function: any sensory deficit is due to other etiology (sensation is unaffected in PPS).
   (6) Respiratory function: examine for dyspnea, difficulty in speaking, weak cough.
   (7) Functional status: functional mobility skills, activities of daily living.
   (8) Endurance, activity levels: fatigue is a primary symptom.
   (9) Aerobic capacity: use ergometer that involves both upper and lower extremities; e.g., Schwinn Air-Dyne, discontinuous protocol, submaximal test (ACSM recommendation).
   (10) EMG to identify prior anterior horn cell (AHC) disease and new motor unit pathology. See denervation changes, fasciculations, fibrillations, increased motor unit amplitude and duration.
   (11) Examine for presence of depression or anxiety.

d. Medical management.
   (1) Antidepressants: e.g., amitriptyline (Elavil), fluoxetine (Prozac).
   (2) Neurotransmitter inhibitors: decreases fatigue and sleep disorders; e.g., serotonin, norepinephrine.

e. Physical therapy goals, outcomes, and interventions.
   (1) Maintain respiratory function: teach breathing exercises, supportive cough maneuvers, postural drainage as indicated.
   (2) Teach energy conservation techniques, activity pacing: balance activity with frequent rest periods to decrease fatigue, prevent overwork damage in weakened, denervated muscle.
      (a) Teach relaxation techniques to maximize rest.
      (b) Avoid unnecessary activities to maximize important work.
   (3) Preserve or increase muscle strength.
      (a) Provide moderate exercise program (nonexhaustive exercise): modified strengthening and conditioning; use low-intensity, discontinuous nonfatiguing exercise with increased rest periods.
      (b) Caution against widespread use of strength training.
      (c) Consider pool programs: minimizes overwork, relieves pain; general body conditioning.
      (d) Foster weight control and reduction.
   (4) Aerobic conditioning: moderate to low-level training depending upon class of disease, discontinuous protocol. In severe atrophic polio, exercise is contraindicated.
   (5) Maintain or increase function: provide recommendations for lifestyle modification; minimize abnormal postures, gait deviations.
   (6) Prescribe appropriate orthoses, mobility aids (motorized cart), assistive devices, environmental modifications.
   (7) Eliminate or control pain: provide options for pain control, foster self-control.
   (8) Teach patient and family all care, activities of daily living; lifestyle modifications.
   (9) Provide psychological support and reassurance.

Pain

The sensory and emotional experience associated with actual or potential tissue damage (International Association for the Study of Pain).

1. Pain pathways/neurophysiology.

a. Fast pain: transmitted over A delta fibers (polymodal, nonmyelinated), processed in spinal cord dorsal horn lamina (I & V), crosses to excite lateral (neo) spinothalamic tract; terminates in brainstem reticular formation and thalamus with projections to cortex; functions for localization, discrimination of pain.

b. Slow pain: transmitted over C fibers, processed in spinal cord lamina (II & III–V), cross to excite anterior (paleo)spinothalamic tract; terminates in brainstem reticular formation; excites RAS, functions for diffuse arousal (protective/aversive reactions), affective and motivational aspects of pain; also terminates in thalamus with projections to cortex.

c. Intrinsic inhibitory mechanisms.
   (1) Gate control theory: transmission of sensation at spinal cord level is controlled by balance between large fibers (A alpha, A beta) and small fibers (A delta, C); activity of large fibers at level of first synapse can block activity of small fibers and pain transmission (counterirritant theory).
   (2) Descending analgesic systems: endogenous opiates (endorphins, enkephalins) produced throughout CNS (e.g., periaqueductal gray, raphe nuclei, pituitary gland/hypothalamus, SC laminae I and II); can depress pain transmission at various sites through mechanisms of presynaptic inhibition.

2. Acute pain. Pain provoked by noxious stimulation, associated with an underlying pathology (injury or acute inflammation/disease); signs include sharp pain and sympathetic changes (increased heart rate, increased blood pressure, pupillary dilation, sweating, hyper-ventilation, anxiety, protective/escape behaviors).

3. **Chronic pain.** Pain that persists beyond the usual course of healing; symptoms present for >6 months, for which an underlying pathology is no longer identifiable or may never have been present.

4. **Pain syndromes.**
   a. Neuropathic pain: pain as a result of lesions in some part of the nervous system (central or peripheral); usually accompanied by some degree of sensory deficit.
      (1) Thalamic pain: continuous, intense, central pain occurring on the contralateral hemiplegic side; the result of a stroke involving the ventral posterolateral thalamus; autonomic and vasomotor dysfunction common.
      (2) Complex regional pain syndrome (CRPS): a complex disorder or group of disorders that develop as a consequence of trauma affecting body part(s) and disuse. The term *regional* indicates that signs and symptoms are present throughout the limb (upper or lower limb) and not occurring in a peripheral nerve or nerve root distribution.
         (a) Typically worse in distal limb than proximal.
         (b) Precipitating trauma can be minor with time of onset of CRPS.
         (c) Pain is severe, out of proportion to original injury.
         (d) Early symptoms include vasodilation in skin, abnormal sweating, edema, and skin atrophy.
         (e) Late changes include atrophy of skin, muscles, and joints; osteoporosis. May develop muscles paresis and spasms.
      (3) Reflex sympathetic dystrophy (RSD) (also known as causalgia, shoulder-hand syndrome, and Sudeck's atrophy): diffuse, persistent pain involving central reorganization of sensory systems. Typically develops as a result of trauma to a peripheral pathway with sympathetic overactivity. Categorized as a syndrome under CRPS. Three stages have been defined.
         (a) Acute or early stage: characterized by diffuse, severe burning or aching pain; increases with emotional stress; allodynia (pain on light touch) and hyperpathia (increased sensitivity to normal stimuli); vasomotor instability with dusky mottling, cool skin, swelling, and edema.
         (b) Dystrophic or middle stage: skin changes with thin, pale, cyanotic skin; cessation of hair and nail growth; hyperhidrosis; muscle atrophy and osteoporosis.
         (c) Atrophic or late stage; decreased hypersensitivity; normal blood flow and temperature; smooth, glossy skin; severe muscles atrophy; pericapsular fibrosis; diffuse osteoporosis; development of claw hand may occur.
      (4) Disorders of peripheral roots and nerves.
         (a) Neuralgia: pain occurring along the branches of a nerve; frequently paroxysmal.
         (b) Radiculalgia: neuralgia of nerve roots.
         (c) Paresthesias, allodynia: with nerve injury or transection.
      (5) Herpes zoster (shingles): an acute, painful mononeuropathy caused by the varicella zoster virus; characterized by vesicular eruption and marked inflammation of the posterior root ganglion of the affected spinal nerve or sensory ganglion of the cranial nerve; ventral root involvement (motor weakness) in 5%–10% of cases; infection can last from 10 days to 5 weeks; postherpetic neuralgia pain may persist for months or years.
      (6) Phantom limb pain: in a limb following amputation of that limb; differentiated from far more common phantom limb sensation.
   b. Musculoskeletal pain.
      (1) Fibromyalgia: widespread pain accompanied by tenderness of muscles and adjacent soft tissues, a nonarticular rheumatic disease of unknown origin.
      (2) Myofascial pain syndrome (MPS): persistent, deep aching pains in muscle, nonarticular in origin; characterized by well-defined, highly sensitive tender spots (trigger points).
      (3) Postural stress syndrome (PSS): postural malalignment produces chronic muscle lengthening and/or shortening and stress to soft tissues.
   c. Pain with psychiatric disorders (psychosomatic pain): the origin of the pain experience is due to mental or emotional disorders.
   d. Headache and craniofacial pain; e.g., temporomandibular joint syndrome (TMJ).
   e. Referred pain: pain arising from deep visceral tissues that is felt in a body region remote from the site of pathology, resulting in tenderness and cutaneous hyperalgesia; e.g., medial left arm pain with heart attack; right subscapular pain from gallbladder attack.

5. **Examine.**
   a. History: determine chief complaints, description of onset, mechanism of injury, localization (chronic pain is poorly localized, not well defined); nature of pain (constant, intermittent); irritating stimuli/activities.
   b. Subjective assessment using pain intensity rating scales.
      (1) Simple descriptive scales: verbal report (e.g., select the words that best describe your pain).

(2) Semantic differentiation scales: McGill Pain Questionnaire.
(3) Numerical rating scales (rate pain on a scale of 1–10; e.g., 8/10).
(4) Visual analog scale (e.g., bisect line where your pain falls, from mild to severe pain).
(5) Spatial distribution of pain: using drawings to plot location, type of pain.

c. For underlying pathology (cause of pain); objective physical findings are usually not readily identified.
   (1) All systems: musculoskeletal, neurological, and cardiopulmonary. Examine for muscle guarding.
   (2) Examine for postural stress syndrome (PSS).
   (3) Examine for movement adaptation syndrome (MAS): habituated movement dysfunction.
   (4) Examine for autonomic changes (sympathetic activity): typically present with acute but not chronic pain.
d. Degree of suffering.
   (1) Verbal complaints are out of proportion to degree of underlying pathology; include emotional content.
   (2) Exhibits a stooped posture, antalgic gait.
   (3) Exhibits facial grimacing.
e. Functional changes, abnormal movements.
   (1) Examine for self-imposed limited activity; disrupted lifestyle; disuse syndrome.
   (2) Examine for avoidance of work, social interactions, or sexual activity.
f. Consequences of pain, behavioral impact, secondary gains.
   (1) Monetary benefits (malingering, insurance claims).
   (2) Sympathy and attention.
   (3) Avoidance of undesirable work.
g. Depression, anxiety.
h. Prescription drug misuse.
i. Dependence on health care system: multiple health care providers, clinical services; "shopping around" behaviors.
j. Responsiveness of pain to physiological interventions/treatments: chronic pain is often unresponsive.
k. Motivational/affective components (sick role).
   (1) Previous experience with pain.
   (2) Learned responses to pain.
   (3) Perception of control over pain.
   (4) Ethnicity/cultural aspects of pain.

6. Physical therapy goals, outcomes, and interventions.
a. Assist patient in identifying pain behaviors, remove behavioral reinforcers, and practice well behaviors.
   (1) Establish a behavior contract: establish consistent level of activity.
   (2) Provide positive reinforcers, educational support.
   (3) Demonstrate change, allow patient to experience success.
b. Teach coping skills.
c. Provide relaxation training.
   (1) Progressive relaxation techniques (e.g., Jacobson's), deep breathing exercises.
   (2) Guided imagery.
   (3) Yoga.
   (4) Biofeedback.
d. Provide direct, time-limited pain control.
   (1) Transcutaneous electrical nerve stimulation (TENS).
   (2) Electrotherapeutic modalities.
   (3) Heat and cold.
   (4) Manipulative procedures: soft tissue massage, mobilization.
   (5) Hydrotherapy.
   (6) Counterirritants; e.g., analgesic balms.
e. Establish a realistic daily exercise program.
   (1) Improve overall level of conditioning: daily walking program. Assistive devices as appropriate.
   (2) Improve overall functional capacity, independence in functional mobility skills, ADLs: ROM, general strengthening, postural training, motor control training.

Interventions for Patients with Neurological Dysfunction

Remediation-Facilitation Intervention

1. General concepts.
a. Includes neuromuscular facilitation, sensory stimulation; exercises/activities designed to reduce impairments, and improve function of involved body segments.
b. Goal is to enhance or improve recovery.
c. Developmental focus: emphasis is on developmental postures/patterns of movement to promote recovery and function.

2. Proprioceptive Neuromuscular Facilitation (PNF).
a. Basic procedures for facilitation.
   (1) The facilitation of total patterns of movement will promote motor learning in synergistic muscle patterns.

(2) Normal movements are spiral and diagonal in character.
(3) Proprioceptive elements.
  (a) Resistance: enhances contraction and motor control, increases strength, and aids motor learning.
  (b) Irradiation and reinforcement: response to stimulation spreads to adjacent muscles working in synergistic patterns.
  (c) Manual contact: increases responses and guides movements.
  (d) Body position and body mechanics: important for control of motion.
  (e) Verbal cues: provide direction for movements and is important for motor learning.
  (f) Vision: use of vision guides movement and is important for motor learning.
  (g) Approximation: compression force applied to joints. Stimulates afferent nerve endings and facilitates extensor muscles, stabilizing patterns.
  (h) Traction: a distraction force applied to joints. Stimulates afferent nerve endings and facilitates flexor muscles, mobilizing patterns.
  (i) Stretch: muscle elongation (stretch reflex) facilitates muscle contraction.
  (j) Timing: goal is to promote normal timing and increase muscle contraction through timing for emphasis.
(4) Total synergistic patterns of movement and posture are important preparatory patterns for advanced functional skills.

b. Techniques, new revised terminology (traditional terminology):
  (1) Rhythmic Initiation: voluntary relaxation followed by passive movements through increasing ROM, followed by active-assisted movements progressing to resisted movements; the patient finishes with active movements. Indications: inability to initiate movement (apraxia); uncoordinated motion (rigidity, ataxia), general tension or tonal impairments (hypertonic muscles); motor learning deficits; communication deficits (aphasia).
  (2) Rhythmic Rotation: voluntary relaxation combined with slow, passive, rhythmic rotations of the body or body part; focus is on gaining ROM. Active holding in the new range is then stressed. Indications: general tension or hypertonia with limitations in function or ROM (hypertonic muscles).
  (3) Stabilizing Reversals (Alternating Isometrics): isometric holding is facilitated first on one side of the joint, followed by alternate holding of the antagonist muscle groups. May be applied in any direction (anterior-posterior, medial-lateral, diagonal). Indications: decreased stability, poor antigravity control, weakness.
  (4) Rhythmic Stabilization: simultaneous isometric contractions of both agonist and antagonist muscles (cocontraction) performed without relaxation using careful grading of resistance; RS emphasizes rotational stability control. Indications: decreased stability in weight bearing and holding, poor antigravity control, weakness, ataxia; also limitations in ROM caused by muscle tightness, painful muscle splinting.
  (5) Dynamic Reversals (Slow Reversals): slow isotonic contractions of first agonist, then antagonist patterns using careful grading of resistance and optimal facilitation; reversals of antagonists without relaxation or pause. An isometric hold can be added at the end of the range at a point of weakness (the hold may be added in both directions or only in one direction). Indications: decreased active ROM, weakness of antagonistic muscles, decreased reciprocal control, hypertonic muscle groups.
  (6) Combination of Isotonics (Agonist Reversals): combines concentric, eccentric, and isometric contractions of one muscle group (agonists: a slow isotonic, shortening contraction through the range, followed by an isometric hold and then an eccentric, lengthening contraction using the same muscle groups). Indications: weak postural muscles, inability to eccentrically control body weight during movement transitions; e.g., sitting down; decreased active ROM, control, weakness.
  (7) Replication (Hold-Relax-Active Motion): an isometric contraction performed in the mid to shortened range followed by voluntary relaxation and passive movement into the lengthened range, and resistance to an isotonic contraction through the range. Indications: an inability to initiate movement, hypotonia, weakness.
  (8) Contract-Relax: a relaxation technique usually performed at a point of limited ROM in the agonist pattern: isotonic movement in rotation is performed followed by an isometric hold of the range-limiting muscles in the antagonist pattern against slowly increasing resistance, then voluntary relaxation, and active contraction (CRAC) into the newly gained range of the agonist pattern. Indications: limitations in ROM caused by muscle tightness, spasticity.
  (9) Hold-Relax: a relaxation technique usually performed at the point of limited ROM in the agonist pattern; an isometric contraction of the range-limiting antagonist pattern is performed against slowly increasing resistance, followed by voluntary relaxation, and passive movement into the newly gained range of the agonist pattern.

Active contraction (HRAC) into the newly gained range of the agonist pattern can also be performed and serves to maintain the inhibitory effects through reciprocal inhibition. Indications: limitations in ROM caused by muscle tightness, muscle spasm, and pain.

(10) Repeated Stretch (Repeated Contractions): repeated stretch linked to voluntary effort to contract stretched muscles; may be repeated without stopping as soon as the contraction weakens or stops. Indications: weakness, fatigue, decreased ability to perform the desired pattern.

c. Diagonal patterns of movement: upper extremity (UE), named for motions occurring at the proximal joint (shoulder); intermediate joint (elbow) may be straight, flexing, or extending (intermediate pivot).
   (1) Flexion-adduction-external rotation (D1F, diagonal 1 flexion)
   Verbal cues (VC) "Close your hand, turn, and pull your arm across your face."
   (2) Extension-abduction-internal rotation (D1E)
   VC: "Open your hand, turn and push your arm down and out."
   (3) Flexion-abduction-external rotation (D2F)
   VC: "Open your hand, turn, and lift your arm up and out."
   (4) Extension-adduction-internal rotation (D2E)
   VC: "Close your hand, turn, and pull your arm down and across your body."

d. Diagonal patterns of movement: lower extremity (LE), named for motions occurring at the proximal joint (hip); intermediate joint (knee) may be straight, flexing, or extending (intermediate pivot).
   (1) Flexion-adduction-external rotation (D1F)
   VC: "Bring your foot up, turn, and pull your leg up and across your body."
   (2) Extension-abduction-internal rotation (D1E)
   VC: "Push your foot down, turn, and push your leg down and out."
   (3) Flexion-abduction-internal rotation (D2F)
   VC: "Lift your foot up, turn, and lift your leg up and out."
   (4) Extension-adduction-external rotation (D2E)
   VC: "Push your foot down, turn, and pull your leg down and in."

e. Diagonal patterns: head and trunk.
   (1) Supine or sitting, chop: upper trunk flexion with rotation to right or left; lead arm moves in D1E, assist arm holds on top of wrist.
   (2) Supine or sitting, lift: upper trunk extension with rotation to right or left; lead arm moves in D2F, assist arm holds beneath the wrist.
   (3) Supine, lower trunk flexion with rotation to right or left; knees flexing.
   (4) Supine or sitting, head and neck flexion with rotation to right or left.

3. Neurodevelopmental Treatment (NDT).

a. Basic concepts.
   (1) Focus is on enhancing motor skills, postural control, and quality of movements through movement experiences. Accurate analysis of the patient's movement patterns is essential.
   (2) Multiple factors contribute to movement dysfunction in patients with neurological dysfunction: sensory and motor deficits (weakness, limited ROM, impaired tone and coordination).
   (4) Focus is on enhancing purposeful relationship between sensory input and motor output; facilitation of normal movement and postural patterns, avoidance (inhibition) of abnormal and compensatory patterns of movement.
   (5) Motor learning (or relearning) of patterns of movement can be facilitated by appropriate handling techniques, a combination of inhibition/facilitation techniques, guided movements, verbal cues, repetition, and experience in the environment.
   (6) Focus is on functional skills with stimulation of critical foundational elements (task components) as well as practice of the whole task. Use of goal directed activities.
   (7) Anticipated goals and outcomes determined in partnership with the family, client, and the interdisciplinary team.

b. Techniques of treatment.
   (1) Therapeutic handling: guided and assisted movements leading to active movements.
      (a) Assistance is given only as needed.
      (b) Task understanding, voluntary control of movement is promoted.
      (c) Low effort: maximizes performance in the presence of tonal disorders; high effort, maximal resistance results in unwanted activity, and is avoided.
      (d) Avoidance of substitution movements.
      (e) Minimizing verbal instructions or feedback during movement.
      (f) Ensuring movement success, avoidance of repeated failures.
   (2) Normalization of postural control.
      (a) Promote appropriate trunk alignment, ability to weight shift, perform transitional movements, and postural control.
      (b) Efforts are made to increase tone if it is too low (hypotonia), or decrease tone if it is too high (spasticity); e.g., rhythmic rotation or tapping.
      (c) Inhibit or prevent abnormal patterns of movements and reflexes.
   (3) Normalization of sensory/perceptual experiences.

c. Patterns of movement.
   (1) Resumption of normal functional activities that are meaningful, goal-oriented; e.g., rolling, sitting up, standing, walking.

CHAPTER 2

(2) Appropriate developmental activities.
(3) Improve timing and synergistic activity of selective limb movements; e.g., UE functional tasks.
(4) Integrated movements utilizing both affected and intact body segments.

4. Sensory stimulation.

a. General concepts.
(1) Indications: patients who demonstrate absent or disordered motor control, i.e., difficulty initiating movement (initial mobility) or sustaining movement (stability), who would benefit from the use of augmented feedback; most useful in the early stages of motor learning.
(2) Contraindications: patients who will not benefit from a hands-on approach, who demonstrate sufficient motor control to perform and refine a motor skill, and the ability to self-correct based on intrinsic feedback mechanisms; e.g., later stages of motor learning.
(3) Response to stimulation is dependent upon multiple factors, including level of intactness of CNS, initial central state/level of CNS arousal, type and amount of stimulation, specific activity of alpha motor neurons pool.
(4) Early use of sensory stimulation techniques should be phased out as soon as possible in favor of active control by the patient; important to avoid feedback/therapist dependence. Can serve as a bridge to active movement control.
(5) Spatial summation (multiple techniques) or temporal summation (repeated application of the same technique) may be necessary to produce the desired response in some low-level patients; e.g., sensory stimulation programs for patients in coma or early recovery following TBI.
(6) Consider cumulative effects: the total environment along with the effects of sensory stimulation techniques.
(a) Avoid bombardment (overload): may prove harmful; CNS shut down is likely in the face of overstimulation or sympathetic fight-or-flight reactions.
(b) Consider what stimuli may yield desired performance and optimum learning.

b. Techniques.
(1) Proprioceptive stimulation techniques.
(a) Quick stretch, tapping of muscle belly or tendon: facilitates agonist muscle, inhibits antagonist.
(b) Prolonged, slowly applied stretch (manual, positioning, inhibitory casts): inhibits agonist muscle, dampens high tone.
(c) Resistance: recruits motor units, both alpha and gamma motor neurons; facilitates, strengthens agonist contraction.
(d) Joint approximation: enhances joint awareness, facilitates cocontraction, action of postural extensors, stabilizing muscles.
(e) Joint traction: enhances joint awareness, action of flexors; relieves muscle spasm (joint mobilization).
(f) Inhibitory pressure (firm pressure on long tendons): inhibits muscle, dampens tone; e.g., weight bearing on an extended open hand (spastic hand) or kneeling (spastic quadriceps).
(2) Exteroceptive stimulation techniques.
(a) Light, quick touch: initiates phasic, withdrawal reactions; e.g., quick stroke to palm of hand can produce withdrawal of the hand away from the stimulus.
(b) Maintained touch (maintained pressure): produces calming effect, generalized inhibition.
(3) Vestibular stimulation techniques.
(a) Slow, maintained vestibular stimulation (slow, repetitive rocking): produces generalized inhibition of tone, relaxation, calming effect.
(b) Fast, irregular vestibular stimulation (spinning, fast rolling): produces generalized facilitation of tone, improved motor coordination, and improved retinal image stability.

Motor Control/Motor Learning Strategies

1. General concepts.

a. Incorporates theories of motor control and motor learning.
b. Used in combination with task-related training.
c. Consideration is given to both intrinsic neuromuscular control processes and environmental constraints.

2. Motor control strategies.

a. General concepts—motor control.
(1) Motor program: a set of prestructured muscle commands that, when initiated, results in the production of a coordinated movement sequence (learned task); can be carried out largely uninfluenced by peripheral feedback.
(2) Motor plan: an overall strategy for movement; an action sequence requiring the coordination of a number of motor programs.
(3) Feedback: afferent information sent by various sensory receptors to control centers.
(a) Feedback updates control centers about the correctness of movement while it progresses; shapes ongoing movement.
(b) Feedback allows motor responses to be adapted to the demands of the environment.
(4) Feedforward: readies the system in advance of movement; anticipatory responses that adjust the system for incoming sensory feedback or for

future movements; e.g., preparatory postural adjustments.

(5) Motor skill acquisition.
  (a) Behavior is organized to achieve a goal-directed task.
  (b) Active problem solving/processing is required for the development of a motor program/motor plan, motor learning; improves retention of skills.
  (c) Adaptive to specific environmental demands (regulatory conditions). Closed environment: fixed, nonchanging. Open environment: variable, changing.

(6) CNS recovery/reorganization is dependent upon experience.

3. Motor learning strategies.

a. General concepts—motor learning.
  (1) A change in the capability of a person to perform a skill; the result of practice or experience.
  (2) Measures of motor learning include:
    (a) Performance: determine overall quality of performance, level of automaticity, level of effort, speed of decision making.
    (b) Retention: the ability to demonstrate the skill after a period of no practice.
    (c) Generalizability: the acquired capability to apply what has been learned to other similar tasks (transfer tests); e.g., transfers wheelchair to mat, to toilet, and to car.
    (d) Resistance to contextual change: acquired capability to apply what has been learned to other environmental contexts; e.g., clinic, home, work.
  (3) Feedback.
    (a) Intrinsic feedback: sensory information normally acquired during performance of a task.
    (b) Augmented feedback: externally presented feedback that is added to that normally acquired during task performance; e.g., verbal cueing.
    (c) Knowledge of results (KR): augmented feedback about the outcome of a movement.
    (d) Knowledge of performance (KP): augmented feedback about the nature of the movement produced; e.g., movement characteristics.
    (e) Feedback schedules: feedback given after every trial; feedback summed (after set number of trials), fading (decreasing), or bandwidth (if responses outside a designated range).
  (4) Practice.
    (a) Blocked practice: practice of a single motor skill repeatedly; repetitive practice.
    (b) Variable practice: practice of varied motor skills in which the performer is required to make rapid modifications of the skill in order to match the demands of the task.
    (c) Random practice: practice of a group or class of motor skills in random order (no predictable order).
    (d) Serial practice: practice of a group or class of motor skills in serial or predictable order.
    (e) Massed practice: relatively continuous practice in which the amount of rest time is small (rest time is less than the practice time).
    (f) Distributed practice: practice in which the rest time is relatively large (practice time is less than rest time).
    (g) Mental practice: cognitive rehearsal of a motor skill without overt physical performance.
  (5) Transfer: the effects of having previous practice of a skill or skills upon the learning of a new skill or upon performance in a new context; transfer may be either positive (assisting learning) or negative (hindering learning).
    (a) Part-whole transfer: a learning technique in which a complex motor task is broken down into its component or subordinate parts for separate practice before practice of the integrated whole.
    (b) Bilateral transfer: improvement in movement skill performance with one limb results from practice of similar movements with the opposite limb.

b. Strategies for effective learning (Table 2–13).
  (1) Feedback given after every trial improves performance, while variable feedback improves learning and retention.
  (2) Early training should focus on visual feedback (cognitive phase of learning), while later training should focus on proprioceptive feedback (associative phase of learning).
  (3) Reduce extraneous environmental stimuli early in learning (e.g., closed environment), while later learning focuses on adaptation to environmental demands (e.g., open environment).
  (4) Supportive feedback (reinforcement) can be used to shape behavior, motivate patient.
  (5) Assist learner in recognizing/pairing intrinsic feedback with movement responses.
  (6) Provide augmented feedback: knowledge of results, knowledge of performance.
    (a) Early in learning, focus feedback on correct aspects of performance.
    (b) Later in learning, focus feedback on errors as they become consistent.
    (c) Feedback after every trial improves performance, useful during early learning.
    (d) Use variable feedback (summed, fading, bandwidth) to improve retention, increase depth of cognitive processing.

Table 2-13 ➤ STAGES OF MOTOR LEARNING AND TRAINING STRATEGIES

COGNITIVE STAGE CHARACTERISTICS	TRAINING STRATEGIES
The learner • develops an understanding of task, *cognitive mapping* • assesses abilities, task demands • identifies stimuli, contacts memory • selects response, performs initial approximations of task • structures motor program • modifies initial responses ***"What to do"*** decision	Highlight purpose of task in functionally relevant terms. Demonstrate ideal performance of task to establish a *reference of correctness* Have patient verbalize task components and requirements. Point out similarities to other learned tasks Direct attention to critical task elements **Select appropriate feedback** • Emphasize intact sensory systems, intrinsic feedback systems • Carefully pair extrinsic feedback with intrinsic feedback • High dependence on vision: have patient watch movement • Provide ***Knowledge of Performance (KP):*** focus on errors as they become consistent; do not cue on large number of random errors • Provide ***Knowledge of Results (KR):*** focus on success of movement outcome Ask learner to evaluate performance, outcomes; identify problems, solutions Use reinforcements (praise) for correct performance and continuing motivation **Organize feedback schedule** • *Feedback* after every trial improves performance during early learning • *Variable feedback* (summed, fading, bandwidth designs) increases depth of cognitive processing, improves retention; may decrease performance initially **Organize initial practice** • Stress controlled movement to minimize errors • Provide adequate rest periods using *distributed practice* if task is complex, long, or energy costly or if learner fatigues easily, has short attention, or has poor concentration • Use manual guidance to assist as appropriate • Break complex tasks down into component parts, teach both parts and integrated whole • Use *bilateral transfer* as appropriate • Use *blocked (repeated) practice* of same task to improve performance • Use *variable practice* (serial or random practice order) of related skills to increase depth of cognitive processing and retention; may decrease performance initially • Use *mental practice* to improve performance and learning, reduce anxiety **Assess, modify arousal levels as appropriate** • High or low arousal impairs performance and learning • Avoid stressors, mental fatigue **Structure environment** • Reduce extraneous environmental stimuli, distractors to ensure attention, concentration • Emphasize closed skills initially gradually progressing to open skills
ASSOCIATED STAGE CHARACTERISTICS	**TRAINING STRATEGIES**
The learner • practices movements • refines motor program • spatial and temporal organization • decreases errors • extraneous movements Dependence on visual feedback decreases, increases for use of proprioceptive feedback; cognitive monitoring decreases ***"How to do"*** decision	**Select appropriate feedback** • Continue to provide KP; intervene when errors become consistent • Emphasize proprioceptive feedback, "feel of movement" to assist in establishing an internal reference of correctness • Continue to provide KR; stress relevance of functional outcomes • Assist learner to improve self-evaluation, decision-making skills • Facilitation techniques, guided movements are counterproductive during this stage of learning **Organize feedback schedule** • Continue to provide feedback for continuing motivation; encourage patient to self-assess achievements • Avoid excessive augmented feedback • Focus on use of variable feedback (summed, fading, bandwidth) designs to improve retention **Organize practice** • Encourage consistency of performance • Focus on variable practice order (serial or random) of related skills to improve retention **Structure environment** • Progress toward open, changing environment • Prepare the learner for home, community, work environments

Table 2-13 ➤ continued

AUTONOMOUS STAGE CHARACTERISTICS	TRAINING STRATEGIES
The learner • practices movements • continues to refine motor responses • spatial and temporal highly organized • movements are largely error-free • minimal level of cognitive monitoring ***"How to succeed"*** decision	Assess need for conscious attention, automaticity of movements **Select appropriate feedback** • Learner demonstrates appropriate self-evaluation, decision-making skills • Provide occasional feedback (KP, KR) when errors evident **Organize practice** • Stress consistency of performance in variable environments, variations of tasks (open skills) • High levels of practice (massed practice) are appropriate **Structure environment** • Vary environments to challenge learner • Ready the learner for home, community, and work environments Focus on competitive aspects of skills as appropriate; e.g., wheelchair sports

From: O'Sullivan S, Schmitz T. Physical Rehabilitation. 5th ed, Philadelphia, FA Davis, 2007, with permission.

(e) Avoid feedback dependence: reduce augmented feedback as soon as possible; foster active introspection, decision making by learner.

(7) Establish practice schedule: use distributed practice when superior performance is desired, when motivation is low, or when the learner has short attention, poor concentration, or fatigues easily.

(8) Use variable practice of a group of functional tasks rather than constant practice to improve learning (promotes retention and generalizability).

(9) Use random or serial practice order rather than blocked practice to improve learning (retention).

(10) Use mental practice to improve learning; have patient verbalize task components, requirements for performance; effective when task has a large cognitive component or to decrease fear and anxiety.

(11) Use parts to whole transfer when task is complex, has highly independent parts or when learner has limited memory or attention, or difficulty with a particular part. Practice both the parts and the integrated whole.

(12) Limit information with learners who have attention deficits, mentally fatigue easily; focus on key task elements; give frequent rest periods.

(13) Tasks that have highly integrated components should be practiced as a whole; e.g., gait.

(14) Transfer of learning is optimized when tasks are highly similar (similar stimuli, similar responses); e.g., bilateral transfer, one arm to the other.

(15) Use guided movement early in learning, not late; most effective for slow postural or positioning tasks.

(16) Optimal arousal is necessary for optimal learning; low arousal or intense arousal yield poor performance and learning (inverted U theory).

(17) Involve learner in goal setting; task should be desirable, functionally relevant, important to learn.

Task-Specific Training Strategies

1. General concepts.

a. Emphasis is on use of the affected body segments/limbs using task-specific experiences and training.
   (1) Patients practice important functional tasks essential to independence; e.g., stand up and sit down; balance, walking and stair climbing, reaching and manipulation.
   (2) Patients practice tasks in appropriate and safe environments; focus is on anticipated environments for daily function.
   (3) Repetition and extensive practice are required, including both in therapy and out of therapy time.

b. Patients practice under therapist's supervision and independently.
   (1) Therapists can provide initial assistance through guided movement and verbal cueing. Progression is to active movements.
   (2) Therapists serve as motor learning coaches, encouraging correct performance.
   (3) Exercise/activity logs help organize the patient's self-monitored practice.
   (4) This approach represents a shift away from the traditional neuromotor approaches that utilize an extensive hands-on approach (e.g., guided or facilitated movements).

c. Motor learning strategies are utilized, including *behavioral shaping techniques* that use reinforcement and reward to promote skill development.

d. Activity-based, task-oriented training effectively counteracts the effects of immobility and the development of indirect impairments such as muscle weakness and loss of flexibility. It prevents *learned nonuse* of the more involved segments while promoting recovery of the central nervous system (neuroplasticity).

e. Box 2–1 presents a summary of strategies for effect activity-based, task-oriented training.

2. **Locomotor training.** Using a motorized treadmill (TT) and partial body weight support (BWS) provides a means of early task training (e.g., for patients with stroke or incomplete spinal cord injury). Tasks are continually altered to increase the level of difficulty.

Box 2-1 ➤ ACTIVITY/TASK-ORIENTED INTERVENTION STRATEGIES TO PROMOTE FUNCTION-INDUCED RECOVERY

- Focus on early activity as soon as possible after injury or insult to utilize specific windows of opportunity, challenge brain functions, and avoid *learned nonuse:* "Use it or lose it."
- Consider the individual's past history, health status, age, and experience in designing appropriate, interesting, and stimulating functional activities.
- Involve the patient in goal setting and decision making, thereby enhancing motivation and promoting active commitment to recovery and functional training.
- Structure practice utilizing activity-based, task-oriented interventions.
- Select tasks important for independent function; include tasks that are important to the patient.
- Identify the patient's abilities/strengths and level of recovery/learning; choose tasks that have potential for patient success.
- Target active movements involving affected body segments; constrain or limit use of less involved segments.
- Avoid activities that are too difficult and result in compensatory strategies or abnormal, stereotypical movements.
- Provide adequate repetition and extensive practice as appropriate.
- Assist (guide) the patient to successfully carry out initial movements as needed; reduce assistance in favor of active movements as quickly as possible.
- Provide explicit verbal feedback to improve movement accuracy and learning and correct errors; promote the patient's own error detection and correction abilities.
- Provide verbal rewards for small improvements in task performance to maintain motivation.
- Provide modeling (demonstrations) of ideal task performance as needed.
- Increase the level of difficulty over time.
- Promote practice of task variations to promote adaptation of skills.
- Maximize practice: include both supervised and unsupervised practice; use an activity log to document practice outside of scheduled therapy sessions.
- Structure context-specific practice.
- Promote initial practice in a supportive environment, free of distracters to enhance attention and concentration.
- Progress to variable practice in real-world environments.
- Maintain focus on therapist's role as *coach* while minimizing hands-on therapy.
- Continue to monitor recovery closely and document progress using valid and reliable functional outcome measures.
- Be cautious about timetables and predictions, as recovery and successful outcomes may take longer than expected.

From: O'Sullivan S, Schmitz T (2010). Improving Functional Outcomes in Physical Rehabilitation. Philadelphia, FA Davis, with permission.

3. **Initial tasks are selected to ensure patient success and motivation.** (E.g., grasp and release of a cup, forward reach for upper extremity dressing).

4. **Tasks are continually altered to increase the level of difficulty.**
   a. Therapists target the functional requirements of walking: a reciprocal stepping pattern, dynamic equilibrium during propulsion, and adaptability.
   b. Verbal cueing and manual assistance are provided as needed to assist in good stepping and posture (e.g., manually assisted trunk/pelvis and the paretic limb(s) movements). Assistance is decreased as skill and control progresses.
   c. Progression is from treadmill speeds in the range of normal walking speeds (minimum of 2 mph) and increased as tolerated.
   d. Progression is from body weight support to no support (e.g., 40%–30% to 20%–10%–0%).
   e. Training is high frequency (3–4 days/week) and moderate duration (20–30 minutes); typically for 8–12 weeks.
   f. Progression is from treadmill walking to overground walking. Community ambulation skills and adaptability are targeted.

5. **Constraint-Induced Movement Therapy (CI Therapy)**
   a. The less affected UE is restrained by the use of a protective hand mitt.
   b. Task practice is focused on using the more affected UE.
      (1) Repetitive practice of functional tasks.
      (2) Shaping: a functional task is selected and is progressively made more difficult. Goal is for the participant to accomplish the task with effort.
   c. Adherence-enhancing behavioral strategies are used, including use of:
      (1) Daily administration of Motor Activity Log.
      (2) Home diary.
      (3) Problem-solving to overcome barriers to use of the more affected UE.
      (4) Behavioral contract.
      (5) Caregiver contract.
      (6) Home skill assignment, home practice, and daily schedule.
   d. Therapist provides feedback, coaching, modeling, and encouragement.
   e. Training is intense (several hours/day), high frequency (daily) for a period of 2-3 consecutive weeks.
   f. Modified CI Therapy is less intense, using lower intensity and frequency over a longer period of time (e.g., 1 hour/day, 3 days per week for 8 weeks).
   g. Progression is to functional skills performed in the home environment.

Compensatory Training Approach

1. General concepts.
   a. Indications: to offset or adapt to residual impairments and disabilities.
   b. Focus is on early resumption of functional independence with reliance on uninvolved segments for function; e.g., functional training with an individual with complete spinal cord injury.
   c. Changes are made in the patient's overall approach to tasks.
      (1) Patient is made aware of movement deficiencies, alternate ways to accomplish tasks.
      (2) Patient relearns functional patterns and habitual ways of moving.
      (3) Patient practices functional skills in a variety of environments.

2. Issues with the compensation approach.
   a. Focus on uninvolved segments to accomplish daily tasks (e.g., stroke, traumatic brain injury) may suppress recovery and contribute to *learned nonuse* of the impaired segments.
   b. Focus on task specific learning may lead to the development of *splinter skills* in patients with brain damage; skills cannot be easily generalized to other tasks or environmental situations.
   c. May be the only approach possible.
      (1) If no additional recovery is anticipated (e.g., complete spinal cord injury).
      (2) If severe motor deficits are present or if sensorimotor recovery has plateaued (e.g., stroke).
      (3) If patient exhibits extensive comorbidities and poor health.

3. Strategies.
   a. Simplify activities.
   b. Establish a new functional pattern; identify key task elements, residual segments available for control of movements.
   c. Repeated practice; work toward consistency, efficiency.
   d. Energy conservation and activity pacing techniques are important to ensure completion of all daily movement requirements.
   e. Adapt environment to facilitate relearning of skills, ease of movement.
      (1) Simplify; set up for optimal performance.
      (2) Use environmental adaptations to enhance performance; e.g., color code stairs, grab bars.

Specific references for Outcome Measures Organized by the International Classification of Functioning, Disability and Health (ICF) Categories can be found in Chapter 12, Appendix E:

- Coma, Cognitive Scales
- Balance & Gait Scales
- TBI Scales
- Wheelchair skills
- MS Scales
- PD Scales

chapter 3 Cardiovascular Physical Therapy

SUSAN B. O'SULLIVAN

Anatomy and Physiology of the Cardiovascular System

The Heart and Circulation

1. **Heart tissue.**
   a. Pericardium: fibrous protective sac enclosing heart.
   b. Epicardium: inner layer of pericardium.
   c. Myocardium: heart muscle, the major portion of the heart.
   d. Endocardium: smooth lining of the inner surface and cavities of the heart.

2. **Heart chambers.**
   a. Right atrium (RA): receives blood from systemic circulation, from the superior and inferior vena cavae.
   b. Right ventricle (RV): receives blood from the RA and pumps blood via the pulmonary artery to the lungs for oxygenation; the low-pressure pulmonary pump.
   c. Left atrium (LA): receives oxygenated blood from the lungs and the four pulmonary veins.
   d. Left ventricle (LV): receives blood from the LA and pumps blood via the aorta throughout the entire systemic circulation; the high-pressure systemic pump. The walls of the LV are thicker and stronger than the RV and form most of the left side and apex of the heart.

3. **Valves.** Provide one-way flow of blood.
   a. Atrioventricular valves: prevent backflow of blood into atria during ventricular systole; anchored by chordae tendineae to papillary muscles; valves close when ventricular walls contract.
      (1) Tricuspid valve (three cusps or leaflets): right heart valve.
      (2) Bicuspid or mitral valve (two cusps or leaflets): left heart valve.
   b. Semilunar valves: prevent backflow of blood from aorta and pulmonary arteries into the ventricles during diastole.
      (1) Pulmonary valve: prevents right backflow.
      (2) Aortic valve: prevents left backflow.

4. **Cardiac cycle.** (Figure 3-1).
   a. The rhythmic pumping action of the heart.
   b. Systole: the period of ventricular contraction. End-systolic volume is the amount of blood in the ventricles after systole; about 50 mL.
   c. Diastole: the period of ventricular relaxation and filling of blood. End-diastolic volume is the amount of blood in the ventricles after diastole; about 120 mL.
   d. Atrial contraction occurs during the last third of diastole and completes ventricular filling.

5. **Coronary circulation.**
   a. Arteries: arise directly from aorta near aortic valve; blood circulates to myocardium during diastole.
      (1) Right coronary artery (RCA): supplies right atrium, most of right ventricle, and in most individuals, the inferior wall of left ventricle, atrioventricular (AV) node, and bundle of His; supplies the sinoatrial (SA) node 60% of the time.
      (2) Left coronary artery (LCA): supplies most of the left ventricle; has two main divisions.
         (a) Left anterior descending (LAD): supplies the left ventricle and the interventricular septum, and in most individuals, the inferior areas of the apex; it may also give off branches to the right ventricle.

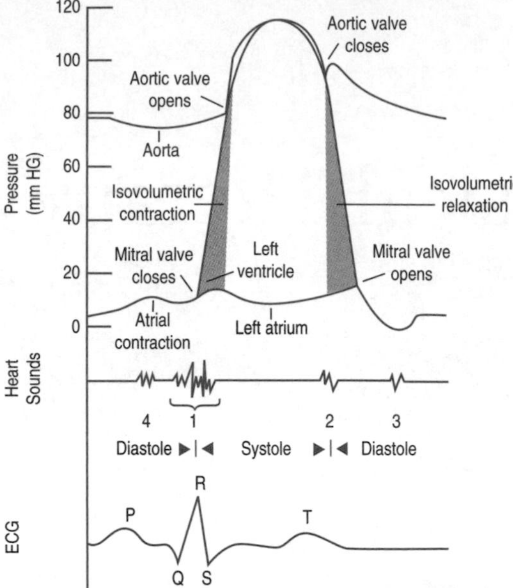

Figure 3-1 • Events of the cardiac cycle. Electrical depolarization of the ventricle (represented by QRS) precedes mechanical systole (contraction), which begins with the first heart sound (S_1) and ends with the second heart sound (S_2). The amount of blood ejected with one contraction (stroke volume) times the number of contractions per minute (heart rate) determines the cardiac output for 1 minute.

(From Stillwell, S, Randall, E. Pocket Guide for Cardiovascular Care. St. Louis, Mosby, 1990, p 2).

(b) Circumflex (Circ): supplies blood to the lateral and inferior walls of the left ventricle and portions of the left atrium; supplies SA node 40% of the time.

b. Veins: parallel arterial system; the coronary sinus receives venous blood from the heart and empties into the right atrium.

c. Distribution of blood supply is variable from individual to individual.

d. Myocardial oxygen supply and myocardial oxygen demand (MVO_2) should be in balance.

6. Conduction.

a. Specialized conduction tissue: allows rapid transmission of electrical impulses in the myocardium (normal sinus rhythm, NSR).
   (1) Nodal tissue.
   (2) Purkinje fibers: specialized conducting tissue of both ventricles.

b. Sinoatrial (SA) node.
   (1) Located at junction of superior vena cava and right atrium.
   (2) Main pacemaker of the heart; initiates the impulse.
   (3) Has sympathetic and parasympathetic innervation affecting both heart rate and strength of contraction.

c. Atrioventricular (AV) node.
   (1) Located at the junction of the right atrium and the right ventricle.
   (2) Has sympathetic and parasympathetic innervation.
   (3) Merges with bundle of His.

d. Purkinje tissue.
   (1) Right and left bundle branches of the AV node are located on either side of intraventricular septum.
   (2) Terminate in Purkinje fibers, specialized conducting tissue of the ventricles.

e. Conduction of heart beat.
   (1) Origin is in the SA node; impulse spreads throughout both atria, which contract together.
   (2) Impulse stimulates AV node, is transmitted down bundle of His to the Purkinje fibers; impulse spreads throughout the ventricles, which contract together.

7. Myocardial fibers.

a. Muscle tissue: striated muscle fibers with more numerous mitochondria; exhibits rhythmicity of contraction; fibers contract as a functional unit (sliding filament theory of contraction).

b. Myocardial metabolism is essentially aerobic, sustained by continuous O_2 delivery, from the coronary arteries.

c. Smooth muscle tissue is found in the walls of blood vessels.

8. Hemodynamics.

a. Stroke volume (SV): the amount of blood ejected with each myocardial contraction; normal range is 55–100 mL/beat. Influenced by:
   (1) Left ventricular end diastolic volume (LVEDV): the amount of blood left in the ventricle at the end of diastole. Also known as preload. The greater the diastolic filling (preload), the greater the quantity of blood pumped (Frank-Starling law).
   (2) Contractility: the ability of the ventricle to contract.
   (3) Afterload: the force the LV must generate during systole to overcome aortic pressure to open the aortic valve.

b. Cardiac output (CO): the amount of blood discharged from the left or right ventricle per minute.
   (1) For average adult at rest, normal range is 4–5 L per minute.
   (2) Determined by multiplying stroke volume times heart rate.
   (3) Cardiac index is CO divided by body surface area; normal range is 2.5 to 3.5 L/min.

c. Left ventricular end-diastolic pressure (LVEDP): pressure in the left ventricle during diastole. Normal range is 5–12 mm Hg.

d. Ejection fraction (EF): percentage of blood emptied from the ventricle during systole; a clinically useful measure of LV function.
   (1) EF = stroke volume (SV)/left ventricular end diastolic volume (LVEDV).

(2) Normal EF averages 60–70%; the lower the EF, the more impaired the LV.

e. Atrial filling pressure: the difference between the venous and atrial pressures.
   (1) Right atrial filling pressure is decreased during strong ventricular contraction and atrial filling is enhanced.
   (2) Right atrial filling pressure is affected by changes in intrathoracic pressure; decreases during inspiration and increases during coughing or forced expiration.
   (3) Venous return increases when blood volume expands and decreases during hypovolemic shock.

f. Diastolic filling time decreases with increased heart rate and with heart disease.

g. Myocardial oxygen demand (MVO_2) represents the energy cost to the myocardium.
   (1) Clinically measured by the product of heart rate (HR) and systolic blood pressure (SBP), known as the rate pressure produce (RPP).
   (2) MVO_2 increases with activity and with HR and/or BP.

Peripheral Circulation

1. Arteries.

a. Transport oxygenated blood from areas of high pressure to lower pressures in the body tissues.
b. Arterial circulation maintained by heart pump.
c. Influenced by elasticity and extensibility of vessel walls, and by peripheral resistance, amount of blood in body.

2. Capillaries.

a. Include small blood vessels that connect the ends of arteries (arterioles) with the beginning of veins (venules); form an anastomosing network.
b. Function for exchange of nutrients and fluids between blood and tissues.
c. Capillary walls are thin, permeable.

3. Veins.

a. Transport dark, unoxygenated blood from tissues back to the heart.
b. Larger capacity, thinner walls than arteries, greater number.
c. One-way valves to prevent backflow.
d. Venous system includes both superficial and deep veins (deep veins accompany arteries, while superficial ones do not).
e. Venous circulation is influenced by muscle contraction, gravity, respiration (increased return with inspiration), compliancy of right heart.

4. Lymphatic system.

a. Includes lymphatics (superficial, intermediate, and deep), lymph fluid, lymph tissues, and organs (lymph nodes, tonsils, spleen, thymus, and the thoracic duct).
b. Drains lymph from bodily tissues and returns it to venous circulation.
c. Lymph travels from lymphatic capillaries to lymphatic vessels to ducts to left subclavian vein. Lymphatic contraction occurs by:
   (1) Parasympathetic, sympathetic, and sensory nerve stimulation.
   (2) Contraction of adjacent muscles.
   (3) Abdominal and thoracic cavity pressure changes during normal breathing.
   (4) Mechanical stimulation of dermal tissues.
   (5) Volume changes within each lymphatic vessel.
d. Major lymph nodes are submaxillary, cervical, axillary, mesenteric, iliac, inguinal, popliteal, and cubital.
e. Contributes to immune system function: lymph nodes collect cellular debris and bacteria, remove excess fluid, blood waste, and protein molecules, and produce antibodies.

Neurohumoral Influences

1. Parasympathetic stimulation (cholinergic).

a. Control located in medulla oblongata, cardioinhibitory center.
b. Via vagus nerve (CN X), cardiac plexus; innervates all myocardium; releases acetylcholine.
c. Slows rate and force of myocardial contraction; decreases myocardial metabolism.
d. Causes coronary artery vasoconstriction.

2. Sympathetic stimulation (adrenergic).

a. Control located in medulla oblongata, cardioacceleratory center.
b. Via cord segments T1–T4, upper thoracic to superior cervical chain ganglia; innervates all but ventricular myocardium; releases epinephrine and norepinephrine.
c. Causes an increase in the rate and force of myocardial contraction and myocardial metabolism.
d. Causes coronary artery vasodilation.
e. The skin and peripheral vasculature receive only postganglionic sympathetic innervation. Causes vasoconstriction of cutaneous arteries; sympathetic inhibition must occur for vasodilation.
f. Drugs that increase sympathetic functioning are sympathomimetics; drugs that decrease sympathetic functioning are sympatholytics.

3. Additional control mechanisms.

a. Baroreceptors (pressoreceptors): main mechanisms controlling heart rate.
   (1) Located in walls of aortic arch and carotid sinus; via vasomotor center.
   (2) Circulatory reflex: respond to changes in blood pressure.
      (a) Increased BP results in parasympathetic stimulation, decreased rate and force of cardiac

contraction; sympathetic inhibition, decreased peripheral resistance.

(b) Decreased BP results in sympathetic stimulation, increased heart rate, blood pressure and vasoconstriction of peripheral blood vessels.

(c) Increased right atrial pressure causes reflex acceleration of heart rate.

b. Chemoreceptors.

(1) Located in the carotid body.

(2) Sensitive to changes in blood chemicals: O_2, CO_2, lactic acid.

(a) Increased CO_2 or decreased O_2, or decreased pH (elevated lactic acid) results in an increase in heart rate.

(b) Increased O_2 levels result in a decrease in heart rate.

c. Body temperature.

(1) Increased body temperature causes heart rate to increase.

(2) Decreased body temperature causes heart rate to decrease.

d. Ion concentrations.

(1) Hyperkalemia: increased concentration of potassium ions decreases the rate and force of contraction, produces electrocardiographic (ECG) changes (widened PR interval and QRS, tall T waves).

(2) Hypokalemia: decreased concentration of potassium ions produces ECG changes (flattened T waves, prolonged PR and QT intervals); arrhythmias, may progress to ventricular fibrillation.

(3) Hypercalcemia: increased calcium concentrations increases heart actions.

(4) Hypocalcemia: decreased calcium concentrations depresses heart actions.

4. Peripheral resistance.

a. Increased peripheral resistance increases arterial blood volume and pressure.

b. Decreased peripheral resistance decreases arterial blood volume and pressure.

c. Influenced by arterial blood volume: viscosity of blood and diameter of arterioles and capillaries.

Cardiovascular Examination: History, Systems Review, Tests, and Measures

Patient Interview

1. History.

a. Presenting symptoms. Note onset, progression, nature of symptoms, insight into medical condition.

(1) Chest pain, palpitations, shortness of breath.

(2) Fatigue: generalized feeling of tiredness, weakness.

(3) Palpitations: awareness by patient of heart rhythm abnormalities; e.g., pounding, fluttering, racing heart beat, skipped beats.

(4) Dizziness, syncope (transient loss of consciousness) due to inadequate cerebral blood flow.

(5) Edema: retention of fluid in tissues; swelling, especially in dependent body parts/lower extremities; sudden weight gain.

b. Positive risk factors (See Table 3–1).

c. Negative risk factors.

(1) High serum, high-density lipoprotein (HDL) cholesterol: > 60 mg/dL.

2. Past medical history.

a. Other diagnoses, surgeries.

b. Medications.

3. Social history.

a. Current living situation, family/social support.

b. Education level, employment.

c. Lifestyle, risk factors.

4. Quality-of-life issues.

a. Functional mobility in home, community

b. Activities of daily living (ADLs); sleep.

5. Risk factors. (See Table 3-1).

a. Focus on social habits: smoking, diet.

b. Past and present level of activity.

Physical Examination—Cardiovascular System

1. Examine pulse.

a. Rhythmical throbbing of arterial wall as a result of each heartbeat; note rate and rhythm.

b. Influenced by force of contraction, volume and viscosity of blood, diameter and elasticity of vessels; emotions, exercise, blood temperature, and hormones.

c. Determine pulses; palpate for 30 seconds with regular rhythm, 1–2 minutes with irregular rhythm (Table 3–2).

(1) Apical pulse or point of maximal impulse (PMI): patient is supine, palpate at 5th interspace, midclavicular vertical line (apex of the heart; may be displaced upward by pregnancy or high diaphragm; may be displaced laterally in congestive heart failure, cardiomyopathy, ischemic heart disease.

TABLE 3-1 ➤ CORONARY ARTERY DISEASE RISK FACTORS THRESHOLDS FOR USE WITH ACM RISK STRATIFICATION

POSITIVE RISK FACTORS	DEFINING CRITERIA
Age	Men > 45 yr; Women > 55 yr
Family History	Myocardial infarction, coronary revascularization or sudden death before 55 years of age in father or other male first-degree relative, or before 65 years of age in mother or other female first-degree relative
Cigarette Smoking	Current cigarette smoker or those who quit within the previous 6 months or exposure to environmental tobacco smoke
Sedentary Lifestyle	Not participating in at least 30 min of moderate intensity (40%-60%VO_2R) physical activity on at least three days of the week for at least three months
Obesity	Body mass index >30 kg.m^{-2} or Waist girth: >102 cm (40 inches) for men and > 88 cm (35 inches) for women
Hypertension	Systolic blood pressure ≥140 mm Hg and/or diastolic ≥90 mm Hg, confirmed by measurements on at least two separate occasions, or on antihypertension medication
Dyslipidemia	Low-density lipoprotein (LDL-C) cholesterol ≥130 mg.dL^{-1} (3.37 mmol.L^{-1}) or high-density lipoprotenin (HDL-C) cholesterol < 40 mg.dL^{-1} (1.04 mmol.L^{-1}), or on lipid-lowering medication. If total serum cholesterol is all that is available, use ≥ 200 mg.dL^{-1} (5.18 mmol.L^{-1})
Prediabetes	Impaired fasting blood glucose (IFG) = fasting plasma glucose >100 mg.dL^{-1} (5.50 mmol.L^{-1}) but < 126 mg.dL^{-1} or impaired glucose tolerance (IGT) = 2-hour values in oral glucose tolerance test (OGTT) > 140 mg.dL L^{-1} (7.70 mmol. L^{-1}) but < 200 mg.dL L^{-1} (11.00 mmol.L^{-1}) confirmed by measurements on two separate occasions
NEGATIVE RISK FACTOR	
High-serum HDL cholesterol	≥ 60 mg.dL^{-1} (1.55 mmol.L^{-1})

From American College of Sports Medicine, *Guidelines for Exercise Testing and Prescription*, 8th edition, Philadelphia, Lippincott Williams & Wilkins, 2010, p. 28, with permission..

(2) Radial: palpate radial artery, radial wrist at base of thumb; most common monitoring site.

(3) Carotid: patient is lying down with head of bed elevated; palpate over carotid artery, on either side of anterior neck between sternocleidomastoid muscle and trachea.

(a) Assess one side at a time to reduce the risk of bradycardia through stimulation of the carotid sinus baroreceptor which produces a reflex drop in pulse rate or blood pressure.

(4) Brachial: palpate over brachial artery, medial aspect of the antecubital fossa; used to monitor blood pressure. Best in infants.

(5) Femoral: palpate over femoral artery in inguinal region.

(6) Popliteal: palpate over popliteal artery, behind the knee with the knee flexed slightly.

(7) Pedal: palpate over dorsalis pedis artery, dorsal medial aspect of foot; used to monitor lower extremity circulation.

d. Determine heart rate (HR).

(1) Normal adult HR is 60-100 beats per minute (bpm); <60 bpm in aerobically trained.

(2) Pediatric: newborn average is 120 bpm; normal range 115–140 bpm.

(3) Tachycardia: greater than 100 bpm. Exercise commonly results in tachycardia. Compensatory tachycardia can be seen with volume loss (surgery, dehydration).

(4) Bradycardia: less than 60 bpm.

e. Pulse abnormalities.

(1) Irregular pulse: variations in force and frequency; may be due to arrhythmias, myocarditis.

(2) Weak, thready pulse: may be due to low stroke volume, cardiogenic shock.

(3) Bounding, full pulse: may be due to shortened ventricular systole and decreased peripheral pressure; aortic insufficiency.

Table 3-2 ➤ GRADING SCALE FOR PERIPHERAL PULSES

0	Absent pulse, not palpable
1+	Pulse diminished, barely perceptible
2+	Easily palpable, normal
3+	Full pulse, increased strength
4+	Bounding pulse

2. Examine heart sounds.

a. Auscultation: the process of listening for sounds within the body; stethoscope is placed directly on chest. Note intensity and quality of heart sounds.

b. Auscultation landmarks.

(1) Aortic valve: locate the 2nd right intercostal space at the sternal border.

(2) Pulmonic valve: locate the 2nd left intercostal space at the sternal border.

(3) Tricuspid valve: locate the 4th left intercostal space at the sternal border.

(4) Mitral valve: locate the 5th left intercostal space at the midclavical area.

c. S1 sound ("lub"): normal closure of mitral and tricuspid valves; marks beginning of systole. Decreased in first-degree heart block.

d. S2 sound ("dub"): normal closure of aortic and pulmonary valves; marks end of systole. Decreased in aortic stenosis.

e. Murmurs: extra sounds.

(1) Systolic: falls between S1 and S2. May indicate valvular disease (e.g., mitral valve prolapse) or may be normal.

(2) Diastolic: falls between S2 and S1. Usually indicates valvular disease.

(3) Grades of heart murmurs: grade 1 (softest audible murmur) to grade 6 (audible with stethoscope off the chest).
(4) Thrill: an abnormal tremor accompanying a vascular or cardiac murmur; felt on palpation.

f. Bruit: an adventitious sound or murmur (blowing sound) of arterial or venous origin; common in carotid or femoral arteries; indicative of atherosclerosis.

g. Gallop rhythm: an abnormal heart rhythm with three sounds in each cycle; resembles the gallop of a horse.
(1) S3; associated with ventricular filling; occurs soon after S2; in older individuals may be indicative of congestive (LV) heart failure.
(2) S4: associated with ventricular filling and atrial contraction; occurs just before S1. S4 is indicative of pathology; e.g., coronary heart disease (CAD), myocaridal infarction (MI), aortic stenosis, or chronic hypertension.

3. Examine heart rhythm.

a. Electrocardiogram (ECG): 12-lead ECG provides information about rate, rhythm, conduction, areas of ischemia and infarct, hypertrophy, electrolyte imbalances.

b. Normal cardiac cycle (normal sinus rhythm).
(1) P wave: atrial depolarization.
(2) P-R interval: time required for impulse to travel from atria through conduction system to Purkinje fibers.
(3) QRS wave: ventricular depolarization.
(4) ST segment: beginning of ventricular repolarization.
(5) T wave: ventricular repolarization.
(6) QT interval: time for electrical systole.

c. Calculate heart rate: count number of intervals between QRS complexes in a 6-second strip and multiply by 10.

d. Assess rhythm: regular or irregular.

e. Identify arrhythmias (dysrhythmias): abnormal, disordered rhythms.
(1) Etiology: ischemic conditions of the myocardium, electrolyte imbalance, acidosis or alkalosis, hypoxemia, hypotension, emotional stress, drugs, alcohol, caffeine.
(2) Ventricular arrhythmias: originate from an ectopic focus in the ventricles (outside the normal conduction system).
(a) Significant in adversely affecting cardiac output; ventricular fibrillation is a pulseless, emergency situation requiring emergency medical treatment: cardiopulmonary resuscitation (CPR), defibrillation, medications.
(b) Premature ventricular contractions (PVCs): a premature beat arising from the ventricle; occurs occasionally in the majority of the normal population. On ECG: no P wave; a bizarre and wide QRS that is premature, followed by a long compensatory pause. Serious PVCs: > 6 per minute, paired or in sequential runs, multifocal, very early PVC (R on T phenomena).
(c) Ventricular tachycardia: a run of three or more PVCs occurring sequentially; very rapid rate (150–200 bpm); may occur paroxysmally (abrupt onset); usually the result of an ischemic ventricle. On ECG: wide, bizarre QRS waves, no P waves. Seriously compromised cardiac output.
(d) Ventricular fibrillation: chaotic activity of ventricle originating from multiple foci; unable to determine rate. On ECG: bizarre, erratic activity without QRS complexes. No effective cardiac output; clinical death within 4–6 minutes.
(3) Atrial arrhythmias (supraventricular): rapid and repetitive firing of one or more ectopic foci in the atria (outside the sinus node).
(a) On ECG, P waves are abnormal (variable in shape) or not identifiable (atrial fibrillation).
(b) Rhythm may be irregular: chronic or occurring paroxysmally.
(c) Rate: rapid with atrial tachycardia (140–250 bpm), atrial flutter (250–350 bpm); fibrillation (> 300 bpm).
(d) Cardiac output is usually maintained; may precipitate ventricular failure.
(4) Atrioventricular blocks: abnormal delays or failure to conduct through normal conducting system.
(a) First, second, or third (complete) degree atrioventricular blocks; bundle branch blocks.
(b) If ventricular rate is slowed, cardiac output decreased.
(c) Third degree, complete heart block is life threatening: requires medications (atropine), surgical implantation of pacemaker.

f. Determine ST segment changes.
(1) With impaired coronary perfusion (ischemia or injury), the ST segment becomes depressed.
(2) ST segment depression can be upsloping, horizontal, or downsloping.
(3) ST segment depression or elevation greater than 1 mm measured 0.8 second from the J point is considered abnormal.

g. ECG changes with MI: present in leads over the infarcted area (see Figure 3-2).
(1) Abnormal Q waves or (central zone of infarction).
(a) Anterior infarction: Q or Qs in leads V1 to V4
(b) Lateral infarction: Q or QS in lead 1, aVL
(c) Inferior infarction: Q or QS in leads II, III, aVF
(d) Posterior infarction: Large R waves in V1–V3, ST depression V1, V2, or V3
(2) ST elevation (zone of injury).
(3) T wave inversion (zone of ischemia).

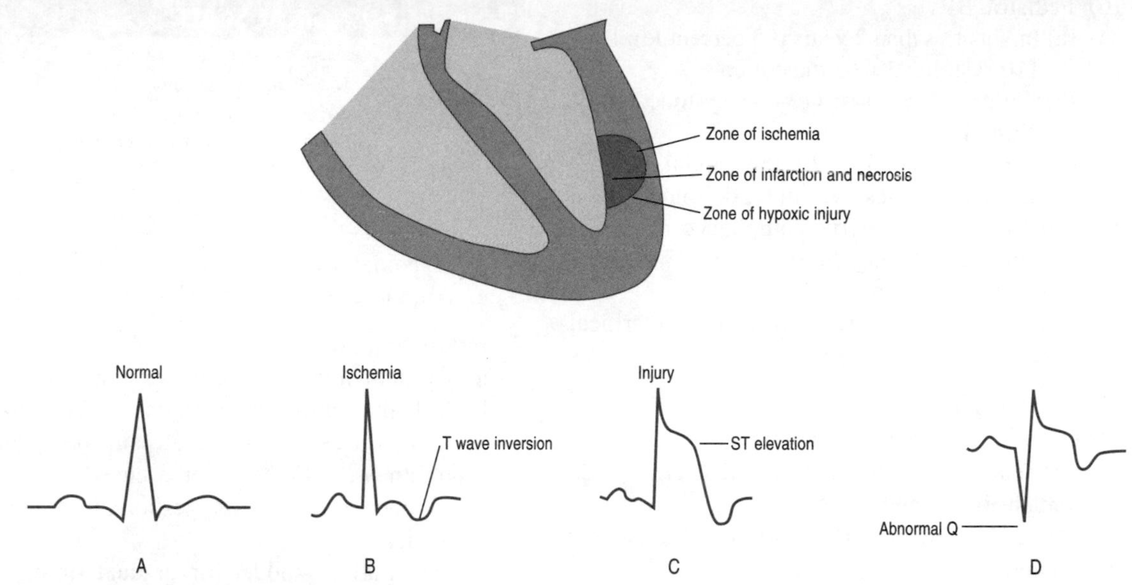

Figure 3-2 • ECG changes after myocardial infarction.
From: Goodman, C, Boissonnault. Pathology Implications for the Physical Therapist. Philadelphia, Saunders, 1998, p 282, with permission.

h. Metabolic and drug influences on the ECG.
   (1) Potassium levels.
      (a) Hyperkalemia: widens QRS, flattens P wave, T wave becomes peaked.
      (b) Hypokalemia: flattens T wave (or inverts), produces a U wave.
   (2) Calcium levels.
      (a) Hypercalcemia: widens QRS, shortens QT interval.
      (b) Hypocalcemia: prolongs QT interval.
   (3) Hypothermia: elevates ST segment; slows rhythm.
   (4) Digitalis: depresses ST segment, flattens T wave (or inverts), QT shortens.
   (5) Quinidine: QT lengthens, T wave flattens (or inverts), QRS lengthens.
   (6) Beta blockers (e.g., propranolol [Inderal]): decreases heart rate, blunts heart rate response to exercise.
   (7) Nitrates (nitroglycerin): increases heart rate.
   (8) Antiarrhythmic agents: may prolong QRS and QT intervals.

i. Holter monitoring: continuous ambulatory ECG monitoring via tape recording of cardiac rhythm for up to 24 hours.
   (1) Used to evaluate cardiac rhythm, transient symptoms, pacemaker function, effect of medications.
   (2) Allows correlation of symptoms with activities (activity diary).

4. Examine blood pressure (BP).

a. Determine blood pressure (2003 Joint National Committee on Prevention, Detection, Evaluation, and Treatment of High Blood Pressure Guidelines).
   (1) Normal adult BP: <120 mm Hg systolic; < 80 mm Hg diastolic.
   (2) Prehypertension: 120–130 mm Hg systolic; 80–89 mm Hg diastolic.
   (3) Hypertension.
      (a) Stage 1: 130–140 mm Hg systolic; 90–100 mm Hg diastolic.
      (b) Stage 2: 140–160 mm Hg systolic; 100–110 mm Hg diastolic.
      (c) Stage 3: >160 mm Hg systolic; > 110 mm Hg diastolic.
      (d) Primary or essential hypertension: no identifiable cause for elevated BP.
      (e) Secondary hypertension: cause can be determined; may be related to arteriosclerosis and vascular disorders, renal disease, endocrine disorders, pregnancy, drug-related.
      (f) Majority of patients with hypertension are asymptomatic.
   (4) Hypotension: a decrease in BP below normal; blood pressure is not adequate for normal perfusion/oxygenation of tissues. May be related to bed rest, drugs, arrhythmias, blood loss/shock, or myocardial infarction.
   (5) Orthostatic hypotension: sudden drop in BP that accompanies change in position.
      (a) Take BP in lying (5 minutes). Repeat BP at 1 and 3 minutes after moving into sitting position, then standing position.
      (b) Common symptoms include lightheadedness, dizziness, loss of balance.
      (c) Drop in systolic BP of more than 20 mm Hg or standing BP less than 100 mm Hg systolic BP is significant and should be reported.

(6) Pediatric BP.
(a) Infants less than 2 years (95 percentile): 106–110 systolic; 59–63 diastolic.
(b) Children 3–5 years: 113–116 systolic, 67–74 diastolic.

b. Mean arterial pressure (MAP): the arterial pressure within the large arteries over time; dependent upon mean blood flow and arterial compliance.
(1) Calculated by taking the sum of SBP and twice the DPR, divided by 3.
(2) An important clinical measure in critical care.

5. Examine respiration.

a. Determine rate, depth of breathing.
(1) Normal adult respiratory rate (RR) is 12 to 20 breaths per minute.
(2) Pediatric: newborn RR is 30 to 40 breaths per minute.
(3) Tachypnea: an increase in RR ≥ 22 breaths per minute.
(4) Bradypnea: a decrease of RR ≤ 10 breaths per minute.
(5) Hyperpnea: an increase in depth and rate of breathing.

b. Dyspnea: shortness of breath.
(1) Dyspnea on exertion (DOE): brought on by exercise or activity.
(2) Orthopnea: inability to breathe when in a reclining position.
(3) Paroxysmal nocturnal dyspnea (PND): sudden inability to breathe occurring during sleep.
(4) Dyspnea scale (Table 3-3).

c. Auscultation of the lungs: assess respiratory sounds.
(1) Normal breath sounds.
(2) Assess for adventitious sounds.
(a) Crackles (rales): rattling, bubbling sounds; may be due to secretions in the lungs.
(b) Wheezes: whistling sounds.

d. Assess cough: productive or nonproductive.

Table 3-3 ➤ DYSPNEA SCALE

+1	Mild, noticeable to patient but not to observer
+2	Mild, some difficulty, noticeable to observer
+3	Moderate difficulty, but can continue
+4	Severe difficulty, patient cannot continue

6. Examine oxygen saturation.

a. Use pulse oximetry, an electronic device that measures the degree of saturation of hemoglobin with oxygen (SaO_2). Normal values are between 95–100% oxygen.

b. Provides an estimate of PaO_2 (partial pressure of oxygen) based on the oxyhemoglobin desaturation curve.

c. Hypoxemia: abnormally low amount of oxygen in the blood (saturation levels below 90%).

Table 3-4 ➤ ANGINAL SCALE

1+	Light, barely noticeable
2+	Moderate, bothersome
3+	Severe, very uncomfortable
4+	Most severe pain ever experienced

d. Hypoxia: low oxygen level in the tissues.

e. Anoxia: complete lack of oxygen.

7. Examine pain.

a. Chest pain may be cardiac or noncardiac in origin.

b. Ischemic cardiac pain (angina or myocardial infarction): diffuse, retrosternal pain; or a sensation of tightness, achiness, in the chest; associated with dyspnea, sweating, indigestion, dizziness, syncope, anxiety.
(1) Angina: sudden or gradual onset; occurs at rest or with activity; precipitated by physical or emotional factors, hot or cold temperatures; relieved by rest or nitroglycerin.
(2) Myocardial infarction pain: sudden onset; pain lasts for more than 30 minutes; may have no precipitating factors; not relieved by medications.
(3) Anginal scale (Table 3-4).

c. Referred pain.
(1) Cardiac pain can refer to shoulders, arms, neck, or jaw.
(2) Pain referred to the back can occur from dissecting aortic aneurysm.

Physical Examination—Peripheral Vascular System

1. Examine condition of extremities.

a. Examine for diaphoresis: excess sweating associated with decreased cardiac output.

b. Examine arterial pulses: decreased or absent pulses associated with peripheral vascular disease (PVD); examine bilaterally.
(1) Lower extremity: position patient supine, check femoral, popliteal, dorsalis pedis, posterior tibial pulses.
(2) Upper extremity: check radial, brachial, and carotid pulses.

c. Examine skin color.
(1) Cyanosis: bluish color related to decreased cardiac output or cold; especially lips, fingertips, nail beds.
(2) Pallor: absence of rosy color in light-skinned individuals, associated with decreased peripheral blood flow, PVD.
(3) Rubor: dependent redness with PVD.

d. Examine skin temperature.

e. Examine for skin changes.

(1) Clubbing: curvature of the fingernails with soft tissue enlargement at base of nail: associated with chronic oxygen deficiency, heart failure.
(2) Trophic changes: pale, shiny, dry skin, with loss of hair is associated with PVD.
(3) Fibrosis: tissues are thick, firm, and unyielding.
(a) Stemmer's sign: dorsal skin folds of the toes or fingers are resistant to lifting; indicative of fibrotic changes and lymphedema.
(4) Abnormal pigmentation, ulceration, dermatitis, gangrene is associated with PVD.
(5) Temperature: decrease in superficial skin temperature is associated with poor arterial perfusion.

f. Examine for pain: intermittent claudication with: pain, cramping, and fatigue occurring during exercise, and relieved by rest, associated with PVD.
(1) Related to arterial insufficiency: pain is typically in calf; may also be in thigh, hips, or buttocks.
(2) Patient may experience pain at rest with severe decrease in arterial blood supply; typically in forefoot, worse at night.

g. Examine for edema.
(1) Measure girth measurements using a tape, or volumetric measurements using a volumeter (useful with irregular body parts, such as hand or foot).
(2) Pitting edema (indentation): depression is maintained when finger is pressed firmly; grading scale (see Table 3-5).
(3) Peripheral causes of edema include chronic venous insufficiency and lymphedema.
(4) Bilateral edema is associated with congestive heart failure.

2. Tests of peripheral venous circulation.

a. Examine venous system before arterial; venous insufficiency can invalidate some arterial tests.

b. Percussion test: determines competence of greater saphenous vein.
(1) In standing, palpate one segment of vein while percussing vein approximately 20 cm higher.
(2) If pulse wave is felt by lower hand, the intervening valves are incompetent.

Table 3-5 ➤ GRADING SCALE FOR EDEMA

1+	Mild, barely perceptible indentation; 0 to 1/4 inch pitting
2+	Moderate, easily identified depression; returns to normal within 15 seconds; 1/4 to 1/2 inch pitting
3+	Severe, depression takes 15–30 seconds to rebound; 1/2 to 1 inch pitting
4+	Very severe, depression lasts for 30 seconds or more; > 1 inch pitting

c. Trendelenburg's test (retrograde filling test): determines competence of communicating veins and saphenous system.
(1) Patient is positioned in supine with legs elevated to 60 degrees (empties venous blood).
(2) Tourniquet is then placed on proximal thigh (occludes venous flow in the superficial veins).
(3) Patient is then asked to stand.
(4) Examiner notes if veins fill in normal pattern. Should take approximately 30 seconds.

d. Venous filling time: Examine time necessary to refill veins after emptying.
(1) With patient supine, passively elevate lower extremity to approximately 45 degrees for 1 minute, then place in dependent position. Note time for veins to refill.
(2) Delayed filling (>15 seconds) is indicative of venous insufficiency.

e. Doppler ultrasound: examination using an ultrasonic oscillator connected to earphones.
(1) Determines blood flow within a vessel; useful in both venous and arterial diseases.
(2) Doppler probe placed over large vessel; ultrasound signal given transcutaneously; movement of blood causes an audible shift in signal frequency.
(3) Useful in locating nonpalpable pulses and measuring systolic BP in extremities.

f. Air plethysmography (APG): pneumatic device calibrated to measure patency of venous system; volume.
(1) Cuff is inflated around calf, attached to a pressure transducer and microprocessor.
(2) Occludes venous return, permits arterial inflow; recorder registers increasing volume with cuff; time to return to baseline with cuff deflation.
(3) Comparison tests performed in sitting, standing, and up onto toes.

3. Tests of peripheral arterial circulation.

a. Ankle brachial indices (ABI): the ratio of lower extremity (LE) pressure divided by upper extremity (UE) pressure.

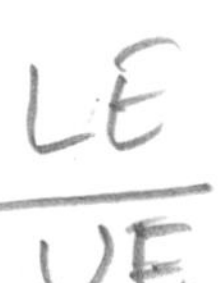

(1) BP cuff is inflated to occlude blood flow temporarily, then deflated.
(2) Examiner listens for return of flow.
(3) Performed in UE at brachial artery; LE at posterior tibial and dorsalis pedis arteries.
(4) ABI indices (Table 3-6).

b. Rubor of dependency. Examine color changes in skin during elevation of foot followed by dependency (seated, hanging position).
(1) With insuffiency, pallor develops in elevated position; reactive hyperemia (rubor of dependency) develops in dependent position.

Table 3-6 ➤ SIGNIFICANCE OF ANKLE-BRACHIAL INDEX VALUES

ABI 1.0 or higher	Normal, ankle systolic pressure is at least as high as brachial pressure
0.8 to 1.0	Mild peripheral artery disease Compression therapy with caution
0.5 to 0.8	Moderate peripheral artery disease, + for intermittent claudication Compression therapy contraindicated
< 0.5	Severe arterial disease, critical limb ischemia, + for rest pain Compression therapy contraindicated

(2) Changes that take longer than 30 seconds are also indicative of arterial insufficiency.

c. Examine for intermittent claudication: exercise-induced pain or cramping in the legs that is absent at rest. Usually calf pain, but may also occur in buttock, hip, thigh, or foot.
   (1) Have the patient walk on level grade, 1 mile/hour; e.g., treadmill. Test is stopped with claudicatory pain.
   (2) Note time of test. Use subjective ratings of pain scale to classify degree of claudication (Table 3-7).
   (3) Examine for coldness, numbness, or pallor in the legs or feet; loss of hair over anterior tibial area.
   (4) Leg cramps may also result from diuretic use with hypokalemia.

4. Examine lymphatic system.
   a. Palpate superficial lymph nodes: cervical, axillary, epitrochlear, superficial inguinal.
   b. Examine for edema.
      (1) Visual inspection: note swelling, decreased range of motion, loss of functional mobility.
      (2) Measure girth.
   c. Examine skin.
      (1) Changes in skin texture, fibrotic tissue changes.
      (2) Presence of papules, leakage, wounds.
   d. Changes in function (ADL, functional mobility, sleep).
   e. Paresthesias may be present.
   f. Lymphangigiography oscintigraphy (x-ray of lymph vessels) using radioactive agents (x-ray of lymph vessels): provides information about lymph flow, lymph node uptake, and backflow.

Table 3-7 ➤ SUBJECTIVE RATINGS OF PAIN WITH INTERMITTENT CLAUDICATION

Grade I	Minimal discomfort or pain
Grade II	Moderate discomfort or pain; patient's attention can be diverted
Grade III	Intense pain; patient's attention cannot be diverted
Grade IV	Excruciating and unbearable pain

Diagnostic Tests

1. Chest x-ray.
   a. Will reveal abnormalities of lung fluids, overall cardiac shape and size (cardiomegaly), aneurysm.

2. Myocardial perfusion imaging.
   a. Used to diagnose and evaluate ischemic heart disease, myocardial infarction.
   b. Thallium-201 scan: thallium (or other radioisotope) is injected into blood via IV; radioisotopes concentrate in normal tissue but not in ischemic or infarcted tissues (cold spots).
   c. Used to identify myocardial blood flow, areas of stress-induced ischemia (exercise test), old infarcts.
   d. Thallium stress test: used with exercise test (treadmill or bicycle ergometer); injected at peak exercise.
   e. Positron emission tomography (PET); uses radioactive marker (18F-fluorodeoxyglucose (FDG).

3. Echocardiogram.
   a. Noninvasive test that uses ultrasound to visualize internal structures (size of chambers, movement of valves, septum, abnormal wall movement).

4. Cardiac catheterization.
   a. Passage of a tiny tube through heart into blood vessels with introduction of a contrast medium into coronary arteries and subsequent x-ray.
   b. Provides information about anatomy of heart and great vessels, ventricular function, abnormal wall movements.
   c. Allows determination of ejection fraction (EF).

5. Central line (Swan-Ganz catheter).
   a. Catheter inserted through vessels into right side of heart.
   b. Measures central venous pressure (CVP), pulmonary artery pressure (PA), pulmonary capillary wedge pressures (PCWP).

Laboratory Tests and Values

1. See Table 3-8.

2. Enzyme changes associated with myocardial infarction.
   a. Elevations in SGOT (serum glutamic-oxaloacetic transaminase) (peaks 24–48 hr).
   b. Elevations CK or CPK (serum creatine phosphokinase) (peaks at 24 hr), CK-MB (serum creatine kinase MB) (peaks 12–24 hr).

TABLE 3-8 ➤ LABORATORY TESTS & VALUES

NORMAL VALUES	CLINICAL SIGNIFICANCE
Arterial Blood Gases (ABGs)	
SaO_2 95%–100%	SaO_2 below 88–90% usually requires supplemental O_2
PaO_2 80–100 mm Hg	↑ in hyperventilation ↓ in cardiac decompensation, COPD and some neuromuscular disorders
$PaCO_2$ 35–45 mm Hg	↑ in COPD ↓ in pregnancy, pulmonary embolism and anxiety
pH, whole blood 7.35–7.45	below 7.35 is acidotic, above 7.45 is alkalotic ↑ in respiratory alkalosis : hyperventilation, sepsis, liver disease, fever ↑ in metabolic alkalosis : vomiting, potassium depletion, diuretics, volume depletion ↓ in respiratory acidosis : COPD, respiratory depressants, myasthenia ↓ in metabolic acidosis (bicarbonate deficit): increased acids (diabetes, alcohol, starvation); renal failure, increased acid intake and loss of alkaline body fluids
Hemostasis (Clotting/Bleeding times)	
Prothrombin time (PT) 11–15 sec	Prolonged in factor X deficiency, hemorrhagic disease, cirrhosis, hepatitis drugs (warfarin) If clotting time is ↑ 2.5 times or more normal: physical therapy is contraindicated
Partial Thromboplastin Time (PTT) 25–40 sec	↑ in factor VIII, IX, and X deficiency
International normalized ratio (INR): Ratio of individual's PT to reference range 0.9–1.1 (ratio)	INR < 2 desirable INR > 2: consult with M.D. for ↑ risk of bleeding INR > 3 ↑ risk of hemarthrosis
Bleeding time 2–10 min	↑ in platelet disorders, thrombocytopenia
-C-reactive protein (CRP) -CRP < 10 mg/L	↑ levels associated with (up arrow) risk of atherosclerosis. ↑ (100 mg/L or more) with inflammation and infection

NORMAL VALUES	CLINICAL SIGNIFICANCE
Complete Blood Cell Count (CBC), adult values	
White Blood Cells (WBCs) Male & Female: 4,300–10,800 cells/mm³	Indicative of status of immune system. ↑ in infection: bacterial, viral; inflammation, hematologic malignancy, leukemia, lyphoma, drugs (corticosteroids) ↓ in aplastic anemia, B_{12} or folate deficiency With immunosuppression: ↑ risk of infection *Exercise considerations:* > 5000: use light exercise only < 5000: with fever, exercise is contraindicated < 1000: use mask, standard precautions
Red Blood Cells (RBCs) Male: 4.6–6.2 10^6/uL Female: 4.2–5.9 10^6/L	↑ in polycythemia ↓ in anemia
Erythrocyte Sedimentation Rate (ESR) Male up to 15 mm/hr Female up to 20 mm/hr	↑ in infection and inflammation: rheumatic or pelvic inflammatory disease, osteomyelitis Used to monitor effects of treatment; e.g., RA, SLE, Hodgkin's disease
Hematocrit (Hct) % of RBC of the whole blood vol. Male 45–52% Female 37–48% (age dependent)	↑ in erythrocytosis, dehydration, shock ↓ in severe anemias, acute hemorrhage *Exercise considerations:* > 25% but less than normal: light exercise only < 25% exercise is contraindicated
Hemoglobin (Hgb) Male: 13–18 g/dL Female: 12–16 g/dL (age-dependent)	↑ polycythemia, dehydration, shock ↓ in anemias, prolonged hemorrhage, RBC destruction (cancer, sickle cell disease) *Exercise considerations:* Low values (8–10 g/dL) result in ↓ exercise tolerance, ↑ fatigue, and tachycardia: use light exercise only < 8 g/dL: exercise contraindicated
Platelet count 150,000–450,000 cells/mm³	↑ chronic leukemia, hemoconcentration ↓ thrombocytopenia, acute leukemia, aplastic anemia, cancer chemotherapy *Exercise considerations:* < 20,000: AROM, ADLs only 20,000–30,000: use light exercise only 30,000–50,000: use moderate exercise
Fibrinogen, plasma 175–433 mg/dL	↑ in inflammatory states, pregnancy, oral contraceptives ↓ in cirrhosis, hereditary diseases

Adapted from: Hopkins, T; Lab Notes, 2nd Ed. Philadelphia, FADavis, 2009.

CHAPTER 3

c. Elevations in LDH (serum lactate dehydrogenase) (peaks 3–6 days).

3. Serum lipids (lipid panel) (mg/dL). Used to determine coronary risk (see Table 3-1).

Coronary Artery Disease (CAD)

Atherosclerosis

1. Characteristics.
   a. Disease of moderate and large arteries.
   b. Thickening of the intimal layer of the blood vessel wall from focal accumulation of lipids, platelets, monocytes, plaque, and other debris.

2. Risk factors.
   a. Nonmodifiable risk factors: age, sex, race, family history of CAD.
   b. Modifiable risk factors: cigarette smoking, high blood pressure, elevated cholesterol levels and LDL levels, elevated blood homocystine, obesity, inactivity, stress.
   c. Contributory diseases: diabetes.
   d. Two or more risk factors multiplies the risk of CAD.

Main Clinical Syndromes of CAD

1. Angina pectoris.
   a. Substernal chest pain or pressure; may be accompanied by Levine's sign (patient clenches fist over sternum).
   b. Represents imbalance in myocardial oxygen supply and demand; brought on by:
      (1) Increased demands on heart: exertion, emotional stress, smoking, extremes of temperature, especially cold, overeating, tachyarrhythmias.
      (2) Vasospasm: symptoms may be present at rest.
   c. Types of angina.
      (1) Stable angina: classic exertional angina; occurs at a predictable rate-pressure product, RPP (HR × BP), relieved with rest and/or nitroglycerin.
      (2) Unstable angina (preinfarction, crescendo angina): coronary insufficiency with risk for myocardial infarction or sudden death; pain is difficult to control; doesn't occur at predictable RPP.

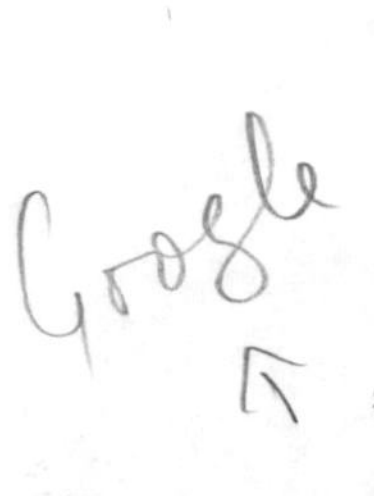

2. Myocardial infarction, MI.
   a. Prolonged ischemia, injury, and death of an area of the myocardium caused by occlusion of one or more of the coronary arteries.
   b. Precipitating factors: atherosclerotic heart disease with thrombus formation, coronary vasospasm or embolism; cocaine toxicity.
   c. Zones of infarction. (Figure 3-2).
      (1) Central zone: consists of necrotic, noncontractile tissue; electrically inert; on ECG, see pathological Q waves.
      (2) Zone of injury: area immediately adjacent to central zone, tissue is noncontractile, cells undergoing metabolic changes; electrically unstable; on ECG, see elevated ST segments in leads over injured area.
      (3) Zone of ischemia: outer area, cells also undergoing metabolic changes, electrically unstable; on ECG, see T wave inversion.
   d. Infarction sites.
      (1) Transmural (Q wave infarctions): full thickness of myocardium.
      (2) Nontransmural (non Q wave infarctions): subendocardial, subepicardial, intramural infarctions.
      (3) Sites of coronary artery occlusion. (Figure 3-3).
         (a) Inferior MI, right ventricle infarction, disturbances of upper conduction system: right coronary artery.
         (b) Lateral MI, ventricular ectopy: circumflex artery.
         (c) Anterior MI, disturbances of lower conduction system: left anterior descending artery.
   e. Impaired ventricular function results in:
      (1) Decreased stroke volume, cardiac output and ejection fraction.
      (2) Increased end diastolic ventricular pressures.
   f. Electrical instability: arrhythmias, present in injured and ischemic areas.

3. Heart failure, H.F.
   a. A condition in which the heart is unable to maintain adequate circulation of the blood to meet the metabolic needs of the body. Termed congestive heart failure (CHF) when edema is present. (Table 3-9).

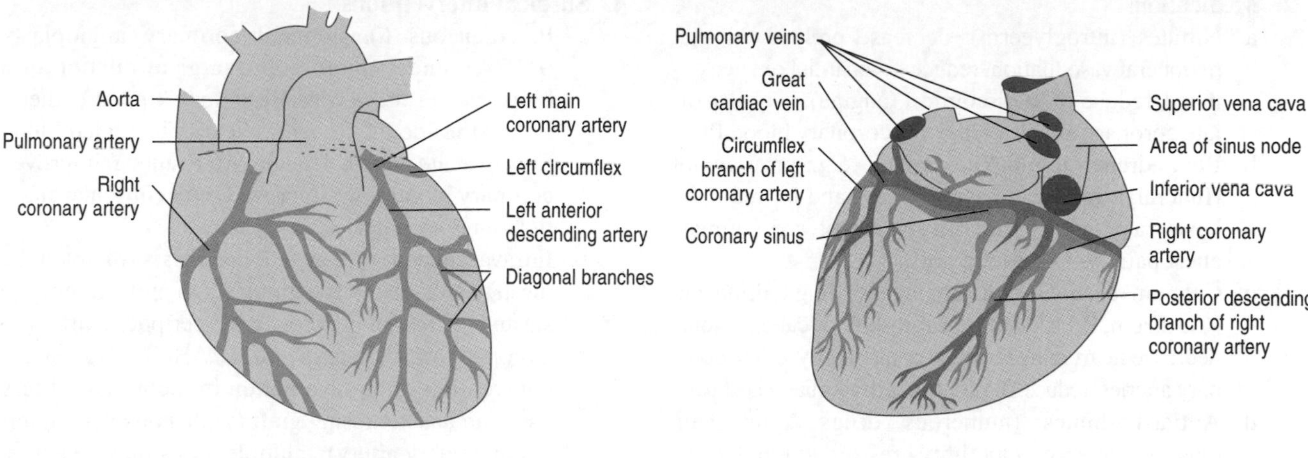

Figure 3-3 • Areas of myocardium affected by arterial insufficiency of specific coronary arteries.
From: Goodman, C, Boissonnault. Pathology Implications for the Physical Therapist. Philadelphia, Saunders, 1998, p 280, with permission.

b. Etiology: results from impairment of left ventricular functioning; from coronary artery disease, valvular disease, congenital heart disease, hypertension, or infection.

TABLE 3-9 ➤ POSSIBLE CLINICAL MANIFESTATIONS OF CARDIAC FAILURE

SIGNS ASSOCIATED WITH RIGHT-SIDED HEART FAILURE	
Nausea	Increase in RAP, CVP
Anorexia	Jugular venous distention
Weight gain	+ hepatojugular reflex
Ascites	Right ventricular heave
Right upper quadrant pain	Murmur of tricuspid insufficiency
	Hepatomegaly
	Peripheral edema
SIGNS ASSOCIATED WITH LEFT-SIDED HEART FAILURE	
Fatigue	Tachycardia
Cough	S_3 gallop
Shortness of breath	Crackles
DOE	Increased PAP, PAWP, SVR
Orthopnea	Laterally displaced PMI
PND	Left ventricular heave
Diaphoresis	Pulsus Alternans
	Confusion
	Decreased urine output
	Cheyne-Stokes respirations (advanced failure)
	Murmur of mitral insufficiency

RAP, right atrial pressure. CVP, central venous pressure. PAP, pulmonary artery pressure. PAWP, pulmonary artery wedge pressure. SVR, systemic vascular resistance. DOE, dyspnea on exertion. PND, paroxysmal nocturnal dyspnea. PMI, point of maximal impulse.
From: Stillwell, S, Randall, E. Pocket Guide to Cardiovascular Care. St. Louis, Mosby, 1990, p 19, with permission.

c. Physiological abnormalities: decreased cardiac output, elevated end-diastolic pressures (preload); increased heart rate; impaired ventricular function which, over time, may progress to cardiomyopathy.

d. Left heart failure (forward HF): blood is not adequately pumped into systemic circulation; due to an inability of left ventricle to pump, increases in ventricular end-diastolic pressure and left atrial pressures, with:
   (1) Increased pulmonary artery pressures and pulmonary edema.
   (2) Pulmonary signs and symptoms: cough, dyspnea, orthopnea.
   (3) Weakness, fatigue.

e. Right heart failure (backward HF): blood is not adequately returned from the systemic circulation to the heart; due to failure of right ventricle, increased pulmonary artery pressures, with:
   (1) Peripheral edema: weight gain, venous stasis.
   (2) Nausea, anorexia.

f. Compensated heart failure: symptoms are controlled by medical therapy.

g. Sympathetic stimulation results in tachycardia.

h. Decreased cardiac output results in pre-renal failure.

4. Sudden death.

Medical and Surgical Management of Cardiovascular Disease

1. Diet.

a. Low salt
b. Low cholesterol.
c. Weight reduction.

2. Medications.

a. Nitrates (nitroglycerin): decrease preload through peripheral vasodilation, reduce myocardial oxygen demand, reduce chest discomfort (angina); may also dilate coronary arteries, improve coronary blood flow.
b. Beta-adrenergic blocking agents (e.g., propranolol [Inderal]): reduce myocardial demand by reducing heart rate and contractility; control arrhythmias, chest pain; reduce blood pressure.
c. Calcium channel blocking agents (e.g., diltiazem [Cardizem, Procardia]): inhibit flow of calcium ions, decrease heart rate, decrease contractility, dilate coronary arteries, reduce BP, control arrhythmias, chest pain.
d. Antiarrhythmics (numerous drugs, four main classes): alter conductivity, restore normal heart rhythm, control arrhythmias, improve cardiac output, (e.g., quinidine, procainamide).
e. Antihypertensives (numerous drugs, four main types): control hypertension; goal is to maintain a diastolic pressure < 90 mm Hg; decrease afterload, reduce myocardial oxygen demand, (e.g., propranolol, reserpine).
f. Digitalis (cardiac glycosides): increases contractility and decreases heart rate; mainstay in the treatment of CHF (e.g., digoxin).
g. Diuretics: decrease myocardial work (reduce preload and afterload), control hypertension, (e.g., furosemide [Lasix], hydrochlorothiazide [Esidrix]).
h. Aspirin: decreases platelet aggregation; may prevent myocardial infarction.
i. Tranquilizers: decrease anxiety, sympathetic effects.
j. Hypolipidemic agents (six major cholesterol-lowering drugs): reduce serum lipid levels when diet and weight reduction are not effective, (e.g., cholestyramine [Questran], colestipol [Colestid], simvastatin [Zocor], lovastatin [Mevacor]).

3. Activity restriction.

a. Acute MI, CHF.
b. Limited, generally to first 24 hours; or until patient is stable for 24 hours.

4. Surgical interventions.

a. Percutaneous transluminal coronary angioplasty (PTCA): under fluoroscopy, surgical dilation of a blood vessel using a small balloon-tipped catheter inflated inside the lumen; relieves obstructed blood flow in acute angina or acute MI; results in improved coronary blood flow, improved left ventricular function, anginal relief.
b. Intravascular stents: an endoprosthesis (pliable wire mesh) implanted postangioplasty to prevent restenosis and occlusion in coronary or peripheral arteries.
c. Coronary artery bypass graft (CABG): surgical circumvention of an obstruction in a coronary artery using an anastomosing graft (saphenous vein, internal mammary artery); multiple grafts may be necessary; results in improved coronary blood flow, improved left ventricular function, anginal relief.
d. Transplantation: used in end-stage myocardial disease; e.g., cardiomyopathy, ischemic heart disease, valvular heart disease.
   (1) Heteroptics: involves leaving the natural heart and piggy-backing the donor heart.
   (2) Orthotopic: involves removing the diseased heart and replacing it with a donor heart.
   (3) Heart and lung transplantation: involves removing both organs and replacing them with donor organs.
   (4) Major problems posttransplantation are rejection, infection, complications of immunosuppressive therapy.
e. Ventricular assist devices (VADs): an implanted device (accessory pump) that improves tissue perfusion and maintains cardiogenic circulation; used with severely involved patients; e.g., cardiogenic shock unresponsive to medications, severe ventricular dysfunction.

5. Thrombolytic therapy.

a. Administered for acute myocardial infarction.
b. Medications activate body's fibrinolytic system, dissolve clot, and restore coronary blood flow, (e.g., streptokinase, tissue plasminogen activator [TPA], urokinase).

Peripheral Vascular Disease (PVD)

Arterial Disease

1. Arteriosclerosis obliterans.

a. Chronic, occlusive arterial disease of medium- and large-sized vessels, the result of peripheral atherosclerosis.
b. Associated with hypertension and hyperlipidemia; patients may also exhibit CAD, cerebrovascular disease, diabetes.
c. Pulses: decreased or absent.
d. Color: pale on elevation, dusky red on dependency.
e. Early stages, patients exhibit intermittent claudication. Pain is described as burning, searing, aching, tightness, or cramping.
f. Late stages, patients exhibit ischemia and rest pain; ulcerations and gangrene, trophic changes.
g. Affects primarily the lower extremities.

TABLE 3-10 ➤ DIFFERENTIAL DIAGNOSIS: PERIPHERAL VASCULAR DISEASES

	CHRONIC ARTERIAL INSUFFICIENCY	CHRONIC VENOUS INSUFFICIENCY
Etiology	Arteriosclerosis obliterans atheroembolism	Thrombophlebitis Trauma, vein obstruction
Risk factors	Smoking Diabetes mellitus Hyperlipoproteinemia Hypertension	Venous hypertension Varicose veins Inherited trait
Signs & Symptoms: determined by location and degree of vascular involvement		
Pain	Severe muscle ischemia/intermittent claudication. Worse with exercise, relieved by rest Rest pain indicates severe involvement Muscle fatigue, cramping, numbness Paresthesias over time	Minimal to moderate steady pain Aching pain in lower leg with prolonged standing or sitting (dependency) Superficial pain along course of vein
Location of pain	Usually calf, lower leg or dorsum of foot May occur in thigh, hip or buttock	Muscle compartment tenderness
Vascular	Decreased or absent pulses Pallor of forefoot on elevation Dependent rubor	Venous dilatation or varicosity edema: moderate to severe
Skin changes	Pale, shiny, dry Loss of hair Nail changes Coolness of extremity	Liposclerosis: Dark, cyanotic Thickened, brown May lead to stasis dermatitis, cellulitis
Acute	Acute arterial obstruction: distal pain, paresthetic, pale, pulseless, sudden onset	Acute thrombophlebitis (DVT): Calf pain, aching, edema, muscle tenderness, 50% asymptomatic
Ulceration	May develop in toes, feet or areas of trauma; gangrene may develop	May develop at sides of ankles, especially medial malleolus; gangrene absent

Adapted from Bickley, L, Szilagyi, P. Bates Guide to Physical Examination and History Taking, 8th ed., Philadelphia, Lippincott Williams & Wilkins, 2003, pp 460–464.

2. **Thromboangiitis obliterans (Buerger's disease).**
   a. Chronic, inflammatory vascular occlusive disease of small arteries and also veins.
   b. Occurs commonly in young adults, largely males, who smoke.
   c. Begins distally and progresses proximally in both upper and lower extremities.
   d. Patients exhibit paresthesias or pain, cyanotic cold extremity, diminished temperature sensation, fatigue, risk of ulceration and gangrene.

3. **Diabetic angiopathy.**
   a. An inappropriate elevation of blood glucose levels and accelerated atherosclerosis.
   b. Neuropathy a major complication.
   c. Neurotrophic ulcers, may lead to gangrene and amputation.

4. **Raynaud's disease or phenomenon.**
   a. Episodic spasm of small arteries and arterioles.
   b. Abnormal vasoconstrictor reflex exacerbated by exposure to cold or emotional stress; tips of fingers develop pallor, cyanosis, numbness, and tingling.
   c. Affects largely females.
   d. Occlusive disease is not usually a factor.

Venous Disease

1. **Varicose veins.**
   a. Distended, swollen superficial veins; tortuous in appearance.
   b. May lead to varicose ulcers.

2. **Superficial vein thrombophlebitis.**
   a. Clot formation and acute inflammation in a superficial vein.
   b. Localized pain; usually in saphenous vein.

3. **Deep vein thrombophlebitis (DVT).**
   a. Clot formation and acute inflammation in a deep vein.
   b. Usually occurs in lower extremity, associated with venous stasis (bed rest, lack of leg exercise), hyperactivity of blood coagulation, and vascular trauma; early ambulation is prophylactic, helps eliminate venous stasis.
   c. Signs and symptoms: may be asymptomatic early; progressive inflammation, tenderness, pain, swelling, warmth, skin discoloration.
   d. Homan's sign (test for DVT of calf veins).
      (1) Supine with knee flexed. Pain with forceful dorsiflexion of ankle.
      (2) Produces calf pain. Limited diagnostic reliability (poor sensitivity and specificity).
   e. May precipitate pulmonary embolism: presents abruptly, with chest pain and dyspnea, also

CHAPTER 3

diaphoresis, cough, apprehension; requires emergency treatment, may be life threatening.
f. Medical management: anticoagulation therapy (e.g., heparin), thrombolytic agents (e.g., streptokinase); bed rest.

3. **Chronic venous insufficiency (deep).**
   a. Pain: none to aching pain on dependency.
   b. Pulses: normal; difficult to take with edema.
   c. Color: normal or cyanotic on dependency.
   d. Venous valvular insufficiency: from fibroelastic degeneration of valve tissue, venous dilation.
   e. Muscle pump dysfunction.
   f. Edema, impairment of fibrinolysis; may lead to venous ulcer formation.
   g. Classification.
      Grade I: mild aching, minimal edema, dilated superficial veins.
      Grade II: increased edema, multiple dilated veins, changes in skin pigmentation.
      Grade III: venous claudication, severe edema, cutaneous ulceration.

Lymphatic Disease

1. **Lymphadenopathy.**
   a. Enlargement of nodes, with or without tenderness.
2. **Lymphedema.**
   a. Chronic disorder with excessive accumulation of fluid due to obstruction of lymphatics.
   b. Causes swelling of the soft tissues in arms and legs.
   c. Results from mechanical insufficieny of the lymphatic system.
   d. Primary lymphedema: congential condition with abnormal lymph node or lymph vessel formation (hypoplasia).
   e. Secondary lymphedema: acquired, due to injury of one or more parts of the lymphatic system.
      (1) Results from surgery (radical mastectomy, femoropopliteal bypass, lymphnode removal), radiation therapy for breast cancer management, or disease (malignancy, infection).
      (2) Can also occur as a result of paralysis and disuse.
      (3) In tropical and subtropical areas, results from filariasis (nematode worm larvae in the lymphatic system).
3. **Acute lymphangitis.**
   a. Acute bacterial infection spreading throughout lymph system.
   b. Usually streptococcal.

Cardiac Rehabilitation

Cardiovascular/pulmonary practice patterns are presented in Table 3-11.

Exercise Tolerance Testing

1. **Exercise tolerance test (ETT).** (Graded exercise test).
   a. Purpose: to determine physiological responses during a measured exercise stress (increasing workloads); allows the determination of functional exercise capacity of an individual.
      (1) Serves as a basis for exercise prescription. Symptom-limited ETT is typically administered prior to start of Phase II outpatient cardiac rehabilitation program and following cardiac rehabilitation as an outcome measure.
      (2) Used as a screening measure for CAD in asymptomatic individuals.
      (3) ETT with radionuclide perfusion: assists in the diagnosis of suspected or established cardiovascular disease.
   b. Testing modes.
      (1) Treadmill and cycle ergometry (leg or arm tests) allow for precise calibration of the exercise workload.
      (2) Step test (upright or sitting) can also be used for fitness screening, healthy population.
   c. ETT may be maximal or submaximal.
      (1) Maximal ETT: defined by target endpoint heart rate.
         (a) Age-adjusted maximum heart rate (AAMHR): 220 minus age of individual.
         (b) Heart-rate range (Karvonen's formula): 60–80% (HR max – resting HR) + resting HR = target HR.
      (2) Submaximal ETT: symptom-limited; used to evaluate the early recovery of patients after MI, coronary bypass, or coronary angioplasty.
   d. Continuous ETT: workload is steadily progressed, usually in 2- or 3-minute stages.
   e. Discontinuous ETT: allows rest in between workloads/stages; used for patients with more pronounced CAD.

TABLE 3-11 ➤ CARDIOVASCULAR/PULMONARY PRACTICE PATTERNS

Pattern A:	Primary Prevention/Risk Reduction for Cardiovascular/Pulmonary Disorders
Pattern B:	Impaired Aerobic Capacity/Endurance Associated with Deconditioning
Pattern C:	Impaired Ventilation, Respiration/Gas Exchange, and Aerobic Capacity/Endurance Associated with Airway Clearance Dysfunction
Pattern D:	Impaired Aerobic Capacity/Endurance Associated with Cardiovascular Pump Dysfunction or Failure
Pattern E:	Impaired Ventilation, Respiration/Gas Exchange Associated with Ventilatory Pump Dysfunction or Failure
Pattern F:	Impaired Ventilation, Respiration/Gas Exchange Associated with Respiratory Failure
Pattern G:	Impaired Ventilation, Respiration/Gas Exchange, and Aerobic Capacity/Endurance Associated with Respiratory Failure in the Neonate
Pattern H:	Impaired Circulation and Anthropometric Dimensions Associated with Lymphatic System Disorder

From: Guide for Physical Therapist Practice, 2nd ed., Phys Ther 81:9, 2001.

2. Monitoring during exercise and recovery.

a. Patient appearance, signs and symptoms of excessive effort and exertional intolerance; examine for:
   (1) Persistent dyspnea.
   (2) Dizziness or confusion.
   (3) Anginal pain.
   (4) Severe leg claudication.
   (5) Excessive fatigue.
   (6) Pallor, cold sweat.
   (7) Ataxia, incoordination.
   (8) Pulmonary rales.

b. Changes in HR: HR increases linearly as a function of increasing workload and oxygen uptake (VO_2), plateaus just before maximal oxygen uptake (VO_2max).

c. Changes in BP: systolic BP should rise with increasing workloads and VO_2; diastolic BP should remain about the same.

d. Rate-pressure product (RPP): the product of systolic BP and HR (the last two digits of a 5-digit number are dropped) is often used an index of myocardial oxygen consumption (MVO_2).
   (1) Increased MVO_2 is the result of increased coronary blood flow.
   (2) Angina is usually precipitated at a given RPP.

e. Ratings of perceived exertion (RPE): developed by Gunnar Borg. Allows subjective rating of feelings during exercise and impending fatigue. Important to use standardized instructions to reduce misinterpretation.
   (1) RPE increases linearly with increasing exercise intensity and correlates closely with exercise heart rates and work rates.
   (2) Variability in accurate use of RPE between individuals exists. Ratings can be influenced by psychological factors, mood states, environmental conditions, exercise modes, and age.
   (3) RPE is an important measure for individuals who do not exhibit the typical rise in HR with exercise (e.g., patients on medications that depress HR, such as beta blockers).
   (4) Category Scale (original Borg scale): rates exercise intensity using numbers from 6 to 20, with descriptors from very, very light (7) to somewhat hard (13) to very, very hard (19).
   (5) Category-Ratio Scale (Borg): rates exercise intensity using numbers from 1 to 11 with descriptors from very weak (1) to moderate (3) to strong (5) to extremely strong (10).

f. Pulse oximetry: measure arterial oxygen saturation levels (SaO_2) before, during, and after exercise.

g. ECG changes with exercise: healthy individual.
   (1) Tachycardia: heart rate increase is directly proportional to exercise intensity and myocardial work.
   (2) Rate-related shortening of QT interval.
   (3) ST segment depression, upsloping, less than 1 mm.
   (4) Reduced R wave, increased Q wave.
   (5) Exertional arrhythmias: rare, single PVCs.

h. ECG changes with exercise: an individual with myocardial ischemia and CAD.
   (1) Significant tachycardia: occurs at lower intensities of exercise.
   (2) Exertional arrhythmias: increased frequency of ventricular arrhythmias during exercise and/or recovery.
   (3) ST segment depression; horizontal or downsloping depression, greater than 1 mm below baseline is indicative of myocardial ischemia.

i. Delayed, abnormal responses to exercise, occur hours later.
   (1) Prolonged fatigue.
   (2) Insomnia.
   (3) Sudden weight gain due to fluid retention.

3. Ambulatory monitoring (telemetry).

a. Continuous 24-hour ECG monitoring.

b. Allows documentation of ST segment depression or elevation, silent ischemia, arrhythmias associated with daily activity.

4. Transtelephonic ECG monitoring.

a. Used to monitor patients as they exercise at home.

5. Activity levels: METs (metabolic equivalents).

a. MET: the amount of oxygen consumed at rest (sitting); equal to 3.5 mL/kg per minute.

b. MET levels (multiples of resting VO_2) can be directly determined during ETT: using collection and analysis of expired air; not routinely done.

c. MET levels can be estimated during ETT during steady state exercise; the max VO_2 achieved on ETT

CHAPTER 3

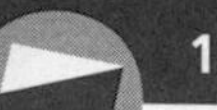

TABLE 3-12 ➤ METABOLIC EQUIVALENT (MET) ACTIVITY CHART

INTENSITY (70-KG PERSON)	ENDURANCE PROMOTING	OCCUPATIONAL	RECREATIONAL
1.5–2 METs	Too low in energy level	Desk work, driving auto, calculating machine operation, light housework, polishing furniture, washing clothes	Standing, strolling (1 mph), flying, motorcycling, playing cards, sewing, knitting
2–3 METs	Too low in energy level unless capacity is very low	Auto repair, radio and television repair, janitorial work, bartending, riding lawn mower, light woodworking	Level walking (2 mph), level bicycling (5 mph), billiards, bowling, skeet shooting, shuffleboard, powerboat driving, golfing with power cart, canoeing, horseback riding at a walk
3–4 METs	Yes, if continuous and if target heart rate is reached	Brick laying, plastering, wheelbarrow (100-lb load), machine assembly, welding (moderate load), cleaning windows, mopping floors, vacuuming, pushing light power mower	Walking (3 mph), bicycling (6 mph), horseshoe pitching, volleyball (six-person, noncompetitive), golfing (pulling bag cart), archery, sailing (handling small boat), fly fishing (standing in waders), horseback riding (trotting), badminton (social doubles)
4–5 METs	Recreational activities promote endurance; occupational activities must be continuous, lasting longer than 2 min	Painting, masonry, paperhanging, light carpentry, scrubbing floors, raking leaves, hoeing	Walking (3⅓ mph), bicycling (8 mph), table tennis, golfing (carrying clubs), dancing (foxtrot), badminton (singles), tennis (doubles), many calisthenics, ballet
5–6 METs	Yes	Digging garden, shoveling light earth	Walking (4 mph), bicycling (10 mph), canoeing (4 mph), horseback riding (posting to trotting), stream fishing (walking in light current in waders), ice or roller skating (9 mph)
6–7 METs	Yes	Shoveling 10 times/min (4.5 kg or 10 lb), splitting wood, snow shoveling, hand lawn mowing	Walking (5 mph), bicycling (11 mph), competitive badminton, tennis (singles), folk and square dancing, light downhill skiing, ski touring (2.5 mph), water skiing, swimming (20 yd/min)
7–8 METs	Yes	Digging ditches, carrying 36 kg or 80 lb, sawing hardwood	Jogging (5 mph), bicycling (12 mph), horseback riding (gallop), vigorous downhill skiing, basketball, mountain climbing, ice hockey, canoeing (5 mph), touch football, paddleball
8–9 METs	Yes	Shoveling 10 times/min (5.5 kg or 14 lb)	Running (5.5 mph), bicycling (13 mph), ski touring (4 mph), squash (social), handball (social), fencing, basketball (vigorous), swimming (30 yd/min), rope skipping
10+ METs	Yes	Shoveling 10 times/min (7.5 kg or 16 lb)	Running (6 mph = 10 METs, 7 mph = 11.5 METs, 8 mph = 13.5 METs, 9 mph = 15 METs, 10 mph = 17 METs), ski touring (5+ mph), handball (competitive), squash (competitive), swimming (> 40 yd/min)

From: Fox, Naughton, Gorman. Mod Concepts Cardiovas Dis 1972, 4:25. American Heart Association, with permission.

is divided by resting VO_2; highly predictable with standardized testing modes.

d. Can be used to predict energy expenditure during certain activities (Table 3-12).

Exercise Prescription

1. **Guidelines for exercise prescription.**
   a. Type (modality).
      (1) Cardiorespiratory endurance activities: walking, jogging, or cycling recommended to improve exercise tolerance; can be maintained at a constant velocity; very low interindividual variability.
      (2) Dynamic arm exercise (arm ergometry): uses a smaller muscle mass, results in lower VO_2 max (60–70% lower) than leg ergometry; at a given workload, HR will be higher, stroke volume lower; systolic and diastolic BPs will be higher.
      (3) Other aerobic activities: swimming, cross-country skiing; less frequently used due to high inter-individual variability, energy expenditure related to skill level.
      (4) Dancing, basketball, racquetball, competitive activities should not be used with high-risk, symptomatic, and low-fit individuals.
      (5) Early rehabilitation: activity is discontinuous (interval training), with frequent rest periods; continuous training can be used in later stages of rehabilitation.
      (6) Warm-up and cool-down activities.

(a) Gradually increase or decrease the intensity of exercise, promote circulatory and muscular adjustment to exercise.
(b) Type: low intensity cardiorespiratory endurance activities, flexibility (ROM) exercises, functional mobility activities.
(c) Duration: 5–10 minutes.
(d) Abrupt beginning or cessation of exercise is not safe or recommended.

(7) Resistive exercises: to improve strength and endurance in clinically stable patients.
(a) Usually prescribed in later rehabilitation, after a period of aerobic conditioning.
(b) Moderate intensities are typically used (e.g., 40% of maximal voluntary contraction).
(c) Monitor responses to resistive training using rate-pressure product (incorporates BP, a safer measure).
(d) Precautions: carefully monitor BP, avoid breath-holding, Valsalva's response (may dramatically increase BP and work of heart).
(e) Contraindicated for patients with: poor left ventricular function, ischemic changes on ECG during ETT, functional capacity less than 6 METs, uncontrolled hypertension or arrhythmias.

(8) Relaxation training: relieves generalized muscle tension and anxiety.
(a) Usually incorporated following an aerobic training session and cool-down.
(b) Assists in successful stress management and life-style modification.

b. Intensity: prescribed as percentage of functional capacity revealed on ETT, within a range of 40–85% depending upon initial level of fitness; typical training intensity is 60–70% of functional capacity; lower training intensities may necessitate an increase in training duration; most clinicians use a combination of HR, RPE, and METs to prescribe exercise intensity (eliminates problems that may be associated with individual measures).

(1) Heart rate.
(a) Percentage of maximum heart rate achieved on ETT; without an ETT, 220 minus age is used (for upper extremity work, 220 minus age minus 11 is used). 70–85% HRmax closely corresponds to 60–80% of functional capacity or VO_2max.
(b) Estimated HR max is used in cases where submaximal ETT has been given.
(c) Heart rate range or reserve (Karvonen's formula, see previous description). More closely approximates the relationship between HR and VO_2 max. Problems associated with use of HR alone to prescribe exercise intensity.
(d) Beta blocking or calcium channel blocking medications: affects ability of HR to rise in response to an exercise stress.
(e) Pacemaker: affects ability of HR to rise in response to an exercise stress.
(f) Environmental extremes, heavy arm work, isometric exercise, and Valsalva may affect HR and BP responses.

(2) Rating of perceived exertion, the original Borg RPE scale (6–20).
(a) RPE values of 12–13 (somewhat hard) correspond to 60% of HR range.
(b) RPE of 16 (hard) corresponds to 85% of HR range.
(c) Useful along with other measures of patient effort if beta blockers or other HR suppressers are used.
(d) Problems with use of RPE alone to prescribe exercise intensity.
- Individuals with psychological problems (e.g., depression).
- Unfamiliarity with RPE scale; may affect selection of ratings.

(3) METs, or estimated energy expenditure (VO_2).
(a) 40–85% of functional capacity (maximal METs) achieved on ETT.
(b) Problems associated with use of METs alone to prescribe exercise intensity.
- With high intensity activities (e.g., jogging), need to adopt a discontinuous work pattern: walk 5 minutes, jog 3 minutes to achieve the desired intensity.
- Varying skill level or stress of competition may affect the known metabolic cost of an activity.
- Environmental stresses (heat, cold, high humidity, altitude, wind, changes in terrain such as hills) may affect the known metabolic cost of an activity.

c. Duration.
(1) Conditioning phase may vary from 15 to 60 minutes, depending upon intensity; the higher the intensity, the shorter the duration.
(2) Average conditioning time is 20–30 minutes for moderate intensity exercise.
(3) Severely compromised individuals may benefit from multiple, short exercise sessions spaced throughout the day (e.g., 3- to 10-minute sessions).
(4) Warm-up and cool-down periods are kept constant; e.g., 5–10 minutes each.

d. Frequency.
(1) Frequency of activity is dependent upon intensity and duration; the lower the intensity, the shorter the duration, the greater the frequency.
(2) Average: three to five sessions/week for exercise at moderate intensities and duration, e.g., > 5 METs.

(3) Daily or multiple daily sessions for low intensity exercise; e.g., < 5 METS.

e. Progression.

(1) Modify exercise prescription if:

(a) HR is lower than target HR for a given exercise intensity.

(b) RPE is lower (exercise is perceived as easier) for a given exercise.

(c) Symptoms of ischemia (e.g., angina) do not appear at a given exercise intensity.

(2) Rate of progression depends on age, health status, functional capacity, personal goals, preferences.

(3) As training progresses, duration is increased first, then intensity.

f. Consider reduction in exercise/activity with

(1) Acute illness: fever, flu.

(2) Acute injury, orthopedic complications.

(3) Progression of cardiac disease: edema, weight gain, unstable angina.

(4) Overindulgence: e.g., food, caffeine, alcohol.

(5) Drugs: e.g., decongestants, bronchodilators, atropine, weight reducers.

(5) Environmental stressors: extremes of heat, cold, humidity, air pollution.

g. Exercise prescription for post-PTCA (percutaneous transluminal coronary angioplasty).

(1) Wait to exercise approximately 2 weeks post-PTCA to allow inflammatory process to subside.

(2) Use post-PTCA ETT to prescribe exercise.

h. Exercise prescription post-CABG (coronary artery bypass grafting).

(1) Limit upper extremity exercise while sternal incision is healing.

(2) Avoid lifting, pushing, pulling for 4–6 weeks postsurgery.

2. (See Box 3-1).

Box 3-1 ➤ CLINICAL INDICATIONS AND CONTRAINDICATIONS FOR INPATIENT AND OUTPATIENT CARDIAC REHABILITATION

Indications

- Medically stable postmyocardial infarction (MI)
- Stable angina.
- Coronary artery bypass graft surgery (CABG)
- Percutaneous transluminal coronary angioplasty (PTCA) or other transcatheter procedure
- Compensated congestive heart failure (CHF)
- Cardiomyopathy
- Heart or other organ transplantation
- Other cardiac surgery including valvular and pacemaker insertion (including implantable cardioverter defibrillator [ICD])
- Peripheral arterial disease (PAD)
- High-risk cardiovascular disease (CVD) ineligible for surgical intervention
- Sudden cardiac death syndrome
- End-stage renal disease
- At risk for coronary artery disease (CAD), with diagnoses of diabetes mellitus, dyslipidemia, hypertension, obesity, or other diseases and conditions
- Other patients who may benefit from structured exercise and/or patient education, based on physician referral and consensus of the rehabilitation team

Contraindications

- Unstable angina
- Resting systolic BP (SBP) > 200 mm Hg or resting diastolic BP (DBP) > 110 mm Hg that should be evaluated on a case by case basis
- Orthostatic BP drop of > 20 mm Hg with symptoms
- Critical aortic stenosis (i.e., peak SBP gradient of > 50 mm Hg with an aortic valve orifice area of < 0.75 cm² in an average size adult)
- Acute systemic illness or fever
- Uncontrolled atrial or ventricular dysrhythmias.
- Uncontrolled sinus tachycardia (> 120 bpm)
- Uncompensated congestive heart failure (CHF)
- Third degree atrioventricular (AV) heart block without pacemaker
- Active pericarditis or myocarditis
- Recent embolism
- Thrombophlebitis
- Resting ST segment depression or elevation (> 2 mm)
- Uncontrolled diabetes
- Severe orthopedic problems that would prohibit exercise
- Other metabolic conditions, such as acute thyroiditis, hypokalemia, hyperkalemia, or hypovolemia.

From: American College of Sports Medicine, Guidelines for Exercise Testing and Prescription, 8th ed., Philadelphia, Lippincott Williams & Wilkins, 2010, p 209, with permission.

Phase 1: Inpatient Cardiac Rehabilitation (Acute)

Length of hospital stay is commonly 3–5 days for uncomplicated MI (no post-MI angina, malignant arrhythmias, or heart failure).

1. Exercise/activity goals and outcomes.
   a. Initiate early return to independence in activities of daily living; typically after 24 hours or until the patient is stable for 24 hours; monitor activity tolerance.
   b. Counteract deleterious effects of bed rest: reduce risk of thrombi, maintain muscle tone, reduce orthostatic hypotension, maintain joint mobility.
   c. Help allay anxiety and depression.
   d. Provide medical surveillance.
   e. Provide patient and family education.
   f. Promote risk factor modification.

2. Exercise/activity guidelines.
   a. Program components: ADLs, selected arm and leg exercises, early supervised ambulation.
   b. Initial activities: are low intensity (2–3 METs) progressing to 3–5 METs by discharge; RPE in fairly light range; HR increase of 10–20 bpm above resting, depending on medications.
   c. Short exercise sessions, two to three times a day; gradually duration is lengthened and frequency is decreased.
   d. Postsurgical patients.
      (1) Typically are progressed more rapidly than post-MI.
      (2) Greater emphasis is placed on upper extremity ROM.
      (3) Lifting activities are restricted, generally for 6 weeks.
   e. ETT (thallium scan or symptom-limited ETT): may be used to determine functional capacity prior to discharge, safely progress exercise intensity greater than 5 METs.

3. Patient and family education goals.
   a. Improve understanding of cardiac disease, support risk factor modification.
   b. Teach self-monitoring procedures, warning signs of exertional intolerance; e.g., persistent dyspnea, anginal pain, dizziness.
   c. Teach general activity guidelines, activity pacing, energy conservation techniques; home exercise program (HEP).
   d. Teach cardiopulmonary resuscitation (CPR).
   e. Provide emotional support.

4. Home exercise program (HEP).
   a. Low-risk patients may be safe candidates for unsupervised exercise at home.
      (1) Gradual increase in ambulation time: goal of 20–30 minutes, one to two times per day at 4–6 weeks post-MI.
      (2) Upper and lower extremity mobility exercises.
   b. Elderly, homebound patients with multiple medical problems may benefit from a home cardiac rehabilitation program.
   c. Patients should be skilled in self-monitoring procedures.
   d. Family training in CPR and AED (automated external defibrillator); emergency lifeline for some patients.

5. (See Box 3-2).

Box 3-2 ➤ Adverse Responses to Inpatient Exercise Leading to Exercise Termination

- Rise in diastolic BP ≥110 mm Hg
- Decrease in systolic BP > 10 mm Hg
- Significant ventricular or atrial dysrhythmias
- Second- or third-degree heart block
- Signs/symptoms of exercise intolerance, including angina, marked dyspnea, and electrocardiogram changes suggestive of ischemia.

Adapted from American Association of Cardiovascular and Pulmonary Rehabilitation. Guidelines for Cardiac Rehabilitation and Secondary Prevention Programs. 4th ed. Champaign, IL, Human Kinetics, 2004.

Phase 2: Outpatient Cardiac Rehabilitation (Subacute)

1. Exercise/activity goals and outcomes.
   a. Improve functional capacity.
   b. Progress toward full resumption of activities of daily living, habitual and occupational activities.
   c. Promote risk-factor modification, counseling as to lifestyle changes.
   d. Encourage activity pacing, energy conservation; stress importance of taking proper rest periods.

2. Exercise/activity guidelines.
   a. Outpatient program.
      (1) Patients at risk for arrhythmias with exercise, angina, other medical problems benefit from outpatient programs with availability of ECG monitoring, trained personnel, and emergency support.
      (2) Group camaraderie and support of program participants may assist in risk-factor modification and lifestyle changes.
      (3) Frequency: three to four sessions/week.
      (4) Duration: 30–60 minutes with 5–10 minutes of warm-up and cool-down.
      (5) Programs may offer a single mode of training (e.g., walking) or multiple modes using a circuit

training approach (e.g., treadmill, cycle ergometer, arm ergometer); strength training.
   (6) Patients are gradually weaned from continuous monitoring to spot checks and self-monitoring.
   (7) Suggested exit point: 9 MET functional capacity (5 MET capacity is needed for safe resumption of most daily activities).
 b. Strength training in Phase 2 programs.
   (1) Guidelines: after 3 weeks cardiac rehab; 5 weeks post-MI or 8 weeks post-CABG.
   (2) Begin with use of elastic bands and light weights (1–3 lb).
   (3) Progress to moderate loads, 12–15 comfortable repetitions.

3. Patient and family education goals. Progression from Phase 1 goals.

Phase 3: Community Exercise Programs (Post-Acute, Post-Discharge from Phase 2 Program)

1. Exercise/activity goals and outcomes.
 a. Improve and/or maintain functional capacity.
 b. Promote self-regulation of exercise programs.
 c. Promote life-long commitment to risk-factor modification.

2. Exercise/activity guidelines.
 a. Location: community centers, YMCA, or clinical facilities.
 b. Entry level criteria: functional capacity of 5 METs, clinically stable angina, medically controlled arrhythmias during exercise.
 c. Progression is from supervised to self-regulation of exercise.

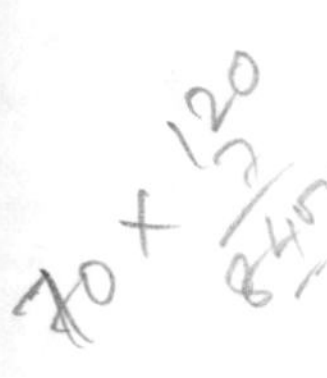

 d. Progression to 50–85% of functional capacity, three to four times/week, 45 minutes or more/session.
 f. Regular medical check-ups and periodic ETT generally required.
 g. Utilize motivational techniques to maintain compliance with exercise programs, life-style modification.
 h. Discharge typically in 6–12 months.

3. Patient and family education goals. Progression from Phase 1 goals.

Resistance Exercise Training

1. Goals and outcomes.
 a. Improve muscle strength and endurance.
 b. Enhance functional independence.
 c. Decrease cardiac demands during daily activities.

2. Patient criteria for resistance training. American Association of Cardiovascular and Pulmonary Rehabilitation Guidelines.
 a. Post-MI or cardiac surgery: minimum of 5 weeks after insult or surgery and 4 weeks of consistent participation in a supervised CR endurance training program.
 b. Post-transcatheter procedure (PTCA, other): minimum of 3 weeks following procedure and 2 weeks of consistent participation in a supervised CR endurance training program.
 c. No evidence of the following conditions: congestive heart failure, uncontrolled dysrhythmias, severe valvular disease, uncontrolled hypertension, and unstable symptoms.

3. Exercise prescription.
 a. Start with low resistance (one set of 10–15 repetitions) and progress slowly.
 b. Resistance can include:
   (1) Weights, 50% or more of maximum weight used to complete one repetition (1 RM).
   (2) Elastic bands.
   (3) Light (1- to 5-lb) cuff and hand weights.
   (4) Wall pulleys.

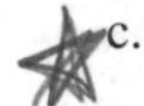

 c. Perceived exertion (RPE–Borg Scale) should range from 11 to 13 ("light" to "somewhat hard").
 d. Rate-pressure product should not exceed that prescribed during endurance exercise.

Exercise Prescription for Patients Requiring Special Considerations

1. Congestive heart failure (CHF).
 a. Patients demonstrate significant ventricular dysfunction, decreased cardiac output, low functional capacities. Classification (New York Heart Association):
   (1) Class I: mild CHF; no limitation in physical activity (up to 6.5 METs); comfortable at rest, ordinary activity does not cause undue fatigue, palpitation, dyspnea, or anginal pain.
   (2) Class II: slight CHF; slight limitation in physical activity (up to 4.5 METs); comfortable at rest, ordinary physical activity results in fatigue, palpitation, dyspnea, or anginal pain.
   (3) Class III: marked CHF; marked limitation of physical activity (up to 3.0 METs); comfortable at rest, less than ordinary activity causes fatigue, palpitation, dyspnea, or anginal pain.
   (4) Class IV: severe CHF; unable to carry out any physical activity (1.5 METs) without discomfort; symptoms of ischemia, dyspnea, anginal pain present even at rest; increasing with exercise.

b. Criteria for exercise training.
   (1) Medically stable.
   (2) Exercise capacity greater than 3 METs.
   (3) Exercise-induced ischemia and arrhythmias poor prognostic indicators.

c. Exercise training.
   (1) Use low intensities: (40–60% functional capacity); gradually increasing durations, with frequent rest periods (interval training).
   (2) Monitor with RPE (ratings of 12–14), ECG, BP, signs of exertional intolerance (dyspnea, fatigue); HR response may be impaired (most patients on digoxin); heart rate limited to resting HR + 10–20 bpm; exercise HR >115 bpm generally contraindicated.
   (3) Exercise may exacerbate CHF: check for for delayed responses of weight gain, edema lower extremities.
   (4) Patients with CHF (capacities under 6 METs) are not candidates for resistance training.
   (5) Respiratory muscle training. Monitoring SaO_2 via pulse oximetry is advisable in some cases.

d. Emphasis on training in energy conservation, self-monitoring techniques.

2. Cardiac transplant.

a. Patients may present with:
   (1) Exercise intolerance due to extended inactivity and convalescence.
   (2) Side effects from immunosuppressive drug therapy: hyperlipidema, hypertension, obesity, diabetes, leg cramps.
   (3) Decreased lower extremity strength.
   (4) Increased fracture risk due to long-term corticosteroid use.

b. Heart rate alone is not an appropriate measure of exercise intensity (heart is denervated). Use RPE, METs, dyspnea scale.

c. Use longer periods of warm-up and cool-down because the physiological responses to exercise and recovery take longer.

3. Pacemakers and automatic implantable cardioverter defibrillators (AICDs).

a. Devices programmed to pace heart rate (pacemaker) and/or deliver an electric shock if HR exceeds set limit (defibrillator).

b. Should know setting for HR limit.

c. ST segment changes may be common.

d. Avoid UE aerobic or strengthening exercises initially after implant.

e. Electromagnetic signals (antitheft devices) may cause devices to fire (defibrillator), or slow down or speed up (pacemaker).

4. Diabetes.

a. Patients demonstrate problems controlling blood glucose, with associated cardiovascular disease, renal disease, neuropathy, peripheral vascular disease and ulceration, and/or autonomic dysfunction.

b. Exercise testing.
   (1) May need to use submaximal ETT tests; maximal tests precluded with autonomic neuropathy.
   (2) With PVD/peripheral neuropathy, may need to shift to arm ergometry.

c. Exercise prescription and training. See discussion in Chapter 6 on Diabetes Mellitus.

Box 3-3 ➤ Possible Effects of Physical Training/Cardiac Rehabilitation

- Decreased HR at rest and during exercise; improved HR recovery after exercise.
- Increased stroke volume.
- Increased myocardial oxygen supply and myocardial contractility; myocardial hypertrophy.
- Improved respiratory capacity during exercise.
- Improved functional capacity of exercising muscles.
- Reduced body fat, increased lean body mass; successful weight reduction requires multifactorial interventions.
- Decreased serum lipoproteins (cholesterol, triglycerides).
- Improved glucose tolerance.
- Improved blood fibrinolytic activity and coagulability.
- Improvement in measures of psychological status and functioning: self-confidence and sense of well-being.
- Increased participation in exercise; improved outcomes with adherence to rehabilitation programming.
  - Decreased angina in patients with CAD: anginal threshold is raised secondary to decreased myocardial oxygen consumption.
  - Reduced total and cardiovascular mortality in patients following myocardial infarction.
  - Decreased symptoms of heart failure, improved functional capacity in patients with left ventricular systolic dysfunction.
  - Improved exercise tolerance and function in patients with cardiac transplantation.

Basic Life Support and Cardiopulmonary Resuscitation (CPR)

1. **Key changes: 2010 CPR Guidelines.**
   a. Compressions come first, then focus on airway and breathing (CAB). Only exception is newborn babies. (ABC)
   b. No more looking, listening, and feeling. Call 911 immediately.
   c. Push a little harder for adult CPR: at least 2 inches deep on chest.
   d. Push a little faster: about 100 compressions/min.
   e. Hands-only CPR for untrained lay rescuers.
   f. Don't stop pushing, no interruptions.
2. **See Table 3-13.**

TABLE 3-13 ➤ SUMMARY OF KEY BASIC LIFE SUPPORT (BLS) COMPONENTS FOR ADULTS, CHILDREN AND INFANTS

	RECOMMENDATIONS		
COMPONENT	**ADULTS**	**CHILDREN**	**INFANTS**
Recognition	Unresponsive (all ages) No breathing, not breathing normally (eg. only gasping)	Same as for adults	Same as for adults
CPR Sequence	CAB	CAB	CAB
Compression Rate	At least 100/min	Same as for adults	Same as for adults
Compression Depth	At least 2 inches (5cm)	At least 1/3 AP depth, about 2 inches (5 cm)	At least 1/3 AP depth, about 1 1/2 inches (4 cm)
Chest Wall Recall	Allow complete recoil between compressions, HCPs rotate compressors every 2 minutes	Same as for adults	Same as for adults
Compression Interruption	30:2 (1 or 2 rescuers)	30:2 Single Rescuer, 15:2 2 HCP Rescuers	30:2 Single Rescuer, 15:2 2 HCP Rescuers
Airway	Head tilt-chin lift (HCP suspected trauma: jaw thrust)	Same as for adults	Same as for adults
Compression to Ventilation Ratio (until advanced airway placed)	30:2 (1 or 2 rescuers)	30:2 single rescuer or 15:2 2 HCP rescuers	30:2 single rescuer or 15:2 2 HCP rescuers
Ventilations: when rescuer untrained or trained and not proficient	Compressions only	Compressions only	Compressions only
Ventilations with Advanced Airway (HCP)	1 breath every 6-8 seconds (8-10 breaths/min) Asynchronous with chest compressions About 1 second per breath Visible chest rise	Same as for adults	Same as for adults
Defibrillation	Attach and use AED as soon as available. Minimize interruptions in chest compressions before and after shock, resume CPR, beginning with compressions immediately after each shock	Same as for adults	Same as for adults

Key: CAB: compressions, airway, breathing; HCP: health care provider; CPR: cardiopulmonary resuscitation; AED: automatic electronic defibrillator
From 2010 American Heart Association Guidelines for CPR and ECG.
Downloaded from circ.ahajournals.org on July 5, 2011.

First Aid

1. **External bleeding.**
   a. Minor bleeding.
      (1) Usually clots within 10 minutes.
      (2) If patient/client is taking aspirin or nonsteroidal anti-inflammatory drugs (NSAIDS), clotting may take longer.
   b. Severe bleeding characteristics.
      (1) Blood spurting from a wound.
      (2) Blood fails to clot even after measures to control bleeding have been taken.
      (3) Arterial bleed: high pressure, spurting, red blood.
      (4) Venous bleed: low pressure, steady flow, dark red or maroon-colored blood.
      (5) Capillary bleed: low pressure, oozing, dark red blood.
   c. Controlling external bleeding.
      (1) Use standard precautions such as wearing gloves.

(2) Apply gauze pads using firm pressure. If no gauze available, use a clean cloth, towel, a gloved hand, or patient's own hand. If blood soaks through, do not remove any gauze, add additional layers.
(3) Elevate the part if possible unless it is deformed or it causes significant pain when elevated.
(4) Apply a pressure bandage, such as roller gauze, over the gauze pads.
(5) If necessary, apply pressure with the heel of your hand over pressure points. The femoral artery in the groin and the brachial artery in the medial aspect of the upper arm are two such points.
(6) Monitor A, B, Cs and overall status of the patient. Administer supplemental oxygen if nearby. Seek more advanced care as necessary.

2. Internal bleeding.

a. The possible result of a fall, blunt force, trauma, or a fracture rupturing a blood vessel or organ.
b. Severe internal bleeding may be life-threatening.
c. Severe internal bleeding characteristics.
(1) Ecchymosis (black and blue) in the injured area.
(2) Body part, especially the abdomen, may be swollen, tender and firm.
(3) Skin may appear blue, gray, or pale and may be cool or moist.
(4) Respiratory rate is increased.
(5) Pulse rate is increased and weak.
(6) Blood pressure is decreased.
(7) Patient may be nauseated or vomit.
(8) Patient may exhibit restlessness or anxiety.
(9) Level of consciousness may decline.
d. Management of internal bleeding.
(1) If minor, follow RICE procedure: rest, ice, compression, elevation.
(2) Major internal bleeding.
(a) Summon advanced medical personnel.
(b) Monitor A, B, Cs and vital signs.
(c) Keep the patient comfortable and quiet. Keep them from getting chilled or overheating.
(d) Reassure patient or victim.
(e) Administer supplemental oxygen if available and nearby.

3. Shock (hypoperfusion).

a. Failure of the circulatory system to perfuse vital organs.
b. At first, blood is shunted from the periphery to compensate.
(1) The victim may lose consciousness as the brain is affected.
(2) The heart rate increases resulting in increased oxygen demand.
(3) Organs ultimately fail when deprived of oxygen.
(4) Heart rhythm is affected, ultimately leading to cardiac arrest and death.
c. Types and causes of shock.
(1) Hemorrhagic: severe internal or external bleeding.
(2) Psychogenic: emotional stress causes blood to pool in body away from the brain.
(3) Metabolic: loss of body fluids from heat or severe vomiting or diarrhea.
(4) Anaphylactic: allergic reaction from drugs, food, or insect stings.
(5) Cardiogenic: MI or cardiac arrest results in pump failure.
(6) Respiratory: respiratory illness or arrest results in insufficient oxygenation of the blood.
(7) Septic: severe infections cause blood vessels to dilate.
(8) Neurogenic: traumatic brain injury (TBI), spinal cord injury (SCI), or other neural trauma causes disruption of autonomic nervous system resulting in disruption of blood vessel dilation/constriction.
d. Signs and symptoms.
(1) Pale, gray, or blue, cool skin.
(2) Increased, weak pulse.
(3) Increased respiratory rate.
(4) Decreased blood pressure.
(5) Irritability or restlessness.
(6) Diminishing level of consciousness.
(7) Nausea or vomiting.
e. Care for shock.
(1) Obtain a history if possible.
(2) Examine the victim for airway, breathing, circulation and bleeding.
(3) Assess level of consciousness.
(4) Determine skin characteristics and perform capillary refill test of finger tips.
(a) Capillary refill test: squeeze fingernail for 2 seconds.
(b) In healthy individuals, the nail will blanch and turn pink when pressure is released.
(c) If nail bed does not refill and turn pink within 2 seconds, the cause could be that blood is being shunted away from the periphery to vital organs or to maintain core temperature.
(5) Treat any specific condition if possible: control bleeding, splint a fracture, Epi-Pen for anaphylaxis, and so on.
(6) Keep the victim from getting chilled or overheated.
(7) Elevate the legs 12 inches unless there is suspected spinal injury or painful deformities of the lower extremities.
(8) Reassure the victim and continue to monitor A, B, Cs.
(9) Administer supplemental oxygen if nearby.
(10) Do not give any food or drink.
(11) Summon advanced medical care.

Peripheral Vascular Disease Management

Rehabilitation Guidelines for Arterial Disease

1. Risk factor modification.
   a. Cessation of smoking, weight control, glucose and lipid control.

2. Limb protection.
   a. Avoid excessive strain, protection of extremities from injury and extremes of temperature.
   b. Bed rest may be required if gangrene, ulceration, acute arterial disease are present.

3. Exercise training for patients with PVD.
   a. May result in improved functional capacity, improved peripheral blood flow, and muscle oxidative capacity.
   b. Consider interval training (multistage discontinuous protocol) with frequent rests.
   c. Walking program, moderate intensity (40–70% VO_2max) and duration, two to three times/day, 3–7 days/week.
   d. Exercise to the point of pain, not beyond. Use scale for subjective ratings for pain. Record time of pain onset.
   e. Non–weight-bearing exercise (cycle ergometry, arm ergometry) may be necessary in some patients; less effective in producing a peripheral conditioning effect.
   f. Well-fitting shoes essential; with insensitive feet, teach techniques of proper foot inspection and care.
   g. Beta blockers for treatment of hypertension or cardiac disorders may decrease time to claudication or worsen symptoms.
   h. Pentoxifylline, dipyridamole, aspirin, and warfarin may improve time to claudication.
   i. High risk for CAD.

5. Lower extremity exercise.
   a. Modified Buerger-Allen exercises: postural exercises plus active plantar and dorsiflexion of the ankle; active exercises improve blood flow during and after exercise; effects less pronounced in patients with PVD.
   b. Resistive calf exercises: most effective method of increasing blood flow.

6. Medical treatment.
   a. Medications to decrease blood viscosity, prevent thrombus formation; e.g., heparin.
   b. Vasodilators: controversial.
   c. Calcium channel blockers in vasospastic disease.

7. Surgical management.
   a. Atherectomy, thromboembolectomy, laser therapy.
   b. Revascularization: angioplasty or bypass grafting.
   c. Sympathectomy: results in permanent vasodilation, improvement of blood flow to skin.
   d. Amputation when gangrene is present.

Rehabilitation Guidelines for Venous Disease

1. Deep vein thrombophlebitis (DVT).
   a. Early stages may be asymptomatic; symptomatic patients demonstrate dull ache, pain, tenderness in calf; may also see slight edema or fever.
   b. Acute: patient is placed on bed rest until signs of inflammation have subsided; elevation of involved leg.
   c. Anticoagulation medications.
   d. Exercise therapy contraindicated during acute phase; increases pain, potential to dislodge clot, progress to pulmonary embolism, potentially fatal.
   e. Ambulation permitted (with elastic stockings) after local tenderness and swelling resolve.

2. Chronic venous insufficiency (CVI).
   a. Management of edema.
      (1) Positioning: extremity elevation, minimum of 18 cm above heart. Encourage patients to elevate leg as much as possible and avoid the dependent position.
      (2) Compression therapy.
         (a) Bandages (elastic, tubular); applied within 20 minutes of rising.
         (b) Paste bandages (Unna boot). Gauze impregnated with zinc oxide, gelatin, and glycerine; applied for 4–7 days.
         (c) Graduated compression stockings (Jobst®).
         (d) Compression pump therapy, used for a 1- to 2-hour session twice daily.
         (e) **Red Flag:** do not apply compression therapy to a limb with an ankle-brachial index (ABI) < 0.8 or with evidence of active cellulitis or infection.
      (3) Exercise.
         (a) Active ankle exercises: emphasis on muscle pump exercises (dorsiflexion/plantarflexion, foot circles.
         (b) Cycle ergometry in sitting or attached to foot of bed.
         (c) Early ambulation as soon as patient is able to get out of bed, three to four times/day.

b. Patient education: meticulous skin care.
c. Severe conditions with dermal ulceration may require surgery (ligation and vein stripping, vein grafts, valvuloplasty).

Rehabilitation Guidelines for Lymphatic Disease

1. **Phase I Management: edema secondary to lymphatic dysfunction.**
   a. Short-stretch compression bandages, worn 24 hours/day.
      (1) Bandages have low resting pressure and high working pressure.
      (2) Bandages maintain limb after techniques applied to reduce limb.
   b. Manual lymph drainage (MLD).
      (1) Massage and passive range of motion (PROM) to assist lymphatic flow (Vodder techniques, modifications by Asdonk, Leduc, Fodi).
      (2) Emphasis is on decongesting proximal segments first, then extremities, directing flow distal to proximal.
   c. Skin care: stress good hygiene.
   d. Exercise.
      (1) Activate muscles in extremity. Work trunk and limb girdle muscles first, then limb muscles from proximal to distal. Performed with compression bandages on.
      (2) Walking program, cycling.
      (3) Water-based programs: swimming.
      (4) Tai Chi and balance activities.
      (5) ADL training.
      (6) Red Flag: strenuous activities, jogging, and ballistic movements are contraindicated, as they are likely to exacerbate lymphedema.
      (7) Signs of lymph overload: discomfort, aching or pain in proximal lymph areas (axilla or inguinal areas, change in skin color. If any of these are present, discontinue activity, elevate the limb, and apply cold packs.
   e. Compression garments at end of Phase 1.
   Red Flag: excessively high pressures will occlude superficial lymph capillaries and restrict fluid absorption.

2. **Phase II Management (self-management).**
   a. Skin care.
   b. Compression garment.
   c. Exercise.
   d. Lymphedema bandaging at night.
   e. MLD as needed.
   f. Compression pumps.
   Red Flag: pressures higher than 45 mm Hg are contraindicated, as they can cause lymphatic collapse; contraindicated with soft tissue injury.

3. **Education.**
   a. Skin and nail care.
   b. Self-massage.
   c. Self-bandaging, garment care.
   d. Infection management.
   e. Maintain exercise while preventing lymph overload.

4. **Specialized education for complete decongestive therapy, including manual lymphatic drainage:**
   a. National Lymphedema Network at http:// www.lymphnet.org
   b. Lymphology Association of North America at http://www.clt-lana.org

5. **Surgery to assist in lymph drainage (severe cases).**

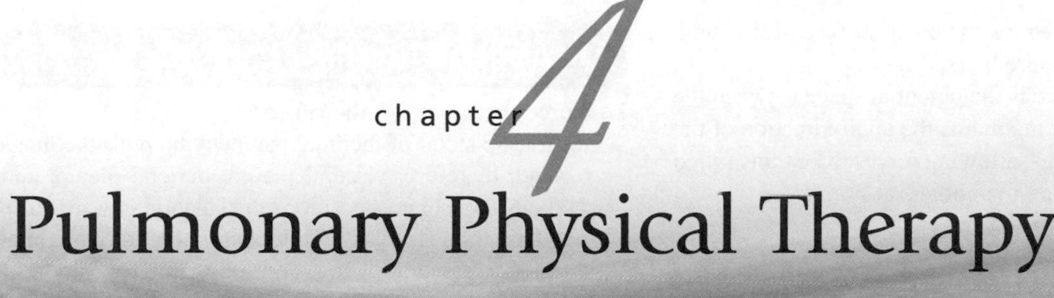

chapter 4 Pulmonary Physical Therapy

JULIE ANN STARR

Pulmonary Anatomy and Physiology

Bony Thorax

1. **Anterior border: the sternum (manubrium, body, xiphoid process).**
   a. The lateral borders of the trachea run perpendicularly into the suprasternal notch.
   b. The angle of Louis (sternal angle), the bony ridge between the manubrium and body, is point of anterior attachment of the second rib and tracheal bifurcation.

2. **Lateral border: the rib cage.**
   a. Ribs 1–6, termed true or costosternal ribs, have a single anterior costochondral attachment to the sternum.
   b. Ribs 7–10, termed false or costochondral ribs, share costochondral attachments before attaching anteriorly to the sternum.
   c. Ribs 11 and 12 are termed floating or costovertebral ribs, as they have no anterior attachment.

3. **Posterior border.**
   a. The vertebral column, from T1 through T12.

4. **Shoulder girdle.**
   a. Can affect the motion of the thorax.
   b. Provides attachments for accessory muscles of ventilation.

Internal Structures

1. **Upper airways.**
   a. Nose or mouth: entry point into the respiratory system. The nose filters, humidifies, and warms air.
   b. Pharynx: common area used for both respiratory and digestive systems.
   c. Larynx: connects the pharynx to trachea, including the epiglottis and vocal cords.

2. **Lower airways.**
   a. The conducting airways, trachea to terminal bronchioles, transport air only. No gas exchange occurs.
   b. The respiratory unit: respiratory bronchioles, alveolar ducts, alveolar sacs, and alveoli. Diffusion of gas occurs through all of these structures.

3. **Lung structures.**
   a. Right lung divides into three lobes by the oblique and horizontal fissure lines. Each lobe divides into segments, totaling 10 segments.
   b. Left lung divides into two lobes by a single oblique fissure line. Each lobe divides into segments, totaling 8 segments.

4. **Pleura.**
   a. Parietal pleura covers the inner surface of the thoracic cage, diaphragm, and mediastinal border of the lung.

b. Visceral pleura wraps the outer surface of the lung, including the fissure lines.
c. Intrapleural space is the potential space between the two pleurae that maintains the approximation of the rib cage and lungs, allowing forces to be transmitted from one structure to another.

Muscles of Ventilation

1. **Primary muscles of inspiration.**
   a. Produce a normal resting tidal volume.
   b. Primary muscle of inspiration is the diaphragm. The diaphragm is made of two hemidiaphragms, each with a central tendon. When the diaphragm is at rest, the hemidiaphragms are arched high into the thorax. When the muscle contracts, the central tendon is pulled downward, flattening the dome. The result is a protrusion of the abdominal wall during inhalation.
   c. Additional primary muscles of inspiration are portions of the intercostals.
2. **Accessory muscles of inspiration.**
   a. Used when a more rapid or deeper inhalation is required or in disease states.
   b. The upper two ribs are raised by the scalenes and sternocleidomastoid. The rest of the ribs are raised by levator costarum and serratus. By fixing the shoulder girdle, the trapezius, pectorals, and serratus can become muscles of inspiration.
3. **Expiratory muscles of ventilation.**
   a. Resting exhalation results from a passive relaxation of the inspiratory muscles and the elastic recoil tendency of the lung. Normal abdominal tone holds the abdominal contents directly under the diaphragm, assisting the return of the diaphragm to the normal high domed position.
   b. Expiratory muscles, used when a quicker and/or fuller expiration is desired, as in exercise or in disease states. These are quadratus lumborum, portions of the intercostals, muscles of the abdomen, and triangularis sterni.
4. **Patients who lack abdominal musculature (e.g., spinal cord injury).**
   a. Have a lower resting position of the diaphragm, decreasing inspiratory reserve.
   b. The more upright the body position, the lower the diaphragm and the lower the inspiratory capacity.
   c. The more supine the body position, the more advantageous the position of the diaphragm.
   d. An abdominal binder may be helpful in providing support to the abdominal viscera, assisting ventilation. Care must be taken not to constrict the thorax with the abdominal binder.

Mechanics of Breathing

1. **Forces acting upon the rib cage.**
   a. Elastic recoil of the lung parenchyma pulls the lungs and, therefore, visceral pleura, parietal pleura, and bony thorax into a position of exhalation (inward pull).
   b. Bony thorax pulls the thorax and, therefore, parietal pleura, visceral pleura, and lungs into a position of inspiration (outward pull).
   c. Muscular action pulls either outward or inward, depending on the muscles used.
   d. Resting end expiratory pressure (REEP) is the point of equilibrium where these forces are balanced. Occurs at end tidal expiration.

Ventilation

1. **Movement of gas in and out of the pulmonary system.**
2. **Volumes.** (Figure 4-1).
   a. Tidal volume (TV): volume of gas inhaled (or exhaled) during a normal resting breath.
   b. Inspiratory reserve volume (IRV): volume of gas that can be inhaled beyond a normal resting tidal inhalation.
   c. Expiratory reserve volume (ERV): volume of gas that can be exhaled beyond a normal resting tidal exhalation.
   d. Residual volume (RV): volume of gas that remains in the lungs after ERV has been exhaled.
3. **Capacities.** Two or more lung volumes added together.
   a. Inspiratory capacity (IRV + TV): the amount of air that can be inhaled from REEP.
   b. Vital Capacity (IRV + TV + ERV): the amount of air that is under volitional control; conventionally measured as a forced expiratory vital capacity (FVC).

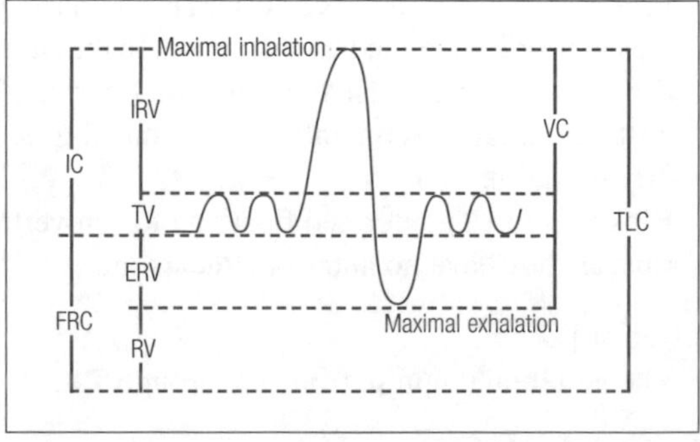

Figure 4-1 • Lung volumes and capacities. IRV = inspiratory reserve volume; TV = tidal volume; ERV = expiratory reserve volume; RV = residual volume; IC = inspiratory capacity; FRC = functional residual capacity, VC = vital capacity; TLC = total lung capacity. From: O'Sullivan S, Schmidt T: Physical Rehabilitation: Assessment and Treatment, 4th ed. Davis, 2001, p 447, with permission.

c. Functional residual capacity (ERV + RV): the amount of air that resides in the lungs after a normal resting tidal exhalation.
d. Total lung capacity (IRV + TV + ERV + RV): the total amount of air that is contained within the thorax during a maximum inspiratory effort.

4. Flow rates.
a. Forced expiratory volume in 1 second (FEV_1): the amount of air exhaled during the first second of FVC. In the healthy person, at least 70% of the FVC is exhaled within the first second ($FEV_1/FVC \times 100 > 70\%$).
b. Forced expiratory flow rate (FEF 25%–75%) is the slope of a line drawn between the points 25% and 75% of exhaled volume on a forced vital capacity exhalation curve. This flow rate is more specific to the smaller airways, and shows a more dramatic change with disease than FEV_1.

Respiration

1. Diffusion of gas across the alveolar-capillary membrane.

2. Arterial oxygenation. The ability of arterial blood to carry oxygen.
a. Partial pressure of oxygen in the atmosphere (PaO_2) at sea level is 760 mm Hg (barometric pressure) × 21% = 159.6 mm Hg.
b. The partial pressure of oxygen in the arterial blood, PaO_2, depends on the integrity of the pulmonary system, the circulatory system, and the PaO_2. PaO_2 at room air is 95–100 mm Hg in a young, healthy individual. Hypoxemia: PaO_2 decreases with age, but in a young healthy individual, mild hypoxemia would be considered at < 90. Hyperoxemia: PaO_2 > 100.
c. Fraction of oxygen in the inspired air (FiO_2) is the percentage of oxygen in air, based on a total of 1.00. The FiO_2 of room air, approximately 21% oxygen, is written as 0.21. Supplemental oxygen increases the percentage (> 21%) of oxygen in the patient's atmosphere. Supplemental oxygen is usually prescribed when the PaO_2 falls below 55 mm Hg.

3. Alveolar ventilation. Ability to remove carbon dioxide from the pulmonary circulation and maintain pH.
a. pH indicates the concentration of free floating hydrogen ions within the body. Normal range for pH is 7.35–7.45.
b. $PaCO_2$: the partial pressure of carbon dioxide within the arterial blood, in health, 35 to 45 mm Hg. Hypercapnea is a $PaCO_2$ > 45 mm Hg. Hypocapnea is a $PaCO_2$ below 35 mm Hg. Removal or retention of CO_2 by the respiratory system alters the pH of the body in an inverse relationship. An increase in the $PaCO_2$ decreases the body's pH. A decrease in the $PaCO_2$ raises the body's pH.
c. HCO_3: amount of bicarbonate ions within the arterial blood, normally 22–28 mEq/mL. Removal or retention of HCO_3 alters the pH of the body in a direct relationship. An increase in bicarbonate ions increases the body's pH. A decrease in bicarbonate ions decreases the body's pH.

Ventilation (V_E) and Perfusion (Blood Flow, or Q)

1. Optimal respiration occurs when ventilation and perfusion (blood flow to the lungs) are matched. Different ventilation and perfusion relationships exist.

2. Dead space.
a. Anatomical (conducting airways) or physiological (diseases such as pulmonary emboli).
b. Dead space is a space that is well-ventilated, but in which no respiration (gas exchange) occurs.

3. Shunt.
a. No respiration occurs because of a ventilation abnormality.
b. Complete atelectasis of a respiratory unit allows the blood to travel through the pulmonary capillary without gas diffusion.

4. Effects of body position on the ventilation perfusion relationship. Gravity affects the distribution of ventilation and perfusion.
a. Upright position.
(1) Perfusion is gravity-dependent; i.e., more pulmonary blood is found at the base of the lung in the upright position.
(2) Ventilation. At the static point of REEP, the apical alveoli are fuller than those at the base. During the dynamic phase of inspiration, more air will be delivered to the less filled alveoli at the bases, causing a greater change in V_E at the bases.
(3) Ventilation perfusion ratio (V/Q ratio): the ratio of pulmonary alveolar ventilation to pulmonary capillary perfusion. In the upright position, the apices are gravity independent, with the lowest blood flow, or Q. Although is relatively low, there is still more air than blood, resulting in a high V/Q ratio (dead space). Perfusion and ventilation of the middle zone of the lung are evenly matched. The bases are gravity-dependent and, therefore, have the most Q. Although V_E is relatively high, there is more blood than air, resulting in a (relatively) low V/Q ratio (shunt).
b. Other body positions. Every body position creates these zones: gravity-independent, middle, and gravity-dependent. The gravity-independent area of the lung, despite the position of the body, acts as dead space. The gravity-dependent area of the lung acts as a shunt. Body positions can be used for a variety of treatment goals: draining secretions, increasing ventilation, or to optimize ventilation perfusion relationships.

Control of Ventilation

1. **Receptors.**
   a. Baroreceptors, chemoreceptors, irritant receptors, stretch receptors within the body assist in adjusting the ventilatory cycle by sending information to the controller.
2. **Central control centers.**
   a. Cortex, pons, medulla, and autonomic nervous system evaluate the receptors' information.
   b. Send a message out to the ventilatory muscles to alter the respiratory cycle in order to maintain adequate alveolar ventilation and arterial oxygenation.
3. **Ventilatory muscles.**
   a. Institute the changes deemed necessary by the central controllers.

Physical Therapy Examination

Patient Interview

1. **Information from the patient, the patient's family, and the medical record.**
2. **Chief complaint.**
   a. Usually involves the loss of function (decreased ability to perform activities of daily living [ADLs]) or discomfort (shortness of breath [dyspnea]).
3. **Present illness.**
   a. Initial onset (sudden vs. insidious) and progression of primary problem.
   b. Anything that worsens or improves condition: positions, rest, medications.
4. **Review the patient's history.**
   a. Occupational history. Past occupational exposures for diseases such as asbestosis, silicosis, and pneumoconiosis. Present occupational exposure to antigens within the workplace (hypersensitivity pneumonitis).
   b. Past medical history that would alter physical exam or treatment plans (e.g., heart disease, long-term steroid use).
   c. Current medications that can mask (steroids) or alter (beta blockers, bronchodilators) vital signs.
   d. Social habits.
      (1) Smoking in pack years (number of packs per day × number of years smoked).
      (2) Alcohol consumption.
      (3) Street drugs.
   e. Functional and exertional activity level during periods of wellness, as well as with present illness.
   f. Cough and sputum production. Record any changes from baseline because of present illness.
   g. Family history of pulmonary disease (e.g., cystic fibrosis).

Tests and Measures

1. **Vital signs.** See Table 4-1 for normal values.

Table 4-1 ➤ NORMAL VALUES FOR INFANTS AND ADULTS

PARAMETER	INFANT	ADULT
Heart Rate	120 bpm	60–100 bpm
Blood Pressure	75/50 mmHg	<120/80 mmHg
Respiratory Rate	40 br/min	12–20 br/min
PaO_2	75–80 mmHg	80–100 mmHg
$PaCO_2$	34–54 mmHg	35–45 mmHg
pH	7.26–7.41	7.35–7.45
Tidal Volume	20 ml	500 ml

   a. Temperature: normal (afebrile) 98.6°F (37°C). Core temperature increase indicates infection.
   b. Heart rate (HR): normal 60–100 bpm; tachycardia: HR > 100 bpm; bradycardia: HR < 60 bpm.
   c. Respirations.
      (1) Rate: in health is 12–20 breaths/bpm. Tachypnea is a rate > 20 bpm. Apnea means no respirations.
      (2) Rhythm: regular or irregular.
      (3) Amplitude: shallow, deep.
   d. Blood pressure.
2. **Observation.**
   a. Peripheral edema seen in gravity-dependent areas and jugular venous distension indicates possible heart failure. Right ventricular hypertrophy and dilation (cor pulmonale) are common sequelae to chronic lung disease.
   b. Body positions. Stabilizing the shoulder girdle (e.g., sitting, hands placed on seat, arms extended, body leaning forward) places the thorax in the inspiratory position and allows the additional recruitment of muscles for inspiration (pectorals).
   c. Color: cyanosis, an acute sign of hypoxemia, is a bluish tinge to nail beds and the areas around eyes and mouth.
   d. Digital clubbing: a sign of chronic hypoxemia. The configuration of the distal phalanx of fingers or toes becomes bulbous.

3. **Inspection and palpation.**
   a. Standard precautions should be used when the therapist may come in contact with a patient's body fluids. See Box 6-1. Gloves are usually all that is needed during a routine physical exam.
   b. Neck.
      (1) Observe the trachea: it should be in midline, superior to the suprasternal notch.
      (2) Note the use of accessory muscles of ventilation.
   c. Thorax.
      (1) Changes in bony thorax (pectus excavatum, carinatum).
      (2) Observe anterior-posterior:lateral dimension. In health, there is a 1:2 ratio. With obstructive pulmonary disease, the lung recoil force is decreased, resulting in a barreled chest and an increase in the A-P dimension.
      (3) The right and left thorax should be symmetrical.
         (a) Symmetry, static and/or dynamic, may be altered by changes in the bony thorax (scoliosis, scapular immobility, pain), changes in the underlying lung and pleura (a patient with pleuritic pain or pneumothorax), or changes in the overlying skin (thoracic burn).
         (b) Thoracic excursion in health, measured at the base of the lungs from full inspiration to full expiration, is between 2 and 3 inches.
         (c) Inspect for scars, indicating potential adhesions to underlying soft tissue or surgical removal of structures within the thorax.

4. **Auscultation.**
   a. Intensity of inspiration and expiration is quieter at the bases than the apex.
      (1) Vesicular (normal breath sound): a soft rustling sound heard throughout all of inspiration and the beginning of expiration.
      (2) Bronchial: a more hollow, echoing sound normally found only over the right superior anterior thorax. This corresponds to an area over the right main stem bronchus. All of inspiration and most of expiration are heard with bronchial breath sounds.
      (3) Decreased: a very distant sound not normally heard over a healthy thorax; allows only some of the inspiration to be heard. Often associated with obstructive lung diseases.
   b. Adventitious (extra) sounds. According to the American Thoracic Society, there are only two adventitious breath sounds:
      (1) Crackles (also termed rales, crepitations): a crackling sound heard usually during inspiration that indicates pathology (atelectasis, fibrosis, pulmonary edema).
      (2) Wheezes: a musically pitched sound, usually heard during expiration, caused by airway obstruction (asthma, chronic obstructive pulmonary disease [COPD], foreign body aspiration). With severe airway constriction, as with croup, wheezes may be heard on inspiration as well.
   c. Vocal sounds.
      (1) Normal transmission of vocal sounds.
         (a) As with breath sounds, vocal transmission is loudest near trachea and main-stem bronchi.
         (b) Words should be intelligible, though softer and less clear at the more distal areas of the lungs.
      (2) Abnormal transmission of vocal sounds may be heard through fluid-filled areas of consolidation, cavitation lesions, or pleural effusions.
         (a) Egophony is a nasal or bleating sound heard during auscultation. "E" sounds are transmitted to sound like "A."
         (b) Bronchophony, characterized by an intense, clear sound during auscultation, even at the lung bases.
         (c) Whispered pectoriloquy occurs when whispered sounds are heard clearly during auscultation.

5. **Radiographic examination.**
   a. Chest x-rays (CXR): a two-dimensional radiographic film to detect the presence of abnormal material (exudate, blood) or a change in pulmonary parenchyma (fibrosis, collapse).
   b. Computed tomographic (CT) scan: computer-generated picture of a cross-sectional plane of the body.
   c. Ventilation perfusion (V/Q) scan: matches the ventilation pattern of the lung to the perfusion pattern to identify the presence of pulmonary emboli.
   d. Fluoroscopy: continuous x-ray beam allows observation of diaphragmatic excursion.

6. **Laboratory tests.** (See Table 4-1 for normal values).
   a. Arterial blood gas (ABG) analysis indicates the adequacy of:
      (1) Alveolar ventilation by determining pH, bicarbonate ion, and partial pressure of carbon dioxide. Table 4-2 presents the four basic conditions of acid-base balance and the $PaCO_2$, pH, and HCO_3- values that accompany each condition.
      (2) Arterial oxygenation by determining the partial pressure of oxygen in relation to the fraction of inspired oxygen.
   b. Electrocardiogram: see Chapter 3 (Cardiovascular Physical Therapy) for discussion.
   c. Sputum studies.
      (1) Gram stain: immediate identification of the category of bacteria (gram negative or gram positive) and its appearance (e.g., pairs, chains).
      (2) Culture and sensitivity: identifies the specific bacteria as well as the organism's susceptibility to various antibiotics. Results available within a few days.

Table 4-2 ➤ INTERPRETATION OF ABNORMAL ACID-BASE BALANCE

TYPE	pH	$PaCO_2$	HCO_3^-	CAUSES	SIGNS AND SYMPTOMS
Respiratory alkalosis	↑	↓	WNL	Alveolar hyperventilation	Dizziness, syncope, tingling, numbness, early tetany
Respiratory acidosis	↓	↑	WNL	Alveolar hypoventilation	Early: anxiety, restlessness, dyspnea, headache Late: confusion, somnolence, coma
Metabolic alkalosis	↑	WNL	↑	Bicarbonate ingestion, vomiting, diuretics, steroids, adrenal disease	Vague symptoms: weakness, mental dullness, possibly early tetany
Metabolic acidosis	↓	WNL	↓	Diabetic, lactic, or uremic acidosis, prolonged diarrhea	Secondary hyperventilation (Kussmaul breathing), nausea, lethargy, and coma

From: Rothstein, J, Wolf S. The four basic conditions of acid-base balance. The Rehabilitation Specialist's Handbook. 2nd ed. Davis, Philadelphia, 1998, p 529, with permission.

(3) Cytology: reports the presence of cancer cells in sputum.

d. Pulmonary function tests (PFTs): evaluate lung volumes, capacities, and flow rates. Used to diagnose disease, monitor progression, and determine the benefits of medical management. See Figure 4-2 for changes with disease states. See Table 4-3 for classification of respiratory impairments including PFT predicted values.

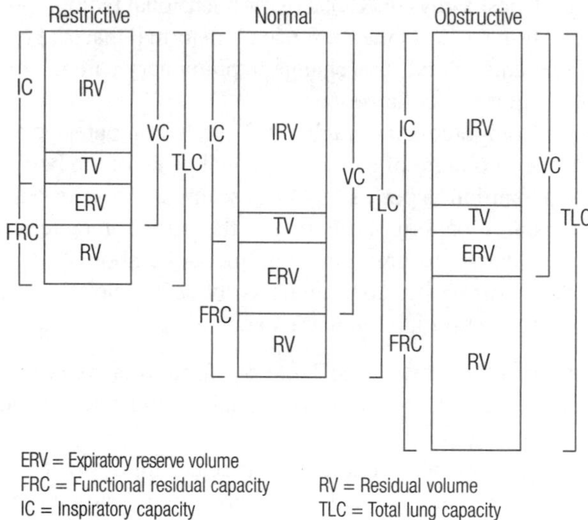

Figure 4-2 • Lung volumes of a healthy pulmonary system compared with the lung volumes and capacities found in restrictive and obstructive pulmonary disease.
From: Rothstein J, Roy S, and Wolf S: The Rehabilitation Specialist's Handbook, 2nd ed. Davis, Philadelphia, 1998, p 509, with permission.

e. Blood values.
   (1) White blood cell count (WBC) normal values: 4,000–11,000.
   (2) Hematocrit (Hct) normal values: 35%–48%.
   (3) Hemoglobin (Hgb) normal values: 12–16 g/dL.

7. Bronchoscopy.

a. Endoscope used to view, biopsy, wash, suction, and/or brush the interior aspects of the tracheobronchial tree.

8. Exercise tolerance tests (ETT) (Graded Exercise Test). (See also Chapter 3, Cardiovascular Physical Therapy.

a. Evaluates an individual's cardiopulmonary response to gradually increasing exercise.
b. Determines the presence of exercise-induced bronchospasm by testing pulmonary function, particularly FEV_1 before and after ETT.
c. Documents the need for supplemental oxygen during an exercise program by analyzing arterial blood gas values throughout the ETT. ABGs also provide a criterion for test termination. If arterial blood sampling is unavailable, pulse oximetry can be used to monitor the percent saturation of oxygen within the arterial blood. Table 4-4 presents criteria for test termination for patients with pulmonary disease.

Table 4-3 ➤ CLASSES OF RESPIRATORY IMPAIRMENT

	CLASS 1 0% IMPAIRMENT	CLASS 2 20–30% IMPAIRMENT	CLASS 3 40–50% IMPAIRMENT	CLASS 4 60–90% IMPAIRMENT
Roentgenographic appearance	Usually normal, but there may be evidence of healed or inactive chest disease including, for example, minimal nodular silicosis or pleura scars.	May be normal or abnormal	May be normal, but usually is not	Usually is abnormal
Dyspnea	When it occurs, it is consistent with the circumstances or activity.	Does not occur at rest and seldom occurs during the performance of the usual activities of daily living. The patient can keep pace with persons of same age and body build on level ground without breathlessness but not on hills or stairs.	Does not occur at rest but does occur during the usual activities of daily living. However, the patient can walk a mile at his own pace without dyspnea, although he cannot keep pace on level ground with others of the same age and body build.	Occurs during such activities as climbing one flight of stairs or walking 100 yards on level ground, on less exertion, or even at rest.
Tests of ventilatory function				
FEV_1, FCV, MMV	Not less than 85% of predicted	70–85% of predicted	55–70% of predicted	Less than 55% of predicted
Arterial oxygen saturation	Not applicable	Not applicable	Usually 88%* or greater at rest and after exercise	Usually less than 88% at rest and after exercise

*88% saturation corresponds to an arterial PO_2 of 58mmHg, assuming the arterial pH is in the normal range.
From: Guides to the Evaluator of Permanent Impairment; The Respiratory System. JAMA 1965, 194: 919, with permission.

Physical Dysfunction/Impairments

Acute Diseases

1. **Bacterial pneumonia.**
   a. An intra-alveolar bacterial infection. Gram-positive bacteria is usually acquired in the community. Pneumococcal pneumonia (streptococcal) is the most common type of gram-positive pneumonia. Gram-negative bacteria usually develop in a host with underlying, chronic, debilitating conditions, severe acute illness, and recent antibiotic therapy. Gram-negative infections result in early tissue necrosis and abscess formation. Common infecting organisms: *Klebsiella, Haemophilus influenzae, Pseudomonas aeruginosa, Proteus, Serratia.*
   b. Pertinent physical findings.
      (1) Shaking chills.
      (2) Fever.
      (3) Chest pain if pleuritic involvement.
      (4) Cough becoming productive of purulent, blood streaked, or rusty sputum.
      (5) Decreased or bronchial breath sounds and/ or crackles.
      (6) Tachypnea.
      (7) Increased white blood cell count.
      (8) Hypoxemia, hypocapnea initially, hypercapnea with increasing severity.
      (9) CXR confirmation of infiltrate.

2. **Viral pneumonia.**
   a. An interstitial or intra-alveolar inflammatory process caused by viral agents (influenza, adenovirus, cytomegalovirus, herpes, parainfluenza, respiratory syncytial virus, measles).
   b. Pertinent physical findings.
      (1) Recent history of upper respiratory infection.
      (2) Fever.
      (3) Chills.
      (4) Dry cough.
      (5) Headaches.
      (6) Decreased breath sounds and/or crackles.
      (7) Hypoxemia and hypercapnea.

Table 4-4 ➤ GRADED EXERCISE TEST TERMINATION CRITERIA

1. Maximal shortness of breath.
2. A fall in PaO_2 of greater than 20 mmHg or a PaO_2 less than 55 mmHg.
3. A rise in $PaCO_2$ of greater than 10 mmHg or greater than 65 mmHg.
4. Cardiac ischemia or arrhythmias.
5. Symptoms of fatigue.
6. Increase in diastolic blood pressure readings of 20 mmHg, systolic hypertension greater than 250 mmHg, decrease in blood pressure with increasing workloads.
7. Leg pain.
8. Total fatigue.
9. Signs of insufficient cardiac output.
10. Reaching a ventilatory maximum.

From: Brannon, F, et al: Cardiopulmonary Rehabilitation: Basic Theory and Application, 3rd ed. Davis, 1998, p 300, with permission.

(8) Normal white blood cell count.
(9) CXR confirmation of interstitial infiltrate.

3. Aspiration pneumonia.

a. Aspirated material causes an acute inflammatory reaction within the lungs. Usually found in patients with impaired swallowing (dysphagia), fixed neck extension, intoxication, impaired consciousness, neuromuscular disease, recent anesthesia.

b. Pertinent physical findings.
(1) Symptoms begin shortly after aspiration event (hours).
(2) Cough may be dry at the onset, progresses to produce putrid secretions.
(3) Dyspnea.
(4) Tachypnea.
(5) Cyanosis.
(6) Tachycardia.
(7) Wheezes and crackles with decreased breath sounds.
(8) Hypoxemia, hypercapnea in severe cases.
(9) Chest pain over the involved area.
(10) Fever.
(11) WBC count shows varying degrees of leukocytosis.
(12) CXR initially shows pneumonitis. Chronic aspiration shows necrotizing pneumonia with cavitation.

4. Tuberculosis (TB).

a. *Mycobacterium tuberculosis* infection spread by aerosolized droplets from an untreated infected host. Incubation period: 2–10 weeks. Primary disease lasts approximately 10 days to 2 weeks.

b. Postprimary infection is reactivation of dormant tuberculous bacillus, which can occur years after the primary infection.

c. Two weeks on appropriate antituberculin drugs renders the host noninfectious. During the infectious stage, the patient must be isolated from others in a negative-pressure room. Anyone entering the room must wear a protective TB mask and follow universal precautions. If the patient leaves the negative-pressure room, he or she must wear a specialized mask to keep from infecting others.

d. Medication is taken for prolonged periods: 3–12 months.

e. There is an increased incidence of TB in patients with HIV.

f. Pertinent physical findings of primary disease can go unnoticed, as it causes only mild symptoms: slight nonproductive cough, low-grade fever, and possible CXR changes consistent with primary disease.

g. Pertinent physical findings of postprimary infection:
(1) Fever.
(2) Weight loss.
(3) Cough.
(4) Hilar adenopathy: enlargement of the lymph nodes surrounding the hilum.
(5) Night sweat.
(6) Crackles.
(7) Hemoptysis: blood-streaked sputum.
(8) WBC shows increased lymphocytes.
(9) CXR shows upper lobe involvement with air space densities, cavitation, pleural involvement, and parenchymal fibrosis.

5. Pneumocystis pneumonia (PCP).

a. Pulmonary infection caused by a fungus (*Pneumocystis carinii*) in immunocompromised hosts. Most often found in patients following transplantation, neonates, or patients infected with HIV.

b. Pertinent physical findings.
(1) Insidious progressive shortness of breath.
(2) Nonproductive cough.
(3) Crackles.
(4) Weakness.
(5) Fever.
(6) Chest x-ray shows interstitial infiltrates.
(7) Complete blood count (CBC) shows no evidence of infection.

6. SARS (severe acute respiratory syndrome).

a. An atypical respiratory illness caused by a coronovirus. Initial outbreak in southern mainland China with worldwide spread to other areas such as Singapore, Toronto, Vietnam, and Hong Kong.

b. Pertinent physical findings.
(1) High temperature.
(2) Dry cough.
(3) Decreased white blood cells, decreased platelets, decreased lymphocytes.
(4) Increased liver function tests.

(5) Abnormal CXR with borderline breath sounds changes.

7. **See Box 6-1, Standard Precautions.**

Chronic Obstructive Diseases

1. **Chronic obstructive pulmonary disease (COPD).**
   a. According to the Global Initiative for Obstructive Lung Disease (GOLD), COPD is a disease state characterized by airflow limitation that is not fully reversible. The airflow limitation is usually both progressive and associated with an abnormal inflammatory response of the lungs to noxious particles or gases.
   b. Stages.
      (1) Stage 1 (mild).
         (a) $FEV_1/FVC < 70\%$.
         (b) $FEV_1 >= 80\%$ predicted.
         (c) With or without chronic symptoms.
      (2) Stage 2 (moderate).
         (a) $FEV_1/FVC < 70\%$.
         (b) $50\% < FEV_1 < 80\%$ predicted.
         (c) Often with symptoms of shortness of breath with exertion.
      (3) Stage 3 (severe).
         (a) $FEV_1/FVC < 70\%$.
         (b) $30\% < FEV_1 < 50\%$.
         (c) With greater shortness of breath, decreased exercise capacity, and exacerbations of their disease.
      (4) Stage 4 (very severe).
         (a) $FEV_1/FVC < 70\%$.
         (b) $FEV_1 < 30\%$ predicted.
         (c) $FEV_1 < 50\%$ with chronic respiratory failure symptoms.
         (d) Impaired quality of life.
         (e) Exacerbations of their disease may be life threatening.
   c. Physical findings: increase in severity as the stage of disease advances:
      (1) Cough/sputum production/ hemoptysis.
      (2) Dyspnea on exertion.
      (3) Breath sounds decreased with adventitious sounds.
      (4) Increased respiratory rate [RR].
      (5) Weight loss/anorexia.
      (6) Increased A-P diameter of chest wall.
      (7) Cyanosis.
      (8) Clubbing.
      (9) Postures to structurally elevate shoulder girdle.
      (10) CXR showing hyperinflation, flattened diaphragms, hyperlucency.
      (11) ABG changes of hypoxemia, hypercapnea.
      (12) PFTs showing obstructive disease, such as decreased FEV_1, decreased FVC, increased FRC and RV, and decreased FEV_1/FVC ratio.

2. **Asthma.**
   a. Increased reactivity of the trachea and bronchi to various stimuli (allergens, exercise, cold); reversible in nature; manifests by widespread narrowing of the airways due to inflammation, smooth muscle constriction, and increased secretions. Even during remission, some degree of airway inflammation is present.
   b. Pertinent physical findings during exacerbation.
      (1) Wheezing, possible crackles, and decreased breath sounds.
      (2) Increased secretions of variable amounts.
      (3) Dyspnea.
      (4) Increased accessory muscle use.
      (5) Anxiety.
      (6) Tachycardia.
      (7) Tachypnea.
      (8) Hypoxemia.
      (9) Hypocapnea. Responding to hypoxemia, there is an increased respiratory rate and minute ventilation. This will decrease $PaCO_2$. With severe airway constriction, an increase in minute ventilation cannot occur and hypercapnea can be found.
      (10) Cyanosis.
      (11) PFTs show impaired flow rates.
      (12) CXR shows hyperlucency and flattened diaphragms during exaccerbation.

3. **Cystic fibrosis (CF).**
   a. A genetically inherited disease characterized by thickening of secretions of all exocrine glands, leading to obstruction (e.g. pancreatic, pulmonic, gastrointestinal). CF may present as an obstructive, restrictive, or mixed disease. Clinical signs include meconium ileus, frequent respiratory infections, especially *Staphylococcus aureus* and *Pseudomonas aeruginosa*, and inability to gain weight despite adequate caloric intake. Diagnosis is made postnatally by a blood test indicating trypsinogen, or later by a positive sweat electrolyte test.
   b. Pertinent physical findings with exacerbation of disease.
      (1) Onset of symptoms usually in early childhood.
      (2) Dyspnea, especially on exertion.
      (3) Productive cough.
      (4) Hypoxemia, hypercapnea.
      (5) Cyanosis.
      (6) Clubbing.
      (7) Use of accessory muscles of ventilation.
      (8) Tachypnea.
      (9) Crackles, wheezes, and/or decreased breath sounds.

(10) Abnormal PFTs showing an obstructive pattern, restrictive pattern or both.
(11) CXR shows increased markings, findings of bronchiectasis, and/or pneumonitis.

4. **Bronchiectasis.**
   a. A chronic congenital or acquired disease characterized by abnormal dilatation of the bronchi and excessive sputum production.
   b. Pertinent physical findings.
      (1) Cough and expectoration of large amounts of mucopurulent secretions.
      (2) Frequent secondary infections.
      (3) Hemoptysis.
      (4) Crackles, decreased breath sounds.
      (5) Cyanosis.
      (6) Clubbing.
      (7) Hypoxemia.
      (8) Dyspnea.
      (9) CXR shows increased bronchial markings with interstitial changes. Bronchograms can outline bronchial dilatation, but are rarely needed.

5. **Respiratory distress syndrome (RDS).** Formerly known as hyaline membrane disease.
   a. Alveolar collapse in a premature infant resulting from lung immaturity, inadequate level of pulmonary surfactant.
   b. Pertinent physical findings within a few hours of birth.
      (1) Respiratory distress.
      (2) Crackles.
      (3) Tachypnea.
      (4) Hypoxemia.
      (5) Cyanosis.
      (6) Accessory muscle use.
      (7) Expiratory grunting, flaring nares.
      (8) CXR shows a classic granular pattern ("ground glass") caused by distended terminal airways and alveolar collapse.
   c. Physical therapy considerations: Increased breathing effort caused by handling a premature infant must be carefully weighed against possible benefits of physical therapy.

6. **Bronchopulmonary dysplasia.**
   a. An obstructive pulmonary disease, often a sequela of premature infants with respiratory distress syndrome; results from high pressures of mechanical ventilation, high fractions of inspired oxygen (FiO_2), and/or infection. Lungs show areas of pulmonary immaturity and dysfunction due to hyperinflation.
   b. Pertinent physical findings.
      (1) Hypoxemia, hypercapnea.
      (2) Crackles, wheezing, and/or decreased breath sounds.
      (3) Increased bronchial secretions.
      (4) Hyperinflation.
      (5) Frequent lower respiratory infections.
      (6) Delayed growth and development.
      (7) Cor pulmonale.
      (8) CXR shows hyperinflation, low diaphragms, atelectasis, and/or cystic changes.

Chronic Restrictive Diseases

1. **Different etiologies.**
   a. Typified by difficulty expanding the lungs, causing a reduction in lung volumes.

2. **Restrictive disease due to alterations in lung parenchyma and pleura.**
   a. Fibrotic changes within the pulmonary parenchyma or pleura due to idiopathic pulmonary fibrosis, asbestosis, radiation pneumonitis, oxygen toxicity.
   b. Pertinent physical findings.
      (1) Dyspnea.
      (2) Hypoxemia, hypocapnea (hypercapnea appears with severity).
      (3) Crackles.
      (4) Clubbing.
      (5) Cyanosis.
      (6) PFTs reveal a reduction in vital capacity, functional residual capacity, and total lung capacity.
      (7) CXR show reduced lung volumes, diffuse interstitial infiltrates, and/or pleural thickening.

3. **Restrictive disease due to alterations in the chest wall.**
   a. Restricted motion of bony thorax, with diseases such as ankylosing spondylitis, arthritis, scoliosis, pectus excavatum, arthrogryposis, or the integumentary changes of the chest wall such as thoracic burns or scleroderma.
   b. Pertinent physical findings.
      (1) Shallow, rapid breathing.
      (2) Dyspnea.
      (3) Hypoxemia, hypocapnea (hypercapnea with increasing severity).
      (4) Cyanosis.
      (5) Clubbing.
      (6) Crackles.
      (7) Reduced cough effectiveness.
      (8) PFTs show reduced vital capacity, functional residual capacity, and total lung capacity.
      (9) CXR show reduced lung volumes, atelectasis.

4. **Restrictive disease due to alterations in the neuromuscular apparatus.**
   a. Decreased muscular strength results in an inability to expand the rib cage, seen in disease states such as multiple sclerosis, muscular dystrophy, Parkinson's disease, spinal cord injury, or cerebrovascular accident (CVA).
   b. Pertinent physical findings.

(1) Dyspnea.
(2) Hypoxemia, hypocapnea (hypercapnea with increasing severity).
(3) Decreased breath sounds, crackles.
(4) Clubbing.
(5) Cyanosis.
(6) Reduced cough effectiveness.
(7) PFTs show reduced vital capacity and total lung capacity.
(8) CXR show reduced lung volumes, atelectasis.

Bronchogenic Carcinoma

1. A tumor that arises from the bronchial mucosa.

2. Characteristics.
   a. Smoking and occupational exposures are the most frequent causal agents.
   b. Cell types: small cell carcinoma (oat cell) and non–small cell carcinoma (squamous cell, adenocarcinoma, and large cell undifferentiated).
   c. Secondary changes due to the tumor: obstruction or compression of an airway, blood vessel, or nerve.
   d. Local metastases in the pleura, chest wall, mediastinal structures. Common distant metastases in lymph nodes, liver, bone, brain, and adrenals.

3. Pertinent physical findings with pulmonary involvement.
   a. Unexplained weight loss.
   b. Hemoptysis.
   c. Dyspnea.
   d. Weakness.
   e. Fatigue.
   f. Wheezing.
   g. Pneumonia with productive cough due to airway compression.
   h. Hoarseness with compression of the laryngeal nerve.
   i. Atelectasis or bacterial pneumonia with nonproductive cough due to airway obstruction.

4. Management of bronchogenic cancer.
   a. Chemotherapy.
   b. Radiation therapy.
   c. Surgical resection if possible.

5. Physical therapy considerations.
   a. Pneumonias that develop behind a completely obstructed bronchus cannot be cleared with physical therapy techniques. Hold treatment until palliative therapy reduces = tumor size and relieves bronchial obstruction.
   b. Possible fractures from thoracic bone metastasis with chest compressive maneuvers and coughing.
   c. Ecchymosis (bruising) in patients with low platelet count.
   d. Fatigue that restricts necessary activities.

Trauma

1. Rib fracture, flail chest.
   a. Fracture of the ribs, usually due to blunt trauma. Flail chest is two or more fractures in two or more adjacent ribs.
   b. Pertinent physical findings.
      (1) Shallow breathing.
      (2) Splinting due to pain (especially with deep inspiration or cough).
      (3) Crepitation may be felt during the ventilatory cycle over fracture site.
      (4) Paradoxical movement of a flail section during the ventilatory cycle (inspiration, the flail section is pulled inward; exhalation, the flail moves outward).
      (5) Confirmation by chest x-ray.

2. Pleural injury.
   a. Pneumothorax.
      (1) Air in the pleural space, usually through a lacerated visceral pleura from a rib fracture or ruptured bullae.
      (2) Pertinent physical findings all increase with severity of injury.
         (a) Chest pain.
         (b) Dyspnea.
         (c) Tracheal and mediastinal shift away from injured side.
         (d) Absent or decreased breath sounds.
         (e) Increased tympany with mediate percussion.
         (f) Cyanosis.
         (g) Respiratory distress.
         (h) Confirmation by CXR.
   b. Hemothorax.
      (1) Blood in the pleural space, usually from a laceration of the parietal pleura.
      (2) Pertinent physical findings increase with severity of injury.
         (a) Chest pain.
         (b) Dyspnea.
         (c) Tracheal and mediastinal shift away from side of injury.
         (d) Absent or decreased breath sounds.
         (e) Cyanosis.
         (f) Respiratory distress.
         (g) Confirmation by CXR.
         (h) Possible signs of blood loss.

3. Lung contusion.
   a. Blood and edema within the alveoli and interstitial space due to blunt chest trauma with or without rib fractures.
   b. Pertinent physical findings increase with severity of injury.

(1) Cough with hemoptysis.
(2) Dyspnea.
(3) Decreased breath sounds and/or crackles.
(4) Cyanosis.
(5) Confirmation by CXR of ill-defined patchy densities.

Other Pulmonary Conditions

1. **Pulmonary edema.**
   a. Excessive seepage of fluid from the pulmonary vascular system into the interstitial space; may eventually cause alveolar edema.
      (1) Cardiogenic: results from increased pressure in pulmonary capillaries associated with left ventricular failure, aortic valvular disease, or mitral valvular disease.
      (2) Non-cardiogenic: results from increased permeability of the alveolar capillary membranes due to inhalation of toxic fumes, hypervolemia, narcotic overdose, or adult respiratory distress syndrome (ARDS).
   b. Pertinent physical findings.
      (1) Crackles.
      (2) Tachypnea.
      (3) Dyspnea.
      (4) Hypoxemia.
      (5) Peripheral edema if cardiogenic.
      (6) Cough with pink, frothy secretions.
      (7) CXR shows increased vascular markings, hazy opacities in gravity-dependent areas of the lung in a typical butterfly pattern. Atelectasis is possible if the surfactant lining is removed by alveolar edema.
2. **Pulmonary emboli.**
   a. A thrombus from the peripheral venous circulation becomes embolic and lodges in the pulmonary circulation. Small emboli do not necessarily cause infarction.
   b. Pertinent physical findings without infarction.
      (1) History consistent with pulmonary emboli: deep vein thrombosis, oral contraceptives, recent abdominal or hip surgery, polycythemia, prolonged bed rest.
      (2) Sudden onset of dyspnea.
      (3) Tachycardia.
      (4) Hypoxemia.
      (5) Cyanosis.
      (6) Auscultatory findings may be normal or show crackles and decreased breath sounds.
      (7) Ventilation-perfusion scan showing perfusion defects with concomitant normal ventilation.
   c. Added pertinent physical findings consistent with pulmonary infarction.
      (1) Chest pain.
      (2) Hemoptysis.
      (3) CXR shows decreased vascular markings, high diaphragm, pulmonary infiltrate, and/ or pleural effusion.
3. **Pleural effusion.**
   a. Excessive fluid between the visceral and parietal pleura, caused mainly by increased pleural permeability to proteins from inflammatory diseases (pneumonia, rheumatoid arthritis, systemic lupus), neoplastic disease, increased hydrostatic pressure within pleural space (CHF), decrease in osmotic pressure (hypoproteinemia), peritoneal fluid within the pleural space (ascites, cirrhosis) or interference of pleural reabsorption from a tumor invading pleural lymphatics.
   b. Pertinent physical findings.
      (1) Decreased breath sounds over effusion; bronchial breath sounds around the perimeter. Pleural friction rub may be possible with inflammatory process.
      (2) Mediastinal shift away from large effusion.
      (3) Breathlessness with large effusions.
      (4) CXR shows fluid in the pleural space in gravity-dependent areas of the thorax if > 300 mL.
      (5) Pain and fever only if the pleural fluid is infected (empyema).
4. **Atelectasis.**
   a. Collapsed or airless alveolar unit, caused by hypoventilation secondary to pain during the ventilatory cycle (pleuritis, postoperative pain, or rib fracture), internal bronchial obstruction (aspiration, mucus plugging), external bronchial compression (tumor or enlarged lymph nodes), low tidal volumes (narcotic overdose, inappropriately low ventilator settings), or neurologic insult.
   b. Pertinent physical findings.
      (1) Decreased breath sounds.
      (2) Dyspnea.
      (3) Tachycardia.
      (4) Increased temperature.
      (5) CXR with platelike streaks.

Physical Therapy Intervention

See Table 3-4 for Preferred Cardiopulmonary Practice Patterns.

Manual Secretion Removal Techniques

1. **Postural drainage.**
   a. Placing the patient in varying positions for optimal gravity drainage of secretions and increased expansion of the involved segment (Figure 4-3).
   b. Indications for use of postural drainage.
      (1) Increased pulmonary secretions.
      (2) Aspiration.
      (3) Atelectasis or collapse.
   c. Considerations prior to use of the postural drainage positions (Table 4-5). These considerations are not intended to imply absolute danger, but rather a possible need for position modification.
   d. Procedure.
      (1) Explain procedure to the patient.
      (2) Place patient in appropriate postural drainage position.
      (3) Observe for signs of intolerance.
      (4) Duration of procedure can be up to 20 minutes per postural drainage position. Typically, duration equals the duration of other manual techniques used in conjunction with postural drainage.
2. **Percussion.**
   a. A force rhythmically applied with the therapist's cupped hands to the specific area of the chest wall that corresponds to the involved lung segment.
   b. Percussion is used to increase the amount of secretions cleared from the tracheobronchial tree; usually used in conjunction with postural drainage. Indications for use of percussion.
      (1) Excessive pulmonary secretions.
      (2) Aspiration.
      (3) Atelectasis or collapse due to mucous plugging obstructing the airways.
   c. Considerations to weigh possible benefits of percussion against possible detriments prior to the application of this technique are listed in Table 4-6. Modification of the technique may be necessary for patient tolerance.
   d. Procedure.
      (1) Explain procedure to the patient.
      (2) Place patient in the appropriate postural drainage position.
      (3) Cover the area to be percussed with a lightweight cloth to avoid erythema.
      (4) Percuss over area of thorax which corresponds to the involved lung segment. The duration of percussion depends on the patient's needs and tolerance. Three to five minutes of percussion per postural drainage position with clinically assessed improvement is a guideline.
      (5) The force of percussion causes the patient's voice to quiver.
3. **Shaking (vibration).**
   a. Following a deep inhalation, a bouncing maneuver is applied to the rib cage throughout exhalation; to hasten the removal of secretions from the tracheobronchial tree.
   b. Commonly used following percussion in the appropriate postural drainage position. Modification may be necessary for patient tolerance.
   c. Indications for the use of shaking.
      (1) Excessive pulmonary secretions.
      (2) Aspiration.

Table 4-5 ➤ CONSIDERATIONS PRIOR TO THE USE OF POSTURAL DRAINAGE

Precautions to the use of Trendelenburg position (Head of bed tipped down 15 to 18 degrees)	
Circulatory system	Pulmonary edema, congestive heart failure, hypertension.
Abdominal problems	Obesity, ascites, pregnancy, hiatal hernia, nausea and vomiting, recent food consumption.
Neurologic system	Recent neurosurgery, increased intracranial pressure, aneurysm precautions.
Pulmonary system	Shortness of breath.
Precautions to the use of sidelying position	
Circulatory system	Axillo-femoral bypass graft
Musculoskeletal system	Humeral fractures, need for hip abduction brace, other situations that make sidelying uncomfortable, e.g., arthritis, shoulder bursitis.

Table 4-6 ➤ CONSIDERATIONS PRIOR TO THE USE OF PERCUSSION AND SHAKING

General guidelines	Pain made worse by the technique.
Circulatory system	Aneurysm precautions, hemoptysis.
Coagulation disorders	Increased partial thromboplastin time (PTT), increased prothrombin time (PT), decreased platelet count (below 50,000), or medications that interfere with coagulation.
Musculoskeletal system	Fractured rib, flail chest, degenerative bone disease, bone metastases.

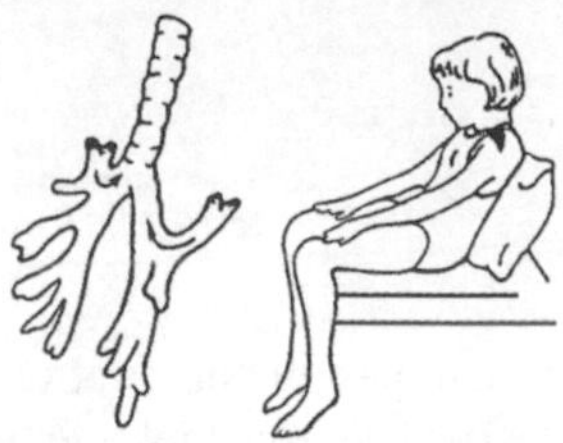

UPPER LOBES Apical Segments

Bed or drainage table flat.

Patient leans back on pillow at 30° angle against therapist.

Therapist claps with markedly cupped hand over area between clavicle and top of scapula on each side.

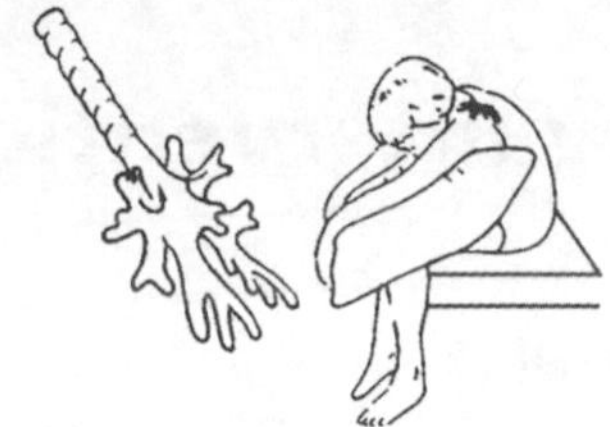

UPPER LOBES Posterior Segments

Bed or drainage table flat.

Patient leans over folded pillow at 30° angle.

Therapist stands behind and claps over upper back on both sides.

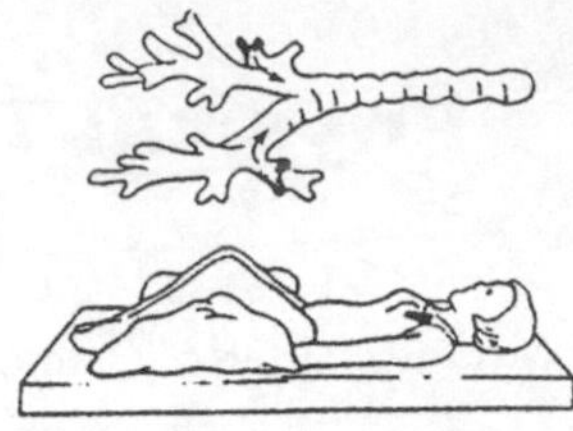

UPPER LOBES Anterior Segments

Bed or drainage table flat.

Patient lies on back with pillow under knees.

Therapist claps between clavicle and nipple on each side.

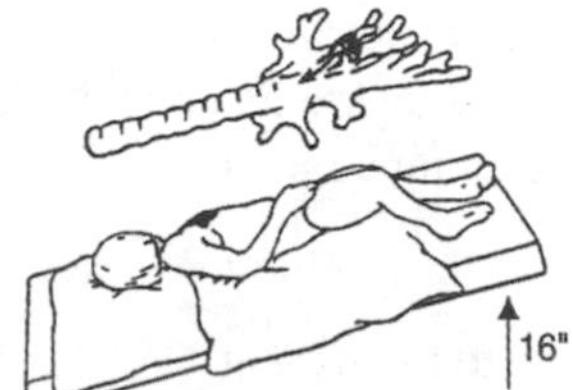

RIGHT MIDDLE LOBE

Foot of table or bed elevated 16 inches.

Patient lies head down on left side and rotates ¼ turn backward. Pillow may be placed behind from shoulder to hip. Knees should be flexed.

Therapist claps over right nipple area. In females with breast development or tenderness, use cupped hand with heel of hand under armpit and fingers extending forward beneath the breast.

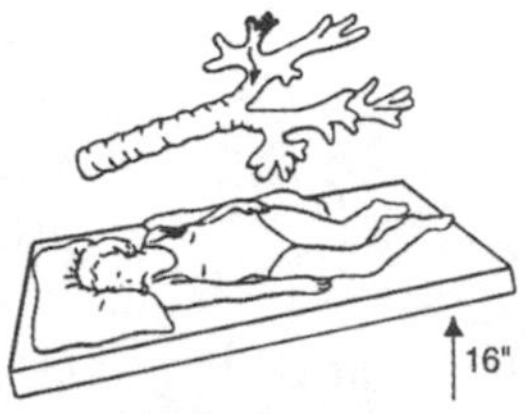

LEFT UPPER LOBE Lingular Segments

Foot of table or bed elevated 16 inches.

Patient lies head down on right side and rotates 1/4 turn backward. Pillow may be placed behind from shoulder to hip. Knees should be flexed.

Therapist claps with moderately cupped hand over left nipple area. In females with breast development or tenderness, use cupped hand with heel of hand under armpit and fingers extending forward beneath the breast.

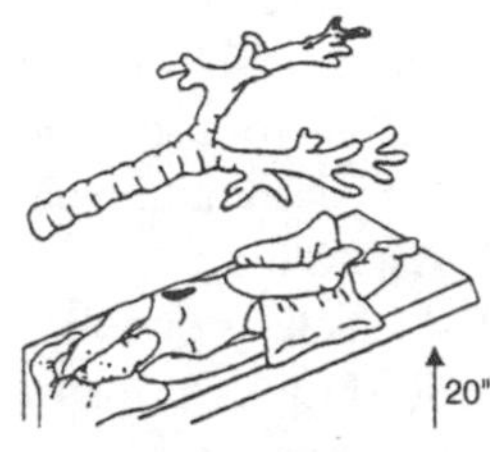

LOWER LOBE Anterior Basal Segments

Foot of table or bed elevated 20 inches.

Patient lies on side, head down, pillow under knees.

Therapist claps with slightly cupped hand over lower ribs. (Position shown is for drainage of **left** anterior basal segment. To drain the right anterior basal segment, patient should lie on his left side in same posture).

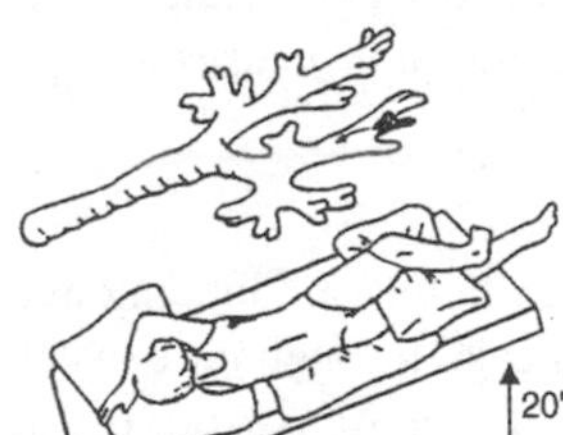

LOWER LOBES Lateral Basal Segments

Foot of table or bed elevated 20 inches.

Patient lies on abdomen, head down, then rotates ¼ turn upward. Upper leg is flexed over a pillow for support.

Therapist claps over uppermost portion of lower ribs. (Position shown is for drainage of right lateral basal segment. To drain the left lateral basal segment, patient should lie on his right side in the same posture).

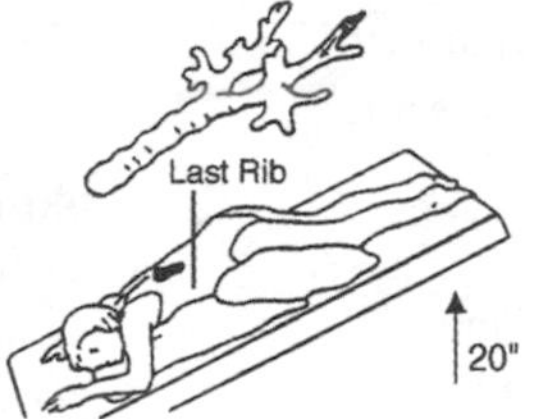

LOWER LOBES Posterior Basal Segments

Foot of table or bed elevated 20 inches.

Patient lies on abdomen, head down, with pillow under hips. Therapist claps over lower ribs close to spine on each side.

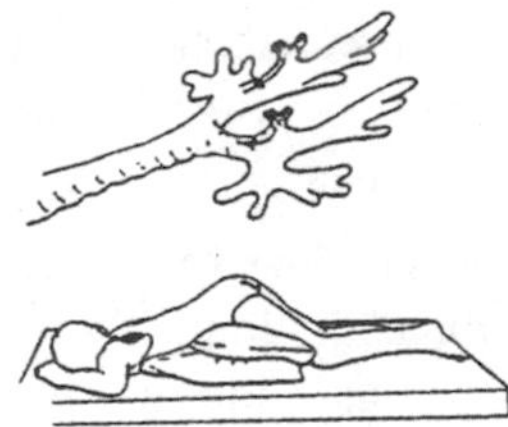

LOWER LOBES Superior Segments

Bed or table flat.

Patient lies on abdomen with two pillows under hips.

Therapist claps over middle of back at tip of scapula on either side of spine.

Figure 4-3 • Positions used for postural drainage.
From: Rothstein J, Roy S, and Wolf S: The Rehabilitation Specialist's Handbook, 2nd ed. Davis, Philadelphia, 1998, p 534–535, with permission.

(3) Atelectasis or collapse of an airway from mucous plugging.

d. Considerations prior to the application of shaking are similar to those of percussion (see Table 4-6).

e. Procedure.
   (1) Explain procedure to the patient.
   (2) Place patient in appropriate postural drainage position.
   (3) Perform percussion if appropriate.
   (4) As patient inhales deeply, the therapist's hands are placed with fingers parallel to the ribs.
   (5) As patient exhales, the therapist's hands provide a jarring, bouncing motion to the rib cage below.
   (6) The duration of shaking depends on the patient's needs, tolerance, and clinical improvement. Five to 10 deep inhalations with the shaking technique is generally acceptable practice. Any more than 10 would risk hyperventilation (increased V_E resulting in decreased $PaCO_2$), and less than 5 may be ineffective.

4. Airway clearance techniques.

a. Cough: patient should be asked to cough in the upright sitting position, if possible, after each area of lung has been treated. Coughing clears secretions from the major central airways.

b. Huffing: more effective in patients with collapsible airways, (e.g., chronic obstructive diseases) prevents the high intrathoracic pressure that causes premature airway closure.
   (1) Ask patient to inhale deeply.
   (2) Immediately, the patient forcibly expels the air, saying "Ha, ha."

c. Assisted cough: the therapist's hand(s) or fist become the force behind the patient's exhaled air. Used when the patient's abdominal muscles cannot generate an effective cough (e.g., spinal cord injury). The amount of force by the therapist depends on patient tolerance and abdominal sensation.
   (1) Position the patient against a solid surface; supine with head of bed flat or in a Trendelenburg position, or sitting with wheelchair against the wall or against the therapist.
   (2) The therapist's hand is placed below the patient's subcostal angle (similar to hand placement for the Heimlich maneuver).
   (3) Patient inhales deeply.
   (4) As the patient attempts to cough, the therapist's hand pushes inward and upward, assisting the rapid exhalation of air.
   (5) Any secretions raised should be removed by a suction catheter if expectoration is problematic.

d. Tracheal stimulation: used with patients who are unable to cough on command, such as infants or patients with brain injury or stroke.
   (1) The therapist's finger or thumb is placed just above the suprasternal notch, and a quick inward and downward pressure on the trachea elicits the cough reflex.

e. Endotracheal suctioning: used only when the above airway clearance techniques fail to adequately remove secretions.
   (1) Standard precautions are employed, since contact with a patient's body fluid is expected.
   (2) Equipment: suction catheters come in sizes of 14 French gauge (Fr), usually for an adult, 10 Fr for older children, 8 and 5–6 Fr for young children and infants. Suction system set at approximately 120 mm Hg of suction. Sterile glove/clean glove.
   (3) Procedure: a catheter is fed through either an artificial airway, oral airway, or the nares through the pharynx, larynx to the carina. When resistance is felt at the carina, the catheter is rotated and withdrawn. Suction is applied intermittently so as not to damage the inner lining of the trachea. The usual suctioning time is 10 to 15 seconds.
   (4) Complications associated with suctioning: hypoxemia, bradycardia or tachycardia, hypotension or hypertension, increased intracranial pressure, atelectasis, tracheal damage, infections.

CHAPTER 4

Independent Secretion Removal Techniques

1. Active cycle of breathing.

a. An independent program to assist in the removal of more peripheral secretions that coughing may not clear.

b. Breathe in a controlled, diaphragmatic fashion.

c. Perform thoracic expansion exercises with or without percussion and shaking. These are deep inhalations with a hold at the top, if possible.

d. Controlled, diaphragmatic breathing. The patient decides what is needed next. If no secretions seem to be mobilized the patient returns to step b, then c, and reassesses his or her situation. If the patient believes secretions can be cleared, the patient moves on to steps d, e, and f.

e. Inhale at a resting tidal volume. Contract the abdominal muscles to produce one or two forced expiratory huffs from mid to low lung volume to raise secretions.

f. Huff from high lung volume or cough to clear.

g. Controlled diaphragmatic breathing.

h. Repeat these cycles until secretions are in large airways.

2. Autogenic drainage.

a. An independent program used to sense peripheral secretions and clear them without the tracheobronchial irritation from coughing.

b. Amount of time spent in each of the following phases is determined by where the patient feels the secretions.
   (1) Unstick phase: quiet breathing at low lung volumes to affect peripheral secretions.
   (2) Collect phase: breathing at mid lung volumes to affect secretions in the middle airways.
   (3) Evacuation phase: breathing from mid to high lung volumes to clear secretions from central airways; replaces coughing as the means to clear secretions.
   (4) Repeat the steps corresponding to the area of retained secretions until all secretions are removed from the airways.

3. **FLUTTER or Acapella device.**
   a. The patient uses an external device that vibrates the airways on exhalation to improve airway clearance with intermittent, positive expiratory pressure.
   b. Patient breathes in a normal tidal volume through the nose or around the mouthpiece of the flutter device.
   c. Patient then exhales through the device, setting up a vibration within the airways. Experimentation in the tipped position of the device may provide the most vibration possible with exhalation.
   d. Repeat between 5 and 10 times.
   e. Patient then breathes in a full inhalation through the nose or around the mouthpiece.
   f. This is followed by a 3-second hold at the top of inhalation and rapid, forced exhalations through the FLUTTER device.
   g. Repeat 2 or 3 times.
   h. Huff or cough to clear secretions.
   i. Repeat steps a–g until all secretions are removed from the airways.

4. **Low-pressure positive expiratory pressure (PEP) mask.**
   a. The patient uses positive expiratory resistance via face mask to help remove airway secretions. Low-pressure PEP measures 10–20 cm H_2O.
   b. Seated patient breathes at tidal volumes with mask in place.
   c. After approximately 10 breaths, the mask is removed for coughing or huffing to clear secretions.
   d. The sequence is repeated until all secretions are removed from the airways.

5. **High-pressure positive expiratory pressure (PEP) mask.**
   a. The patient with an unstable airway uses high expiratory pressures via face mask to assist in the removal of airway secretions. High pressure PEP uses the point of PEP between 50 and 120 cm H_2O, where the patient is able to exhale a larger FVC with the mask than without.
   b. Seated patient breathes at tidal volumes with mask in place.
   c. After approximately 10 breaths, huffing from high to low lung volumes is performed with the mask in place.
   d. The sequence is repeated until all secretions are removed from the airways.

Breathing Exercises

1. **Diaphragmatic breathing.**
   a. Used to increase ventilation, improve gas exchange, decrease work of breathing, facilitate relaxation, and maintain or improve mobility of chest wall.
   b. Used with postoperative patients, posttrauma patients, and patient's with obstructive or restrictive pulmonary lung diseases.
   c. Procedure.
      (1) Explain procedure to patient.
      (2) Position patient in semireclined (e.g., semi-Fowler's position).
      (3) Place therapist's hand gently over subcostal angle of the thorax.
      (4) Apply gentle pressure throughout the exhalation phase.
      (5) Increase to firm pressure at end of exhalation.
      (6) Ask patient to inhale against resistance of the therapist's hand.
      (7) Release pressure, allowing a full inhalation.
      (8) Progress to independence of therapist's hand, in upright sitting, standing, walking, and stair climbing.

2. **Segmental breathing.**
   a. Used to improve ventilation to hypoventilated lung segments, alter regional distribution of gas, maintain or restore functional residual capacity, maintain or improve mobility of chest wall, and prevent pulmonary compromise.
   b. Used for patients with pleuritic, incisional, or post-trauma pain that causes decreased movement in a portion of the thorax (splinting), and those at risk of developing atelectasis.
   c. Inappropriate for intractable hypoventilation until medical situation is resolved; palliative therapy to reduce bronchogenic tumor size or chest tube to reduce a pneumothorax.
   d. Procedure.
      (1) Explain procedure to patient.
      (2) Position patient to facilitate inhalation to a certain segment, such as postural drainage positions, upright sitting.
      (3) Apply gentle pressure to the thorax over area of hypoventilation during exhalation.
      (4) Increase to firm pressure just prior to inspiration.

(5) Ask patient to breathe in against the resistance of therapist's hands.
(6) Release resistance, allowing a full inhalation.

3. Sustained maximal inspiration (SMI).

a. Used to increase inhaled volume, sustain or improve alveolar inflation, maintain or restore functional residual capacity.

b. Used in acute situations; e.g., patients with post-trauma pain, postoperative pain, acute lobar collapse.

c. Procedure.
(1) Inspire slowly through nose or pursed lips to maximal inspiration.
(2) Hold maximal inspiration for 3 seconds.
(3) Passively exhale the volume.
(4) Incentive spirometers (devices used to measure and encourage deep inspiration) can help patient in achieve maximal inspiration during SMI.

4. Pursed lip breathing.

a. Used to reduce respiratory rate, increase tidal volume, reduce dyspnea, decrease mechanical disadvantages of impaired ventilatory pump, improve gas mixing at rest for patients with COPD, and facilitate relaxation.

b. Primarily used for patients with obstructive disease who experience dyspnea at rest or with minimal activity/exercise, or with ineffective breathing patterns during activity/exercise.

c. Procedure.
(1) Slowly inhale through nose or mouth.
(2) Passively exhale through pursed lips (position mouth as if blowing out candles).
(3) Additional hand pressure from the therapist applied to abdomen can gently prolong expiration.
(4) Abdominal muscle contraction can be used judiciously to increase exhaled volume. Care must be taken not to increase intrathoracic pressure, which may cause airway collapse.

5. Abdominal strengthening.

a. Used when abdominal muscles are too weak to provide an effective cough. Abdominal splinting: used when the abdominal muscles cannot provide the necessary support needed for passive exhalation, e.g., in high thoracic and cervical spinal cord injuries. It is important to ensure that the binder does not restrict inspiration.

b. Glossopharyngeal breathing (air gulping) can also be taught to assist coughing.

Postsurgical Care

1. Postoperative physical therapy sessions.

a. Decrease the number and severity of pulmonary complications.

b. Prevent postoperative pulmonary complications.
(1) Remove residual secretions.
(2) Improve aeration.
(3) Gradually increase activity.
(4) Return to baseline pulmonary functioning.

c. Pertinent physical findings of postoperative pulmonary complications.
(1) Increased temperature.
(2) Increase in white blood cell count.
(3) Change in breath sounds from the preoperative evaluation.
(4) Abnormal chest x-ray.
(5) Decreased expansion of the thorax.
(6) Shortness of breath.
(7) Change in cough and sputum production.

d. Physical therapy considerations.
(1) Determine need for pain management.
(2) Choose appropriate intervention based on patient's needs.
(a) Secretion removal techniques.
(b) Breathing exercises to improve aeration, incentive spirometry.
(c) Early mobilization.

Activities for Increasing Functional Abilities

1. General conditioning.

a. A prescription for exercise can be written to improve cardiopulmonary fitness based on results of exercise tolerance test. (See Chapter 3 for discussion).

b. Mode. Any aerobic activity that allows a graded workload; usually, a circuit program of multiple activities (e.g., bike, walking, arm ergometry) since patients with pulmonary disease may be deconditioned. Patient preference should be considered.

c. Intensity. Patients with mild or moderate lung disease will likely reach their cardiovascular endpoint with an exercise test. Using the test data in Karvonen's formula ([maximum heart rate – resting heart rate] [40%–85%] + resting heart rate) results in safe range for exercise intensity. Patients with severe and very severe pulmonary disorders will likely reach a pulmonary endpoint before a cardiovascular end point. Intensity for these patients should be at or near maximum heart rate. Ratings of Perceived Exertion scale is used to monitor exercise intensity.

d. Duration. With high-intensity exercise, the patient may need an intermittent exercise program with rest periods for tolerance. Progression is directed first toward a duration of 20–30 minutes of continuous exercise before an increase in intensity is considered.

e. Frequency. The goal is 20–30 minutes of exercise three to five times per week. With durations of less than 20–30 minutes, exercise should occur more frequently (five to seven times per week).

2. Inspiratory muscle trainer (IMTs).

a. Used to load muscles of inspiration by breathing through a series of graded aperture openings. By increasing strength and endurance of muscles of ventilation, the patient will develop more efficient ventilatory muscles, less effort in breathing, and decreased possibility of respiratory muscle fatigue. However, evidence is inconclusive for improved functional ability. Whether or not this translates into improved functional abilities has been cause for debate, and has yet to be conclusively proven.

b. IMT is appropriate for patients with decreased compliance, decreased intrathoracic volume, resistance to airflow, alteration in length tension relationship of ventilatory muscles, decreased strength of the respiratory muscles.

c. Procedure.

(1) Explain procedure to patient with emphasis on maintenance of respiratory rate and tidal volume during training sessions.

(2) Determine maximum inspiratory pressure (MIP).

(3) Choose an aperture opening that requires 30%–50% of MIP (intensity) and allows 10–15 minutes of training per session.

(4) Ask patient to inhale through device while maintaining their usual respiratory rate and tidal volume for at least 10–15 minutes.

(5) Progression initially focuses on increasing duration to 30 minutes, then increasing intensity with smaller apertures.

3. Paced breathing (activity pacing).

a. Used to spread out the metabolic demands of an activity over time by slowing its performance.

b. Indications: patients who become dyspneic during the performance of an activity or exercise.

c. Procedure.

(1) Break down any activity into manageable components that can be performed within the patient's pulmonary system's abilities.

(2) Inhale at rest.

(3) Upon exhalation with pursed lips, complete the first component of the desired activity.

(4) Stop the activity and inhale at rest.

(5) Upon exhalation with pursed lips, complete next component of activity.

(6) Repeat steps (4) and (5) until activity is accomplished in full without shortness of breath. For example, stair climbing can be done by ascending one or more stairs on exhalation, and then resting, inhaling at rest, then more stairs on exhalation, and so on.

4. Energy conservation.

a. The energy consumption of many activities of daily living can be decreased with some careful thought and planning, making seemingly impossible tasks possible.

b. For example, showering is difficult for the patient with pulmonary disease, given the activity and the hot, humid environment. With a shower seat, hand-held shower, and use of a terry cloth robe after showering, the patient does not have to stand, hold his or her breath as often, or dry off in the humid environment, thus reducing the energy cost of the activity.

Medical and Surgical Management of Pulmonary Disease

Surgical Management

1. Types of surgeries to remove diseased lung portions.

a. Pneumonectomy: removal of a lung.

b. Lobectomy: removal of a lobe of a lung.

c. Segmental resection: removal of a segment of a lobe.

d. Wedge resection: removal of a portion of a lung without anatomical divisions.

e. Lung volume reduction surgery (LVRS), or pneumectomy, removes large emphysematous, nonfunctioning areas of the lung to normalize thoracic mobility and improve gas exchange of the remaining lung.

2. Types of incisions.

a. Midsternotomy: sternum is cut in half lengthwise and rib cage is retracted; used in most heart surgeries. The sternum is wired together at the close of surgery; therefore, physical therapy should encourage full upper-extremity range of motion postoperatively.

b. Thoracotomy; used for most lung resections; incision follows the path of the fourth intercostal space; full range of motion should be encouraged postoperatively.

Medical Management

1. Rescue drugs.

a. Used for immediate relief of break-through symptoms of tightness, wheezing, and shortness of breath.

b. Short-acting beta-2 agonists (sympathomimetics): mimic the activity of the sympathetic nervous system that produce bronchodilation; can increase heart rate and blood pressure.

c. Given topically through a metered-dose inhaler (MDI), unwanted systemic effects are reduced. Examples of rescue beta-2 agonists are Ventolin (albuterol), Alupent (metaproterenol), Maxair (pirbuterol).

2. **Maintenance drugs.**
   a. Taken on a regular schedule to maintain optimal airway diameter.
   b. Long-acting beta-2 agonists (sympathomimetics): Mimic activity of sympathetic nervous system, allowing for bronchodilation; may decrease need for rescue drugs and inhaled anti-inflammatories. An example of this type of beta-2 maintenance drug is Serevent (salmeterol xinafoate).
   c. Anticholinergics: inhibit the parasympathetic nervous system; increase heart rate, blood pressure, and bronchodilation. Side effects can include lack of sweating, dry mouth, and delusions. Administered by MDI with minimal side effects. Should be used on a regular schedule to maintain bronchodilation. An example of this category of drug is Atrovent (ipratropium).
   d. Methylxanthines: produce smooth muscle relaxation, but use is limited due to serious toxicity, increased blood pressure, increased heart rate, arrhythmias, gastrointestinal distress, nervousness, headache, and seizures. Blood levels should be drawn to ensure medication effect without toxicity. Examples are aminophylline and theophylline.
   e. Leukotriene receptor antagonists: block leukotrienes released in allergic reactions. Inhibit airway edema and smooth muscle contraction; additive benefits when used in conjunction with other anti-inflammatories. An example of this drug is montelukast (Singulair).
   f. Cromolyn sodium: antiallergic drug; prevents release of mast cells (i.e., histamine) after contact with allergens; used prophylactically to prevent exercise-induced bronchospasm and severe bronchial asthma via oral inhalation. Not to be used as a rescue drug during acute situations. Frequent inhalation can result in hoarseness, cough, dry mouth, and bronchial irritation. Symptoms of overdosage include paradoxical bronchospasm. Brand names include Intal.
   g. Anti-inflammatory agents: used to decrease mucosal edema, inflammation, and airway reactivity. Steroids can be administered systemically or topically (MDI). Side effects of systemic administration: increased blood pressure, sodium retention, muscle wasting, osteoporosis, GI irritation, and hypercholesteremia. The main side effect of inhaled steroids is thrush, a fungal infection of the mouth and throat. Examples are Vanceril (beclomethasone, MDI), Azmacort (triamcinolone, MDI).
   h. Vaccinations. It is recommended that patients with pulmonary disorders routinely receive the influenza and the pneumonia vaccinations.

3. **Crisis drugs.**
   a. May be used in a crisis situation, such as in an emergency room. Often, drugs that might be given topically are given systemically, and potentially in larger doses. For example, anti-inflammatory agents usually administered via MDI will now be prescribed as prednisone (po) or SoluMedral (methylprednisolone, IV).
   b. Antibiotics are not recommended for maintenance, but only for treatment of infection, such as an infectious exacerbation.
      (1) Categories: culture and sensitivity results are used to prescribe the most effective antibiotic.
         (a) Penicillins.
         (b) Erythromycins.
         (c) Tetracyclines.
         (d) Cephalosporins.
         (e) Aminoglycosides.
      (2) Side effects. Include allergic reactions, stomach cramps, nausea, vomiting, and diarrhea.

Intensive Care Unit Management

1. **Physical therapy in the ICU.**
   a. Employed for pulmonary care (secretion removal or improved aeration) and early mobility (range of motion, positioning, therapeutic exercise, transfers, ambulation). The following equipment is frequently encountered when treating patients in the ICU.

2. **Mechanical ventilation.**
   a. Maintains an adequate V_E for patients who cannot do so independently.
   b. Requires intubation with an endotracheal (oral), nasotracheal (nasal) or tracheal (through a tracheostomy directly into the trachea) tube. Endotracheal and nasotracheal tubes are taped in place, while tracheal tubes may be sutured in place.
   c. Tubes or mechanical ventilation pose no contraindications to physical therapy treatment. A patient who is intubated can ambulate using a mechanical resuscitator bag to maintain ventilation. It is sometimes easier to use a stationary device, e.g., peddler, to exercise a patient who needs a ventilator.
   d. When moving a patient who is intubated, avoid placing excessive tension on the tube. Alteration in the placement of the tube (either a drop inward or a pull outward) could reduce optimal ventilation. If tube movement is suspected, a nurse or respiratory therapist should check tube placement. If the tube is dislodged, a physician, often an anaesthesiologist, should replace the tube.

3. **Chest tubes.**
   a. Used to evacuate air or fluid trapped in the intrapleural space. Chest tubes are sutured in place to make them secure.

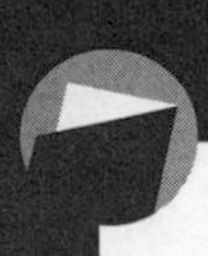

b. There are no contraindications to physical therapy treatment with a chest tube. If the chest tube is connected to a suction device, mobility is limited only by the length of the tubing. Portable suction machines can be used for increased mobility.
c. If the tube is dislodged during treatment, cover the defect and seek assistance.

4. **IVs.**
   a. Intravenous catheters used to deliver medications.
   b. There are no contraindications to physical therapy treatment with IV lines; however, the upper extremity should not be raised above the level of the IV medication for any length of time or backflow of blood may occur.
   c. Rolling IV poles allow for mobility. Most IV pumps have a battery back-up system to allow patient mobility.

5. **Arterial lines.**
   a. Catheters that are placed within the arterial system, usually the radial artery. The tubing is connected to a pressure pack that exceeds arterial pressure so the line does not back up with blood.
   b. Caution to maintain patency during moving is warranted. These lines may be capped off by nursing for a short time to allow mobility. For out-bed activity for prolonged periods, mobility is limited only by the length of the tubing.
   c. If this line becomes dislodged, immediate, firm pressure must be applied to or above the arterial insertion site to stop bleeding.

6. **Monitors/Oscilloscopes.**
   a. Continuous electrocardiogram (ECG) with a reported heart rate.
   b. Blood pressure reading, either periodic using noninvasive cuff (NIBP), or continuous using a transducer attached to the arterial line (ABP).
   c. Continuous oxygen saturation (SaO_2) with pulse wave. SaO_2 is the percent saturation of oxygen in the arterial blood. This noninvasive measurement relates to the PaO_2 on an S-shaped curve, called the oxyhemoglobin desaturation curve. Normal levels are 98%–100% saturated. The pulse oximeter utilizes a finger sensor (or an ear sensor) to obtain a consistent reading.

7. **Supplemental oxygen.**
   a. Increases the FiO_2 (up to 1) of the patient's environment. A portable oxygen cylinder attached to the oxygen delivery device (cannula, mask, or a manual resuscitator bag attached to the endotracheal tube) can be used during mobility training to provide supplemental oxygen for the patient.
   b. Supplemental oxygen is indicated if SaO_2 is $< 88\%$ or PaO_2 is < 55 mm Hg, regardless of activity level. Monitor the patient's SaO_2 to assure adequate oxygenation with increased activity.
   c. Oxygen must be prescribed by a physician, since it is considered a form of medication.

Integumentary Physical Therapy

SUSAN B. O'SULLIVAN

Integumentary System

Skin or Integument

1. **External covering of the body.** The largest organ system of the body (15%–20% of body weight).
2. **Functions of skin.**
   a. Protection of underlying body structures against injury or invasion.
   b. Insulation of body.
   c. Maintenance of homeostasis: fluid balance, regulation of body temperature.
   d. Aids in elimination: small amounts of urea and salt are excreted in sweat.
   e. Synthesizes vitamin D.
   f. Receptors in dermis give rise to cutaneous sensations.
3. **Layers of skin.** (See Table 5-1).
4. **Appendages of the skin.**
   a. Hair.
      (1) Terminal hair: coarse, thick, pigmented; e.g., scalp, eyebrows.
      (2) Vellus hair: short, fine; e.g., arms, chest
   b. Nails: nail plate, lunula (whitish moon), proximal nail fold/cuticle, lateral nail folds.
   c. Sebaceous glands: secrete fatty substance through hair follicles; on all skin surfaces except palms and soles.
   d. Sweat glands.
      (1) Eccrine glands: widely distributed, open on skin; help control body temperature.
      (2) Apocrine glands: found in axillary and genital areas, open into hair follicles; stimulated by emotional stress.

Circulation

1. **Blood flow to capillaries of the skin.**
   a. Increased blood flow with an increase in oxyhemoglobin to skin capillaries causes reddening of the skin.

Table 5-1 ➤ LAYERS OF SKIN

Epidermis	Outer, most superficial layer; contains no blood vessels Comprised of two layers of stratified epithelium: 1 Stratum corneum is outermost, horny layer, comprised of nonliving cells 2 Stratum lucidum, comprised of living cells; produces melanin responsible for skin color
Dermis (corium)	Inner layer comprised primarily of collagen and elastin fibrous connective tissues Mucopolysaccharide matrix and elastin fibers provide elasticity, strength to skin Contains lymphatics, blood vessels, nerves and nerve endings, sebaceous and sweat glands
Subcutaneous tissues	Underneath dermis Consists of loose connective and fat tissues Provides insulation, support, and cushion for skin; stores energy for skin Muscles and fascia lie underneath subcutaneous layer

b. Peripheral cyanosis is due to reduced blood flow to skin and loss of oxygen to tissues (changes to deoxyhemoglobin) and results in a darker, somewhat blue color.

c. Central cyanosis is due to reduced oxygen level in the blood; causes include advanced lung disease, congenital heart disease, and abnormal hemoglobins.

Common Skin Disorders

Dermatitis (Eczema)

1. **Inflammation.** Causes itching, redness, skin lesions.
2. Causes:
   a. Allergic or contact dermatitis; e.g., poison ivy, harsh soaps, chemicals, adhesive tape.
   b. Actinic: photosensitivity, reaction to sunlight, ultraviolet.
   c. Atopic: etiology unknown, associated with allergic, hereditary, or psychological disorders.
3. Stages.
   a. Acute: red, oozing, crusting rash; extensive erosions, exudate, pruritic vesicles.
   b. Subacute: erythematous skin, scaling, scattered plaques.
   c. Chronic: thickened skin, increased skin marking secondary to scratching; fibrotic papules, and nodules; postinflammatory pigmentation changes. Course can be relapsing.
4. **Precautions or contraindications.**
   a. Some physical therapy modalities.
   b. Avoid use of alcohol.
5. **Medical management aimed at inflammation.** Topical or systemic therapy.
6. **Daily care includes hydration and lubrication of skin.**

Bacterial Infections

1. **Enter through portals in the skin.** (E.g., abrasions or puncture wounds).
2. **Impetigo.**
   a. Superficial skin infection caused by staphylococci or streptococci.
   b. Associated with inflammation, small pus-filled vesicles, itching.
   c. Contagious; common in children and the elderly.
3. **Cellulitis.**
   a. Suppurative inflammation of cellular or connective tissue in or close to the skin.
   b. Tends to be poorly defined and widespread.
   c. Streptococcal or staphylococcal infection common; can be contagious.
   d. Skin is hot, red, and edematous.
   e. Management: antibiotics; elevation of the part; cool, wet dressings.
   f. If untreated, lymphangitis, gangrene, abscess, and sepsis can occur.
   g. The elderly and individuals with diabetes, wounds, mal-nutrition, or on steroid therapy are at increased risk.
4. Abscess.
   a. A cavity containing pus and surrounded by inflamed tissue.
   b. The result of a localized infection.
   c. Commonly a staphylococcal infection.
   d. Healing typically facilitated by draining or incising the abscess.

Viral Infections

1. **Herpes 1 (herpes simplex).**
   a. Itching and soreness, followed by vesicular eruption of the skin on the face or mouth; a cold sore or fever blister.
2. Herpes 2.
   a. Common cause of vesicular genital eruption.
   b. Spread by sexual contact.
   c. In newborns, may cause meningoencephalitis; may be fatal.
3. **Herpes zoster (shingles).**
   a. Caused by varicella-zoster virus (chickenpox); reactivation of virus lying dormant in cerebral ganglia or ganglia of posterior nerve roots.
   b. Pain and tingling affecting spinal or cranial nerve dermatome; progresses to red papules along distribution of infected nerve; red papules progressing to vesicles develop along a dermatome.
   c. Usually accompanied by fever, chills, malaise, gastrointestinal (GI) disturbances.
   d. Ocular complications with cranial nerve (CN) III involvement: eye pain, corneal damage; loss of vision with CN V involvement.

e. Postherpetic neuralgic pain: may be intermittent or constant; lasts weeks; occasionally, intractable pain lasts months or years.
f. Management: no curative agent, antiviral drugs slow progression; symptomatic treatment for itching and pain; e.g., systemic corticosteroids.
g. Contagious to individuals who have not had chickenpox.
h. Heat or ultrasound contraindicated: can increase severity of symptoms.

4. Warts.
a. Common, benign infection by human papilloma viruses (HPVs).
b. Transmission is through direct contact; autoinoculation is possible.
c. Common warts: on skin, especially hands and fingers.
d. Plantar wart: on pressure points of feet.
e. Management: cryotherapy, acids, electrodessication and curettage; over-the-counter medications.

Fungal Infections

1. Ringworm (tinea corporis).
a. Fungal infection involving the hair, skin, or nails.
b. Forms ring-shaped patches with vesicles or scales.
c. Itchy; transmission is through direct contact.
d. Treated with topical or oral antifungal drugs (e.g., griseofulvin).

2. Athlete's foot (tinea pedis).
a. Fungal infection of foot, typically between the toes.
b. Causes erythema, inflammation, pruritus, itching, and pain.
c. Treated with antifungal creams.
d. Can progress to bacterial infections, cellulitis if untreated.

3. Transmission.
a. Person-to-person or animal-to-person.
b. Observe *standard precautions.*

Parasitic Infections

1. Caused by insect and animal contacts.

2. Scabies (mites).
a. Burrow into skin, causing inflammation, itching, and possibly pruritus.
b. Treated with scabicide.

3. Lice (pediculosis).
a. A parasite that can affect head, body, genital area with bite marks, redness, and nits.
b. Treatment with special soap or shampoo.

4. Transmission.
a. Person-to-person or sexually transmitted.
b. Avoid direct contact; observe *standard precautions.*

Immune Disorders of the Skin

1. Psoriasis.
a. Chronic disease of skin characterized by erythematous plaques covered with a silvery scale; common on ears, scalp, knees, elbows, and genitalia.
b. Common complaints: itching and pain from dry, cracked lesions.
c. Variable course: exacerbations and remissions are common.
d. May be associated with psoriatic arthritis, joint pain, particularly of small distal joints.
e. Etiological factors: hereditary, associated immune disorders, certain drugs.
f. Precipitating factors: trauma, infection, pregnancy and endocrine changes; cold weather, smoking, anxiety, and stress.
g. Management: no cure; topical preparations (corticosteroids, occlusive ointments, coal tar); systemic drugs (methotrexate).
h. Physical therapy intervention: long-wave ultraviolet (UV) light; combination UV light with oral photosensitizing drugs (psoralens).

2. Lupus erythematosus.
a. Chronic, progressive inflammatory disorder of connective tissues; characteristic red rash with raised, red, scaly plaques.
b. Discoid lupus erythematosus (DLE): affects only skin; flare-ups with sun exposure; lesions can resolve or cause atrophy, permanent scarring, hypopigmentation or hyperpigmentation.
c. Systemic lupus erythematosus (SLE): chronic, systemic inflammatory disorder affecting multiple organ systems, including skin, joints, kidneys, heart, nervous system, mucous membranes; can be fatal; commonly affects young women. Symptoms can include fever, malaise, characteristic butterfly rash across bridge of nose, skin lesions, chronic fatigue, arthralgia, arthritis, skin rashes, photosensitivity, anemia, hair loss, Raynaud's phenomenon.
d. Management: no cure; topical treatment of skin lesions (corticosteroid creams); salicylates, or indomethacin with fever and joint pain; immunosuppressive agents (cytotoxic agents) with life-threatening disease.
e. Observe for side effects of corticosteroids: edema, weight gain, acne, hypertension, bruising, purplish stretch marks; long-term use of corticosteroids is associated with increased susceptibility to infection (immunosuppressed patient); osteoporosis, myopathy, tendon rupture, diabetes, gastric irritation, low potassium.

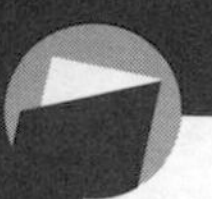

3. **Scleroderma.**
   a. Chronic, diffuse disease of connective tissues causing fibrosis of skin, joints, blood vessels, and internal organs (GI tract, lungs, heart, kidneys). Usually accompanied by Raynaud's phenomenon. Progressive systemic sclerosis (PSS) is a relatively rare autoimmune form.
   b. Skin is taut, firm, edematous, firmly bound to subcutaneous tissues.
   c. Limited disease/skin thickening: symmetrical skin involvement of distal extremities and face; slow progression of skin changes; late visceral involvement.
   d. Diffuse disease/skin thickening: symmetrical, widespread skin involvement of distal and proximal extremities, face, trunk; rapid progression of skin changes with early appearance of visceral involvement.
   e. Management: no specific therapy; supportive therapy can include corticosteroids, vasodilators, analgesics, immunosuppressive agents.
   f. Physical therapy slows development of contracture and deformity.
   g. Precautions with sclerosed skin, sensitive to pressure; acute hypertension may occur, stress regular blood pressure checks.

4. **Polymyositis (PM).**
   a. A disease of connective tissue characterized by edema, inflammation, and degeneration of the muscles; dermatitis is associated with some forms.
   b. Affects primarily proximal muscles: shoulder and pelvic girdles, neck, pharynx; symmetrical distribution.
   c. Etiology unknown; autoimmune reaction affecting muscle tissue with degeneration and regeneration, fiber atrophy; inflammatory infiltrates.
   d. Rapid, severe onset: may require ventilatory assistance, tube feeding.
   e. Cardiac involvement: may be fatal.
   f. Management: medication (corticosteroids and immunosuppressants).
   g. Precautions: additional muscle fiber damage with too much exercise; contractures and pressure ulcers from inactivity, prolonged bed rest.

Skin Cancer

1. **Benign tumors.**
   a. Seborrheic keratosis: proliferation of basal cells leading to raised lesions, typically multiple lesions on trunk of older individuals; untreated unless causing irritation, pain; can be removed with cryotherapy.
   b. Actinic keratosis: flat, round or irregular lesions, covered by dry scale on sun-exposed skin. Precancerous: can lead to squamous cell carcinoma.
   c. Common mole (benign nevus): proliferation of melanocytes, round or oval shape, sharply defined borders, uniform color, < 6 mm, flat or raised. Can change into melanoma: signs include new swelling, redness, scaling, oozing, or bleeding.

Table 5-2 ➤ CLINICAL EXAMINATION OF MALIGNANT MELANOMA "ABCDEs."

Asymmetry	Uneven edges, lopsided
Borders	Irregular, poorly defined edges, notching
Color	Variations, especially mixtures of black, blue, or red
Diameter	Larger than 6 mm.
Elevation	Usually elevated, but may be flat

2. **Malignant tumors.**
   a. Basal cell carcinoma: slow-growing epithelial basal cell tumor, characterized by raised patch with ivory appearance; has rolled border with indented center. Rarely metastasizes, common on face, in fair-skinned individuals. Associated with prolonged sun exposure.
   b. Squamous cell carcinoma: has poorly defined margins; presents as a flat red area, ulcer, or nodule. Grows more quickly, common on sun-exposed areas, face and neck, back of hand. Can be confined (in situ) or invasive to surrounding tissues; can metastasize.
   c. Malignant melanoma: tumor arising from melanocytes (cells that produce melanin); superficial spreading melanoma (SSM) most common type.
      (1) Clinical manifestations of Melanoma (Table 5-2)
      (2) Melanoma risk factors: family history, intense year-round sun exposure, fair skin and freckles, nevi that are changing or atypical, especially if > 50.
      (3) Lesions may have swelling or redness beyond the border, oozing or bleeding, or sensations of itching, burning, or pain.
      (4) Red Flags: Suspicious lesions should be referred to a dermatologist for further evaluation and biopsy. Treatment is surgical resection. Prognosis depends on extent of invasion.
   d. Kaposi's sarcoma (KS): lesions of endothelial cell origin with red or dark purple/blue macules that progress to nodules or ulcers; associated with itching and pain.
      (1) Common on lower extremities; may involve internal structures producing lymphatic obstruction.
      (2) Increased incidence in individuals of central European descent and with AIDS-associated immunodeficiency.

Skin Trauma

1. **Contusion.**
   a. Injury in which skin is not broken; a bruise.
   b. Characterized by pain, swelling, and discoloration.
   c. Immediate application of cold may limit effects.

2. **Ecchymosis.**
   a. Bluish discoloration of skin caused by extravasation of blood into the subcutaneous tissues.
   b. The result of trauma to underlying blood vessels or fragile vessel walls.

3. **Petechiae.**
   a. Tiny red or purple hemorrhagic spots on the skin.

4. **Abrasion.**
   a. Scraping away of skin due to injury or mechanical abrasion (e.g., dermabrasion).

5. **Laceration.**
   a. An irregular tear of the skin that produces a torn, jagged wound.

Examination of Integumentary Integrity

Patient/Client History

1. **Complete history.**
   a. Age, sex, race/ethnicity, social/ health habits, work, living, general health status, medical/surgical.
2. **Current condition(s)/chief complaint(s).**
3. **Functional status/activity level.**
4. **Medications.**
5. **Clinical tests.**
6. **Risk factor assessment.**

Examination of Skin

1. **Techniques.** Observation, palpation, photographic assessment, and thermography.

2. **Pruritus.**
   a. Itching.
   b. Common in diabetes, drug hypersensitivity, hyperthyroidism.

3. **Urticaria.**
   a. Smooth, red, elevated patches of skin, hives.
   b. Indicative of an allergic response to drugs or infection.

4. **Rash.**
   a. Local redness and eruption on the skin, typically accompanied by itching.
   b. Seen in inflammation, skin diseases, chronic alcoholism, vasomotor disturbances, pyrexia, medications; e.g., diaper rash, heat rash, drug rash.

5. **Xeroderma**
   a. Excessive dryness of skin with shedding of epithelium.
   b. Can indicate deficiency of thyroid function, diabetes.

6. **Edema.**
   a. Can indicate anemia, venous or lymphatic obstruction, inflammation; cardiac, circulatory, or renal decompensation.
   b. Determine activities and postures that aggravate or relieve edema.
   c. Palpation, volume, and girth measurements.

7. **Changes in nails.**
   a. Clubbing: thickened and rounded nail end with spongy proximal fold; indicative of chronic hypoxia secondary to heart disease, lung cancer, cirrhosis.
   b. White spots seen with trauma to nails.

8. **Changes in skin.** Pigmentation, tissue mobility, skin turgor and texture.
   a. Wrinkling may be due to aging or prolonged immersion in water, dehydration.
   b. Blistering.

9. **Changes in skin color.**
   a. Cherry red: indicative of carbon monoxide poisoning.
   b. Cyanosis: slightly bluish, grayish, slate-colored discoloration.
      (1) Indicative of lack of oxygen (hemoglobin); can indicate congestive heart failure, advanced lung disease, congenital heart disease, venous obstruction.
      (2) Examine lips, oral mucosa, tongue for blue color (central causes) or nails, hands, feet (peripheral causes).
   c. Pallor (lack of color, paleness).
      (1) Can indicate anemia, internal hemorrhage, lack of exposure to sunlight.
      (2) Temporary pallor seen with arterial insufficiency and syncope, chills, shock, vasomotor instability, or nervousness.
   d. Yellow: indicates jaundice, liver disease: look for yellow color in sclera of eyes, lips, skin. With increased carotene intake (carotenemia), look for yellow color of palms, soles, and face.
   e. Liver spots: brownish yellow spots may be due to aging, uterine and liver malignancies, pregnancy.

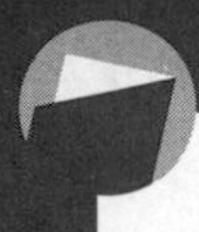

f. Brown: increased pigmentation sometimes associated with venous insufficiency.

10. Changes in skin temperature.

a. Correlate with internal temperature, unless skin is exposed to local heat or cold.

b. Examine with backs of fingers for generalized warmth or coolness.

(1) Abnormal heat can indicate febrile condition, hyperthyroidism, mental excitement, excessive salt intake.

(2) Abnormal cold can indicate poor circulation or obstruction; e.g., vasomotor spasm, venous or arterial thrombosis, hypothyroidism.

c. Examine temperature of reddened areas: local warmth may indicate inflammation or cellulitis.

11. Hydrosis.

a. Moist skin (hyperhidrosis), increased perspiration: can indicate fevers, pneumonic crisis, drugs, hot drinks, exercise.

b. Dry skin (hypohidrosis): can indicate dehydration, ichthyosis, or hypothyroidism.

c. Cold sweats: can indicate great fear, anxiety, depression or disease (AIDS).

12. Changes in hair.

a. Examine quality, texture, distribution.

b. Alopecia: hair loss.

c. Hypothyroidism sees thinning hair; hyperthyroidism sees silky hair.

13. Presence of lesions, unusual growths.

a. Determine anatomical location and distribution; i.e., generalized or localized, exposed or nonexposed surface symmetrical or asymmetrical.

b. Type.

(1) Flat spot: macule (small, up to 1 cm), patch (1 cm or greater).

(2) Palpable elevated solid mass: papule (small, up to 1cm), plaque (elevated, 1 cm or larger), nodule (marble-like lesion), wheal (irregular, localized skin edema; e.g., hives).

(3) Elevated lesions with fluid cavities: vesicle (up to 1 cm, contains serous fluid; e.g., herpes simplex); bulla or blister (1 cm or larger, contains serous fluid; e.g., second-degree burn); pustule (contains pus; e.g., acne).

c. Color.

Other Systems

1. Body Composition.

a. Height, weight.

b. Body mass index; skinfold thickness.

2. Circulation (arterial, venous, lymphatic).

a. Heart rate, rhythm, sounds.

b. Blood pressures and flow.

c. Superficial vascular responses.

3. Respiratory.

a. Respiratory rate.

b. Respiratory pattern.

4. Sensory.

a. Superficial sensations: sharp/dull discrimination, temperature, light touch, pressure.

b. Deep sensations: proprioception, kinesthesis.

c. Pain and soreness.

5. Musculoskeletal.

a. Gross range of motion (ROM) including muscle length.

b. Gross strength.

6. Neuromuscular.

a. Coordination.

b. Gait, locomotion, balance.

7. Functional.

a. Activities, positions, postures that produce or reduce trauma to skin.

b. Safety during functional activities.

c. Assistive, adaptive, protective, orthotic or prosthetic devices that produce or reduce skin trauma.

d. Likelihood of trauma to skin.

Physical Therapy Intervention for Impaired Integumentary Integrity

Interventions

1. Patient/client-related instruction.

a. Enhance disease awareness, healthy behaviors.

b. Assist patient to avoid harsh soaps, known irritants, temperature extremes, exacerbating factors or triggers.

c. Enhance activities of daily living (ADLs), functional mobility and safety.

d. Enhance self-management of symptoms.

2. Infection control practices. (See Box 6-1).

3. Therapeutic exercise.

a. Strengthening and ROM exercises.

b. Aerobic conditioning.

Table 5-3 ➤ PREFERRED PRACTICE PATTERNS: INTEGUMENTARY

PATTERN A:	Primary Prevention/Risk Reduction for Integumentary Disorders
PATTERN B:	Impaired Integumentary Integrity Associated with Superficial Skin Involvement
PATTERN C:	Impaired Integumentary Integrity Associated with Partial Thickness Skin Involvement and Scar Formation
PATTERN D:	Impaired Integumentary Integrity Associated with Full-Thickness Skin Involvement and Scar Formation
PATTERN E:	Impaired Integumentary Integrity Associated with Skin Involvement Extending into Fascia, Muscle, or Bone and Scar Formation

From: Guide to Physical Therapist Practice, ed., 2. Phys Ther 81: 595–688, 2001.

c. Body mechanics, postural awareness training.
d. Gait, locomotion, and balance training.
e. Aquatic therapy.

4. **Functional training.**
   a. ADL training (basic and instrumental).
   b. Activity pacing and energy conservation; stress management.
   c. Skin and joint protection techniques.
   d. Instruct in safe use of assistive and adaptive devices.
   e. Prescription, application, and training in use of orthotic, protective, or supportive devices.

5. **Manual lymphatic drainage, therapeutic massage.** (See Chapter 3).

6. **Dressings and topical agents.** (See Wound Care).

7. **Electrotherapeutic modalities.** (See Chapter 10).
   a. Electrical muscle stimulation (EMS).
   b. High voltage pulsed current (HVPC).
   c. Transcutaneous electrical nerve stimulation (TENS): relief of pain.

8. **Therapeutic modalities.** (See Chapter 10).
   a. Sound agents: ultrasound, phonophoresis.
   b. Hydrotherapy: aquatic therapy, whirlpool tanks.
   c. Light agents: ultraviolet.
   d. Mechanical modalities: compression therapies.

Burns

Pathophysiology

1. **Burn injury.** Results from thermal, chemical, electrical, or radioactive agents.

2. **Burn wound, consists of three zones:**
   a. Zone of coagulation: cells are irreversibly injured, cell death occurs.
   b. Zone of stasis: cells are injured; may die without specialized treatment, usually within 24-48 hours.
   c. Zone of hyperemia: minimal cell injury; cells should recover.

3. **Degree of burn.**
   a. Burns are classified by severity, layers of skin damaged (Table 5-4).
   b. Extent of burned area.
      (1) Rule of Nines for estimating burn area (estimates are for adult patients).
      - Head and neck: 9%.
      - Anterior trunk: 18%.
      - Posterior trunk: 18%.
      - Arms: 9% each.
      - Legs: 18% each.
      - Perineum: 1%.

      (2) Percentages vary by age (growth) for children: use Lund-Browder charts for estimating body areas.
   c. Classification by percentage of body area burned.
      (1) Critical: 10% of body with third-degree burns and 30% or more with second-degree burns; complications common (e.g., respiratory involvement, smoke inhalation).
      (2) Moderate: less than 10% with third-degree burns and 15–30% with second-degree burns.
      (3) Minor: less than 2% with third-degree burns and 15% with second-degree burns.

Complications of Burn Injury

1. **Infection.** Leading cause of death; gangrene may develop.

2. **Shock.**

3. **Pulmonary complications.**
   a. Smoke inhalation injury from inhalation of hot gases, smoke poisoning; results in pulmonary edema and airway obstruction; suspect with burns of the face, singed nose hairs.
   b. Restrictive lung disease from burns of the trunk.
   c. Pneumonia.

Table 5-4 ➤ BURN WOUND CLASSIFICATION

DEPTH OF BURN	CHARACTERISTICS	HEALING/SCARRING
Superficial Burn (first degree)	Damage is to epidermis only Pink or red appearance; no blistering (dry surface) Minimal edema Tenderness, delayed pain	Spontaneous healing in 3–7 days No scarring
Superficial Partial-thickness Burn	Epidermis and upper layers of dermis are damaged Bright pink or red appearance Blisters, moist surface, weeping Moderate edema Painful, sensitive to touch, temperature changes	Spontaneous healing, typically in 7–21 days Minimal scarring; discoloration
Deep Partial–thickness Burn (second degree)	Severe damage to epidermis and dermis with injury to nerve endings, hair follicles, and sweat glands Mixed red or waxy white appearance with slow capillary refill Broken blisters, wet surface Marked edema Sensitive to pressure but insensitive to light touch or soft pin prick	Healing is slow and occurs through scar formation and reepithelialization Excessive scarring without preventive treatment
Full-thickness Burn (third degree)	Complete destruction of epidermis, dermis, and subcutaneous tissues; may extend into muscle. White, gray, charred, or black appearance; no blanching; poor distal circulation Parchment-like, dry leathery surface; depressed Little pain; nerve endings are destroyed	Removal of eschar and skin grafting are necessary due to destruction of dermal and epidermal tissue Risk of infection is increased Hypertrophic scarring and wound contracture are likely to develop without preventive measures
Subdermal Burn (fourth-degree)	Complete destruction of epidermis, dermis, subcutaneous tissues with muscle damage Charred appearance Destruction of vascular system, may lead to additional necrosis. From electrical burns; prolonged contact with flame Additional complications likely with electrical burns: ventricular fibrillation, acute kidney damage, spinal cord damage	Heals with skin grafting and scarring Requires extensive surgery; amputation may be necessary.

4. **Metabolic complications.** Increased metabolic and catabolic activity results in weight loss, negative nitrogen balance, and decreased energy.
5. **Cardiac and circulatory complications.** Fluid and plasma loss results in decreased cardiac output.

Burn Healing

1. **Epidermal healing.** Retention of viable cells allows for epithelialization to occur (epithelial cells grow and proliferate, migrate to cover the wound).
   a. Protection of epithelial cells is critical.
   b. Loss of sebaceous glands can result in drying and cracking of wound; protection with moisturizing creams important.
2. **Dermal healing.**
   a. Results in scar formation (injured tissue is replaced by connective tissue).
   b. Scars are initially red or purple, later become white.
3. **Phases.**
   a. Inflammatory phase: characterized by redness, edema, warmth, pain, decreased range of motion; lasts 3–5 days.
   b. Proliferative phase: fibroblasts form scar tissue (deeper tissues); characterized by wound contraction; reepithelialization may occur at wound surface if viable cells remain.
   c. Maturation phase: scar tissue remodeling lasts up to 2 years.
      (1) Hypertrophic scar may result: a raised scar that stays within the boundaries of the burn wound and is characteristically red, raised, firm.
      (2) Keloid scar may result: a raised scar that extends beyond the boundaries of the original burn wound and is red, raised, firm. More common in young women and those with dark skin.

Burn Management

1. **Emergency care.**
   a. Immersion in cold water. If less than half the body is burned and injury is immediate; cold compresses may also be used.
   b. Cover burn with sterile bandage or clean cloth; no ointments or creams.

2. **Medical management.**
   a. Asepsis and wound care.
      (1) Removal of charred clothing.
      (2) Wound cleansing.
      (3) Topical medications (antibacterial agents): can be applied without dressings (open technique); reapplied daily.
         (a) Silver nitrate: acts only on surface organisms; applied with wet dressings; requires frequent dressing changes.
         (b) Silver sulfadiazine: common topical agent.
         (c) Sulfamylon (mafenide acetate): penetrates through eschar.
      (4) Occlusive dressings (closed technique): dressings are applied on top of a topical agent.
         (a) Prevents bacterial contamination, prevents fluid loss, and protects the wound.
         (b) May additionally limit ROM.
   b. Establish and maintain airway, adequate oxygenation, and respiratory function.
   c. Monitor.
      (1) Arterial blood gases, serum electrolyte levels, urinary output, vital signs.
      (2) Gastrointestinal function: provide nutritional support.
   d. Pain relief; e.g., morphine sulfate.
   e. Prevention and control of infection.
      (1) Tetanus prophylaxis.
      (2) Antibiotics.
      (3) Isolation, sterile techniques.
   f. Fluid replacement therapy.
      (1) Prevention and control of shock.
      (2) Post shock fluid and blood replacement.
   g. Surgery.
      (1) Primary excision: surgical removal of the eschar.
      (2) Grafts: closure of the wound.
         (a) Allograft (homograft): use of other human skin; e.g., cadaver skin; temporary grafts for large burns, used until autograft is available.
         (b) Xenograft (heterograft): use of skin from other species; e.g., pigskin; a temporary graft.
         (c) Biosynthetic grafts: combination of collagen and synthetics.
         (d) Cultured skin: laboratory grown from patient's own skin.
         (e) Autograft: use of the patient's own skin.
         (f) Split-thickness graft: contains epidermis and upper layers of dermis from donor site.
         (g) Full-thickness graft: contains epidermis and dermis from donor site.
      (3) Surgical resection of scar contracture; e.g., Z-plasty (a surgical incision in the form of the letter Z used to lengthen a burn scar).

Physical Therapy Goals, Outcomes, and Interventions

1. **Burn wound care.** Infection control techniques at all times.
   a. Immersion in hydrotherapy tank.
      (1) Débridement: the excision of loose, charred, dead skin.
      (2) Wet removal of dressings.
      (3) ROM exercises, early mobilization.
      (4) Anti-infection agents are added to assist in infection control.
   b. Sharp debridement: excision of eschar using sterilized surgical instruments (forceps, scalpel, scissors).
   c. Autolytic dressings or enzyme use are other selective means to help remove eschar.

2. **Rehabilitation.** Prevent or reduce the complications of immobilization.
   a. Exercises to promote deep breathing and chest expansion; ambulation to prevent pneumonia.
   b. Positioning and splinting to prevent or correct deformities.
      (1) Anterior neck: common deformity is flexion; stress hyperextension; position with firm (plastic) cervical orthosis.
      (2) Shoulder: common deformity is adduction and internal rotation; stress abduction, flexion, and external rotation; position with an axillary splint (airplane splint).
      (3) Elbow: common deformity is flexion and pronation; stress extension and supination; position in extension with posterior arm splint.
      (4) Hand: common deformity is a claw hand (intrinsic minus position); stress wrist extension (15°), MP flexion (70°), PIP, and DIP extension, thumb abduction (intrinsic plus position); position in intrinsic plus position with resting hand splint.
      (5) Hip: common deformity is flexion and adduction; stress hip extension and abduction; position in extension, abduction, neutral rotation.
      (6) Knee: common deformity is flexion; stress extension; position in extension with posterior knee splint.
      (7) Ankle: common deformity is plantar flexion; stress dorsiflexion; position with foot-ankle in neutral with splint or plastic ankle-foot orthosis.
   c. Edema control: elevation of extremities, active ROM.
   d. Active and passive exercise to promote full ROM.
      (1) Combine with dressing changes, hydrotherapy; medication doses.
      (2) Postgrafting: discontinue exercise for 3–5 days to allow grafts to heal.
   e. Massage to help reduce scar formation; e.g., deep friction massage.
   f. Resistive and strengthening exercises to correct loss of muscle mass and strength.

g. Increase activity tolerance and cardiovascular endurance; e.g., ambulation.
h. Promote independence in ADLs, all functional mobility skills.
i. Elastic supports to help control edema; pressure garments to help prevent hypertrophic scarring or keloid formation.
j. Management of chronic pain.

3. **Provide emotional support.**

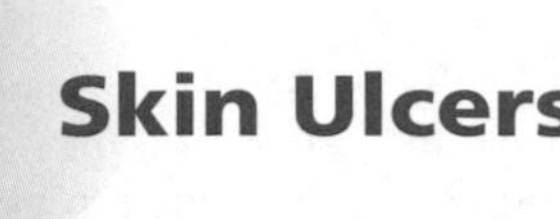

Skin Ulcers

Venous Ulcer

1. **Etiology.** Associated with chronic venous insufficiency; valvular incompetence history of deep venous thrombosis (DVT), venous hypertension.

2. **Clinical features.**
   a. Can occur anywhere in lower leg; common over area of medial malleolus, sometimes lateral.
   b. Pulses: normal.
   c. Pain: none to aching pain in dependent position.
   d. Color: normal or cyanotic in dependent position. Dark pigmentation may appear, liposclerosis (thick, tender, indurated, fibrosed tissue).
   e. Temperature: normal.
   f. Edema: present, often marked.
   g. Skin changes: pigmentation, stasis dermatitis may be present; thickening of skin as scarring develops.
   h. Ulceration: may develop, especially medial ankle; wet, with large amount of exudate.
   i. Gangrene: absent.

3. **Staging for venous, arterial, and diabetic ulcers.** Uses partial- and full-thickness classifications.

Table 5-5 ➤ DIFFERENTIAL DIAGNOSIS: ARTERIAL VERSUS VENOUS ULCERS

ULCERS	ARTERIAL	VENOUS
Etiology	Arteriosclerosis obliterans Atheroembolism	Valvular incompetance Venous hypertension
Appearance	Irregular, smooth edges Minimum to no granulation Usually deep	Irregular: dark pigmentation, sometimes fibrotic Good granulation Usually shallow
Location	Distal lower leg: toes, feet Lat. malleolus Ant. tibial area	Distal lower leg Med. malleolus
Pedal Pulses	Decreased or absent	Usually present
Pain	Painful, especially if legs elevated	Little pain, comfortable with legs elevated
Drainage		Moderate to large amounts of exudate
Associated Gangrene	May be present	Absent
Associated Signs	Trophic changes Pallor on foot elevation Dusky rubor on dependency	Edema Stasis dermatitis Possible cyanosis on dependency

Arterial Ulcer

1. **Etiology.** Associated with chronic arterial insufficiency; arteriosclerosis obliterans; atheroembolism; history of minor nonhealing trauma.

2. **Clinical features.**
   a. Can occur anywhere in lower leg; common in small toes, feet, on bony areas of trauma (shin).
   b. Preceded by signs of arterial insufficiency; pulses poor or absent.
   c. Pain: often severe, intermittent claudication, progressing to pain at rest.
   d. Color: pale on elevation; dusky rubor on dependency.
   e. Temperature: cool.
   f. Skin changes: trophic changes (thin, shiny, atrophic skin); loss of hair on foot and toes; nails thickened.
   g. Ulceration: of toes or feet; can be deep.
   h. Gangrene: black, gangrenous skin adjacent to ulcer can develop.

Diabetic Ulcer

1. **Etiology.**
   a. Diabetes is associated with arterial disease and peripheral neuropathy.
   b. Caused by repetitive trauma on insensitive skin.

2. **Clinical features.**
   a. Occurs where arterial ulcers usually appear; or where peripheral neuropathy appears (plantar aspect of foot).
   b. Pain: typically not painful; sensory loss usually present.
   c. Pulses: may be present or diminished.
   d. Absent ankle jerks with neuropathy.
   e. Sepsis common; gangrene may develop.

Pressure Ulcer (Decubitus Ulcer)

1. **Etiology.**
   a. Lesions caused by unrelieved pressure resulting in ischemic hypoxia and damage to underlying tissue.
2. **Risk factors.**
   a. Prolonged pressure, shear forces, friction, repetitive stress.
   b. Nutritional deficiency.
   c. Maceration (softening associated with excessive moisture).
   d. Common in:
      (1) Elderly, debilitated, or immobilized individuals.
      (2) Decrease blood flow from hypotension or microvascular disease: diabetes, atherosclerosis.
      (3) Neurologically impaired skin: decreased sensation.
      (4) Cognitive impairment.
3. **Clinical features.**
   a. Location: occurs over bony prominences; i.e., sacrum, heels, trochanter, lateral malleoli, ischial areas, elbows.
   b. Color: red, brown/black, or yellow.
   c. Localized infection.
   d. Pain: can be painful if sensation intact.
   e. Inflammatory response with necrotic tissue: hyperemia, fever, increased white blood cell count (WBC).
   f. If left untreated, will progress from superficial simple erosion to involvement of deep layers of skin and underlying muscle and bone.
5. **Graded by stages of severity (tissue damage).** (See Table 5-6).

Examination of Wounds

1. **Complete history, risk factor assessment.**

Table 5-6 ➤ STAGING OF PRESSURE ULCERS

STAGE	CHARACTERISTICS
Stage I	Nonblanchable erythema of intact skin. May include changes in: skin temperature (warm or cool), tissue consistency (firm or boggy), and/or sensation (pain, itching).
Stage II	Partial-thickness skin loss: involves epidermis, dermis, or both. Ulcer is superficial. Presents clinically as an abrasion, blister, or shallow crater.
Stage III	Full-thickness skin loss: involves damage to or necrosis of subcutaneous tissue. May extend down to, but not through, underlying fascia. Presents clinically as a deep crater.
Stage IV	Full-thickness skin loss: involves extensive destruction, tissue necrosis, or damage to muscle, bone, or supporting structures. Undermining and sinus tracts may be present.

From: Consortium for Spinal Cord Medicine: Pressure Ulcer Prevention and Treatment Following Spinal Cord Injury, Paralyzed Veterans of America, August 2000, with permission.

2. **Physical examination.**
   a. Determine location of wound: use anatomical landmarks.
   b. Assess size: (length, width, depth, wound area).
      (1) Use clear film grid superimposed on wound for size.
      (2) Insert sterile cotton tip applicator into deepest part of wound for depth; indicate gradations of depth from shallow to deep.
   c. Examine for tunneling (rimming or undermining): underlying tissue destruction beneath intact skin.
      (1) Evaluate for sinus tracts (communication with deeper structures); associated with unusual or irregular borders.
      (2) Sinogram (radiographic imaging studies).
   d. Determine wound exudate (drainage).
      (1) Type: serous (watery-like serum), purulent (containing pus), sanguineous (containing blood).
      (2) Amount: dry, moderate, or high exudate.
      (3) Odor.
      (4) Consistency: e.g., macerated ulcer (softened tissues due to high fluid environment).
   e. Identify color and tissues involved.
      (1) Clean red wounds: healthy granulating wounds (in need of protection); absence of necrotic tissue.
      (2) Yellow wounds: include slough (necrotic or dead tissue), fibrous tissue.
      (3) Black wounds: covered with eschar (dried necrotic tissue).
      (4) Indolent ulcer: ulcer that is slow to heal; is not painful.
      (5) Check to see if fascia, muscle, tendons, or bone involved.
   f. Determine temperature: indicative of inflammation. Use temperature probe (thermistor) to detect surface temperature.
   g. Determine girth.
      (1) Use circumferential measurements of both involved and noninvolved limbs; referenced to bony landmarks.
      (2) Use volumetric measurements: measure water displacement from filled volumeter.
   h. Examine viability of periwound tissue.
      (1) Halo of erythema, warmth, and swelling may indicate infection (cellulitis).
      (2) Maceration of surrounding tissues due to moisture (urine, feces) or wound drainage increases risk for wound deterioration and enlargement.
      (3) Trophic changes may indicate poor arterial nutrition.
      (4) Cyanosis may indicate arterial insufficiency.
   i. Determine sensory integrity, risk for trauma or pressure breakdown.
   j. Examine for signs of infection.
      (1) Bacterial culture: to identify colonization and infection; culture wound site only.
      (2) Observations, palpation.

k. Wound scar tissue characteristics: banding, pliability, texture.
l. Photographic records of wound appearance aid narrative descriptions. Use marker pen to outline wound edges on transparent dressing with a calibrated grid to provide a measuring scale.

Wound Care

1. Infection control.

a. Wounds are cultured; antibiotic treatment regimen prescribed.
  (1) Topical antimicrobial agents: e.g., silver nitrate, silver sulfadiazine, erythromycin, gentamicin, neomycin, triple antibiotic.
  (2) Anti-inflammatory agents: e.g., corticosteroids, hydrocortisone, ibuprofen, indomethacin.
  (3) Topical anesthetics and analgesics: e.g., lidocaine, lignocaine.
b. Hand washing of health care practitioners.
c. Sterile technique.
d. Vacuum-assisted closure (VAC).
  (1) An open-cell foam dressing placed into the wound.
  (2) Controlled subatmospheric pressure (typically 125 mm Hg below ambient pressure) is applied via specialized device.
  (3) Helps to control chronic edema, increases localized blood flow, and removes infectious material.

2. Surgical intervention.

a. Indicated for excising of ulcer, enhancing vascularity and resurfacing wound (grafts), and preventing sepsis and osteomyelitis.
b. May be indicated for stage III and IV ulcers.

3. Hyperbaric oxygen therapy (HBO).

a. Patient breathes 100% oxygen in a sealed, full-body chamber with elevated atmospheric pressure (between 2.0 and 2.5 atmospheres absolute, ATA).
b. Hyperoxygenation reverses tissue hypoxia and facilitates wound healing due to enhanced solubility of oxygen in the blood.
c. Contraindicated in untreated pneumothorax and some antineoplastic medications (e.g., doxorubicin, disulfiram, cisplatin, mafenide acetate).

4. Wound cleansing.

a. Removal of loose cellular debris, metabolic wastes, bacteria, and topical agents that retard wound healing.
b. Cleanse wounds initially and at each dressing change.
c. Normal saline (0.9% NaCl) recommended for most ulcers; nontoxic effects in wound.
d. Cleansing topical agents: contain surfactants that lower surface tension. Limited use, may be toxic to healing tissues; e.g., povidone-iodine solution, sodium hypochlorite solution, Dakin's solution, acetic acid solution, hydrogen peroxide.
e. Delivery systems.
  (1) Minimal mechanical force: cleansing with gauze, cloth or sponge.
  (2) Irrigation.
    (a) Using syringe, squeezable bottle with tip or battery-powered irrigation device (pulsatile lavage); loosens wound debris and removes it by suction.
    (b) Safe and effective irrigation pressures range from 4 to 15 psi.
  (3) Hydrotherapy (i.e., whirlpool).
    (a) Indicated for ulcers with large amounts of exudate, slough, and necrotic tissue.
    (b) Increases circulation; assists in debridement of wounds or removal of dressings.
    (c) Discontinue whirlpool when ulcer is clean.
f. Do not use harsh soaps, alcohol-based products, or harsh antiseptic agents; may erode skin.

5. Wound debridement.

a. Removal of necrotic or infected tissue that interferes with wound healing. (Table 5-7).
b. Allows examination of ulcer, determination of extent of wound.
c. Decreases bacterial concentration in wound; improves wound healing.
d. Decreases spread of infection; i.e., cellulitis or sepsis.

6. Wound dressings.

a. Topical products that protect the wound from contamination and trauma; permit application of medications; absorb drainage; débride necrotic tissue; and enhance healing. (Table 5-8).
b. Moisture-retentive (occlusive) wound dressings: maintain a moist environment; wound tissue fluid is maintained in contact with tissues and cells; facilitates autolytic debridement, wound healing (reepithelialization) with less pain.
  (1) Alginate dressings: e.g., Sorbsan, Kaltostat.
  (2) Transparent film dressings: e.g., Bioclusive, OpSite.
  (3) Foam dressings: e.g., LYOfoam, Flexzan.
  (4) Hydrogel dressings: e.g., Second Skin, Clearsite.
  (5) Hydrocolloid dressings: e.g., DuoDerm, Curaderm.
c. Gauze dressings.
  (1) Standard gauze (not impregnated).
  (2) Impregnated gauze: e.g., Telfa pad, Vaseline Petroleum Gauze.
d. Semirigid dressings: Unna boot is a pliable, nonstretchable dressing impregnated with ointments; e.g., zinc oxide, calamine, and gelatin.

7. Edema management.

a. Leg elevation and exercise (ankle pumps).

Table 5-7 ➤ METHODS OF PRESSURE ULCER DEBRIDEMENT

METHOD	DEFINITION	INDICATIONS	CONTRAINDICATIONS
Autolytic	A selective method of natural debridement promoted under occlusive or semiocclusive moisture-retentive dressings that results in solubilization of necrotic tissue only by phagocytic cells and by proteolytic and collagenolytic enzymes inherent in the tissues.	• Individuals on anticoagulant therapy • Individuals who cannot tolerate other forms of debridement • All necrotic wounds in people who are medically stable	• Infected wounds • Wounds of immunosupressed individuals • Dry gangrene or dry ischemic wounds
Enzymatic	A selective method of chemical debridement that promotes liquefication of necrotic tissue by applying topical preparations of proteolytic or collagenolytic enzymes to those tissues. Proteolytic enzymes help loosen and remove slough or eschar while collagenolytic enzymes digest denatured collagen in necrotic tissue.	• All moist necrotic wounds • Eschar after cross-hatching • Homebound individuals • People who cannot tolerate surgical debridement	• Ischemic wounds unless adequate vascular status has been determined • Dry gangrene • Clean, granulated wounds
Mechanical	A nonselective method of debridement that removes foreign material and devitalized or contaminated tissue by physical forces (wet-to-dry gauze dressing, dextranomers, pulsatile lavage with suction or whirlpool), and may remove healthy tissue as well.	• Wounds with moist necrotic tissue or foreign material present	• Clean, granulated wounds
Sharp	A selective method of debridement using sterile instruments (scalpel, scissors, forceps, silver nitrate stick) that sequentially removes only necrotic wound tissue without anesthesia and with little or no bleeding induced in viable tissue.	• Scoring and/or excision of leathery eschar • Excision of moist necrotic tissue	• Clean wounds • Advancing cellulitis with sepsis • When infection threatens the individual's life • Individual on anticoagulant therapy or has coagulopathy
Surgical	For deep (stage III or IV) or complicated pressure ulcer, the most efficient method of debridement. It is selective and is performed by a physician or surgeon using sterile instruments (scalpel, scissors, forceps, hemostat, silver nitrate sticks) in a one-time operative procedure. The procedure usually removes most, if not all, necrotic tissue, but may also remove some healthy tissue in what is termed wide excision. Because there may be associated pain and/or bleeding, the individual may require anesthesia, and the procedure will likely require an operating or special procedures room.	• Advancing cellulitis with sepsis • Immunocompromised individuals • When infection threatens the individual's life • Clean wounds as a preliminary procedure to surgical wound closure line. • Granulation and scar tissue may be excised	• Cardiac disease, pulmonary disease, or diabetes • Severe spasticity • Individuals who cannot tolerate surgery • Individuals with a short life expectancy • Quality of life cannot be improved

From: Consortium for Spinal Cord Medicine: Pressure Ulcer Prevention and Treatment Following Spinal Cord Injury, Paralyzed Veterans of America, August 2000, with permission.

b. Compression therapy: to facilitate movement of excess fluid from lower extremity.
   (1) Compression wraps: elastic or tubular bandages.
   (2) Paste bandages; e.g., Unna boot.
   (3) Compression stockings; e.g., Jobst.
   (4) Compression pump therapy.

8. **Electrical stimulation for wound healing.** (See Chapter 10).
   a. Uses capacitive coupled electrical current to transfer energy to a wound, improve circulation, facilitate debridement, enhance tissue repair.
   b. Continuous waveform application with direct current.
   c. High-voltage pulsed current (HVPC).
   d. Microcurrent electrical stimulation (MENS).
   e. Alternating/biphasic current.

9. **Nutritional considerations.**
   a. Delayed wound healing associated with malnutrition and poor hydration.
   b. Provide adequate hydration: eight 8-oz glasses of no caffeine fluids per day unless contraindicated.
   c. Provide adequate nutrition: frequent highcalorie/high-protein meals; energy intake (25 to 35 kcal/kg/body weight) and protein (1.5–2.5 gm/kg body weight).
   d. Patients with trauma stress and burns require higher intakes.

10. **Injury prevention or reduction.**
   a. Daily, comprehensive skin inspection, paying particular attention to bony prominences (e.g., sacrum, coccyx, trochanter, ischial tuberosities, medial or lateral malleolus).

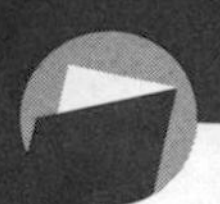

Table 5-8 ➤ CHARACTERISTICS OF SOME MAJOR DRESSING CATEGORIES

DRESSING CATEGORY AND DEFINITION	INDICATIONS	ADVANTAGES
Transparent Films Clear, adhesive, semipermeable membrane dressings. Permeable to atmospheric oxygen and moisture vapor yet impermeable to water, bacteria, and environmental contaminants.	• Stage I and II pressure ulcers • Secondary dressing in certain situations • For autolytic debridement • Skin donor sites • Cover for hydrophilic powder and paste preparations and hydrogels	• Visual evaluation of wound without removal • Impermeable to external fluids and bacteria • Transparent and comfortable • Promote autolytic debridement • Minimize friction
Hydrocolloids Adhesive wafers containing hydroactive/absorptive particles that interact with wound fluid to form a gelatinous mass over the wound bed. May be either occlusive or semi-occlusive. Available in paste form that can be used as a filler for shallow cavity wounds.	• Protection of partial-thickness wounds • Autolytic debridement of necrosis or slough • Wounds with mild exudate	• Maintain a moist wound environment • Nonadhesive to healing tissue • Conformable • Impermeable to external bacteria and contaminants • Support autolytic debridement • Minimal to moderate absorption • Waterproof • Reduce pain • Easy to apply • Time-saving • Thin forms diminish friction
Hydrogels Water- or glycerine-based gels. Insoluble in water. Available in solid sheets, amorphous gels, or impregnated gauze. Absorptive capacity varies.	• Partial- and full-thickness wounds • Wounds with necrosis and slough • Burns and tissue damaged by radiation	• Soothing and cooling • Fill dead space • Rehydrate dry wound beds • Promote autolytic debridement • Provide minimal to moderate absorption • Conform to wound bed • Transparent to translucent • Many are nonadherent • Amorphous form can be used when infection is present
Foams Semipermeable membranes that are either hydrophilic or hydrophobic. Vary in thickness, absorptive capacity, and adhesive properties	• Partial- and full-thickness wounds with minimal to moderate exudate • Secondary dressing for wounds with packing to provide additional absorption • Provide protection	• Insulate wounds • Provide some padding • Most are nonadherent • Conformable • Manage light or moderate exudate • Easy to use • Some newer products are designed for deep cavities
Alginates Soft, absorbant, nonwoven dressings derived from seaweed that have a fluffy cottonlike appearance. React with wound exudate to form a viscous hydrophilic gel mass over the wound area. Available in ropes and pads.	• Wounds with moderate to large amounts of exudate • Wounds with combination exudate and necrosis • Wounds that require packing and absorbtion • Infected and noninfected exuding wounds	• Absorb up to 20 times their weight in drainage • Fill dead space • Supports debridement in presence of exudate • Easy to apply
Gauze Dressings Made of cotton or synthetic fabric that is absorptive and permeable to water and oxygen. May be used wet, moist, dry, or impregnated with petrolatum, antiseptics, or other agents. Come in varying weaves and with different size interstices.	• Exudative wounds • Wounds with dead space, tunneling, or sinus tracts • Wounds with combination exudate or necrotic tissue WET TO DRY • Mechanical debridement of necrotic tissue and slough CONTINUOUS DRY • Heavily exudating wounds CONTINUOUS MOIST • Protection of clean wounds • Autolytic debridement of slough or eschar • Delivery of topical needs	• Readily available • Can be used with appropriate solutions such as gels, normal saline, or topical antimicrobials to keep wounds moist • Can be used on infected wounds • Good mechanical debridement if properly used • Cost-effective filler for large wounds • Effective delivery of topicals if kept moist

Table 5-8 ➤ CHARACTERISTICS OF SOME MAJOR DRESSING CATEGORIES (continued)

DISADVANTAGES	CONSIDERATIONS
Transparent Films • Nonabsorptive • Application can be difficult • Channeling or wrinkling occurs • Not to be used on wounds with fragile surrounding skin or infected wounds	• Allow 1–2 inch wound margin around bed • Shave surrounding hair • Secondary dressing not required • Dressing change varies with wound condition and location • Avoid in wounds with infection, copious drainage, or tracts
Hydrocolloids • Nontransparent • May soften and change shape with heat or friction • Odor and yellow drainage on removal (melted dressing material) • Not recommended for wounds with heavy exudate, sinus tracts, or infections; wounds that expose bone or tendon; or wounds with fragile surrounding skin • Dressing edges may curl	• Characteristic odor with yellow exudate similar to pus; normal when dressing is removed • Allow 1–1$^1/_2$ inch margin of healthy tissue around wound edges • Taping edges will help prevent curling • Frequency of changes depends on amount of exudate • Change every 3–7 days and as needed with leakage • Avoid in wounds with infection or tracts
Hydrogels • Most require a secondary dressing • Not used for heavily exudating wounds • May dry out and then adhere to wound bed • May macerate surrounding skin	• Sheet form works well on partial-thickness ulcers • Do not use sheet form on infected ulcers • Sheet form can promote growth of pseudomonas and yeast • Dressing changes every 8–48 hours • Use skin barrier wipe on surrounding intact skin to decrease risk of maceration.
Foams • Nontransparent • Nonadherent foams require secondary dressing, tape, or net to hold in place • Some newer foams have tape on edges • Poor conformability to deep wounds • Not for use with dry eschar or wounds with no exudate	• Change schedule varies from 1–5 days or as needed for leakage • Protect intact surrounding skin with skin sealant to prevent maceration
Alginates • Require secondary dressing • Not recommended for dry or lightly exudating wounds • Can dry wound bed	• May use dry gauze pad or transparent film as secondary dressing • Change schedule varies (with type of product used and amount of exudate) from every 8 hours to every 2–3 days
Gauze Dressings • Delayed healing if used improperly • Pain on removal (wet to dry) • Labor-intensive • Require secondary dressing	• Change schedule varies with amount of exudate • Pack loosely into wounds; tight packing compromises blood flow and delays wound closure • Use continuous roll of gauze for packing large wounds (ensures complete removal) • If too wet, dressings will macerate surrounding skin • Use wide mesh gauze for debridement and fine mesh gauze for protection • Protect surrounding skin with moisture barrier ointment or skin sealant as needed

From: Consortium for Spinal Cord Medicine: Pressure Ulcer Prevention and Treatment Following Spinal Cord Injury, Paralyzed Veterans of America, August 2000, with permission.

b. Therapeutic positioning to relieve pressure and allow tissue reperfusion.
   (1) In bed: turning or repositioning schedule every 2 hours during acute and rehabilitation phases.
   (2) In wheelchair: wheelchair push-ups every 15 minutes.
c. Use techniques to ensure skin protection, avoid friction, shear or abrasion injury.
   (1) Lifting, not dragging.
   (2) Use of turning and draw sheets; trapeze, manual or electric lifts.
   (3) Use of cornstarch, lubricants, pad protectors, thin film dressings, or hydrocolloid dressings over friction risk sites.
   (4) Use of transfer boards for sliding wheelchair transfers.
d. Pressure-relieving devices (PRDs).
   (1) Reduce tissue interface pressures.
   (2) Static devices: use if patient can assume a variety of positions; examples include foam, air, or gel mattress overlays; water-filled mattresses; pillows or foam wedges, protective padding (heel relief boots).

CHAPTER 5

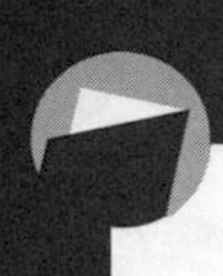

(3) Dynamic devices: use if patient cannot assume a variety of positions; examples include alternating pressure air mattresses, fluidized air or high-air-loss bed.
(4) Seating supports: use for chair-bound or wheelchair-bound patients; examples include cushions made out of foam, gel, air, or some combination.

e. Avoid restrictive clothing, e.g., with rough textures, hard fasteners, and studs. Avoid tight-fitting shoes, socks, splints, and orthoses.

f. Avoid maceration injury.
(1) Prevent moisture accumulation and temperature elevation where skin contacts support surface.
(2) Incontinence management strategies: use of absorbent pads, brief or panty pad; scheduled toileting and prompted voiding; ointments, creams, and skin barriers prophylactically in perineal and perianal areas.

g. Patient and caregiver education.
(1) Mechanisms of pressure ulcer development.
(2) Daily skin inspection.
(3) Avoidance of prolonged positions.
(4) Repositioning, weight shifts, lifts.
(5) Safety awareness during self-care.
(6) Safety awareness with use of devices and equipment.
(7) Importance of ongoing activity/exercise program.

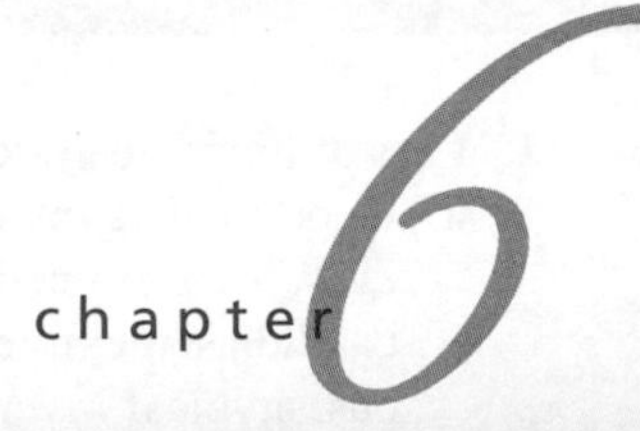

chapter 6

Other Systems: Immune, Hematological, Gastrointestinal, Genital/Reproductive, Renal and Urological, Endocrine and Metabolic

SUSAN B. O'SULLIVAN

Immune System

Overview

1. **Anatomy and physiology of the immune system.**
   a. The immune system consists of immune cells, central immune structures where immune cells are produced (the bone marrow and thymus), and the peripheral immune structures (lymph nodes, spleen, and other accessory structures).
   b. There are several different types of immune cells.
      (1) An antigen (immunogen) is a foreign molecule that elicits the immune response. Antibodies or immunoglobulins are the proteins that are engaged to tag antigens.
      (2) Lymphocytes (T and B lymphocytes) are the primary cells of the immune system.
      (3) Macrophages are the accessory cells that process and present antigens to the lymphocytes.
      (4) Cytokines are molecules that link immune cells with other tissues and organs.
      (5) CD molecules (e.g., CD4 helper cells) serve as master regulators of the immune response by influencing the function of all other immune cells.
      (6) Recognition of foreign threat from self (autoimmune responses) is mediated by major histocompatibility complex (MHC) membrane molecules.
   c. The thymus is the primary central gland of the immune system. It is located behind the sternum above the heart and extends into the neck region to the lower edge of the thyroid gland.
      (1) It is fully developed at birth and reaches maximum size at puberty. It then decreases in size and is slowly replaced by adipose tissue.
      (2) It produces mature T lymphocytes.
   d. The lymph system is a vast network of capillaries, vessels, valves, ducts, nodes, and organs that function to produce, filter, and convey various lymph and blood cells.
      (1) Lymph nodes are small areas of lymphoid tissue connected by lymphatic vessels throughout the body. High concentrations are found in the axillae, groin, and along the great vessels of the neck, thorax, and abdomen.
      (2) Lymph nodes function to filter the lymph and trap antigens. Lymphocytes, monocytes, and plasma cells are formed in lymph nodes.
   e. The spleen is a large lymphoid organ located in the upper left abdominal cavity between the stomach and the diaphragm.
      (1) It functions to filter antigens from the blood and produce leukocytes, monocytes, lymphocytes, and plasma cells in response to infection.

(2) In the embryo, the spleen produces red and white blood cells; after birth, only lymphocytes are produced unless severe anemia exists.

2. The immune response.
   a. A coordinated response of the body's cells and molecules that provides protection from infectious disease (bacteria, viruses, fungi, parasites) and foreign substances (plant pollens, poison ivy resin, insect venom, transplanted organs). It also defends against abnormal cells produced by the body (cancer cells).
   b. Provides natural resistance to disease and consists of rapidly activated phagocytes (macrophages, neutrophils, natural killer cells, dendritic cells). Barriers also provide a natural defense (skin, mucous membranes) as do inflammation and fever (antimicrobial molecules).
   c. The adaptive immune response includes the slower acting defenses mediated by the lymphocytes.
   d. Repeat exposure activates immunological memory, producing more rapid and efficient responses.
   e. Excessive immune response causes allergies or autoimmune reactions.

3. Immunodeficiency diseases.
   a. Characterized by depressed or absent immune responses.
   b. Primary immunodeficient disorders result from a defect in T cells, B cells, or lymphoid tissues.
      (1) Congenital disorders are a failure of organs to develop and produce mature lymphocytes.
      (2) Severe combined immunodeficiency disease (SCID).
   c. Secondary immunodeficiency disorders are caused by underlying pathology or treatment that depresses the immune system, resulting in failure of the immune response.
      (1) Diseases include leukemia, bone marrow tumor, chronic diabetes, renal failure, cirrhosis, cancer treatment (chemotherapy, radiation therapy).
      (2) Organ transplant, graft-versus-host disease.

4. Autoimmune diseases.
   a. Characterized by immune system responses directed against the body's normal tissues; self-destructive processes impair body function.
   b. Can be organ-specific: Hashimoto's thyroiditis.
   c. Can be systemic (non–organ specific): systemic lupus erythematosus (SLE), fibromy algia.
   d. Etiology is unknown; possible factors include genetic predisposition, hormonal changes, environment, viral infection, and stress.

Acquired Immunodeficiency Syndrome (AIDS)

1. Caused by the human immunodeficiency virus (HIV-1 or HIV-2).

2. Loss of immune system function.
   a. Opportunistic infections: most common is *Pneumocystis carinii* pneumonia; also oral and esophageal candidiasis, cytomegalovirus infection, cryptococcus, atypical mycobacteriosis, chronic herpes simplex, toxoplasmosis, *Mycobacterium tuberculosis*.
   b. Malignancies: most common is Kaposi's sarcoma; also non-Hodgkin's lymphoma; primary brain lymphoma.
   c. Neurological disease: focal encephalitis (central nervous system [CNS] toxoplasmosis); cryptococcal meningitis; AIDS dementia complex; herpes zoster.

3. Pathophysiology.
   a. Reduction of $CD4^+$ helper T cells, resulting in $CD4^+$ T lymphocytopenia; a major defect in the immune system.
   b. A retrovirus: replicates in reverse fashion, the RNA code is transcribed into DNA.

4. Transmission.
   a. Through contact with infected body fluids (blood, saliva, semen, cerebrospinal fluid, breast milk, vaginal/cervical secretions).
   b. High-risk behaviors for HIV transmission.
      (1) Unprotected sexual contact.
      (2) Contaminated needles: sharing, frequent injection of IV drugs; transfusions (exposure to contaminated blood is no longer a major risk).
      (3) Maternal-fetal transmission in utero or at delivery; contaminated breast milk.
   c. Low-risk behaviors for HIV transmission.
      (1) Occupational transmission: needle sticks.
      (2) Casual contact: kissing.
   d. AIDS cannot be contacted through respiratory inhalation, skin contact, or human waste (urine, feces, sweat, or vomit).

5. Diagnosis.
   a. Based on clinical findings and systemic evidence of HIV infection and absence of other known causes of immunodeficiency.
   b. AIDS-related complex (ARC): presence of acute symptoms secondary to immune system deficiency; early/middle AIDS.
      (1) May include recurrent fever and chills, night sweats, swollen lymph glands, loss of appetite, weight loss, diarrhea, persistent fatigue, infections, apathy, and depression.
      (2) May last weeks or months; a precursor to full-blown AIDS.
   c. AIDS: exhibits some or all of the symptoms of ARC, general failure to thrive, and:
      (1) Opportunistic infections.
      (2) Headaches, blurred vision, dyspnea, dry cough, oral or skin lesions, dysphagia, dementia, seizures, and focal neurological signs.

d. Deconditioning, anxiety, and depression are common.
e. Laboratory evidence.
   (1) HIV-1 antibody test (enzyme-linked immunosorbent assay [ELISA]): 30,000–50,000 copies of HIV per milliliter.
   (2) Absolute T4 (CD4) cell counts per deciliter of blood: normal CD4 counts: 800–1200/ mL; symptomatic AIDS CD4 counts: 200–500/mL.
   (3) Western blot (WB) and immunofixation methods (IFA methods).

6. Clinical course.
a. May exhibit brief, early, nonspecific viral infection, and then remain asymptomatic for many years.
b. There is no cure. Combination therapies may extend life. Prognosis is poor without treatment or with long-standing disease with secondary infections.

7. Medical interventions.
a. Multidrug (antiviral) therapy; three main groups of anti-AIDS drugs:
   (1) Nucleoside reverse transcriptase inhibitors (NRTIs), e.g., zidovudine (formerly azidothymidine [AZT]).
   (2) Protease inhibitors.
   (3) Nonnucleoside reverse transcriptase inhibitors (NNRTIs).
   (4) Initiated for symptomatic patients with AIDS, patients with CD4 counts fewer than 500; newly infected individuals.
   (5) Red Flags: Common adverse effects of antiviral therapy include rash, nausea, headaches, dizziness, muscle pain, weakness, fatigue, and difficulty sleeping. With hepatotoxicity, signs of carpal tunnel syndrome may be seen.
b. Symptomatic treatment.
   (1) Education to prevent the spread of infection and disease.
   (2) Treat opportunistic infections; prophylactic vaccinations.
   (3) Maintain nutritional status.
   (4) Provide supportive care for management of fatigue, e.g., energy-conservation techniques, self-care.
   (5) Respiratory management as needed.
   (6) Provide skin care.
   (7) Maintain functional mobility and safety; prevent disability.
   (8) Provide supportive care, e.g., emotional support for patients and families.

8. Physical therapy goals, outcomes, and interventions.
a. Observe standard AIDS/HIV precautions for health-care workers (see Box 6-1).
b. Exercise has a positive effect on the immune system; reduces stress level and pain; improves cardiovascular endurance and strength (disuse effects common).
c. Exercise recommendations.
   (1) Moderate aerobic exercise training.
   (2) Strength training.
   (3) Avoid exhaustive exercise with symptomatic individuals.
   (4) During acute stages of opportunistic infections: reduce exercise to mild levels.
d. Teach activity pacing: balancing rest with activity; scheduling strenuous activities during periods of high energy.
e. Teach energy conservation: analysis and modification of daily activities to reduce energy expenditure.
f. Teach stress management, relaxation training (e.g., meditation and mindfulness, tai chi chuan, yoga).
g. Neurological rehabilitation for patients with involvement of the CNS: See Chapter 2.

Chronic Fatigue Syndrome (CFS)

1. Characteristics.
a. A complex syndrome characterized by disabling fatigue accompanied by various other complaints.
b. Also called chronic fatigue and immune dysfunction syndrome (CFIDS)

2. Pathophysiology.
a. Etiology: unknown, viral cause suspected; often preceded by flu-like symptoms.
b. Immunological abnormalities present.
c. Neuroendocrine changes.

3. Diagnosis by exclusion.
a. Must have the two major criteria and either eight symptom criteria or six symptom criteria with at least two physical criteria (CDC case definition).
b. Major criteria.
   (1) New onset of persistent or relapsing fatigue; must be present for at least 6 months; does not resolve with bed rest and reduces daily activity by at least 50%.
   (2) Exclusion of other chronic conditions.
c. Symptom criteria.
   (1) Profound or prolonged fatigue; inability to recover from normal exercise.
   (2) Low-grade fever or chills.
   (3) Sore throat: nonexudative pharyngitis.
   (4) Lymph node pain and tenderness.
   (5) Muscle weakness.
   (6) Muscle discomfort or myalgia.
   (7) Sleep disturbances (insomnia or hypersomnia).
   (8) Headaches.
   (9) Migratory arthralgias without joint swelling or redness.
   (10) Cognitive impairments: photophobia, impaired memory, difficulty thinking, inability to concentrate, irritability, confusion.
   (11) Main symptom complex develops over a few hours or days.
d. Deconditioning, anxiety, and depression are common.
e. More common in women than men; younger ages (20s and 30s).
f. Limited recovery: only 5%–10% recover completely.

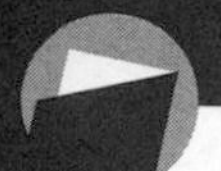

Box 6-1 ➤ STANDARD PRECAUTIONS*

Standard Precautions combine the major features of Universal Precautions (UP) and Body Substance Isolation (BSI) and are based on the principle that all blood, body fluids, secretions, excretions except sweat, nonintact skin, and mucous membranes may contain transmissible infectious agents. Standard Precautions include a group of infection prevention practices that apply to all patients, regardless of suspected or confirmed infection status, in any setting in which health care is delivered. These include hand hygiene; use of gloves, gown, mask, eye protection, or face shield, depending on the anticipated exposure; and safe injection practices. Also, equipment or items in the patient environment likely to have been contaminated with infectious body fluids must be handled in a manner to prevent transmission of infectious agents (e.g., wear gloves for direct contact, contain heavily soiled equipment, properly clean and disinfect or sterilize reusable equipment before use on another patient). The application of Standard Precautions during patient care is determined by the nature of the health care worker (HCW)–patient interaction and the extent of anticipated blood, body fluid, or pathogen exposure. For some interactions (e.g., performing venipuncture), only gloves may be needed; during other interactions (e.g., intubation), use of gloves, gown, and face shield or mask and goggles is necessary. Education and training on the principles and rationale for recommended practices are critical elements of Standard Precautions because they facilitate appropriate decision-making and promote adherence when HCWs are faced with new circumstances. An example of the importance of the use of Standard Precautions is intubation, especially under emergency circumstances when infectious agents may not be suspected, but later are identified (e.g., severe acute respiratory syndrome [SARS]–coronavirus [CoV], Neisseria meningitides). Standard Precautions are also intended to protect patients by ensuring that health-care personnel do not carry infectious agents to patients on their hands or via equipment used during patient care.

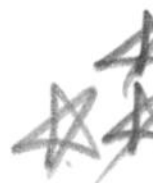

A.1. New Elements of Standard Precautions Infection control problems that are identified in the course of outbreak investigations often indicate the need for new recommendations or reinforcement of existing infection control recommendations to protect patients. Because such recommendations are considered a standard of care and may not be included in other guidelines, they are added here to Standard Precautions. Three such areas of practice that have been added are Respiratory Hygiene/Cough Etiquette, safe injection practices, and use of masks for insertion of catheters or injection of material into spinal or epidural spaces via lumbar puncture procedures (e.g., myelogram, spinal or epidural anesthesia). While most elements of Standard Precautions evolved from Universal Precautions that were developed for protection of health-care personnel, these new elements of Standard Precautions focus on protection of patients.

A.1.a. Respiratory Hygiene/Cough Etiquette The transmission of SARS-CoV in emergency departments by patients and their family members during the widespread SARS outbreaks in 2003 highlighted the need for vigilance and prompt implementation of infection control measures at the first point of encounter within a health-care setting (e.g., reception and triage areas in emergency departments, outpatient clinics, and physician offices). The strategy proposed has been termed Respiratory Hygiene/Cough Etiquette and is intended to be incorporated into infection control practices as a new component of Standard Precautions. The strategy is targeted at patients and accompanying family members and friends with undiagnosed transmissible respiratory infections, and applies to any person with signs of illness including cough, congestion, rhinorrhea, or increased production of respiratory secretions when entering a health-care facility. The term cough etiquette is derived from recommended source control measures for Mycobacteria tuberculosis. The elements of Respiratory Hygiene/Cough Etiquette include (1) education of health-care facility staff, patients, and visitors; (2) posted signs, in language(s) appropriate to the population served, with instructions to patients and accompanying family members or friends; (3) source control measures (e.g., covering the mouth/nose with a tissue when coughing and prompt disposal of used tissues, using surgical masks on the coughing person when tolerated and appropriate); (4) hand hygiene after contact with respiratory secretions; and (5) spatial separation, ideally > 3 feet, of persons with respiratory infections in common waiting areas when possible. Covering sneezes and coughs and placing masks on coughing patients are proven means of source containment that prevent infected persons from dispersing respiratory secretions into the air. Masking may be difficult in some settings (e.g., pediatrics, in which case, the emphasis by necessity may be on cough etiquette. Physical proximity of < 3 feet has been associated with an increased risk for transmission of infections via the droplet route (e.g., N. meningitidis and group A streptococcus and therefore supports the practice of distancing infected persons from others who are not infected. The effectiveness of good hygiene practices, especially hand hygiene, in preventing transmission of viruses and reducing the incidence of respiratory infections both within and outside health-care settings is summarized in several reviews.

These measures should be effective in decreasing the risk of transmission of pathogens contained in large respiratory droplets (e.g., influenza virus, adenovirus, Bordetella Pertussis, and Mycoplasma pneumoniae. Although fever will be present in many respiratory infections, patients with pertussis and mild upper respiratory tract infections are often afebrile. Therefore, the absence of fever does not always exclude a respiratory infection. Patients who have asthma, allergic rhinitis, or chronic obstructive lung disease also may be coughing and sneezing. While these patients often are not infectious, cough etiquette measures are prudent.

Health-care personnel are advised to observe Droplet Precautions (i.e., wear a mask) and hand hygiene when examining and caring for patients with signs and symptoms of a respiratory infection. Health-care personnel who have a respiratory infection are advised to avoid direct patient contact, especially with high-risk patients. If this is not possible, then a mask should be worn while providing patient care.

Recommendations

IV. Standard Precautions

Assume that every person is potentially infected or colonized with an organism that could be transmitted in the health-care setting and apply the following infection control practices during the delivery of health care.

IV.A. Hand Hygiene

IV.A.1. During the delivery of health care, avoid unnecessary touching of surfaces in close proximity to the patient to prevent both contamination of clean hands from environmental surfaces and transmission of pathogens from contaminated hands to surfaces.

IV.A.2. When hands are visibly dirty, contaminated with proteinaceous material, or visibly soiled with blood or body fluids, wash hands with either a nonantimicrobial soap and water or an antimicrobial soap and water.

IV.A.3. If hands are not visibly soiled, or after removing visible material with nonantimicrobial soap and water, decontaminate hands in the clinical situations described in IV.A.3.a–f. The preferred method of hand decontamination is with an alcohol-based hand rub. Alternatively, hands may be washed with an antimicrobial soap and water. Frequent use of an alcohol-based hand rub immediately following hand washing with nonantimicrobial soap may increase the frequency of dermatitis. Perform hand hygiene:

IV.A.3.a. Before having direct contact with patients.

IV.A.3.b. After contact with blood, body fluids or excretions, mucous membranes, nonintact skin, or wound dressings.

IV.A.3.c. After contact with a patient's intact skin (e.g., when taking a pulse or blood pressure or lifting a patient).

IV.A.3.d. If hands will be moving from a contaminated body site to a clean body site during patient care.

IV.A.3.e. After contact with inanimate objects (including medical equipment) in the immediate vicinity of the patient.

IV.A.3.f. After removing gloves.

Box 6-1 ➤ continued

IV.A.4. Wash hands with nonantimicrobial soap and water or with antimicrobial soap and water if in contact with spores (e.g., Clostridium difficile or Bacillus anthracis) is likely to have occurred. The physical action of washing and rinsing hands under such circumstances is recommended because alcohols, chlorhexidine, iodophors, and other antiseptic agents have poor activity against spores.

IV.A.5. Do not wear artificial fingernails or extenders if duties include direct contact with patients at high risk for infection and associated adverse outcomes (e.g., those in intensive care units [ICUs] or operating rooms).

IV.A.5.a. Develop an organizational policy on the wearing of non-natural nails by health-care personnel who have direct contact with patients outside of the groups specified above.

IV.B. Personal protective equipment (PPE)

IV.B.1. Observe the following principles of use:

IV.B.1.a. Wear PPE, as described in IV.B.2–4, when the nature of the anticipated patient interaction indicates that contact with blood or body fluids may occur.

IV.B.1.b. Prevent contamination of clothing and skin during the process of removing PPE.

IV.B.1.c. Before leaving the patient's room or cubicle, remove and discard PPE.

IV.B.2. Gloves

IV.B.2.a. Wear gloves when it can be reasonably anticipated that contact with blood or other potentially infectious materials, mucous membranes, nonintact skin, or potentially contaminated intact skin (e.g., of a patient incontinent of stool or urine) could occur.

IV.B.2.b. Wear gloves with fit and durability appropriate to the task.

IV.B.2.b.i. Wear disposable medical examination gloves for providing direct patient care.

IV.B.2.b.ii. Wear disposable medical examination gloves or reusable utility gloves for cleaning the environment or medical equipment.

IV.B.2.c. Remove gloves after contact with a patient and/or the surrounding environment (including medical equipment) using proper technique to prevent hand contamination. Do not wear the same pair of gloves for the care of more than one patient. Do not wash gloves for the purpose of reuse since this practice has been associated with transmission of pathogens.

IV.B.2.d. Change gloves during patient care if the hands will move from a contaminated body site (e.g., perineal area) to a clean body site (e.g., face).

IV.B.3. Gowns

IV.B.3.a. Wear a gown that is appropriate to the task to protect skin and prevent soiling or contamination of clothing during procedures and patient-care activities when contact with blood, body fluids, secretions, or excretions is anticipated.

IV.B.3.a.i. Wear a gown for direct patient contact if the patient has uncontained secretions or excretions.

IV.B.3.a.ii. Remove gown and perform hand hygiene before leaving the patient's environment.

IV.B.3.b. Do not reuse gowns, even for repeated contacts with the same patient.

IV.B.3.c. Routine donning of gowns upon entrance into a high-risk unit (e.g., ICU, neonatal intensive care unit [NICU], hematopoietic stem cell transplantation [HSCT] unit) is not indicated.

IV.B.4. Mouth, nose, eye protection.

IV.B.4.a. Use PPE to protect the mucous membranes of the eyes, nose, and mouth during procedures and patient-care activities that are likely to generate splashes or sprays of blood, body fluids, secretions, and excretions. Select masks, goggles, face shields, and combinations of each according to the need anticipated by the task performed.

IV.B.5. During aerosol-generating procedures (e.g., bronchoscopy, suctioning of the respiratory tract [if not using in-line suction catheters], endotracheal intubation) in patients who are not suspected of being infected with an agent for which respiratory protection is otherwise recommended (e.g., M. tuberculosis, SARS, or hemorrhagic fever viruses), wear one of the following: a face shield that fully covers the front and sides of the face, a mask with attached shield, or a mask and goggles (in addition to gloves and gown).

IV.C. Respiratory Hygiene/Cough Etiquette

IV.C.1. Educate health-care personnel on the importance of source control measures to contain respiratory secretions to prevent droplet and fomite transmission of respiratory pathogens, especially during seasonal outbreaks of viral respiratory tract infections (e.g., influenza, respiratory syncytial virus [RSV], adenovirus, parainfluenza virus) in communities.

IV.C.2. Implement the following measures to contain respiratory secretions in patients and accompanying individuals who have signs and symptoms of a respiratory infection, beginning at the point of initial encounter in a health-care setting (e.g., triage, reception and waiting areas in emergency departments, outpatient clinics, and physician offices).

IV.C.2.a. Post signs at entrances and in strategic places (e.g., elevators, cafeterias) within ambulatory and inpatient settings with instructions to patients and other persons with symptoms of a respiratory infection to cover their mouths/noses when coughing or sneezing, use and dispose of tissues, and perform hand hygiene after hands have been in contact with respiratory secretions.

IV.C.2.b. Provide tissues and no-touch receptacles (e.g., foot pedal–operated lid or open, plastic-lined waste basket) for disposal of tissues.

IV.C.2.c. Provide resources and instructions for performing hand hygiene in or near waiting areas in ambulatory and inpatient settings; provide conveniently located dispensers of alcohol-based hand rubs and, where sinks are available, supplies for hand washing.

IV.C.2.d. During periods of increased prevalence of respiratory infections in the community (e.g., as indicated by increased school absenteeism, increased number of patients seeking care for a respiratory infection), offer masks to coughing patients and other symptomatic persons (e.g., persons who accompany ill patients) upon entry into the facility or medical office and encourage them to maintain special separation, ideally a distance of at least 3 feet, from others in common waiting areas.

IV.C.2.d.i. Some facilities may find it logistically easier to institute this recommendation year-round as a standard of practice.

IV.D. Patient placement

IV.D.1. Include the potential for transmission of infectious agents in patient placement decisions. Place patients who pose a risk for transmission to others (e.g., uncontained secretions, excretions or wound drainage, infants with suspected viral respiratory or gastrointestinal infections) in a single-patient room when available.

(Continued on following page)

CHAPTER 6

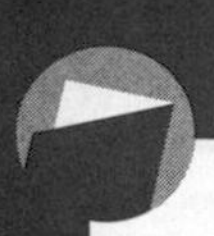

Box 6-1 ➤ continued

IV.D.2. Determine patient placement based on the following principles:

- Route(s) of transmission of the known or suspected infectious agent
- Risk factors for transmission in the infected patient
- Risk factors for adverse outcomes resulting from a hospital-acquired infection (HAI) in other patients in the area or room being considered for patient placement
- Availability of single-patient rooms
- Patient options for room sharing (e.g., cohorting patients with the same infection)

IV.E. Patient-care equipment and instruments/devices

IV.E.1. Establish policies and procedures for containing, transporting, and handling patient-care equipment and instruments/devices that may be contaminated with blood or body fluids.

IV.E.2. Remove organic material from critical and semicritical instrument/devices, using recommended cleaning agents before high-level disinfection and sterilization to enable effective disinfection and sterilization processes.

IV.E.3. Wear PPE (e.g., gloves, gown), according to the level of anticipated contamination, when handling patient-care equipment and instruments/devices that are visibly soiled or may have been in contact with blood or body fluids.

IV.F. Care of the environment

IV.F.1. Establish policies and procedures for routine and targeted cleaning of environmental surfaces as indicated by the level of patient contact and degree of soiling.

IV.F.2. Clean and disinfect surfaces that are likely to be contaminated with pathogens, including those that are in close proximity to the patient (e.g., bed rails, over bed tables) and frequently touched surfaces in the patient-care environment (e.g., door knobs, surfaces in and surrounding toilets in patients' rooms) on a more frequent schedule compared to that for other surfaces (e.g., horizontal surfaces in waiting rooms).

IV.F.3. Use Environmental Protection Agency (EPA)–registered disinfectants that have microbiocidal (i.e., killing) activity against the pathogens most likely to contaminate the patient-care environment. Use in accordance with manufacturer's instructions.

IV.F.3.a. Review the efficacy of in-use disinfectants when evidence of continuing transmission of an infectious agent (e.g., rotavirus, C. difficile, norovirus) may indicate resistance to the in-use product and change to a more effective disinfectant as indicated.

IV.F.4. In facilities that provide health care to pediatric patients or have waiting areas with child play toys (e.g., obstetric/gynecology offices and clinics), establish policies and procedures for cleaning and disinfecting toys at regular intervals. Category IA

Use the following principles in developing this policy and procedures:

- Select play toys that can be easily cleaned and disinfected.
- Do not permit use of stuffed furry toys if they will be shared.
- Clean and disinfect large stationary toys (e.g., climbing equipment) at least weekly and whenever visibly soiled.
- If toys are likely to be mouthed, rinse with water after disinfection; alternatively wash in a dishwasher.
- When a toy requires cleaning and disinfection, do so immediately or store in a designated labeled container separate from toys that are clean and ready for use.

IV.F.5. Include multiuse electronic equipment in policies and procedures for preventing contamination and for cleaning and disinfection, especially those items that are used by patients, those used during delivery of patient care, and mobile devices that are moved in and out of patient rooms frequently (e.g., daily).

IV.F.5.a. No recommendation for use of removable protective covers or washable keyboards. Unresolved issue

IV.G. Textiles and laundry

IV.G.1. Handle used textiles and fabrics with minimum agitation to avoid contamination of air, surfaces, and persons.

IV.G.2. If laundry chutes are used, ensure that they are properly designed, maintained, and used in a manner to minimize dispersion of aerosols from contaminated laundry.

IV.H. Safe injection practices: see CDC website

IV.I. Infection control practices for special lumbar puncture procedures: see CDC website

IV.J. Worker safety. Adhere to federal and state requirements for protection of health-care personnel from exposure to bloodborne pathogens.

***Date last modified:** October 12, 2007.

*Excerpt with modifications from Centers for Disease Control and Prevention, Guideline for Isolation Precautions: Preventing Transmission of Infectious Agents in Healthcare Settings, 2007. PDF (1.33MB/219 pages), downloaded 9.15.08. http://www.cdc.gov/ncidod/dhqp/gl_isolation_standard.html

4. **Medical interventions.**
   a. Antiviral agents in clinical trials.
   b. Supportive and symptomatic treatment; symptoms may persist for months or years.
      (1) Analgesics and anti-inflammatory nonsteroidal medications for myalgia and arthralgia.
      (2) Nutritional support.
      (3) Psychological support and counseling; antidepressants.
5. **Physical therapy examination.**
   a. Examine exercise tolerance levels. Vital signs may reveal fluctuations in heart rate (HR) and blood pressure (BP); orthostatic hypotension is common. If deconditioned, dyspnea with exercise.
   b. Examine posture. Postural stress syndrome (poor posture) and movement adaptation syndrome (inefficient movement patterns) may be present and can contribute to chronic pain.

c. Examine activity levels and degree of fatigue. Objective measure: Modified Fatigue Impact Scale.
d. Examine for depression. Determine degree of emotional support present.

6. Physical therapy goals, outcomes, and interventions.
a. Activities are reduced when fatigue is maximal; bed rest contraindicated other than for sleep.
b. Graded exercise program: short duration, gradually increasing intensity; components include stretching, strengthening, aerobic training (e.g., walking).
c. Avoid overexertion.
d. Teach activity pacing: balancing rest with activity; scheduling strenuous activities during periods of high energy.
e. Teach energy conservation: analysis and modification of daily activities to reduce energy expenditure.
f. Teach stress management, relaxation training (e.g., meditation and mindfulness, tai chi chuan, yoga).
g. Refer to support group.

Fibromyalgia Syndrome (FMS)

1. A chronic pain syndrome affecting muscles and soft tissues (nonarticular rheumatism).

2. Pathophysiology.
a. Etiology unknown; viral cause suspected, multifactoral.
b. Immunological and neurohormonal abnormalities are present; genetic factor (autosomal dominant).
c. More common in women (75%-80% of cases) than men.

3. Characteristics.
a. Myalgia (muscle pain).
b. Generalized aching, persistent fatigue (mental and physical)
c. Sleep disturbances with generalized morning stiffness.
d. Multiple tender points (trigger points).
e. Additional signs and symptoms: visual problems, mental and physical fatigue, spasm, cold intolerance, headaches, irritable bladder or bowel, cognitive problems (impaired memory, decreased attention and concentration), restless legs, atypical patterns of numbness and tingling (sensitivity amplification).
f. Anxiety and depression are common.
g. Triggering events: emotional stress/anxiety trauma, hyperthyroidism, infection.

4. Medical management.
a. Diagnosis by exclusion. Presence of 11 of 18 specified tender points (Copenhagen Fibromyalgia Syndrome definition).
b. Anti-inflammatory agents, muscle relaxants, pain medications.
c. Nutritional support.
d. Psychological support and counseling; antidepressants.

5. Physical therapy goals, outcomes, and interventions.
a. See recommendations for chronic fatigue syndrome (section I.C).
b. Patient typically demonstrates exercise intolerance. Daily exercise is important. Focus is on aerobic training, mild to moderate intensities.
c. Teach protection strategies to avoid overuse syndromes.
d. Aquatic therapy is ideal to decrease pain and increase cardiovascular conditioning and strength.
e. Teach techniques for taking control: self-responsibility for own health, education, coping strategies, keeping a journal.
f. Work and work environment adjustments.
g. Refer to support group.

Infectious Diseases

Staphylococcal Infections

1. *Staphylococcus aureus* (SA).
a. A common bacterial pathogen.

2. Pathophysiology.
a. Typically begins as localized infection; entry is through skin portal, e.g., wounds, ulcers, burns.
b. Bacterial invasion and spread is through bloodstream or lymphatic system to almost any body location, e.g., heart valves, bones (acute staphylococcal osteomyelitis), joints (bacterial arthritis), skin (cellulitis, furuncles and carbuncles, ulcers), respiratory tract (pneumonia), bowel (enterocolitis).
c. Infection produces suppuration (pus formation) and abscess.

3. Medical interventions.
a. Laboratory diagnosis to confirm pathogen.
b. Antibiotic therapy; determine antibiotic sensitivity. Antibiotic resistance is common.
c. Drainage of abscesses.
d. Skin infections that are untreated can become systemic; sepsis can be lethal.

4. **Methicillin-resistant Staphylococcus aureus (MRSA).**
   a. An antibiotic-resistant strain.
   b. MRSA is resistant to all penicillins (especially methicillin) and cephalosporins.
   c. It is found in about 1% of the population.
   d. Hospitalized patients with MRSA infections are isolated and standard mask-gown-gloves precautions required.

5. **Vancomycin-resistant Staphylococcus aureus (VRSA).**
   a. Resistant to vancomycin.
   b. Can be a life-threatening infection.

Streptococcal Infections

1. **Characteristics.**
   a. A common bacterial pathogen.
   b. Types.
      (1) Group A streptococcus (*S. pyogenes*): pharyngitis, rheumatic fever, scarlet fever, impetigo, necrotizing fasciitis (gangrene), cellulitis, myositis.
      (2) Group B streptococcus (*S. agalactiae*): neonatal and adult streptococcal B infections.
      (3) Group C streptococcus (*S. pneumoniae*): pneumonia, otitis media, meningitis, endocarditis.

2. **Medical interventions.**
   a. Laboratory diagnosis to confirm pathogen.
   b. Antibiotic therapy; antibiotic resistance common.
   c. Skin infections that are untreated can become systemic.

Hepatitis

1. **Characteristics.**
   a. Inflammation of the liver; may be caused by viral or bacterial infection; chemical agents (alcohol, drugs, toxins).
   b. Types.
      (1) Hepatitis A virus (HAV, acute infectious hepatitis).
         (a) Transmission is primarily through fecal-oral route; contracted through contaminated food or water, infected food handlers.
         (b) Prevention: good personal hygiene, hand washing, sanitation; immunization (vaccine).
      (2) Hepatitis B virus (HBV, serum hepatitis).
         (a) Transmission from blood, body fluids, or body tissues, through blood transfusion, oral or sexual contact, or contaminated needles.
         (b) Prevention: education, use of disposable needles, screening of blood donors; precautions for health-care workers; immunization (vaccine).
      (3) Hepatitis C virus (HCV, non-A, non-B).
         (a) Transmission is same as for HBV (posttransfusion is most common route).

2. **Clinical signs and symptoms.**
   a. Initial (preicteric phase): low-grade fever, anorexia, nausea, vomiting, fatigue, malaise, headache, abdominal tenderness and pain.
   b. Jaundice (icteric) phase: fever, jaundice, enlarged liver with tenderness; abatement of earlier symptoms.
   c. Elevated lab values: hepatic transaminases and bilirubin.
   d. Course: variable.
      (1) Acute: may last from several weeks to months.
      (2) Chronic: HBV and HCV may lead to chronic liver infection, including necrosis, cirrhosis, and liver failure.

3. **Medical interventions.**
   a. No specific treatment for acute viral hepatitis; treatment is symptomatic, e.g., IV fluids, analgesics.
   b. Chronic hepatitis: interferon is the main therapy.

Tuberculosis (TB)

1. **Characteristics.**
   a. An airborne infectious disease caused by the bacillus *Mycobacterium tuberculosis.*
   b. Most commonly affects the respiratory system; may also affect the gastrointestinal and genitourinary systems, bones, joints, the nervous system, and skin.
   c. Course: may be acute, generalized or chronic, localized.

2. **Signs and symptoms.**
   a. Pulmonary: productive cough, rales, dyspnea, pleuritic pain, and hemoptysis.
   b. Systemic: fatigue, low-grade fever, night sweats, anorexia, and weight loss.

3. **Medical interventions.**
   a. Chemotherapy: a combination of daily drugs; incidence of drug-resistant strains is increasing.
   b. Isolation and bed rest (limited with advent of chemotherapy).
   c. Adequate diet.

4. **Pulmonary precautions.**
   a. Instruct patient in infection control measures.
   b. Transmission is through:
      (1) Respiratory droplets or sputum: use tissues to cover nose and mouth when coughing or sneezing; disposable containers for sputum, tissues.
      (2) Soiled dressings.

Centers for Disease Control and Prevention (CDC) Standard Precautions

Standard Precautions

1. A group of infection prevention practices that apply to all patients, regardless of suspected or confirmed infection status. (See Box 6-1).

2. Standard Precautions combine major features of:
   a. Universal Precautions.
   b. Body Substance Isolation.
   c. Based on the principle that all blood, body fluids, secretions, excretions except sweat, nonintact skin, and mucous membranes may contain transmissible infectious agents.

Physical Therapy–Related Infection Control

1. Purpose: to destroy bacteria, infectious organisms.

2. Sterilization.
   a. The total destruction of all microorganisms by exposure to chemical or physical agents; required for all objects introduced to the body; e.g., scalpels, catheters.
   b. Methods:
      (1) Autoclaving: sterilization of instruments by heat (250–270°F) and water pressure; contraindicated with heat-sensitive articles.
      (2) Boiling water (212°F): kills organisms that do not form spores.
      (3) Ionizing radiation: used to sterilize some medications, plastics, or sutures.
      (4) Dry heat: prolonged exposure to high heat in ovens.
      (5) Gaseous: ethylene oxide, formaldehyde gas.

3. Disinfection.
   a. The reduction of the number of microorganisms; typically used on surfaces or equipment, e.g., respiratory and hydrotherapy equipment.
   b. Methods:
      (1) Ultraviolet light: used for air and surface disinfection; harmful to unprotected skin and eyes.
      (2) Filtration: used for water or air purification.
      (3) Physical cleaning.
         (a) Ultrasonic: disinfects instruments.
         (b) Washing with an antimicrobial product: used to disinfect hands and surfaces.
      (4) Chemicals.
         (a) Chlorination: used for water disinfection, filtration systems; also used for food surface sanitizing.
         (b) Iodines: used in hydrotherapy when filtering system not possible; provides full bactericidal activity when organic matter (skin, feces, urine) is present.
         (c) Phenols: general disinfectants.
         (d) Quaternary ammonia compounds, e.g., benzalkonium chloride (Zephiran).
         (e) Formaldehyde (5%).
      (5) Hydrotherapy disinfection.
         (a) Drain and clean tanks after every patient.
         (b) Scrub pumps and equipment (e.g., drains, agitator unit) with a germicidal detergent, e.g., sodium hypochlorite (bleach), povidone-iodine, chloramine-T (Chlorazene).
         (c) Rinse before refilling.

Hematological System

Overview

1. Composition of blood. (See Table 3-8 for normal values).
   a. Plasma comprises about 55% of total blood volume and is the liquid part of blood and lymph; it carries the cellular elements of blood through the circulation.
      (1) Plasma is composed of about 91% water, 7% proteins, and 2%–3% other small molecules.
      (2) Electrolytes in plasma determine osmotic pressure and pH balance and are important in the exchange of fluids between capillaries and tissues.
      (3) Carries nutrients and waste products and hormones.
      (4) Plasma proteins include albumin, globulins, and fibrinogen.
      (5) Serum is plasma without the clotting factors.
   b. Erythocytes, or red blood cells (RBCs), comprise about 45% of the total blood volume and contain the oxygen-carrying protein hemoglobin responsible for transporting oxygen.
      (1) RBCs are produced in the marrow of the long bones and controlled by hormones (erythropoietin). RBCs are time-limited, surviving for approximately 120 days.

CHAPTER 6

(2) RBC count varies with age, activity, and environmental conditions.

c. Leukocytes, or white blood cells (WBCs), comprise about 1% of total blood volume and circulate through the lymphoid tissues.

(1) Leukocytes function in immune processes as phagocytes of bacteria, fungi, and viruses. They also aid in capturing toxic proteins resulting from allergic reactions and cellular injury.

(2) Leukocytes are produced in the bone marrow.

(3) There are five types of leukocytes: lymphocytes and monocytes (agranulocytes) and neutrophils, basophils, and eosinophils (granulocytes).

2. Hematopoiesis.

a. The normal function and generation of blood cells in the bone marrow.

b. Production, differentiation, and function of blood cells is regulated by cytokines and growth factors (chemical messengers) acting on blood-forming cells (pluripotent stem cells).

c. Disorders of hematopoiesis include aplastic anemia and leukemias.

3. Blood screening tests.

a. Complete blood count (CBC) determines the number of red blood cells, white blood cells, and platelets per unit of blood.

b. White cell differential count determines the relative percentages of individual white cell types.

c. Erythrocyte sedimentation rate (ESR) is the rate of red blood cells that settle out in a tube of unclotted blood; expressed in millimeters per hour.

(1) Elevated ESR indicates the presence of inflammation.

(2) Normal values (see Table 3-8).

4. Hemostasis.

a. The termination or arrest of blood flow by mechanical or chemical processes. Mechanisms include vasospasm, platelet aggregation, and thrombin and fibrin synthesis.

b. Blood clotting requires platelets produced in bone marrow, von Willebrand's factor produced by the endothelium of blood vessels, and clotting factors produced by the liver using vitamin K.

c. Fibrinolysis is clot dissolution that prevents excess clot formation.

5. Hypercoaguability disorders are caused by:

a. Increased platelet function as seen in atherosclerosis, diabetes mellitus, elevated blood lipids, and cholesterol.

b. Accelerated activity of the clotting system as seen in congestive heart failure, malignant diseases, pregnancy and use of oral contraceptives, immobility.

6. Hypocoagulopathy (bleeding) disorders are caused by:

a. Platelet defects as seen in bone marrow dysfunction, thrombocytopenia, thrombocytopathia,

b. Coagulation defects as seen in hemophilia, and von Willebrand's disease.

c. Vascular disorders as seen in hemorrhagic telangiectasia, vitamin C deficiency, Cushing's disease; senile purpura.

7. Shock.

a. An abnormal condition of inadequate blood flow to the body tissues. It is associated with hypotension, inadequate cardiac output, and changes in peripheral blood flow resistance.

b. Hypovolemic shock is caused by hemorrhage, vomiting, or diarrhea. Loss of body fluids also occurs with dehydration, Addison's disease, burns, pancreatitis, or peritonitis.

c. Orthostatic changes may develop, characterized by a drop in systolic blood pressure of 10–20 mm Hg or more. Pulse and respiration increase.

d. Progressive shock is associated with restlessness and anxiety, weakness, lethargy, pallor with cool, moist skin and fall in body temperature.

e. Vital functions must be carefully monitored and restored as quickly as possible. The patient should be placed supine or in a modified Trendelenburg's position to aid venous return.

8. Signs and symptoms of hematological disorders.

a. Easy bruising with spontaneous petechiae and purpura of the skin.

b. External hematomas may also be present (e.g., thrombocytopenia).

9. Medications.

a. Long-term use of certain drugs (steroids, nonsteroidal anti-inflammatory drugs [NSAIDs]) can lead to bleeding and anemia.

10. Red Flags: Physical therapy interventions.

a. Use extreme caution with manual therapy and use of some modalities (e.g., mechanical compression).

b. Strenuous exercise is contraindicated due to the risk of increased hemorrhage.

Anemia

1. Characteristics.

a. Decrease in hemoglobin levels in the blood.

b. Normal range: (see Table 3-8).

2. Etiology.

a. Decrease in RBC production: nutritional deficiency (iron, vitamin B, folic acid); cellular maturation defects, decreased bone marrow stimulation (hypothyroidism), bone marrow failure (leukemia, aplasia, neoplasm), and genetic defect.

b. Destruction of RBCs: autoimmune hemolysis, sickle cell disease, enzyme defects, parasites (malaria), hypersplenism, chronic diseases (rheumatoid arthritis, tuberculosis, cancer).
c. Loss of blood (hemorrhage): trauma, wound, bleeding, peptic ulcer, excessive menstruation.

3. Clinical symptoms.
   a. Fatigue and weakness with minimal exertion.
   b. Dyspnea on exertion.
   c. Pallor or yellow skin of the face, hands, nail beds, and lips.
   d. Tachycardia.
   e. Bleeding of gums, mucous membranes, or skin in the absence of trauma.
   f. Severe anemia can produce hypoxic damage to liver and kidney, heart failure.

4. Medical intervention.
   a. Variable, depends on causative factors.
   b. Transfusion.
   c. Nutritional supplements.

5. Physical therapy intervention.
   a. Red Flags: Patients with anemia exhibit decreased exercise tolerance.
      (1) Exercise should be instituted gradually with physician approval.
      (2) Perceived exertion levels should be used (rate of perceived exertion [RPE] ratings).

Sickle Cell Disease

1. Characteristics.
   a. Group of inherited, autosomal recessive disorders; erythrocytes, specifically hemoglobin S (Hb S), are abnormal. RBCs are crescent or sickle-shaped instead of biconcave.
   b. Sickle cell trait: heterozygous form of sickle cell anemia characterized by abnormal red blood cells. Individuals are carriers and do not develop the disease. Counseling is important, especially if both parents have the trait.
   c. Chronic hemolytic anemia (sickle cell anemia): hemoglobin is released into plasma with resultant reduced oxygen delivery to tissues; results from bone marrow aplasia, hemolysis, folate deficiency, or splenic involvement.
   d. Vaso-occlusion from misshapen erythrocytes: results in ischemia, occlusion, and infarction of adjacent tissue.
   e. Chronic illness that can be fatal.

2. Sickle cell crisis.
   a. Acute episodic condition occurring in children with sickle cell anemia.
   b. Symptoms.
      (1) Pain: acute and severe from sickle cell clots formed in any organ, bone, or joint.
         (a) Acute abdominal pain from visceral hypoxia.
         (b) Painful swelling of soft tissue of the hands and feet (hand-foot syndrome).
         (c) Persistent headache.
      (2) Bone and joint crises: migratory, recurrent joint pain; extremity and back pain.
      (3) Neurological manifestations: dizziness, convulsions, coma, paresthesias, cranial nerve palsies, blindness, nystagmus.
      (4) Coughing, dyspnea, tachypnea may occur.
      (5) Vascular complications: stroke, chronic leg ulcers, bone infarcts, avascular necrosis of femoral head.
      (6) Renal complications: enuresis, nocturia, hematuria, renal failure.
      (7) Anemic crisis: characterized by rapid drop in hemoglobin levels.
      (8) Aplastic crisis: characterized by severe anemia; associated with acute viral, bacterial, or fungal infection. Increased susceptibility to infection.
      (9) Splenic sequestration crisis: liver and spleen enlargement, spleen atrophy.

3. Medical interventions.
   a. Immediate transfusion of packed red cells in acute anemic crisis.
   b. Analgesics or narcotics as needed for pain.
   c. Short-term oxygen therapy in severe anoxia.
   d. Hydration, electrolyte replacement.
   e. Antibiotics for infection control.
   f. Oral anticoagulants to relieve pain of vaso-occlusion; associated with increased risk of bleeding.
   g. Splenectomy may be considered.
   h. Bone marrow transplant in severe cases.
   i. Uremia may require renal transplantation or hemodialysis.

4. Physical therapy goals, outcomes, and interventions.
   a. Pain control: application of warmth is soothing (e.g., hydrotherapy).
   b. Red Flags: Cold is contraindicated, as it increases vasoconstriction and sickling.
   c. Relaxation techniques.
   d. Emotional support and counseling of family.
   e. Patient and family education: avoidance of stressors that can precipitate a crisis.

Hemophilia

1. Pathophysiology. A group of hereditary bleeding disorders.
   a. Inherited as a sex-linked recessive disorder of blood coagulation; affects males, females are carriers.
   b. Clotting factor VIII deficiency (hemophilia A) is most common; classic hemophilia.
   c. Clotting factor IX deficiency (hemophilia B or Christmas disease).

d. Level of severity and rate of spontaneous bleeds varies by percentage of clotting factor in blood: mild, moderate, severe.
e. Bleeding is spontaneous or a result of trauma; may result in internal hemorrhage and hematuria.
f. Hemarthrosis (bleeding into joint spaces) most common in synovial joints: knees, ankles, elbows, hips.
   (1) Joint becomes swollen, warm, and painful with decreased range of motion (ROM).
   (2) Long-term results can include chronic synovitis and arthropathy leading to bone and cartilage destruction.
g. Hemorrhage into muscles often affects forearm flexors, gastrocnemius/soleus, and iliopsoas.
   (1) Produces pain.
   (2) Decreases movement.

2. Medical interventions.
a. Blood infusion, factor replacement therapy.
b. Use of acetaminophen (Tylenol), not aspirin, for pain management.
c. Rest, ice, elevation, functional splinting, and no weight-bearing during an acute bleed.
d. HIV or hepatitis transmission was a possible transfusion result prior to current purification techniques.

3. Complications.
a. Joint contractures.
   (1) Hip, knee, elbow flexion; ankle plantar flexion.
b. Muscle weakness around affected joints.
c. Leg-length discrepancies.
d. Postural scoliosis.
e. Decreased aerobic fitness.
f. Gait deviations.
   (1) Equinus gait.
   (2) Lack of knee extensor torque.
g. Activities of daily living (ADL) deficiencies, e.g., elbow contractures could affect dressing ability.

4. Physical therapy examination.
a. Clinical signs and symptoms of acute bleeding episodes: decreased ROM, stiffening, pain, swelling, tenderness, heat, prickling or tingling sensations.
b. Goniometry.
c. Joint deformities, e.g., genu valgum, rearfoot/forefoot.
d. Muscle strength; girth.
e. Functional mobility skills, gait.
f. Pain.
g. Activities of daily living.

5. Physical therapy interventions. Acute stage.
a. RICE: rest, ice, compression, elevation.
b. Maintain position, prevent deformity.

6. Physical therapy interventions. Subacute stage after hemostasis.
a. Factor replacement best done just before treatment.
b. Isometric exercise and aquatic therapy early.
c. Pain management: transcutaneous electrical nerve stimulation (TENS), massage, relaxation techniques, ice, biofeedback.
d. Active assistive exercise progressing to active, isokinetic, and open chain resistive exercises.
   (1) Passive ROM rarely, if ever, used.
   (2) Closed chain exercise may put too much compressive force through joint.
   (3) Important to strengthen hip, knee, elbow extensors, and ankle dorsiflexors.
e. Contracture management.
   (1) Manual traction, mobilization techniques, serial casting, dynamic splinting during the day, resting splints at night.
   (2) Red Flags: Passive stretching is rarely used, due to risk of myositis ossificans.
f. Functional and gait training as needed.
   (1) Protective use of helmets or pads for very young boys during ambulation and play.
   (2) Temporary use of ambulatory aids as needed.
   (3) Foot orthoses, shoe inserts, and adhesive taping for ankle or foot problems.

7. Physical therapy interventions. Chronic stage.
a. Daily home exercise program to maintain or increase joint function, aerobic fitness, and strength.
b. Outpatient physical therapy as necessary.
c. Appropriate recreational activities or adaptive physical education if at school.

8. Emotional support for patients and families.

Cancer

Overview

1. Cancer is a broad group of diseases characterized by rapidly proliferating anaplastic cells.

2. Characteristics. Involves all body organs; invasive.
a. Etiology: unknown; multiple factors are implicated.
   (1) Carcinogens: chemical (e.g., asbestos, smoking or oral tobacco), radiation (e.g., x-rays, sun exposure), or viral (e.g., herpes simplex, AIDS/immune system depression).

(2) Genetic factors: hereditary.
(3) Dietary factors: obesity, high-fat diet, diet low in vitamins A, C, E.
(4) Psychological factors: chronic stress.

b. Early warning signs.
(1) Unusual bleeding or discharge.
(2) A lump or thickening of any area, e.g., breast.
(3) A sore that does not heal.
(4) A change in bladder or bowel habits.
(5) Hoarseness or persistent cough.
(6) Indigestion or difficulty swallowing.
(7) Change in size or appearance of a wart or mole.
(8) Unexplained weight loss.

c. Classification (staging): delineates extent and prognosis of disease.

d. Incidence: second leading cause of death in United States.

e. Prognosis: aggressive treatments have resulted in higher cure rates, increased survival times.

f. Quality of life (maintaining normal function and lifestyle) is an important issue.

3. Pathophysiology.

a. Tumor or neoplasm: an abnormal growth of new tissue that is nonfunctional and competes for vital blood supply and nutrients.

b. Benign tumor (neoplasm): localized, slow-growing, usually encapsulated; not invasive.

c. Malignant tumors (neoplasms): invasive, rapid growth giving rise to metastases; can be life-threatening.
(1) Carcinoma: a malignant tumor originating in epithelial tissues, e.g., skin, stomach, colon, breast, rectum. Carcinoma in situ is a premalignant neoplasm that has not invaded the basement membrane.
(2) Sarcoma: a malignant tumor originating in connective and mesodermal tissues, e.g., muscle, bone, fat.
(3) Lymphoma: affecting the lymphatic system, e.g., Hodgkin's disease, lymphatic leukemia.
(4) Leukemias and myelomas: affecting the blood (unrestrained growth of leukocytes) and blood-forming organs (bone marrow).

d. Metastasis: movement of cancer cells from one body part to another; spread is via lymphatic system or bloodstream.

4. Staging. Describes extent of disease.

a. Primary tumor (T).
b. Regional lymph node involvement (N).
c. Metastasis (M).
d. Numbers used to denote extent of involvement, from 1 to 4 (least involvement to most involvement, e.g., T2, N1, M1).

5. Medical interventions.

a. Curative versus palliative (relief of symptoms, e.g., pain); can be used alone or in combination.

b. Surgery.
(1) Can be curative (tumor removal following biopsy) or palliative (to relieve pain, correct obstruction).
(2) Often used in combination with chemotherapy or radiation therapy.
(3) Can result in significant functional deficits and weakness; edema.

c. Radiation therapy.
(1) Destroys cancer cells, inhibits cell growth and division.
(2) Can be used preoperatively to shrink tumors, prevent spread.
(3) Can be used postoperatively to kill/prevent residual cancer cells from metastasizing.

d. Chemotherapy.
(1) Drugs can be given orally, subcutaneously, intramuscularly, intravenously, intrathecally (within the spinal canal).
(2) Usually intermittent doses to allow for bone marrow recovery.

e. Biotherapy (immunotherapy).
(1) Strengthens host's ability to fight cancer cells.
(2) Agents can include interferons, interleukin-2, and cytokines.
(3) Bone marrow (stem cell) transplant; follows high doses of chemotherapy or radiation that destroys both cancer cells and bone marrow cells.
(4) Monoclonal antibodies.
(5) Hormonal therapy.

f. Red Flags: Local and systemic effects of cancer therapy.
(1) With radiation therapy, can see radiation sickness, immunosuppression, fibrosis, burns, delayed wound healing, edema, hair loss, CNS effects.
(2) With chemotherapy, can see gastrointestinal symptoms (anorexia, nausea, vomiting, diarrhea, ulcers, hemorrhage), bone marrow suppression, skin rashes, neuropathies, phlebitis, and hair loss.
(3) With biotherapy (immunotherapy), can see fever, chills, nausea, vomiting, anorexia, fatigue, fluid retention.
(4) With hormonal therapy, can see gastrointestinal symptoms, hypertension, steroid-induced diabetes and myopathy, weight gain, hot flashes and sweating, altered mental status, impotence.

6. Hospice care. For the terminally ill patient and family.

a. Multidisciplinary focus.
b. Palliative care provided at home or in a hospice center.
c. Provision of supportive services: emotional, physical, social, spiritual, financial.

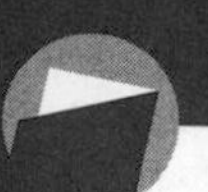

Physical Therapy Examination

1. **Detailed systems assessment.** Dependent upon cancer history.
2. **Pain.**
   a. Cancer pain syndrome: cancer-related pain is a common experience, e.g., nerve or nerve root compression, ischemic response to blockage of blood supply, bone pain. Sympathetic signs and symptoms may accompany moderate to severe pain, e.g., tachycardia, hypertension, tachypnea, nausea, vomiting.
   b. Pain at site distal to initial tumor site may suggest metastasis.
   c. Iatrogenic pain may result from surgery, radiation, or chemotherapy.
3. **Metastasis.**
   a. Lung, breast, prostate, thyroid, and lymphatic cancers commonly metastasize to bone.
   b. Pathological fractures, pain, and muscle spasms may result.
4. **Red Flags.**
   a. Paraneoplastic syndrome: signs and symptoms are produced at a site distant from the tumor or its metastasized sites, from ectopic hormone production by tumor cells or metabolic abnormalities from secretion of tumor-vasoactive products.
   b. Cushing's syndrome can result from small cell cancer of the lung.
   c. Symptoms can result from cancer stimulation of antibody production, e.g., anorexia, malaise, diarrhea, weight loss, fever, progressive muscle weakness (type II atrophy), diminished deep tendon reflexes (DTRs), myositis, joint pain.
   d. Neurological syndromes can include cerebellar degeneration, peripheral neuropathy, and myasthenia gravis.
5. **Red Flags: Adverse side effects of cancer treatment.**
   a. With immunosuppressed patient, monitor vital signs, physiological responses to exercise carefully; may see elevated HR and BP, dyspnea, pallor, sweating, fatigue. Patient is easily fatigued with minimal exertion.
   b. Muscle atrophy and weakness: secondary to high doses of steroids in many chemotherapy protocols; weakness may also result from disuse or tumor compression/invasion.
   c. ROM deficits: particularly with high-dose radiation around joints.
   d. Hematological disruptions.
      (1) White blood cell suppression (leukopenia); increased susceptibility to infection.
      (2) Platelet suppression (thrombocytopenia): increased bleeding.
      (3) Red blood cell suppression (anemia): diminished aerobic capacity.

Physical Therapy Goals, Outcomes, and Interventions

1. **Educate patient and family about disease process, rehabilitation goals, process, and expected outcomes.**
2. **Identify and support patient and family.**
   a. Assist in coping mechanisms.
   b. Assist through the grieving process.
3. **Positioning.**
   a. Provide for proper positioning to prevent or correct deformities, maintain skin integrity.
   b. Provide for overall patient comfort.
4. **Edema control.**
   a. Elevation of extremities, active ROM.
   b. Massage.
   c. Postoperative compression (elastic bandages, pressure garments).
5. **Pain control.**
   a. TENS stimulation: may not control deep cancer pain; effective for postoperative pain.
   b. Massage.
6. **Maintain or correct loss of ROM.**
   a. Active-assisted/ stretching.
   b. Active ROM exercises.
7. **Maintain or correct loss of muscle mass and strength.**
   a. Isometric and lightweight isotonic strengthening exercises safe for most patients with cancer.
   b. Red Flags: Patients with significant bony metastases, osteoporosis, or low platelet counts (< 20,000).
      (1) AROM, ADL exercise only.
      (2) Weight bearing may be restricted; provide appropriate ambulatory aids, orthoses.
      (3) High risk of vertebral compression and other fractures with metastatic disease. Use light exercise only.
8. **Maintain or increase activity tolerance and cardiovascular endurance.**
   a. Following prolonged bed rest or inactivity: careful examination, gradual exercise and activity progression; submaximal aerobic exercise is indicated.
   b. Monitor fatigue levels. Use activity pacing, carefully balance activity and rest periods; use short sessions throughout the day. Teach energy-conservation techniques.
   c. Precaution with patients who are anemic: may experience decreased aerobic capacity.
   d. Precaution with certain types of chemotherapy (e.g., doxorubicin [Adriamycin]): may experience cardiac side effects.
   e. Precaution with severe bony metastases, weakness: light aerobic exercise (cycling, swimming) may be indicated.

9. Maintain or increase functional independence.
   a. Activities of daily living, e.g., self-care.
   b. Functional mobility skills, e.g., bed mobility, transfers, and ambulation.
   c. Coordination, balance, and safety.

10. Specific considerations for exercise programs.
   a. Postmastectomy.
      (1) Focus is on restoration of pain-free full ROM of the shoulder, prevention/reduction of edema, restoration of function.
      (2) Early postoperative exercise is stressed: some protocols as early as Day 1.
   b. Post–bone marrow transplant.
      (1) Experience prolonged hospitalization and inactivity: average is 30 days; prolonged chemotherapy and radiotherapy, strict isolation.
      (2) Focus is on restoration of function, overcoming the effects of deconditioning.
      (3) Red Flags: Exercise is contraindicated in patients with platelet counts 20,000 or less; use caution with counts 20,000–50,000. See Table 3-12.

11. Physical agents. (See Chapter 10).
   a. Thermal agents (hot packs, paraffin baths, fluidotherapy, infrared lamps) and deep heating agents (ultrasound, diathermy).
      Red Flags:
      (1) Do not use directly over tumor.
      (2) Do not use over dysvascular tissue: tissue exposed to radiation therapy.
      (3) Do not use with individuals with decreased sensitivity to temperature or pain in affected area.
      (4) Do not use in areas of increased bleeding or hemorrhage, typically the result of corticosteroid therapy.
      (5) Do not use with acute injury, inflammation, open wounds.
   b. Cryotherapy.
      Red Flags:
      (1) Do not use with patients with insensitivity to cold or delayed wound healing.
      (2) Do not use over dysvascular tissue: tissue exposed to radiation therapy.
   c. Hydrotherapy with agitation.
      Red Flags:
      (1) Do not use over dysvascular tissue: tissue exposed to radiation therapy.
      (2) Do not use with individuals with decreased sensitivity to temperature or pain in affected area.
      (3) Do not use in areas of increased bleeding or hemorrhage or open wounds.
      (4) Risk of cross infection is high with immunosuppressed patients.

Gastrointestinal System

Overview

1. Anatomy/Physiology.
   a. The gastrointestinal (GI) tract is a long hollow tube extending from the mouth to the anus. Ingested foods and fluids are broken down into molecules that are absorbed and used by the body while waste products are eliminated.
      (1) The upper GI tract consists of the mouth, esophagus, stomach and functions for ingestion and initial digestion of food.
      (2) The middle GI tract is the small intestine (duodenum, jejunum, and ileum). The major digestive and absorption processes occur here.
      (3) The lower GI tract consists of the large intestine (cecum, colon, and rectum), with primary functions that include absorption of water and electrolytes, storage and elimination of waste products.
      (4) Accessory organs aid in digestion by producing digestive secretions and include the salivary glands, liver, and pancreas.
   b. GI motility propels food and fluids through the GI system and is provided by rhythmic, intermittent contractions (peristaltic movements) of smooth muscle (except for pharynx and upper one third of the esophagus).
   c. Neural control is achieved by the autonomic nervous system (ANS). Both sympathetic and parasympathetic plexuses extend along the length of the GI wall. Vagovagal (mediated by the vagus nerve) reflexes control the secretions and motility of the GI tract.
   d. Major GI hormones include cholecystokinin, gastrin, and secretin.

2. Signs and symptoms common to many types of GI disorders:
   a. Nausea and vomiting. Nausea is an unpleasant sensation that signals stimulation of medullary vomiting center and often precedes vomiting. Vomiting is the forceful oral expulsion of abdominal contents.
      (1) Nausea and vomiting can be triggered by many different causes including food, drugs, hypoxia,

CHAPTER 6

shock, inflammation of abdominal organs, distention, irritation of the GI tract, and motion sickness.

(2) Prolonged vomiting can produce fluid and electrolyte imbalance, and can result in pulmonary aspiration and mucosal or GI damage.

b. Diarrhea is the passage of frequent, watery, unformed stools. The amount of fluid loss determines the severity of the illness.

(1) Dehydration, electrolyte imbalance, dizziness, thirst, and weight loss are common complications of prolonged diarrhea.

(2) Numerous conditions can trigger diarrhea including infectious organisms (*Escherichia coli*, rotavirus, *Salmonella*), dysentery, diabetic enteropathy, irritable bowel syndrome, hyperthyroidism, neoplasm, and diverticulitis. Diet, medications, and strenuous exercise can also cause diarrhea.

c. Constipation is a decrease in normal elimination with excessively hard, dry stools and difficult elimination.

(1) Constipation causes increased bowel pressure and lower abdominal discomfort.

(2) Many different factors can trigger constipation, including a diet lacking in bulk and fiber, inadequate consumption of fluids, sedentary lifestyle, increasing age, and drugs (opiates, antidepressants, calcium channel blockers, anticholinergics).

(3) Numerous conditions can cause constipation including hypothyroidism, diverticular disease, irritable bowel syndrome, Parkinson's disease, spinal cord injury, tumors, bowel obstruction, and rectal lesions.

(4) Obstipation is intractable constipation with resulting fecal impaction, the retention of hard, dry stools in the rectum and colon. Impaction can cause partial or complete bowel obstruction. The patient may exhibit a history of watery diarrhea, fecal soiling, and fecal incontinence. Removal of the fecal mass is indicated.

(5) Red Flags: Constipation can cause abdominal pain and tenderness in the anterior hip, groin, or thigh regions.

(6) Constipation may develop as a result of muscle guarding and splinting; e.g., in the patient with low back pain.

d. Anorexia is the loss of appetite with an inability to eat. It is associated with anxiety, fear, and depression along with a number of different disease states and drugs.

(1) Anorexia nervosa is a disorder characterized by prolonged loss of appetite and inability to eat. Individuals exhibit emaciation, emotional disturbance concerning body image, and fear of gaining weight. It is common in adolescent girls, who may also exhibit amenorrhea.

e. Dysphagia refers to difficulty in swallowing.

(1) Patients experience choking, coughing, or abnormal sensations of food sticking in the back of the throat or esophagus.

(2) Numerous conditions can cause dysphagia including lesions of the CNS (stroke, Alzheimer's disease, Parkinson's disease), strictures and esophageal scarring, swelling, cancer, and scleroderma.

(3) Achalasia is a condition in which the lower esophageal sphincter fails to relax and food is trapped in the esophagus.

f. Heartburn is a painful burning sensation felt in the esophagus in the mid epigastric area behind the sternum or in the throat.

(1) It is typically caused by reflux of gastric contents into the esophagus.

(2) Certain foods (fatty foods, citrus foods, chocolate, peppermint, alcohol, coffee, caffeine), increased abdominal pressure (food, tight clothing, back supports, pregnancy), and certain positions/movements (bending over or laying down after a large meal) can aggravate heartburn.

g. Abdominal pain is common in GI conditions. It is the result of inflammation, ischemia, and mechanical stretching. Visceral pain can occur in the epigastric region (T3–T5 sympathetic nerve distribution, the periumbilical region (T10 sympathetic nerve distribution), and the lower abdominal region (T10–L2 sympathetic nerve distribution).

h. Red Flags: Referred GI pain patterns.

(1) Visceral pain from the esophagus can refer to the mid back.

(2) Mid thoracic spine pain (nerve root pain) can appear as esophageal pain.

(3) Visceral pain from the liver, diaphragm, or pericardium can refer to the shoulder.

(4) Visceral pain from the gallbladder, stomach, pancreas, or small intestine can refer to the mid back and scapular regions.

(5) Visceral pain from the colon, appendix, or pelvic viscera can refer to the pelvis, low back, or sacrum.

i. GI bleeding is evidenced by blood appearing in vomitus or feces.

(1) It can result from erosive gastritis, peptic ulcers, prolonged use of NSAIDs, and chronic alcohol use.

(2) Occult or hidden blood can only be revealed by stool testing.

j. Abdominal pain is generally aggravated by coughing, sneezing, or straining.

Esophagus

1. Gastroesophageal reflux disease (GERD).

a. Caused by reflux or backward movement of gastric contents of the stomach into the esophagus, producing heartburn.

b. Results from failure of the lower esophageal sphincter to regulate flow of food from the esophagus into the stomach and increased gastric pressure.

c. The diaphragm that surrounds the esophagus and oblique muscles also contribute to antireflux function.

d. Over time, acidic gastric fluids (pH < 4) damage the esophagus producing reflux esophagitis.

e. Heartburn commonly occurs 30–60 minutes after eating and at night when lying down (nocturnal reflux).

f. Red Flags.

(1) Atypical pain may present as head and neck pain.

(2) Chest pain is sometimes mistaken for heart attack; it is unrelated to activity.

(3) Respiratory symptoms can occur, including wheezing and chronic cough due to microaspiration, laryngeal injury, and vagus-mediated bronchospasm. Hoarseness can also result from chronic inflammation of the vocal cords.

g. Complications include strictures and Barrett's esophagus (a precancerous state).

h. Physical therapy interventions.

(1) Positional changes from full supine to modified, more upright positions are indicated.

(2) Valsalva's maneuver is contraindicated.

i. Lifestyle modifications include avoiding large meals and certain foods; sleeping with head elevated; medications include acid-suppressing proton pump inhibitors (PPIs) (e.g., Prilosec), H_2 blockers (e.g., ranitidine [Zantac], cimetidine [Tagamet]), and antacids (e.g., Tums). In severe cases, surgery is an option.

2. Hiatal hernia.

a. Is the protrusion of the stomach upward through the diaphragm (rolling hiatal hernia) or displacement of both the stomach and gastroesophageal junction upward into the thorax (sliding hiatal hernia).

b. May be congenital or acquired.

c. Symptoms include heartburn from GERD.

d. Conservative or symptomatic treatment is the same as for GERD. Surgery may be indicated.

Stomach

1. Gastritis.

a. Inflammation of the stomach mucosa. Gastritis can be acute or chronic.

b. Acute gastritis is caused by severe burns, aspirin or other NSAIDs, corticosteroids, food allergies, or viral or bacterial infections. Hemorrhagic bleeding can occur.

c. Symptoms include anorexia, nausea, vomiting, and pain.

d. Chronic gastritis occurs with certain diseases such as peptic ulcer, bacterial infection caused by *Helicobacter pylori*, stomach cancer, pernicious anemia, or with autoimmune disorders (thyroid disease, Addison's disease).

e. Red Flags: Patients taking NSAIDs long-term should be monitored carefully for stomach pain, bleeding, nausea, or vomiting.

f. Management is symptomatic and includes avoiding irritating substances (caffeine, nicotine, alcohol), dietary modification, and medications include acid-suppressing PPIs, H_2 blockers, and antacids.

2. Peptic ulcer disease.

a. Refers to ulcerative lesions that occur in the upper GI tract in areas exposed to acid-pepsin secretions. It can affect one or all layers of the stomach or duodenum.

b. Caused by a number of factors, including bacterial infection (*H. pylori*), acetylsalicylic acid (aspirin) and NSAIDs, excessive secretion of gastric acids, stress, and heredity.

c. Symptoms include epigastric pain, which is described as a gnawing, burning, or cramp-like. Pain is aggravated by change in position and absence of food in the stomach and relieved by food or antacids.

d. Complications include hemorrhage. Bleeding may be sudden and severe or insidious with blood in vomitus or stools. Symptoms can include weakness, dizziness, or other signs of circulatory shock.

e. Management includes use of antibiotics for treatment of *H. pylori* along with acid-suppressing drugs (PPIs, H_2 blockers, and antacids). Dietary modification including avoidance of stomach irritants is indicated. Surgical intervention is indicated for perforation and uncontrolled bleeding.

f. Red Flags:

(1) Pain from peptic ulcers located on the posterior wall of the stomach can present as radiating back pain. Pain can also radiate to the right shoulder.

(2) Stress and anxiety can increase gastric secretions and pain.

Intestines

1. Malabsorption syndrome.

a. A complex of disorders characterized by problems in intestinal absorption of nutrients (fat, carbohydrates, proteins, vitamins, calcium, and iron).

b. Can be caused by gastric or small bowel resection (short-gut syndrome) or a number of different diseases including cystic fibrosis, celiac disease, Crohn's disease, chronic pancreatitis, and pernicious anemia. Malabsorption can also be drug-induced (NSAID gastroenteritis).
c. Deficiencies of enzymes (pancreatic lipase) and bile salts are contributing factors.
d. Symptoms can include anorexia, weight loss, abdominal bloating, pain and cramps, indigestion, and steatorrhea (abnormal amounts of fat in feces). Diarrhea can be chronic and explosive.
e. Red Flags:
   (1) Iron-deficiency anemia.
   (2) Easy bruising and bleeding due to lack of vitamin K.
   (3) Muscle weakness and fatigue due to lack of protein, iron, folic acid, and vitamin B.
   (4) Bone loss, pain, and predisposition to develop fractures from lack of calcium, phosphate, and vitamin D.
   (5) Neuropathy including tetany, paresthesias, numbness, and tingling from lack of calcium, vitamins B and D, magnesium, potassium.
   (6) Muscle spasms from electrolyte imbalance and lack of calcium.
   (7) Peripheral edema.

2. Inflammatory bowel disease (IBD).

a. Refers to two related chronic inflammatory intestinal disorders, Crohn's disease (CD) and ulcerative colitis (UC). Both diseases result in inflammation of the bowel and are characterized by remissions and exacerbations.
b. Symptoms include abdominal pain, frequent attacks of diarrhea, fecal urgency, and weight loss.

Red Flags:
   (1) Joint pain (reactive arthritis) and skin rashes can occur. Pain can be referred to the low back.
   (2) Complications can include intestinal obstruction and corticosteroid toxicity (low bone density, increased fracture risk).
   (3) Intestinal absorption is disrupted and nutritional deficiencies are common.
   (4) Chronic IBD can lead to anxiety and depression.

c. Crohn's disease involves a granulomatous type of inflammation that can occur anywhere in the GI tract. Areas of adjacent normal tissue called skip lesions are present.
d. Ulcerative colitis involves an ulcerative and exudative inflammation of the large intestine and rectum. It is characterized by varying amounts of bloody diarrhea, mucus, and pus. Skip lesions are absent.

3. Irritable bowel syndrome (IBS).

a. Characterized by abnormally increased motility of the small and large intestines. IBS is also known as spastic colon, nervous or irritable colon.
b. IBS is associated with emotional stress and certain foods (high fat content or roughage, lactose intolerance). No structural or biochemical abnormalities have been identified.
c. Symptoms include persistent or recurrent abdominal pain that is relieved by defecation. Patients may experience constipation or diarrhea, bloating, abdominal cramps, flatulence, nausea, and anorexia.
d. Stress reduction and medications to reduce anxiety or depression are important components of treatment.
e. Regular physical activity is effective in reducing stress and improving bowel function.

4. Diverticular disease.

a. Characterized by pouch-like herniations (diverticula) of the mucosal layer of the colon through the muscularis layer.
b. Diverticulosis refers to pouch-like herniations of the colon, especially the sigmoid colon.
   (1) Symptoms are minimal but can include rectal bleeding.
   (2) Dietary factors (lack of dietary fiber), lack of physical activity, and poor bowel habits contribute to its development.
   (3) Diverticulosis can lead to diverticulitis.
c. Diverticulitis refers to inflammation of one or more diverticula. Fecal matter penetrates diverticula and causes inflammation and abscess.
   (1) Symptoms include pain and cramping in the lower left quadrant, nausea and vomiting, slight fever, and an elevated WBC.
   (2) Complications include bowel obstruction, perforation with peritonitis, and hemorrhage.
d. Red Flags: Patients may complain of back pain.
e. Regular exercise is an important component of treatment.

5. Appendicitis.

a. An inflammation of the vermiform appendix. As the condition progresses, the appendix becomes swollen, gangrenous, and perforated. Perforation can be life threatening and lead to the development of peritonitis.
b. Pain is abrupt at onset, localized to the epigastric or periumbilical area, and increases in intensity over time.
c. Rebound tenderness (Blumberg's sign) is present in response to depression of the abdominal wall at a site distant from the painful area.
d. Point tenderness is located at McBurney's point, the site of the appendix located 1-1/2 to 2 inches above the anterior superior iliac spine in the right lower quadrant.
e. Red Flags: Immediate medical attention is required.
f. Elevations in WBC count (> 20,000/mm^3) are indicative of perforation. Surgery is indicated.

6. Peritonitis.

a. Inflammation of the peritoneum, the serous membrane lining the walls of the abdominal cavity.

b. Peritonitis results from bacterial invasion and infection of the peritoneum. Common agents include *E. coli, Bacteroides, Fusobacterium,* and streptococci.
c. A number of different factors can introduce infecting agents including penetrating wounds, surgery, perforated peptic ulcer, ruptured appendix, perforated diverticulum, gangrenous bowel, pelvic inflammatory disease, and gangrenous gallbladder.
d. Symptoms include abdominal distension, severe abdominal pain, rigidity from reflex guarding, rebound tenderness, decreased or absent bowel sounds, nausea and vomiting, and tachycardia.
e. Elevated WBC count, fever, electrolyte imbalance, and hypotension are common.
f. Peritonitis can lead to toxemia and shock, circulatory failure, and respiratory distress.
g. Treatment is aimed at controlling inflammation and infection and restoring fluid and electrolyte imbalances. Surgical intervention may be necessary to remove an inflamed appendix or close a perforation.

Rectum

1. **Rectal fissure.**
   a. A tear or ulceration of the lining of the anal canal.
   b. Constipation and large, hard stools are contributing factors.
2. **Hemorrhoids (piles).**
   a. Varicosities in the lower rectum or anus caused by congestion of the veins in the hemorrhoidal plexus.
   b. Hemorrhoids can be internal or external (protruding from the anus).
   c. Symptoms include local irritation, pain, rectal itching.
   d. Prolonged bleeding can result in anemia.
   e. Straining with defecation, constipation, and prolonged sitting contribute to discomfort.
   f. Pregnancy increases the risk of hemorrhoids.
   g. Treatment includes topical medications to shrink the hemorrhoid, dietary changes, sitz baths, local hot or cold compresses, and ligation or surgical excision.

Genital/Reproductive System

Overview: Female Reproductive System

1. **Anatomy/Physiology.**
   a. External genitalia, located at the base of the pelvis, consist of the mons pubis, labia majora, labia minora, clitoris, and perineal body.
   b The urethra and anus are in close proximity to the external genital structures, and cross-contamination is possible.
   c The internal genitalia consist of the vagina, the uterus and cervix, the fallopian tubes, and paired ovaries.
2. **Sexual and reproductive functions.**
   a. The ovaries store female germ cells (ova) and produce female sex hormones (estrogens and progesterone) under control of the hypothalamus (gonadotropin-releasing hormone) and the anterior pituitary gland (gonadotropic follicle–stimulating and luteinizing hormones).
   b. Sex hormones influence the development of secondary sex characteristics, regulate the menstrual cycle (ovulation), maintain pregnancy (fertilization and implantation, gestation), and influence menopause (cessation of the menstrual cycle).
      (1) Estrogens decrease the rate of bone resorption.
      Red Flags: Osteoporosis and risk of bone fracture increase dramatically after menopause.
      (2) Estrogens increase production of the thyroid and increase high-density lipoproteins (a protective effect against heart disease).
      Red Flags: Heart disease and stroke risk increases after menopause.
3. **Breasts.**
   a. Mammary tissues located on the anterior chest wall between the 3rd and 7th ribs.
   b. Breast function is related to production of sex hormones and pregnancy, producing milk for infant nourishment.

Pregnancy: Normal

1. **Pregnancy weight gain.** Average 20–30 lb.
2. **Physical therapists teach childbirth education classes.**
   a. Relaxation training: e.g., Jacobsen's progressive relaxation, relaxation response, mental imagery, yoga.
   b. Breathing management: slow, deep, diaphragmatic breathing; Lamaze techniques; avoidance of Valsalva's maneuver.
   c. Provide information about pregnancy and childbirth.
3. **Common changes with pregnancy and physical therapy interventions.**
   a. Postural changes: kyphosis with scapular protraction, cervical lordosis and forward head; lumbar lordosis;

CHAPTER 6

postural stress may continue into postpartum phase with lifting and carrying the infant.
(1) Postural evaluation.
(2) Teach postural exercises to stretch, strengthen, and train postural muscles.
(3) Teach pelvic stabilization exercises, e.g., posterior pelvic tilt.
(4) Teach correct body mechanics, e.g., sitting, standing, lifting, ADLs.
(5) Limit certain activities in the third trimester, e.g., supine position to avoid inferior vena cava compression, bridging.

b. Balance changes: center of gravity shifts forward and upward as the fetus develops; with advanced pregnancy, there will be a wider base of support, increased difficulty with walking and stair climbing, rapid challenges to balance.
(1) Teach safety strategies.

c. Ligamentous laxity secondary to hormonal influences (relaxin).
(1) Joint hypermobility (e.g., sacroiliac joint), pain.
(2) Predisposition to injury especially in weight-bearing joints of lower extremities and pelvis.
(3) May persist for some time after delivery; teach joint protection strategies.

d. Muscle weakness: abdominal muscles are stretched and weakened as pregnancy develops; pelvic floor weakness with advanced pregnancy and childbirth. Stress incontinence secondary to pelvic floor dysfunction (experienced by 80% of women).
(1) Teach exercises to improve control of pelvic floor, maintain abdominal function.
(2) Stretching exercises to reduce muscle cramping.
(3) Avoid Valsalva's maneuver: may exacerbate condition.

e. Urinary changes: pressure on bladder causes frequent urination; increased incidence of reflux, urinary tract infections.

f. Respiratory changes: elevation of the diaphragm with widening of thoracic cage; hyperventilation, dyspnea may be experienced with mild exercise during late pregnancy.

g. Cardiovascular changes: increased blood volume; increased venous pressure in the lower extremities; increased heart rate and cardiac output, decreased blood pressure due to venous distensibility.
(1) Teach safe progression of aerobic exercises.
(a) Exercise in moderation, with frequent rests.
(b) Stress use of familiar activities; avoidance of unfamiliar.
(c) Postpartum: emphasize gradual return to previous level of activity.
(2) Stress gentle stretching, adequate warm-ups and cool-downs.
(3) Teach ankle pumps for lower extremity edema (late-stage pregnancy); elevate legs to assist in venous return.
(4) Wear loose, comfortable clothing.

h. Altered thermoregulation: increased basal metabolic rate; increased heat production.

Pregnancy-Related Pathologies

1. Diastasis recti abdominis.

a. Lateral separation or split of the rectus abdominis; separation from midline (linea alba) greater than 2 cm is significant; associated with loss of abdominal wall support, increased back pain.

b. Physical therapy interventions.
(1) Teach protection of abdominal musculature: avoid abdominal exercises, e.g., full sit-ups or bilateral straight leg raising.
(2) Resume abdominal exercises when separation is less than 2 cm: teach safe abdominal strengthening exercises, e.g., partial sit-ups (knees bent), pelvic tilts; utilize hands to support abdominal wall.

2. Pelvic floor disorders.

a. The result of weakening of pelvic floor muscles (pubococcygeal [PC] muscles).

b. PC muscles normally function to support the vagina, urinary bladder, and rectum and help maintain continence of the urethra and rectum.

c. Weakness or laxity of PC muscles typically results from overstretching during pregnancy and childbirth. Further loss of elasticity and muscle tone during later life can result in partial or total organ prolapse. Examples include:
(1) Cystocele: the herniation of the bladder into the vagina.
(2) Rectocele: the herniation of the rectum into the vagina.
(3) Uterine prolapse: the bulging of the uterus into the vagina.

d. PC muscles can also go into spasm.

e. Symptoms include pelvic pain (perivaginal, perirectal, lower abdominal quadrant), urinary incontinence, and pain with sexual intercourse.

Red Flags: Pain can radiate down the posterior thigh.

f. Surgical correction is often required, depending on degree of prolapse.

g. Physical therapy intervention (pelvic floor rehabilitation).
(1) Observe for: urinary frequency and urgency, painful urination, painful defecation; low back and perineal pain with prolapse.
(2) Teach pelvic floor exercises (Kegel's exercises) to strengthen the PC muscles is indicated.
(3) Postural education and muscle reeducation, pelvic mobilization, and stretching of tight lower extremity (LE) muscles are also important components.

3. **Low back and pelvic pain.**
   a. Physical therapy interventions
      (1) Teach proper body mechanics.
      (2) Balance rest with activity.
      (3) Emphasize use of a firm mattress.
      (4) Massage, modalities for pain (no deep heat).

4. **Sacroiliac dysfunction.**
   a. Secondary to postural changes, ligamentous laxity.
   b. Symptoms include posterior pelvic pain; pain in buttocks, may radiate into posterior thigh or knee.
   c. Associated with prolonged sitting, standing, or walking.
   d. Physical therapy interventions.
      (1) External stabilization, e.g., sacroiliac support belt, may help reduce pain.
      (2) Avoid single-limb weight bearing: may aggravate sacroiliac dysfunction.

5. **Varicose veins.**
   a. Physical therapy interventions.
      (1) Elevate extremities; avoid crossing legs which may press on veins.
      (2) Use of elastic support stockings may help.

6. **Preeclampsia.**
   a. Pregnancy-induced, acute hypertension after the 24th week of gestation.
   b. May be mild or severe.
   c. Evaluate for symptoms of hypertension, edema, sudden excessive weight gain, headache, visual disturbances, or hyperreflexia.
   d. Initiate prompt physician referral.

7. **Cesarean childbirth.**
   a. Surgical delivery of the fetus by an incision through the abdominal and uterine walls; indicated in pelvic disproportion, failure of the birth process to progress, fetal or maternal distress, or other complications.
   b. Physical therapy interventions.
      (1) Postoperative TENS can be used for incisional pain; electrodes are placed parallel to the incision.
      (2) Prevent postsurgical pulmonary complications: assist patient in breathing, coughing.
      (3) Postcesarean exercises.
         (a) Gentle abdominal exercises; provide incisional support with pillow.
         (b) Pelvic floor exercises: labor and pushing is typically present before surgery.
         (c) Postural exercises; precautions about heavy lifting for 4–6 weeks.
      (4) Ambulation.
      (5) Prevent incisional adhesions: friction massage.

Disorders of the Female Reproductive System

1. **Endometriosis.**
   a. Characterized by ectopic growth and function of endometrial tissue outside of the uterus. Common sites include ovaries, fallopian tubes, broad ligaments, uterosacral ligaments, pelvis, vagina, or intestines.
      (1) The ectopic tissue responds to hormonal influences but is not able to be shed as uterine tissue is during menstruation.
      (2) Endometrial tissue can lead to cysts and rupture, producing peritonitis and adhesions as well as adhesions and obstruction.
   b. Symptoms include pain, dysmenorrheal, dyspareunia (abnormal pain during sexual intercourse), and infertility.
   c. Red Flags: Patients may complain of back pain. Endometrial implants on muscle (e.g., psoas major, pelvic floor muscles) may produce pain with palpation or contraction.
   d. Treatment involves pain management, endometrial suppression, and surgery.

2. **Pelvic inflammatory disease (PID.)**
   a. An inflammation of the upper reproductive tract involving the uterus (endometritis), fallopian tubes (salpingitis), or ovaries (oophoritis).
   b. PID is caused by a polymicrobial agent that ascends through the endocervical canal.
   c. Symptoms include lower abdominal pain that typically starts after a menstrual cycle, purulent cervical discharge, and painful cervix. Fever, elevated WBC count, and increased ESR (erythrocyte sedimentation rate) are present.
   d. Complications can include pelvic adhesions, infertility, ectopic pregnancy, chronic pain, and abscesses.
   e. Treatment involves antibiotic therapy to treat the infection and prevent complications.

Overview: The Male Reproductive System

1. **Anatomy/Physiology.**
   a. The male reproductive system is composed of paired testes, genital ducts, accessory glands, and penis.
   b. The testes, or male gonads, are located in the scrotum, paired egg-shaped sacs located outside the abdominal cavity. They produce male sex hormones (testosterone) and spermatozoa (male germ cells).
   c. The accessory glands (seminal vesicles, prostate gland, and bulbourethral glands) prepare sperm for ejaculation.
   d. The ductal system (epididymides, vas deferens, and ejaculatory ducts) stores and transports sperm.
   e. The urethra, enclosed in the penis, functions in the elimination of urine and semen.
   f. Sperm production requires an environment that is 2°–3°C lower than body temperature.
   g. Testosterone and other male sex hormones (androgens).

(1) During development, induce differentiation of the male genital tract.
(2) Stimulate development of primary and secondary sex characteristics during puberty and maintains them during life.
(3) Promote protein metabolism, musculoskeletal growth, and subcutaneous fat distribution (anabolic effects).

h. The hypothalamus and anterior pituitary gland maintain endocrine via gonadotropic hormones (follicle-stimulating hormone [FSH] and luteinizing hormone [LH]).
(1) FSH initiates spermatogenesis.
(2) LH regulates testosterone production.

Disorders of the Male Reproductive System

1. Erectile dysfunction (ED) (impotence).

a. The inability to achieve and maintain erection for sexual intercourse.

b. Organic causes.
(1) Neurogenic causes: stroke, cerebral trauma, spinal cord injury, multiple sclerosis, Parkinson's disease.
(2) Hormonal causes: decreased androgen levels with hypogonadism, hypothyroidism, and hypopituitarism.
(3) Vascular causes: hypertension, coronary heart disease, hyperlipidemia, cigarette smoking, diabetes mellitus, pelvic irradiation.
(4) Drug-induced: antidepressants, antipsychotics, antiandrogens, antihypertensives, amphetamines, alcohol.
(5) Aging increases risk of ED.

c. Psychogenic causes.
(1) Performance anxiety.
(2) Depression and psychiatric disorders (schizophrenia).

d. Surgical causes.
(1) Transurethral procedures.
(2) Radical prostatectomy.
(3) Proctocolectomy.
(4) Abdominoperineal resection.

e. Advancing age.

f. Treatment requires accurate identification and remediation of specific causes of ED.

g. Medications are available to improve function (e.g., sildenafil [Viagra]).

2. Prostatitis.

a. infection and inflammation of the prostate gland.

b. Types include acute bacterial, chronic prostatitis, and nonbacterial.
(1) Acute bacterial prostatitis involves bacterial urinary tract infection (UTI) and is associated with catheterization and multiple sex partners. Symptoms include urinary frequency, urgency, nocturia, dysuria, urethral discharge, fever and chills, malaise, myalgia and arthralgia, and pain.
Red Flags: Dull, aching pain may be found in the lower abdominal, rectal, lower back, sacral, or groin regions.
(2) Chronic prostatitis can also be bacterial in origin and is associated with recurrent UTI. Symptoms include urinary frequency and urgency, myalgia and arthralgia, and pain in the low back or perineal region.
(3) Nonbacterial inflammatory prostatitis produces pain in the penis, testicles, and scrotum; painful ejaculation; low back pain or pain in the inner thighs; urinary symptoms; decreased libido; and impotence.

c. Because the prostate encircles the urethra, obstruction of urinary flow can result.

Renal and Urological Systems

Overview

1. Anatomy.

a. Kidneys are paired, bean-shaped organs located outside of the peritoneal cavity (retroperitoneal) in the posterior upper abdomen on each side of the vertebral column at the level of T12–L2.

b. Each kidney is multilobular; each lobule is composed of more than a million nephrons (the functional units of the kidney).

c. Each nephron consists of a glomerulus that filters the blood and nephron tubules. Water, electrolytes, and other substances vital for function are reabsorbed into the bloodstream, while other waste products are secreted into the tubules for elimination.

d. The renal pelvis is a wide, funnel-shaped structure at the upper end of the urethra that drains the kidney into the lower urinary tract (bladder and urethra).

e. The bladder is a membranous sac that collects urine and is located behind the symphysis pubis.

f. The ureter extends from the renal pelvis to the bladder and moves urine via peristaltic action.
g. The urethra extends from the bladder to an external orifice for elimination of urine from the body.
h. In females, proximity of the urethra to vaginal and rectal openings increases the likelihood of UTI.

2. Functions of the kidney

a. Regulates the composition and pH of body fluids through reabsorption and elimination; controls mineral (sodium, potassium, hydrogen, chloride, and bicarbonate ions) and water balance.
b. Eliminates metabolic wastes (urea, uric acid, creatinine) and drugs/drug metabolites.
c. Assists in blood pressure regulation through renninangiotensin-aldosterone mechanisms and salt and water elimination.
d. Contributes to bone metabolic function by activating vitamin D and regulating calcium and phosphate conservation and elimination.
e. Controls the production of red blood cells in the bone marrow through the production of erythropoietin.
f. The glomerular filtration rate (GFR) is the amount of filtrate that is formed each minute as blood moves through the glomeruli and serves as an important gauge of renal function.
   (1) Regulated by arterial blood pressure and renal blood flow.
   (2) Measured clinically by obtaining creatinine levels in blood and urine samples.
   (3) Normal creatinine clearance is 115–125 mL/min.
g. Blood urea nitrogen (BUN) is urea produced in the liver as a by-product of protein metabolism that is eliminated by the kidneys.
   (1) BUN levels are elevated with increased protein intake, gastrointestinal bleeding, and dehydration.
   (2) BUN-creatinine ratio is abnormal in liver disease.

3. Normal values of urine (urinalysis findings).

a. Color: yellow-amber.
b. Clarity: clear.
c. Specific gravity: 1.010–1.025 with normal fluid intake.
d. pH: 4.6–8.0; average is 6 (acid).
e. Protein: 0–8 mg/dL.
f. Sugar: 0.

Urinary Regulation of Fluids and Electrolytes

1. Homeostasis. Regulated through thirst mechanisms and renal function via circulating antidiuretic hormone (ADH).

2. Fluid imbalances.

a. Daily fluid requirements vary based on presence or absence of such factors as sweating, air temperature, and fever.
b. Dehydration: excessive loss of body fluids; fluid output exceeds fluid intake.
   (1) Causes: poor intake; excess output: profuse sweating, vomiting, diarrhea, and diuretics; closely linked to sodium deficiency.
   (2) Observe for: poor skin turgor, dry mucous membranes, headache, irritability, postural hypotension, incoordination, lethargy, disorientation.
   (3) May lead to uremia and hypovolemic shock (stupor and coma).
   (4) Decreased exercise capacity, especially in hot environments.
c. Edema: an excess of body fluids with expansion of interstitial fluid volume.
   (1) Causes.
      (a) Increased capillary pressure: heart failure, kidney disease, premenstrual retention, pregnancy, environmental heat stress; venous obstruction (liver disease, acute pulmonary edema, venous thrombosis).
      (b) Decreased colloidal osmotic pressure: decreased production or loss of plasma proteins (protein-losing kidney disease, liver disease, starvation, malnutrition).
      (c) Increased capillary permeability: inflammation, allergic reactions, malignancy, tissue injury, burns.
      (d) Obstruction of lymphatic flow.
   (2) Observe for swelling of the ankles and feet, weight gain; headache, blurred vision; muscle cramps and twitches.
      (a) Edema can be restrictive, producing a tourniquet effect.
      (b) Tissues are susceptible to injury and delayed healing.
      (c) Pitting edema occurs when the amount of interstitial fluid exceeds the absorptive capacity of tissues.

3. Potassium.

a. Normal serum level is 3.5–5.5 mEq/L.
b. Hypokalemia
   (1) Causes: deficient potassium or excessive loss due to diarrhea, vomiting, metabolic acidosis, renal tubular disease, alkalosis.
   (2) Observe for: muscle weakness, aches, fatigue; cardiac arrhythmias; abdominal distention; nausea and vomiting.
c. Hyperkalemia
   (1) Causes: inadequate secretion with acute renal failure, kidney disease, metabolic acidosis, diabetic ketoacidosis, sickle cell anemia, SLE.
   (2) Often symptomless until very high levels. Observe for: muscle weakness, arrhythmias, ECG changes (tall T wave, prolonged P-R interval and QRS duration).

4. Sodium.

a. Normal serum level is 135–146 mEq/L.
b. Hyponatremia

(1) Causes: water intoxication (excess extracellular water) associated with excess intake or excess ADH (Tumors, endocrine disorders).

(2) Observe for: confusion, decreased mental alertness can progress to convulsions, signs of increased intracerebral pressure; poor motor coordination; sleepiness; anorexia.

c. Hypernatremia

(1) Causes: occurs with water deficits (not salt excesses) with dehydration, insufficient water intake.

(2) Observe for: circulatory congestion (pitting edema, excessive weight gain); pulmonary edema with dyspnea; hypertension, tachycardia; agitation, restlessness, convulsions.

5. Calcium.

a. Normal total calcium in blood is 8.4-10.4 mg/dL.

b. Hypocalcemia

(1) Causes: reduced albumin levels, hyperphosphatemia, hypoparathyroidism, malabsorption of calcium and vitamin D, alkalosis, acute pancreatitis, vitamin D deficiency.

(2) Observe for: muscle cramps, tetany, spasms; paresthesias; anxiety, irritability, twitching convulsion; arrhythmias, hypotension.

c. Hypercalcemia

(1) Causes: hyperparathyroidism, tumors, hyperthyroidism, vitamin A intoxication.

(2) Observe for: fatigue, depression, mental confusion, nausea/vomiting, increased urination, occasional cardiac arrhythmias.

6. Magnesium.

a. Normal serum level is 1.8-2.4 mg/dL.

b. Hypomagnesemia

(1) Causes; hemodialysis, blood transfusions, chronic renal disease, hepatic cirrhosis (alchololism), chronic pancreatitis, hypoparathyroidism, malabsorption syndromes, severe burns, excess loss of body fluid.

(2) Observe for: hyperirritability, confusion; leg and foot cramps.

c. Hypermagnesemia

(1) Causes: renal failure, diabetic acidosis, hypothyroidism, Addison's disease, with dehydration and with use of antacids.

(2) Observe for: hyporeflexia, muscle weakness, drowsiness, lethargy, confusion, bradycardia, hypotension.

7. Acid-base balance.

a. Balance of acids and bases in the body (normally a ratio of 20 base to 1 acid; normal serum pH is 7.35–7.45 [slightly alkaline]); regulated by blood buffer systems (the lungs and the kidneys).

b. Metabolic acidosis: a depletion of bases or an accumulation of acids; blood pH falls below 7.35.

(1) Causes: diabetes, renal insufficiency or failure, diarrhea.

(2) Observe for: hyperventilation (compensatory), deep respirations; weakness, muscular twitching; malaise, nausea, vomiting and diarrhea; headache; dry skin and mucous membranes, poor skin turgor.

(3) May lead to stupor and coma (death).

c. Metabolic alkalosis: an increase in bases or a reduction of acids; blood pH rises above 7.45.

(1) Causes: excess vomiting, excess diuretics, hypokalemia; peptic ulcer, and excessive intake of antacids.

(2) Observe for: hypoventilation (compensatory), depressed respirations; dysrhythmias; prolonged vomiting, diarrhea; weakness, muscle twitching; irritability, agitation, convulsions, and coma (death).

d. Respiratory acidosis: CO_2 retention, impaired alveolar ventilation.

(1) Causes: hypoventilation, drugs/oversedation, chronic pulmonary disease (e.g., emphysema, asthma, bronchitis, pneumonia) or hypermetabolism (sepsis, burns).

(2) Observe for: dyspnea, hyperventilation cyanosis; restlessness, headache.

(3) May lead to disorientation, stupor and coma, death.

e. Respiratory alkalosis: diminished CO_2, alveolar hyperventilation.

(1) Causes: anxiety attack with hyperventilation, hypoxia (emphysema, pneumonia), impaired lung expansion, congestive heart failure (CHF), pulmonary embolism, diffuse liver or CNS disease, salicylate poisoning, extreme stress (stimulation of respiratory center).

(2) Observe for: tachypnea, dizziness, anxiety, difficulty concentrating, numbness and tingling, blurred vision, diaphoresis, muscle cramps, twitching or tetany, weakness, arrhythmias, convulsions.

Renal and Urological Disorders

1. Urinary tract infections (UTIs).

a. Infection of the urinary tract with microorganisms.

b. Lower UTI: cystitis (inflammation and infection of the bladder) or urethritis (inflammation and infection of the urethra).

(1) Usually secondary to ascending urinary tract infections; may also involve kidneys and ureters.

(2) Associated with symptoms of urinary frequency, urgency, burning sensation during urination. Urine may be cloudy and foul smelling. Pain is noted in suprapubic, lower abdominal, or groin area, depending on site of infection.

c. Upper UTI: pyelonephritis (inflammation and infection of one or both kidneys).
   (1) Associated with symptoms of systemic involvement: fever, chills, malaise, headache, tenderness and pain over kidneys (back pain), tenderness over the costovertebal angle (Murphy's sign). Symptoms also include frequent and burning urination; nausea and vomiting may occur.
   (2) Palpitation or percussion over the kidney typically causes pain.
   (3) Can be acute or chronic; generally more serious than lower UTI.

d. Increased risk of UTI in persons with autoimmunity, urinary obstruction and reflux, neurogenic bladder and catheterization, diabetes, and kidney transplantation. Older adults and women are also at increased risk for UTI.

2. Renal cystic disease.

a. Renal cysts are fluid-filled cavities that form along the nephron and can lead to renal degeneration or obstruction.

b. Types include polycystic, medullary sponge, acquired, and simple renal cysts.

c. Symptoms can include pain, hematuria, and hypertension. Fever can occur with associated infection, Cysts can rupture producing hematuria. Simple cysts are generally asymptomatic.

3. Obstructive disorders.

a. Developmental defects, renal calculi, prostatic hyperplasia or cancer, scar tissue from inflammation, tumors, and infection.

b. Pressure build-up backwards from site of obstruction; can result in kidney damage. Dilation of ureters and renal pelves may be used to reduce obstruction. Observe for pain, signs and symptoms of UTI, and hypertension.

c. Renal calculi (kidney stones): crystalline structures formed from normal components of urine (calcium, magnesium ammonium phosphate, uric acid, and cystine).
   (1) Etiological influences include concentration of stone components in urine and a urinary environment conducive to stone formation.
   (2) Symptoms include renal colic pain (pain from a stone lodged in the ureter made worse by stretching the collecting system). Pain may radiate to the lower abdominal quadrant, bladder area, and perineal area (scrotum in the male and labia in the female). Nausea and vomiting are common and the skin may be cool and clammy.
   (3) Extracorporeal shock wave lithotripsy (ESWL) is used to break up stones into fragments to allow for easy passage.
   (4) Treatment/prevention can also include increased fluid intake, thiazide diuretics, dietary restriction of foods high in oxalate, acidification or alkalinization of urine depending on type of stone.

4. Renal failure.

a. Acute renal failure: sudden loss of kidney function with resulting elevation in serum urea and creatinine.
   (1) Etiology: may be due to circulatory disruption to kidneys, toxic substances, bacterial toxins, acute obstruction, or trauma.

b. Chronic renal failure: progressive loss of kidney function leading to end-stage failure.
   (1) Etiology: may result from prolonged acute urinary tract obstruction and infection, diabetes, systemic lupus erythematosus, uncontrolled hypertension.
   (2) Uremia: an end-stage toxic condition resulting from renal insufficiency and retention of nitrogenous wastes in blood; symptoms can include anorexia, nausea, and mental confusion.
   (3) Red Flags: May lead to multisystem abnormalities and failure.
      (a) Dizziness, headaches, anxiety, memory loss, inability to concentrate, convulsions, and coma.
      (b) Hypertension, dyspnea on exertion, heart failure.
      (c) Chronic pain: ischemic leg pain, painful cramps.
      (d) Edema: peripheral edema, pulmonary edema.
      (e) Muscle weakness: peripheral neuropathy, cramping, restless legs.
      (f) Skeletal: osteomalacia, osteoporosis, bone pain, fracture.
      (g) Skin: pallor, ecchymosis, pruritus, dry skin.
      (h) Anemia, tendency to bleed easily.
      (i) Decreased endurance; functional losses.
      (j) Autonomic nervous system dysfunction: decreased heart rate, blood pressure; orthostatic hypotension.

c. Dialysis: process of diffusing blood across a semipermeable membrane for the purposes of removal of toxic substances; maintains fluid, electrolyte, and acid-base balance in presence of renal failure; peritoneal, or renal (hemodialysis).
   (1) Dialysis disequilibrium: symptoms of nausea, vomiting, drowsiness, headache, and seizures; the result of rapid changes after beginning dialysis.
   (2) Dialysis dementia: signs of cerebral dysfunction (e.g., speech difficulties, mental confusion, myoclonus, seizures, eventually death); the result of long-standing years of dialysis treatment.
   (3) Locate dialysis shunts: taking BP at the shunt site is contraindicated.
   (4) Locate peritoneal catheters (if used): avoid trauma to area.

(5) Examine for multisystem dysfunction: vital signs, strength, sensation, ROM, function, and endurance.

d. Transplantation is a major treatment choice (renal allograft).

5. Urinary incontinence.

a. Inability to retain urine; the result of loss of sphincter control; may be acute (due to transient causes, e.g., cystitis) or persistent (e.g., stroke, dementia).

b. Types.

(1) Stress incontinence: sudden release of urine due to:

(a) Increases in intra-abdominal pressure, e.g., coughing, laughing, exercise, straining, obesity.

(b) Weakness and laxity of pelvic floor musculature, sphincter weakness, e.g., postpartum incontinence, menopause, damage to pudendal nerve.

(2) Urge incontinence: bladder begins contracting and urine is leaked after sensation of bladder fullness is perceived; an inability to delay voiding to reach toilet due to:

(a) Detrusor muscle instability or hyperreflexia, e.g., stroke.

(b) Sensory instability: hypersensitive bladder.

(3) Overflow incontinence: bladder continuously leaks secondary to urinary retention (an overdistended bladder or incomplete emptying of bladder) due to:

(a) Anatomical obstruction, e.g., prostate enlargement.

(b) Acontractile bladder, e.g., spinal cord injury, diabetes.

(c) Neurogenic bladder, e.g., multiple sclerosis, suprasacral spinal lesions.

(4) Functional incontinence: leakage associated with inability or unwillingness to toilet due to:

(a) Impaired cognition (dementia); depression, e.g., Alzheimer's disease.

(b) Impaired physical functioning, e.g., stroke.

(c) Environmental barriers.

c. Management.

(1) Dietary management: control of food and beverages that aggravate the bladder or incontinence (e.g., citrus fruit or juices, caffeine, chocolate); control fluid intake.

(2) Medical management.

(a) Identify and treat acute, reversible problems, e.g., cystometry.

(b) Drug therapy for urge, stress, and overflow incontinence, e.g., estrogen with phenylpropanolamine.

(c) Control of medications that may aggravate incontinence, e.g., diuretics for CHF, anticholinergic or psychotropic drugs.

(d) Catheterization: used for overflow incontinence and other types if unresponsive to other treatments and skin integrity is threatened; associated with high rates of urinary tract infection.

(e) Surgery: bladder neck suspension, removal of prostate obstructions; suprapubic cystostomy.

(3) Bladder training: prompted voiding to restore a pattern of voiding.

(a) Involves toileting schedule: taking patient to bathroom at regular intervals.

(b) May also include intermittent catheterization, e.g., for patients with overdistention, persistent retention (e.g., multiple sclerosis).

d. Examination.

(1) Symptoms of incontinence: onset and duration, urgency, frequency, timing of episodes/causative factors.

(2) Strength of pelvic floor muscles using a perineometer.

(3) Functional mobility, environmental factors.

e. Physical therapy goals, outcomes, and interventions for stress and urge incontinence.

(1) Teach pelvic floor muscle exercises (pubococcygeus muscle): used to treat stress incontinence.

(a) Kegel's exercises: active, strengthening exercises; type 1 works on holding contractions, progressing to 10-second holds, rest 10 seconds between contractions; type 2 works on quick contractions to shut off flow of urine, 10–80 repetitions a day. Avoid squeezing buttocks or contracting abdominals (bearing down).

(b) Functional electrical stimulation: for muscle reeducation if patient is unable to initiate active contractions.

(c) Biofeedback: uses pressure recordings to reinforce active contractions, relax bladder.

(d) Progressive strengthening: use of weighted vaginal cones for home exercises or pelvic floor exerciser.

(e) Incorporating Kegel's exercise into everyday life: e.g., with lifting, coughing, changing positions.

(2) Provide behavioral training.

(a) Record keeping: patients are asked to keep a history of their voiding (voiding diary).

(b) Education: regarding anatomy, physiology, reasons for muscle weakness, incontinence; avoidance of Valsalva's maneuver, heavy resistance exercises.

(3) Functional mobility training as needed. Ensure independence in sit-to-stand transitions, ambulation, and safe toilet transfers.

(4) Environmental modifications as needed: e.g., toilet rails, raised toilet seat, or commode.

(5) Maintain adequate skin condition.

(a) Teach appropriate skin care, maintain toileting schedule.
(b) Adequate protection: adult diapers, underpads.

(6) Provide psychological support: emotional and social consequences of incontinence are significant.

Endocrine and Metabolic Systems

Overview of the Endocrine System

1. **Hormonal regulation.**
   a. The endocrine system uses hormones (chemical messengers) to relay information to cells and organs and regulate many of the body functions (digestion, use of nutrients, growth and development, electrolyte and water balance, and reproductive functions).
   b. The hypothalamus and pituitary gland along with the nervous system comprise the central network that exerts control over many other glands in the body with wide-ranging functions. Endocrine functions are also closely linked with the immune system.
   c. Hormones bind to specific receptor sites which are linked to specific systems and functions.
   d. The hypothalamus controls release of pituitary hormones (corticotropin-releasing hormone [CRH], thyrotropin-releasing hormone [TRH], growth hormone–releasing hormone [GHRH], and somatostatin).
   e. The anterior pituitary gland controls the release of growth hormone (GH), adrenocorticotropic hormone (ACTH), follicle-stimulating hormone (FSH), luteinizing hormone (LH), and prolactin.
   f. The posterior pituitary gland controls the release of antidiuretic hormone (ADH) and oxytocin.
   g. The adrenal cortex controls the release of mineral corticosteroids (aldosterone), glucocorticoids (cortisol), adrenal androgens (dehydroepiandrosterone (DHEA), and androstenedione.
   h. The adrenal medulla controls the release of epinephrine and norepinephrine.
   i. The thyroid controls the release of triiodothyronine and thyroxine. Thyroid C cells control the release of calcitonin.
   j. The parathyroid glands control the release of parathyroid hormone (PTH).
   k. The pancreatic islet cells control the release of insulin, glucagons, and somatostatin.
   l. The kidney controls the release of 1, 25-dihydroxy vitamin D.
   m. The ovaries control the release of estrogen and progesterone.
   n. The testes control the release of androgens (testosterone).

Overview of the Metabolic System

1. **Normal glucose control.** The result of nutrient, neural, and hormonal regulation.
2. **Hormones.** Released by islets of Langerhans in pancreas.
   a. Insulin: allows uptake of glucose from the bloodstream; suppresses hepatic glucose production, lowering plasma glucose levels. Secreted by the beta cells.
   b. Glucagon: stimulates hepatic glucose production to raise glucose levels, especially in fasting state. Secreted by the alpha cells.
   c. Amylin: modulates rate of nutrient delivery (gastric emptying); suppresses release of glucagon. Secreted by the beta cells.
   d. Somatostatin: acts locally to depress secretion of both insulin and glycogen; decreases motility of stomach, duodenum, and gall bladder; decreases secretion and absorption of GI tract. Secreted by the delta cells.

Diabetes Mellitus (DM)

1. **Characteristics.**
   a. A complex disorder of carbohydrate, fat, and protein metabolism caused by deficiency or absence of insulin secretion by the beta cells of the pancreas or by defects of the insulin receptors.
   b. May be acquired, familial, idiopathic, neurogenic, or nephrogenic. Possible viral/autoimmune and genetic etiology. Represents 5%–10% of DM.
   c. Types.
      (1) Type 1 diabetes mellitus (T1DM); also known as insulin-dependent, juvenile-onset diabetes. Characteristics include:
         (a) Decrease in size and number of islet cells resulting in absolute deficiency in insulin secretion.
         (b) Usually occurs in children and young adults. Long preclinical period, often with abrupt onset of symptoms around the age of puberty.
         (c) Etiology: caused by autoimmune abnormalities, genetic causes, or environmental causes.

CHAPTER 6

(d) Insulin-dependent: requires insulin delivery by injection, insulin pump, or inhalation.
(e) Prone to ketoacidosis. Presence of ketone bodies in the urine, the by-products of fat metabolism (ketonuria).

(2) Type 2 diabetes mellitus (T2DM) results from inadequate utilization of insulin (insulin resistance) and progressive beta cell dysfunction; also known as adult-onset or maturity-onset diabetes. Represents 90%–95% of DM cases. Characteristics include:
(a) Gradual onset; may have familial pattern.
(b) Usually not insulin dependent.
(c) Individual is not prone to ketoacidosis (may form ketones with stress).
(d) Etiology: a progressive disease caused by a combination of factors, including:
- Insulin resistance in muscle and adipose tissue.
- Progressive decline in pancreatic insulin production.
- Excessive hepatic glucose production.
- Inappropriate glucagon secretion.
- Decreased production of gastrointestinal incretins.

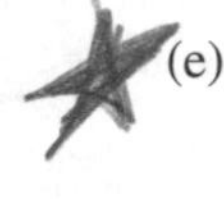

(e) Linked to obesity and older adults (typically over the age of 40). Can occur in nonobese individuals with increased percentage of body fat in the abdominal region.

d. Insulin resistance and metabolic syndrome (insulin resistance syndrome, syndrome X).
(1) A group of risk factors that increase the likelihood of developing heart disease, stroke, and type 2 diabetes. Criteria for diagnosis include three or more of the following:
(a) Abdominal obesity: waist circumference > 40 inches in men or > 35 inches in women.
(b) Elevated triglycerides: triglyceride level of 150 mg/dL or higher.
(c) Low HDL cholesterol or being on medicine to treat low HDL: HDL level lower than 40 mg/dL in men or 50 mg/dL in women.
(d) Elevated blood pressure: systolic BP 130 mm Hg or higher and/or diastolic pressure 85 mm Hg or higher.
(e) Fasting plasma glucose level > 110 mg/dL. A level between 100 and 125 mg/dL is considered prediabetes.
(2) Lifestyle changes can reverse or reduce the chance of developing metabolic syndrome: weight loss, exercise, medications to control triglycerides, cholesterol, blood pressure, or glucose.

e. Secondary diabetes: associated with other conditions (pancreatic disease or removal of pancreatic tissue), endocrine disease (e.g., acromegaly, Cushing's syndrome, pheochromocytoma), drugs (e.g., some diuretics, diazoxide, glucocorticoids, levodopa), and chemical agents.

f. Impaired glucose tolerance (IGT): asymptomatic or borderline diabetes with abnormal response to oral glucose test. Ten to 15% of individuals will convert to type 2 diabetes within 10 years.

g. Gestational diabetes mellitus (GDM): glucose intolerance associated with pregnancy; most likely in third trimester.

2. Classic signs and symptoms of DM.
a. Elevated blood sugar (hyperglycemia).
b. Elevated sugar in urine (glycosuria).
c. Excessive excretion of urine (polyuria).
d. Excessive thirst (polydipsia).
e. Excessive hunger (polyphagia) and unexplained weight loss (usually type 1).

3. Complications of DM.
a. Microvascular disease.
(1) Retinopathy.
(2) Renal disease.
(3) Polyneuropathy.
b. Macrovascular disease: dyslipidemia (accelerated atherosclerosis).
(1) Stroke (CVA).
(2) Myocardial infarction (MI).
(3) Peripheral arterial disease (PAD).
c. Integumentary impairments: including degenerative connective tissue changes; anhidrosis; increased risk of ulcers and infections.
d. Musculoskeletal impairments.
(1) Joint stiffness and increased risk of contractures.
(2) Increased risk of adhesive capsulitis of shoulder, tenosynovitis, plantar fasciitis.
(3) Increased risk of osteoporosis.
e. Neuromuscular impairments.
(1) Diabetic polyneuropathy.
(a) Symmetrical; stocking and glove distribution.
(b) Distal (long nerves first) progressing to proximal.
(c) Altered sensations; paresthesias, shooting pain; loss of protective sensations.
(d) Motor weakness: foot/ankle weakness initially with balance and gait impairments.
(2) Diabetic autonomic neuropathy (DAN).
(a) Cardiovascular autonomic neuropathy (CAN): resting tachycardia; exercise intolerance with abnormal HR, BP, and cardiac output responses; exercise-induced hypoglycemia; postural hypotension.
(b) Integumentary: anhidrosis, abnormal sweating, dry skin, heat intolerance.
(c) Gastrointestinal: gastroparesis, GERD, diarrhea, constipation.
(d) Metabolic: abnormal or delayed responses to hypoglycemia; lack of awareness of hypoglycemia.

(3) Mononeuropathies: focal nerve damage resulting from vasculitis with ischemia and infarction.
(4) Entrapment neuropathies: resulting from repetitive trauma to superficial nerves.

f. Kidney impairments including kidney failure.
g. Vision impairments including diabetic retinopathy (associated with chronic hyperglycemia) and diabetic macular edema.
h. Liver impairments including fatty liver disease (steatosis).

4. Diagnostic criteria for DM.

a. Symptoms of diabetes plus casual plasma glucose concentration ≥ 200 mg/dL (11.1 mmol/L). "Casual" is defined as any time of day, without regard to time since last meal.
b. Fasting plasma glucose test (FPG) ≥ 126 mg/dL (7 mmol/L). Fasting is defined as no caloric intake for at least 8 hours).
c. 2-hour postload glucose ≥ 200 mg/dL (11.1 mmol/L) during an oral glucose tolerance test (OGTT). OGTT, as described by the World Health Organization, uses a glucose load containing the equivalent of 75 g anhydrous glucose dissolved in water.

5. Medical goals and interventions.

a. Maintain insulin glucose homeostasis.
(1) Frequent monitoring of blood glucose levels.
(2) Dietary control: weight reduction, control of carbohydrate, protein, fat, and calorie intake.
(3) Oral hypoglycemic agents to lower blood glucose; indicated for type 2 diabetes.
(4) Insulin to lower blood glucose via injections, infusion pump, or intraperitoneal dialysis for patients with renal failure. Indicated for type 1 diabetes or for more severe type 2 diabetes.
(5) Maintenance of normal lipid levels.
(6) Control of hypertension.

b. Exercise and physical fitness.
c. Health promotion.

6. Physical therapy goals, outcomes, and interventions.

a. Exercise.
(1) Outcomes of exercise include improved glucose tolerance, increased insulin sensitivity, decreased glycosylated hemoglobin, and decreased insulin requirements. Additional outcomes include improved lipid profiles, BP reduction, weight management, increased physical work capacity, and improved well-being.
(2) Response to exercise is dependent upon adequacy of disease control.

b. Exercise testing is recommended prior to exercise due to increased cardiovascular risk.
c. Exercise prescription—Cardiovascular training (American College of Sports Medicine [ACSM] Guidelines, 2006).
(1) Intensity: 50%–80% of VO_2 max or heart rate reserve (HRR).
(2) Frequency: 3–4 days/week.
(3) Duration: 20–60 minutes.

d. Exercise prescription—Resistance training (ACSM Guidelines, 2006).
(1) Lower resistance, 40%–60% of one repetition max.
(2) One set of exercises for major muscle groups with 10–15 repetitions (progress to 15–20 repetitions).
(3) Minimum frequency 2 days/week; at least 48 hours between sessions.
(4) Proper technique: minimize sustained gripping, static work, and Valsalva's maneuver (essential to decrease risk of hypertensive response).

e. Flexibility exercises.
f. Balance exercises.
g. Red Flags: Exercise precautions.
(1) Monitor glucose levels prior to and following exercise.
(2) Hypoglycemia is the most common problem for patients with diabetes who exercise.
(a) Observe for signs and symptom of hypoglycemia (Box 6-2). Do not exercise if blood glucose is < 70 mg/dL. Provide carbohydrate snack initially (15 g of carbohydrate); have readily available during exercise (15 g carbohydrate for every hour of intense activity).

Box 6-2 ➤ SIGNS AND SYMPTOMS OF HYPOGLYCEMIA (LOW BLOOD SUGAR)

Glucose is low: < 70 mg/dL or a rapid drop in glucose. Onset is rapid (minutes)

Early signs and symptoms:
Pallor
Shakiness/trembling
Sweating
Excessive hunger
Tachycardia and palpitations
Fainting or feeling faint
Dizziness
Fatigue and weakness
Poor coordination and unsteady gait

Late signs and symptoms:
Nervousness and irritability
Headache
Blurred or double vision
Slurred speech
Drowsiness
Inability to concentrate, confusion, delusions
Loss of consciousness and coma

Response: If patient is awake, provide sugar (juice, candy bar, glucose tablets and gel).
If patient unresponsive, seek immediate medical treatment; glucagon injection or intravenous glucose is required.

(b) Hypoglycemia associated with exercise may last as long as 48 hours after exercise. To prevent postexercise hypoglycemia, monitor plasma glucose levels and ingest carbohydrates as needed.

(3) Hyperglycemia: Do not exercise when blood glucose levels are high (fasting glucose > 300 mg/dL) or poorly controlled (ketosis is present with urine test) (Box 6-3).

(4) Do not exercise without eating at least 2 hours before exercise.

(5) Do not exercise without adequate hydration. Maintain hydration during exercise session.

(6) Do not exercise alone. Exercise with a partner or under supervision.

(7) Do not inject short-acting insulin in exercising muscles or sites close to exercising muscles as insulin is absorbed more quickly. Abdominal injection site is preferred.

(8) Do not exercise patients with poorly controlled complications.

(a) Cardiovascular disease, hypertension. May see chronotropic incompetence, blunted systolic BP response, blunted oxygen uptake and anhidrosis. RPE may be used to regulate exercise intensity.

(b) Retinopathy. Avoid activities that dramatically increase BP (> 170 mm Hg systolic BP); avoid pounding or jarring activities.

(c) Neuropathy, nephropathy. Limit weight-bearing exercise for patients with significant neuropathy. There is increased fall risk with balance and gait abnormalities.

(d) Autonomic neuropathy is associated with sudden death and silent ischemia. Monitor for signs and symptoms of silent ischemia due to patient's inability to perceive angina.

Box 6-3 ➤ SIGNS AND SYMPTOMS OF HYPERGLYCEMIA (ABNORMALLY HIGH BLOOD SUGAR)

Glucose is high: > 300 mg/dL. Gradual onset (days).
Weakness
Increased thirst
Dry mouth
Frequent, scant urination
Decrease appetite, nausea/vomiting, abdominal tenderness
Dulled senses, confusion, diminished reflexes, paresthesias.
Flushed, signs of dehydration
Deep, rapid respirations
Pulse: rapid, weak
Fruity odor to the breath (acetone breath)
Hyperglycemic coma

Response: seek immediate medical treatment.

(e) Nephropathy. Limit exercise to low to moderate intensities; discourage strenuous intensities.

(9) Do not exercise in extreme environmental temperatures (very hot or cold).

h. Emphasize proper diabetic foot care: good footwear, hygiene.

i. Patient and family education.

(1) Control of risk factors (obesity, physical inactivity, prolonged stress, and smoking).

(2) Dietary intervention strategies.

(3) Injury prevention strategies.

(4) Self-management strategies.

Obesity

1. Obesity.

a. A condition characterized by excess body fat.

2. Body Mass Index (BMI).

a. Formula for determining obesity.

b. BMI is calculated by dividing an individual's weight in kilograms by the square of the person's height in meters.

c. Criteria: World Health Organization Classification (adopted by National Institutes of Health):

(1) Overweight is defined as a BMI ranging from 25 to 29.9.

(2) Obesity is defined as a BMI ≥ 30.

(3) Morbidly obese is defined as a BMI > 40.

d. Measurement by skin calipers using a fold of skin and subcutaneous fat from various body locations (mid biceps, mid triceps, and subscapular or inguinal areas). Greater than 1 inch is indicative of excess body fat.

3. Scope of problem.

a. A national health problem: overweight (65% of Americans) and obesity (31% of Americans).

b. Health risks associated with obesity: hypertension, hyperlipidemia, type 2 diabetes, cardiovascular disease, stroke, glucose intolerance, type 2 diabetes, gallbladder disease, menstrual irregularities and infertility, and cancer (endometrium, breast, prostate, colon).

c. Waist circumference is used to determine distribution of body fat. Abdominal obesity (central accumulation of fat) is an independent predictor of morbidity and mortality.

d. Childhood obesity: most prevalent nutritional disorder affecting children in United States.

4. Causes.

a. An imbalance when energy intake exceeds energy consumption. Excess calories are consumed, exceeding those expended through exercise and activity.

b. Interaction of psychological and environmental factors (behavioral, cultural, social, economic factors).

Observe for depression, smoking cessation, yo-yo dieting with fluctuations in weight.

c. Genetic factors (biochemical defects): may account for about 30%–40% of BMI.

d. Endocrine and metabolic disorders (e.g., metabolic syndrome).

5. Prevention and management.

a. Lifestyle modification: combination of dietary changes to reduce body weight combined with increased physical activity.

(1) Personalized diet with reduced caloric intake: fat intake of < 30% of total energy intake, emphasis on fruits, vegetables, whole grains, and lean protein.

(2) Personalized exercise program, including stretching exercises, resistance exercises, and aerobic exercises.

(3) Instruction in self-monitoring of exercise responses (heart rate, perceived exertion).

b. Behavior therapy: self-monitoring of eating habits and physical activity (use of a food and exercise diary); stress management, relapse prevention, and social support.

c. Pharmacology: over-the-counter (OTC) and prescriptive weight loss therapy (e.g., sibutramine, orlistat).

d. Surgery (bariatric surgery): limited to persons with BMI over 40 (or individuals with comorbid conditions and a BMI over 35). Procedures include gastric banding and gastric bypass.

6. Exercise evaluation (ACSM guidelines).

a. Individuals are typically sedentary with low physical work capacities.

b. Interviews should include goals, past exercise history, perceived barriers to exercise participation, and exercise likes and dislikes.

c. Exercise testing: submaximal, low initial workload (typically 2–3 METs), small workload increments per test stage (0.5–1.0 METs).

d. Use of leg or arm ergometry may enhance testing performance.

e. Use of proper size equipment: wide seat ergometer, large-size BP cuff.

7. Exercise prescription (ACSM Guidelines).

a. Start slowly, provide adequate warm-ups and cool-downs. Initial exercise intensity should be moderate (40%–60% VO_2R or HRR).

b. Increase intensity gradually in order to prevent injury: moderate-intensity activity (50%–70% VO_2R or HRR).

c. Frequency: 5–7 days/week.

d. Duration: 45–60 minutes.

e. Use of circuit training in order to combine resistive training with aerobic training activities. Provide with short rests between activities/exercise bouts.

f. Involve the patient in activity selection, incorporating individual preferences and likes.

g. Select adequate footwear and orthotic devices as needed.

h. Aquatic exercise programs can assist in reducing musculoskeletal strain and injury.

i. Use of special bariatric equipment: wide seats on ergometers, bariatric lifts.

8. Red Flags: Exercise precautions and risks.

a. Typically exhibit cardiopulmonary compromise: shortness of breath, elevated blood pressure, and angina.

b. Typically exhibit altered biomechanics affecting hips, knees, ankle/foot; back and joint pain; and increased risk of orthopedic injury.

c. Increased risk of skin breakdown due to shear forces.

d. Increased heat intolerance, risk of hyperthermia and heat exhaustion.

e. Increased risk of therapist injury: poor body mechanics, inadequate assistance during transfers and lifts.

Thyroid Disorders

1. Hypothyroidism. Decreased activity of the thyroid gland with deficient thyroid secretion.

a. Metabolic processes are slowed.

b. Etiology: decreased thyroid-releasing hormone secreted by the hypothalamus or by the pituitary gland; atrophy of the thyroid gland; chronic autoimmune thyroiditis (Hashimoto's disease); overdosage with antithyroid medication.

c. Symptoms include weight gain, mental and physical lethargy, dry skin and hair, low blood pressure, constipation, intolerance to cold, and goiter.

d. If untreated, leads to myxedema (severe hypothyroidism) with symptoms of swelling of hands, feet, face. Can lead to coma and death.

e. Treatment: life-long thyroid replacement therapy.

f. Red Flags: Can result in exercise intolerance, weakness, apathy; exercise-induced myalgia; reduced cardiac output.

2. Hyperthyroidism. Hyperactivity of the thyroid gland.

a. Etiology unknown.

b. Thyroid gland is typically enlarged and secretes greater than normal amounts of thyroid hormone (thyroxine), e.g., Graves' disease, thyroid storm, thyrotoxicosis.

c. Metabolic processes are accelerated.

d. Symptoms include nervousness, hyperreflexia, tremor, hunger, weight loss, fatigue, heat intolerance, palpitations, tachycardia, and diarrhea.

e. Treatment: antithyroid drugs.

f. Radioactive iodine may also be prescribed or surgical ablation may be necessary.

g. Red Flags: Can result in exercise intolerance; fatigue is associated with hypermetabolic state.

Adrenal Disorders

1. Primary adrenal insufficiency (Addison's disease).

a. Partial or complete failure of adrenocortical function; results in decreased production of cortisol and aldosterone.

b. Etiology: autoimmune processes, infection, neoplasm, or hemorrhage.

c. Signs and symptoms.

(1) Increased bronze pigmentation of skin.
(2) Weakness, decreased endurance.
(3) Anorexia, dehydration, weight loss, gastrointestinal disturbances.
(4) Anxiety, depression.
(5) Decreased tolerance to cold.
(6) Intolerance to stress.

d. Medical interventions.

(1) Replacement therapy: glucocorticoid, adrenal corticoids.
(2) Adequate fluid intake, control of sodium and potassium.
(3) Diet high in complex carbohydrates and protein.

2. Secondary adrenal insufficiency.

a. Can result from prolonged steroid therapy (ACTH); rapid withdrawal of drugs; and hypothalamic or pituitary tumors.

3. Cushing's syndrome.

a. Metabolic disorder resulting from chronic and excessive production of cortisol by the adrenal cortex.

b. From drug toxicity (overadministration of glucocorticoids).

c. Etiology: most common cause is a pituitary tumor with increased secretion of ACTH.

d. Signs and symptoms.

(1) Decreased glucose tolerance.
(2) Round "moon" face.
(3) Obesity: rapidly developing fat pads on chest and abdomen; buffalo hump.
(4) Decreased testosterone levels or decreased menstrual periods.
(5) Muscular atrophy.
(6) Edema.
(7) Hypokalemia.
(8) Emotional changes.

e. Medical interventions.

(1) Goal is to decrease excess ACTH: irradiation or surgical excision of pituitary tumor or control medication levels.
(2) Monitor weight, electrolyte, and fluid balance.

Psychiatric Conditions

Psychiatric States/Mechanisms

1. Anxiety.

a. Feelings of apprehension, worry, uneasiness; a normal reaction to tension, conflict, or stress.

b. Degree of anxiety is related to degree of perceived threat and capacity to engage behaviors that can reduce anxiety.

c. Anxiety can be constructive, stimulate an individual toward purposeful activity, or neurotic (pathological).

d. Sympathetic responses (fight or flight) generally accompany anxiety, e.g., increased heart rate, dyspnea, hyperventilation, dry mouth, GI symptoms (nausea, vomiting, diarrhea); palpitations.

2. Depression.

a. Altered mood characterized by morbid sadness, dejection, sense of melancholy. Can be a chronic, relapsing disorder.

b. Red Flags: Clinical manifestations.

(1) Loss of interest in all usually pleasurable outlets, e.g., work, family.
(2) Poor appetite, weight loss, or weight gain.
(3) Insomnia or hypersomnia; decreased energy.
(4) Psychomotor imbalance: agitation or excessive fatigue, irritability.
(5) Feelings of worthlessness, self-reproach, guilt, hopelessness.
(6) Impaired concentration, ability to think.
(7) Recurrent thoughts of suicide or death.

c. Management.

(1) Treatment is pharmacological: tricyclic antidepressant drugs.

Red Flags: Patients on these medications may exhibit disturbed balance, postural hypotension, falls and fractures, increased HR, dysrhythmias, ataxia, seizures.

(2) Cognitive therapy may help.

d. Physical therapy interventions.

(1) Maintain a positive attitude, consistently demonstrate warmth and interest.
(2) Acknowledge depression, provide hope.
(3) Use positive reinforcement, build in successful treatment experiences.
(4) Involve the patient in treatment decisions.
(5) Avoid excessive cheerfulness.
(6) Take all suicidal thoughts and acts seriously.

3. Coping and adapting mechanisms.
   a. typically unconscious behaviors by which the individual resolves or conceals conflicts or anxieties.
   b. Compensation: covering up a weakness by stressing a desirable or strong trait, e.g., a learning disabled child becomes an outstanding athlete.
   c. Denial: a refusal to recognize reality, e.g., refusal to acknowledge a fatal disease.
   d. Repression: refusal or inability to recall undesirable past thoughts or events.
   e. Displacement: the transferring of an emotion to a less dangerous substitute, e.g., yelling at your child instead of your boss.
   f. Reaction formation: a defensive reaction in which behavior is exactly opposite what is expected, e.g., a messy individual becomes neat.
   g. Projection: the attributing of your own undesirable behavior to another, e.g., "He made me do it."
   h. Rationalization: the justification of behaviors using reasons other than the real reason, e.g., presenting an attitude of not caring.
   i. Regression: resorting to an earlier, more immature pattern of functioning, e.g., in traumatic brain injury; common under high stress situations.

4. General adaptation syndrome (GAS).
   a. Total body coping/adaptation to a catastrophic event (illness, trauma).
   b. Alarm stage, or "fight-or-flight" response: activation of the sympathetic system.
   c. Sustained resistance.
   d. Chronic resistance, exhaustion leading to stress-related illnesses.

Pathologies

1. Anxiety disorders (anxiety neurosis).
   a. Excessive anxiety not associated with realistically threatening specific situations, e.g., generalized anxiety.
   b. Panic attacks: acute, intense anxiety or terror; may be uncontrollable, accompanied by sympathetic signs, loss of mental control, sense of impending death.
   c. Phobias: excessive and unreasonable fear leads to avoidance behaviors, e.g., agoraphobia (fear of being alone or in public places).
   d. Obsessive-compulsive behavior: persistent anxiety is manifested by repetitive, stereotypic acts; behaviors interfere with social functioning, e.g., hand washing, counting, and touching.

2. Posttraumatic stress disorder (PTSD).
   a. Exposure to a traumatic event produces a variety of stress-related symptoms.
   b. PTSD symptoms.
      (1) Reexperiencing the traumatic event.
      (2) Psychic numbing with reduced responsiveness.
      (3) Detachment from the external world; survival guilt.
      (4) Exaggerated autonomic arousal, hyperalertness.
      (5) Disturbed sleeping.
      (6) Ongoing irritability.
      (7) Impaired memory and concentration.
   c. PTSD can be acute (symptoms last < 3 months) or chronic (3 months or longer); onset can also be delayed.
   d. Symptoms should not be ignored. A mental health consultation is indicated.

3. Psychosomatic disorders (somatoform disorders).
   a. Physical signs or diseases that are related to emotional causes, e.g., psychosocial stress.
   b. Characteristics.
      (1) Cannot be explained by identifiable disease process or underlying pathology.
      (2) Not under voluntary control; provides a means of coping with anxiety and stress.
      (3) Patient is frequently indifferent to symptoms.
   c. Types.
      (1) Conversion disorder (hysterical paralysis): loss or altered physical functioning representing psychosocial conflict or need, e.g., can result in paralysis, hemiplegia.
      (2) Hypochondria: abnormal or heightened concerns about health or body functions; false beliefs about suffering from some disease or condition.
   d. Management.
      (1) Physical symptoms are real: treat the patient as you would any other patient with similar symptoms.
      (2) Provide a supportive environment.
      (3) Identify primary gain (internal conflicts); assist patient in learning new, alternate methods of stress management.
      (4) Identify secondary gains (additional advantages, e.g., attention, sympathy); do not reinforce.
      (5) Provide encouragement and support for the total person.

4. Schizophrenia.
   a. A group of disorders characterized by disruptions in thought patterns; of unknown etiology; a biochemical imbalance in the brain.
   b. Symptoms.
      (1) Disordered thinking: fragmented thoughts, errors of logic, delusions, poor judgment, memory.
      (2) Disordered speech: may be coherent but unintelligible, incoherent, or mute.
      (3) Disordered perception: hallucinations and delusions.
      (4) Inappropriateness of affect: withdrawal of interest from other people and from the outside world; loss of self-identity, self-direction; disordered interpersonal relations.

(5) Functional disturbances: inability to function in daily life, work.
(6) Little insight in to problems and behavior.

c. Paranoia: a type of schizophrenic disorder characterized by feelings of extreme suspiciousness, persecution, grandiosity (feelings of power or great wealth), or jealousy; withdrawal of all emotional contact with others.
d. Catatonia: a type of schizophrenic disorder characterized by mutism or stupor; unresponsiveness; catatonic posturing (remains fixed, unable to move or talk for extended periods).

5. Bipolar disorder (manic-depressive illness).
   a. A disorder characterized by mood swings from depression to mania; a biochemical dysfunction.
   b. Often intense outbursts, high energy and activity, excessive euphoria, decreased need for sleep, unrealistic beliefs, distractibility, poor judgment, denial.
   c. Followed by extreme depression (see depression symptoms).
   d. Treatment is pharmacological, e.g., lithium carbonate.

6. Perseveration.
   a. The continued repetition of a movement, word, or expression, e.g., patient gets stuck and repeats the same activity over and over again; often accompanies traumatic brain injury or stroke.

Grief Process

1. Emotional process. By which an individual deals with loss, e.g., of a significant loved one, body part, or function.

2. Characteristics.
   a. Somatic symptoms: e.g., fatigue, sighing, hyperventilation, anorexia, insomnia.
   b. Psychological symptoms: e.g., sorrow, discomfort, regret, guilt, anger, irritability, depression.
   c. Resolution may take months or years.

3. Stages.
   a. Shock and disbelief; inability to comprehend loss.
   b. Increased awareness and anguish; crying or anger is common.
   c. Mourning.
   d. Resolution of loss.
   e. Idealization of lost person or function.

4. Management.
   a. Provide support and understanding of the grief process.
   b. Encourage expression of feelings, memories.
   c. Respect privacy, cultural or religious customs.

Death and Dying

1. Characteristics: decreasing physical and mental functioning, gradual loss of consciousness.

2. Stages (Kübler-Ross).
   a. Denial: patients insist they are fine, joke about themselves, are not motivated to participate in treatment.
      (1) Allow denial: denial is a protective compensatory mechanism necessary until such time as the patient is ready to face his/her illness.
      (2) Provide opportunities for patient to question, confront illness and impending death.
   b. Anger, resentment: patients may become disruptive, blame others.
      (1) Be supportive: allow patient to express anger, frustration, resentment.
      (2) Encourage focus on coping strategies.
   c. Bargaining: patients bargain for time to complete life tasks; turn to religion or other individuals, make promises in return for function.
      (1) Provide accurate information, honest, truthful answers.
   d. Depression: patients acknowledge impending death, withdraw from life; demonstrate an overwhelming sense of loss, low motivation.
      (1) Observe closely for suicidal ideation.
      (2) Allay fears and anxieties, especially loneliness and isolation.
      (3) Assist in providing for comfort of the patient.
   e. Acceptance and preparation for death: acceptance of their condition; relate more to their family, make plans for the future.

3. Management.
   a. Support patient and family during each stage.
   b. Maintain hope without supporting unrealistic expectations.

Interventions

1. Physical therapist's role.
   a. Motivate patients, manage the human side of rehabilitation
   b. Establish boundaries of the professional relationship: identify problems, expectations, purpose, roles, and responsibilities.
   c. Provide empathic understanding: the capacity to understand what your patient is experiencing from that patient's perspective.
      (1) Recognize losses; allow opportunity to mourn "old self."
      (2) Ask open-ended questions that reflect what the patient is feeling.

(a) Empathetic response; e.g., "It sounds like you are worried and anxious about your pain and are trying your best."

(b) Nonempathetic response; e.g., "Don't worry about your pain", "You're overreacting."

(3) Sympathy is not helpful or therapeutic; caregiver is closely affected by the patient's behaviors, e.g., therapist cries when the patient cries.

d. Set realistic, meaningful goals; involve the patient and family in the goal-setting process; self-determination is important.

e. Set realistic time frames for the rehabilitation program; recognize symptoms, stages of the grief process, or death and dying and adjust accordingly.

f. Recognize and reinforce healthy, positive, socially appropriate behaviors; allow the patient to experience success.

g. Recognize secondary gains, unacceptable behaviors; do not reinforce (e.g., malingering behaviors such as avoidance of work).

h. Provide an environment conducive to the patient's emotional state, learning, and optimal function.

(1) Provide a message of hope tempered with realism.

(2) Keep patients informed.

(3) Lay adequate groundwork or preparation for expected changes or discharge.

(4) Help to reestablish personal dignity and self-worth; acknowledge whole person.

i. Help patients identify feelings, successful coping strategies, recognize successful conflict resolution, and rehabilitation gains.

(1) Stress ability to overcome major obstacles.

(2) Stress that recovery is unique and highly individual.

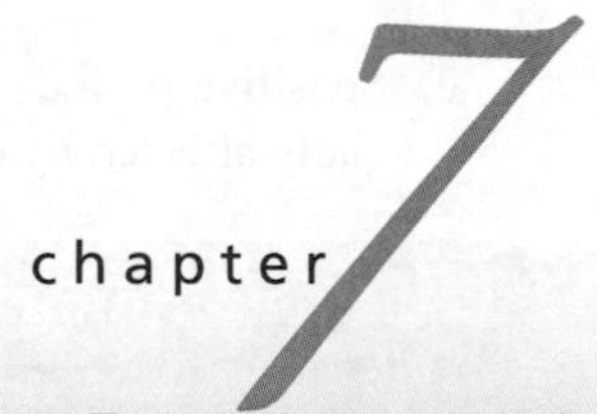

chapter 7 Pediatric Physical Therapy

LINDA KAHN-D'ANGELO

Theories of Development, Motor Control, and Motor Learning

Development

1. **The sequence of events through which the individual grows, changes, evolves and matures.** (See Table 7-2).
2. **Theories of development.**
   a. Maturationist theories.
      (1) Individual genetically and biologically determined.
      (2) Aspects of human behavior are preformed and innate.
   b. Empiricist theories.
      (1) Source of human behavior is the environment.
   c. Behavioral theory.
      (1) Environmental reinforcement motivates and shapes cognitive and motor behavior.
      (2) Used in behavior modification treatment where desired behaviors are positively reinforced and unwanted behaviors are ignored.
   d. Interactionist theory.
      (1) Child is an active social being who contributes to his development.
   e. Piagetian theory.
      (1) Interaction of environment and neural maturation results in spiraling of development with equilibrium and disequilibrium resulting.

Motor Control

1. **The study of postures and movement, and the parts of the mind and body that control them.**
2. **Theories of motor control.**
   a. Neuromaturationist theory.
      (1) Cortex is command center, with descending control and inhibition of lower centers by higher one in central nervous system (CNS).
   b. Systems theory.
      (1) Command center changes from cortex to other levels, depending on the task.
      (2) Stresses interaction between brain, body, and environment including biomechanics and body geometry.
      (3) Sensory systems mature, become integrated and connected to muscle coordination patterns, starting with the visual system.
      (4) Immature postures involve cocontraction of agonists and antagonists; cocontraction decreases with maturation.
   c. Neuronal group selection theory.
      (1) Genetic code of species outlines limits of neural network formation.
      (2) Actual network formation results from individual experience.
      (3) Cell death of unexercised synaptic and strengthening of synaptic connections selectively activated.

Early Motor Learning

1. **Motor skill.** Any motor activity which becomes better organized, more effective and efficient as a result of practice.

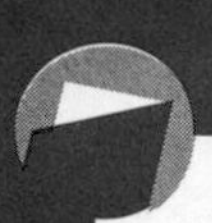

2. **Enhancement of early motor skills development.**
   a. Use of goal-oriented tasks.
   b. Internal feedback via corollary discharge and effector organ feedback (i.e., visual, somatosensory vestibular feedback).
   c. External feedback through knowledge of results and knowledge of performance feedback from instructor; i.e., every other time and after a delay.
   d. Practice of high intensity and duration as tolerated.

3. **Principles of motor development.**
   a. Occurs in cephalocaudal direction.
   b. Unrefined to refined movement.
   c. Stability to controlled mobility.
   d. Occurs in spiraling manner, with periods of equilibrium and disequilibrium.
   e. Sensitive periods occur when infant/child is especially affected by environmental input.

Fetal Sensorimotor Development

1. **Gestational age.**
   a. Age of fetus or newborn, in weeks, from first day of mother's last normal menstrual period.
   b. Normal gestational period is 38–42 weeks.
   c. Gestational period is divided into three equal trimesters (Table 7-1).

2. **Conceptional age.**
   a. Age of a fetus or newborn in weeks since conception.

Table 7-1 ➤ FETAL SENSORIMOTOR DEVELOPMENT

	FIRST TRIMESTER	SECOND TRIMESTER	THIRD TRIMESTER
Muscle Spindle	• Muscle starts to differentiate • Tissue becomes specialized	• Motor end plate forms • Clonus response to stretch	• Some muscles are mature and functional, others still maturing
Touch and Tactile System	• First sensory system to develop • Response to tactile stimulus	• Receptors differentiate	• Touch functional • Actual temperature discrimination at end of third trimester • Most mature sensory system at birth
Vestibular System	• Functioning at the end of the first trimester (not completely developed)		
Vision	• Eyelids fused • Optic nerve and cup being formed	• Startle to light • Visual processing occurs	• Fixation occurs • Able to focus (fixed focal length)
Auditory		• Turns to auditory sounds	• Debris in middle ear, loss of hearing
Olfactory			• Nasal plugs disappear, some olfactory perception
Taste	• Taste buds develop		• Responds to different tastes (sweet, sour, bitter, salt)
Movement	• Sucking, hiccuping • Fetal breathing • Quick, generalized limb movement • Positional changes • 71/2 weeks: bends neck and trunk	• Quickening • Sleep states • Grasp reflex • Reciprocal and symmetrical limb movements	• 28 weeks: primitive motor reflexes • Rooting, suck, swallow • Palmar grasp • Plantar grasp • MORO away from perioral stroke • Crossed extension

Table 7-2 ➤ DEVELOPMENTAL SEQUENCE SUMMARY

Age	Milestones
1 Month	• Decreased flexion • Momentary head elevation with minimal forearm support • Tracks a moving object • Head usually to side • Reciprocal and symmetrical kicking • Positive support and primary walking reflexes in supported standing • Hands fisted with indwelling thumb most of the time • Neonatal reaching • Alert, brightening expression
2 Months	• Head elevation to 45 degrees in prone, prone on elbows with elbows behind shoulders • Head bobs in supported sitting • Does not accept weight on lower extremities (astasia-abasia) • Responds to friendly handling
3 Months	• Prone on elbows, weight bearing on forearms • Elbows in line with shoulders, head elevated to 90 degrees • Head in midline in supine, hands on chest • Increased back extension with scapular adduction in supported sitting • Takes some weight with toes curled in supported standing • Coos, chuckles • Optical and labyrinthine head-righting present
4 Months	• Rolls prone to side, supine to side • Sits with support • No head lag in pull-to-sit • Bilateral reaching with forearm pronated when trunk supported • Ulnarpalmar grasp • Laughs out loud
5 Months	• Rolls from prone to supine • Weight shifting from one forearm to the other in prone • Head control in supported sitting
6 Months	• Prone on hands with elbows extended, weight shifting from hand to hand • Rolls supine to prone • Independent sitting • Pulls-to-stand, bounces
7 Months	• Can maintain quadruped • Pivots on belly; moves body in circle while prone • Pivot prone (prone extension) position • Assumes sitting from quadruped • Trunk rotation in sitting • Recognizes tone of voice • May show fear of strangers
8-9 Months	• Belly crawls • Quadruped creeping • Moves quadruped to sitting • Side-sitting • Pulls-to-stand through kneeling • Cruises sideways, can stand alone • Reaches with closest arm, radial digital grasp, radial palmar, 3 jaw chuck grasp, and inferior pincer grasp with thumb and forefinger • Can transfer objects from one hand to the other
10-15 Months	• Begins to walk unassisted • Begins self-feeding • Reaches with supination, neat pincer grasp, can release, build a tower of 2 cubes • Searches for hidden toys • Suspicious of strangers • Plays patty-cake and peek-a-boo • Imitates
20 Months	• Ascends stairs step-to pattern (2 feet on each step) • Running more coordinated • Jumps off of bottom step • Plays make-believe
2 Years	• Runs well • Can go up stairs foot-over-foot (reciprocal stair climbing) • Active, restless, tantrums
3 Years	• Rides tricycle • Stands on one foot briefly • Jumps with two feet • Hops on one foot • Kicks ball • Understands sharing
4 years	• Hops on one foot several times • Stands on tiptoes • Throws ball overhand • Relates to friends
5 years	• Skips • Kicks ball well • Dresses self

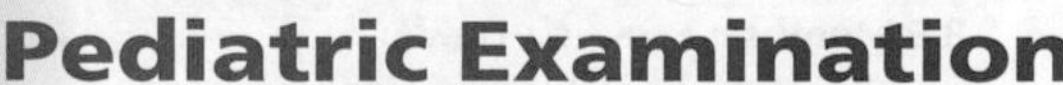

Pediatric Examination

Patient Interview

1. **Mother's pregnancy and birth history.** Prematurity, fetal distress, difficult labor, umbilical cord around neck.
2. **Medical history.** Special care unit admission, diagnoses, intubated and on ventilator, surgeries, medications.
3. **Family history.** Caretakers, current home situation, support to family, socioeconomic status.

Preterm Infant Examination

1. **Neurological assessment.** Preterm and full-term newborn infants.
   a. Neurological items include newborn reflexes, infant states of alertness.
   b. Neurobehavioral items from Neonatal Behavioral Assessment Scale (NBAS).
   c. Assessment of gestational age by evaluation of muscle tone, physical characteristics.
2. **Assessment of Premature Infant Behavior (APIB).**
   a. Refinement and extension of the NBAS.
   b. Assesses the organization and balance of infant's physiological, motor, and behavioral states.
   c. Test is lengthy, used mainly for research.
3. **Newborn Individualized Developmental Care and Assessment of Progress (NIDCAP).**
   a. Systematic behavioral observation of preterm or full-term infant in nursery or home during environmental input, caretaking, and treatments.
   b. Note what stresses, consoles infant.
4. **Test of Infant Motor Performance (TIMP).**
   a. Developed for infants from 32 weeks postconceptual age to 3½ months postterm.
   b. Evaluates spontaneous and elicited movements to analyze postural alignment and selective control for functional movements.

Full-Term Newborn, Infant, and Child Examination

1. **APGAR screening test.** Administered to newborn at 1, 5, 10 minutes after birth.
   a. Five items: heart rate, respiration, reflex irritability, muscle tone, color each scored 0, 1, or 2.
   b. Score of 7 and above considered good.
2. **Neurological examination of the newborn.**
   a. Assigns states of consciousness.
   b. Tests newborn reflexes.
3. **Neonatal Behavioral Assessment Scale.**
   a. Tests interactive, self-organizational abilities, and newborn reflexes and muscle tone.
4. **Skeletal system examination.**
   a. Fractured clavicle.
   b. Dislocated hip: asymmetrical gluteal folds, hip click.
   c. Spine: curved, inflexible, kyphosis, scoliosis; spinal bifida occulta: dimple, patch of hair, pigmentation visible, and x-ray verify.
   d. Talipes equinovarus (clubfoot): ankle in plantar flexion, forefoot adduction.
5. **Range of motion (ROM).**
   a. Newborn has decreased ROM into extension due to physiological flexion, but increased dorsiflexion of ankles.
6. **Posture.**
   a. Physiological flexion of all four limbs due to position in utero.
   b. Head to one side.
7. **Movements.**
   a. Spontaneous and reflexive.
   b. Occasional tremulousness normal.
8. **Neonatal reflexes.** Primary motor patterns and infant reflexes and reactions.
   a. Present at birth and become "integrated" or inhibited, or not evident later in development.
   b. In CNS lesions, they may persist and interfere with motor milestone attainment or cause deformities.
   c. Babinski reflex: stroke lateral aspect of the plantar surface of foot, get extension and fanning of toes (0–12 months).
   d. Flexor withdrawal: sharp, quick pressure stimulus to sole of foot or palm of hand causes withdrawal of stimulated extremity (0–2 months, although some sources say present throughout life).
   e. Crossed extension: sharp, quick pressure stimulus to sole of foot results in withdrawal of stimulated lower extremity and extension of opposite leg (0–2 months).
   f. Galant or trunk incurvation reaction: sharp stoke along paravertebral line from scapula to top of iliac crest results in lateral trunk flexion toward stimulated side (0–2 months).
   g. Moro reflex: sudden extension of neck results in flexion, abduction of shoulders, extension of elbows,

followed by shoulder adduction and elbow flexion. Usually also results in crying. Test last! (0–4 months).

h. Primary standing reaction: infant held in supported standing position supports some weight and extends lower extremities. If this reflex persists, will interfere with walking by causing extension of all joints of the lower extremity and preventing disassociation of flexion and extension.

i. Primary walking: hold infant in supported standing, tilt trunk forward slightly, reciprocal stepping motions in lower extremities (0–2 months unless practiced).

j. Neonatal neck righting (neck righting on body, NOB): Turn head with infant in supine position; body log-rolls toward same side (0–6 months).

k. Rooting: stroking of perioral region results in head turning to that side with mouth opening (0–3 months). Important feeding reflex.

l. Sucking: touch to lips, tongue, palate results in automatic sucking (0–6 months). Important feeding reflex.

m. Startle: loud noise, sudden light, or cold stimulus causes a sudden jerking of whole body or extension and abduction of upper extremities, followed by adduction of shoulders (0–6 months).

n. Tonic labyrinthine reflex (classic): prone position results in maximal flexor tone and supine position results in maximal extensor tone. If reflex persists and is strong, may block rolling from supine position, due to increased extensor tone (0–6 months).

o. Asymmetrical tonic neck reflex: rotation of head results in extension of face side extremities and flexion of skull side extremities. Stronger in lower extremities of neonates (0–5 months). If reflex persists, may result in scoliosis or hip dislocation and interfere with grasping and hand-mouth activities.

p. Palmar grasp: pressure stimulus against palm results in grasping of object with slow release (0–4 months).

q. Plantar grasp: pressure stimulus to sole or lowering of feet to floor results in curling of toes. Must be integrated before walking occurs (0–9 months).

r. Placing reactions: drag dorsum of foot or back of hand against edge of table, get placing of foot or hand onto table top (0–6 months).

s. Traction or pull-to-sit: Pull infant to sitting from supine position; upper extremities will flex, and head will lag until about 4–5 months.

t. Optical and labyrinthine righting: head orients to a vertical position when body is tilted. Test labyrinthine righting with the eyes blindfolded (1 month–throughout life).

u. Protective extension: Quick displacement of trunk in downward direction while held or while sitting in forward, sideward, or backward direction results in extension of legs downward and extension of arms in sitting position to catch weight. Downward begins at 4 months, sideward sitting at 6 months, forward sitting at 7 months, backwatard sitting 9 months; these reactions persist through life.

v. Body-righting reaction acting on the head (BOH): contact of body with solid surface results in head righting with respect to gravity, interacts with labyrinthine righting reaction on head to maintain orientation of head in space. Begins at 4–6 months and persists through life.

w. Body-righting reaction acting on the body (BOB): rotation of head or thorax results in rolling over, with rotation between trunk and pelvis. Begins at 6–8 months and persists.

x. Symmetrical tonic neck reflex: extension of cervical joints produces extension of upper extremities and flexion of lower extremities; flexion of cervical joints products flexion of upper extremities and extension of lower extremities (6–8 months). If reflex persists, it may interfere with development of stable quadruped position and creeping.

y. Landau's reaction: Infant held in ventral suspension will extend neck, trunk, and hips (4–18 months).

z. Tilting reactions: slow shifting of base of support or slow displacement of body in space will result in lateral flexion of spine toward elevated side of support, abduction of extremities on elevated side, and sometimes trunk rotation toward elevated side. Prone begins at 5 months; supine begins at 7 months; sitting at 8 months; quadruped at 12 months. These reactions persist throughout life.

9. Screening tests.

a. Denver Developmental Screening Test II.
   (1) To screen for developmental delay.
   (2) Tests social, fine, gross motor, and language skills from birth to 6 years of age.

b. Alberta Infant Motor Scale (AIMS): observational scale for assessing gross motor milestones in infants from birth through independent walking.

10. Standardized motor tests.

a. Movement Assessment of Infants.
   (1) To identify motor dysfunction and changes in the status of motor dysfunction and establishing an intervention program for infants from birth to 1 year.
   (2) Criterion-referenced exam of muscle tone, reflexes, automatic reactions, and volitional movements.

b. Peabody Developmental Motor Scales.
   (1) Assesses gross and fine motor development from birth to 42 months.
   (2) Includes spontaneous, elicited, reflexes, and automatic reactions.

c. Gross motor function test.

(1) Developed to measure change in gross motor function over time in children with cerebral palsy.
(2) All items on the test could be accomplished by a 5 year-old with typical motor development.
(3) Focuses on voluntary movement in five developmental dimensions: prone and supine, sitting, crawling and kneeling, standing, walking and jumping.

11. Sensory Integration and Praxis Test.
    a. Sensorimotor assessment for children between ages of 4 and 9 with mild to moderate learning impairment.
    b. Includes tests of balance, proprioceptive and tactile sensation, and control of specific movements.

12. **Comprehensive developmental assessments.**
    a. Bayley Scales of Infant Development revision: Norm-referenced motor and mental scales for children from birth to 42 months of age.

13. **Pediatric functional assessments.**
    a. Pediatric Evaluation of Disability Inventory (PEDI): interview or questionnaire scale of activities of daily living (ADL), with or without modification completed by caregiver.
    b. Functional Independence Measure for children (WeeFIM): assesses function in self-care, mobility, locomotion, and communication and social cognition.

Overview of Pediatric Physical Therapy Intervention

Roles of the Pediatric Physical Therapist

1. **Direct care provider.**
    a. In children's hospital settings.
    b. In special care nurseries, neonatal intensive care units.
    c. Pediatric rehabilitation settings.
    d. In early intervention programs (EIPs) (0–3 years).
    e. In educational settings.

2. **Consultant/indirect care provider.**
    a. Pediatric PT may be consultant in educational settings, instructing teachers and teacher's assistants in facilitating attainment of educational goals.
    b. Pediatric PT may work with physical therapist assistant in delivery of care in many settings.

3. **Parent education.** Pediatric PT is always involved in parent/family or caretaker education.

Goals, Outcomes, and Intervention

1. **Primary prevention of disability through education and treatment.**

2. **Prevention and/or improvement of secondary disabilities.** (E.g., contractures/deformities).

3. **Attainment of maximal functional goals of child and family.**

Pediatric Therapies

1. **Developmental activities to facilitate development of functional motor skills.** These activities use postures and movements from the developmental sequence to increase strength, ROM, coordination. Remember, play is the work of the child; make activities fun.

2. **Neurodevelopmental Treatment (NDT).**
    a. Utilizes reflex-inhibiting patterns (RIPs) which are active/passive movements or postures opposite to the spastic flexion or extension synergies.
    b. Encourages active, functional movements appropriate for the developmental level and individual needs of the child and goals of the child and family.

3. **Motor control/motor learning approaches.** Utilize principles of motor control and early motor learning appropriate for individual child.

4. **Sensory integration.**
    a. Goal is to facilitate child's organization and processing of proprioceptive, tactile, and vestibular input.
    b. Facilitation will influence postural responses, environmental awareness, and motor planning.

Pediatric Conditions & Interventions

Prematurity Physical Therapy Practice

1. A subspecialty of pediatrics. Requires advanced didactic and supervised practical experience.
2. Definition and categories.
   a. Birth of infant before 37 weeks gestation.
   b. Categorized by birth weight.
3. Preterm postural and movement profile.
   a. Preterm infant does not develop the physiological flexion of full-term newborn.
   b. May exhibit hyperextended neck and trunk (may be partially a result of supine and intubation positions).
   c. Shoulders may be elevated, abducted, extended with scapular retraction.
   d. Hips abducted and extended.
   e. Pelvis tipped anteriorly (increased lumbar lordosis).
   f. Decreased midline arm movement.
   g. May bear weight on toes when in supported standing position.
4. Medical complications and medical surgical treatment in prematurity.
   a. Complications depend on severity of prematurity and birth weight.
   b. Respiratory distress syndrome (RDS) or hyaline membrane disease.
      (1) Respiratory distress due to atelectasis caused by insufficient surfactant in premature lungs.
      (2) May lead to acute respiratory failure and death.
      (3) Treatment includes oxygen supplementation, assisted ventilation, and surfactant administration.
      (4) Chronic RDS may lead to bronchopulmonary dysplasia.
   c. Bronchopulmonary dysplasia.
      (1) Chronic lung disease as a result of damage to lungs from mechanical ventilation, oxygen administration, and chronic RDS.
      (2) Predisposes child to frequent respiratory infections and developmental disability.
      (3) Treatment includes respiratory support, infection control, and bronchodilator administration.
   d. Periventricular leukomalacia (PVL).
      (1) Necrosis of white matter adjacent to ventricles of brain due to systemic hypotension or ischemia.
      (2) May result in cerebral palsy.
   e. Periventricular-intraventricular hemorrhage.
      (1) Bleeding into immature vascular matrix.
      (2) Bleeds graded I–IV; grades II–IV may result in cerebral palsy.
   f. Retinopathy of prematurity (ROP).
      (1) Due to combination of low birth weight and high oxygen levels.
      (2) Sequelae may range from nonsignificant to detachment of retinas and blindness.
   g. Necrotizing enterocolitis.
      (1) Ischemia results in inflammatory, infected bowel.
   h. Increased fragility of skin.
   i. Thermoregulation problems.
   j. Feeding problems.
   k. Interaction/attachment problems with caregivers.
5. Physical therapy examination in prematurity.
   a. Medical history review.
   b. Autonomic functions.
   c. Neurobehavioral organization (interactive items after infant is 32 weeks conceptional age).
   d. Muscle tone.
   e. Postural control.
   f. Spontaneous movements.
   g. Reflexes including feeding.
   h. Musculoskeletal evaluation.
   i. Family needs.
   j. Test of Infant Motor Performance (TIMP), Newborn Individualized Developmental Care Plan (NIDCAP), Assessment of Premature Infant Behavior (APIB).
6. Intervention/activities to teach parents.
   a. Play activities and positioning to facilitate shoulder protraction and adduction such as supported side-lying while doing visual (use black, white, and red objects 9 inches away) and auditory tracking, and reaching.
   b. Midline positioning of head.
   c. Encourage reaching for toys, parent's face if infant is over 32 weeks conceptional age.
   d. Supervised side-lying and prone positioning (tummy time) for periods during the day. Academy of Pediatrics recommends sleeping in the supine position to decrease possibility of sudden infant death syndrome (SIDS).
   e. Avoid activities which may increase extensor tone, such as use of infant jumpers and walkers.

Note: This is a subspecialty of pediatrics, and requires advanced didactic and supervised clinical practice.

Cerebral Palsy (CP)

1. **Pathology.**
   a. Group of disorders which are prenatal, perinatal, or postnatal in origin.
   b. Major causes include hemorrhage below lining of ventricles, hypoxic encephalopathy, malformations and trauma of CNS.
   c. Preterm birth associated with CP.

2. **Classifications of CP.**
   a. By area of body showing impairment.
      (1) One limb—monoplegia.
      (2) Two lower limbs—diplegia.
      (3) Upper and lower limbs of one side of the body—hemiplegia.
      (4) All four limbs—quadriplegia.
   b. Type of most obvious impairment.
      (1) Spastic—increased tone, lesion of motor cortex or projections from motor cortex.
      (2) Athetosis—fluctuating muscle tone, lesion of basal ganglia.
      (3) Ataxia—instability of movement, lesion of the cerebellum.
   c. Gross motor function classification system for CP (Table 7-3).

3. **Impairments for all classifications of CP.**
   a. Insufficient force generation.
   b. Tone abnormality.
   c. Poor selective control of muscle activity.
   d. Poor regulation of muscle activity in anticipation of postural changes.
   e. Decreased ability to learn unique movements.
   f. Abnormal patterns of movement in total flexion and extension.
   g. Persistence of primitive reflexes.
      (1) Interfere with normal posture and movement.
      (2) May cause contractures and deformities.

4. **Impairments by classification of CP.**
   a. Spastic cerebral palsy.
      (1) Increased muscle tone in antigravity muscles.

Table 7-3 ➤ GROSS MOTOR CLASSIFICATION FOR CEREBRAL PALSY

Level I	• Walk without restrictions, limitations in more advanced gross motor skills.
Level II	• Walk without assistive devices; limitations walking outdoors and in the community.
Level III	• Walk with assistive mobility devices; limitations walking outdoors and in the community.
Level IV	• Self-mobility with limitations; children are transported or use power mobility outdoors and in the community.
Level V	• Self-mobility is severely limited, even with the use of assistive technology.

      (2) Abnormal postures and movements with mass patterns of flexion/extension.
      (3) Imbalance of tone across joints may cause contractures and deformities, especially of hip flexors, adductors, internal rotators, and knee flexors, ankle plantarflexors in lower extremities; scapular retractors, glenohumeral extensors, and adductors, elbow flexors, forearm pronators.
      (4) Visual, auditory, cognitive, and oral motor deficits may be associated with spastic CP.
   b. Athetoid cerebral palsy.
      (1) Generalized decreased muscle tone, floppy baby syndrome.
      (2) Poor functional stability especially in proximal joints.
      (3) Ataxia and incoordination when child assumes upright position, with decreased base of support and muscle tone fluctuations.
      (4) Poor visual tracking, speech delay, and oral motor problems.
      (5) Tonic reflexes such as asymmetrical tonic neck reflex (ATNR), symmetrical tonic neck reflex (STNR), and tonic labyrinthine reflex (TLR) may be persistent, blocking functional postures and movement.
   c. Ataxia cerebral palsy.
      (1) Low postural tone with poor balance.
      (2) Stance and gait are wide based.
      (3) Intention tremor of hands.
      (4) Uncoordinated movement.
      (5) Ataxia follows initial hypotonia.
      (6) Poor visual tracking, nystagmus.
      (7) Speech articulation problems.
      (8) May occur with spastic or athetoid CP.

5. **Functional limitations.**
   a. Dependent on classification of CP.
   b. Spasticity may lead to decreased ROM, which may limit mobility.
   c. Ambulation.
      (1) Ambulation without use of assistive devices may be attained by children with hemiplegia, and by some with diplegia and ataxia.
      (2) Ambulation may be attained with use of rollator walkers or crutches by some children with diplegia, athetosis, and a few with mild quadriplegia.

6. **Interventions and goals in CP.**
   a. Very individualized, depending on abilities, age, type of CP. Incorporate child and family in intervention planning, implementation and goal setting.
   b. Focus on prevention of disability by minimizing effects of impairment, preventing or limiting secondary impairment such as contractures, scoliosis.
      (1) Utilize static positioning and dynamic patterns of movement opposite to habitual abnormal spastic patterns.
      (2) Facilitate symmetry in postures.

(3) Elongate spastic hamstrings and heel cords.
(4) Serial casting may be used to increase length of muscle and decrease tone.

c. Maximize the gross motor functional level.
(1) Use principles of motor learning and motor control; facilitate functional motor skills, including voluntary movement, anticipatory and reactive postural adjustments. Use toys, fun activities, balls, and bolsters to facilitate postural control and developmental activities.
(2) Use weight-bearing and postural challenge to increase muscle tone and strength.
(3) Incorporate orthoses as necessary.
(a) Ankle-foot orthosis (AFO) most commonly used; may be rigid or with articulated ankle.
(b) Submalleolar orthosis for forefoot and midfoot malalignment; e.g., pronated foot.
(4) Utilize adaptive equipment as necessary.
(a) Seating should maintain head in neutral position, trunk upright, hips, knees, and ankles at 90 degrees flexion (hips in abduction if spastic adductors). Wheelchair or seat may be tilted posteriorly to decrease extensor tone and maintain hip flexion.
(b) Prone or supine standers and parapodium will promote weight-bearing through lower extremities and encourage bone mineralization, gastrointestinal function, tone, strengthening of lower extremity muscles, and social interaction. TLR will elicit more extensor tone in supine, more flexor tone in prone.
(c) Side-lying will help decrease effect of TLR.
(d) Rollator walkers often used. Posterior rollator walker helps child maintain upright position, and arm position helps decrease extensor tone.

7. Prognosis for CP.

a. Prognosis depends on severity of brain lesion.
b. Most children with spastic hemiplegia, mild to moderate spastic CP, and mild ataxia will be able to ambulate.

8. Medical-surgical, pharmacological interventions for CP.

a. Management of spasticity.
(1) Oral medications—presynaptic inhibition of acetylcholine release.
(a) Benzodiazepines, diazepam (Valium).
(b) Baclofen (Lioresal).
(c) Side effects include sedation, weakness, drowsiness, dry mouth.
(2) Intrathecal baclofen pump (ITB). Delivers drug directly to spinal cord, producing muscle relaxation with less medication and decreased side effects. Pump is implanted subcutaneously in abdomen with catheter to spinal cord. Programmable doses released. Reservoir holds 1 to 4-month supply.
(3) Selective dorsal rhizotomy (SDR).
(a) Surgical transection of electromyography (EMG)–selected dorsal sensory rootlets with the goals of facilitating or maintaining ambulation or improving ease of caregiving.
(b) Intensive strengthening program after surgery when ambulation is goal.
(4) Peripheral nerve block.
(a) Injection of phenol/alcohol into peripheral nervous system from nerve root to motor endplate.
(b) Lasts 3–6 months.
(5) Botox injections—minute amounts of botulinum toxin injected into muscle, paralyzing it for 4–6 months.

9. Orthopedic management of CP.

a. Lengthening procedures.
(1) Muscle/tendon lengthening to correct deformity or weak muscle prevents hip subluxation/dislocation.
(2) Muscles most often lengthened include Achilles' tendon, hamstrings, iliopsoas, and hip adductors.

b. Muscle transfers.
(1) Muscle attachments moved to change direction of force in order to increase function and decrease spasticity.
(2) Most often done with hip adductors transferred to hip abductor.

c. Osteotomies.
(1) Cutting, removing, or repositioning bone to facilitate normal alignment, prevent subluxation/dislocation.
(2) Most often performed at hip (femoral or pelvic osteotomy).

Myelodysplasia/Spina Bifida

1. Pathology.

a. Neural tube defect resulting in vertebral and/or spinal cord malformation. Elevated serum or amniotic alpha-fetoprotein, amniotic acetylcholinesterase in prenatal period, and sonogram are used for detection.
b. Spina bifida occulta—no spinal cord involvement, may be indicated by a tuft of hair, dimple, or sinus.
c. Spina bifida cystica—visible or open lesion.
(1) Meningocele—cyst includes cerebrospinal fluid; cord intact.
(2) Myelomeningocele—cyst includes cerebrospinal fluid (CSF) and herniated cord tissue.
d. Neural tube defects linked to maternal decreased folic acid, infection, hot tub soaks, and exposure to teratogens such as alcohol and valproic acid.

e. Hydrocephalus significantly related to closure of neural tube defect. Shunting relieves pressure of hydrocephalus.
f. Meningitis common if defect not closed soon after birth.
g. Foot deformities such as talipes equinovarus (club-foot) common, especially with L4, L5 level.
h. Tethered cord may lead to increased severity of problems as child grows.
i. Latex sensitivity/allergy.

2. Impairments.

a. Depends on level of lesion and amount of malformation of cord (Table 7-2).
b. Muscle paralysis and imbalance resulting from spinal and lower limb deformities and joint contractures.
 (1) Kyphoscoliosis.
 (2) Shortened hip flexors and adductors.
 (3) Flexed knees.
 (4) Pronated feet.
c. L4, L5 lesion results in bowel and bladder dysfunction.
d. Sensory loss.
e. Developmental delays.
f. Abnormal tone: may have low tone, leading to poor strength and/or spasticity in upper extremities.
g. Osteoporosis.
h. Cognitive impairments including mental retardation, learning and perceptual disabilities, language disorders.

3. Functional limitations.

a. Highly variable, depending on level of lesion (see Table 7-2).
b. Weakness or paralysis of hip flexors (high lumbar level lesion) makes ambulation possible only with reciprocating gait orthosis (RGO).
c. Problems with learning, communication.

4. Medical-surgical management of spina bifida.

a. If open defect, surgical closure within 24–48 hours.
b. Ventriculoperitoneal shunt performed for hydrocephalus.
c. Orthopedic surgeries similar to cerebral palsy.

5. Physical therapy examination for spina bifida.

a. Physiological homeostasis in infants, breathing, oxygenation.
b. Gross and fine motor development including reflex and behavioral examination of infant.
c. Communicate with parents, family members about concerns, goals for intervention.
d. Functional abilities using PEDI or WeeFIM.
e. Active and passive ROM.
f. Muscle strength: may observe developmental abilities if child under 3 years of age.
g. Sensation: stroke skin and note response; record by dermatome.
h. Skin: check for skin breakdown, suture of closure, skin over shunt line.

6. Interventions, goals, and prognosis for spina bifida.

a. Teach parents proper positioning, handling, and exercise, keeping physiological flexion of the newborn. Include prone positioning to avoid shortening of hip flexors, as well as hip ROM, low tone, and osteoporosis.
b. Use adaptive equipment/orthoses, such as spinal orthoses for alignment, adaptive chairs for sitting (if needed), parapodium for early standing, lower extremity (LE) orthoses and ambulation assistive devices and/or wheelchair as needed.
c. Facilitate functional motor development, including appropriate developmental activities, primary or voluntary movement as well as reactive and anticipatory postural adjustments.
d. Educate parents regarding shunt malfunction. Signs include increased irritability, decreased muscle tone, seizures, vomiting, bulging fontanels, headache, and redness along shunt tract.
e. (See Table 7-4).

Brachial Plexus Injury

1. Pathology.

a. Traction or compression injury to unilateral brachial plexus during birth process or due to cervical rib abnormality.
 (1) Erb's palsy involves C5-6, upper arm paralysis, may involve rhomboids, levator scapulae, serratus anterior, deltoid, supraspinatus, infraspinatus, biceps brachii, brachioradialis, brachialis, supinator, and long extensors of wrist, fingers, and thumb.
 (2) Klumpke's palsy involves C8-T1, lower arm paralysis, involves intrinsic muscles of hand, flexors and extensors of wrist and fingers.
 (3) Erb-Klumpke palsy, whole-arm paralysis.
b. Nerve sheath is torn and nerve fibers compressed by hemorrhage and edema, although total avulsion of nerve is possible.

2. Impairments.

a. Sensory deficits of upper extremity.
b. Paralysis or paresis of upper extremity.
c. Characteristic position for Erb's palsy of upper extremity is adduction, internal rotation of shoulder with extension of elbow, pronation of forearm and flexion of wrist.

3. Functional limitations.

a. Dependent on severity of injury.
 (1) Erb's palsy results in decreased shoulder girdle function with 1:1 humeroscapular movement.

Table 7-4 ➤ IMPAIRMENT AND FUNCTION IN MYELODYSPLASIA

NEUROSEGMENTAL LEVEL	MUSCLES INNERVATED	PREAMBULATION ORTHOSES	AMBULATION ORTHOSES	ASSISTIVE DEVICES	FUNCTIONAL PROGNOSIS	MUSCULOSKELETAL PROBLEMS
Thoracic	Abdominal	Standing frame	Reciprocating gait orthosis	Parallel bars	Wheelchair	Spinal deformity
				Walker		Decubiti
				Forearm crutches		
Upper lumbar	Above & hip flexors	Standing frame	Reciprocating gait orthosis	Parallel bars	Wheelchair	Hip flexion contractures
				Walker	Possible household or therapeutic ambulation	
				Forearm crutches	Standing transfers	
Mid-lumbar	Above & knee extensors, hip adductors	None	HKAFO	Parallel bars	Wheelchair for community, Orthoses for house-hold ambulation	Hip dislocation, subluxation
			KAFO	Walker		
			AFO (depending on quad strength)	Forearm crutches		
Low-lumbar	Above & hip abductors, knee flexors, ankle & foot dorsiflexors, evertors, invertors, toe flexors	None	KAFO	Parallel bars	Household or community ambulators	Foot deformities
			AFO	Walker		
				Forearm crutches		
				None		
Lumbosacral	Above & ankle plantar flexors, foot intrinsic muscles	None	AFO or none	Walker	Community ambulators	Foot pressure sores
			AFO recommended to maintain gait quality & decrease compensatory overactivity of muscles	None		

From: Ryan, K., Eman, J., Ploski, C. Goal Attainment and Habilitation of Infants and Children with Spinal Bifida, APTA National Conference, 1991.

(2) Klumpke's palsy results in decreased wrist and hand function.

b. Traction injuries resolve spontaneously.

c. Avulsion injuries may require surgical nerve repair if not resolved within three months.

d. Shoulder subluxation and contractures of muscles may develop.

4. Physical therapy examination for brachial plexus injury.

a. Observe infant posture, as well as arm position and movement.

b. Test reflexes: Moro's, biceps, radial reflexes are not present; grasp is intact.

c. Sensory testing of affected upper extremity (UE).

5. Physical therapy intervention and prognosis.

a. Partial immobilization of limb across upper abdomen for 1–2 weeks to avoid further injury.

b. Gentle ROM after initial immobilization to avoid contractures.

c. Elicit muscle activity with age-appropriate functional movements of UE.

d. May use gentle constraint of unaffected arm to facilitate use of affected UE.

e. Prognosis depends on severity of nerve injury, favorable in most instances. If recovery does not occur, surgery is indicated.

Down Syndrome (Trisomy 21)

1. Pathology.

a. Chromosomal abnormality caused by breakage and translocation of a piece of chromosome onto normal chromosome.

b. Milder form with some normal cells interspersed with abnormal cells, called mosaic type.
c. Brain weight less than normal.
d. Cerebellum and brain stem lighter than normal.
e. Smaller convolutions of cortex.

2. Impairments.
a. Hypotonia.
b. Decreased force generation of muscles.
c. Congenital heart defects.
d. Visual and hearing losses.
e. Atlantoaxial subluxation/dislocation could be due to laxity of transverse odontoid ligament.
   (1) Signs include decreased strength, ROM, deep tendon reflexes (DTRs), and sensation in extremities. This is a medical emergency.
f. Cognitive deficit (mental retardation).

3. Functional limitations.
a. Gross motor developmental delay.
b. Difficulties in eating and speech development due to low tone.
c. Forceful neck flexion and rotation activities should be limited, due to atlantoaxial ligament laxity.
d. Cognitive and perceptual deficits may result in delay of fine motor and psychosocial development.

4. Physical therapy examination for Down syndrome.
a. Developmental test of gross and fine motor skills.
b. Test of tone by passive ROM.
c. Active and passive ROM.
d. Muscle testing; may use observation of developmental postures and movements if child under 3 years of age.
e. Functional level.

5. Physical therapy interventions, goals, and prognosis for Down syndrome.
a. Minimize gross motor delay.
   (1) Facilitate gross and fine motor development through appropriate positioning, posture, and movement activities.
   (2) Increase strength and stability by manipulating gravity and resistance in a graded manner.
b. Encourage oral motor function.
   (1) Facilitate lip closure and tongue retrusion.
   (2) Short, frequent feeding sessions for energy conservation.
c. Avoid hyperextension of elbows and knees during weight-bearing activities.
d. Prognosis may be correlated with tone; the lower the tone, the more significant the motor delay.
e. All children with Down syndrome will eventually become ambulatory.

6. Medical-surgical management of Down syndrome.
a. Yearly radiographs to rule out atlantoaxial subluxation.
b. Medical-surgical correction of cardiac problems.

Traumatic Brain Injury (TBI)

1. Pathology.
a. Primary brain injury due to mechanical forces of initial impact.
   (1) Acceleration-dependent injuries when force is applied to movable head such as coup-contrecoup and rotational injury.
   (2) Nonacceleration-dependent injuries include skull depression into brain tissue and vibration.
   (3) May be accidental or due to child abuse such as "shaken baby syndrome."
b. Secondary brain injury due to processes initiated as a result of initial trauma.
   (1) Cerebral edema increases intracranial pressure and may lead to herniation, cerebral infarctions, brain stem injury, and coma.
   (2) Epidural hematoma due to bleeds of middle meningeal artery, vein, or venous sinus bleeds into epidural space.
   (3) Subdural hematoma due to lacerated cortical blood vessels.
c. Evaluation of traumatic brain injury.
   (1) Imaging such as computed tomography (CT) scan and magnetic resonance imaging (MRI) to determine extent of initial and secondary injury.
   (2) Monitoring intracranial pressure.
   (3) Behavioral scales such as the Glasgow Coma Scale and the Rancho Los Amigos scale assess the child's orientation to time and place and the ability to respond to various stimuli. Infant coma scale used for nonverbal infants.

2. Impairments.
a. Depend on the severity and location of the initial and secondary injuries.
b. Level of consciousness and cognitive level may be temporarily or permanently impaired.
c. Spasticity, loss of functional ROM, contractures, and deformities.
d. Weakness, balance, and coordination problems.
e. Heterotopic ossification—pathological bone formation around joint due to increased tone around joint, immobility, and coma.

3. Functional limitations.
a. Decreased mobility skills.
b. Cognitive and perceptual difficulties.
c. Developmental process may be affected, resulting in abnormal development or developmental delay.

4. Physical therapy examination of traumatic brain injury.
a. History, MRI, CT, electroencephalographic (EEG) results, current medications.
b. Level of consciousness (Children's Coma Scale, Rancho Los Amigos Coma Scale).

c. Active and passive ROM.
d. Muscle strength: observe spontaneous movements if manual muscle test (MMT) is not possible.
e. Sensory testing.
f. Balance and coordination testing, developmental testing if appropriate.
g. Determination of muscle tone (modified Ashworth Scale).
h. Cranial nerve testing.
i. Functional level testing.
j. Integumentary examination to check for pressure sores.

5. **Interventions, goals, and prognosis.**
a. Maintain or improve joint flexibility by positioning, serial casting, ROM.
b. Stimulate/arouse level of consciousness through sensory stimuli.
c. Minimize gross and fine motor delay.
(1) Facilitate gross and fine motor development through appropriate positioning, postures, and movement activities.
(2) Increase strength and stability by manipulating gravity and resistance in a graded manner.
d. Parent/family or caregiver education.
e. Prognosis depends on severity of injury, rate of recovery, social and physical supports available.

6. **Medical-surgical management for TBI.**
a. Mechanical ventilation, if needed.
b. Pharmacological agents to control intracranial pressure, including sedatives, paralytics, diuretics, and barbiturates.
c. Intracranial pressure monitored by intracranial pressure bolt.
d. Surgical evacuation of hematoma.

Duchenne's Muscular Dystrophy (Pseudohypertrophic Muscular Dystrophy)

1. **Pathology.**
a. X-linked recessive, inherited by boys, carried by recessive gene of mother. Diagnosis confirmed by clinical examination, EMG, muscle biopsy, DNA analysis, and blood enzyme levels.
b. Dystrophin gene missing results in increased permeability of sarcolemma and destruction of muscle cells.
c. Collagen, adipose laid down in muscle leading to pseudohypertrophic calf muscles.

2. **Impairments.**
a. Progressive weakness from proximal to distal beginning at 3 years of age to death in late adolescence or early adulthood.
b. Positive Gower's sign due to weak quadriceps and gluteal muscles; child must use upper extremities to "walk up legs" and rise from prone to standing.
c. Cardiac tissue also involved.
d. Contractures and deformities develop due to muscle imbalance, especially of heel cords and tensor fascia latae, as well as lumbar lordosis and kyphoscoliosis.

3. **Functional impairments.**
a. Developmental milestones may be delayed.
b. Ambulation ability will be lost, necessitating eventual use of wheelchair.
c. Progressive cardiopulmonary limitations.

4. **Examination for muscular dystrophy.**
a. Muscle strength—MMT, dynamometer.
b. Active and passive ROM.
c. Functional testing.
d. Skeletal alignment (check for lordosis, scoliosis, kyphosis).
e. Respiratory function, chest excursion during breathing or spirometer.
f. Assess need for adaptive equipment.

5. **Interventions, goals, and prognosis.**
a. Maintain mobility as long as possible by encouraging recreational and functional activities to maintain strength and cardiopulmonary function.
b. Maintain joint ROM with active and passive ROM exercises, and positioning devices, such as prone standers or standing frames. Gastrocnemius and tensor fascia lata shorten first. Night splints may be used.
c. Electrical stimulation of muscles for younger children may increase contractile ability.
d. Educate and support parents and family in a sensitive manner.
e. Do not exercise at maximal level; may injure muscle tissue (overwork injury).
f. Supervise use of adaptive equipment as needed.
g. Disease is progressive, leading to respiratory insufficiency and death in young adulthood.

6. **Medical-surgical management.**
a. Palliative and supportive, treating symptoms as they occur.
b. Steroids (prednisone) increase life expectancy by decreasing pulmonary dysfunction. Antibiotics for pulmonary infections.
c. Orthopedic surgery for scoliosis (spinal instrumentation), muscle lengthening of gastrocnemius.

Note: See Chapter 1, Musculoskeletal Physical Therapy for additional pediatric conditions, e.g., deformities; disorders of the hip, knee, ankle/foot, and spine.

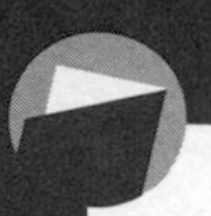

Pediatric Adaptive Equipment

1. **Positioning equipment.** Used to maintain skeletal alignment, prevent or reduce development of contractures and deformities, and facilitate functional abilities.
   a. Standers give the child weight-bearing experience, which maintains hips, knees, ankles, and trunk in optimal position, facilitates formation of acetabulum, and aids bowel and bladder function.
   b. Side-lyers decrease effects of TLR, put hands in visual field.
   c. Adaptive seating is customized to meet the specific support and posture needs of the individual.
   d. Abductor pad at hips often used in positioning equipment to decrease scissoring extension pattern of hip extension, adduction, with knee extension and plantar flexion of ankles.

2. **Equipment for therapeutic exercise.**
   a. Balls of different sizes to promote strengthening, balance, coordination, and make motor learning fun.
   b. Wedges to facilitate or increase muscle contraction needed, depending on position of wedge.
   c. Bolsters combine characteristics of ball and wedge.
   d. Swings to promote sensory integration.
   e. Scooter boards for prone stability/mobility work.
   f. Others include toys, modified tricycles, music, pets, and family members.

3. **Lower extremity orthotics.**
   a. AFOs to provide support to foot, ankle, and knee, to provide a stable base of support, and to reduce the effects of spasticity and hypoextensibility of muscles.
      (1) Ankle set at 5–10 degrees dorsiflexion to decrease genu recurvatum.
      (2) Articulating ankle AFO controls amount of dorsiflexion and plantar flexion.
      (3) Tone-reducing AFO may be polypropylene or plaster cast, bivalved.
         (a) Decreases effects of spasticity, including scissoring by maintained stretch.
         (b) Stretches and maintains length of heel cord to prevent or lessen contracture.
         (c) Provides good mechanical base of support for standing and ambulation.
   b. Knee-ankle-foot orthosis (KAFO).
      (1) For standing or ambulation.
      (2) Reciprocal or swing-through gait.
      (3) Knee may be solid at 0–5 degrees flexion or hinged.
      (4) Used by children with spina bifida or muscular dystrophy.
   c. Hip-knee-ankle-foot orthosis (HKAFO).
      (1) For standing and ambulation.
      (2) Swing-through gait.
      (3) Used by children with spina bifida or spinal cord injuries.
   d. Reciprocating gait orthosis (RGO).
      (1) HKAFO with molded body jacket.
      (2) Cable system allows forward step with lateral weight shift.
      (3) Used by children with thoracic level spinal bifida or spinal cord injuries.
   e. Pavlik harness.
      (1) For infants with congenital hip dysplasia.
      (2) Hips held in flexion and abduction to maintain femoral head in acetabulum.

4. **Mobility aids.**
   a. Wheelchairs.
      (1) Must be the correct size for the child.
      (2) Posture, movement, strength, endurance, abnormal tone, contractures are important in determining custom features of a wheelchair, including method of mobility, seating stability.
      (3) Stroller-type chairs limit independence of child.
      (4) Scooter/three wheelers require fair (3/5) sitting balance and upper extremity control.
   b. Walkers.
      (1) Rollator walkers with wheels usually used.
      (2) Forward walker (anterior rollator walker).
         (a) Encourages forward trunk leaning.
         (b) Provides maximum anterior stability.
      (3) Posterior walker (posture control walker).
         (a) Encourages trunk extension.
         (b) Encourages shoulder depression, elbow extension, neutral wrist which may decrease scissoring in lower extremities.
      (4) Gait trainers offer maximum support to upper extremities and trunk.
   c. Crutches.
      (1) Require more postural control than walkers.
      (2) Axillary and Lofstrand crutches available.

Family, Early Intervention, and the Education Setting

1. **Family.** The single most important constant and environmental factor.
   a. PT must collaborate with child and family.
   b. Family-centered approach begins with child's and family's strengths, needs, and hopes, and results in a service plan which responds to the needs of the whole family. Role of PT is to support, encourage,

and enhance the competence of parents or caretakers in their role as caregivers.

c. Parents of children with developmental disabilities often suffer from chronic sorrow due to the loss of the typical potential of their child.

2. Early Intervention Programs (EIPs).

a. Mandated by public law.
   (1) To provide comprehensive, multidisciplinary EIP.
   (2) For infants and children from birth to 3 years.
   (3) Multidisciplinary assessment.
   (4) Individual Family Service Plan (IFSP) developed.
   (5) Family is a member of the team.

3. School System: Individual Education Plan (IEP).

a. Mandated by public law.
   (1) Free and appropriate public education for all children with disabilities.
   (2) For children 3 to 21 years.
   (3) Multidisciplinary assessment.
   (4) Right to related services such as PT is related to educational need.
   (5) Least restrictive environment.

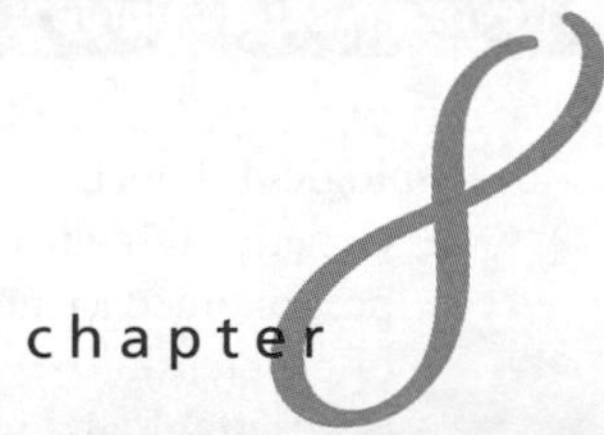

chapter 8

Geriatric Physical Therapy

SUSAN B. O'SULLIVAN

Foundations of Geriatric Physical Therapy

General Concepts and Definitions of Aging

1. **Aging.** The process of growing old; describes a wide array of physiological changes in the body systems; complex and variable.
   a. Common to all members of a given species.
   b. Progressive with time.
   c. Evidenced by:
      (1) Decline in homeostatic efficiency.
      (2) Increasing probability that reaction to injury will not be successful.
   d. Varies among and within individuals.

2. **Gerontology.** The scientific study of the factors impacting the normal aging process and the effects of aging.

3. **Geriatrics.** The branch of medicine concerned with the illnesses of old age and their care.

4. **Life span.** Maximum survival potential, the inherent natural life of the species; in humans, 110–120 years.

5. **Life expectancy.** The number of years of life expectation from year of birth, 75.8 years in the United States; women live 6.6 years longer than men.

6. **Senescence.** Last stages of adulthood through death.

7. **Categories of elderly.**
   a. Young elderly: ages 65–74 (60% of elderly population).
   b. Old elderly: ages 75–84.
   c. Old, old elderly or old & frail elderly: ages > 85.

8. **Ageism.** Discrimination and prejudice leveled against individuals on the basis of their age.

Demographics, Mortality, and Morbidity

1. **Persons over 65.**
   a. A rapidly growing segment of the population with lengthening of life expectancy; 13% of US. population in year 2000; by year 2030, expected to be 22% of US population.
   b. Older women outnumber older men; 145 women for every 100 men.
   c. Whites represent about 90% of persons over 65; only 10% are nonwhite (8% black).

2. **Increased life expectancy.**
   a. Aging of the population due to:
   b. Advances in health care, improved infectious disease control.
   c. Advances in infant/child care, decreased mortality rates.
   d. Improvements in nutrition and sanitation.

3. **Leading causes of death (mortality) in persons over 65, in order of frequency.**
   a. Coronary heart disease (CHD); accounts for 31% of deaths.
   b. Cancer, accounts for 20% of deaths.
   c. Cerebrovascular disease (stroke).

d. Chronic obstructive pulmonary disease (COPD).
e. Pneumonia/flu.

4. Leading causes of disability/chronic conditions (morbidity) in persons over 65, in order of frequency.
a. Arthritis, 49%.
b. Hypertension, 37%.
c. Hearing impairments, 32%.
d. Heart impairments, 30%.
e. Cataracts and chronic sinusitis, 17% each.
f. Orthopedic impairments, 16%.
g. Diabetes and visual impairments, 9% each.
h. Most older persons (60–80%) report one or more chronic conditions.

5. Socioeconomic factors.
a. Half of all older women are widows; older men are twice as likely to be married as older women.
b. Most live on fixed incomes: social security is the major source of income; poverty rate for persons over 65 is 11.4%; another 8% live near the poverty rate.
c. About half of older persons have completed high school.
d. Noninstitutionalized elderly: most live in family settings.
e. Institutionalized elderly: about 5% of persons over 65 reside in nursing homes; percentage increases dramatically with age (22% of persons over 85).

6. Health care costs.
a. Older persons account for 12% of population and 36% of total health care expenditures.
b. Older persons account for 33% of all hospital stays, 44% of all hospital days of care.

Theories of Aging

1. Aging is developmental, occurs across the life span.

2. Aging changes.
a. Cellular changes.
(1) Increase in size; fragmentation of Golgi apparatus and mitochondria.
(2) Decrease in cell capacity to divide and reproduce.
(3) Arrest of DNA synthesis and cell division.
b. Tissue changes.
(1) Accumulation of pigmented materials, lipofuscins.
(2) Accumulation of lipids and fats.
(3) Connective tissue changes: decreased elastic content, degradation of collagen; presence of pseudoelastins.
c. Organ changes.
(1) Decrease in functional capacity.
(2) Decrease in homeostatic efficiency.

3. Biological theories.
a. Genetic: aging is intrinsic to the organism; genes are programmed to modulate aging changes, overall rate of progression.
(1) Individuals vary in the expression of aging changes; e.g., graying of hair, wrinkles.
(2) Polygenic controls exist (multiple genes are involved): no one gene can modulate rate of development in all aspects of aging.
(3) Premature aging syndromes (progeria) provide evidence of defective genetic programming; individuals exhibit premature aging changes; i.e., atrophy and thinning of tissues, graying of hair, arteriosclerosis.
(a) Hutchinson-Gilford syndrome: progeria of childhood.
(b) Werner's syndrome: progeria of young adults.
b. Doubling/biological clock (Hayflick's limit theory): functional deterioration within cells is due to limited number of genetically programmed cell doublings (cell replication).
c. Free radical theory: free radicals are highly reactive, toxic forms of oxygen produced by cell mitochondria; the released radicals.
(1) Cause damage to cell membranes and DNA cell replication.
(2) Interfere with cell diffusion and transport, resulting in decreased O_2 delivery and tissue death.
(3) Decrease cellular integrity, enzyme activities.
(4) Result in cross-linkages: chemical bonding of elements not generally joined together; interfere with normal cell function.
(5) Result in accumulation of aging pigments, lipofuscins.
(6) Can trigger pathological changes: atherosclerosis in blood vessel wall; cell mutations and cancer.
d. Cell mutation (intrinsic mutagenesis): errors in the synthesis of proteins (DNA, RNA) lead to exponential cascade of abnormal proteins and aging changes.
e. Hormonal theory: functional decrements in neurons and their associated hormones lead to aging changes.
(1) Hypothalamus, pituitary gland, adrenal gland are the primary regulators, timekeepers of aging.
(a) Thyroxine is the master hormone of the body; controls rate of protein synthesis and metabolism.
(b) Secretion of regulatory pituitary hormones influence thyroid.
(2) Decreases in protective hormones: estrogen, growth hormone, adrenal DHEA (dehydroepiandrosterone).
(3) Increases in stress hormones (cortisol) can damage brain's memory center, the hippocampus, and destroy immune cells.

f. Immunity theory: thymus size decreases, shrivels by puberty, becomes less functional; bone marrow cell efficiency decreases; results in steady decrease in immune responses during adulthood.
   (1) Immune cells, T cells, become less able to fight foreign organisms; B cells become less able to make antibodies.
   (2) Autoimmune diseases increase with age.

4. **Environmental theories (stochastic or nongenetic theories).**
   a. Aging is caused by an accumulation of insults from the environment.
   b. Environmental toxins include ultraviolet, cross-linking agents (saturated fats), toxic chemicals (metal ions, Mg, Zn), radiation, and viruses.
   c. Can result in errors in protein synthesis and DNA synthesis/genetic sequences (error theory), cross-linkage of molecules, mutations.

5. **Psychological theories.**
   a. Stress theory: homeostatic imbalances alter structural and chemical composition.
      (1) General adaptation syndrome (Selye's): initial alarm reaction, progressing to stage of resistance, progressing to stage of exhaustion.
      (2) Closely linked to hormonal theory.
   b. Erickson's bipolar theory of lifespan development. Stages of later adulthood.
      (1) Integrity: individual exhibits full unification of personality; life is viewed with satisfaction (productive life), remains optimistic, continues to grow.
      (2) Despair: individual lacks ego integration; life is viewed with despair (fear of death, feelings of regret and disappointment, missed opportunities).

6. **Sociological theories.**
   a. Life experience/lifestyles influence aging process.
   b. Activity theory: older persons who are socially active exhibit improved adjustment to the aging process; allows continued role enactment essential for positive self-image and improved life satisfaction.
   c. Disengagement theory: distancing of an individual or withdrawal from society; reduction in social roles leads to further isolation and life dissatisfaction.
   d. Dependency: increasing reliance on others for meeting physical and emotional needs; focus is increasingly on self.

7. **An integrated model of aging.**
   a. Assumes that aging is a complex, multifactorial phenomenon in which some or all of the above processes may contribute to the overall aging of an individual; aging is not adequately explained by any single theory.

Physiological Changes and Adaptation in the Older Adult

Muscular

1. **Age-related changes.**
   a. Changes may be due more to decreased activity levels (hypokinesis) and disuse than from aging process.
   b. Loss of muscle strength: peaks at age 30, remains fairly constant until age 50, after which there is an accelerating loss (20–40% loss by age 65 in the nonexercising adult).
   c. Loss of power (force/unit time): significant declines due to losses in speed of contraction, changes in nerve conduction and synaptic transmission.
   d. Loss of skeletal muscle mass (atrophy): both size and number of muscle fibers decrease; by age 70, loss of 33% of skeletal muscle mass.
   e. Changes in muscle fiber composition: selective loss of type II, fast-twitch fibers, with increase in proportion of type I fibers.
   f. Changes in muscular endurance: muscles fatigue more readily.
      (1) Decreased muscle tissue oxidative capacity.
      (2) Decreased peripheral blood flow, oxygen delivery to muscles.
      (3) Altered chemical composition of muscle: decreased myosin adenosine triphosphatase (ATPase) activity, glycoproteins, and contractile protein.
      (4) Collagen changes: denser, irregular due to cross-linkages, loss of water content and elasticity; affects tendons, bone, cartilage.

2. **Clinical implications.**
   a. Movements become slower.
   b. Movements fatigue easier; increased complaints of fatigue.
   c. Connective tissue becomes denser and stiffer.
      (1) Increased risk of muscle sprains, strains, tendon tears.

(2) Loss of range of motion (ROM): highly variable by joint and individual; activity level.
(3) Increased tendency for fibrinous adhesions, contractures.

d. Decreased functional mobility, limitations to movement.

e. Gait changes.
(1) Stiffer, fewer automatic movements.
(2) Decreased amplitude and speed, slower cadence.
(3) Shorter steps, wider stride, increased double support to ensure safety, compensate for decreased balance.
(4) Decreased trunk rotation, arm swing.
(5) Gait may become unsteady due to changes in balance, strength; increased need for assistive devices.

f. Clinical risk of falls.

3. Interventions to slow or reverse changes.

a. Improve health.
(1) Correction of medical problems that may cause weakness: hyperthyroidism, excess adrenocortical steroids (e.g., Cushing's disease, steroids); hyponatremia (low sodium in blood).
(2) Improve nutrition.
(a) Correction of hyponatremia.
(b) Increased fatigue associated with diarrhea, prolonged use of diuretics.
(3) Address alcoholism.

b. Increase levels of physical activity, stress functional activities and activity programs.
(1) Gradual increase in intensity of activity to avoid injury.
(2) Adequate warm-up and cool-down; appropriate pacing and rest periods.

c. Provide strength training.
(1) Significant increases in strength noted in older adults with isometric and progressive resistive exercise programs.
(2) High-intensity training programs (70%–80% of one-repetition maximum) produce quicker and more predictable results than moderate-intensity programs; both have been successfully used with the elderly.
(3) Age not a limiting factor: significant improvements noted in frail, institutionalized 80 and 90 year-olds.
(4) Improvements in strength correlate to improved functional abilities.

d. Provide flexibility, ROM exercises.
(1) Utilize slow, prolonged stretching, maintained for 20–30 seconds.
(2) Tissues heated prior to stretching are more distensible; e.g., warm pool.
(3) Maintain newly gained range: incorporate into functional activities.
(4) Mobility gains are slower with older adults.

Skeletal System

1. Age-related changes.

a. Cartilage changes: decreased water content, becomes stiffer, fragments, and erodes; by age 60, more than 60% of adults have degenerative joint changes, cartilage abnormalities.

b. Loss of bone mass and density: peak bone mass at age 40; between ages 45 and 70, bone mass decreases (in women, by about 25%; in men, by 15%); decreases another 5% by age 90.
(1) Loss of calcium and bone strength, especially trabecular bone.
(2) See discussion of osteoporosis under pathological manifestations of aging.
(3) Decreased bone marrow red blood cell production.

c. Intervertebral discs: flatten, less resilient due to loss of water content (30% loss by age 65) and loss of collagen elasticity; trunk length, overall height decreases.

d. Senile postural changes.
(1) Forward head.
(2) Kyphosis of thoracic spine.
(3) Flattening of lumbar spine.
(4) With prolonged sitting, tendency to develop hip and knee flexion contractures.

2. Clinical implications.

a. Maintenance of weight-bearing is important for cartilaginous/joint health.

b. Clinical risk of fractures.

3. Interventions to slow or reverse changes.

a. Postural exercises: stress components of good posture.

b. Weight-bearing (gravity-loading) exercise can decrease bone loss in older adults; e.g., walking; stair climbing; weight belts can increase load.

c. Nutritional, hormonal, and medical therapies: see discussion of osteoporosis.

Neurological System

1. Age-related changes.

a. Atrophy of nerve cells in cerebral cortex: overall loss of cerebral mass/brain weight of 6%–11% between ages of 20 and 90; accelerating loss after age 70.

b. Changes in brain morphology.
(1) Gyral atrophy: narrowing and flattening of gyri with widening of sulci.
(2) Ventricular dilation.
(3) Generalized cell loss in cerebral cortex: especially frontal and temporal lobes, association areas (prefrontal cortex, visual).

(4) Presence of lipofuscins, senile or neuritic plaques, and neurofibrillary tangles (NFT): significant accumulations associated with pathology; e.g., Alzheimer's dementia.
(5) More selective cell loss in basal ganglia (substantia nigra and putamen), cerebellum, hippocampus, locus coeruleus; brainstem minimally affected.

c. Decreased cerebral blood flow and energy metabolism.

d. Changes in synaptic transmission.
(1) Decreased synthesis and metabolism of major neurotransmitters; e.g., acetylcholine, dopamine.
(2) Slowing of many neural processes, especially in polysynaptic pathways.

e. Changes in spinal cord/peripheral nerves.
(1) Neuronal loss and atrophy: 30%–50% loss of anterior horn cells, 30% loss of posterior roots (sensory fibers) by age 90.
(2) Loss of motoneurons results in increase in size of remaining motor units (development of macromotor units).
(3) Slowed nerve conduction velocity: sensory greater than motor.
(4) Loss of sympathetic fibers: may account for diminished, autonomic stability, increased incidence of postural hypotension in older adults.

f. Age-related tremors (essential tremor, ET).
(1) Occur as an isolated symptom, particularly in hands, head, and voice.
(2) Characterized as postural or kinetic, rarely resting.
(3) Benign, slowly progressive; in late stages, may limit function.
(4) Exaggerated by movement and emotion.

2. Clinical implications.

a. Effects on movement.
(1) Overall speed and coordination are decreased; increased difficulty with fine motor control.
(2) Slowed recruitment of motoneurons contributes to loss of strength.
(3) Both reaction time and movement time increase.
(4) Older adults are affected by the speed/ accuracy tradeoff.
(a) The simpler the movement, the less the change.
(b) More complicated movements require more preparation, longer reaction and movement times.
(c) Faster movements decrease accuracy, increase errors.
(5) Older adults typically shift in motor control processing from open to closed loop; e.g., demonstrate increased reliance on visual feedback for movement.
(6) Demonstrate increased cautionary behaviors, an indirect effect of decreased capacity.

b. General slowing of neural processing: learning and memory may be affected.

c. Problems in homeostatic regulation: stressors (heat, cold, excess exercise) can be harmful, even life-threatening.

3. Interventions to slow or reverse changes.

a. Correction of medical problems: improve cerebral blood flow.

b. Improve health: diet, smoking cessation.

c. Increase levels of physical activity to encourage neuronal branching, slow rate of neural decline, improve cerebral circulation.

d. Provide effective strategies to improve motor learning and control.
(1) Allow for increased reaction and movement times to improve motivation, accuracy of movements.
(2) Allow for limitations of memory by avoiding long sequences of movements.
(3) Allow for increased cautionary behaviors: provide adequate explanation, demonstration when teaching new movement skills.
(4) Stress familiar, well-learned skills, and repetitive movements.

Sensory Systems

1. Age-related changes.

a. May lead to sensory deprivation, isolation, disorientation, confusion, appearance of senility.

b. May strain social interactions.

c. May lead to decreased functional mobility, risk of injury.

2. Vision.

a. Aging changes: there is a general decline in visual acuity; gradual prior to sixth decade, rapid decline between ages 60 and 90; visual loss as high as 80% by age 90.
(1) Presbyopia: visual loss in middle and older ages characterized by inability to focus properly and blurred images due to loss of accommodation, elasticity of lens.
(2) Decreased ability to adapt to dark and light.
(3) Increased sensitivity to light and glare.
(4) Loss of color discrimination, especially for blues and greens.
(5) Decreased pupillary responses, size of resting pupil increases.
(6) Decreased sensitivity of corneal reflex: less sensitive to eye injury or infection.
(7) Oculomotor responses diminished: restricted upward gaze, reduced pursuit eye movements; ptosis may develop.

b. Additional vision loss with pathology.
(1) Cataracts: opacity, clouding of lens due to changes in lens proteins; results in gradual

loss of vision: central first, then peripheral; increased problems with glare; general darkening of vision; loss of acuity, distortion.

(2) Glaucoma: increased intraocular pressure, with degeneration of optic disc, atrophy of optic nerve; results in early loss of peripheral vision (tunnel vision), progressing to total blindness.

(3) Senile macular degeneration: loss of central vision associated with age-related degeneration of the macula, compromised by decreased blood supply or abnormal growth of blood vessels under the retina; initially, patients retain peripheral vision; may progress to total blindness.

(4) Diabetic retinopathy: damage to retinal capillaries, growth of abnormal blood vessels and hemorrhage leads to retinal scarring and finally retinal detachment; central vision impairment; complete blindness is rare.

(5) Cerebrovascular accident (CVA), homonymous hemianopsia: loss of one half visual field in each eye (nasal half of one eye and temporal half of other eye); produces an inability to receive information from right or left side; corresponds to side of sensorimotor deficit.

(6) Medications: impaired or fuzzy vision may result with antihistamines, tranquilizers, antidepressants, steroids.

c. Clinical implications/compensatory strategies.

(1) Examine vision: acuity, peripheral vision, light and dark adaptation, depth perception; diplopia, eye fatigue, eye pain.

(2) Maximize visual function: assess for use of glasses, need for environmental adaptations.

(3) Sensory thresholds are increased: allow extra time for visual discrimination and response.

(4) Work in adequate light, reduce glare; avoid abrupt changes in light; e.g., light to dark.

(5) Decreased peripheral vision may limit social interactions, physical function: stand directly in front of patient at eye level when communicating with patient.

(6) Assist in color discrimination: use warm colors (yellow, orange, red) for identification and color coding.

(7) Provide other sensory cues when vision is limited; e.g., verbal descriptions to new environments, touching to communicate you are listening.

(8) Provide safety education; reduce fall risk.

3. Hearing.

a. Aging changes: occur as early as fourth decade; affect a significant number of elderly (23% of individuals aged 65–74 have hearing impairments and 40% over age 75 have hearing loss; rate of loss in men is twice the rate of women, also starts earlier).

(1) Outer ear: build-up of cerumen (earwax) may result in conductive hearing loss; common in older men.

(2) Middle ear: minimal degenerative changes of bony joints.

(3) Inner ear: significant changes in sound sensitivity, understanding of speech, and maintenance of equilibrium may result with degeneration and atrophy of cochlea and vestibular structures, loss of neurons.

b. Types of hearing loss.

(1) Conductive: mechanical hearing loss from damage to external auditory canal, tympanic membrane, or middle ear ossicles; results in hearing loss (all frequencies); tinnitus (ringing in the ears) may be present.

(2) Sensorineural: central or neural hearing loss from multiple factors; e.g., noise damage, trauma, disease, drugs, arteriosclerosis.

(3) Presbycusis: sensorineural hearing loss associated with middle and older ages; characterized by bilateral hearing loss, especially at high frequencies at first, then all frequencies; poor auditory discrimination and comprehension, especially with background noise; tinnitus.

c. Additional hearing loss with pathology.

(1) Otosclerosis: immobility of stapes results in profound conductive hearing loss.

(2) Paget's disease.

(3) Hypothyroidism.

d. Clinical implications/compensatory strategies.

(1) Examine hearing: acuity, speech discrimination/comprehension; tinnitus, dizziness, vertigo, pain.

(2) Measure air and bone conduction: Rinne's test, Weber's test. See Chapter 2.

(3) Determine use of hearing aids; check for proper functioning.

(4) Minimize auditory distractions: work in quiet environment.

(5) Speak slowly and clearly, directly in front of patient at eye level.

(6) Use nonverbal communication to reinforce your message; e.g., gesture, demonstration.

(7) Orient person to topics of conversation they cannot hear to reduce paranoia, isolation.

4. Vestibular/balance control.

a. Aging changes: degenerative changes in otoconia of utricle and saccule; loss of vestibular hair-cell receptors; decreased number of vestibular neurons; vestibular ocular reflex (VOR) gain decreases; begins at age 30, accelerated decline at ages 55–60 results in diminished vestibular sensation.

(1) Diminished acuity, delayed reaction times, longer response times.

(2) Reduced function of VOR; affects retinal image stability with head movements, produces blurred vision.

(3) Altered sensory organization: older adults more dependent on somatosensory inputs for balance.
(4) Less able to resolve sensory conflicts when presented with inappropriate visual or proprioceptive inputs due to vestibular losses.
(5) Postural response patterns for balance are disorganized: characterized by diminished ankle torque, increased hip torque, increased postural sway.

b. Additional loss of vestibular sensitivity with pathology.
(1) Ménière's disease: episodic attacks characterized by tinnitus, dizziness, and a sensation of fullness or pressure in the ears; may also experience sensorineural hearing loss.
(2) Benign paroxysmal positional vertigo (BPPV): brief episodes of vertigo (<1 minute) associated with position change; the result of degeneration of the utricular otoconia that settle on the cupula of the posterior semicircular canal; common in older adults.
(3) Medications: antihypertensives (postural hypotension), anticonvulsants, tranquilizers, sleeping pills, aspirin, nonsteroidal anti-inflammatory drugs (NSAIDs).
(4) Cerebrovascular disease: vertebrobasilar artery insufficiency (TIAs, strokes); cerebellar artery stroke, lateral medullary stroke.
(5) Cerebellar dysfunction: hemorrhage, tumors (acoustic neuroma, meningioma); degenerative disease of brainstem and cerebellum; progressive supranuclear palsy.
(6) Migraine.
(7) Cardiac disease.

c. Clinical implications/compensatory strategies.
(1) Increased incidence of falls in older adults.
(2) Refer to section on falls and instability.

5. Somatosensory.

a. Aging changes.
(1) Decreased sensitivity of touch associated with decline of peripheral receptors, atrophy of afferent fibers; lower extremities more affected than upper.
(2) Proprioceptive losses, increased thresholds in vibratory sensibility, beginning around age 50: greater in lower than in upper extremities, greater in distal than proximal extremities.
(3) Loss of joint receptor sensitivity; losses in lower extremities, cervical joints may contribute to loss of balance.
(4) Cutaneous pain thresholds increased: greater changes in upper body areas (upper extremities, face) than in lower extremities.

b. Additional loss of sensation with pathology.
(1) Diabetes, peripheral neuropathy.
(2) CVA, central sensory losses.
(3) Peripheral vascular disease, peripheral ischemia.

c. Clinical implications/compensatory strategies.
(1) Examine sensation: check for increased thresholds to stimulation, sensory losses by modality, area of body.
(2) Allow extra time for responses with increased thresholds.
(3) Use touch to communicate: maximize physical contact; e.g., rubbing, stroking.
(4) Highlight, enhance naturally occurring intrinsic feedback during movements; e.g., stretch, tapping.
(5) Provide augmented feedback through appropriate sensory channels; e.g., walking on carpeted surfaces may be easier than on smooth floors.
(6) Teach compensatory strategies to prevent injury to anesthetic limbs, falls.
(7) Provide assistive devices as needed to prevent falls.
(8) Provide biofeedback devices as appropriate (e.g., limb-load monitor).

6. Taste and smell.

a. Aging changes.
(1) Gradual decrease in taste sensitivity.
(2) Decreased smell sensitivity.

b. Additional loss of sensation.
(1) Smokers.
(2) Chronic allergies, respiratory infections.
(3) Dentures.
(4) CVA, involvement of hypoglossal nerve.

c. Clinical implications/compensatory strategies.
(1) Examine ability to identify odors, tastes (sweet, sour, bitter, salty); somatic sensations (temperature, touch).
(2) Decreased taste, enjoyment of food leads to poor diet and nutrition.
(3) Older adults frequently increase use of taste enhancers: e.g., salt or sugar.
(4) Decreased home safety: e.g., gas leaks, smoke.

Cognition

1. Age-related changes.

a. No uniform decline in intellectual abilities throughout adulthood.
(1) Changes do not typically show up until mid-60s; significant declines affecting everyday life do not show up until early 80s.
(2) Most significant decline in measures of intelligence occurs in the years immediately preceding death (termed terminal drop).

b. Tasks involving perceptual speed show early declines (by age 39); require longer times to complete tasks.

c. Numeric ability (tests of adding, subtracting, multiplying) peaks in mid-40s, well-maintained until 60s.
d. Verbal ability peaks at age 30, well-maintained until 60s.
e. Memory.
   (1) Impairments typically noted in short-term memory; long-term memory retained.
   (2) Impairments are task-dependent; e.g., deficits primarily with novel conditions, new learning.
f. Learning. All age groups can learn; learning in older adults affected by:
   (1) Increased cautiousness.
   (2) Anxiety.
   (3) Pace of learning: fast pace is problematic.
   (4) Interference from prior learning.

2. Clinical implications.
a. Older adults utilize different strategies for memory (context-based strategies) than young adults (memorization).
b. Stress relationship, importance for function.

3. Interventions to slow or reverse changes.
a. Improve health.
   (1) Correction of medical problems: imbalances between oxygen supply and demand to central nervous system (CNS); e.g., cardiovascular disease, hypertension, diabetes, hypothyroidism.
   (2) Pharmacological changes: drug reevaluation; decreased use of multiple drugs; monitor closely for drug toxicity.
   (3) Reduction in chronic use of tobacco and alcohol.
   (4) Correction of nutritional deficiencies.
b. Increase physical activity.
c. Increase mental activity.
   (1) Keep mentally engaged—"Use it or Lose it"; e.g., chess, crossword puzzles, high level of reading.
   (2) Engaged lifestyle: socially active; e.g., clubs, travel, work.
   (3) Cognitive training activities.
d. Auditory processing may be decreased: provide written instructions.
e. Provide stimulating, "enriching" environment; avoid environmental dislocation; e.g., hospitalization or institutionalization may produce disorientation and agitation in some elderly.
f. Stress reduction counseling and family support.

Cardiovascular System

1. Age-related changes.
a. Changes due more to inactivity and disease than aging.
b. Degeneration of heart muscle with accumulation of lipofuscins (characteristic brown heart); mild cardiac hypertrophy, left ventricular wall.
c. Decreased coronary blood flow.
d. Cardiac valves thicken and stiffen.
e. Changes in conduction system: loss of pacemaker cells in sinoatrial node (SA) node.
f. Changes in blood vessels: arteries thicken, less distensible; slowed exchange capillary walls; increased peripheral resistance.
g. Resting blood pressures rise: systolic greater than diastolic.
h. Decline in neurohumoral control: decreased responsiveness of end-organs to beta-adrenergic stimulation of baroreceptors.
i. Decreased blood volume, hemopoietic activity of bone.
j. Increased blood coagulability.

2. Clinical implications.
a. Changes at rest are minor: resting heart rate and cardiac output relatively unchanged; resting blood pressures increase.
b. Cardiovascular responses to exercise: blunted, decrease in heart rate acceleration, decrease maximal oxygen uptake and heart rate; reduced exercise capacity, increased recovery time.
c. Decreased stroke volume due to decreased myocardial contractility.
d. Maximum heart rate declines with age (HR max = 220 – age).
e. Cardiac output decreases 1% per year after age 20 due to decreased heart rate and stroke volume.
f. Orthostatic hypotension: common problem in elderly due to reduced baroreceptor sensitivity and vascular elasticity.
g. Increased fatigue; anemia common in elderly.
h. Systolic ejection murmur common in elderly.
i. Possible electrocardiographic (ECG) changes: loss of normal sinus rhythm; longer PR and QT intervals; wider QRS; increased arrhythmias.

Pulmonary System

1. Age-related changes.
a. Chest wall stiffness. Declining strength of respiratory muscles results in increased work of breathing.
b. Loss of lung elastic recoil, decreased lung compliance.
c. Changes in lung parenchyma: alveoli enlarge, become thinner; fewer capillaries for delivery of blood.
d. Changes in pulmonary blood vessels: thicken, less distensible.
e. Decline in total lung capacity: residual volume increases, vital capacity decreases.
f. Forced expiratory volume (airflow) decreases.
g. Altered pulmonary gas exchange: oxygen tension falls with age, at a rate of 4 mm Hg/decade; PaO_2 at age 70 is 75, compared to 90 at age 20.

h. Blunted ventilatory responses of chemoreceptors in response to respiratory acidosis: decreased homeostatic responses.
i. Blunted defense/immune responses: decreased ciliary action to clear secretions, decreased secretory immunoglobulins, alveolar phagocytic function.

2. Clinical implications.

a. Respiratory responses to exercise: similar to younger adults at low and moderate intensities; at higher intensities, responses include increased ventilatory cost of work, greater blood acidosis, increased likelihood of breathlessness, and increased perceived exertion.
b. Clinical signs of hypoxia are blunted; changes in mentation and affect may provide important cues.
c. Cough mechanism is impaired.
d. Gag reflex is decreased, increased risk of aspiration.
e. Recovery from respiratory illness: prolonged in the elderly.
f. Significant changes in function with chronic smoking, exposure to environmental toxic inhalants.

3. Interventions.

a. To slow or reverse changes in cardiopulmonary systems.
b. Complete cardiopulmonary examination before beginning an exercise program is essential in older adults, due the high incidence of cardiopulmonary pathologies.
   (1) Selection of appropriate exercise tolerance testing (ETT) protocol is important.
   (2) Absence of standardized test batteries and norms for elderly.
   (3) Many elderly cannot tolerate maximal testing; submaximal testing commonly used.
   (4) Testing and training modes should be similar.
c. Individualized exercise prescription essential.
   (1) Choice of training program based on: fitness level, presence or absence of cardiovascular disease, musculoskeletal limitations, individual's goals and interests.
   (2) Prescriptive elements (frequency, intensity, duration, mode) are the same as for younger adults. See Chapter 3.
   (3) Walking, chair and floor exercises, modified strength/flexibility calisthenics well-tolerated by most elderly.
   (4) Consider pool programs (exercises, walking, and swimming) with bone and joint impairments.
   (5) Consider multiple modes of exercise (circuit training) on alternate days to reduce likelihood of muscle injury, joint overuse, pain, and fatigue.
d. Aerobic training programs can significantly improve cardiopulmonary function in the elderly.
   (1) Decrease heart rate at a given submaximal power output.
   (2) Improve maximal oxygen uptake (VO_2max).
   (3) Greater improvements in peripheral adaptation, muscle oxidative capacity than central changes; major difference from training effects in younger adults.
   (4) Improves recovery heart rates.
   (5) Decreases systolic blood pressure, may produce a small decrease in diastolic blood pressure.
   (6) Increases maximum ventilatory capacity: vital capacity.
   (7) Reduces breathlessness, lowers perceived exertion.
   (8) Psychological gains: improved sense of well-being, self-image.
   (9) Improves functional capacity.
e. Improve overall daily activity levels for independent living.
   (1) Lack of exercise is an important risk factor in the development of cardiopulmonary diseases.
   (2) Lack of exercise contributes to problems of immobility and disability in the elderly.

Integumentary System

1. Changes in skin composition.

a. Dermis thins with loss of elastin.
b. Decreased vascularity; vascular fragility results in easy bruising (senile purpura).
c. Decreased sebaceous activity and decline in hydration.
d. Appearance: skin appears dry, wrinkled, yellowed, and inelastic; age spots appear (clusters of melanocyte pigmentation); increase with sun exposure.
e. General thinning and graying of hair due to vascular insufficiency and decreased melanin production.
f. Nails grow more slowly, become brittle and thick.

2. Loss of effectiveness as protective barrier.

a. Skin grows and heals more slowly, less able to resist injury and infection.
b. Inflammatory response is attenuated.
c. Decreased sensitivity to touch, perception of pain and temperature; increased risk for injury from concentrated pressures or excess temperatures.
d. Decreased sweat production with loss of sweat glands results in decreased temperature regulation and homeostasis.

Gastrointestinal System

1. Age-related changes.

a. Decreased salivation, taste, and smell. Along with inadequate chewing (tooth loss, poorly fitting dentures), poor swallowing reflex may lead to poor dietary intake, nutritional deficiencies.
b. Esophagus: reduced motility and control of lower esophageal sphincter; acid reflux and heartburn, hiatal hernia common.

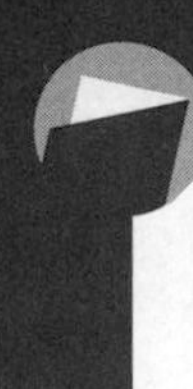

c. Stomach: reduced motility, delayed gastric emptying; decreased digestive enzymes and hydrochloric acid; decreased digestion and absorption; indigestion common.
d. Decreased intestinal motility; constipation common.

Renal System

1. **Age-related changes.**
   a. Kidneys: loss of mass and total weight with nephron atrophy, decreased renal blood flow, decreased filtration.
      (1) Blood urea rises.
      (2) Decreased excretory and reabsorptive capacities.
   b. Bladder: muscle weakness; decreased capacity, causing urinary frequency; difficulty with emptying, causing increased retention.
      (1) Urinary incontinence common (affects over 10 million adults; over half of nursing home residents and one third of community-dwelling elders); affects older women with pelvic floor weakness and older men with bladder or prostate disease.
      (2) Increased likelihood of urinary tract infections.

Pathological Conditions Associated with the Elderly

Musculoskeletal Disorders and Diseases

1. **Osteoporosis.**
   a. Disease process that results in reduction of bone mass; a failure of bone formation (osteoblast activity) to keep pace with bone reabsorption and destruction (osteoclast activity).
   b. WHO diagnostic criteria.
      (1) Osteoporosis is defined by bone mineral density (BMD) at the hip or spine that is ≥ 2.5 standard deviations (SD) below the young, normal mean reference population.
      (2) Osteopenia is defined by a BMD between 1.0 and 2.5 SD below the young, normal mean reference population.
   c. Etiological factors.
      (1) Hormonal deficiency associated with menopause and hypogonadism: loss of estrogens or androgens.
      (2) Age-related deficiencies.
      (3) Nutritional deficiency: inadequate calcium, impaired absorption of calcium; excessive alcohol, caffeine consumption.
      (4) Decreased physical activity: inadequate mechanical loading.
      (5) Diseases that affect bone loss: hyperthyroidism, diabetes, hyperparathyroidism, rheumatic disease (lupus), celiac disease, gastric bypass, pancreatic disease, multiple myeloma, sickle cell disease, end-stage renal disease, Paget's disease, cancer, and chemotherapeutic drugs.
      (6) Medications that affect bone loss: corticosteroids, thyroid hormone, anticonvulsants, catabolic drugs, some estrogen antagonists, chemotherapy.
      (7) Additional risk factors: family history, Caucasian/Asian race, early menopause, thin/small build, smoking.
   d. Characteristics.
      (1) Estimated 10 million Americans with osteoporosis; additional 33.6 million with low bone density (osteopenia). Eighty percent are women (will affect about one in two women); one third will experience major orthopedic problems related to osteoporosis.
      (2) Bone loss is about 1% per year (starting at ages 30–35 in women, and at ages 50–55 in men), accelerating loss in postmenopausal women, approximately 5% per year for 3–5 years.
      (3) Structural weakening of bone.
      (4) Decreased ability to support loads.
      (5) High risk of fractures.
      (6) Trabecular bone more involved than cortical bone; common areas affected:
         (a) Vertebral column.
         (b) Femoral neck.
         (c) Distal radius/wrist, humerus.
   e. Examination.
      (1) Medical record review.
         (a) History, physical exam, nutritional history.
         (b) BMD testing.
         (c) X-rays for known or suspected fractures.
         (d) Check for secondary causes.
      (2) Physical activity/fall history.
      (3) Assess dizziness: Dizziness Handicap Inventory.
      (4) Sensory integrity: vision, hearing, somatosensory, vestibular; sensory integration.
      (5) Motor function: strength, endurance, motor control.
      (6) ROM/flexibility.
      (7) Postural deformity.
         (a) Feet: hammer toes, bunions lead to antalgic gait.
         (b) Postural kyphosis, forward head position.
         (c) Hip and knee flexion contractures.

(8) Postural hypotension.
(9) Gait and balance assessment.

f. Goals, outcomes, and interventions.
   (1) Medical therapy: initiated with BMD T-scores ≤–2.5 at the femoral neck or spine by dual-energy x-ray absorptiometry (DXA) or individuals > 50 years with low bone mass (T-score between −1.0 and +2.5, osteopenia). Current Food and Drug Administration (FDA)–approved pharmacological options include:
      (a) Biphosphonates (alendronate, ibandronate, risedronate, and zoledronic acid).
      (b) Calcitonin.
      (c) Estrogens and/or hormone therapy.
      (d) Parathyroid hormone (teriparatide).
      (e) Estrogen agonist/antagonist (raloxifene).
   (2) Promote health; provide counseling on risk of osteoporosis and related fractures, health behaviors.
      (a) Daily calcium intake, individuals age 50 or older: 1200 mg per day.
      (b) Daily vitamin D intake, individuals age 50 or older: 800–1000 IU per day.
      (c) Avoid tobacco smoking and excessive alcohol intake.
      (d) Diet: low in salt; avoid excess protein, since it inhibits body's ability to absorb calcium.
   (3) Maintain bone mass: regular weight-bearing exercise.
      (a) Walking (30 min/day); stair-climbing; use of weight belts to increase loading.
      (b) Muscle-strengthening (resistance) exercises to reduce risk of falls and fractures.
   (4) Postural/balance training.
      (a) Postural reeducation, postural exercises to reduce kyphosis, forward head position.
      (b) Flexibility exercises.
      (c) Functional balance exercises; e.g., chair rises, standing/kitchen sink exercises (e.g., toe raises, unilateral stance, hip extension, hip abduction, partial squats).
      (d) Tai Chi.
      (e) Gait training.
   (5) Safety education/fall prevention.
      (a) Advise patients to avoid forward bending and exercising with trunk in flexion, especially in combination with twisting.
      (b) Avoid long-term bed rest.
      (c) Proper shoes: thin soles, flat shoes enhance balance abilities (no heels).
      (d) Assistive device to decrease fall risk: cane; walker as needed.
      (e) Fracture prevention: counseling on safe activities; avoid sudden forceful movements, twisting, standing, bending over, lifting, supine sit-ups.
      (f) Hip protectors for patients with significant risk for falls or who have previously fractured a hip.
      (g) Evaluate home environment for fall risk.

2. Fractures.

a. High risk of fractures in the elderly: associated with low bone density and multiple risk factors; e.g., age, comorbid diseases, dementia, psychotropic medications.

b. Hip fracture: common orthopedic problem of older adults, with more than 270,000 hip fractures annually in the United States; rate doubles each decade after age 50; by age 90, affects 32% of women and 17% of men.
   (1) Mortality rate: 20%, associated with complications.
   (2) About 50% will not resume their premorbid level of function; e.g., walk independently.
   (3) May result in dependency; continued institutionalization occurs in as many as one third of patients with hip fractures.
   (4) Majority of hip fractures are treated surgically: 95% are femoral neck or intertrochanteric fractures; remaining 5% are subtrochanteric fractures.
   (5) Intensive interdisciplinary rehabilitation program with early mobilization may improve outcome.
   (6) Treatment protocols based on type of fracture and surgical procedure used: internal fixation versus prosthetic replacement.

c. Vertebral compression fractures.
   (1) Usually occur in lower thoracic, lumbar regions (T8–L3).
   (2) Typically result from routine activity: bending, lifting, rising from chair.
   (3) Chief complaints: immediate, severe local spinal pain, increased with trunk flexion.
   (4) Lead to shortening of spine, progressive loss of height; spinal deformity (kyphosis), can progress to respiratory compromise.
   (5) Goals, outcomes, and interventions: acute phase.
      (a) Horizontal bed rest, out of bed 10 minutes every hour.
      (b) Emphasis on proper posture, extension in sleeping, sitting, and standing.
      (c) Isometric extension exercises in bed.
   (6) Goals, outcomes, and interventions: chronic phase.
      (a) Teach patient extension exercises; avoid flexion activities.
      (b) Postural training.
      (c) Modalities for relief of pain.
      (d) Safety education/modify environment.
      (e) Decrease vertebral loading; e.g., use soft-soled shoes.

(f) Spinal orthotics: may provide pain relief; long-term use may lead to muscle weakness and further deconditioning.

(7) **Red Flag:** use caution with pain medications that can cause disorientation or sedation, increasing risk of falls.

(8) Surgery: Kyphoplasty or vertebroplasty can be performed for individuals with painful vertebral fractures.

d. Stress fractures: fine, hairline fracture (insufficiency fracture) without soft tissue injury.

(1) In elderly, common in pelvis, proximal tibia, distal fibula, metatarsal shafts, foot.

(2) May be unsuspected source of pain.

(3) Observe for signs of local tenderness and swelling; e.g., postexercise.

(4) Goals, outcomes, and interventions.

(a) Rest.

(b) Correction of exercise excesses or faulty exercise program.

(c) Reduction of vertical loading; e.g., soft-sole shoes.

e. Upper extremity fractures: humeral head, Colles' fractures common.

f. For discussion of fracture assessment and management; see Chapter 1.

g. Clinical implications of fracture management in the elderly.

(1) Fractures heal more slowly.

(2) Older adults are prone to complications; e.g., pneumonia, decubitus ulcers, mental status complications with hospitalization.

(3) Rehabilitation may be complicated or prolonged by lack of support systems; comorbid conditions, decreased vision, poor balance.

3. Degenerative arthritis (osteoarthritis).

a. A noninflammatory, progressive disorder of joints; typically affects hips, knees, fingers, and spine.

b. Affects more than 16 million in the United States.

(1) Incidence increases with age: at age 55, affects 57% of population; by age 75, affects 70% of population.

(2) Prevalence higher in men up to age 45; by age 65, women five times more likely to be affected.

c. Moderate to severe limitation in functional daily activities seen in 24% of individuals.

d. Characteristics.

(1) Pain, swelling, and stiffness, worse early morning or with over-use; e.g., knee pain, hip pain.

(2) Muscle spasm.

(3) Loss of ROM and mobility; crepitus.

(4) Bony deformity.

(5) Muscle weakness secondary to disuse.

e. Goals, outcomes, and interventions.

(1) Medical management: NSAIDs, corticosteroid injections, topical analgesics, joint replacements.

(2) Reduction of pain and muscle spasm: modalities, relaxation training.

(3) Exercises.

(a) Maintain or improve ROM.

(b) Correct muscle imbalances: strengthening exercises to support joints, improve balance and ambulation.

(c) Aerobic conditioning: walking programs are associated with decreased joint symptoms, improved function, and sense of well-being.

(d) Aquatic programs; e.g., pool walking, Arthritis Foundation program: produces beneficial effects similar to aerobic conditioning; enhances ease of movement.

(4) Patient education and empowerment.

(a) Teach patients about disease, taking an active role in care.

(b) Teach joint protection, energy conservation strategies.

(5) Provide assistive devices for ambulation and activities of daily living; e.g., canes, walkers, shoe inserts, reachers.

(6) Promote healthy lifestyle: weight reduction to relieve stress on joints.

Neurological Disorders and Diseases

1. Stroke (CVA).

a. Sudden, focal neurological deficit resulting from ischemic or hemorrhagic lesions in the brain.

b. Most common cause of adult disability in the United States.

(1) Incidence of stroke increases dramatically with age; most strokes (43%) occur in persons over the age of 74.

(2) Approximately 30% die during the acute phase, and another 30%–40% will have severe disability.

c. Clinical signs and symptoms; examination and intervention; see Chapter 2.

2. Degenerative diseases.

a. Parkinson's disease: chronic, progressive disease of nervous system.

(1) Parkinson's symptoms afflict about 20% of individuals over the age of 65; frequency of symptoms increases with age, affecting 50% of individuals over the age of 85.

(2) Parkinson's disease affects about 1% of individuals over age 55, reaching proportions of 2.6 percent by age 85; in the United States. Affects approximately 1.5 million individuals, with 50,000 new cases annually; mean age of onset is between 59 and 62.

(3) Clinical signs and symptoms; examination and intervention; see Chapter 2.

3. Clinical implications.

a. Older adults are prone to complications/indirect impairments; e.g., contracture and deformity, decubitus ulcers, mental status complications.

b. Rehabilitation may be complicated or prolonged by lack of support systems, co-morbid conditions, decreased sensorimotor function, poor balance.

c. With irreversible neurological disease, it is important to address the impairments and functional limitations responsive to interventions; overall focus should be on improved function and safety.

d. Compensatory treatment strategies should be considered when impairments cannot be remediated; strategies can include environmental modifications, assistive devices, use of home health aides.

Cognitive Disorders

1. Delirium

a. Fluctuating attention state causing temporary confusion and loss of mental function; an acute disorder, potentially reversible. (Table 8-1).

b. Etiology: drug toxicity and/or systemic illness, oxygen deprivation to brain; environmental changes and sensory deprivation; e.g., recent hospitalization, institutionalization.

c. Characteristics.

(1) Acute onset, often at night; fluctuating course with lucid intervals; worse at night.

(2) Duration: hours to weeks.

(3) May be hypoalert or hyperalert, distractible; fluctuates over course of day.

(4) Orientation usually impaired.

(5) Illusions/hallucinations, periods of agitation.

Table 8-1 ➤ DIFFERENTIAL DIAGNOSIS: ORGANIC BRAIN SYNDROMES

	MULTI-INFARCT DEMENTIA	SENILE DEMENTIA ALZHEIMER'S TYPE (SDAT)	PRESENILE DEMENTIA ALZHEIMER'S TYPE (PDAT)
Age of Onset	55–70	60+	40–60
Gender Distribution	M:W = 3:1	M:W = 2:3	M:W = 2:3
Duration	Varies: days>years	Varies: months>years; mean survival 7–11 yr.	Rapid Mean survival: 4 years
Mode of Onset	Sudden	Gradual	Less gradual than SDAT
Course	Intermittent step-wise	Slowly or rapidly progressive	Rapidly progressive
Prognosis	Varies	Poor: mod. or severe cases	Very poor
Outcome	Death from CVA, CAD, or infection	Death from general system failure, infection	
Hereditary	Atherosclerosis	Multifactorial: age	
Precipitating Factors	Some familial tendency	Genetic: chromosome 21 abnormality; APOE4 gene; traumatic brain injury, Down Syndrome	
Neuropathology	Small or large areas of infarction secondary gliosis, senile plaques not common	Neuronal degeneration, neurofibrillary tangles, amyloid deposits, senile plaques, decreased cholinergic neuronal activity	
Clinical Signs of Brain Damage	Diffuse or focal, areas of preserved function	Diffuse, generalized	Diffuse, generalized, more severe than SDAT
Impairment of Higher Cortical Functions	Isolated impairments, focal signs, episodes of confusion with lucid intervals, some insight	Progressive dementia, progressive disorientation, memory loss, impaired cognition, judgment, abstract thinking, visuospatial deficits, apraxia, delusions, hallucinations; late stages: disorders of sleep, eating, sexual behavior, no insight	
Affect	Emotional lability, anxious, depressed	Variable: depressed, anxious, paranoid, hostile, restlessness, agitation, wandering, "sundowning" Late: apathy Personality changes: egocentricity, impulsivity, irritability, inappropriate social behaviors	
Neuromuscular	Focal signs: may see hemiparesis, hemisensory loss	Occasional tremors, generalized weakness, unsteady gait, increased tone: rigid postures, decreased postural reflexes, increased fall risk, repetitive behaviors	
Seizures	Yes	Rare	Occasional
Medical	TIAs, CVA, hypertension, headaches	Infections, contractures, fractures, decubitus ulcers, urinary and fecal incontinence	

(6) Memory deficits: immediate and recent.
(7) Disorganized thinking, incoherent speech.
(8) Sleep/wake cycles always disrupted.

2. Dementia.

a. Loss of intellectual functions and memory, causing dysfunction in daily living (see Table 8-1).

b. Criteria for dementia.
(1) Deterioration of intellectual functions: impoverished thinking, impaired judgment; disorientation, confusion; impaired social functioning.
(2) Disturbances in higher cortical functions: language (aphasia), motor skills (apraxia), perception (agnosia).
(3) Memory impairment: recent and remote.
(4) Personality changes: alteration or accentuation of premorbid traits; behavioral changes.
(5) Alertness (consciousness) usually normal.
(6) Sleep often fragmented.

c. Reversible dementias: (10%–20% of dementias); multiple causes.
(1) Drugs: sedatives, hypnotics, antianxiety agents, antidepressants, antiarrhythmics, antihypertensives, anticonvulsants, antipsychotics, drugs with anticholinergic side effects.
(2) Nutritional disorders: vitamin B_6 deficiency, thiamine deficiency, vitamin B_{12} deficiency/pernicious anemia, folate deficiency.
(3) Metabolic disorders: hyper/hypothyroidism, hypercalcemia, hyper/hyponatremia, hypoglycemia, kidney or liver failure, Cushing's syndrome, Addison's disease, hypopituitarism, carcinoma.
(4) Psychiatric disorders: depression, anxiety, psychosis.
(5) Toxins: air pollution, alcohol.

d. Primary degenerative dementia, Alzheimer's type: (50%–70% of dementias).
(1) Affects estimated 1.6 million individuals, 10%–20% of the over 65 population; third costliest disease in United States; fourth leading cause of death.
(2) Leading cause of institutionalization; affects up to 50% of nursing home population.
(3) Etiology unknown.
(a) Evidence of chromosomal abnormalities.
(b) Predisposing factors: family history, Down syndrome, traumatic brain injury, aluminum toxicity.
(4) Pathophysiology.
(a) Generalized atrophy of brain with decreased synthesis of neurotransmitters, diffuse ventricular dilation.
(b) Histopathological changes: neurofibrillary tangles; neuritic senile plaques: build-up of beta-amyloid protein.
(5) Types.
(a) Senile dementia, Alzheimer's type (SDAT): onset after the age of 60 (average age 75).
(b) Presenile dementia Alzheimer's type (PDAT): onset between ages of 40–60.
(6) Characteristics.
(a) Dementia: insidious onset with generally progressive deteriorating course; irreversible, mean survival time postdiagnosis is 4 years.
(b) May have periods of agitation and restlessness, wandering.
(c) Sundowning syndrome: confusion and agitation increases in late afternoon.

e. Multi-infarct dementias (MIDs), (20%–25% of dementias).
(1) Etiology: large and small vascular infarcts in both gray and white matter of brain, producing loss of brain function.
(2) Characteristics.
(a) Sudden onset rather than insidious; stepwise progression.
(b) Spotty and patchy distribution of deficits: areas of preserved ability along with impairments.
(c) Focal neurological signs and symptoms; e.g., gait and balance abnormalities, weakness, exaggerated deep tendon reflexes (DTRs).
(d) Emotional lability common.
(e) Associated with history of stroke, cardiovascular disease, hypertension.

f. Other types of dementias.
(1) Parkinson's disease: dementia estimated in 10%–35% of cases, in late stages of the disease.
(2) Alcohol-related: chronic alcoholism with prolonged nutritional (vitamin B_1) deficiency; e.g., Korsakoff's psychosis.

g. Examination.
(1) History: determine onset of symptoms, progression, triggering events; common problems, social history.
(2) Examine cognitive functions: orientation, attention, calculation, recall, language. Standardized test: Mini-Mental State Examination (MMSE); score of < 24 out of possible 30 is indicative of mental decline/dementia.
(3) Examine for impairments in higher cortical functions: inability to communicate, perceptual dysfunction.
(4) Examine for behavioral changes: restless, agitated, distracted, paranoid, wandering, inappropriate social behaviors, repetitive behaviors.
(5) Examine self-care: ability to carry out activities of daily living; e.g., limitations in grooming and hygiene, continence.
(6) Examine motor function: dyspraxia, gait, and balance instability.
(7) Examine environment for safety, optimal function.

h. Goals, outcomes, and interventions.

(1) Environment.
(a) Provide safe environment: prevent falls, injury or further dysfunction, safety from wandering; utilize safety monitoring devices as needed; e.g., alarm device.
(b) Provide soothing environment with reduced environmental distractions: reduces agitation, increases attention.
(2) Support individual's remaining function.
(a) Approach the patient in a friendly, supportive manner; model calm behavior.
(b) Use consistent, simple commands; speak slowly.
(c) Use nonverbal communication: sensory cues and demonstration.
(d) Provide reorienting information: use prompts; e.g., wall calendars, daily schedules, memory aids whenever possible.
(e) Avoid stressful tasks, emphasize familiar, well-learned skills; provide redirection.
(f) Approach learning in a simple, repetitious way, proceed slowly, and provide adequate rest time.
(g) Provide mental stimulation: utilize simple, well-liked activities, games.
(3) Provide regular physical activity.
(a) Safe walking program.
(b) Balance activities for fall prevention.
(c) Activities to promote body awareness and sensory stimulation.
(4) Participate in restraint reduction program.
(5) Educate/support family, caregivers.
(6) Present a realistic, consistent team approach to management.

3. Depression.
a. A disorder characterized by depressed mood and lack of interest or pleasure in all activities, and other associated symptoms, lasting for at least 2 weeks.
b. Incidence.
(1) Community-dwelling elderly: 5% have clinically diagnosed major depression (exhibit at least five symptoms); another 10%–20% have depressive symptoms.
(2) Institutionalized elderly: 12% have major depression; another 15%–20% have depressive symptoms.
c. Determine predisposing factors.
(1) Family history, prior episodes of depression.
(2) Illness, drug side effects; hormonal.
(3) Chronic condition: loss of physical functions, pain; e.g., stroke.
(4) Sensory deprivation (loss of vision or hearing).
(5) History of losses: death of family and friends, job, income, independence.
(6) Social isolation: lack of family support.
(7) Psychological losses: memory, intellectual functions.
d. Examine for depressive symptoms.
(1) Nutritional problems: significant weight loss or weight gain; dehydration.
(2) Sleep disturbances: insomnia or hypersomnia.
(3) Psychomotor changes: inactivity with resultant functional impairments, weakness or agitation.
(4) Fatigue or loss of energy.
(5) Feelings of worthlessness, low self-esteem, guilt.
(6) Inability to concentrate, slowed thinking, impaired memory, indecisiveness.
(7) Withdrawal from family and friends, self-neglect.
(8) Recurrent thoughts of death, suicidal ideation: document and immediately report all threats of suicide.
(9) Decline in cognitive function; i.e., document with MMSE.
(10) Standardized test: Geriatric Depression Scale; 30-item yes/no scale; score > 8 indicates depression.
e. Goals, outcomes, and interventions.
(1) Medical treatment.
(a) Pharmacotherapy; tricyclic antidepressants (e.g., Chlorpromazine, fluoxetine [Prozac]) widely used.
(b) Psychotherapy.
(c) Electroconvulsive shock therapy (ECT) may be used if drug treatment is unsuccessful or contraindicated.
(2) Avoid excessive cheerfulness; provide support and encouragement.
(3) Assist patient in adjustment process to losses, coping strategies.
(4) Encourage activities, exercise program: aerobic training is associated with increased feelings of well-being.
(5) Assist in improving/maintaining independence; emphasize mastery by patient, achievement of short-term rather than long-term goals.

Cardiopulmonary & Integumentary Disorders and Diseases

1. Hypertension.
a. Significant risk factor in cardiovascular disease, stroke, renal failure, and death.

2. Coronary artery disease (CAD).
a. Affects 40% of individuals aged 65–74 and 50% over age 75.
b. Angina.
(1) Angina pain not always a consistent indicator of ischemia in elderly; shortness of breath, ECG ST segment depression may be more reliable indicators.
c. Acute myocardial infarction.
(1) Clinical presentation may vary from younger adults: may present with sudden dyspnea, acute confusion, syncope.

(2) Clinical course often more complicated in the elderly, mortality rates twice that of younger adults.

d. Congestive heart failure.
e. Conduction system diseases: pacemaker dysfunction results in low cardiac output.

3. Peripheral vascular disease.

4. Clinical signs and symptoms.

a. Examination and intervention. See Chapter 3.

5. Chronic bronchitis.

6. Chronic obstructive pulmonary disease (COPD).

7. Asthma.

8. Pneumonia.

a. Initial symptoms may vary: instead of high fever and productive cough, may see altered mental status, tachypnea, dehydration.

9. Lung cancer.

10. Clinical signs and symptoms.

a. Examination and intervention. See Chapter 4.

11. Pressure ulcers (decubitus ulcers).

a. Characteristics.

(1) Affects 10%–25% of hospitalized, ill elderly patients.
(2) Risk factors: immobility and inactivity, sensory impairment, cognitive deficits, decreased circulation, poor nutritional status, incontinence, and moisture.
(3) Common over bony prominences: ischial tuberosities, sacrum, greater trochanter, heels, ankles, elbows, and scapulae.
(4) If not treated promptly, can progress to damage of deep structures.
(5) Potentially fatal in frail elderly and chronically ill.

b. Clinical signs and symptoms; examination and intervention. See Chapter 5.

Metabolic Pathologies

1. Diabetes mellitus.

a. Aging is associated with deteriorating glucose tolerance; type 2 diabetes affects as many as 10%–20% of individuals over age of 60.
b. Associated with obesity and sedentary lifestyle.
c. Clinical signs and symptoms; examination and intervention. See Chapter 6.

Patient Care Concepts

General Principles of Geriatric Rehabilitation

1. Recognize variability of older adults.

a. Uniqueness of the individual.
b. Developmental issues unique to the elderly.

2. Focus on careful and accurate clinical examination.

a. To identify remediable problems.
b. Determine capacity for safe function.
c. Determine effects of inactivity versus activity.
d. Determine effects of normal aging versus disease pathologies.

3. Focus on functional goals.

a. Determine priorities, remediable problems.
b. Develop goals, plan of care in conjunction with patient/caregiver.

4. Promote optimal health.

a. Focus on increasing health-conducive behaviors, prevention of disability.
b. Minimize and compensate for health-related losses and impairments of aging.

5. Restore/maintain.

a. Individual's highest level of function and independence within the care environment.
b. Determine how patient autonomy can be maximized by appropriate assistance and environmental manipulations.
c. Empower elders: ensure they are in control of their own decisions whenever possible.
d. Be sensitive to cultural and ethnicity issues; losses, fears, and insecurities; provide comfort and sustenance.
e. Enhance coping skills.
f. Recognize functional abilities, limitations of caregivers.

6. Holism.

a. Consider the whole person; integrate all facets of an individual's life.
b. Determine social support systems, effects of social isolation.
c. Determine effects of losses.
d. Determine effects of depression, dementia.

7. Recognize demands.

a. For continuity of care, interactions in a complex health-care delivery system.

b. Advocate for needed services.
c. Provide effective documentation.

Reimbursement Issues

1. **Benefits from government programs.**
   a. Cover about two thirds (63%) of health-care expenditures of older persons.
   b. Medicare: Federal government–sponsored insurance for persons over age 65, disabled persons of all ages.
      (1) Part A covers inpatient hospital care, skilled nursing facility care, home health care provided by agencies, hospice care.
         (a) No premiums; eligibility under social security.
         (b) Must pay deductibles and coinsurance.
      (2) Part B covers physician services, outpatient services, durable medical equipment.
         (a) Must pay premiums to be eligible.
         (b) Must pay deductibles and coinsurance.
   c. Medicaid (Federal-state funding): covers long-term care of frail and aged patients in nursing homes, impoverished adults, and children.
      (1) Must spend down or exhaust income to qualify for low-income status.
      (2) Administered by individual states that set qualification guidelines; specific requirements vary by state.

2. **Supplemental insurance.**
   a. May be purchased from private insurance companies.
   b. Copayments that elderly must pay under Medicare (Medex), termed Medigap policies.
   c. Long-term care insurance.
   d. Enrollment in Health Maintenance Organizations (HMOs).

3. **Documentation and reimbursement.**
   a. Requirements specific to type of insurance program.
      (1) Medicare requirements for physical therapy services.
         (a) Must be prescribed by a physician.
         (b) Must include a determination of need: reasonable and necessary for individual's illness or injury according to acceptable standards of practice.
         (c) Requires the skilled services of a licensed physical therapist to establish the plan of care (POC) (signature and professional identity is required).
         (d) The physician should review and sign and date the POC (certification). The POC should be certified for the first 30 days of treatment and recertified every 30 days (signed and dated).
         (e) If the service is not covered under Medicare statutes (e.g., exceeding therapy cap, maintenance care, prevention and wellness), the patient can be billed directly.
      (2) Private insurance requirements: vary by specific carrier; most adopt Medicare requirements (e.g. physician certification).
   b. Baseline data must be described in functional and measurable terms.
   c. Goals and outcomes should be measurable, objective, specific to patient, and indicate a predicted time frame.
   d. Plan of Care (POC).
      (1) Address findings, relate impairments to functional performance.
      (2) Include frequency and duration of treatment, projected end date, and disposition.
   e. Progress report.
      (1) Focuses on improvements, objective changes; subjective statements by patient.
      (2) Documents remaining deficits, lack of progress, or declining status.
      (3) Must be completed at least once during each Progress Report period.

Ethical and Legal Issues

1. **Professional practice.**
   a. Affirms patient rights and dignity (professional ethical standards, APTA Code of Ethics).

2. **Informed consent.**
   a. Respect for personal autonomy; competent patients have the right to refuse treatment; e.g., do not resuscitate (DNR) orders.
   b. Legal right to self-determination. Information must be provided to patient that outlines:
      (1) The nature and purpose of treatment.
      (2) Treatment alternatives.
      (3) Risks and consequences of treatment.
      (4) Likelihood of success or failure of treatment.
   c. Consent must be obtained from a legal guardian if the individual is judged incompetent.
      (1) Older adults with fluctuating mental abilities must be carefully evaluated for periods of lucidity.
      (2) Documentation with a mental status exam is essential.

3. **Advance Care Medical Directive (Living Will).**
   a. Established by Federal Patient Self-Determination Act of 1990.
   b. Health Care Proxy (Durable Power of Attorney): identifies a valid agent who is granted authority to make health-care decisions for an individual, should that individual become incapacitated.

c. Requirements.
   (1) Regulated by individual states; specific requirements vary by state.
   (2) Must be in writing, signed by principal, witnessed by two adults.
   (3) Empowers health-care agent: includes specific guidelines on which treatment options will and will not be allowed, e.g., artificial life support, feeding tubes.
   (4) Defines conditions/scope of agent's authority.

Common Problem Areas for Geriatric Clients

Immobility-Disability

1. Impaired mobility and disability.
   a. Can result from a host of diseases and problems.

2. Limitations in function.
   a. Increase with age in persons over age 65.
   b. 23% report difficulty with one or more personal care activities.
   c. 27% report difficulty with one or more home management activities.

3. Immobility.
   a. Can result in additional problems.
   b. Immobility can lead to complications in almost every major organ system; e.g., pressure sores, contractures, bone loss, muscular atrophy, deconditioning.
   c. Metabolic changes can include negative nitrogen and calcium balance, impaired glucose tolerance, decreased plasma volume, altered drug pharmacokinetics.
   d. Psychological changes can include loss of positive self-image, depression.
   e. Behavioral changes can include confusion, dementia secondary to sensory deprivation, egocentricity.
   f. Loss of independence and dependency.

4. Examination.
   a. To identify the source of immobility or disability.

5. Goals, outcomes, interventions.
   a. Establish a supportive relationship and promote self-determination of goals.
   b. Focus on optimal function, gradual progression of physical daily activities.
   c. Prevent further complications or injury.
   d. A team approach of health professionals to address all aspects of the patient's problems; patient participation in decision-making.

Falls and Instability

1. Falls and fall injury.
   a. Are a major public health concern for the elderly.
   b. Each year, approximately 30% of persons over the age of 65 fall.
   c. 24% of falls result in severe soft tissue injury and fractures.
      (1) Mortality rate associated with falls is 6%.
      (2) Falls are a factor in 40% of admissions to nursing homes.
   d. Fall results.
      (1) Increased caution and fear of falling.
      (2) Loss of confidence to function independently.
      (3) Reduced motivation and levels of activity.
      (4) Increased risk of recurrent falls.

2. Fall etiology.
   a. Most falls are multifactorial, the result of multiple intrinsic and extrinsic factors and their cumulative effects on mobility; e.g., disease states, age-related changes.
   b. Intrinsic/physiological factors.
      (1) Age: incidence of falls increases with age.
      (2) Sensory changes.
         (a) Reduced vision, hearing, cutaneous proprioceptive, and vestibular function.
         (b) Altered sensory organization for balance, reduced resolution of sensory conflict situations, increased dependence on support surface somatosensory inputs.
      (3) Musculoskeletal changes.
         (a) Weakness.
         (b) Decreased ROM.
         (c) Altered postural synergies.
      (4) Neuromotor changes.
         (a) Dizziness, vertigo common.
         (b) Timing and control problems: impaired reaction and movement times; slowed onset.
      (5) Cardiovascular changes.
         (a) Orthostatic hypotension.
         (b) Hyperventilation, coughing, arrhythmias.
      (6) Drugs.
         (a) Strong evidence linking psychotropic agents.
         (b) Some evidence linking certain cardiovascular agents, especially those that cause peripheral vasodilation.
         (c) Conflicting evidence linking analgesics, hypoglycemics.
   c. Intrinsic/psychosocial factors.
      (1) Mental status/cognitive impairment.
      (2) Depression.

(3) Denial of aging.
(4) Fear of falling: associated with self-imposed activity restriction.
(5) Relocation.

d. Extrinsic/environmental factors.
(1) Setting: three times as many falls for institutionalized or hospitalized elderly than for community-dwelling elderly.
(2) Consider ground surfaces, lighting, doors/ doorways, stairs.
(3) At home, most falls occur in bedroom (42%); bathroom (34%).

e. Activity-related risk factors.
(1) Most falls occur during normal daily activity: getting up from bed/chair, turning head/body, bending, walking, climbing/descending stairs.
(2) Only a small percentage (5%) occur during clearly hazardous activities; e.g., climbing on ladder.
(3) Improper use of assistive device: e.g., walker, cane, wheelchair.

3. Fall prevention.

a. Examination.
(1) Accurate fall history: location, activity, time, symptoms; previous falls.
(2) Physical examination of patient: cognitive, sensory, neuromuscular, and cardiopulmonary.
(3) Standardized tests and measures for functional balance and instability; see Table 2-7.

b. Identify fall risk: determine all intrinsic and/or extrinsic factors.

c. Goals, outcomes, and interventions.
(1) Eliminate or minimize all fall risk factors; stabilize disease states, medications.
(2) Exercise to increase strength, flexibility.
(3) Sensory compensation strategies.
(4) Balance and gait training.
(5) Functional training.
(a) Focus on sit-to-stand transitions, turning, walking, and stairs.
(b) Modify activities of daily living for safety; provide assistive devices, adaptive equipment as appropriate.
(c) Allow adequate time for activities; instruct in gradual position changes.
(6) Safety education.
(a) Identify risks.
(b) Provide instructions in writing.
(c) Communicate with family and caregivers.
(7) Modify environment to reduce falls and instability: use environmental checklist.
(a) Ensure adequate lighting.
(b) Use contrasting colors to delineate hazardous areas.
(c) Simplify environment, reduce clutter.

d. When the patient falls.
(1) Check for fall injury.
(a) Hip fracture: complaints of pain in hip, especially on palpation; external rotation of leg, inability to bear weight on leg, changes in gait, weight-bearing.
(b) Head injury: loss of consciousness, mental confusion.
(c) Stroke, spinal cord injury: loss of sensation or voluntary movement.
(d) Cuts, bruises, painful swelling.
(2) Check for dizziness that may have preceded the fall.
(3) Provide reassurance.
(4) Do not attempt to lift patient by yourself; get help, provide first aid, and call emergency services if necessary.
(5) Solicit witnesses of fall event.

Medication Errors

1. Scope of the problem.

a. Most elderly (60%–85%) utilize prescription drugs to address a chronic medical problem.

b. One third have three or more medical problems requiring multiple medications and complex dosage schedules.

c. Average older person takes between four and seven prescription drugs each day; takes an additional three over-the-counter drugs.

d. Adverse drug reactions.
(1) 4%–10% of hospital admissions in the elderly.
(a) Affects approximately 25% of all hospitalized patients over the age of 80.
(b) Adverse effects are potentially disabling or life-threatening.
(2) High incidence of falls/hip fractures; e.g., psychotropic agents.
(3) Motor vehicle accidents.

2. Older adults are at increased risk for drug toxicity.

a. Factors include age-related changes in pharmacokinetics.
(1) Alterations in drug absorption, distribution to tissues, oxidative metabolism.
(2) Alterations in excretion associated with a decline in hepatic and renal function: decreased clearance in certain drugs; e.g., digoxin, lithium.
(3) Altered sensitivity to the effects of drugs.
(a) Increased with certain drugs; e.g., narcotic analgesics, benzodiazepines.
(b) Decreased with certain drugs; e.g., drugs mediated by beta-adrenergic receptors, isoproterenol, propranolol.
(4) Drugs may interfere with brain function, cause confusion; e.g., psychoactive drugs: sedatives, hypnotics, antidepressants, anticonvulsants, antiparkinsonism agents.

(5) Older adults have less homeostatic reserve; e.g., are more susceptible to orthostatic hypotension with vasodilating drugs due to dampened compensatory baroreceptor response.

(6) Drug processing effects: multiple drugs compete for binding sites.

(a) Drug-to-drug interactions; e.g., levodopa and monamine oxidase inhibitors (MAOIs) may result in hypertensive response.

(b) Most drugs exert more than one specific action in the body (polypharmacological effects); e.g., prednisone prescribed for anti-inflammatory action may benefit arthritic symptoms but aggravate a coexisting diabetic state (augments blood glucose levels).

b. Physicians may prescribe inappropriate medications for elderly; estimated in 17.5% of Medicare prescriptions.

c. Most patients are not knowledgeable about drug actions, drug side effects.

d. Drug-food interactions can interfere with effectiveness of medications; e.g., efficacy of levodopa is compromised if ingested too close to a high-protein meal; potential vitamin/drug interactions.

e. Polypharmacy phenomena: multiple drug prescriptions.

(1) Exacerbated by elderly who visit multiple physicians, use different pharmacies.

(2) Lack integrated care; e.g., computerized system of drug monitoring.

f. Health status influences/socioeconomic factors.

(1) Older adults have a high rate of medication dosage errors; associated with memory impairment, visual impairments, incoordination, and low literacy.

(2) Older adults are targeted for aggressive marketing by drug companies: may result in self-administration of medications for uninvestigated symptoms.

(3) Financial issues: due to high costs, fixed incomes, elderly may skip dosages, stop taking medications.

g. Common adverse effects.

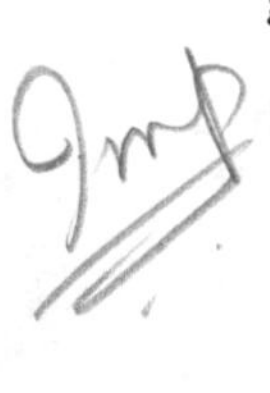

(1) Confusion/dementia: e.g., tranquilizers, barbiturates, digitalis, antihypertensives, anticholinergic drugs; analgesics, antiparkinsonians, diuretics, beta-blockers.

(2) Sedation/immobility: e.g., psychotropic drugs, narcotic analgesics.

(3) Weakness: e.g., antihypertensives, vasodilators, digitalis, diuretics, oral hypoglycemics.

(4) Postural hypotension: e.g., antihypertensives, diuretics, tricyclic antidepressants, tranquilizers, nitrates, narcotic analgesics.

(5) Depression: e.g., antihypertensives, anti-inflammatories, antimycobacterials, antiparkinsonians, diuretics, H_2 receptor antagonists, sedative-hypnotics, vasodilators.

(6) Drug-induced movement disorders.

(a) Dyskinesias (involuntary, stereotypic and repetitive movements; i.e., lip smacking, hand movements, etc.) associated with long-term use of neuroleptic drugs and anticholinergic drugs, levodopa.

(b) Akathisia (motor restlessness) associated with antipsychotic drugs.

(c) Essential tremor associated with tricyclic antidepressants, adrenergic drugs.

(d) Parkinsonism: associated with antipsychotics, sympatholytics.

(7) Incontinence: caused or exacerbated by a variety of drugs; e.g., barbiturates, benzodiazepines, antipsychotic drugs, anticholinergic drugs.

3. Goals, outcomes, and interventions.

a. Assist in adequate monitoring of drug therapy.

(1) Recognize drug-related side effects, adverse reactions to drugs, potential drug interactions in the elderly.

(2) Carefully document patient responses to medications, exercise, and activity.

b. Assist in patient and family drug education/compliance: e.g., understanding of purpose of drugs, dosage, potential side effects.

c. Encourage centralization of medications through one pharmacy.

d. Assist in simplification of drug regimen and instructions.

(1) Administration of drugs; e.g., daily pill box, drug calendar.

(2) Check to see if patient is taking medications on schedule.

(3) Time doses in conjunction with daily routine.

e. Coordinate physical therapy with drug schedule/optimal dose; e.g., exercise during peak dose with individual on Parkinson's disease medications (levodopa).

f. Recognize potentially harmful interaction effects: modalities that cause vasodilatation in combination with vasodilating drugs.

Nutritional Deficiency

1. Many older adults have primary nutritional problems.

a. Nutritional problems in elderly are linked to health status and poverty rather than to age itself.

(1) Chronic diseases alter the overall need for nutrients/energy demands, the ability to take in and utilize nutrients, and overall activity levels; e.g., Alzheimer's disease, CVA, diabetes.

(2) Limited, fixed incomes severely limit food choices and availability.

b. Both undernourishment and obesity exist in the elderly and contribute to decreased levels of vitality and fitness.
c. Contributing factors to poor dietary intake.
   (1) Decreased sense of taste and smell.
   (2) Poor teeth or poorly fitting dentures.
   (3) Reduced gastrointestinal function.
      (a) Decreased saliva.
      (b) Gastromucosal atrophy.
      (c) Reduced intestinal mobility; reflux.
   (4) Loss of interest in foods.
   (5) Lack of social support, socialization during meals.
   (6) Lack of mobility.
      (a) Inability to get to grocery store, shop.
      (b) Inability to prepare foods.
d. There is an age-related slowing in basal metabolic rate and a decline in total caloric intake; most of the decline is associated with a concurrent reduction in physical activity.
e. Dehydration is common in the elderly, resulting in fluid and electrolyte disturbances.
   (1) Thirst sensation is diminished.
   (2) May be physically unable to acquire/ maintain fluids.
   (3) Environmental heat stresses may be life threatening.
f. Diets are often deficient in nutrients, especially vitamins A and C, B_{12}, thiamine, protein, iron, calcium/vitamin D, folic acid, and zinc.
g. Increased use of taste enhancers, e.g., salt and sugar, or alcohol influences nutritional intake.
h. Drug/dietary interactions influence nutritional intake; e.g., reserpine, digoxin, antitumor agents, excessive use of antacids.

2. Examination.
a. Dietary history: patterns of eating, types of foods.
b. Psychosocial: mental status, desire to eat/depression, social isolation.
c. Body composition.
   (1) Weight/height measures.
   (2) Skin fold measurements: triceps/subscapular skin fold thickness.
   (3) Upper arm circumference.
d. Sensory function: taste and smell.
e. Dental and periodontal disease, fit of dentures.
f. Ability to feed self: mastication, swallowing, hand/mouth control, posture, physical weakness and fatigue.
g. Integumentary: skin condition, edema.
h. Compliance to special diets.
i. Functional assessment: basic activities of daily living, feeding; overall exercise/activity levels.

3. Goals, outcomes, and interventions.
a. Assist in monitoring adequate nutritional intake.
b. Assist in health promotion.
   (1) Maintain adequate nutritional support.
      (a) Nutritional consults as necessary.
      (b) Nutritional educational programs.
      (c) Assistance in grocery shopping, meal preparation; e.g., recommendations for home health aides.
      (d) Elderly food programs: home-delivered/Meals on Wheels; congregate meals/senior center daily meal programs; federal food stamp programs.
   (2) Maintain physical function, adequate activity levels.

chapter 9 Therapeutic Exercise Foundations

THOMAS BIANCO and SUSAN B. O'SULLIVAN

Training Programs

Strength Training

1. **Concepts of muscle function and strength.**
   a. Strength is the force output of a contracting muscle and is directly related to the amount of tension a contracting muscle can produce.
   b. Contractile elements of muscle.
      (1) Muscles are composed of fibers, which are made up of myofibrils. Myofibrils are composed of sarcomeres that are connected in series. The overlapping cross-bridges of actin and myosin make up a sarcomere.
      (2) When a muscle contracts, the actin-myosin filaments slide together and the muscle shortens. The cross bridges slide apart when the muscle relaxes and returns to its resting length.
   c. Motor unit nerve supply to the muscle.
      (1) Slow-twitch (ST) fibers (type I).
         (a) Slow contraction speed.
         (b) Low force (tension) production.
         (c) Highly resistant to fatigue.
      (2) Fast-twitch (FT) fibers (type IIa).
         (a) Fast contraction speed.
         (b) Fatigue resistant.
         (c) Characteristics can be influenced by the type of training.
      (3) Fast-twitch (FT) fibers (type IIb).
         (a) Fast contraction speed.
         (b) High force production.
         (c) Susceptible to quick fatigue.
      (4) Hereditary influences and fiber type distribution.
         (a) The percentage of either FT or ST fibers in the body is determined by genetics. This ratio cannot be changed via normal exercise.
         (b) Specific training can modify metabolic characteristics of all fiber types; e.g., high-intensity, anaerobic strength training will stimulate optimal FT adaptation.
      (5) Order of fiber type recruitment.
         (a) Recruitment order depends upon type of activity, force required, movement pattern, and position of the body.
         (b) ST motor units have the lowest functional thresholds and are recruited during lighter, slower efforts such as low-intensity, long-duration endurance activities.
         (c) Higher forces with greater velocity cause the activation of more powerful, higher threshold FT motor units.
         (d) Order of recruitment is ST, followed by FT IIa, and finally followed by FT IIb motor units.
   d. Length-tension.
      (1) As the muscle shortens or lengthens through the available range of motion (ROM), the tension it produces varies. Maximum tension is generated at some midpoint in the ROM; less tension is developed in either shortened or lengthened ROM.

(2) The weight lifted or lowered cannot exceed that which the muscle is able to control at its weakest point in the ROM.
(3) When a muscle is stretched beyond the resting length, there is a mechanical disruption of the cross-bridges as the microfilaments slide apart and the sarcomeres lengthen. Releasing the stretch allows the sarcomeres to return to their resting length. This change in ratio of length to tension is called elasticity.
(4) Once released, a muscle stretched into the elastic range will contract and produce a force or tension as the muscle returns to its original length.

2. Adaptations to strength training.

a. Muscle.
   (1) Hypertrophy is an increase in muscle size as a result of resistance training and can be observed after at least 6–8 weeks of training.
   (2) Remodeling: individual muscle fibers are enlarged, contain more actin and myosin, and have more, larger myofibrils; sarcomeres are increased.
   (3) An increase in motor unit recruitment and synchronization of firing facilitates contraction and maximizes force production.
   (4) The average person has a ratio of 50% fast to slow-twitch motor units. Performing workloads of low intensity will challenge half of the body's muscle mass. High-intensity exercises for shorter durations (less than 20 repetitions) are needed to train the highly adaptable fast-twitch IIa fibers.
   (5) Disuse atrophy occurs when a muscle loses both size and strength from lack of use or when a limb is immobilized.
   (6) Cross-section area of a muscle highly correlates with strength gains. The larger the muscle, the greater the strength of that muscle.

b. Positive changes in impairments. Improvement in:
   (1) Strength.
   (2) Bone mass.
   (3) Body composition: fat to lean body composition.
   (4) Weight control and weight maintenance; decreased risk of adult-onset diabetes.
   (5) Reaction time.
   (6) Metabolism, calorie burning during and after exercise.
   (7) Cardiovascular status: reduction in resting blood pressure.
   (8) Immunological function.

c. Positive changes in function and quality of life.
   (1) Improved balance and coordination.
   (2) Improved gait and functional mobility.
   (3) Improved activities of daily living.
   (4) Improved job/recreational/athletic performance.
   (5) Improved sense of well-being, posture and self-image.

3. Guidelines to develop strength.

a. Overload principle: to increase strength, the muscle must be loaded or challenged beyond its current force capability. Higher levels of tension will cause hypertrophy and recruitment of muscle fibers. This level will change with each adaptation.

b. Specificity of training: adaptations in the metabolic and physiological systems of the body depending on the type of overload imposed. Specific modes of exercise elicit specific adaptations creating specific training effects.

c. Reversibility: benefits of training are not sustained unless muscles are continuously challenged. Detraining effects include decreased muscle recruitment and muscle fiber atrophy.

d. Metabolic effects of strength training.
   (1) Muscle contraction to about 60% of its force-generating capacity causes a blockage of blood flow to the working muscle due to increased intramuscular pressure. The energy source for this level of muscle contraction is mainly anaerobic and does not improve with aerobic conditioning.
   (2) Strength training of specific muscles has a brief activation period and uses a relatively small muscle mass, producing less cardiovascular metabolic demands than vigorous exercise, e.g., walking, running, swimming.
   (3) Rhythmic activities increase blood flow to exercising muscles via a contraction and relaxation "milking action." The primary energy source is aerobic.
   (4) Circuit training (cross-training) with high repetitions and low weights incorporates all modes of training and provides more general conditioning to improve body composition, muscular strength, and some cardiovascular fitness.

e. Common errors associated with resistance or strength training.
   (1) Valsalva's maneuver: forcible exhalation with the glottis, nose, and mouth closed while contraction is being held. Valsalva's maneuver increases intrathoracic pressure, slows heart rate (HR), decreases return of blood to the heart, and increases venous pressure and cardiac work.
   (2) Inadequate rest after vigorous exercise. Three to 4 minutes are needed to return the muscle to 90%–95% of preexercise capacity. Most rapid recovery occurs in the first minute.
   (3) Increasing exercise progression too quickly (intensity, duration, frequency) can overwork muscles and cause injuries.

(4) Substitute motions occur from too much resistance, incorrect stabilization, and when muscles are weak from fatigue, paralysis, or pain.

4. Exercises to improve strength and range.

a. Manual resistance: a type of active exercise in which another person provides resistance.
  (1) Advantages.
    (a) Useful in the early stages of an exercise program when the muscle is weak. The therapist can judge the capability of muscle to safely meet demands of exercise.
    (b) Can be modified for a painful arc in the joint range of motion.
    (c) Safe resistance exercise when the joint movement needs to be carefully controlled and the resistance is mild to moderate.
    (d) Can be easily changed to include diagonal or functional patterns of movement, (e.g., proprioceptive neuromuscular facilitation [PNF]) or appropriate facilitation techniques (e.g., quick stretch).
  (2) Disadvantages.
    (a) The amount of resistance cannot be measured quantitatively.
    (b) It may be difficult to maintain the same resistance during the full joint ROM and to consistently repeat the same resistance.
    (c) The amount of resistance is limited by the strength of the therapist or caregiver.

b. Mechanical resistance: a type of active exercise in which resistance is applied through the use of equipment or mechanical apparatus.
  (1) Advantages.
    (a) The amount of resistance can be measured quantitatively and increased over time.
    (b) Can be used when amounts of resistance are greater than the therapist can apply manually.
  (2) Disadvantages.
    (a) Not easily modified to exercise in diagonal or functional patterns.
    (b) May not be safe if resistance needs to be carefully controlled or maintained at low levels.

c. Goals and indications for resistance exercise.
  (1) Increase strength in a muscle group that lifts, lowers, or controls heavy loads for relatively low number of repetitions.
  (2) Increase muscular endurance by performing low-intensity repetitive exercise over a prolonged period.
  (3) Improve muscular performance related to strength and speed of movement.

d. Precautions.
  (1) Local muscle fatigue is a normal response of the muscle from repeated dynamic or static contractions over a period of time. Fatigue is due to depleted energy stores, insufficient oxygen, and build-up of lactic acid. It is characterized by a decline in peak torque and increased muscle pain with occasional spasm and decreased active ROM (AROM).
  (2) General muscular fatigue affects the whole body after prolonged activities such as walking or jogging; usually due to low blood sugar, decreased glycogen stores in muscle and liver, depletion of potassium.
  (3) Fatigue may be associated with specific clinical diseases; e.g., multiple sclerosis, cardiac disease, peripheral vascular dysfunction, and pulmonary diseases. These patients fatigue more rapidly and require longer rest periods.
  (4) Overwork or overtraining causes temporary or permanent loss of strength as a result of exercise. In normal individuals, fatigue causes discomfort, so overtraining and muscle weakness does not usually occur. Patients with lower motor neuron disease who participate in vigorous resistance exercise programs can have a deterioration of strength; e.g., postpolio syndrome. Overwork can be avoided with slow progression of the exercise intensity, duration, and progression.
  (5) Osteoporosis makes the bone unable to withstand normal stresses and highly susceptible to pathological fracture. May develop as a result of prolonged immobilization, bed rest, inability to bear weight on an extremity, and nutritional or hormonal factors.
  (6) Acute muscle soreness develops during or directly after strenuous anaerobic exercise performed to the point of fatigue. Decreased blood flow and reduced oxygen (ischemia) creates a temporary build-up of lactic acid and potassium. A cool-down period of low-intensity exercise can facilitate the return of oxygen to the muscle and reduce soreness.
  (7) Delayed-onset muscle soreness (DOMS) can begin 12–24 hours after vigorous exercise or muscular overexertion. Peaks at 24–48 hours after exercise. Muscle tenderness and stiffness can last up to 5–7 days. Usually greater after muscle lengthening or eccentric exercise. Severity of soreness can be lessened by gradually increasing the intensity and duration of exercises.

e. Contraindications.
  (1) Inflammation: resistance exercises can increase swelling and cause damage to muscles or joints.
  (2) Pain: severe joint or muscle pain during exercise or for more than 24 hours after exercise requires elimination or reduction of the exercise.

f. Types of resistance exercise.
   (1) Isometric exercise is static and occurs when a muscle contracts without a length change. Resistance is variable and accommodating. Contractions should be held for at least 6 seconds to obtain adaptive changes in the muscle.
      (a) Strengthening of muscles is developed at a point in the ROM, not over the entire length of the muscle.
      (b) This type of resistance exercise can increase blood pressure, and should be used cautiously with the patient with a cardiac condition.
      (c) Monitor for potential Valsalva's maneuver.
   (2) Isotonic exercise is dynamic and can have a constant (free weights) or variable (machine) load as the muscle lengthens or shortens through the available ROM. Speed can be variable for this type of exercise.
      (a) Weight-lifting machines have an oval shaped cam or wheel that mimics the length-tension curve of the muscle; e.g., Nautilus or Cybex. These machines vary resistance as the muscle goes through the ROM, providing resistance that the muscle can safely complete at various points of the ROM.
      (b) Free weights do not vary the resistance through the ROM of a muscle. The weakest point along the length-tension curve of each muscle limits the amount of weight lifted.
      (c) Weight-lifting machines are safer than free weights; used early in a resistance exercise or rehabilitation program.
   (3) Isokinetic exercise is dynamic and has a speed control for muscle shortening and lengthening. Resistance is accommodating and variable.
      (a) Peak torque, the maximum force generated through the ROM, is inversely related to angular velocity, the speed, the body segment moves through its ROM; e.g., increasing angular velocity decreases peak torque production.
      (b) Concentric or eccentric resistance exercise can be performed on isokinetic equipment.
      (c) Isokinetic exercise provides maximum resistance at all points in the ROM as the muscle contracts.
      (d) During isokinetic testing, the weight of a body segment creates a torque output around the joint; e.g., the lower leg around the knee joint in sitting knee flexion. This gravity-produced torque adds to the force generated by the muscle when it contracts and gives a higher torque output than is actually created by the muscle. The higher value can affect the testing values of the muscle group and which muscle group needs to be strengthened. Software can correct for the effects of gravity.
   (4) Eccentric (lengthening) versus concentric (shortening).
      (a) Maximum eccentric contraction produces more force than maximal concentric contraction.
      (b) Resistance training performed concentrically improves concentric muscle strength, and eccentric training improves eccentric muscle strength (specificity of training).
      (c) Eccentric contractions occur in a wide variety of functional activities, such as lowering the body against gravity; e.g., sitting down or descending stairs.
      (d) Eccentric contractions provide a source of shock absorption during closed-chain functional activities.
      (e) Eccentric contractions consume less oxygen and fewer energy stores than concentric contractions against similar loads.

g. Range of motion.
   (1) Short-arc exercise: resistance exercise performed through a limited ROM; e.g., initial exercise post–knee surgery (anterior cruciate repair), painful full-range movement.
   (2) Full arc exercise: resistance exercise performed through full ROM.

h. Open versus closed-chain exercises.
   (1) Open-chain exercise occurs when the distal segment (hand or foot) moves freely in space; e.g., when an arm lifts or lowers a hand-held weight.
   (2) Resistance exercises usually are open chain, which may be the only option if weight bearing is contraindicated.
   (3) Open-chain exercise does not adequately prepare a patient for functional weight-bearing activities.
   (4) Closed-chain exercise occurs when the body moves over a fixed distal segment; e.g., stair climbing or squatting activities.
   (5) Closed-chain exercise loads muscles, bones, joints, and noncontractile soft tissues such as ligaments, tendons, and joint capsules.
   (6) Mechanoreceptors are stimulated by closed-chain exercises, adding to joint stability, balance, coordination, and agility in functional weight-bearing postures.

5. Specific exercise regimens.

a. Progressive resistive exercise (PRE): uses the repetition maximum (RM), or the greatest amount of weight a muscle can move through the ROM a specific number of times (e.g., DeLorme used 10 RM as baseline). Three sets of 10 repetitions are completed with brief rests (1–2 minutes) between sets. Progression (DeLorme): exercise begins with 10 repetitions at 50% RM, followed by 10 repetitions at 75% RM, and finally 10 repetitions at 100% RM. (Table 9-1).

b. Circuit weight training: a sequence of exercises for total-body conditioning. A rest period of usually 30

Table 9-1 ➤ RESISTANCE TRAINING SPECIFICITY CHART

RELATIVE LOADING	OUTCOME	% 1 RM	REPETITION RANGE	# OF SETS	REST BETWEEN SETS
Light	Muscular Endurance	<70	12–20	1–3	20–30 seconds
Moderate	Hypertrophy and Strength	70–80	8–12	1–6	30–120 seconds
Heavy	Maximum Strength	80–100	1–8	1–5+	2–5 minutes

seconds to 1 minute is taken between each exercise. Exercises can be done with free weights or weight-training machines.

c. Plyometric training, or stretch-shortening activity: an isotonic exercise that combines speed, strength, and functional activities. Used in later stages of rehabilitation to achieve high level of performance; e.g., jumping off of a platform, then up onto the platform at a rapid pace to improve vertical jumping abilities.

d. Brief, repetitive isometric exercise: occurs with up to 20 maximum contractions held for 5–6 seconds and performed daily. A 20-second rest after each contraction is recommended to prevent increases in blood pressure. Strength gains occur in 6 weeks.

Endurance Training

1. Training strategies to develop muscular endurance.

a. Muscular endurance: the ability of an isolated muscle group to perform repeated contractions over time.

b. Muscular endurance is improved by performing low-load resistance exercise for many repetitions. Exercise programs that increase strength also increase muscular endurance.

c. Muscular endurance programs are indicated after injuries to joints and soft tissues. Dynamic exercises at a high number of repetitions against light resistance are more comfortable and create less joint irritation than heavy resistance exercises.

d. Early in a strength-training program, high repetitions and low-load exercises cause less muscle soreness and reduce the risk of muscle injury.

2. Training strategies to develop cardiovascular endurance.

a. Cardiovascular endurance: the ability to perform large-muscle, dynamic exercise, such as walking, swimming, and/or biking, for long periods of time.

b. Overload principle: used to enhance physiological improvement and bring about a training change. Specific exercise overload must be applied.

(1) Training adaptation occurs by exercising at a level above normal.

(2) The appropriate overload for each person can be achieved by manipulating combinations of training frequency, intensity, and duration.

c. Specificity principle: adaptations in the metabolic and physiological systems, depending on the type of overload imposed.

(1) Specific exercise elicits specific adaptations, creating specific training effects; e.g., swim training will increase cardiovascular conditioning only when tested in swimming. There is no crossover for conditioning from swimming to running.

d. Individual differences principle: training benefits are optimized when programs are planned to meet the individual needs and capacities of the participants.

e. Reversibility principle: detraining occurs rapidly, after only 2 weeks, when a person stops exercising. Beneficial effects of exercise training are transient and reversible.

f. FITT equation: includes factors that affect training; frequency, intensity, time, and type. Intensity is interrelated with both duration (time) and frequency.

(1) Frequency is the number of exercise sessions per week. If training at a lower intensity, then more frequent exercise is indicated.

(a) If the intensity is constant, the benefit from two versus four or three versus five times per week is the same.

(b) For weight loss, 5–7 days per week increases the caloric expenditure more than 2 days per week.

(c) Less than 2 days per week does not produce adequate changes in aerobic capacity or body composition.

(2) Intensity (overload) is the primary way to improve cardiovascular endurance.

(a) Relative intensity for an individual is calculated as a percentage of the maximum function, e.g. maximum oxygen consumption (VO_{2max}) or maximum heart rate (HR_{max}).

(b) The VO_{2max} or HR_{max} can be measured directly or indirectly based on different methods; e.g., 3-minute step, 12-minute run, or 1-mile walk test.

(c) HR_{max} can be estimated using 220 minus the age of individual. Training level or target heart rate (THR) can be established at 70% of maximum to increase aerobic capacity.

(d) The Karvonen formula is used to predict heart rate reserve (HRR) or HR_{max} minus the resting heart rate (RHR) and correlates directly to VO_{2max}. THR = (HR_{max} – RHR) × % of desired training intensity + RHR.

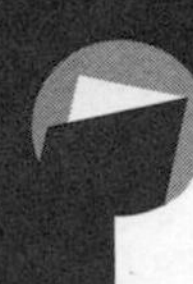

(e) Rating of perceived exertion (RPE) can be used to evaluate training at submaximal levels. A cardiorespiratory training effect can be achieved at a rating of "somewhat hard" or "hard" (13–16 on the original Borg scale of 6–19). An appropriate level of training should result in conversational exercise or "talk test"; moderate exercise that is not too strenuous and can improve endurance.

(3) Duration (time).

(a) Duration is increased when intensity is limited; e.g., by initial fitness level. Improvements in aerobic capacity, therefore, depend on increasing exercise duration and frequency, e.g., 3–5 minutes per day produces training effects in poorly conditioned individuals, whereas 20–30 minutes, three to five times per week is optimal for conditioned people.

(b) Multiple sessions of short durations are also indicated when intensity is limited by environmental conditions, such as heat and humidity or by medical conditions, such as intermittent claudication or congestive heart failure.

(c) Obese individuals should exercise at longer durations and lower intensities. At this exercise level, the person can speak without gasping and does not have muscle ache or burn from lactic acid accumulation.

(d) Obesity increases the mechanical work of the heart and can lead to cardiac and left ventricular dysfunction.

(4) Type of exercise needed to increase cardiovascular endurance should involve large muscle groups activated in rhythmic aerobic nature. Specificity of training should be considered.

(5) See Chapter 3.

3. Training strategies to develop pulmonary endurance.

a. Pulmonary endurance is related to the ventilation of the lungs and oxygen consumption.

b. Ventilation is the process of air exchange in the lungs. The volume of air breathed each minute, or minute, ventilation (V_e), is 6 liters. V_e = breathing rate × tidal volume. In maximum exercise, increases in breathing rate and depth may produce ventilation as high as 200 liters per minute.

c. Energy is produced aerobically as oxygen is supplied to exercising muscles. Oxygen consumption rises rapidly during the first minutes of exercise, and then levels off as the aerobic metabolism supplies the energy required by the working muscles (steady state).

d. The more fit a person is, the more capable their respiratory system is of delivering oxygen to sustain aerobic energy production at increasingly higher levels of intensity.

(1) Obesity can impair pulmonary function because of the added effort to move the chest wall.

e. In severe pulmonary disease, the cost of breathing can reach 40% of the total exercise oxygen consumption. This decreases the oxygen available to the exercising nonrespiratory muscles and limits exercise capabilities. Obesity can significantly increase the level of impairments.

f. Exercise-induced asthma (EIA) can occur when the normal initial bronchodilatation is followed by bronchoconstriction. The reduction in airflow from airway obstruction affects the ability of the lungs to provide oxygen to exercising muscles.

(1) EIA is an acute, reversible airway obstruction that develops 5–15 minutes after strenuous exercise when a person does not breathe through the nose, which warms and humidifies the air.

(2) When a person mouth-breathes, the air is cold and dry, contributing to the bronchoconstriction.

(3) Lowering the intensity level and allowing the person to breathe through the nose can allow prolonged aerobic exercise to continue.

(4) The problem is rare in activities that require only short bursts of activity such as baseball, and is more likely to occur in endurance activities such as soccer.

(5) When exercising in humid versus dry environments, the exercise-induced asthmatic response is considerably reduced. See Chapter 4.

4. Aerobic training.

a. Aerobic training (cardiorespiratory endurance training) can result in higher fitness levels for healthy individuals, slow the decrease in functional capacity in the elderly, and recondition those with illness or chronic disease.

b. Positive effects of aerobic training on the cardiovascular and respiratory systems.

(1) Improve breathing volumes and increased VO_{2max}.

(2) Increase heart weight and volume; cardiac hypertrophy is normal with long-term aerobic training.

(3) Increase total hemoglobin and oxygen delivery capacity.

(4) Decrease resting and submaximal exercise heart rates. Can be utilized to measure improvements from aerobic training.

(5) Increase cardiac output and stroke volume.

(6) Improve distribution of blood to working muscles and enhanced capacity of trained muscles to extract and use oxygen.

(7) Reduce resting blood pressure.

c. Continuous training at a submaximal energy requirement can be prolonged for 20–60 minutes without exhausting the oxygen transport system.

(1) Work rate is increased progressively as training improvements are achieved; overload can be accomplished by increasing the exercise duration.
(2) In healthy individuals, continuous training is the most effective way to improve endurance.

d. Circuit training uses a series of exercise activities that are repeated several times.
(1) Several exercise modes can be utilized, involving large and small muscle groups both statically and dynamically.
(2) Circuit training improves endurance and strength by stressing the aerobic and anaerobic energy systems.

e. Interval training includes an exercise period followed by a prescribed rest interval. It is perceived to be less demanding than continuous training, and tends to improve strength and power more than endurance.
(1) The relief interval can be passive or active; its duration ranges from a few seconds to several minutes. Active or work recovery involves doing the exercise at a reduced level. During the relief period, a portion of the adenosine triphosphate (ATP) and oxygen used by the muscles during the work period is replenished by the aerobic system.
(2) The longer the work interval, the more the aerobic system is stressed.
(3) With appropriate spacing of work-relief intervals, a significant amount of high-intensity work can be achieved. The total amount of work completed with interval training is greater than the amount of work accomplished with continuous training.

f. Warm-up and cool-down periods: each exercise session includes a 5- to 15-minute warm-up and a 5- to 15-minute cool-down period.
(1) The warm-up period prevents the heart and circulatory system from being suddenly taxed. It includes low-intensity cardiorespiratory activities and flexibility exercises.
(2) The cool-down period also consists of exercising at a lower intensity. It reduces abrupt physiological alterations that can occur with sudden cessation of strenuous exercise; e.g., venous pooling in the lower extremities, which causes decreased venous return to the heart.
(3) Longer warm-up and cool-down periods may be needed for deconditioned or older individuals.

5. Common errors associated with muscular, cardiovascular, and pulmonary endurance training.

a. Lack, of exercise tolerance testing (ETT) before the exercise prescription is determined could result in a training program set too high or too low for that individual.
b. Starting out at too high a level can overly stress the cardiorespiratory and muscular systems and potentially cause injuries.
c. Increasing intensity too fast can create a problem for an individual during endurance training.
d. Exercising at too intense a level can use the anaerobic energy system, not the aerobic system; this increases strength and power, not endurance.
e. Insufficient warm-up or cool-down results in inadequate cardiorespiratory and muscular adaptation; there is inadequate time to prepare for or recover from higher intense activity.
f. Inconsistent training frequency, duration, or intensity does not properly stress or overload the aerobic system to create training effects.

6. Exercise at high altitude.

a. At altitudes of 6,000 feet (1,829 meters [m]) or higher there can be a noticeable drop in performance of aerobic activities.
b. The partial pressure of oxygen is reduced, resulting in poor oxygenation of hemoglobin.
c. This hypoxia at altitude can result in immediate compensatory hyperventilation (stimulation of the baroreceptors) and increased heart rate.
d. Reduction in CO_2 from hyperventilation results in more alkaline body fluids.
e. Adjustments or acclimatization to higher altitude.
(1) Takes 2 weeks at 2,300 m and an additional week for every additional 600 m in altitude.
(2) There is a decrease in plasma volume (concentrating red blood cells) and an increase in total red blood cells and hemoglobin improving oxygenation.
(3) Changes in local circulation may facilitate oxygen transport.
(4) Adjustments do not fully compensate for altitude. Max VO_2 is decreased 2% for every 300 m above 1,500 m. Thus, there is a drop in performance for endurance activities.
(5) Training at altitude does not provide any improvement in sea-level performance.

f. The air in mountainous regions tends to be cool and dry. Body fluids can be rapidly lost through evaporation and result in dehydration.
(1) Ensure adequate hydration for those exercising or engaged in sports at altitude.

7. Exercise in hot weather.

a. When exercising in the heat, muscles require oxygen to produce energy.
b. To decrease metabolic heat, blood is shunted to the periphery; thus, working muscles are deprived of needed oxygen.
c. Core temperature increases and sweating increases. Fluids must be continually replaced or core temperatures can rise to dangerous levels.

d. Hot, humid environments diminish the evaporative cooling component, even with profuse sweating. Excess fluid loss can compromise cardiovascular function.
e. Fluid replacement.
   (1) Maintain plasma volume.
   (2) Colder fluids are emptied from the stomach more rapidly than room-temperature fluids.
   (3) Concentrated carbohydrate drinks impair gastric emptying and slow fluid replacement.
   (4) Glucose-polymer drinks do not impair physiological functioning. They may also resupply lost electrolytes.
f. Repeated heat stress results in acclimatization in about 10 days of exposure.
   (1) Exercise capacity is increased.
   (2) Cardiac output is better regulated.
   (3) Sweating is more efficient.
   (4) Acclimatization to heat stress does not seriously deteriorate with age.
g. Men and women can adapt equally well to heat, even though the mechanisms of thermoregulation differ slightly. The menstrual cycle is not a factor.
h. Obesity is a major consideration when exercising in the heat.

8. Exercise recommendations for individuals with obesity. (See Chapter 6).

Mobility and Flexibility Training

1. Flexibility.

a. Flexibility refers to the ability to move a joint through an unrestricted, pain-free ROM; the musculotendinous unit elongates as the body segment moves through the ROM.
b. Dynamic flexibility refers to the active ROM of a joint, and is dependent upon the amount of tissue resistance met during active movement.
c. Passive flexibility is the degree to which a joint can be passively moved through the available ROM, and is dependent upon the extensibility of the muscle and connective tissue around the joint.

2. Stretching.

a. Stretching involves any therapeutic technique that lengthens shortened soft-tissue structures and increases ROM.
b. Type of stretching is determined by the type of force applied, the intensity of stretch, and duration of stretch to contractile and noncontractile tissues.
   (1) Manual, passive stretching takes the structures beyond the free ROM to elongate tissues beyond their resting length.
      (a) The stretch force is applied for at least 15–30 seconds and repeated several times during a session.
      (b) Manual stretching is considered a short-duration stretch, and is maintained statically for less time than mechanical stretching.
      (c) Intensity and duration depend on patient tolerance and therapist strength and endurance.
      (d) Low-intensity manual stretch, applied as long as possible, is better tolerated and results in optimal improvement in tissue length with minimal risk of injury to any weakened tissue.
   (2) Ballistic stretching is a high-intensity, very short-duration "bouncing" stretch. By contracting the opposite muscle group, the patient uses body weight and momentum to elongate the tight muscle.
      (a) It is considered unsafe because of poor control and the potential of rupturing weakened tissues. It should not be performed after an injury or surgery.
      (b) Ballistic stretch facilitates the stretch reflex, causing an increase in tension in the muscle that is being stretched. It is contraindicated in spastic muscles.
   (3) Prolonged mechanical stretching is a low-intensity, external force (5–15 lb to 10% of body weight) applied over a prolonged period by positioning a patient with weighted pulley and traction systems. Dynamic splints or serial casts may also be used.
      (a) Prolonged stretch may be maintained for 20–30 minutes or as long as several hours.
      (b) Dynamic splints are applied for 8–10 hours to increase ROM.
      (c) Low-intensity, prolonged mechanica stretching has been shown to be more effective than manual, passive stretching with long-standing flexion contractures.
   (4) Active stretching occurs when voluntary, unassisted movement by the patient provides the stretch force to a joint. It requires strength and muscular contraction of the prime mover to actively stretch the antagonist muscle group.
      (a) The force is controlled by the patient and is considered low-intensity (to tolerance). The risk of tissue injury is low.
      (b) Duration is equal to passive, manual stretching, or about 15–30 seconds, and is limited by prime mover muscular endurance.
   (5) Facilitated stretching (active inhibition) refers to techniques in which the patient reflexively relaxes the muscle to be elongated prior to or during the stretching technique; e.g., PNF.
      (a) Hold-relax (HR): a relaxation technique usually performed at the point of limited ROM in the agonist pattern; an isometric contraction of the range-limiting antagonist is performed against slowly increasing resistance,

followed by voluntary relaxation, and passive movement by the therapist into the newly gained range of the agonist pattern. The muscle relaxes as a result of autogenic inhibition, possibly from the Golgi tendon organ (GTO) firing and decreasing muscular tension.

(b) Hold-relax-active contraction (HRAC): following hold-relax technique, active contraction into the newly gained range of the agonist pattern is performed. The muscle is further relaxed through the inhibitory effects of reciprocal inhibition.

(c) Contract-relax-active contraction (CRAC): a relaxation technique usually performed at a point of limited ROM in the agonist pattern; isotonic movement in rotation is performed followed by an isometric hold of the range-limiting muscles in the antagonist pattern against slowly increasing resistance, voluntary relaxation, and active movement into the new range of the agonist pattern.

(d) Indications for active inhibition techniques include limitations in ROM caused by muscle tightness or muscle spasm. CR techniques may be more painful, especially if muscle cocontraction is present.

c. Contractile tissue.
   (1) A muscle that is lengthened over a prolonged period will have an increase in the number of sarcomeres in series. The muscle will adjust its length over time.
   (2) A muscle immobilized in a shortened position will have a decrease in the number of sarcomeres and an increase in connective tissue.
   (3) The sarcomere adaptation is transient. A muscle allowed to resume its normal length will produce or absorb sarcomeres (lengthen or shorten).

d. Neurophysiological properties of contractile tissue.
   (1) The muscle spindle monitors the velocity and length changes in muscle.
   (2) A quick stretch to a muscle stimulates the alpha motoneurons and facilitates muscle contraction via the monosynaptic stretch reflex. This can increase tension in a muscle to be lengthened.
   (3) The GTO inhibits contraction of the muscle. When excessive tension develops, the GTO fires, inhibiting alpha motoneuron activity and decreasing tension in the muscle.
   (4) Slow stretching, especially applied at end range, causes the GTO to fire and inhibit the muscle (autogenic inhibition), allowing the muscle to lengthen (stretch-protection reflex).

e. Noncontractile connective tissue, including ligaments, tendons, joint capsules, fasciae and skin, can affect joint flexibility and requires remodeling to increase length.
   (1) Low-magnitude loads over long periods increase the deformation of noncontractile tissue, allowing a gradual rearrangement of collagen bonds (remodeling). This type of stretch is better tolerated by the patient.
   (2) 15–20 minutes of low-intensity sustained stretch, repeated on 5 consecutive days, can cause a change in the length of muscles and connective tissue.
   (3) Intensive stretching is usually not done every day in order to allow time for healing. Without healing time, a breakdown of tissue will occur, as in overuse syndromes and stress fractures.
   (4) With aging, collagen loses its elasticity and tissue blood supply is decreased, reducing healing capability. Stretching in older adults should be performed cautiously.

f. Overstretch is a stretch well beyond the normal joint ROM resulting in hypermobility. If the supporting structures of a joint are insufficient and weak, they cannot hold a joint in a stable, functional position during functional activities. This is known as stretch weakness.

g. Contracture is the adaptive shortening of muscle or other soft tissues that cross a joint; contracture results in decreased ROM.
   (1) Myotatic contracture (pertaining to muscle) involves a musculotendinous unit that has adaptively shortened with loss of ROM. Usually occurs without specific tissue pathology and in two-joint muscles such as the hamstrings, rectus femoris, or gastrocnemius. Can typically be resolved in a short time with gentle stretching exercises, and active inhibition techniques.
   (2) Adhesions can occur if tissue is immobilized in a shortened position for extended periods of time, resulting in a loss of mobility.
   (3) Scar tissue adhesions develop due to injury and the inflammatory response. Initially, new fibers develop in a disorganized pattern and will restrict motion unless remodeled along lines of stress; e.g., the patient with burns.
   (4) Irreversible contracture: a permanent loss of soft tissue extensibility that cannot be released by nonsurgical treatment. Occurs when normal soft tissue is replaced by an excessive amount of nonextensible tissue, such as bone or fibrotic tissue.

3. Relaxation of muscles.

a. Local relaxation techniques can assist in the lengthening of contractile and noncontractile tissue.

b. Heat increases the extensibility of the shortened tissues. Warm muscles relax and lengthen more easily, reducing the discomfort of stretching. Connective tissue stretches with less force and shorter duration.
   (1) GTO sensitivity is increased, making it more likely to fire and inhibit muscle tension.

(2) Low-intensity active exercise performed prior to stretching will increase circulation to soft tissue and warm the tissues to be stretched.
(3) Heat without stretching has little or no effect on long-term improvement in muscle flexibility. The combination of heat and stretching produces greater long-term gains in tissue length than stretching alone.

c. Massage increases local circulation to the muscle and reduces muscle spasm and stiffness.
d. Biofeedback helps the patient reduce the amount of tension in a muscle and improves flexibility while decreasing pain. Increased level of feedback signals (auditory, visual) assists the patient in recognizing tense muscles.

4. Common errors associated with mobility and flexibility training.

a. Passively forcing a joint beyond its normal ROM.
b. Aggressively stretching a patient with a newly united fracture or osteoporosis may result in fracture.
c. Using high-intensity, short-duration (ballistic) stretching procedures on muscles and connective tissues that have been immobilized over a long time or recovering from injury or surgery.
d. Stretching muscles around joints without using strengthening exercises to develop an appropriate balance between flexibility and strength.
e. Overstretching of weak muscles, especially postural muscles that support the body against gravity.

Postural Stability Training

1. Stability (static postural control).

a. Refers to the synergistic coordination of the neuromuscular system that enables an individual to maintain a stable position in an antigravity, weight-bearing position.
b. Postural stability control involves prolonged holding of core muscles.

2. Dynamic stabilization, controlled mobility.

a. Proximal segments and trunk provide a stable base for functional movements.
   (1) An individual maintains postural stability of the trunk while weight shifting.
   (2) Distal segments are fixed, while proximal segments are moving.
   (3) Movement normally occurs through increments of range (small range to large range).
b. Patients with hyperkinetic movement disorders (e.g., ataxia) should be progressed from large range to small range movements, and finally to holding steady (stability control).

3. Dynamic stabilization, static-dynamic control.

a. An individual maintains postural stability of the trunk during dynamic extremity movements (e.g., reaching, kicking a ball).
b. Strength, endurance, flexibility, and coordination are needed for static and dynamic stabilization.

4. Guidelines to develop postural stability.

a. Consider exercise protocols that effectively challenge core muscle groups and create adequate stability to perform functional activities. Stability requires the recruitment of tonic, slow-twitch muscle fibers for sustained periods of time.
b. Start training by teaching safe spinal ROM in a variety of basic postures. Teach chin tucking with axial extension of the cervical spine and pelvic tilting with ROM of the lumbar spine.
c. Incorporate procedures to retrain kinesthetic awareness of postural position. Teach the neutral pelvis position first to ensure a stable base.
   (1) Emphasis is placed on strength and endurance of back multifidi and oblique abdominals rather than erector spinae.
   (2) Focus patient's awareness on normal alignment of the spine and pelvis, and on muscles required to maintain that position.
   (3) Visual, verbal, and proprioceptive cues, e.g., resistance of elastic bands or light manual resistance, can be used to improve postural awareness.
d. To safely develop strength and endurance in the stabilizing muscles, practice maintained holding in a variety of postures. The higher the center-of-mass and smaller the base-of-support, the greater the degree of postural challenge; e.g., sitting versus standing.
e. Movements of the extremities challenge trunk and neck stabilization; functional position must be maintained as movements are carried out.
f. Resistance can be applied to the trunk or the moving extremities; functional position must be maintained as resistance is increased.
g. Alternating isometric contractions between antagonists can enhance stabilizing contractions and develop postural control; e.g., PNF techniques of stabilizing reversals and rhythmic stabilization.
   (1) Stabilizing reversals: isometric holding is facilitated first on one side of the joint, followed by alternate holding of the antagonist muscle groups. May be applied in a variety of directions; i.e. anterior-posterior, medial-lateral, diagonal.
   (2) Rhythmic stabilization (RS): simultaneous isometric contractions of both agonist and antagonist patterns performed without relaxation, using careful grading of resistance; results in cocontraction of opposing muscle groups; RS emphasizes rotational stability control.

h. During early training, emphasize muscles needed for trunk support in the upright posture, for performing basic body mechanics, and for upper extremity lifting.
i. Teach control of functional positions while moving from one position to another. This is called transitional stabilization and requires graded contractions and adjustments between the trunk flexors and extensors. Consider moving out of a posture (eccentric control) before moving into a posture (concentric control).
j. Introduce simple patterns of motion that develop safe body mechanics and movement.
k. Closed-chain tasks are good choices to enhance postural stabilization (e.g., partial squats and controlled lunges) add arm motions and weights as tolerated.
l. More complex patterns of movement (e.g., rotation and diagonal motions) can be added (e.g., PNF trunk patterns of chop/reverse chop, or lift/reverse lift). Postures can be progressed to add difficulty (e.g., supine to sitting to standing).
m. Incorporate stretching into the postural exercise program. Adequate flexibility is necessary for postural muscles to hold body parts in proper alignment.

5. Common errors associated with postural stability training.

a. Inadequate stretching of tight muscles (e.g., tight hip flexors that hold the pelvis in an anterior pelvic tilt or tight hamstrings that hold the pelvis in a posterior tilt); both prevent a stable postural base (neutral pelvis and spine position).
b. Inadequate control of core muscles could place excessive stress on proximal structures during functional activities; e.g., the vertebrae and discs of the spine during sitting.
c. Progressing too quickly or starting at too high a functional level for the patient to maintain postural stability.
d. Exercising past the point of fatigue, which is determined by the inability of the trunk or neck muscles to stabilize the spine in its functional position.
e. Attempting to force a patient into a general neutral position instead of finding the proper and safe position for each individual.

6. Stability ball training. (Swiss ball, physio ball, or therapy ball).

a. Benefits/uses.
   (1) Promotes balance; provides an unstable base of support, requiring continuous adjustments in balance. Moving the feet and/or the ball changes the base of support and challenges balance. Allows safe practice of falling.
   (2) Works muscles in functional, synergistic patterns.
      (a) Recruits and retrains core muscles (deep spinal and abdominal muscles).
      (b) Promotes postural relearning; e.g., neutral position in sitting, cervical or trunk rotation.
      (c) Enhances coordination, movement combinations; e.g., arm and leg bilateral symmetrical, bilateral asymmetrical movements, four-limb Mexican hat dance.
   (3) Heightens proprioception and sensory perception, awareness of the body moving in space.
   (4) Improves range of motion, allows safe stretching; e.g., total body extension or flexion, upper or lower extremity stretches.
   (5) Allows relaxation training; e.g., gentle bouncing combined with deep breathing. Gentle rocking can be used to decrease tone in hypertonic patient.
   (6) Allows a safe, dynamic cardiovascular workout; e.g., dynamic bouncing with extremity movements.
   (7) Increases strength. Can be combined with resistance training (e.g., lifting the ball with arms or legs), using hand weights or resistive bands while on the ball, or closed chain exercises (e.g., partial squats using the ball).
   (8) Has been used to replace chairs in schools; improves posture and concentration, calms hyperactive children.
b. Advantages: light, portable, durable, and inexpensive.
c. Determining appropriate ball size.
   (1) Sitting on ball with feet flat, the ball height should place the hips and knees at 90° angles.
   (2) Supine with ball under knees, the ball height should equal the distance between the greater trochanter and the knee.
   (3) Quadruped, the ball height should equal the distance between the shoulder and the wrist.
d. Firmness/inflation.
   (1) Ball should be comfortable and have some bounce.
   (2) A firm ball moves more quickly.
   (3) A soft ball moves more slowly, may make patient feel safer, more secure.
   (4) Surface affects movement of the ball: quicker on hard surface, slower on mat or soft surface.
e. Precautions.
   (1) Obese individuals, exceeding ball weight limits.
   (2) Avoid sharp belt buckles, zippers when over the ball; check surface for sharp objects.
   (3) Lack of foot traction, feet slipping: use bare feet, rubber-soled shoes, or yoga sticky mat.
   (4) Requires adequate space around exercising individual.
   (5) Watch for sensory overload: sympathetic signs (e.g., children, adults with traumatic brain injury).

(6) Increased pain with mobility exercises and degenerative joint disease.
(7) Muscle fatigue.

f. Contraindications.
(1) Dizziness or nausea associated with vestibular pathology.
(2) Extreme anxiety or fear of being on the ball.

Coordination and Balance Training

1. Goals and outcomes.

a. Motor function (motor control and learning) is improved.
b. Postural control, biomechanical alignment, and symmetrical weight distribution are improved.
c. Strength, power, and endurance necessary for movement control and balance are improved.
d. Sensory control and integration of sensory systems (somatosensory, visual, and vestibular) necessary for movement control and balance are improved.
e. Performance, independence, and safety are improved in transfers, gait, and locomotion.
f. Performance, independence, and safety are improved in basic activities of daily living (BADL) and instrumental activities of daily living (IADL).
g. Aerobic capacity and endurance are improved.
h. Self-management of symptoms is improved.

2. Training strategies to improve coordination and balance.

a. Motor learning strategies are important to assist the central nervous system (CNS) in adaptation for movement control.
(1) Learning requires repetition. Practice schedules should be carefully organized. Initial practice may feel threatening to patient; e.g., patient may feel in danger of losing control or balance. Progression should be gradual; the therapist should ensure patient confidence and safety, continuing motivation.
(2) Sensory cues are used to enhance motor performance.
(3) Feedback should stress *knowledge of results* (KR). Attention is drawn to the success of the outcome. It is important to establish a reference of correctness during early, cognitive learning.
(4) Feedback should address *knowledge of performance* (KP). Attention is drawn to missing elements, how to recruit, correct responses, and sequence responses.
(5) Feedback schedules: feedback given frequently (after every trial) improves initial performance. Feedback given less frequently (summed after a given number of trials or fading with decreasing frequency) improves retention of skills.
(6) A variety of activities and environments should be used to promote adaptability and generalizability of skills. Practice is from a closed environment (fixed) to open variable environments.
(7) Patient decision-making skills are promoted.

b. Remedial strategies focus on use of involved body segments (e.g., affected extremities in the patient with stroke).
(1) Control is first developed in isolated movements and progressed to more complex movements. Developmental postures/functional activities can be used to isolate body segments and focus on specific body skills; e.g., weight shifts to improve hip control are practiced first in kneeling before standing.
(2) Control is first achieved in holding (stability) before moving in a posture (stability-dynamic control) and skill level function (e.g., gait).
(3) Specific techniques can be used to remediate impairments (weakness, incoordination, and adaptive shortening, abnormal tone); e.g., tapping to improve responses of a weak quadriceps in standing position.
(4) As quality of movement improves, speed of movement and control is increased.
(5) Active responses and active learning should be promoted; progression is to unassisted or unfacilitated movements as soon as possible.

c. Compensatory strategies are utilized as appropriate to promote safety and early resumption of functional skills; e.g., the patient with delayed or absent recovery, multiple comorbidities. Compensatory training may lead to learned nonuse of impaired extremities and delay recovery in those patients with recovery potential; e.g., the patient with stroke.
(1) Safety is improved by substitution: intact segments (sound limbs) for impaired segments; cognitive control for impaired motor control; e.g., the patient with ataxia.
(2) Safety is improved by altering postural strategies; e.g., widening the base of support (BOS) and lowering the center of mass (COM).
(3) Safety is improved by use of appropriate assistive devices and shoes; e.g., weighted walker, athletic shoe.
(4) Safety is improved through environmental adaptations; e.g., handrails, adequate lighting, contrast tape on stairs and removal of throw rugs.

3. Interventions to improve coordination.

a. Functional training.
(1) Initial focus is on postural stability activities: holding.
(a) A number of different weight-bearing postures can be used; e.g., prone-on-elbows, sitting, quadruped, kneeling, plantigrade, and

standing. Progression is to gradually decrease BOS while raising height of COM.
   (b) Specific exercise techniques to enhance stability include stabilizing reversals and rhythmic stabilization.
   (c) Use dynamic reversals by decreasing ROM with ataxic movements.
  (2) Progress to controlled mobility activities: weight shifting through decrements (decreasing) ROM progressing to stability (steady holding); moving in and out of postures (movement transitions).
   (a) Specific exercise techniques include dynamic reversals by increasing ROM.
   (b) PNF patterns can be utilized to enhance synergistic control and reciprocal action of muscles; can be used to modulate timing and force output.
  (3) Aquatic exercises: water increases proprioceptive loading, slows down ataxic movements, provides buoyancy and light resistance.
  (4) Stabilization devices, e.g., air splints, soft neck collars, stabilize body segments and eliminate unwanted movement.
  (5) Environment: patients with ataxia do better in a low-stimulus environment; allows better utilization of cognitive strategies.
 b. Sensory training.
  (1) Patients with proprioceptive losses.
   (a) Visual compensation strategies (e.g., Frenkel's exercises in which position is varied from supine to sitting to standing); movements are guided visually.
   (b) Light weights: wrist cuffs, ankle cuffs, weighted walkers, elastic resistance bands to increase proprioceptive loading.
  (2) Patients with visual losses benefit from cognitive training strategies along with environmental adaptations and assistive devices.

4. Interventions to improve balance.
 a. Exercises to improve ROM, strength, and synergistic responses in order to withstand challenges to balance.
  (1) "Kitchen sink exercises": heel-cord stretches, heel-rises, toe-offs, partial wall squats, single-leg activities (side kicks, back kicks), marching in place, look-arounds (head and trunk rotation), hip circles. Progression from bilateral upper extremity (UE) touch-down support to unilateral UE support to no UE support.
  (2) Postural awareness training: focus on control of body position, centering the COM within the limits of stability (LOS).
  (3) Weight shifts (postural sway): training of ankle strategies, hip strategies. Can include postural sway biofeedback (e.g., Balance Master).
  (4) Training of change-of-support strategies: stepping strategies (forward, backward, sideward, crossed-step); UE reaching and protective extension.
 b. Functional training activities.
  (1) Sit-to-stand (STS) and sit-down (SIT) activities. Practice moving body mass forward over BOS, extending lower extremities (LEs), and raising body mass over feet and reverse. Focus on balance control while pivoting body mass over feet.
  (2) Floor-to-standing rises. Practice rising from floor to standing in the event of a fall; e.g., side-sit to quadruped to kneeling to half-kneeling to standing transitions.
  (3) Gait activities: practice walking forward, backward, sideward; slow to fast; normal BOS to narrowed BOS; wide turns to the right and left; 360° turns; head turns right and left; crossed-step walking and braiding; over and around obstacles.
  (4) Elevation activities: practice step-ups, lateral step-ups, stair climbing, and ramps.
  (5) Dual-task training. In standing or walking, practice simultaneous UE activities (e.g., bouncing a ball, catching or throwing a ball); in standing, practice LE activities (e.g., kicking a ball, tracing letters with one foot).
  (6) Community activities. Practice walking in open (variable) environments; e.g., pushing or pulling doors, car transfers, grocery shopping.
  (7) Practice anticipatory timing activities; e.g., getting on/off elevator, escalator.
 c. Disturbed balance activities, including manual perturbations, moveable BOS devices (stability ball, wobble board, split foam roller, dense foam).
  (1) Carefully grade force of perturbations, range, and speed of movements.
  (2) Stability ball training. Practice sitting, active weight shifts (e.g., pelvic clock), UE movements (e.g., arm circles, reaching), LE movements (e.g., stepping, marching), trunk movements (e.g., head and trunk turns).
  (3) Wobble board/equilibrium boards. Practice both self-initiated and therapist-initiated shifts in sitting or standing. Gradually increase range and speed of shifts.
 d. Sensory training.
  (1) Visual changes. Practice standing and walking, eyes open (EO) to eyes closed (EC); full lighting to reduced lighting.
  (2) Somatosensory changes. Practice standing and walking on tile floor to carpet (low pile to high), dense foam, outside terrain.
  (3) Vestibular changes. Practice standing, walking and moving head side-to-side, up-and-down; on a moving surface (e.g., escalator, elevator, bus).
  (4) Introduce sensory conflict situations (e.g., standing on foam cushion with eyes closed).

e. Safety education/fall prevention.
   (1) Assist patient in identification of fall risk factors; e.g., effect of medications, postural hypotension.
   (2) Lifestyle counseling: assist patient in recognizing unsafe activities, harmful effects of a sedentary lifestyle.
   (3) See Chapter 8.

5. Interventions to improve aerobic capacity and muscular endurance.
   a. Treadmill walking: Focus on velocity control; progression is from slow to fast. Safety harness can be worn to provide partial body weight support (BWS) if patient is unstable; e.g., the patient with ataxia or stroke. Incline and distance can also be modified.
   b. Ergometers. Pace pedaling on a cycle ergometer; progression is from slow to fast. Resistance and distance can also be modified. Can include both LE and UE training.
   c. Strength training.
      (1) Active/active assistive exercise.
      (2) Manual resistance; PNF patterns can be used to promote synergistic control, improve timing.
      (3) Weights, pulleys, hydraulics, elastic resistance bands, mechanical or electromechanical devices.
   d. Stretching exercises.

6. Teach activity pacing and energy conservation strategies as appropriate.
   a. The patient with ataxia has increased energy expenditure and can experience debilitating fatigue.

Relaxation Training

1. Relaxation.
   a. Relaxation refers to a conscious effort to relieve excess tension in muscles.
      (1) Excess muscle tension can cause pain leading to muscle spasm, which in turn produces more pain. To break the pain/spasm cycle, patients must learn to relax tense muscles.
      (2) Excess tension in tissues can result from maintaining a constant posture or sustaining muscle contractions for a period of time. Abnormal shortening or lengthening of muscles and ligaments is termed postural stress syndrome (PSS).
      (3) Habituation of compensatory movement patterns that contribute to the persistence of pain is termed movement adaptation syndrome (MAS).
   b. Awareness of prolonged muscle tension is accompanied by techniques designed to promote relaxation, improve circulation, and maintain flexibility.

2. Training strategies to promote relaxation.
   a. Start with the patient in a comfortable resting position, with all body parts well supported.
   b. Jacobson's progressive relaxation technique includes a systematic distal to proximal progression of conscious contraction and relaxation of musculature.
      (1) A period of reflex relaxation follows active contraction of muscle. The stronger the contraction, the greater the relaxation.
      (2) Breathing control: deep breathing coupled with the progressive relaxation to further promote relaxation. In diaphragmatic breathing, the patient breathes in slowly and deeply through the nose, allowing the abdomen to expand and then relax. This allows air to be expired through the relaxed, open mouth.
   c. Cognitive strategies/guided imagery: the patient is instructed to focus on relaxing the body, visualizing calmness and relaxation.
      (1) Patient focuses on letting go of all muscular effort, letting tension melt away.
      (2) Patient focuses on a relaxing environment or pleasant images to promote relaxation; e.g., lying on a tropical beach in the warm sunshine.
   d. Active range of motion: AROM can be used to reduce tension by moving body segments slowly.
   e. Rhythmic rotation (RRo) involves slow, passive, rotational movements of the limbs or trunk, and can be very effective in relieving muscular tension and spasticity; e.g., hooklying with both feet flat or with the LEs placed on a stability ball, gently rocking the knees from side-to-side.
   f. Slow vestibular stimulation: applied with gentle rocking techniques; can also be used to enhance relaxation, e.g., gentle rocking of the infant with colic.
   g. Biofeedback training can be an effective modality to promote relaxation; e.g., training to reduce the level of tension in the frontalis muscle.
   h. Stress management/lifestyle adaptation techniques.
      (1) Careful identification and evaluation of life stressors (e.g., Life Events Scale, Holmes-Rahe Social Readjustment Scale, Hassles Scale) are critical in developing an appropriate plan of care to reduce chronic stress. Stress-control techniques include both cognitive and physical strategies.
      (2) Lifestyle modification reduces frequency of high-stress situations and events. It is important to ensure adequate rest, activity and nutrition.
      (3) Enhance coping skills: Ensure that the patient maintains some level of control and decision making.
      (4) Maximize effective use of social support systems.

3. **Common errors associated with relaxation training.**
   a. Lack of awareness of the effects of the environment on an individual. Failure to have the patient in a low-stress environment and comfortably positioned.
   b. Lack of awareness of stress factors affecting the patient. Failure to evaluate stressors carefully and incorporate stress-management techniques.
   c. When using progressive relaxation techniques, progressing too fast from one body segment to another; e.g., distal to proximal body parts. Failure to combine slow deep breaths with each contraction and relaxation.
   d. Lack of effective training of kinesthetic awareness. Patients do not recognize when their muscles are tense. They perceive the tense muscle as normal, not needing any relaxation intervention.

Aquatic Exercise

1. **Goals and outcomes.**
   a. Motor function and motor learning are enhanced.
   b. ROM of motion and flexibility are improved.
   c. Postural control, biomechanical alignment, and symmetrical weight distribution are improved.
   d. Strength, power, and endurance are improved.
   e. Sensory control and integration of sensory systems (somatosensory, visual, and vestibular) are improved.
   f. Performance, independence, and safety in balance, gait, and locomotion are improved.
   g. Aerobic capacity and endurance are improved.
   h. Relaxation, reduction of pain, and decreased muscle spasm are enhanced.

2. **Strategies.**
   a. Immersion in pools or tanks is used to facilitate exercise. Water buoyancy, buoyant devices, and various depths of immersion decrease body weight and enhance movement; similar movements on land may be more difficult or impossible to perform.
   b. Allows greater freedom and range of movement than is permitted in whirlpools or Hubbard tanks.
   c. Pools or tanks with a walking track, with or without a treadmill, are used to enhance gait and endurance.

3. **Physics related to aquatic exercise.**
   a. Buoyancy: the upward force of water on an immersed or partially immersed body or body part. Equal to the weight of the water that it displaces (Archimedes' principle). This creates an apparent decrease in the weight and joint unloading of an immersed body part allowing easier movement in water.
   b. Cohesion: the tendency of water molecules to adhere to each other. The resistance encountered while moving through water is due to cohesion; some force is needed to separate water molecules.
   c. Density: the mass per unit volume of a substance. The density of water is proportional to its depth; deeper water must support the water above it.
   d. Hydrostatic pressure: the circumferential water pressure exerted on an immersed body part. A pressure gradient is established between the surface water and deeper water, due to the increase in water density at deeper levels.
      (1) Pascal's law states that the pressure exerted on an immersed body part is equal on all surfaces.
      (2) Increased pressure counteracts effusion and edema, and enhances peripheral blood flow.
   e. Turbulence: movement of a body part through water creates circular motion of the water (eddy current) near the surface of the part producing frictional drag.
      (1) As speed of movement increases, greater resistance is encountered.
      (2) Moving through turbulent water creates greater resistance as compared to calm water.
      (3) Use of equipment (e.g., paddle or boot) increases resistance and drag as the patient moves through water.

4. **Thermodynamics.**
   a. Water temperature affects body temperature and performance.
   b. Water temperature is determined by specific needs of patient and intervention goals.
      (1) Cooler temperatures are used for higher intensity exercise.
      (2) Warmer temperatures are used to enhance mobility, flexibility, and relaxation; e.g., patients with arthritis.
      (3) Ambient air temperature should be close to water temperature (e.g., within 3°C).
   c. There is decreased heat dissipation through sweating with immersion.
   d. At temperatures > 37°C (98.6°F), patients have increased cardiovascular demands at rest and during exercise.
   e. At temperatures < 25°C (77°F), patients have difficulty maintaining core temperature.

5. **Special equipment.**
   a. Buoyancy assistance devices: inflatable cervical collar, flotation rings, buoyancy belt or vest, kickboard.
   b. Buoyant dumbbells (swimmers): used for upright or horizontal support.
   c. Webbed gloves and hand paddles: used to increase resistance to upper extremity movement.
   d. Fins and boots: used to increase resistance to lower extremity movement.

6. **Exercise applications.**
   a. Movement horizontal to or upward toward the water surface (active assistive exercise) is made easier due to the buoyancy of water. A flotation device may be needed to support very weak patients.

b. Movement downward into the water is more difficult because of the buoyancy of water.
   (1) A flotation device or hand-held paddle can be used to increase resistance.
   (2) A paddle turned to slice through the water decreases resistance.
c. Resistance exercise can be controlled by the speed of the movement.
   (1) Resistance increases with increased velocity of movement due to the cohesion and turbulence of the water.
   (2) Slower movements meet less resistance.
   (3) Ataxic movements are slower and more controlled against the resistance of water.
d. Stretching exercises can be assisted by the buoyancy of water.
e. The amount of weight bearing on the lower extremities is determined by the height of the water/level of immersion (buoyancy) relative to the upright patient.
   (1) The greater the water depth, the less the weight/loading on extremities.
   (2) Can be used for partial weight-bearing (PWB) gait training.
f. Lower extremity reciprocal movements are enhanced by use of a kick board and using kicking movements.
g. Aerobic conditioning is enhanced with deep water walking or running, high-step marching. Progresses to reduced water levels and then to land walking/running.
   (1) Immersed equipment (e.g., cycle ergometer, treadmill, or upper body ergometer) can be used to enhance conditioning.
   (2) Swimming is an excellent aerobic training activity.
   (3) Regular monitoring of exercise responses (e.g., heart rate, ratings of perceived exertion) is required.
h. Treatment time varies with the type of activity, patient tolerance, and level of skill.

7. Contraindications.

a. Bowel or bladder incontinence.
b. Severe kidney disease.
c. Severe epilepsy.
d. Severe cardiac or respiratory dysfunction; e.g., cardiac failure, unstable angina, severely reduced vital capacity, unstable blood pressure.
e. Severe peripheral vascular disease.
f. Large open wounds, skin infections, colostomy.
g. Bleeding or hemorrhage.
h. Water and airborne infections; e.g., influenza, gastrointestinal infections.

8. Precautions.

a. Fear of water, inability to swim.
b. Patients with heat intolerance; e.g., patients with multiple sclerosis.
c. Use waterproof dressing on small open wounds and intravenous lines.

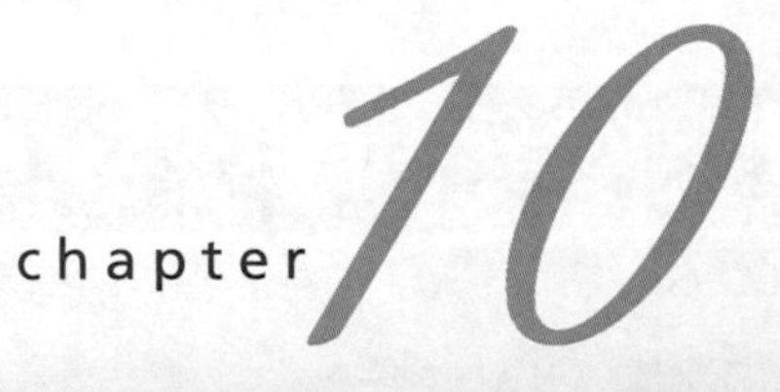

Therapeutic Modalities

JOHN CARLOS, JR. and ELIZABETH OAKLEY

Physical Agents

Superficial Thermotherapy

1. **Physics related to heat transmission.**
   a. Conduction: heat transfer from a warmer object to a cooler object by means of direct molecular interaction of objects in physical contact. Conductive modalities: hot packs, paraffin.
   b. Convection: heat transfer by movement of air or fluid from a warmer area to a cooler area or moving past a cooler body part. Convective modalities: whirlpool, Hubbard tank, fluidotherapy.
   c. Radiation: transfer of heat from a warmer object to a cooler object by means of transmission of electromagnetic energy without heating of an intervening medium. Infrared waves absorbed by cooler body. Radiation modality: infrared lamp.
2. **Physiological effects of general heat application.**
   a. Large areas of the body surface area are exposed to heat modality; e.g., whirlpool (hip and knee immersed), Hubbard tank (lower extremities and trunk immersed) (Table 10-1).

Table 10-1 ➤ PHYSIOLOGICAL EFFECTS OF GENERAL HEAT APPLICATION

INCREASED	DECREASED
Cardiac output	Blood pressure
Metabolic rate	Muscle activity (sedentary effect)
Pulse rate	Blood to internal organs
Respiratory rate	Blood flow to resting muscle
Vasodilation	Stroke volume

3. **Physiological effects of small surface area heat application.**
   a. Heat modality applied to discrete area of body; e.g., low back, hamstring, neck.
   b. Body tissue responses to superficial heat.
      (1) Skin temperature rises rapidly and exhibits greatest temperature change.
      (2) Subcutaneous tissue temperature rises less rapidly and exhibits smaller change.
      (3) Muscles and joints show least temperature change, depending on size of structure.
   c. Physiological effects on body systems and structures to small surface area heat modalities are listed in Tables 10-2 and 10-3.
4. **Goals and indications for superficial thermotherapy.**
   a. Modulate pain; increase connective tissue extensibility; reduce or eliminate soft-tissue inflammation and swelling; accelerate rate of tissue healing; reduce or eliminate soft tissue and joint restriction and muscle spasm.
   b. Preparation for electrical stimulation (ES); massage; passive and active exercise.
5. **Precautions for use of superficial thermotherapy.**
   a. Cardiac insufficiency; edema; impaired circulation; impaired thermal regulation; metal in treatment site; pregnancy; in areas where topical counterirritants have recently been applied; demyelinated nerves and open wounds.
6. **Contraindications to the use of superficial thermotherapy.**
   a. Acute and early subacute traumatic and inflammatory conditions, decreased circulation, decreased

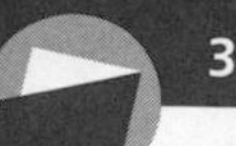

Table 10-2 ➤ INCREASED PHYSIOLOGICAL RESPONSES OF BODY SYSTEMS AND STRUCTURES TO LOCAL HEAT APPLICATION

SYSTEM/STRUCTURE	MECHANISM
a. Blood flow	Dilation of arteries and arterioles
b. Capillary permeability	Increase in capillary pressure
c. Elasticity of nonelastic tissues	Increased extensibility of collagen tissue
d. Metabolism	For every 10°C increase in tissue temperature, the rate of cellular oxidation increases by two to three times (Van't Hoff's Law)
e. Vasodilation	Activation of axon reflex and spinal cord reflex, release of vasoactive agents (bradykinin, histamine, prostaglandin)
f. Edema	Increased capillary permeability

Table 10-3 ➤ DECREASED PHYSIOLOGICAL RESPONSES OF BODY SYSTEMS AND STRUCTURES TO LOCAL HEAT APPLICATION

SYSTEM/STRUCTURE	MECHANISM
a. Joint stiffness	Increased extensibility of collagen tissue and decreased viscosity
b. Muscle strength	Decreased function of glycolytic process
c. Muscle spasm	Decreased firing of II afferents of muscle spindle and increased firing of Ib GTO fibers reduces alpha motor neuron activity, and thus decreases tonic extrafusal activity
d. Pain	Presynaptic inhibition of A delta and C fibers via activation of A beta fibers (Gate Theory), disruption of pain-spasm cycle

sensation, deep vein thrombophlebitis, impaired cognitive function, malignant tumors, tendency toward hemorrhage or edema, very young and very old patients. Additional contraindications are listed with each specific modality.

7. **General treatment preparation for thermotherapy and cryotherapy.**
   a. The application of physical agents must be performed by a qualified physical therapist or personnel supervised by a physical therapist (physical therapist assistant, affiliating physical therapist or physical therapist assistant student). The treatment and expected sensations must be explained to the patient.
   b. Place patient in comfortable position.
   c. Expose treatment area and drape patient properly.
   d. Inspect skin and check temperature sensation prior to treatment.
   e. If patient has good cognitive function, a call bell or other signaling device can be given to patient to alert personnel of any untoward effects of treatment. Check patient frequently during initial treatment.
   f. Dry and inspect skin at conclusion of treatment.
   g. Specific procedures for each physical agent are listed separately.

8. **Superficial heating physical agents.**
   a. Hot pack.
      (1) A canvas pack filled with silica gel, heated by immersion in water between 165° and 170°F.
      (2) Method of heat transmission: conduction.
      (3) Method of application.
         (a) Add 6-8 layers of toweling between the hot pack and the patient. This can be accomplished in the following ways:
         (b) Place pack(s) into a terry cloth cover, which usually equals 4-6 layers of toweling. Place one folded towel between patient and pack for hygienic purposes.
            (1) One-towel method:
               - Fold four towels in half, width-wise.
               - Place each towel on top of the other, forming eight layers of toweling.
               - Place towels on treatment area.
               - Place pack on towels and cover pack with folded towel to retard heat loss.
            (2) Two-towel wrap method:
               - This method is only appropriate for the standard size pack. Typical towels used in the clinic are not wide or long enough for a full-sized pack.
               - Fold two towels lengthwise and place one perpendicular over the other, forming a cross.
               - Place pack in the center of the towels.
               - Fold the ends of the towels over the pack, forming eight layers of toweling on top of the pack. Invert pack, placing the eight layers of toweling on patient.
         (c) Place pack on patient. If patient must be placed on pack, use additional towels to minimize excessive heating of treatment area caused by weight of patient on pack and to

protect bony prominences. Additional pillows may be necessary to support and make the patient comfortable when lying on top of the pack.

(d) Secure the pack to the patient with towels, sandbags or straps, if needed.

(e) Cover pack with folded towel to retard heat loss.

(f) The hot pack reaches peak heat within the first 5 minutes of application; during this time, the patient is at the greatest risk for a burn. Thus, the physical therapist or physical therapist assistant should check the skin within the first 5 minutes of treatment and periodically thereafter, especially if the patient is lying on top of the pack.

(4) Treatment time: 20–30 minutes.

b. Paraffin bath. Therapeutic application of liquid paraffin to a body part for the transmission of heat. Paraffin bath is a thermostatically controlled unit that contains a paraffin wax and mineral oil mixture in a 6:1 or 7:1 ratio. The paraffin/mineral oil mixture melts between 118°–130°F and is normally self-sterilizing at temperatures of 175°–180°F. Paraffin is primarily applied to small, irregularly-shaped areas such as the wrist, hand, and foot.

(1) Method of heat transmission: conduction.

(2) Procedure.

(a) Glove method (dip and wrap).

(1) Remove jewelry, or cover jewelry with several layers of gauze, if jewelry cannot be removed.

(2) Wash the part and check for infection and open areas.

(3) The part is dipped several times to apply 6–12 layers of paraffin.

(4) After the paraffin has solidified, the part is wrapped with plastic wrap or waxed paper, and covered with several layers of toweling, and secured with tape or rubber bands.

(5) The patient places the part in a comfortable or elevated position for 15–20 minutes.

(b) Dip and immersion method: the procedure follows steps (a)–(c) above, except that the part remains comfortably in the bath after the final dip.

(3) Treatment temperature of paraffin: 125°–127°F.

(4) Treatment time: 15–20 minutes.

(5) Indications: painful joints caused by arthritis or other inflammatory conditions in the late subacute or chronic phase, joint stiffness. Most often used on wrists and hands.

(6) Contraindications: allergic rash, open wounds, recent scars and sutures, skin infections.

c. Fluidotherapy is no longer tested on the NPTE.

d. Infrared lamp is no longer tested on the NPTE.

e. Hydrotherapy (whirlpool and Hubbard tank). Partial or total immersion baths in which the water is agitated and mixed with air to be directed against or around the affected part. Patients can move the extremities easily because of the buoyancy and therapeutic effect of the water.

(1) Method of heat transmission: convection.

(2) Physics related to hydrotherapy.

(a) Specific heat is the heat-absorbing capacity of water, representing the amount of heat a gram of water absorbs or gives off to change the temperature 1°C. The specific heat of water is about four times that of air.

(b) Thermal conductivity is the capability of a liquid, gas, or solid to conduct heat.

(c) Buoyancy is the upward force of water on an immersed or partially immersed body or body part which is equal to the weight of the water that it displaced (Archimedes' principle).

(d) Viscosity is the ease at which fluid molecules move with respect to one another. High temperature lowers the viscosity of the fluid.

(e) Hydrostatic pressure is the circumferential water pressure exerted on an immersed body part. A pressure gradient is established between the surface water and deeper water caused by the increase in water density at deeper levels.

(f) Cohesion is the tendency of water molecules to adhere to one another. The resistance encountered while moving through water is partially caused by the cohesion of water molecules and the force needed to separate them.

(g) Density of water is proportional to its depth. Deeper water is denser because it must support the water above it.

(3) Method of application: whirlpool.

(a) Fill the tank with water to the proper level and to the desired temperature. Whirlpool liners may be used for patients with burns, wounds, or those who are infected with blood-borne pathogens (human immunodeficiency virus or hepatitis-B virus).

(b) Add disinfectant if open wounds are present. Common antibacterial agents: sodium hypochlorite (bleach), dilution of 200 parts per million (ppm); Chloramine-T, 100–200 ppm.

(c) Standard precautions (gowns, goggles, masks, and gloves) should be applied when working in infected environment, particularly when working with possibility of splashing. (See Box 6-1).

(d) Assist patient in immersing his or her body or body part into the tank.
(e) Pressure points should be padded for patient comfort and to minimize compression of blood vessels and nerves. Keep towels out of water.
(f) Adjust agitator to desired position.
(g) Turn on agitator and adjust the force, direction, depth, and aeration.
(h) Monitor patient's response and tolerance to the whirlpool.
(i) At end of treatment, dry and inspect skin.

(4) Method of application: Hubbard tank.
(a) Fill the tank with water to the proper level and to the desired temperature.
(b) Add disinfectant, if open wounds are present.
(c) Position and secure patient supine on stretcher or pneumatic lift.
(d) Lift patient over edge of tank and slowly lower to water line to enable patient to get accustomed to the water temperature.
(e) Continue to lower patient into the water with head elevated. Secure head end of stretcher to bracket in the tank. Remove the suspended hoist when stretcher is resting on bottom of tank or halt descent of lift at desired level.
(f) Turn on agitator and adjust the force, direction, depth, and aeration.
(g) Monitor patient's response and tolerance to the whirlpool.
(h) At end of treatment, remove patient onto stretcher or lift. Dry and inspect skin.
(i) Clean and dry whirlpool.

(5) Treatment temperature: varies with size and status of area treated.
(a) 103°–110°F: whirlpool.
(b) 100°F: Hubbard tank.
(c) 95°–100°F: peripheral vascular disease.
(d) 92°–96°F: open wounds.

(6) Treatment time: 20 minutes, or up to 30 minutes, if other therapeutic procedures are also being performed.

(7) General cleaning procedures. Procedures may vary in different settings.
(a) After draining water from tank, rinse the entire tank, including openings in agitator and all drains.
(b) Wipe all areas that were in contact with water with a clean dry towel.
(c) Wash inside of tank, outside of agitators, and the drains with disinfectant diluted in warm water. Also wash agitators, thermometers, and all equipment used in treatment. Some tanks have a hose for spraying the tank. Allow disinfectant to stand for at least 1 minute.
(d) Place agitator in bucket filled with water and disinfectant, covering all openings with solution. Turn on agitator for ~20–30 seconds. Turn off motor and remove agitator from bucket.
(e) Rinse entire tank and all equipment until all residue is removed. Following use with patients with wounds or burns, refill tank with hot water and disinfectant, and allow solution to stand for 5 minutes (with or without agitator).
(f) Repeat step (4) with clean water. You may wish to rinse that tank a second time with hot water (110°–115°F) to hasten drying.
(g) Wipe inside and outside of tank dry with a clean towel.

(8) Indications: decubitus ulcers, open burns and wounds, post-hip fractures, postsurgical conditions of hip, subacute and chronic musculoskeletal conditions of neck, shoulders, and back, rheumatoid arthritis.

(9) Precautions.
(a) Local immersion: decreased temperature sensation; impaired cognition; recent skin graft; confusion/disorientation; deconditioned state.
(b) Full body immersion: confusion/disorientation; decreased strength, endurance, balance or ROM; medications; urinary incontinence; hydrophobia; respiratory problems; alcohol ingestion. Precautions for full immersion in hot or very warm water: pregnancy, multiple sclerosis, impaired thermal regulatory system.

(10) Contraindications.
(a) Local immersion: bleeding; wound maceration.
(b) Full body immersion: cardiac instability; profound epilepsy; suicidal patients, bowel incontinence, infections that can be spread by water.

(11) Electrical safety: safety precautions must be taken with any modality that potentially exposes the patient to electrical hazards from faulty electrical connections.
(a) A ground fault circuit interrupter should be installed at the circuit breaker of receptacle of all whirlpools and Hubbard tanks. The electrical circuit is broken if current is diverted to the patient (macroshock) who is grounded rather than to a grounded modality.
(b) All whirlpool turbines, tanks and motors, and motors used to lift patients should be checked for current leakage (broken or frayed connections).

f. Nonimmersion irrigation device.

(1) Small, hand-held electric water pump that produces a water jet to create a shearing force to loosen tissue debris. Some devices produce a pulsed lavage, and include suction to remove debris.

(2) Procedure.
(a) Treatment should take place in an enclosed area.
(b) Face and eye protection, gloves, and waterproof gown are required.
(c) Sterile, warm saline is used. Antimicrobials may be added.
(d) Select appropriate treatment pressure, usually 4–8 psi. Pressure may be increased in presence of large amounts of necrotic tissue or tough eschar. Pressure should be decreased with bleeding, near a major vessel, or if a patient complains of pain.
(e) Treatment time is usually 5–15 minutes, once a day. Wound size and amount of necrotic tissue may increase treatment parameters.

g. Aquatic therapy.
(1) A form of hydrotherapy used primarily for weightbearing activities, active exercise, or horizontal floating activities. Swimming pools or Hubbard tanks with or without walking troughs and treadmill units are used.
(2) Principles.
(a) Movement horizontal to or upward toward the water surface (active assistive exercise) is facilitated by the buoyancy of the water. A flotation device may be used as well.
(b) Movement downward is more difficult. A flotation device increases resistance.
(c) Increasing speed of movement increases resistance because of turbulence and cohesion of water. Use of hand-held paddles, held width-wise, increases resistance. Streamlining can be achieved by turning the paddle and slicing through the water.
(d) Amount of weightbearing can be determined by water depth. The greater the depth, the less the load on the extremities because of buoyancy.
(3) Water temperature is 92°–98°F.
(4) Treatment time varies with patient tolerance.
(5) Open wounds and skin infections must be covered.
(6) Goals are to improve standing balance: partial weightbearing ambulation; aerobic exercise; improve ROM; increase muscle strength via active assistive, active, or resistive exercise.
(7) Precautions and contraindications.
(a) Additional contraindications are unprotected open wounds and unstable blood pressure.

Cryotherapy

1. Physics related to cryotherapy energy transmission.

a. Abstraction: the removal of heat by means of conduction or evaporation.
(1) Conduction: transfer of heat from a warmer object to a cooler object by means of direct molecular interaction of objects in physical contact. Conductive modalities: cold pack, ice pack, ice massage, cold bath.
(2) Evaporation (heat of vaporization): highly volatile liquids that evaporate rapidly on contact with warm object. Evaporative modality: vapocoolant sprays (Fluori-Methane). Continued use questionable due to environmental concerns.

2. Physiological effects of large surface area cold application. (See Table 10-4).

3. Physiological effects of small surface area cold application.

a. Effects of cold application on body tissues.
(1) Skin temperature falls rapidly and exhibits greatest temperature change.
(2) Subcutaneous temperature falls less rapidly and displays smaller temperature change.
(3) Muscle and joint show least temperature changes, that require longer cold exposure.

b. Vasoconstriction of skin capillaries that results in blanching of skin in the center of contact area and hyperemia due to a decreased rate in oxygen-hemoglobin dissociation, around the edge of contact area in normal tissue.

c. Cold-induced vasodilation: cyclic vasoconstriction and vasodilation following prolonged cold exposure (>15 minutes). Occurs mostly in hands, feet, and face where arteriovenous anastomoses are found. Called the "hunting" reaction. Recent studies have questioned the clinical significance of this reaction.

d. Physiological effects on body systems and structures to small surface area cold modalities (Tables 10-5 and 10-6).

e. Adverse physiological effects of cold due to hypersensitivity.
(1) Cold urticaria: erythema of the skin with wheal formation, associated with severe itching due to histamine reaction.
(2) Facial flush, puffiness of eyelids, respiratory problems, and in severe cases, anaphylaxis (<blood pressure, >heart rate) with syncope are also related to histamine release.

Table 10-4 ➤ PHYSIOLOGICAL EFFECTS OF GENERAL COLD APPLICATION

DECREASED	INCREASED
Metabolic rate	Blood flow to internal organs
Pulse rate	Cardiac output
Respiratory rate	Stroke volume
Venous blood pressure	Arterial blood pressure Shivering (occurs when core temperature drops)

Table 10-5 ➤ DECREASED PHYSIOLOGICAL RESPONSES OF BODY SYSTEMS AND STRUCTURES TO LOCAL COLD APPLICATION

SYSTEM/STRUCTURE	MECHANISM
a. Blood flow	Sympathetic adrenergic activity produces vasoconstriction of arteries, arterioles and venules
b. Capillary permeability	Decreased fluids into interstitial tissue
c. Elasticity of nonelastic tissues	Decreased extensibility of collagen tissue
d. Metabolism	Decreased rate of cellular oxidation
e. Muscle spasm	Decreased firing of II afferents of muscle spindle, increased firing of Ib GTO fibers reduces alpha motor neuron activity and thus decreases tonic extrafusal activity
f. Muscle strength	Decreased blood flow, increase in viscous properties of muscle (long duration: >5–10 min.)
g. Spasticity	Decrease in muscle spindle discharge (afferents: primary, secondary), decreased gamma motor neuron activity
h. Vasoactive agents	Decreased blood flow

Table 10-6 ➤ INCREASED PHYSIOLOGICAL RESPONSES OF BODY SYSTEMS AND STRUCTURES TO LOCAL COLD APPLICATION

SYSTEM/STRUCTURE	MECHANISM
a. Joint stiffness	Decreased extensibility of collagen tissue and increased tissue viscosity
b. Pain threshold	Inhibition of A delta and C fibers via activiaton of A beta fibers (Gate Theory), interruption of pain-spasm cycle, decreased sensory and motor conduction, synaptic transmission slowed or blocked.
c. Increased blood viscosity	Decreased blood flow in small vessels facilitates red blood cells adhering to one another and vessel wall, impeding blood flow.
d. Muscle strength	Facilitation of alpha motor neuron (short duration: 1–5 min)

4. Goals and indications for cryotherapy.

a. Modulate pain; reduce or eliminate soft-tissue inflammation or swelling; reduce muscle spasm; reduce spasticity, cryokinetics; cryostretch; management of symptoms in multiple sclerosis.

5. Precautions.

a. Hypertension; impaired temperature sensation; open wound; over superficial nerve; very old or young and cognitive changes.

6. Contraindications to use of cryotherapy.

a. Cold hypersensitivity (urticaria); cold intolerance; cryoglobulinemia; peripheral vascular disease; impaired temperature sensation; Raynaud's disease; paroxysmal cold hemoglobinuria; over regenerating peripheral nerves.

7. Procedures.

a. Cold packs. Vinyl casing filled with silica gel or sand-slurry mixture.
   (1) Method of heat transmission: conduction.
   (2) Method of application.
      (a) Keep patient warm throughout treatment.
      (b) Dampen a towel with warm water, wring out excessive water, fold in half width-wise, and place cold pack on towel.
      (c) Place pack on patient and cover with dry towel to retard warming.
      (d) Secure pack.
   (3) Treatment temperature: packs are maintained in refrigerated unit at 0°–10°F.
   (4) Treatment time: 10–20 minutes.
   (5) Indications/contraindications: see general information.

b. Ice packs. Crushed ice folded in moist towel or placed in plastic bag covered by moist towel.
   (1) Method of heat transmission: conduction (abstraction).
   (2) Method of application.
      (a) Apply the ice pack to body part.
      (b) Cover pack with dry towel.
   (3) Treatment time: 10–20 minutes.

c. Ice massage. Ice cylinder formed by freezing water in a paper cup or Styrofoam cup. Salt may be added to create a colder slush mixture. A lollipop stick or wooden tongue depressor may or may not be placed in water during freezing process. During the application of ice massage, the patient will usually experience the following sequence of physiological response stages: cold, burning, aching, and numbness.
   (1) Method of heat transmission: conduction.
   (2) Method of application.
      (a) Remove ice from container. Wrap ice with towel or washcloth, if ice has no lollipop stick. If ice is retained in container, tear off bottom half and hold top half.

(b) Apply the ice massage to an area no larger then 4 × 6 inches in slow (2 inches/second) overlapping circles or overlapping longitudinal strokes, each stroke covering one-half of previous circle or stroke. If treating a large area, divide into smaller areas.
(c) Do not massage over bony area or superficial nerve (e.g., peroneal/fibular).
(d) Use a towel to dab excess water from treatment area. Ice will melt rapidly at first, but rate of melting will slow as skin cools.
(e) Continue treatment until anesthesia is achieved.

(3) Treatment time: 5–10 minutes, or until analgesia occurs.

d. Vapocoolant spray. A nontoxic, nonflammable volatile liquid which produces rapid cooling when a fine spray is applied to the skin. Vapocoolant sprays are used primarily to reduce muscle spasm, desensitizing trigger points. The use of vapocoolant sprays is being questioned because of the chlorofluorocarbon ingredients in the spray and their effect on the environment.

(1) Method of heat transmission: evaporation.
(2) Procedure (spray and stretch method).
(a) Invert container, nozzle down, hold ~18–24 inches from treatment area.
(b) Spray at 30° angle and sweep spray over treatment at 4 inches/second.
(c) Allow liquid to completely evaporate before applying next sweep. Caution! Do not frost skin.
(d) The muscle should be passively stretched before and during application.
(e) Cover the entire treatment area, starting at the pain site, and moving to the area of referred pain.
(f) Have patient perform active exercise after spraying.
(3) Treatment time: 10–15 minutes.
(4) Indications: myofascial referred pain, trigger points.
(5) Contraindications: refer to section IIF.

e. Contrast baths. The alternating immersion of a body part in warm and cold water to produce vascular exercise through active vasodilation and vasoconstriction of the blood vessels. The effectiveness of this method to raise deep tissue temperature via increased circulation of deep vessels has been questioned. It may be useful in promoting pain modulation.

(1) Method of heat transmission: conduction.
(2) Procedure.
(a) Treatment usually begins in warm (80°–110°F) water.
(b) Place part in warm water for 4 minutes, and then transfer to cold water for 1 minute.
(c) Immerse part in warm water for 4 minutes.
(d) Continue sequence of 4:1. End in warm water.
(e) Patient's condition may determine the ending temperature. Ending in cold water may be more beneficial if reducing edema is the goal.
(3) Treatment temperature.
(a) Hot water: 100°–110°F.
(b) Cold water: 55°–65°F.
(c) During initial treatment, you may wish to begin with the upper end of the cold range and the lower end of the hot range.
(4) Treatment time: 20–30 minutes.
(5) Indications: any condition requiring stimulation of peripheral circulation in limbs, peripheral vascular disease, sprains, strains, and trauma (after acute condition abates).
(6) Contraindications: advanced arteriosclerosis, arterial insufficiency, loss of sensation to heat and cold.

Acoustic Radiation: Ultrasound (US)

1. Biophysics related to ultrasound.

a. Conversion: mechanical energy produced by sound waves at frequencies between 85 KHz and 3 MHz and delivered at intensities between 1 and 3 w/cm^2 is absorbed by body tissues and changed to thermal energy.

b. Applicator contains a piezoelectric crystal (transducer).

(1) Transducer converts electrical energy into acoustical energy by means of reverse piezoelectric effect.
(2) Alternating voltage causes mechanical deformation of the crystal.
(3) Crystal resonates (vibration) at current frequency.
(4) Oscillating crystal produces sound waves with little dispersion of energy (collimated beam).
(5) Oscillating sound wave produces mechanical pressure waves in the tissue fluid medium. The molecules within the tissue vibrate, and the resulting friction produces heat.

c. Transducer size.

(1) US transducers come in a variety of sizes, from 1 cm^2 to 10 cm^2. The most commonly used is 5 cm^2.
(2) Transducer size should be selected relative to the size of the treatment area (1 cm^2 = wrist; 5 cm^2 = shoulder, leg).
(3) Effective radiating area (ERA).
(a) The ERA is the area of the faceplate (crystal size) which is smaller relative to the soundhead.

d. Spatial characteristics of US.
   (1) During continuous US, spatial characteristics of US are predominant.
   (2) Continuous US is applied to achieve thermal effects (e.g., chronic conditions).
   (3) US energy (intensity) is not uniformly distributed over the surface of the transducer, because the energy is mechanically blocked by the adhesive bonding of the crystal in the transducer and the pressure waves interfere with each other as they radiate from different areas of the crystal.
   (4) Uneven intensity produces a high level of energy in the center of the US beam relative to the surrounding areas. This effect produces a "hot spot" (peak spatial intensity) in the beam. Moving the soundhead or using pulsed US tends to reduce the effect of the hot spot.
   (5) Spatial average intensity. The total power (watts) divided by the area (cm^2) of the transducer head. This is typically the measurement used to document US treatments.
   (6) Beam nonuniformity ratio (BNR). The ratio of spatial peak intensity to spatial average intensity. The lower the BNR, the more uniform the energy distribution, and the less risk of tissue damage. BNR should be between 2:1–6:1. An ideal 1:1 ratio is not technically feasible.

e. Temporal characteristics of US.
   (1) During pulsed US, temporal characteristics of the US are important.
   (2) Pulsed US is applied when nonthermal effects are desired (e.g., acute soft tissue injuries).
   (3) Duty cycle. The fraction of time the US energy is on over one pulse period (time on + time off). For example, a 20% duty cycle could have an on-time of 2 msec and an off-time of 8 msec. A duty cycle of ≤50% is considered pulsed US. A duty cycle of 51%–99% produces less acoustic energy and less heat.
   (4) Temporal peak intensity. The peak intensity of US during the on-time phase of the pulse period.
   (5) Temporal average intensity. The US power averaged over one pulse period.
   (6) Attenuation. The reduction of acoustical energy as it passes through soft tissue. Absorption, reflection and refraction effect attenuation. Absorption is highest in tissues with high collagen and protein content (muscles, tendons, ligaments, capsules). The scattering of sound waves that result from reflection and refraction produces molecular friction that the sound wave must overcome to penetrate tissues.

f. Depth of penetration: 3–5 cm.
   (1) At 3 MHz, greater heat production in superficial layers, caused by greater scatter (attenuation) of sound waves in superficial tissue; e.g., temporomandibular joint.
   (2) Increased heat production in deep layers at 1 MHz, is caused by less scatter in superficial tissues; thus, more US energy is able to penetrate to deeper tissues.

2. Physiological effects of ultrasound.

a. Thermal: produced by continuous sound energy of sufficient intensity. Range: 0.5–3 w/cm^2. US intensity will vary depending upon tissue type and pathology.
   (1) Increased tissue temperature, increased pain threshold, increased collagen tissue extensibility, alteration of nerve conduction velocity, increased enzymatic activity, and increased tissue perfusion.
   (2) Increased temperature at tissue interfaces due to reflection and refraction. Tissue interfaces could be bone/ligament, bone/joint capsule and bone/muscle.
   (3) Excessively high temperatures may produce a sudden, strong ache caused by overheating of periosteal tissue (periosteal pain). Reduce intensity or increase surface area of treatment if periosteal pain is expressed by patient.
   (4) Insufficient coupling agent may produce discomfort caused by a "hot spot," which is the uneven distribution of the acoustical energy through the sound head. However, this is a greater problem if the stationary technique is used.

b. Nonthermal: generated by very low intensity or pulsed (intermittent) sound energy. Pulsed US is related to duty cycle. Typical duty cycles are 20%–50% for nonthermal intervention.
   (1) Cavitation: alternating compression (condensation phase) and expansion (rarefaction phase) of small gas bubbles in tissue fluids caused by mechanical pressure waves.
      (a) Stable cavitation: Gas bubbles resonate without tissue damage. Stable cavitation may be responsible for diffusional changes in cell membranes.
      (b) Unstable cavitation: Severe collapse of gas bubbles during compression phase of US can result in local tissue destruction due to high temperatures.
      (1) Acoustic streaming: movement of fluids along the boundaries of cell membranes resulting from mechanical pressure wave. Acoustic streaming may produce alterations in cell membrane activity, increased cell wall permeability, increased intracellular calcium, increased macrophage response, and in creased protein synthesis; may accelerate tissue healing.

3. Goals and indications.

a. Modulate pain; increase connective tissue extensibility; reduce or eliminate soft-tissue inflammation; accelerate rate of tissue healing; wound healing; reduce or eliminate soft-tissue and joint restriction and muscle spasm.

4. Precautions.

a. Acute inflammation; breast implants; open epiphyses and US over healing fractures.

5. Contraindications.

a. Impaired circulation; impaired cognitive function; impaired sensation; malignant tumors; over or near an area with thrombophlebitis; joint cement; directly over plastic components; over vital areas such as brain, ear, eye, heart, cervical ganglia; carotid sinuses; reproductive organs; exposed or unprotected spinal cord; over or in the area of cardiac pacemakers or in the abdomen, low back, uterus or pelvis during pregnancy.

6. Procedures.

a. Direct contact (transducer/skin interface). Moving sound head in contact with relatively flat body surface.
   (1) Apply generous amount of coupling medium (gel/cream) to skin.
   (2) US requires a homogenous medium (mineral oil, water, commercial gel) for effective sound wave transmission and acts as a lubricating agent.
   (3) Select sound head size (ERA one half the size of the treatment area). Place sound head at right angle to skin surface.
   (4) Move sound head slowly (~1.5 inches/sec) in overlapping circles or longitudinal strokes maintaining sound head to body surface angle.
   (5) Each motion covers one-half of previous circle or stroke.
   (6) Do not cover an area greater than two to three times the size of the effective radiating area (ERA) per 5 minutes of treatment. To cover an area greater than twice the ERA, apply US in two or more sections.
   (7) While sound head is moving and in firm contact, turn up intensity to desired level.
   (8) Treatment intensity: 0.5–2.5 w/cm^2, depending on treatment goal. Lower intensities for acute conditions or thin tissue (wrist joint); for chronic conditions or thick tissue (low back), higher intensities should be considered.
   (9) Periosteal pain occurring during treatment may be caused by high-intensity, momentary slowing, or cessation of moving head. If this occurs, stop treatment and readjust US intensity or add more coupling agent.
   (10) Treatment time: 3–10 minutes, depending on size of area, intensity, condition and frequency.

b. Indirect contact (water immersion). Use with irregular body parts.
   (1) Fill container with water high enough to cover treatment area. A plastic container is preferred because it will reflect less acoustic energy than a metal container.
   (2) Place part in water.
   (3) Place sound head in water, keeping it 1 cm from skin surface and at right angle to body part.
   (4) Move sound head slowly, as in direct contact. If applying stationary technique, reduce intensity or use pulsed US.
   (5) Turn up intensity to desired level.
   (6) Periodically wipe off any air bubbles that may form on sound head or body part during treatment.

c. Indirect contact. A fluid-filled, thin-walled bag such as a balloon, condom, or surgical glove applied over irregular bony surfaces. Not widely used, but may be an alternative to immersion technique.
   (1) Place bag around side of sound head, squeeze out fluid until all air is removed and sound head is immersed in water.
   (2) Apply coupling agent to skin and place bag over treatment area.
   (3) Move sound head slowly within bag to maintain a right angle between sound head and treatment area. Do not slide bag on skin.
   (4) Increase intensity to desired level.

7. Phonophoresis.

a. The use of US to drive medications through the skin into the deeper tissues. Local analgesics (lidocaine) and anti-inflammatory drugs (dexamethasone, salicylates) are often used.

b. Method of application is similar to direct contact technique, except that a medicinal agent is used as part of coupling medium.
   (1) Mode: pulsed 20%
   (2) Treatment intensity: 1–3 w/cm^2.
   (3) Treatment time: 5–10 minutes.
   (4) 0.5-0.75 w/cm^2, using a medication that is prepared in a medium that will allow transmission of the US. Gel mediums or transdermal patches have good transmisivity; avoid pastes and creams.

c. Goals and indications.
   (1) Pain modulation; decrease inflammation in subacute and chronic musculoskeletal conditions.

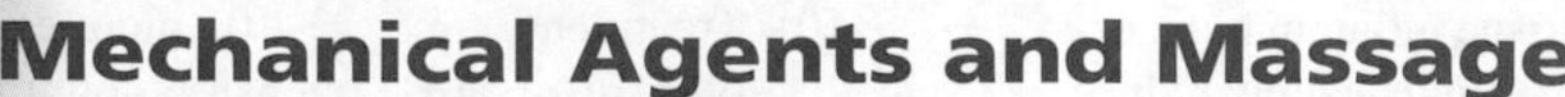

Mechanical Agents and Massage

Mechanical Spinal Traction (Intermittent Traction)

1. **Description.**
   a. A distraction force applied to the spine to separate articular surfaces between vertebral bodies and elongate spinal structures. This force is applied to multiple spinal segments in the cervical and lumbar region. Many types of spinal traction are presently used, such as manual, positional, gravity-assisted, inversion, continuous, and static traction. This section will focus on mechanical traction.

2. **Effects of traction.**
   a. Joint distraction: a separation of the facet joints occurs with sufficient force. This opens up the intervertebral foramen, relieves pressure on the nerve root and decreases compressive forces on the facets. For the lumbar region, a force of 50% of the patient's body weight is required to cause separation. In the cervical region, 7% of the patient's body weight or about 20-30 lbs results in separation. In both instances, lower traction forces (lumbar: 30-40 lbs; cervical: 8-10 lbs) are recommended for initial treatment to decrease reactive muscle spasm and determine patient tolerance. In follow-up treatments, force can be gradually increased to achieve a maximal decrease in symptoms, but not to exceed 7% of body weight in the cervical region and 50% in the lumbar region.
   b. Reduction of disc protrusion: separation of vertebral bodies occurs at higher forces, causing a decrease in intradiscal pressure that creates a suction-like effect on the nucleus, drawing it back in centrally. The surrounding ligamentous structures are stretched taut, which also helps to push the disc in centrally. For the lumbar region, 60-120 lbs or up to 50% of a patient's body weight, and for the cervical region, 12-15 lbs is recommended to achieve these desired effects.
   c. Soft-tissue stretching: The surrounding spinal muscles, ligaments, tendons and discs can be stretched, decreasing the pressure on the facet joints, nerve roots, vertebral bodies and discs without achieving joint separation. Lower traction forces are sufficient to achieve this effect (lumbar region: 25% of body weight; cervical region: 12-15 lbs).
   d. Muscle relaxation: Both intermittent and static traction can decrease muscle tone. Traction can interrupt the pain-muscle spasm cycle by stimulating mechanoreceptors through the motion caused by interrupted traction, and by inhibiting motor neuron firing with static traction. The forces recommended for soft-tissue stretching are also used for muscle relaxation.
   e. Joint mobilization: At lower forces, intermittent traction stimulates the mechanoreceptors to inhibit pain and decrease spasm, while high force traction causes decreased pressure on the joints and stretches the surrounding soft tissue. Unlike manual joint mobilization, traction cannot be isolated to a particular segment and provides general mobilization in the cervical or lumbar region.

3. **Goals and indications.**
   a. Decrease joint stiffness (hypomobility); decrease meniscoid blocking muscle spasm; degenerative disc; disc protrusion; joint disease; modulate discogenic pain; modulate subacute or chronic joint pain; reduce nerve root impingement.

4. **Precautions.**
   a. Claustrophobia, hiatal hernia, vascular compromise, pregnancy, and impaired cognition;. any disease or condition that can compromise the structure of the spine, such as: osteoporosis, tumor, infection, rheumatoid arthritis or protracted steroid use; TMJ; problems with halter use; disc extrusion; medial disc protrusion; complete resolution of severe pain with traction.

5. **Contraindications.**
   a. Acute strains, sprains and inflammation; spondylolisthesis, fractures, post-op spinal surgery, spinal joint instability or hypermobility and spinal cord compression; hypertension; increased peripheralization of pain, numbness or tingling, decreased myotomal strength and decreased reflex response.

6. **Procedure (intermittent traction).**
   a. Cervical traction.
      (1) Can be seated or supine. Supine position is generally preferred.
      (2) Cervical halter.
         (a) Head halter is placed under the occiput and the mandible.
         (b) Head halter is attached to the traction cord directly or to the traction unit through the spreader bar.
         (c) Slack is removed from the traction cord. The neck should be maintained in 20–30 degrees of flexion; a pillow may be used to achieve this angle.

(d) Some target area specificity may be achieved by varying the neck angle approximately 0–5 degrees of cervical flexion to increase intervertebral space and joint separation at C1 through C5; up to 25–30 degrees for C5 through C7; neutral spine (approximately 20 degrees of flexion) for disc dysfunction.

(e) Traction force should be applied to the occipital region and not on the chin. If patient expresses discomfort in the temporomandibular joint area, treatment should stop, and head halter should be readjusted to ensure that the force is properly applied.

(3) Cervical sliding device.

(a) The head is placed on padded headrest, which positions the neck in 20–30 degrees of flexion.

(b) Adjustable neck yoke is tightened to firmly grip just below the mastoid process.

(c) Head strap is secured across the forehead.

(d) Traction rope is then attached to the gliding platform of the device.

(4) Traction force is determined by treatment goals and patient tolerance.

(a) Acute phase.

(1) Disc protrusion, elongation of soft tissue, muscle spasm, ~10-15 pounds or 7%–10% of body weight.

(2) Joint distraction ~20–30 pounds.

(5) Treatment time.

(a) Five to 10 minutes for acute conditions and disc protrusion, 15–30 minutes for other conditions.

(6) Duty cycle.

(a) Static traction is recommended for disc protrusions or when symptoms are aggravated by motion.

(b) Intermittent traction can also be used for disc protrusions and joint distraction, but a 3:1 hold/rest ratio is recommended. A 1:1 ratio is recommended when mobility is desired, i.e. joint mobilization.

b. Lumbar traction.

(1) A split table is usually used to minimize friction between the body and the table.

(2) Supine position, with pillow under the knee or small bench under lower leg, is recommended when the goal is to open up the intervertebral foramen, separate the facet joints, or elongate the muscles. The prone position may be preferable in the case of a posterior herniated lumbar disc. Some target area specificity may be achieved by varying the angle of pull (i.e., to increase intervertebral space at L5-S1 to ~45–60 degrees of hip flexion, or at L3 to L4 up to 75–90 degrees).

(3) Apply the pelvic harness so that the top edge is above the iliac crest.

(4) Attach the thoracic harness so that the inferior margin is slightly below lower ribs.

(5) Secure the harness around the pelvis and attach it to the traction rope or spreader bar.

(6) Thoracic harness provides countertraction to the pull on the pelvis, and is secured at the top of the table.

(7) Treatment force.

(a) Acute phase 30–40 pounds.

(b) Disc protrusion, spasm; elongation of soft tissues, 25% of body weight.

(c) Joint distraction, 50 pounds or 50% of body weight.

(8) Treatment time: 5–10 minutes for herniated disc, 10–30 minutes for other conditions.

Intermittent Mechanical Compression

1. Description.

a. Pneumatic device that applies external pressure to an extremity through an inflatable appliance (sleeve).

b. Appliances are designed in a variety of sizes and lengths to fit either the upper or lower extremity (ankle, ankle and lower leg, or full extremity).

c. The device is attached to an inflatable pneumatic sleeve by rubber tubing.

d. The compression units and appliances are designed to inflate a single compartment to produce uniform, circumferential pressure on the extremity, or multiple compartments by applying pressure in a sequential manner. Pressure is greater in the distal compartments and lesser in the proximal compartments.

e. Cold can be applied simultaneously with intermittent compression in which a coolant (50°–77°F) is pumped through an inflatable sleeve.

2. Physiological effects.

a. External pressure on the extremity increases the pressure in the interstitial fluids, forcing the fluids to move into the lymphatic and venous return systems, thus reducing the fluid volume in the extremity. In addition to mechanical compression, some conditions may require the daily use of compression stockings to counteract the effect of gravity on the vascular and lymph systems in the lower extremities.

3. Goals and indications.

a. Amputation; decrease chronic edema; postmastectomy lymphedema; stasis ulcer; venous insufficiency. Manual massage/drainage techniques have supplanted use of mechanical compression in many instances.

4. Precautions.

a. Impaired sensation; malignancy; uncontrolled hypertension; over an area where there is a superficial peripheral nerve, such as the fibular nerve.

5. **Contraindications.**
   a. Acute inflammation, trauma or fracture; acute deep venous thrombosis (DVT) and thrombophlebitis; obstructed lymph or venous return; arterial disease/insufficiency; arterial revascularization; acute pulmonary edema; diminished sensation; cancer; edema with cardiac or renal impairment; impaired cognition; infection in treatment area; hypoproteinemia (< 2 g/dL); very old or young patients.

6. **Procedure.**
   a. Check patient's blood pressure.
   b. Place patient in comfortable position, with limb elevated approximately 45 degrees and abducted 20–70 degrees.
   c. Apply stockinet over extremity. Be sure all wrinkles are removed.
   d. Place the appliance over the extremity and attach the rubber tube to both the appliance and the compression unit.
   e. Set the inflation and deflation ratio to ~3:1. Generally, for edema reduction 45–90 seconds on/15–30 seconds off. To shape residual limb, a 4:1 ratio is often used.
   f. Turn the power on and slowly increase the pressure to the desired level.
      (1) The patient's blood pressure determines the setting of the device. Some manufacturers recommend that the setting never exceed the patient's diastolic blood pressure. Others advise that the pressure can fall between the diastolic and systolic pressure because the pressure is on for only a short period of time.
      (2) Numbness, tingling, pulse, or pain should not be felt by the patient during the treatment.
   g. At the end of the treatment, turn off the unit, remove the appliance and stockinet. Inspect skin.
   h. Usually an elastic bandage or compression stocking is placed on the extremity to retain the reduction before a dependent position is allowed.
   i. Treatment time.
      (1) The duration may vary, depending on the patient's tolerance. Minimum daily treatment times for lymphedema: 2 hours to two 3-hour sessions; traumatic edema: 2 hours; venous ulcers: 2.5 hours/3×/week to 2-hour periods; residual limb reduction: 1 hour to three 1-hour sessions, totaling 4 hours. Some conditions may warrant shorter treatment times initially.

Continuous Passive Motion (CPM)

1. **Description.**
   a. Uninterrupted passive motion of the joint through a controlled range of motion (ROM). A mechanical device provides continuous movement for extended periods of time.

2. **Physiological effects of CPM.**
   a. Accelerate rate of interarticular cartilage regeneration, tendon and ligament healing.
   b. Decrease edema and joint effusion.
   c. Minimize contractures.
   d. Decrease postoperative pain.
   e. Increase synovial fluid lubrication of the joint.
   f. Improve circulation.
   g. Prevent adhesions.
   h. Improve nutrition to articular cartilage and periarticular tissues.
   i. Increase joint ROM.

3. **Goals and indications.**
   a. Postimmobilization fracture, tendon or ligament repair; total knee or hip replacement.

4. **Precautions.**
   a. Intracompartmental hematoma from anticoagulant use.

5. **Contraindications.**
   a. Increases in pain, edema, or inflammation following treatment.

6. **Procedure (postoperative knee).**
   a. CPM applied immediately postoperatively, with carriages appropriately measured and adjusted.
   b. Rate of motion set at 1- to 4-minute cycles.
   c. If applied at the knee, ROM may be 20–40 degrees of knee flexion initially and increased 5–10 degrees, as tolerated, until optimal range is reached. Usually a goal of 110–120 degrees is acceptable.
   d. Treatment time, as little as 1-hour sessions, three times a day, up to 24 continuous hours. Patient's limb may be removed periodically for active or active assistive exercise, or activities of daily living (ADL) activities.
   e. Duration of treatment: 1 to 3 weeks or until therapeutic goals are attained.

Tilt Table

1. **Description.**
   a. Mechanical or electrical table designed to elevate patient from horizontal (0 degrees) to vertical (90 degrees) position in a controlled, incremental manner.

2. **Physiological effects of tilt table.**
   a. Stimulate postural reflexes to counteract orthostatic hypotension.
   b. Facilitate postural drainage.
   c. Gradual loading of one or both lower extremities.
   d. Begin active head or trunk control.
   e. Provide positioning for stretch of hip flexors, knee flexors, and ankle plantar flexors.

3. **Indications.**
   a. Prolonged bed rest; immobilization; spinal cord injury, traumatic brain injury; orthostatic hypotension; spasticity.

4. **Procedure.**
   a. Patient is placed in supine position.
   b. Abdominal binder, long elastic stockings, or tensor bandaging to counteract orthostatic hypotension (venous pooling) may be used.
   c. Patient secured to table by straps. Knee (just proximal to patella), hip (over pelvis), and trunk (over chest just under the axilla).
   d. Take baseline vitals (blood pressure, heart rate, respiratory rate).
   e. Table raised gradually to given angle. Incremental rise to 30 degrees, 45 degrees, 60 degrees, 80 degrees or 85 degrees, or as tolerated. Position can be maintained for as long as 30–60 minutes.
   f. Vital signs (blood pressure, heart rate, respiratory rate) need to be monitored to assess the patient's tolerance to treatment. Cyanotic lips or fingernail beds may indicate compromised circulation.
   g. Treatment time.
      (1) Initially, the duration of treatment depends on the patient's tolerance, but should not exceed 45 minutes, once or twice daily.

Massage

1. **Description.**
   a. Mechanical manipulation of soft tissue by the hands. (Electrical, mechanical, or hydraulic methods will not be discussed. Alternate forms of massage such as acupressure, shiatsu, or reflexology are beyond the scope of this section).

2. **Physiological effects.**
   a. Increased venous and lymphatic flow.
   b. Stretching and loosening of adhesions.
   c. Edema reduction.
   d. Sedation.
   e. Muscle relaxation.
   f. Modulate pain.

3. **Description of selected techniques.**
   a. Stroking (effleurage): gliding movements of hands over surface of skin. Superficial stroking: light contact. Deep stroking: heavy pressure.
   b. Kneading (petrissage): grasping and lifting of tissues. Similar to kneading bread.
   c. Friction: compression of tissue using small circular or long stroking movements, usually with the palmar surface of hand or fingers. Pressure may be light (superficial) initially, progressing to heavy (deep), moving superficial tissues over deeper tissues.
   d. Tapping (tapotement): rapid striking with palmar surface of hand and/or fingers, cupped hand (clapping, percussion), or ulnar edge of hand and fingers (hacking) in an alternating manner.
   e. Vibration: shaking of tissue using short, rapid quivering motion with hands in contact with the body part.

4. **Procedure.**
   a. Stroking: usually initiates and ends treatment. Hand is molded over body part and movement is usually distal to proximal. Stroking is used to move from one area to another and between other strokes. Superficial strokes make no attempt to move deep tissue. Some passive muscle stretching is performed with deep stroking.
   b. Kneading: milking effect of kneading aids in loosening adhesions and increasing venous return. Technique can be done with one or both hands, fingers, or the thumb and first finger. Wring and lift tissues to break down adhesions. Direction of strokes may vary, depending on body structure; however, to increase venous return, strokes should move from distal to proximal along the extremity.
   c. Friction: heavy compression over soft tissues will stretch scars and loosen adhesions. Ball of fingers or thumb should move in small circular or stroking manner, pressing superficial tissues over deep structures. Pressure gradually increases to the patient's tolerance as technique moves up and down or around the targeted structures. Pressure never abruptly released. Cross-fiber friction consists of deep strokes across the muscle fiber rather than along longitudinal axis of the fibers.
   d. Tapotement: used when stimulation is desired treatment effect.
   e. Cupping: applied to the chest to mobilize bronchial secretions (postural drainage).
   f. Vibration: often used in conjunction with cupping for postural drainage to loosen adherent secretions.

5. **General considerations in the application of massage.**
   a. Place patient in comfortable, relaxed position with treatment part in gravity-eliminated position, or position in which gravity will assist in venous flow.
   b. Body part exposed and well supported, with no clothing restricting circulation.
   c. Begin with superficial stokes. May move to deep stroking.
   d. Deep stroking may be followed by kneading. May alternate between stroking and kneading.
   e. Stroking or kneading should follow friction massage.
   f. Massage should begin in the proximal segment of the extremity, move distally, and return to proximal region. All stroking movements are directed distal to proximal, especially for edema.
   g. Complete treatment with stroking, moving from deep to superficial stroking.

6. Contraindications.
   a. Acute inflammation in area, acute febrile condition, severe atherosclerosis, severe varicose veins, phlebitis, areas of recent surgery, thrombophlebitis, cardiac arrhythmia, malignancy, hypersensitivity, severe rheumatoid arthritis, hemorrhage in area, edema secondary to kidney dysfunction, heart failure, and venous insufficiency.

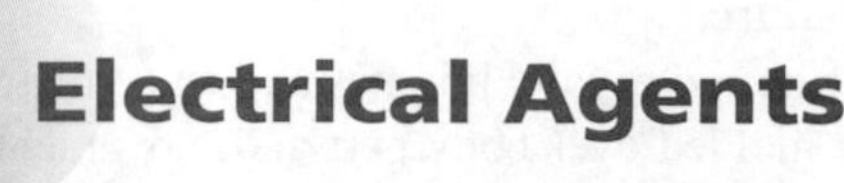

Electrical Agents

Basic Concepts of Nerve and Muscle Physiology

1. Properties of electrically excitable cells. (See Figure 10-1).
   a. Resting membrane potential (RMP).
      (1) The cell membrane is more permeable to potassium (K^+) compared to sodium (Na^+) and negatively-charged proteins (anions).
      (2) Electrical potential is generated across the cell, membrane, due to the higher concentration of K^+ and anions on the inside of the cell relative to the concentration of Na^+ on the outside.
      (3) A negative charge is produced within the cell, and a positive charge develops on the outside of the cell as the positively charged K^+ diffuses from the cell.
      (4) RMP is –60 mV to –90 mV for excitable cells.
      (5) RMP is maintained by an active sodium-potassium pump that takes in K^+ and extrudes Na^+.
   b. Action potential (Figure 10-2).
      (1) A stimulus (e.g., electrical) causes the cell membrane to becomes more permeable to Na^+ ions.
      (2) An action potential (AP) is generated when the influx of Na^+ causes a reduction in RMP, which occurs slowly at first. Reduction in the RMP is called depolarization.
      (3) When transmembrane potential reaches a critical threshold level (approximately –55 mV), the voltage-sensitive Na^+ and K^+ channels open widely. Permeability to Na^+ increases rapidly, whereas the permeability to K^+ increases slowly.
      (4) During depolarization, transmembrane potential may rise as high as +35 mV. A positive charge is generated inside the cell, and a negative charge outside is produced, as a result of the flow of ions.
      (5) The K^+ channels are fully open at about the time that the Na^+ are closed, and K^+ rushes rapidly out of the cell, making the transmembrane potential progressively more negative. This process is called repolarization.

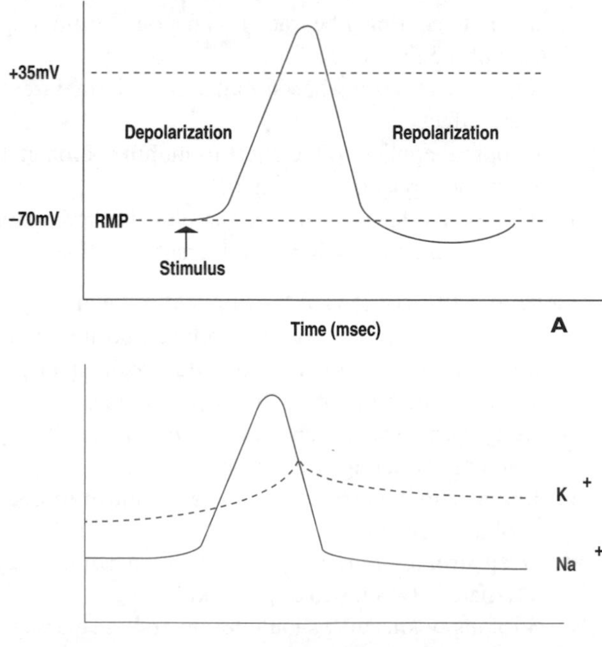

Figure 10-1 • A. Changes in transmembrane potential and B. Changes in membrane permeability of sodium and potassium during an action potential.

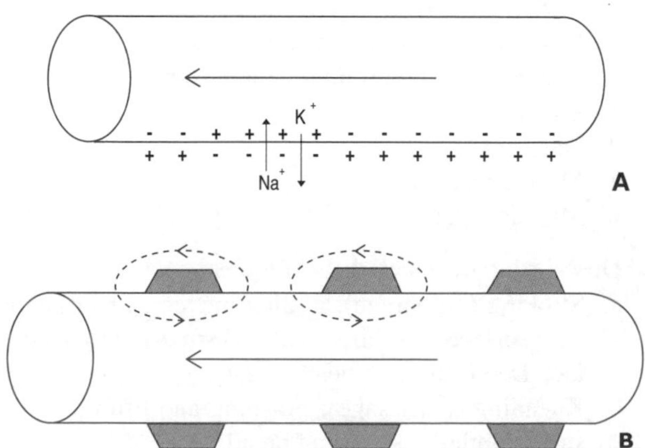

Figure 10-2 • A. Propagation of action potential in unmyelinated axon and B. myelinated axon.

(6) The K^+ channels remain open long enough to repolarize the membrane (10–20 mV <RMP). This is called hyperpolarization.
(7) The K^+ channels close and passive diffusion of the ions rapidly returns the RMP to its initial level.

c. Propagation of the action potential (Figure 10-2).
(1) Opening of the Na^+ and K^+ channels and voltage changes that produce an AP at one segment of the membrane triggers successive depolarization in adjacent regions of the nerve, muscle or membranes.
(2) AP movement occurs along the surface of the nerve or muscle cell.
(3) Movement of the AP along an unmyelinated nerve is generated via sequential depolarization (eddy currents) along neighboring sites in the nerve membrane. Speed of conduction in small diameter fibers is slow due to the greater internal resistance in the small fibers.
(4) In myelinated nerve fibers, saltatory conduction occurs at discrete junctures (nodes of Ranvier) in the myelin sheath which surrounds the nerve.
(5) Na^+ and K^+ ion exchange and current flow is concentrated at these points. The impulse jumps from node to node, conducting nerve impulses at greater rates compared to smaller, unmyelinated nerve fibers.

2. Electrical action of muscle and nerve.

a. Characteristics of ES necessary to initiate excitable cell depolarization.
(1) Amplitude or intensity of the stimulus must be great enough to cause the membrane potential to be lowered sufficiently to reach threshold levels.
(2) Duration of the individual stimulus must be long enough to produce depolarization of the cell membrane. A duration of ≤1 ms is sufficient to stimulate nerve cell membrane, but is too short to stimulate muscle cell membrane.
(3) Rate of rise of the current to peak intensity must be rapid enough to prevent accommodation, which is the rapid adjustment of the membrane to stimuli to prevent depolarization. Square wave delivers instantaneous rise.

3. Strength-duration curve. (See Figure 10-3).

a. Rheobase is the intensity of the current, with a long duration stimulus, required to produce a minimum muscle contraction.
b. Chronaxie is the pulse duration of the stimulus at twice the rheobase intensity. Chronaxie of a denervated muscle is >1 msec.
c. Very short pulse durations (<0.05 msec) with low intensities can depolarize sensory nerves. Longer pulse durations (<1 msec) are required to stimulate motor nerves. Long pulse durations (>10 msec) with high

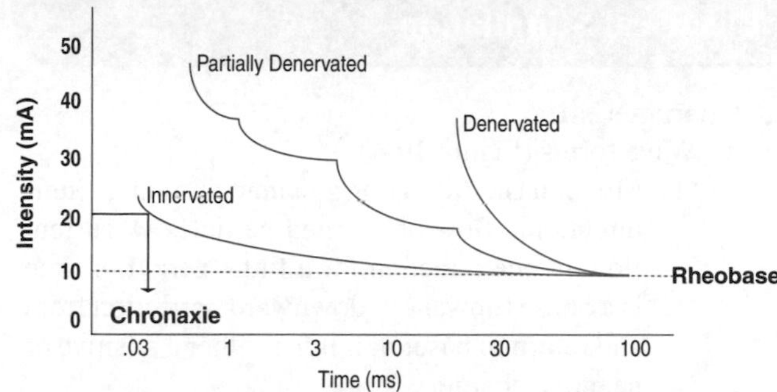

Figure 10-3 • Strength-duration curves for normally innervated, partially denervated, and completely denervated muscle.

intensities are needed to elicit a response from a denervated muscle.
d. Nerve conduction velocity and EMG have rendered strength-duration testing virtually obsolete.

4. Motor point.

a. An area of greatest excitability on the skin surface in which a small amount of current generates a muscle response.
b. In innervated muscle, the motor point is located at or near where the motor nerve enters the muscle, usually over the muscle belly.
c. In denervated muscle, the area of greatest excitability is located over the muscle distally toward the insertion.

5. Types of muscle contraction.

a. A low-frequency pulse (1–10 pulses/sec) produces a brief muscle twitch or muscle contraction with each stimulus.
b. Increasing the number of stimuli (frequency) progressively fuses the individual muscle twitches to a point where individual twitches are not discernible. A tetanic contraction results.
c. An asynchronous or worm-like (vermicular) muscle response is noted in denervated muscle.

6. Basic concepts of electricity.

a. Electrical current is the movement of electrons through a conducting medium.
b. Amperage is the rate of flow of electrons.
c. Voltage is the force that drives electrons through the conductive medium.
d. Resistance is the property of a medium which opposes the flow of electrons. A substance with a high resistance (e.g., rubber) is an insulator, and a substance with a low resistance (e.g., metal) is a conductor.
e. Ohm's law expresses the relationship between amperage, voltage, and resistance. The current is directly proportional to the voltage and inversely proportional to the resistance. The inverse of resistance is called conductance.

Electrical Stimulation

1. **Characteristics.**
   a. Wave forms (Figure 10-4).
      (1) Monophasic (direct or galvanic current): a unidirectional flow of charged particles. A current flow in one direction for a finite period of time is a phase (upward or downward deflection from and return to baseline). It has either a positive or negative charge.
      (2) Biphasic wave (alternating current): a bidirectional flow of charged particles. This type of wave form is illustrated as one half of the cycle above the baseline and the second phase below the baseline. One complete cycle (two phases) equals a single pulse. It has a zero net charge if symmetrical.
      (3) Polyphasic wave: biphasic current modified to produce three or more phases in a single pulse. This waveform in medium frequency may be Russian or interferential current.

2. **Current modulation.**
   a. Continuous mode: uninterrupted flow of current.
   b. Interrupted mode: intermittent cessation of current flow for ≥1 second.
   c. Surge mode: a gradual increase and decrease in the current intensity over a finite period of time.
   d. Ramped mode: a time period with a gradual rise of the current intensity, which is maintained at a selected level for a given period of time, followed by a gradual or abrupt decline in intensity.

3. **Goals and indications.**
   a. Pain modulation.
      (1) Activation of gate mechanisms (Gate theory).

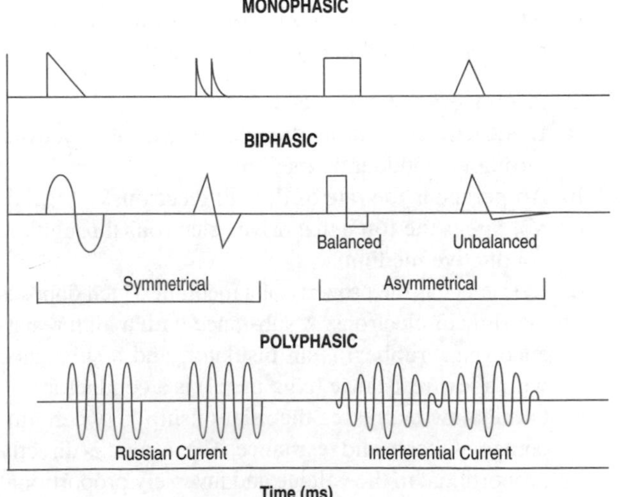

Figure 10-4 • Basic waveform characteristics.

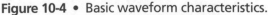

      (2) Initiation of descending inhibition mechanisms (endogenous opiate production).
   b. Decrease muscle spasm.
      (1) Muscle fatigue: tetanic contraction sustained for several minutes by means of continuous modulation.
      (2) Muscle pump: interrupted or surge modulation producing rhythmic contraction and relaxation of the muscle to increase circulation.
      (3) Muscle pump and heat: combination of ES and US to increase tissue temperature and produce muscle pumping at the same time.
   c. Impaired ROM (increase in or maintenance of joint mobility).
      (1) Mechanical stretching of connective tissue and muscles associated with a joint. Used when muscle strength is deficient or neuromuscular dysfunction (e.g., spasticity) prevents adequate joint movement.
      (2) Decrease pain to encourage joint motion.
      (3) Decrease in edema if significant impediment to motion.
   d. Muscle reeducation (training muscles to respond appropriately to volitional effort).
      (1) Acts as active assistive exercise.
      (2) Provides proprioceptive feedback.
      (3) Assists in coordinated muscle movement.
   e. Disuse atrophy (muscle weakness).
      (1) Used as an adjunct to volitional movement.
   f. Soft-tissue repair (wound healing).
      (1) Pulsed currents (monophasic, biphasic, polyphasic) with interrupted modulations. Improved circulation via the muscle pump to improve tissue nutrition and hasten metabolic waste disposal.
      (2) Monophasic currents (low-volt continuous modulations, high-volt pulsed currents).
         (a) Electrical potential theory. Restoration of electrical charges in wound area.
         (b) Bactericidal effect. Disruption of DNA, RNA synthesis or cell transport system of microorganisms.
         (c) Biochemical effects. Increased adenosine triphosphate (ATP) concentration, amino acid uptake, and increased protein and DNA synthesis.
         (d) Galvanotaxic effect. Attraction of tissue repair cells via electrode polarity.
            (1) Inflammation phase: macrophages (positive); mast cells (negative); neutrophils (positive or negative).
            (2) Proliferation phase: fibroblasts (positive).
            (3) Wound contraction phase: alternating positive/negative.
            (4) Epithelialization phase: epithelial cells (positive).

(3) Both low-intensity, continuous nonpulsed low-volt direct current and high-volt pulsed current can be applied for wound healing. Though the current characteristics (continuous versus pulse) differ, the treatment protocols are similar (low amplitude current for 30–60 minutes).

g. Edema reduction.
   (1) Muscle pump to increase lymph and venous flow.
   (2) Electrical field phenomenon for acute edema. By electrostatic repulsion, a monophasic waveform with a negative polarity is set up to surround the injured area and repel the negatively charged proteins attempting to accumulate in the interstitium.

h. Spasticity (ES to reduce hypertonicity).
   (1) Fatigue of the agonist.
   (2) Reciprocal inhibition (stimulate antagonist/inhibit agonist).

i. Denervated muscle.
   (1) Controversy exists relative to the use of ES for denervated muscle. Previous animal and clinical studies indicated that denervated muscle can be stimulated by monophasic or biphasic currents with long pulse duration, producing a vermicular contraction. The goal of stimulation is to retard the effects of disuse atrophy and shorten recovery time.
   (2) Recent animal studies suggest that ES may be deleterious to denervated muscle by:
      (a) Interfering with regeneration of neuromuscular junction and subsequent reinnervation.
      (b) Traumatizing hypersensitive denervated muscle.
   (3) The financial cost and prolonged treatment time required until reinnervation occurs are additional factors for consideration of ES on denervated muscles.

4. Contraindications/Precautions.

a. Contraindications.
   (1) Anywhere in the body for patients with demand-type pacemakers, unstable arrhythmias, suspected epilepsy or seizure disorder.
   (2) Over or in the area of the carotid sinus, thrombosis or thrombophlebitis, eyes, thoracic region, phrenic nerve, urinary bladder stimulators and abdomen or low back during pregnancy.
   (3) Transcerebrally or transthoracically.
   (4) In the presence of active bleeding or infection.
   (5) Superficial metal implants.
   (6) Pharyngeal or laryngeal muscles.
   (7) Motor-level stimulation should not be applied in conditions that prohibit motion.

b. Precautions.
   (1) Cardiac disease.
   (2) Impaired mentation.
   (3) In areas of impaired sensation, malignant tumors, skin irritation or open wounds.
   (4) Applying iontophoresis in the area after the application of another physical agent.
   (5) In patients with hypotension or hypertension, excessive adipose tissue or edema.
   (6) Bleeding disorders.
   (7) Menstruating uterus.
   (8) Pregnancy-during labor and delivery.

c. Procedural cautions.
   (1) Do not use any electrical modality if there is evidence of broken or frayed wires or if the unit is not connected to a ground fault circuit interrupter (see Hydrotherapy section).
   (2) Electrodes that are too small, have uneven contact, or are self-adhesive and no longer stick or conduct well can cause skin irritation or burns.
   (3) Electrical stimulation should not be used while playing sports, driving, operating heavy machinery, near a diathermy device or in conjunction with other electronic monitoring equipment.
      (a) ES should not be placed over:
         (1) Healing fractures (unless specifically used for bone stimulation).
         (2) Areas of active bleeding.
         (3) Malignancies or phlebitis in treatment area.
         (4) Superficial metal implants.
         (5) Pharyngeal or laryngeal muscles.
         (6) ES should not be applied to patients with demand-type pacemaker, myocardial disease.
      (b) Use precaution in applying ES to areas of impaired sensation, during pregnancy, and severe edema.
      (c) Do not use any electrical modality if there is evidence of broken or frayed wires or if the unit is not connected to a ground fault circuit interrupter (see Hydrotherapy section).

5. General guidelines for ES procedures.

a. General muscle stimulation procedure.
   (1) Explain procedure and effects to patient.
   (2) Place patient in comfortable position with treatment area properly exposed.
   (3) Support body part to be treated.
   (4) Assess skin condition and sensation.
   (5) Reduce skin resistance, if necessary (hot pack, alcohol rub, gentle abrasion).
   (6) Check to confirm that all controls are in proper starting position before turning on the modality.
   (7) Electrode selection.
      (a) Electrode size.
         (1) Two electrodes (leads) are required to complete the current circuit. One electrode is generally called the active (stimulating) electrode and is often placed on

the motor point; the second, larger electrode is called the dispersive or inactive electrode.

(2) Current density (the amount of current that is dispersed under the electrode) is relative to the electrode size. A given current intensity passing through the smaller active electrode produces high current density and thus a strong stimulus, while the same current is perceived as less intense under the larger dispersive electrode because of the lesser current density.

(3) Electrode size should be relative to the size of the treatment site. Large electrodes in a small treatment area (i.e., forearm) could result in current overflowing to surrounding muscles and produce undesired effects.

(4) Conversely, small electrodes applied to a large muscle (i.e., quadriceps) could result in high current density under the electrodes that make ES uncomfortable to the patient.

(8) The active electrode is usually placed over the treatment site (motor point), in order to produce a stimulation effect. The dispersive electrode may be placed on the treatment site or at a remote site (see electrode placement).

(9) Electrode preparation.

(a) Metal plate/sponge: moisten sponge, then remove sponge from water and remove excess water.

(b) Carbonized rubber: place small amount of gel in center of electrode. Spread gel to cover entire surface.

(c) Pregelled electrode: remove protective cover and place a small amount of gel (metal mesh/foil electrode) or water (Karaya electrode) on electrode.

(10) Electrode placement.

(a) Unipolar/monopolar placement: one single electrode or multiple (bifurcated) active electrodes placed over treatment area. Usually larger-sized dispersive electrode (inactive) placed ipsilaterally away from treatment area.

(b) Bipolar placement: equal-sized active and dispersive electrodes on same muscle group or in same treatment area. Smaller, bifurcated treatment electrodes may be used to better conform to small treatment areas.

(c) The space between the active and dispersive electrodes should be at least the diameter of the active electrode. The distance between the electrodes should be as great as is practicable. The greater the space between electrodes, the lesser the current density in the intervening superficial tissue, thus minimizing the risk of skin irritation, and burns. If deep penetration causes contraction of undesired muscles, move the electrodes closer together.

(11) Inspect the patient's skin. Vigilant skin inspection and skin care is very important with long-term use of ES. This is especially important during home use of transcutaneous ES and other ES modalities. Long-term repetitive stimulation and electrode placement and removal can irritate the skin and initiate skin breakdown.

(12) Secure electrodes to body part.

(13) Set appropriate frequency, waveform and modulation rate.

(14) Adjust intensity to achieve the optimal treatment effect.

(15) At end of treatment, slowly decrease intensity to zero before lifting the active electrode from skin. Turn all controls to beginning position.

b. Muscle strengthening, muscle spasm or edema (muscle pump), ROM.

(1) Slowly increase intensity until a muscular response is observed.

(2) 10–25 muscle contractions may be sufficient to obtain treatment goal.

(3) Duty cycle.

(a) Interrupted/ramped modulation of current allows the muscle to recover between stimulation periods.

(b) It has been shown that stimulation on/off ratios of ≥1:3 minimize the fatigue effects of ES.

c. Muscle spasm (fatigue).

(1) Procedure as above for innervated muscle. Current applied in continuous mode or 1:1 on/off ratio.

d. Muscle reeducation.

(1) Parameters and procedure similar to muscle strengthening techniques.

(2) Stimulation for multiple sets of singular or multiple muscle repetitions.

(3) Treatment sessions of 10–30 minutes depending on patient's mental and physical tolerance.

Iontophoresis

1. Description.

a. The application of a continuous direct current to transport medicinal agents through the skin or mucous membranes for therapeutic purposes.

2. Physics.

a. Like charges repel like charges.

b. Unlike charges attract unlike charges.

Table 10-7 ➤ INDICATIONS FOR THE USE OF IONTOPHORESIS AND IONS COMMONLY USED

INDICATIONS	ION	POLARITY	SOURCE
Analgesia	Lidocaine, Xylocaine Salicylate	Positive Negative	Lidocaine, Xylocaine Sodium salicylate
Calcium deposits	Acetate	Negative	Acetic acid
Dermal ulcers	Zinc	Positive	Zinc oxide
Edema reduction	Hyaluronidase	Positive	Wyadase
Fungal infections	Copper	Positive	Copper sulfate
Hyperhidrosis	Water	Positive/Negative	Tap water
Muscle spasm	Calcium Magnesium	Positive Positive	Calcium chloride Magnesium sulfate
Musculoskeletal inflammatory conditions	Dexamethasone Hydrocortisone	Negative Positive	

3. Electrochemical effects related to iontophoresis.
   a. Dissolved acids, bases, salts, or alkaloids in an aqueous solution dissociate into positively or negatively charged substances (ions) when electrical current flows through a substance.
   b. Polar effects.
      (1) Positive ions move toward the negative pole (cathode) where a secondary alkaline reaction (NaOH) occurs.
      (2) Negative ions move toward the positive pole (anode) where an acid is produced (HCl).

4. Ion transfer.
   a. The number of ions transferred through the skin is directly related to the:
      (1) Duration of treatment.
      (2) Current density.
      (3) Concentration of ions in the solution.

5. ES characteristics of iontophoresis.
   a. Direct current.
   b. Maximum intensity of 4-5 mA.

6. Procedure.
   a. Clean and inspect skin.
   b. Position patient and support treatment area.
   c. Place appropriate-sized active electrode on treatment area. Active electrode same polarity as the medicinal ion. To reduce the alkaline effect on the skin, the negative electrode should be twice as large as the positive regardless of which is the active electrode.
   d. Dispersive electrode placed at either proximal or distal distant site about 4–6 inches away.
   e. The space between the active and dispersive electrodes should be at least the diameter of the active electrode. However, commercial electrode sets have a fixed distance that limits the spacing between electrodes.
   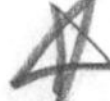
   f. Determine dose. Dosage is product of time and current intensity. Safe limit for active electrode: anode, 1 mA/cm², cathode, 0.5 mA/cm². Duration is 10–40 minutes.
   g. Turn intensity up slowly to selected level unless apparatus automatically adjusts parameters.
   h. Observe treatment area every 3–5 minutes. Report any adverse reactions.
   i. Turn intensity down slowly to zero at completion of treatment. Some units have an automatic cutoff.

7. Indications. (See Table 10-7).

8. Contraindications.
   a. Refer to general rules for ES.
   b. Impaired skin sensation.
   c. Allergy or sensitivity to medicinal agent or direct current.
   d. Denuded area or recent scars.
   e. Cuts, bruises, or broken skin.
   f. Metal in or near treatment area.

Transcutaneous Electrical Nerve Stimulation (TENS)

1. Description.
   a. TENS is designed to provide afferent stimulation for pain management.

2. Physiological effects.
   a. Pain modulation through activation of central inhibition of pain transmission (Gate control theory).
      (1) Large diameter A-beta fibers (Figure 10-5) activate inhibitory interneurons (substantia gelatinosa) located in the dorsal horn (primarily laminae II and III) of the spinal cord, producing inhibition of smaller A-delta and C-fibers (pain fibers).
      (2) Presynaptic inhibition of the T cells closes the "gate" and modulates pain. The gating mechanism also includes release of enkephalins which

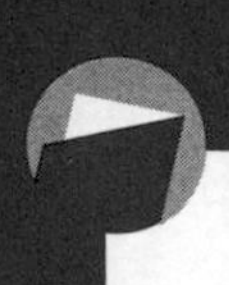

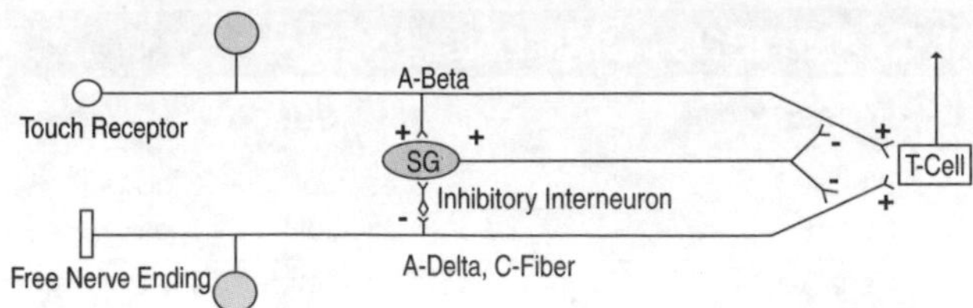

Figure 10-5 • Schematic of Gate control theory. (From Melzack and Wall.)

combine with opiate receptors to depress release of substance P from the A-delta and C-fibers.

b. Pain modulation through descending pathways generating endogenous opiates (Figure 10-6).
   (1) Noxious stimuli generate endorphin production from the pituitary gland and other CNS areas.
   (2) Endogenous opiate-rich nuclei, periaqueductal gray matter (PAG) in the midbrain and thalamus are also activated by strong stimuli.
   (3) Neurotransmitters from the PAG facilitate the cells of the nucleus raphe magnus (NRM) and reticularis gigantocellularis (RGC).
   (4) Efferents from these nuclei travel through the dorsal lateral funiculus, terminating on the enkephalinergic interneurons in the spinal cord and presynaptically inhibiting the release of substance P from the A-delta and C-fibers.

3. ES characteristics.

a. Wave form: typically, asymmetrical biphasic with a zero net direct current component. Other variations including pulsed monophasic current have been used.
b. Current: continuous pulsatile or burst.

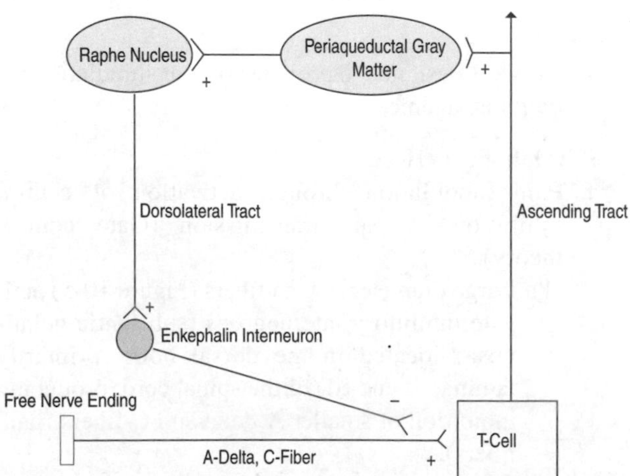

Figure 10-6 • Schematic of descending inhibition mechanisms.

4. Procedures.

a. Conventional (high rate) TENS: this most common mode of TENS can be applied during the acute or chronic phase of pain. Modulation of pain via inhibition of pain fibers by large-diameter fiber activation (gate mechanism). Onset of pain relief is relatively fast and duration of relief is relatively short.
   (1) Amplitude: comfortable tingling sensation, paresthesia. No muscle response.
   (2) Pulse rate 50–80 pps.
   (3) Pulse duration 50–100 μsec.
   (4) Mode: continuous
   (5) Duration of treatment: 20-60 minutes.
   (6) Duration of pain relief: temporary.
b. Acupuncture-like (strong low rate) TENS can be applied during the chronic phase of pain. Analgesia produced through stimulation-evoked production of endogenous opiates. Onset of pain relief may be as long as 20–40 minutes. Duration of relief may be long-lasting (≥1 hour).
   (1) Amplitude: strong, but comfortable rhythmic muscle twitches.
   (2) Pulse rate: 1–5 pps.
   (3) Pulse duration: 150–300 μsec.
   (4) Mode continuous.
   (5) Duration of treatment: 30-40 minutes.
   (6) Duration of pain relief: long-lasting.
c. Brief intense TENS: This mode is used to provide rapid-onset, short-term pain relief during painful procedures (wound debridement, deep friction massage, joint mobilization, or passive stretching).
   (1) Amplitude: to patient's tolerance.
   (2) Pulse rate: 80–150 pps.
   (3) Pulse duration: 50–250 μsec.
   (4) Mode continuous.
   (5) Duration of treatment: 15 minutes.
   (6) Duration of pain relief: temporary (30–60 minutes).
d. Burst-mode (pulse trains) TENS: combines characteristics of both high- and low-rate TENS. Stimulation of endogenous opiates, but current is more tolerable to patient than low-rate TENS. Onset of analgesia similar to low-rate TENS.
   (1) Amplitude: comfortable, intermittent paresthesia.
   (2) Pulse rate: 50–100 pps delivered in packets or bursts of 1–4 pps.
   (3) Pulse duration: 50–200 μsec.
   (4) Mode continuous.
   (5) Duration of treatment: 20–30 minutes.
   (6) Duration of pain relief: long-lasting (hours).
e. Hyperstimulation (point stimulation) TENS: use of a small probe to locate and noxiously stimulate acupuncture or trigger points. Multiple sites may be stimulated per treatment. Onset of pain relief is similar to acupuncture-like TENS.
   (1) Amplitude: strong, to patient's tolerance.

(2) Pulse rate 1–5 pps.
(3) Pulse duration 150–300 μsec.
(4) Duration of treatment: 15 to 30 second increments.
(5) Duration of pain relief: long-lasting.

f. Modulation mode TENS: a method of modulating the parameters of the above TENS modes to prevent neural or perceptual adaptation due to constant ES. Frequencies, intensities or pulse durations can be altered by ≥10%, one or two times per second.

5. Electrode placement.

a. Several options should be considered. Acupuncture site, dermatome distribution of involved nerve, over painful site, proximal or distal to pain site, segmentally related myotomes, or trigger points.

6. Goals and indications.

a. Acute and chronic pain modulation.

7. Contraindications.

a. Patient with demand-type pacemaker or over chest of patient with cardiac disease.
b. TENS not applied over eyes, laryngeal or pharyngeal muscles, head and neck of patient following cerebral vascular accident, or with epilepsy.
c. TENS not applied to mucosal membranes.

High-Voltage Pulsed Galvanic Stimulation

1. Description.

a. High-voltage pulsed current (HVPC). Typically, monophasic, twin-peaked pulses of short duration.

2. Physics.

a. Skin offers high resistance (impedance) to the flow of low-voltage current.
b. Passage of HVPC decreases skin resistance caused by the current flowing toward the skin capacitors (little energy loss) rather than the skin resistors. Thermal effects are negligible (little resistance to current).

3. ES characteristics of HVPC.

a. Wave form: paired monophasic, with instantaneous rise and exponential fall of current.
b. Current: continuous, surged, or interrupted pulsatile current.

4. Procedure.

a. Muscle stimulation protocol: refer to general application procedure.
b. Wound healing concept.
(1) Intact skin surface negative with respect to deeper epidermal layers.
(2) Injury to skin develops positive potentials initially and negative potentials during healing process.
(3) Absent or insufficient positive potentials retard tissue regeneration.
(4) Addition of positive potentials, initially through anode, may promote or accelerate healing.

c. Wound healing parameters.
(1) Amplitude: comfortable tingling sensation, paresthesia, no muscle response.
(2) Pulse rate: 50–200 pps.
(3) Pulse duration: 20–100 μsec.
(4) Mode continuous.
(5) Duration of treatment: 20–60 min.

d. Wound healing procedures.
(1) Inspect wound area.
(2) Position patient and support treatment area.
(3) Clean and débride wound site. Pack with sterile saline-soaked gauze.
(4) Both high-volt pulsed current and low-intensity continuous low-volt direct current can be used for wound healing. Although current characteristics differ, treatment parameters are similar in current intensity and treatment duration.
(5) Place active electrode over gauze.
(6) For bactericidal effect, active electrode should have negative polarity. For culture-free wound, active electrode should be positive.
(7) Turn the intensity up slowly to selected level.
(8) At conclusion of treatment, turn intensity down slowly to zero.

5. Goals and indications.

a. Inflammation phase: free from necrosis and exudates. Promote granulation.
b. Proliferation phase: reduce wound size, including depth, diameter, and tunneling.
c. Epithelialization phase: stimulate epidermal proliferation and capillary growth.

6. Contraindications.

a. See general contraindications for ES.

Concept of Medium Frequency Currents in ES

1. Description.

a. ES frequencies in the range of 2,000–5,000 pps that are modulated to produce physiologically applied frequencies. This concept is utilized in the Russian (time-modulated) and the interferential (amplitude-modulated) ES techniques.

2. Physics related to medium frequency.

a. A decrease in the capacitive skin impedance of the skin is noted relative to the increase in current frequency (Figure 10-7).
b. ES frequency categories:
(1) Low frequency: 1–1,000 pps.

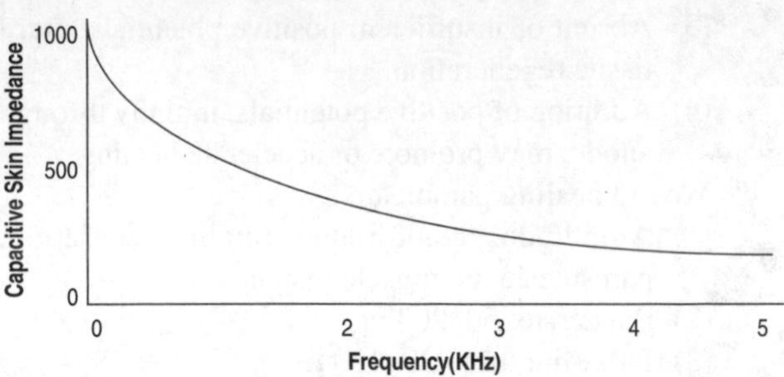

Figure 10-7 • Capacitive skin resistance decreases as current frequency increases.

(2) Medium frequency: 1,000–10,000 pps.
(3) High frequency: >10,000 pps.

Russian Current

1. Description.

a. A 2,500 Hz sine wave (carrier frequency), which is interrupted for 10 milliseconds at 10-millisecond intervals, producing fifty 10-millisecond bursts per second. This type of time interval interruption produces time-modulated current (Figure 10-8). Also known as medium frequency, burst alternating current.

2. ES characteristics of russian current.

a. Wave form: polyphasic sinusoidal burst.
b. Current: time modulated to create a pulsatile burst current.

3. Method of application: muscle-strengthening protocol.

a. Amplitude: tetanic muscle contraction.
b. Pulse rate: 50–70 pps.
c. Pulse duration: 150–200 μsec or 50% duty cycle.

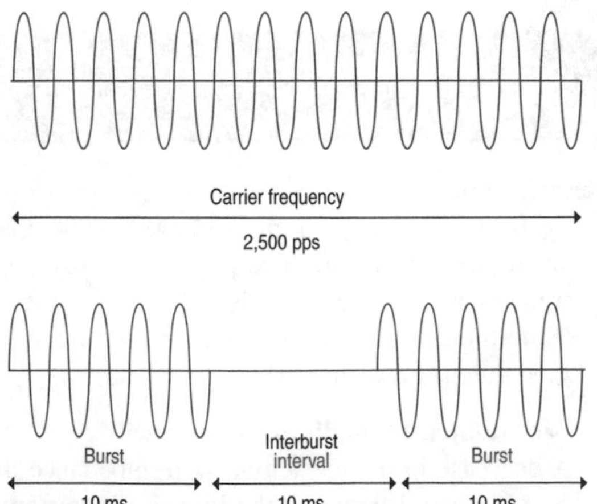

Figure 10-8 • Russian current. Time-modulated polyphasic waveform.

d. Mode: Interrupted.
(1) Ramp: 1–5 seconds, based on patient's tolerance.
(2) Duty cycle: 1:5.
e. Current applied to provide stimulation during the following volitional activities:
(1) Isometric exercise at several points through ROM.
(2) Slow isokinetic exercise; e.g., 5–10 degrees/sec.
(3) Short arc joint movement when ROM is restricted.

4. Muscle spasm protocol.

a. Muscle fatigue using continuous isometric contraction for several minutes to tolerance.
b. If muscle pumping is goal, duty cycle is 1:1.
c. If ROM is goal, duty cycle is 2:5.

5. Contraindications.

a. See general contraindications for ES.

Interferential Current (IFC)

1. Description.

a. This current is characterized by the crossing of two sinusoidal waves with similar amplitudes, but different carrier frequencies which interfere with one another to generate an amplitude-modulated beat frequency. The consequent beat frequency is the net difference between the two superimposed frequencies.

2. Physics related to IFC.

a. Constructive interference: When the two waves are in phase, the sum of the superimposed wave is large (Figure 10-9A).
b. Destructive interference. The sum of the two waves is zero when the waves are 180 degrees out of phase (Figure 10-9B).
c. Beat frequency (amplitude-modulated). Resultant frequency produced by the two frequencies going into and out of phase (Figure 10-9C).
(1) Constant. Both carrier frequencies are fixed. Beat frequency is net difference between both frequencies.
(2) Variable. One carrier frequency is fixed and the other varies in frequency, generating a variable or sweep frequency. Sweep used to minimize accommodation.
d. IFC produces a cloverleaf-like pattern, since the electrical stimulating effect is at a 45 degree angle to the flow of current in the two circuits as interference occurs at the targeted area of the body (Figure 10-10).
(1) Static interferential fields are generated when four electrodes (two circuits) are used and the cloverleaf pattern is produced.

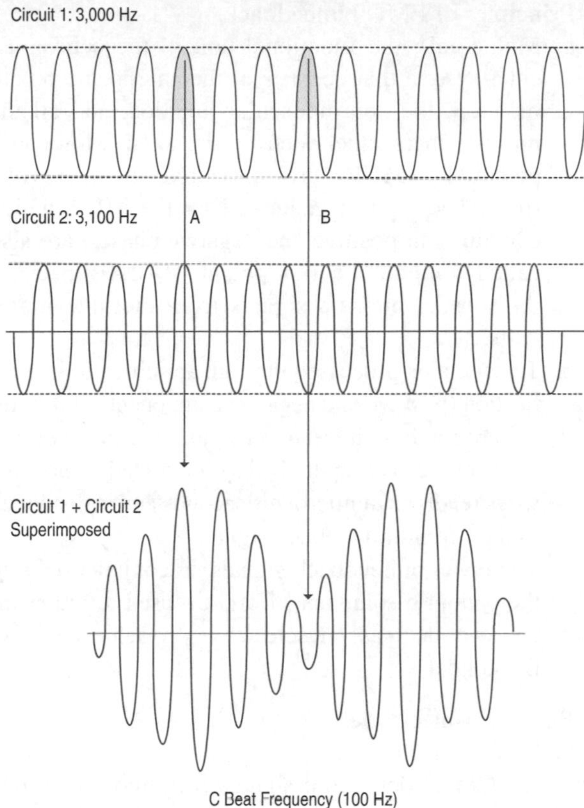

Figure 10-9 • Interferential current. Amplitude modulated polyphasic waveform.

(2) Dynamic (scan) interferential fields occur when the interferential fields are rotated 45 degrees, caused by the vectoring effect of rhythmically unbalancing the IFC to change the position of the stimulation areas. This effect is purported to provide a greater area of stimulation in comparison with static interferential fields.

(3) Full-field scanning produces a similar effect as dynamic interferential fields by bursting the current over the two circuits.

e. Premodulated IFC occurs when two carrier frequencies are crossed in the ES unit. The interference occurs in the unit, and the current can then be delivered through one circuit. This is ideal for small areas that would be amply covered with two electrodes.

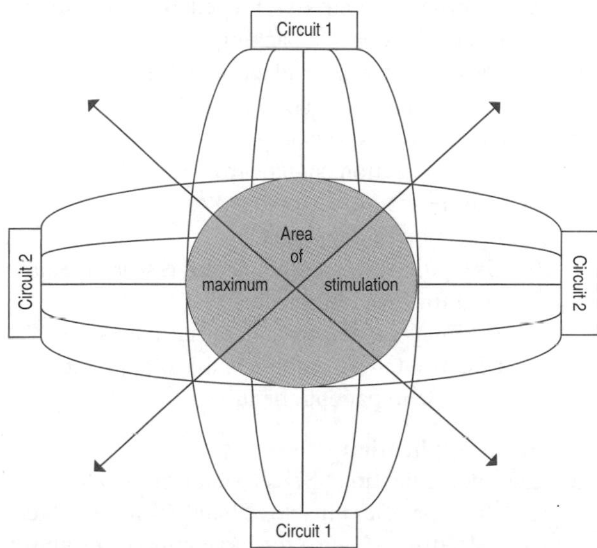

Figure 10-10 • Static interference field depicting the area of maximum stimulation (circle) and the direction of maximal stimulation (arrows).

3. ES characteristics.

a. Wave form: polyphasic, sinusoidal (amplitude-modulated) beats.

b. Current: amplitude modulated continuous (pain); interrupted (muscle exercise).

4. Procedure.

a. Electrode placement (pad or suction cup electrodes).

(1) Bipolar (premodulated IFC). Active and dispersive electrodes placed over or around small area.

(2) Quadripolar (IFC). Two sets of electrodes placed diagonally to one another over large area.

b. Treatment parameters.

(1) Pain protocol.

(a) Similar to high- or low-rate TENS.

(2) Muscle-strengthening protocol.

(a) Similar to low- or medium-frequency ES.

5. Goals and indications.

a. Modulate pain: increase muscle strength or ROM.

6. Contraindications.

a. See general contraindications for ES.

Functional ES (FES)

1. Description.

a. FES encompasses a wide range of stimulator units and techniques for disuse atrophy, impaired ROM, muscle spasm, muscle reeducation, and spasticity management. FES is also called neuromuscular electrical stimulation (NMES) and functional neuromuscular electrical stimulation. This section will describe FES as an alternative or supplement to the use of orthotic devices.

2. Shoulder subluxation.

a. Patients with cerebrovascular accident (CVA) may initially exhibit weakness or flaccid paralysis of the muscles supporting the glenohumeral joint, especially the supraspinatus and posterior deltoid.

b. The force of gravity acting on the unsupported upper extremity tends to stretch the ligamentous structures surrounding the glenohumeral joint that result in severe pain and decreased upper extremity function.

c. ES characteristics of FES.
   (1) Wave form: asymmetrical biphasic square.
   (2) Current: interrupted pulsatile current.
d. Procedure.
   (1) Electrode placement: bipolar. Electrodes on supraspinatus and posterior deltoid.
   (2) Treatment parameters.
      (a) Amplitude: tetanic muscle contraction to patient's tolerance.
      (b) Pulse rate 12–25 pps.
      (c) Duration of treatment: 15–30 minutes. Three times daily, up to 6–7 hours. On/off ratio: 1:3 (2 sec: 6 sec) progressing to 12:1 (24 sec: 2 sec).

3. Dorsiflexion assist in gait training.
   a. Patients with hemiplegia sometimes exhibit paralyzed dorsiflexor, and evertor muscles.
   b. FES controls foot drop, and facilitates dorsiflexors and evertors during swing phase.
   c. ES characteristics.
      (1) Wave form: asymmetric biphasic square.
      (2) Pulse duration: 20–250 μsec.
      (3) Mode: interrupted by foot switch.
   d. Procedure.
      (1) Electrode placement: bipolar. Peroneal (fibular) nerve near head of fibula or anterior tibialis muscle.
      (2) Treatment parameters.
         (a) Amplitude: tetanic muscle contraction sufficient to decrease plantar flexion.
         (b) Pulse rate 30–300 pps.
         (c) Treatment mode: heel switch contains pressure-sensitive contact that stops stimulation during stance phase and activates stimulation during swing phase. Hand switch also allows therapist to control stimulation during gait.

4. Other gait-assisted protocol considerations.
   a. Placement of electrodes on appropriate muscles to control muscles during push-off (plantar flexors, late swing phase (hamstrings), quadriceps, and/or gluteals (stance phase).
   b. ES characteristics: similar to dorsiflexion protocol.
   c. Method of application: similar to dorsiflexion protocol, except for electrode placement.

Electromyographic Biofeedback (EMG Biofeedback)

1. Description.
   a. Electronic instrument used to measure motor unit action potentials (MUAP) generated by active muscles. The signals are detected, amplified, and converted into audiovisual signals that are used to reinforce voluntary control.

2. Principles of EMG biofeedback.
   a. Motor unit: the functional unit of the neuromuscular system that consists of the anterior horn cell, its axon, the neuromuscular junction, and all the muscle fibers innervated by the axon. Motor unit potentials (MUP) are measured in microvolts (μV). The signals generated by the MUP, which contain both positive and negative phases, are also called compound action potentials (CAP) because the sensors pick up signals from multiple motor units.
   b. The signal is processed through amplification, rectification (positive and negative components of the signal are made unidirectional), and integration (area under curve is computed). The integrated signal provides readings in microvolt-seconds and is displayed as the EMG biofeedback signal.
   c. The EMG biofeedback signals, in conjunction with the patient's voluntary effort, are used to either increase or decrease muscle activity to achieve a functional goal.

3. Recording electrodes.
   a. Surface electrodes.
      (1) Global detection: signals from more than one muscle.
      (2) Detection from mostly superficial muscles.
      (3) Advantages: easy to apply, acceptable to patient/client.
      (4) Disadvantages: detection from mostly superficial muscles, frequently from more than one muscle group.
   b. Types of surface electrodes/sensors.
      (1) Metal electrodes (silver-silver chloride): cup-shaped to accommodate conducting gel.
      (2) Disposable electrodes: pregelled center with surrounding adhesive backing.
      (3) Carbonized rubber electrodes (reusable): flexible to conform to body part.
   c. Needle electrodes/sensors.
      (1) Local detection: signals from specific muscle or muscle group.
      (2) Detection of deep muscles.
      (3) Used for EMG diagnosis or research. Rarely used for EMG biofeedback.
      (4) Advantages: detection of specific muscles.
      (5) Disadvantages: requires skill to apply, less acceptable to patient/client.

4. Electrode application.
   a. Electrode selection: Select small electrodes (0.02 cm) for specific muscles (hand, forearm, face); large electrodes (1 cm) for large muscles or muscle groups.
   b. Electrode placement.
      (1) Bipolar technique: two active (positive and negative) and one reference (ground) electrode. The

reference electrode may be placed between or adjacent to active electrodes. This minimizes or eliminates extraneous electrical activity (noise or cross-talk).

(2) Active electrodes are placed on or near motor point of targeted muscle or muscle group.

(3) Generally, active electrodes are placed ~1–5 cm apart and parallel to muscle fibers. Reference electrode is placed near treatment site.

(4) Active electrodes are placed close together; minimizes cross-talk, yield small, more precise signals.

(5) Active electrodes are placed further apart; yield large signals, detection from more than one muscle.

5. Procedure.

a. Begin treatments in quiet setting, if possible.

b. Clean treatment site with alcohol (slight abrasion, if necessary) to remove dirt and oils from skin to reduce skin impedance.

c. Apply conductive gel, if needed.

d. Secure the electrodes.

e. Protocol for increasing muscle activity (motor recruitment).

(1) For weak muscles, begin with electrodes widely spaced and biofeedback instrument sensitivity high, to increase detection.

(a) For a single weak muscle, begin with electrodes close together if a more precise signal is desired.

(2) Instruct patient to try and contract muscle (isometrically for 6–10 sec) to produce an audiovisual signal.

(3) As patient's motor recruitment ability improves, decrease the sensitivity, making it more difficult to produce an audiovisual signal.

(4) Use facilitation techniques (tapping, cross facilitation, vibration) to encourage motor unit recruitment, if necessary.

(5) Progress from simple to more complex/functional movements as patient gains motor control.

(6) Treatment sessions may be from 5–10 minutes to ≥30 minutes, depending on patient tolerance.

(7) At end of session, clean patient's skin and electrodes.

f. Technique for decreasing muscle activity (muscle relaxation).

(1) Begin with electrodes closely spaced and biofeedback instrument sensitivity low to minimize crosstalk.

(2) Instruct patient to relax, using deep breathing or visual imagery to help to lower the audiovisual signal.

(3) Progress from low to high sensitivity as patient gains ability to relax muscle and perform functional activities.

(4) Treatment sessions may be from 5–10 minutes to ≥30 minutes, depending on patient tolerance.

(5) At end of session, clean patient's skin and electrodes.

5. Criteria for patient selection for biofeedback training.

a. Good vision, hearing, and communication abilities.

b. Good comprehension of simple commands, concentration.

c. Good motor planning skills.

d. No profound sensory or proprioceptive loss.

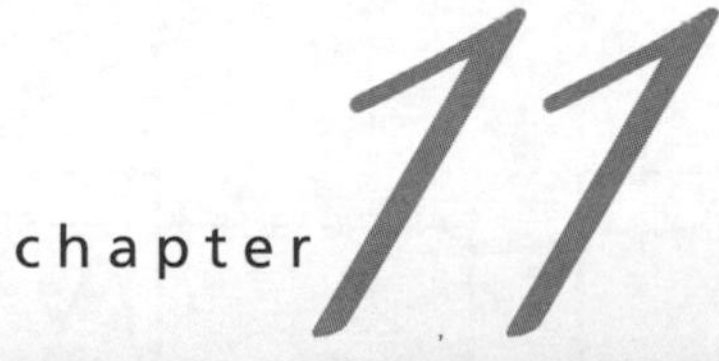

chapter 11

Functional Training, Equipment, and Devices

SUSAN B. O'SULLIVAN

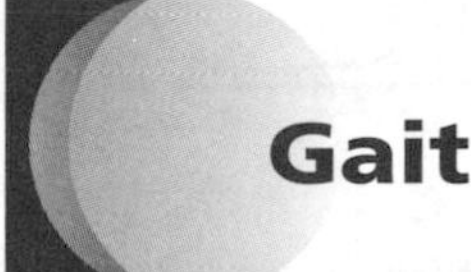

Gait

Phases of the Gait Cycle

Traditional terminology appears first and refers to points in time in the gait cycle; Rancho Los Amigos (RLA) terminology follows and refers to lengths of time in the gait cycle; as both are in clinical use, readers should be familiar with both.

1. **Heel strike:** the point when the heel of the reference or support limb contacts the ground at the beginning of stance phase.
   Initial contact (RLA): the instant that the foot of the lead extremity strikes the ground.
   Muscle activation patterns (Figure 11-1): knee extensors (quadriceps) are active at heel strike through early stance to control small amount of knee flexion for shock absorption; ankle dorsiflexors (anterior tibialis, ext. hallucis longus, ext. digitorum longus) decelerate the foot, slowing the plantarflexion from heel strike to foot flat.

2. **Foot flat:** the point when the sole of the foot of the reference or support limb makes contact with the ground; occurs immediately after heel strike.
   Loading response (RLA): the first period of double support immediately after initial contact until the contralateral leg leaves the ground.
   Muscle activation patterns: gastrocnemius-soleus muscles are active from foot flat through midstance to eccentrically control forward tibial advancement.

3. **Midstance:** the point at which full body weight is taken by the reference or support limb.
   Midstance (RLA): the contralateral limb leaves the ground; body weight is taken and advanced over and ahead of the support limb; a period of single limb support.
   Muscle activation patterns: hip, knee, and ankle extensors are active throughout stance to oppose antigravity forces and stabilize the limb; hip extensors control forward motion of the trunk; hip abductors stabilize the pelvis during unilateral stance.

4. **Heel-off:** occurs after midstance as the heel of the reference or support limb leaves the ground.
   Terminal stance (RLA): the last period of single limb support that begins with heel rise and continues until the contralateral leg contacts the ground.
   Muscle activation patterns: peak activity of plantarflexors occurs just after heel-off to push off and generate forward propulsion of the body.

5. **Toe-off:** the last portion of stance following heel off when only the toe of the reference or support limb is in contact with the ground.
   Preswing (RLA): the second period of double support from initial contact of the contralateral limb to lift off of the support limb.
   Muscle activation patterns: hip and knee extensors (hamstrings and quadriceps) may contribute to forward propulsion with a brief burst of activity.

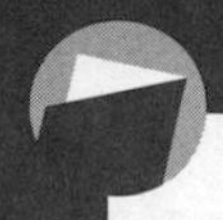

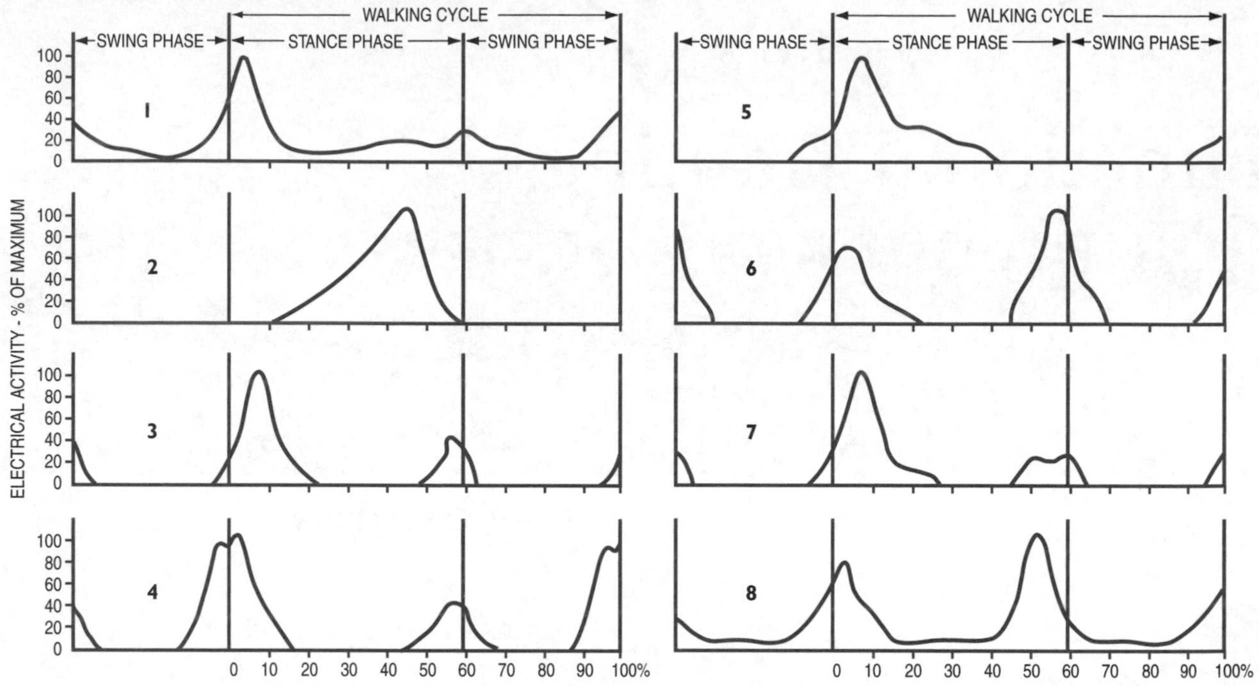

Idealized summary curves representing phasic action of major muscle groups in level walking at 90 steps/min.
1, pretibial group; 2, calf muscles; 3, quadriceps; 4, hamstrings; 5, abductors; 6, adductors; 7, gluteus maximus; 8, erector spinae.

Figure 11-1 • Actions of Major Muscle Groups During Gait.
(From Smith, L., Weiss, E., Lehmkuhl, D. Brunnstrom's Clinical Kinesiology, 5th ed., Philadelphia, Davis, 1996, p 426, with permission.)

6. **Acceleration:** the first portion of the swing phase from toe-off of the reference limb until midswing.
   Initial swing (RLA): the first portion of the swing phase from toe-off of the reference limb until maximum knee flexion of the same extremity.
   Muscle activation patterns: forward acceleration of the limb during early swing is achieved through the brief action of quadriceps; by midswing the quadriceps is silent and pendular motion is in effect; hip flexors (iliopsoas) aid in forward limb propulsion.
7. **Midswing:** the midportion of the swing phase when the reference extremity moves directly below the body.
   Midswing (RLA): the portion of the swing phase from maximum knee flexion of the reference extremity to a vertical tibial position.
   Muscle activation patterns: foot clearance is achieved by contraction of the hip, knee flexors, and ankle dorsiflexors.
8. **Deceleration:** the end portion of the swing phase when the reference extremity is slowing down in preparation for heel strike.
   Terminal swing (RLA): the portion of the swing phase from a vertical tibial position of the reference extremity to just prior to initial contact.
   Muscle activation patterns: hamstrings act during late swing to decelerate the limb in preparation for heelstrike; quadriceps and ankle dorsiflexors become active in late swing to prepare for heelstrike.
9. **Pelvic motion.**
   a. The pelvis moves forward and backward (transverse pelvic rotation).
      (1) Forward rotation occurs on the side of the unsupported or swing extremity; mean rotation is 4 degrees.
      (2) Weight-bearing or stance extremity rotates 4 degrees (a total of 8 degrees).
   b. The pelvis moves up and down on the unsupported or swing side (lateral pelvic tilt): 5 degrees; controlled by hip abductor muscles.
      (1) The high point is at midstance.
      (2) The low point is during the period of double support.
   c. The pelvis moves side to side 4 cm, follows the stance or support limb.
10. **Cadence:** the number of steps taken per unit of time.
    a. Mean cadence is 113 steps/minute.
    b. Increased cadence: shorter step length and decreased duration of period of double support.

c. Running occurs when the period of double support disappears, typically at a cadence of 180 steps/minute.

11. Step.
   a. Step length: the linear distance between point of foot contact (preferably heel strike) of one extremity to the point of heel strike of the opposite extremity (in cm or m).
   b. Step time: the number of seconds that elapse during one step.
   c. Step width: the distance between feet (e.g., base of support); measured from one heel to the same point on the opposite heel (in cm or m).
      (1) Normal step width ranges between 2.54 and 12.7 cm (1 and 5 inches).
      (2) Increases as stability demands rise; e.g., wide-based gait in older adults or very small children.

12. Stride.
   a. Stride length: the linear distance between two consecutive contact points of the same extremity (in cm or m).
   b. Stride time: the number of seconds that elapse during one stride (one complete gait cycle).

13. Velocity (walking speed): the rate of motion in any direction, the distance is divided by the time (in cm/sec or m/min).
   a. Average walking speed is 82 m/min (3 mi/hour).
   b. Affected by physical characteristics: height, weight, gender.
   c. Decreased with age, physical disability, etc.

14. Acceleration: the rate of change of velocity in relation to time.

15. Energy cost of walking.
   a. Average oxygen rate for comfortable walking is 12 mL/kg × min.
   b. Metabolic cost of walking averages 5.5 kcal/min on level surfaces; energy costs may vary widely depending on speed of walking, stride length, body weight, type of surface, gradient, and activity (e.g., stair climbing).
   c. Increased energy costs occur with age, abnormal gait (e.g., disease, muscle weakness or paralysis, physical disability), or with the use of functional devices (e.g., crutches, orthoses, prostheses).

Common Gait Deviations: Stance Phase

1. Trunk and hip.
   a. Lateral trunk bending: the result of weak gluteus medius; will see bending to the same side as the weakness (Trendelenburg gait); also seen with pain in the hip.
   b. Backward trunk lean: the result of weak gluteus maximus; will also see difficulty going up stairs or ramps.
   c. Forward trunk lean: the result of weak quadriceps (decreases flexor movement at the knee), hip and knee flexion contractures.
   d. Excessive hip flexion: the result of weak hip extensors or tight hip and/or knee flexors.
   e. Limited hip extension: the result of tight or spastic hip flexors.
   f. Limited hip flexion: the result of weak hip flexors or tight extensors.
   g. Abnormal synergistic activity (e.g., stroke): excessive hip adduction combined with hip and knee extension, plantarflexion; scissoring, or adducted gait pattern.
   h. Antalgic gait (painful gait): stance time is abbreviated on the painful limb that results in an uneven gait pattern; the uninvolved limb has a shortened step length since it must bear weight sooner than normal.

2. Knee.
   a. Excessive knee flexion: the result of weak quadriceps (knee wobbles or buckles) or knee flexor contracture.
      (1) Will also see difficulty going down stairs or ramps.
      (2) Forward trunk bending can compensate for weak quadriceps.
   b. Hyperextension: the result of a weak quadriceps, plantar flexion contracture, or extensor spasticity (quadriceps and/or plantar flexion).

3. Ankle/foot.
   a. Toe first: toes contact at heel strike; the result of weak dorsiflexors, spastic or tight plantarflexors; may also be caused by a shortened leg (leg length discrepancy); painful heel; or positive support reflex.
   b. Foot slap: the foot makes floor contact with an audible slap; the result of weak dorsiflexors or hypotonia; compensated for with steppage gait.
   c. Foot flat: entire foot contacts ground; the result of weak dorsiflexors, limited range of motion (ROM; immature gait pattern (neonatal).
   d. Excessive dorsiflexion with uncontrolled forward motion of the tibia (calcaneus gait): the result of weak plantarflexors.
   e. Excessive plantarflexion (equinus gait): heel does not touch the ground; the result of spasticity or contracture of the plantar flexors; will see poor eccentric contraction and advancement of the tibia.
   f. Supination: excessive lateral contact of foot during stance with varus position of calcaneus. May occur at initial contact and correct at footflat with weight acceptance or remain throughout stance. Possible causes: spastic invertors, weak evertors, pes varus, genu varum.
   g. Pronation: excessive medial contact of foot during stance with valgus position of calcaneus. Possible causes: weak invertors, spasticity, pes valgus, genu valgum.

h. Toes claw: the result of spastic toe flexors, possibly a hyperactive plantar grasp reflex.
i. Inadequate push off: the result of weak plantar flexors, decreased ROM, or pain in the forefoot.

Common Gait Deviations: Swing Phase

1. **Trunk and hip.**
   a. Insufficient forward pelvic rotation (stiff pelvis, pelvic retraction): the result of weak abdominal muscles, weak flexor muscles (e.g., stroke).
   b. Insufficient hip and knee flexion: the result of weak hip and knee flexors; inability to lift the leg and move it forward.
   c. Circumduction: the leg swings out to the side (abduction/external rotation followed by adduction/internal rotation); the result of weak hip and knee flexors.
   d. Hip hiking (quadratus lumborum action): a compensatory response for weak hip and knee flexors, or extensor spasticity.
   e. Excessive hip and knee flexion (steppage gait): a compensatory response to shorten the leg; the result of weak dorsiflexors (e.g., diabetic neuropathy of the fibular nerve).
   f. Abnormal synergistic activity (e.g., stroke): excessive hip and knee flexion with abduction.
2. **Knee.**
   a. Insufficient knee flexion: the result of extensor spasticity, pain/decreased ROM, or weak hamstrings.
   b. Excessive knee flexion: the result of flexor spasticity; flexor withdrawal reflex.
3. **Ankle/foot.**
   a. Foot drop (equinus): the result of weak or delayed contraction of the dorsiflexors or spastic plantarflexors.
   b. Varus or inverted foot: the result of spastic invertors (anterior tibialis), weak peroneals, or abnormal synergistic pattern (e.g., stroke).
   c. Equinovarus: the result of spasticity of the posterior tibialis and/or gastrocnemius/soleus; developmental abnormality.

Ambulatory Aids

Canes

1. **Indications:**
Widen the base of support to improve balance; provide limited stability and unweighting (can unload forces on involved extremity by 30%); can be used to relieve pain, antalgic gait.

2. **Cane measurement.**
   a. 20–30 degrees of elbow flexion is desirable.
   b. Measure from the greater trochanter to a point 6 inches to the side of the toes.

3. **Types.**
   a. Wood or aluminum (adjustable with push pin lock).
   b. Standard, single point cane: handle and shaft may be standard (J-shaped) or offset.
   c. Quad cane: four contact points with the ground; provides increased stability but slows gait.
      (1) Small-based quad cane (SBQC): useful for stairs.
      (2) Wide-based quad cane (WBQC): does not fit on stairs.

4. **Gait:** cane is held in the hand opposite to the involved extremity; cane and involved extremity are advanced together, followed by the uninvolved extremity.

Crutches

1. **Indications:**
Used to increase the base of support, provide moderate degree of stability, or relieve weight-bearing on the lower extremities.

2. **Crutch measurement.**
   a. 20–30 degrees of elbow flexion is desirable.
   b. For standing patients, subtract 16 inches from the patient's height or measure from a point 2 inches below the axilla to a point 6 inches in front and 2 inches lateral to the foot.
   c. For supine patients, measure from the axilla to a point 6–8 inches lateral to the heel.
   d. Forearm crutches: the cuff should cover the proximal third of the forearm, 1–1$^1/_2$ inches below the elbow.

3. **Types.**
   a. Axillary crutches: wood, or aluminum designs; handgrip height and crutch height adjusted by wing nuts; push button locks with telescoping legs on some aluminum crutches; axillary pads cushion the top of crutch.
      (1) Provide increased upper extremity weight-bearing over forearm crutches.
      (2) May be difficult to use in small areas.

(3) Prolonged leaning on the axillary bar can result in vascular and/or nerve damage (axillary artery/radial nerve).

b. Forearm (Lofstrand) crutches: have a forearm cuff and a hand grip; provide slightly less stability but increased ease of movement; frees hands for use without dropping the crutch (secured by cuff).

c. Forearm platform crutches: allow weight-bearing on the forearm; used for patients who are unable to bear weight through their hands; e.g., patients with arthritis; platforms can also be attached to walkers.

d. Crutch tips: rubber ~1.5 inches in diameter; provide suction, minimize slippage.

Walkers

1. **Indications:**

Widen base of support, provide increased lateral and anterior stability, can reduce weight-bearing on one or both lower extremities; easy to use; frequently prescribed for patients with debilitating conditions, poor balance, or lower extremity injury when use of crutches is precluded; e.g., elderly patients. Negative features include no reciprocal arm swing and increased flexor posture.

2. **Types of walkers.**
   a. Folding (collapsible): facilitate mobility in the community, cars.
   b. Rolling (wheeled): available with either two or four wheels (four wheels require hand brake to provide added stability in stopping); facilitates walking as a continuous movement sequence (step through gait pattern); allows for increased speed.
   c. Stair climbing walker: has two posterior extensions and additional handgrips off of the rear legs for use on stairs.
   d. Reciprocal walkers: hinged, allows advancement of one side of walker at a time; used with reciprocal gait patterns, reciprocating orthoses.
   e. Hemi walker: modified for use with one hand only.
   f. Attachments: fold-down seats, carrying baskets.

3. **Measurement:** same as for cane.

Bariatric Equipment

1. **(See discussion of obesity in Chapter 6)**

2. **Selection:** based on specific patient needs (patient safety, gait pattern, fatigue) and weight capacity.

3. **Typical gait changes:** include greater hip abduction and hip rotation, less knee flexion, difficulty rotating from side-to-side with increased girth.

4. **Heavy duty mechanical lifts:** used to help transfer patients (e.g., sit-to-stand).

5. **Heavy duty, extra wide walkers:** used to assist ambulation.

Gait Patterns: Use of Assistive Devices

1. **Weight-bearing status.**
   a. Nonweight-bearing: no weight-bearing is permitted.
   b. Partial weight-bearing: toes or ball of involved foot contacts with the floor; allows a limited amount of weight-bearing.
   c. Full weight-bearing: full weight is permitted on the involved extremity. Weight can be objectively controlled by means of a limb load monitor.

2. **Two-point gait.**
   a. One crutch and opposite extremity move together, followed by the opposite crutch and extremity; requires use of two assistive devices (canes or crutches).
   b. Allows for natural arm and leg motion during gait, good support and stability from two opposing points of contact.

3. **Three-point gait.**
   a. Both crutches and involved leg are advanced together, then uninvolved leg is advanced forward; requires use of two assistive devices (crutches or canes) or a walker.
   b. Indicated for use with involvement of one extremity; e.g., lower extremity fracture.

4. **Four-point gait.**
   a. A slow gait pattern in which one crutch is advanced forward and placed on the floor, followed by advancement of the opposite leg; then the remaining crutch is advanced forward, followed by the opposite remaining leg; requires the use of two assistive devices (crutches or canes).
   b. Provides maximum stability with three points of support while one limb is moving.

5. **Swing-to gait.**
   a. Both crutches are advanced forward together; weight is shifted onto hands for support and both legs are then swung forward to meet the crutches; requires the use of two crutches or a walker.
   b. Indicated for individuals with limited use of both lower extremities and trunk instability.

6. **Swing-through gait.**
   a. Both crutches are advanced forward together; weight is shifted onto the hands for support and both legs which are swung forward beyond the point of crutch placement; requires the use of two crutches.
   b. Both swing-to and swing-through gaits are used for bilateral lower extremity involvement, and trunk instability; e.g.; patient with paraplegia, spina bifida. Not as safe as swing-to gait.

7. **Stairs.**
   a. Ascent: the uninvolved leg always goes up first, followed by the crutches (or cane) and the involved leg together.
   b. Descent: the crutches (or cane) and involved leg go down first, followed by the uninvolved leg.

c. Mnemonic devices to teach patient: "The good go to heaven, the bad go to hell." "Up with the good, down with the bad."

Guarding

Protects the patient from falling; requires the use of a gait belt for initial training for most patients.

1. **Level surfaces:** stand slightly behind and to one side, typically on the more involved side.
2. **Stairs:** therapist is positioned below the patient.
   a. Ascent: stand behind and slightly to the involved side.
   b. Descent: stand in front and slightly to the involved side.
3. **Sit-to-stand transfers.**
   a. Stand to one side and slightly behind the patient.
   b. Increased levels of assistance may require therapist to stand in front of patient.

Locomotor Training

1. **Body Weight Support (BWS) and motorized treadmill.**
   a. BWS: an overhead harness is used to support body weight.
      (1) Initially, support is high (e.g., 40% of body weight), progresses to less weight support (30%, 20%, 10%), to no body weight support.
      (2) BWS >55% is contraindicated as it interferes with gait cycle (unable to achieve flat foot during stepping).
   b. Motorized treadmill training.
      (1) Progresses from treadmill walking with slow speeds (e.g., 0.6–0.8 mph) to faster, near-normal walking speeds (e.g., 2.6–2.8 mph).
      (2) Progresses from level walking to slight incline walking.
      (3) Progresses from treadmill walking to over-ground walking.
   c. Manual assistance:
      (1) Level of assistance decreases as training progresses (maxA, to modA, to minA, to no assistance).
      (2) Assistance can include hands on pelvis (assisted pelvic motions) and hands on LE (assisted stepping).
2. **Robotic ambulation assistance.**
   a. Can also be used to improve gait pattern and ambulatory status (e.g., Lokomat).
   b. Indications: Patients with paraparesis.
3. **Conventional over-ground training.**

Orthotics

General Concepts

1. **Orthosis is a device used to:**
   a. Correct malalignment and prevent deformity.
   b. Restrict or assist motion.
   c. Transfer load to improve function.
   d. Reduce pain.
2. **Splint.**
   a. A temporary device that may serve the same functions.
   b. Materials generally not as durable, able to withstand prolonged use.
3. **Three-point pressure principle.**
   a. Forms the mechanical basis for orthotic correction.
   b. A single force is placed at the area of deformity or angulation; two additional counterforces act in the opposing direction.
4. **Alignment.**
   a. Correct alignment permits effective function.
   b. Minimizes movement between limb and orthoses (pistoning).
   c. Minimizes compression on pressure sensitive tissues.

Lower-Limb Orthoses: Components/Terminology

1. **Shoes.**
   a. The foundation for an orthosis; shoes can reduce areas of concentrated pressure on pressure-sensitive feet.
   b. Traditional leather orthopedic shoes or athletic sneakers can be worn with orthoses; attachments can be external (to the outer part of a leather shoe's sole) or internal (a molded shoe insert).
   c. Blucher opening: has vamps (the flaps contain the lace stays) that open wide apart from the anterior margin of the shoe for ease of application.
   d. Bal (Balmoral) opening: has stitched down vamps, not suitable for orthotic wear.
2. **Foot orthoses (FO).**
   a. May be attached to the interior of the shoe (e.g., an inserted pad) or the exterior of the shoe (e.g., Thomas heel).
   b. Soft inserts (i.e., viscoelastic plastic or rubber pads or relief cut-outs) reduce areas of high loading, restrict

forces, and protect painful or sensitive areas of the feet.
   (1) Metatarsal pad: located posterior to metatarsal heads; moves pressure from the metatarsal heads to the metatarsal shafts; allows more push-off in weak or inflexible feet.
   (2) Cushion heel: cushions and absorbs forces at heel contact; used to relieve strain on plantar fascia in plantar fasciitis.
   (3) Heel-spur pad.
c. Longitudinal arch supports: prevent depression of the subtalar joint and correct for pes planus (flat foot); flat foot can be flexible or rigid.
   (1) UCBL (University of California Biomechanics Laboratory) insert: a semirigid plastic molded insert to correct for flexible pes planus.
   (2) Scaphoid pad: used to support the longitudinal arch.
   (3) Thomas heel: a heel wedge with an extended anterior medial border used to support the longitudinal arch and correct for flexible pes valgus (pronated foot).
d. Posting.
   (1) Rearfoot posting: alters the position of the subtalar joint (STJ), or rearfoot, from heelstrike to footflat. Must be dynamic, control but not eliminate STJ motion.
      (a) Varus post (medial wedge): limits or controls eversion of the calcaneus and internal rotation of the tibia after heelstrike. Reduces calcaneal eversion during running.
      (b) Valgus post (lateral wedge): controls the calcaneus and subtalar joint that are excessively inverted and supinated at heelstrike.
   (2) Forefoot posting: supports the forefoot.
      (a) Medial wedge prescribed for forefoot varus.
      (b) Lateral wedge prescribed for forefoot valgus.
   (3) Contraindicated in the insensitive foot.
e. Heel lifts (or heel platform).
   (1) Accommodates for leg length discrepancy; can be placed inside the shoe (up to 3/8 inch) or attached to the outer sole.
   (2) Accommodates for limitation in ankle joint dorsiflexion.
f. Rocker bar: located proximal to metatarsal heads; improves weight shift onto metatarsals.
g. Rocker bottom: builds up the sole over the metatarsal heads and improves push-off in weak or inflexible feet. May also be used with insensitive feet.

3. Ankle-foot orthoses, (AFOs).

a. Consist of a shoe attachment, ankle control, uprights, and a proximal leg band.
b. Shoe attachments.
   (1) Foot plate: a molded plastic shoe insert; allows application of the brace before insertion into the shoe, ease of changing shoes of same heel height.
   (2) Stirrup: a metal attachment riveted to the sole of the shoe; split stirrups allow for shoe interchange; solid stirrups are fixed permanently to the shoe and provide for maximum stability.
c. Ankle controls.
   (1) Free motion: provides mediolateral stability that allows free motion in dorsiflexion and plantar flexion.
   (2) Solid ankle: allows no movement; indicated with severe pain or instability.
   (3) Limited motion: allows motion to be restricted in one or both directions.
      (a) Bichannel adjustable ankle lock (BiCAAL): an ankle joint with the anterior and posterior channels that can be fit with pins to reduce motion or springs to assist motion.
      (b) Anterior stop (dorsiflexion stop): determines the limits of ankle dorsiflexion. In an AFO, if the stop is set to allow slight dorsiflexion (5 degrees), knee flexion results; can be used to control for knee hyperextension; if the stop is set to allow too much dorsiflexion, knee buckling could result.
      (c) Posterior stop (plantar flexion stop): determines the limits of ankle plantar flexion. In an AFO, if the stop is set to allow slight plantar flexion (5 degrees), knee extension results; can be used to control for an unstable knee that buckles; if the stop is set to allow too much plantar flexion, recurvatum or knee hyperextension could result.
      (d) Solid AFO: limits all foot and ankle motion.
   (4) Dorsiflexion assistance.
      (a) Spring assist (Klenzak housing): double upright metal AFO with a single anterior channel for a spring assist to aid dorsiflexion.
      (b) Posterior leaf spring (PLS): a plastic AFO that inserts into the shoe; widely used to prevent drop foot.
   (5) Varus or valgus correction straps (T straps): control for varus or valgus forces at the ankle. Medial strap buckles around the lateral upright and corrects for valgus; lateral strap buckles around the medial upright and corrects for varus.
d. Uprights and attachments (bands or shells).
   (1) Conventional AFOs have metal uprights (aluminum, carbon graphite, or steel) and a hinged ankle joint allowing plantarflexion and dorsiflexion. Provides maximum support; if the patient's condition is changing (e.g., peripheral edema), conventional metal AFOs may be easier to alter to accommodate changes than molded AFOs.
      (a) Double metal uprights extend upwards from the ankle on both sides of the leg and attach to a calf band.

(b) Conventional AFO, calf band (metal with leather lining or plastic); provides for proximal stabilization on leg; anterior opening and buckle or Velcro closure.

(2) Molded AFOs are made of molded plastic and are lighter in weight and cosmetically more appealing; contraindicated for individuals with changing leg volume.

(a) Posterior leaf spring (PLS): has a flexible, narrow posterior shell; functions as dorsiflexion assist; holds foot at 90-degree angle during swing; displaced during stance; provides no medial-lateral stability.

(b) Modified AFO: has a wider posterior shell with trimlines just posterior to malleoli; foot plate includes more of medial and lateral borders of foot; provides more medial-lateral stability (control of calcaneal and forefoot inversion and eversion).

(c) Solid ankle AFO: has widest posterior shell with trimlines extending forward to malleoli; controls (prevents) dorsiflexion, plantarflexion, inversion, and eversion.

(d) Spiral AFO: a molded plastic AFO that winds (spirals) around the calf; provides limited control of motion in all planes.

(e) Hinged plastic AFOs are available.

(3) Specialized AFOs.

(a) Patellar-tendon-bearing brim: allows for weight distribution on the patellar shelf similar to patellar-tendon-bearing prosthetic socket; reduces weight-bearing forces through the foot.

(b) Tone-reducing orthosis: molded plastic AFO that applies constant pressure to spastic or hypertonic muscles (plantarflexors and invertors); snug fit is essential to achieve the benefits of reciprocal inhibition.

4. Knee-ankle-foot orthosis (KAFO).

a. Consists of a shoe attachment, ankle control, uprights, knee control, and bands or shells for the calf and thigh.

b. Knee controls.

(1) Hinge joint: provides mediolateral and hyperextension control while allowing for flexion and extension.

(a) Offset: the hinge is placed posterior to the weight-bearing line (trochanter-knee-ankle (TKA) line); assists extension, stabilizes knee during early stance; patients may have difficulty on ramps where knee may flex inadvertently.

(2) Locks.

(a) Drop ring lock: ring drops over joint when knee is in full extension to provide maximum stability; a retention button may be added to hold the ring lock up, permit gait training with the knee unlocked.

(b) Pawl lock with bail release: the pawl is a spring-loaded posterior projection (lever or ring) that allows the patient to unlock the knee by pulling up or hooking the pawl on the back of a chair and pushing it up; adds bulk and may unlock inadvertently with posterior knee pressure.

(3) Knee stability.

(a) Sagittal stability achieved by bands or straps used to provide a posteriorly directed force.

- Anterior band or strap (knee cap): attaches by four buckles to metal uprights; may restrict sitting, increases difficulty in putting on KAFO.
- Anterior bands: pretibial or suprapatellar or both.

(b) Frontal plane controls: for control of genu varum or genu valgum.

- Posterior plastic shell.
- Older braces utilize valgum (medial) or varum (lateral) correction straps which buckle around the opposite metal upright: less effective as controls than plastic shell.

c. Thigh bands.

(1) Proximal thigh band.

(2) Quadrilateral or ischial weight-bearing brim: reduces weight-bearing through the limb.

(a) Patten bottom: a distal attachment added to keep the foot off the floor; provides 100% unweighting of the limb; a lift is required on the opposite leg, e.g., used with Legg-Perthes disease.

d. Specialized KAFOs.

(1) Craig-Scott KAFO: commonly used appliance for individuals with paraplegia; consists of shoe attachments with reinforced foot plates, Bi-CAAL ankle joints set in slight dorsiflexion, pretibial band, pawl knee locks with bail release, and single thigh bands.

(2) Oregon orthotic system: a combination of plastic and metal components allows for triplanar control in three planes of motion (sagittal, frontal, and transverse).

(3) Fracture braces: a KAFO device with a calf or thigh shell that encompasses the fracture site and provides support.

(4) Functional electrical stimulation (FES) orthosis: orthotic use and functional ambulation is facilitated by the addition of electrical stimulation to specific muscles; the pattern and sequence of muscle activation by portable stimulators is controlled by an externally worn miniaturized computer pack; requires full passive range of motion (PROM) good functional endurance; in limited use with individuals with paraplegia, drop foot; also scoliosis.

e. Standing frames.
   (1) Standing frames: allows for standing without crutch support; may be stationary or attached to a wheeled mobility base (e.g., used with some patients with SCI).
   (2) Parapodium: allows for standing without crutch support; also allows for ease in sitting with the addition of hip and knee joints that can be unlocked (e.g., used with children with myelodysplasia).

5. Specialized knee orthoses (KOs).
   a. Articulated KOs: control knee motion and provide added stability.
      (1) Postsurgery KO protects repaired ligaments from overload.
      (2) Functional KO is worn long-term in lieu of surgery or during selected activities (sports competitions).
      (3) Examples include Lenox Hill, Pro-AM, Can-Am, Don Joy.
   b. Swedish knee cage: provides mild control for excessive hyperextension of the knee.
   c. Patellar stabilizing braces.
      (1) Improve patellar tracking; maintain alignment.
      (2) Lateral buttress (often made of felt) or strap positions patella medially.
      (3) A central patellar cutout may help positioning and minimizes compression.
   d. Neoprene sleeves.
      (1) Nylon-coated rubber material.
      (2) Provide compression, protection and proprioceptive feedback.
      (3) Provide little stabilization unless metal or plastic hinges are added.
      (4) Retains body heat, which may increase local circulation.
      (5) A central cutout minimizes patellar compression.
      (6) Can be used in other areas of the body, such as elbow, thigh and so on.

6. Hip-knee-ankle orthoses (HKAFOs).
   a. Contain a hip joint and pelvic band added to a KAFO.
   b. Hip joint: typically a metal hinge joint.
      (1) Controls for abduction, adduction, and rotation.
      (2) Controls for hip flexion when locked, typically with a drop ring lock; a locked hip restricts gait pattern to either a swing-to or swing-through.
   c. Pelvic attachments: a leather-covered, metal pelvic band; attaches the HKAFO to the pelvis between the greater trochanter and iliac crest; adds to difficulty in donning and doffing; adds weight and increases overall energy expenditure during ambulation.

7. Specialized THKAFOs.
   a. Contains a trunk band added to a HKAFO.
   b. Reciprocating gait orthosis (RGO): utilizes plastic molded solid-ankle orthoses with locked knees, plastic thigh shells, a hip joint with pelvic and trunk bands; the hips are connected by steel cables, which allow for a reciprocal gait pattern (either four-point or two-point); when the patient leans on the supporting hip, it forces it into extension, while the opposite leg is pushed into flexion; allows limb advancement.

8. Specialized lower limb devices.
   a. Denis Browne splint: a bar connecting two shoes that can swivel; used for correction of club foot or pes equinovarus in young children.
   b. Frejka pillow: keeps hips abducted; used for hip dysplasia or other conditions with tight adductors in young children.
   c. Toronto hip abduction orthosis: abducts the hip; used in treatment of Legg-Calvé-Perthes disease.

Spinal (Trunk) Orthoses: Components/Terminology

1. Corset.
   a. Provides abdominal compression, increases intraabdominal pressure.
   b. Assists respiration in individuals with spinal cord injury.
   c. Relieves pain in low-back disorders; sacroiliac support; e.g., pregnancy.

2. Lumbosacral orthoses (LSO).
   a. Control or limit lumbosacral motions.
   b. Lumbosacral flexion, extension, lateral control orthoses (LS FEL) (Knight spinal): includes pelvic and thoracic bands to anchor the orthosis with two posterior uprights, two lateral uprights, and an anterior corset.
   c. Plastic lumbosacral jacket: provides maximum support by spreading forces over a larger area; more cosmetic, but hotter.

3. Thoracolumbosacral orthoses (TLSO).
   a. Control or limit thoracic and lumbosacral motions.
   b. Thoracolumbosacral flexion, extension control orthosis (TLS FE) (Taylor brace): includes components of a LS FEL with the addition of axillary shoulder straps to limit upper trunk flexion.
   c. Plastic thoracolumbosacral jacket: provides maximum support and control of all motions; used in individuals recovering from spinal cord injury; allows for early mobilization out-of-bed and functional training.
   d. Jewett (TLSO): limits flexion, but encourages hyperextension (lordosis); used for compression fractures of the spine.

4. Cervical orthoses (CO).
   a. Control or limit cervical motion.
   b. Soft collar: provides minimal levels of control of cervical motions; e.g., cervical pain, whiplash.

c. Four-poster orthosis: has two plates (occipital and thoracic) with two anterior and two posterior posts to stabilize the head; used for moderate levels of control in individuals with cervical fracture/spinal cord injury.
d. Halo orthosis: attaches to the skull with screws; four uprights connect from the halo to a thoracic band or plastic jacket; provides maximal control for patients with cervical fracture/ spinal cord injury; allows for early mobilization out-of-bed and functional training.
e. Minerva orthosis: a rigid plastic appliance that provides maximum control of cervical motion; uses a forehead band without screws.

5. **Specialized trunk orthoses.**
   a. Milwaukee orthosis: a cervical, thoracic, lumbosacral orthosis (CTLSO) used to control scoliosis; it has a molded plastic pelvic jacket with one anterior and two posterior uprights extended to a superior neck or chest ring; pads and straps are used to apply pressure to areas of convexity of spinal curves; bulky, less cosmetic; may be used for all kyphotic and scoliotic curves of ≤40 degrees.
   b. Boston orthosis (TLSO): a low-profile, molded plastic orthosis for scoliosis; more cosmetic, can be worn under clothing; used for midthoracic or lower scoliosis curves of ≤40 degrees; also used to treat spondylolisthesis and conditions of severe trunk weakness; e.g., muscular dystrophy.

Upper-Limb Orthoses: Components/Terminology

1. **Functional considerations:** Most UL orthoses are directed toward creating usable prehension, functional hand position.

2. **Passive (static) positioning devices.**
   a. Generally made out of a variety of low-temperature plastic; i.e., Orthoplast, Hexalite.
   b. Resting splint (cock-up splint): an anterior or palmar splint that positions the wrist and hand in a functional position.
      (1) Wrist can be held in neutral or in 12–20 degrees wrist extension.
      (2) Fingers supported, phalanges slightly flexed, with thumb in partial opposition and abduction.
      (3) Used for patients with rheumatoid arthritis, fractures of carpal bones, Colles' fracture, carpal tunnel syndrome, stroke with paralysis, etc.
   c. Dorsal wrist splint: frees the palm for feeling and grasping through the use of grips that curve around over the second and fifth metacarpal heads; allows for the attachment of dorsal devices (i.e., rubber bands) to form a dynamic device.
   d. Airplane splint: positions the patient's arm out to the side at 90 degrees of abduction, with elbow flexed to 90 degrees; the weight of the outstretched arm is borne on a padded lateral trunk bar and iliac crest band; a strap holds the device across the trunk; used to immobilize the shoulder following fracture or injury when strapping to the chest is not desirable, or with burns.

3. **Dynamic devices.**
   a. Wrist-driven prehension orthosis (flexor hinge orthosis): assists patients in use of wrist extensors to approximate the thumb and forefingers (grip) in the absence of active finger flexion; e.g., facilitates tenodesis grasp in patients with quadriplegia.
   b. Motor-driven flexor hinge orthosis: complex control systems that allow for grasp; not generally in widespread use.

Physical Therapy Intervention

The physical therapist functions as a member of an orthotic clinic team that includes the physician, orthotist, and therapists.

1. **Examination.**
   a. Preorthotic assessment and prescription evaluate:
      (1) Joint mobility.
      (2) Sensation.
      (3) Strength and motor function.
      (4) Functional level.
      (5) Psychological status.
   b. Orthotic prescription: Considerations.
      (1) Patient's abilities and needs.
         (a) Level of impairments, functional limitations, disability.
         (b) Status: Consider if the patient's condition is permanent or changing.
      (2) Level of function, current lifestyle.
         (a) Consider if the patient is going to be a community ambulator versus a household ambulator.
         (b) Consider recreational and work-related needs.
      (3) Overall weight of orthotic devices, energy capabilities of patient. Some individuals abandon their orthoses quickly in favor of wheelchairs because of the high-energy demands of ambulating with orthoses; e.g., patients with high levels of paraplegia.
      (4) Manual dexterity, mental capacity of the individual. The donning and use of devices may be too difficult or complicated for some individuals.
      (5) Pressure tolerance of the skin and tissues.
      (6) Use of a temporary orthosis to assess likelihood of functional independence, reduce costs; e.g., patients with high levels of paraplegia.

c. Orthotic check-out.
  (1) Ensure proper fit and function; construction of the orthosis.
  (2) Static assessment.
    (a) Examine alignments for lower limb orthoses: In midstance, foot should be flat on floor.
      - Orthotic hip joint: 0.8 cm anterior and superior to greater trochanter.
      - Medial knee joint: ~2 cm above joint space, vertically midway between medial joint space and adductor tubercle.
      - Ankle joint: at tip of malleolus.
      - Plastic shells or metal uprights, thigh and calf bands: conform to contours of limb.
      - No undue tissue pressure or restriction of function.
  (3) Dynamic assessment.
    (a) Fit and function during activities of daily living (ADLs), functional mobility skills; e.g., sit-to-stand.
    (b) Fit and function during gait.

2. Orthotic training.

a. Instruct the patient in procedures for orthotic maintenance: routine skin inspection and care.
b. Ensure orthotic acceptance.
  (1) Patient should clearly understand functions, limitations of an orthosis.
  (2) Can use support groups to assist.
c. Teach proper application (donning-doffing) of the orthosis.
d. Teach proper use of the orthosis.
  (1) Balance training.
  (2) Gait training.
  (3) Functional activities training.
e. Reassess fit, function, and construction of the orthosis at periodic intervals; assess habitual use of the orthosis.

3. Selected orthotic gait deviations.

a. Lateral trunk bending: patient leans toward the orthotic side during stance. Possible causes: KAFO medial upright too high; insufficient shoe lift; hip pain, weak or tight abductors on the orthotic side; short leg; poor balance.
b. Circumduction: during swing, leg swings out to the side in an arc. Possible causes: locked knee; excessive plantar flexion (inadequate stop, plantar flexion contractures); weak hip flexors or dorsiflexors. All of these could also cause vaulting (rising up on the sound limb to advance the orthotic limb forward).
c. Anterior trunk bending: patient leans forward during stance. Possible causes: inadequate knee lock; weak quadriceps; hip or knee flexion contracture.
d. Posterior trunk bending: patient leans backward during stance. Possible cases: inadequate hip lock; weak gluteus maximus; knee ankylosis.
e. Hyperextended knee: excessive extension during stance. Possible causes: inadequate plantar flexion stop; inadequate knee lock; poor fit of calf band (too deep); weak quadriceps; loose knee ligaments or extensor spasticity; pes equinus.
f. Knee instability: excessive knee flexion during stance. Possible causes: inadequate dorsiflexion stop; inadequate knee lock; knee and/or hip flexion contracture; weak quadriceps or insufficient knee lock; knee pain.
g. Foot slap: foot hits the ground during early stance. Possible causes: inadequate dorsiflexor assist; inadequate plantarflexor stop; weak dorsiflexors.
h. Toes first: on-toes posture during stance. Possible causes: inadequate dorsiflexor assist; inadequate plantarflexor stop; inadequate heel lift; heel pain, extensor spasticity; pes equinus; short leg.
i. Flat foot: contact with entire foot. Possible causes: inadequate longitudinal arch support; pes planus.
j. Pronation: excessive medial foot contact during stance, valgus position of calcaneus. Possible causes: transverse plane malalignment; weak invertors; pes valgus; spasticity; genu valgum.
k. Supination: excessive lateral foot contact during stance, varus position of the calcaneus. Possible causes: transverse plane malalignment; weak evertors; pes varus; genu varum.
l. Excessive stance width: patient stands or walks with a wide base of support. Possible causes: KAFO height of medial upright too high; HKAFO hip joint aligned in excessive abduction; knee is locked; abduction contracture; poor balance; sound limb is too short.

Adhesive Taping

General Concepts

1. Purpose.

a. Limit ROM of specific joints.
b. Support injured body segment.
c. Secure protective devices such as felt, foam, gel, or plastic padding, orthoplast or plastazote.
d. Keep dressings and bandages in place and secure.
e. Preventive support for a joint that is at risk.

f. Realign position and reduce pain; e.g., McConnell treatment for patellofemoral pain.
g. May enhance proprioception.

2. **Preparation.**
   a. Part to be taped should be properly positioned and supported.
   b. Select appropriate type and width of tape.
   c. Body hair should be shaved, skin should be clean. Foam underwrap or stockinet may be used.
   d. Lubricated pads should be placed over areas of potential blister formation from friction. e.g.; heel and lace-area pads on the foot.
   e. Occlusive dressings should be applied over wounds or skin conditions to be covered by the tape.
   f. Skin adherent such as benzoin should be applied to increase adhesion of the tape and aid in toughening the skin to decrease irritation.

3. **Application.**
   a. If the part has not been previously injured, it should be taped in a neutral position.
   b. Injured ligaments should be held in a shortened position.
      (1) Lateral or inversion ankle sprains should be taped in an everted position.
      (2) Tape should follow body contours and be applied primarily from medial to lateral in the case of an inversion sprain.
   c. Tape should be applied with even pressure, and with overlap of previous tape strip by one-half.
   d. Circular strapping should be applied very cautiously due to potential circulatory compromise.
   e. Avoid creases and folds.
   f. If tape is too tight, adjust by removing or modifying strips or reapply.

4. **Complications.**
   a. Allergic reactions to the tape.
   b. Skin irritation.
   c. Reduced circulation.
   d. If tape is too tight, it might compromise the ability of the patient to perform the skill intended.
   e. Tape may lose its effectiveness in an hour or so, and may need to be reapplied.

Prosthetics

General Concepts

1. **Prosthesis:** a replacement of a body part with an artificial device; an artificial limb.

2. **Levels of amputation.**
   a. Transmetatarsal amputation: partial foot amputation.
   b. Ankle disarticulation (Syme's): amputation through the ankle joint; heel pad is preserved and attached to distal end of tibia for weight-bearing.
   c. Transtibial amputation: below-knee (BK) amputation; ideally, 20%–50% of the tibial length is spared; short transtibial is < 20% of tibial length.
   d. Knee disarticulation: amputation through the knee joint; femur is intact.
   e. Transfemoral amputation: above-knee (AK) amputation; ideally 35%–60% of the femoral length is spared; short transfemoral is < 35% of femoral length.
   f. Hip disarticulation: amputation of entire lower limb, pelvis is preserved.
   g. Hemipelvectomy: amputation of entire lower limb, lower half of the pelvis is resected.
   h. Hemicorporectomy: amputation of both lower limbs and pelvis below L4, L5 level.
   i. Transradial amputation: below-elbow (BE) amputation.
   j. Elbow disarticulation: amputation through the elbow joint.
   k. Transhumeral amputation: above-elbow (AE) amputation.
   l. Shoulder disarticulation: amputation through the shoulder joint.

3. **Components.**
   a. All prosthetic devices contain a socket and terminal device with varying components in between.
   b. Sockets are custom-molded to the residual limb; total contact is desired, with the load distributed to all tissues; assists in circulation and provides maximal sensory feedback.
      (1) Functions to:
         (a) Contain the residual tissues.
         (b) Provide a means to suspend the prosthetic limb.
         (c) Transfer forces from the prosthesis to the residual limb.
      (2) Selective loading: pressure-tolerant areas are built up to increase loading (i.e., build-ups for tendon-bearing areas), while pressure-sensitive areas are

relieved to decrease loading (i.e., relief for bony prominences, nerves, and tendons).

(3) Types.

(a) A socket made of hard plastic with a soft polyethylene foam liner is the most common type; removable liners aid in ease of prosthetic donning and adjustment.

(b) Flexible sockets are made of soft, pliable thermoplastic material within a rigid frame; used for most AK sockets due to better suspension.

(4) Socks.

(a) Used in every suspension system except suction.

(b) Provide a soft interface between the residual limb and the socket; minimize shear forces between socket and skin.

(c) Changing sock thickness or adding more socks can assist in accommodating to changes in volume of residual limb, prevent pistoning.

(d) Excessive thickness of socks (>15 ply) can alter fit and weight-bearing ability of the socket.

c. Terminal device (TD).

(1) Provides an interface between the amputee's prosthesis with the external environment.

(2) Lower limb prosthesis: TD is a foot.

(3) Upper limb prosthesis: TD is a hook or hand.

Lower-Limb Prosthetic Devices (LLPs)

1. Partial-foot prosthesis.

a. Plastic foot replacement: restores foot length, protects amputated stump.

b. Function may be assisted by the addition of a rocker bottom or plastic calf shell.

2. Transtibial (below knee) prosthesis.

a. Foot-ankle assembly.

(1) Functions to:

(a) Absorb shock at heel strike.

(b) Plantarflex in early stance, permits metatarsophalangeal hyperextension in late stance.

(c) Cosmetic replacement of foot.

(2) Solid ankle cushion heel (SACH) foot.

(a) The most commonly prescribed foot; nonarticulated; contains an energy-absorbing cushion heel and internal wooden keel that limits sagittal plane motion, primarily to plantarflexion.

(b) Permits a very small amount of mediolateral (frontal plane) and transverse plane motion.

(c) Assists in hyperextension of knee (knee stability) during stance.

(3) Solid-ankle flexible (SAFE) foot: a flexible, nonarticulated foot (similar to SACH); permits more nonsagittal plane motions; prescribed for more active individuals.

(4) Flex-foot: a leaf-spring shank (not a foot) used with an endoskeletal prosthesis; the long band of carbon fiber originates directly from the shank; stores energy in early stance for later use during push-off; prescribed for more active individuals.

(5) Single axis foot: an articulated foot with the lower shank; motion is controlled by anterior and posterior rubber bumpers that limit dorsiflexion and plantarflexion; more stable (permits only sagittal plane motion); may be prescribed for individuals with bilateral transfemoral amputations.

b. Shank.

(1) Functions to:

(a) Provide leg length and shape.

(b) Connects and transmits weight from socket to foot.

(2) Exoskeletal: conventional components, usually made of wood with a plastic laminated finish; colored for cosmesis; durable.

(3) Endoskeletal: contains a central metal shank (aluminum, titanium, and other high-strength alloys), covered by soft foam and external stocking; offers improved cosmesis; modular components allows for increased ease of prosthetic adjustment.

c. Socket.

(1) PTB socket (patellar tendon-bearing): a total contact socket that allows for moderate loading over the area of the patellar tendon.

(2) Pressure-sensitive areas of the transtibial residual limb include:

(a) Anterior tibia.

(b) Anterior tibial crest.

(c) Fibular head and neck.

(d) Fibular nerve.

(3) Pressure-tolerant areas of the typical transtibial residual limb include:

(a) Patellar tendon.

(b) Medial tibial plateau.

(c) Tibial and fibular shafts.

(d) Distal end (rarely, may be sensitive).

d. Suspension.

(1) Supracondylar leather cuff suspension: buckles over the femoral condyles; widely used, easily adjusted.

(2) Supracondylar socket suspension (SC): medial and lateral walls of the socket extend up and over the femoral condyles; a removable medial wedge assists in donning and removal; more cosmetic (no buckles or straps); provides increased mediolateral stability.

(3) Supracondylar/suprapatellar (SC/SP): similar to SC but with a high anterior wall; assists in suspension of short residual limbs.
(4) Thigh corset suspension: a hinged joint with metal uprights attached to a thigh corset; provides larger surface for weight-bearing; prescribed for individuals with sensitive skin on the residual limb; the knee joint allows for knee control (locks); pistoning may be a problem.

3. Transfemoral (above-knee) prosthesis.

a. Knee unit.
  (1) Axis.
    (a) Single axis: permits knee motions to occur around a fixed axis; knee flexion is needed during late stance and swing, sitting, and kneeling.
    (b) Polycentric systems (multiple axes): changing axis of motion allows for adjustments to the center of knee rotation; more stable than single axis joints; complex; not widely used.
  (2) Friction devices: control knee motions; provide resistance to pendular motion at the knee.
    (a) Constant friction: continuous resistance is provided by a clamp that acts on the knee mechanism; friction device can be easily adjusted by screws; usually prescribed for older individuals who do not vary their gait speeds greatly.
    (b) Variable friction: resistance can be regulated to the demands of the gait cycle; at early swing, high resistance is needed to prevent excessive heel rise; during midswing when the leg swings forward, friction demands are minimal; at late swing, friction is increased to prevent terminal swing impact.
    (c) Hydraulic knee units (fluid-controlled) or pneumatic knee units (air-controlled): adjusts resistance dynamically to the individual's walking speed; prescribed for younger, more active individuals; heavier, more complicated; increased maintenance, cost.
  (3) Knee stabilization in extension achieved by:
    (a) Prosthetic alignment: the knee center is aligned posterior to the TKA line; a knee aligned further posterior will be very stable (will not flex easily); may be prescribed for short residual limbs; an unstable knee may occur if the knee falls anterior to the TKA line.
    (b) Manual lock: prescribed for individuals who require a constantly locked knee; e.g., weakness of hip extensors; difficulty with clearance of the leg during swing can be controlled by shortening the total prosthetic limb length ~1 cm.
    (c) Friction brake: a device that increases friction at midstance to prevent knee flexion, but permits smooth knee motion through the rest of the gait cycle.
    (d) Extension aid: an external elastic strap or internal coiled spring that assists in terminal knee extension during late swing.

b. Socket.
  (1) Quadrilateral socket: most commonly prescribed AK socket; quadrilateral in shape.
    (a) Contains a broad horizontal posterior shelf for seating of the ischial tuberosity and gluteals.
    (b) The medial wall is the same height as the posterior wall, while the anterior and lateral walls are $2^1/_2$–3 inches higher.
    (c) A posterior directed force is provided by the anterior and lateral walls to ensure proper seating.
    (d) Scarpa's bulge: an area built up on the anterior wall to distribute forces across the femoral triangle.
    (e) Reliefs are provided for the adductor longus tendon, hamstring tendons and sciatic nerve, gluteus maximus and rectus femoris.
  (2) Pressure-sensitive areas of the typical transfemoral residual limb.
    (a) Distolateral end of the femur.
    (b) Pubic symphysis.
    (c) Perineal area.
  (3) Pressure-tolerant areas of the typical transfemoral residual limb.
    (a) Ischial tuberosity.
    (b) Gluteals.
    (c) Lateral sides of residual limb.
    (d) Distal end (rarely, may be sensitive).

c. Suspension.
  (1) Suction suspension: suction is employed to maximize contact and suspension; air is pumped out through a one-way air release valve located at the socket's bottom; suction suspension can be total or partial (individual wears a sock).
  (2) Strap suspension: adjustable, readily accommodates to volume changes. Disadvantage: pistoning, when it is the sole type of suspension.
    (a) Silesian bandage: a strap that anchors the TKA prosthesis by reaching around the pelvis (below iliac crest); controls rotatory motions.
  (3) Hinge suspension: hinged hip joint attached to a metal/leather pelvic band, anchored around the pelvis.
    (a) Adds control for medial/lateral stability of hip (rotation, abduction/adduction).
    (b) Reduces Trendelenburg gait deviation.
    (c) Disadvantages: adds extra weight and bulk.

4. **Knee disarticulation prosthesis.**
   a. Functional, allows weight-bearing on the distal end of the femur.
   b. Problems with cosmesis, added thigh length with the knee joint attached, especially noticeable in sitting.
   c. Lower shank is shortened to balance leg length in standing.

5. **Hip disarticulation prosthesis.**
   a. Socket is molded to accommodate the pelvis; weight-bearing occurs on ischial seat, iliac crests.
   b. Endoskeletal components frequently used, decreases weight of prosthesis.
   c. Stability achieved with hip extension aid; posterior placement of knee joint with anterior placement of the hip joint to the weight-bearing line.

6. **Immediate postoperative prosthesis (rigid dressing).**
   a. Plaster of Paris socket is fabricated in the operating room with the capability to attach a foot and pylon.
   b. Advantages.
      (1) Allows early, limited weight-bearing ambulation within days of surgery.
      (2) Limits postoperative sequelae: edema, postoperative pain.
      (3) Enhances wound healing.
      (4) Allows for earlier fit of permanent prosthesis.
   c. Limitations.
      (1) Requires skilled application and close monitoring.
      (2) Does not allow for daily wound inspection; contraindicated for older patients with cardiovascular compromise and increased risk for wounds.

Upper-Limb Prosthetic Devices (ULPs)

1. **Below Elbow (BE) prosthesis:** contains a terminal device (TD), wrist and forearm socket, harness system.

2. **Above Elbow (AE) prosthesis:** in addition, contains an elbow and arm socket.

3. **Conventional system.**
   a. Power for voluntary opening of the TD (hook or hand) is transmitted by a cable from a figure-of-eight shoulder harness to the TD.
   b. Rubber bands are used for closure and prehensile strength.
   c. Forearm rotation is done by manual prepositioning of the TD.
   d. Movement control.
      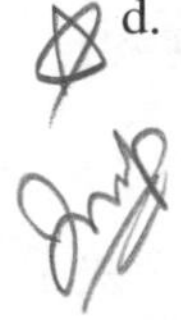
      (1) BE prosthesis: bilateral scapular abduction or ipsilateral flexion of the humerus is used to pull on the cable and force opening of the hook.
      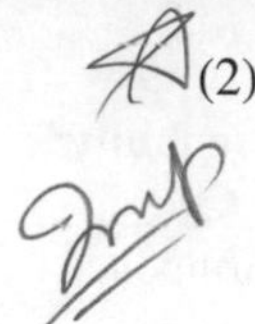
      (2) AE prosthesis (dual control system): the same motions can be used to flex the elbow in the AE prosthesis; when the elbow locks (by scapular depression and humeral extension), the forces are then transmitted to operate the TD.

4. **Externally powered system.**
   a. Microswitches (EMG myoelectric devices) are activated by the same motions as conventional power systems.
   b. Small electric motors (battery-powered) are activated to operate the TD.
      (1) Improves ease of function, prehensile strength.
      (2) Adds weight, increased maintenance, cost.

Physical Therapy Intervention

The physical therapist functions as a member of the prosthetic clinic team that includes physician, prosthetist, and therapist.

1. **Preprosthetic management.**
   a. Preprescription examination.
      (1) Skin: inspect incision for healing; scar tissue; other lesions.
      (2) Residual limb.
         (a) Circumference measurements: check for edema.
         (b) Length: bone, soft tissue length.
         (c) Shape: should be cylindrical or conical; check for abnormalities (i.e., bulbous end, dog ears, adductor roll).
      (3) Vascular status of sound limb, residual limb: examine pulses, color, temperature, trophic changes, pain/intermittent claudication.
      (4) AROM and PROM: examine for contractures that might interfere with prosthetic prescription (e.g., hip and knee flexion contractures).
      (5) Sensation.
         (a) Proprioception, visual, vestibular function, contributions to balance; loss of proprioception in the amputated limb will necessitate a compensatory shift to the other senses for balance control.
         (b) Phantom limb sensation: a feeling of pressure or paresthesia as if coming from the amputated limb. Sensations are normal, not painful; may last for the lifetime of the individual.
         (c) Phantom pain: an intense burning or cramping pain; disabling, frequently interferes with rehabilitation.
      (6) Strength: examine strength of residual limb as tolerated; strength of the sound limb, trunk, and upper extremities needed for function.

(7) Functional status.
  (a) Functional mobility skills: bed mobility, transfers, wheelchair use.
  (b) Activities of daily living: basic, instrumental (use of telephone, shopping, etc.).

(8) Cardiopulmonary function, endurance.
  (a) The shorter the amputation limb, the greater the energy demands; i.e., oxygen consumption is increased 65% over normal walking in the patient with transfemoral amputation; similar to fast walking in those without amputations for the patient with transtibial amputation.
  (b) Functional capacity further limited by: concomitant diseases (e.g., cardiovascular disease, diabetes), individual fitness level, pain.

(9) Neurologic factors.
  (a) Cognitive function.
  (b) Check for neuropathy.
  (c) Check for neuroma: an abnormal growth of nerve cells that occurs in the residual limb after amputation.

(10) Psychosocial factors: motivation, adjustment and acceptance, availability of support systems.

b. Preprosthetic training: goals and interventions.

(1) Ideally begins preoperatively and continues postoperatively.

(2) Facilitate psychological acceptance.

(3) Postoperative dressings: applied to the residual limb; helps to limit edema, accelerate healing, reduce postoperative pain, and shape the residual limb.
  (a) Elastic wraps: flexible, soft bandaging, inexpensive; requires frequent reapplication, with pressure greatest distal to proximal; if wraps are allowed to loosen, may have problems with edema control; avoid circular wrapping, which produces a tourniquet effect.
  (b) Stump shrinkers: flexible, soft, inexpensive, readily available in different sizes.
  (c) Semirigid dressings: Unna paste dressing (zinc oxide, gelatin, glycerin, and calamine); applied in the operating room.
  (d) Rigid dressings: plaster of Paris dressing; applied in the operating room; a component of immediate postoperative fitting; allows for edema reduction and early ambulation with a temporary prosthesis (pylon and foot). Good for young patients who are good candidates for a permanent prosthesis.

(4) Desensitizing activities: pressure, rubbing, stroking, bandaging of the residual limb.

(5) Hygiene: inspection and care of the residual limb.

(6) Positioning for prevention of contracture; positions to avoid include:
  (a) Transtibial: prolonged flexion and external rotation at the hip, knee flexion; counteract with use of a posterior board to keep knee straight while in wheelchair; regularly scheduled time in prone-lying.
  (b) Transfemoral: flexion, abduction, external rotation of hip; counteract with regularly scheduled time in prone-lying time.

(7) Flexibility exercises.
  (a) Full AROM and PROM, active stretching, especially in hip and knee extension.
  (b) Flexibility of sound limb and trunk.

(8) Strengthening: utilize a general strengthening exercise program with special emphasis on:
  (a) Hip extensors: especially for the patient with transfemoral amputation.
  (b) Knee extensors: the patient with transtibial amputation.
  (c) Hip abductors: for stance phase pelvic stability.
  (d) Dynamic exercises: utilize gravity and body weight to provide resistance during functional mat activities.

(9) Functional mobility training.
  (a) Sit-to-stand transitions, transfers, standing.
  (b) Wheelchair independence.
  (c) Hopping on the sound limb; mobility in the seated position; i.e., scooting for patients with bilateral transfemoral amputation.
  (d) Early walking with crutches or walker; consider early ambulation with a temporary prosthesis.

(10) Bilateral lower-extremity amputation.
  (a) Wheelchair training important. Will be primary means of locomotion.
  (b) Prolonged wheelchair time increases likelihood of hip and knee flexion contractures; prone positioning program is important.
  (c) Energy expenditure during prosthetic ambulation is increased dramatically; a trial period with temporary prostheses can be used to evaluate ambulation potential with permanent prostheses; especially useful with the elderly.
  (d) Bilateral transfemoral amputation: ambulation usually requires walker; loss of lower-extremity proprioception increase balance difficulties; loss of knee extensor function will result in significant later difficulties with stair-climbing, curbs, stepping.
  (e) Bilateral transfemoral amputation: patients can be fitted with shortened prostheses (stubbies) consisting of a socket and foot component (modified rocker feet) with no knee joints; increases ease of use and function; generally poor acceptance due to cosmesis.

2. Prosthetic management.

a. Prosthetic check-out.

(1) Prosthesis: delivered as ordered, proper functioning; inspect both on and off the patient.

(2) Static assessment.
(a) Alignment and comfort in standing, sitting.
(b) Leg length discrepancy: pelvis level.
(c) Fit and suspension: pistoning when pelvis is lifted.
(3) Dynamic assessment.
(a) Sit-to-stand transitions.
(b) Gait: smooth, safe gait, absence of gait deviations; gait speeds normally decrease to reduce high levels of energy expenditure.
(c) Stairs and inclines.
(4) Inspection of the residual limb with the prosthesis off.
(a) Proper loading: transient redness is to be expected in pressure tolerant areas after prosthetic use.
(b) No redness should be seen in pressure sensitive areas.

b. Prosthetic training: goals and interventions.
(1) Donning and doffing of the prosthesis: training specific to type of socket and type of suspension.
(2) Strengthening, flexibility exercises.
(a) Emphasis on hip extension and knee extension (transtibial) with the prosthesis on.
(3) Balance and coordination.
(a) Symmetrical stance and weight-bearing on prosthetic limb.
(b) Weight shifting to limits of stability.
(c) Dynamic balance control; e.g., stepping activities.
(4) Gait training.
(a) Conventional training: focus on smooth weight transfer from sound limb to prosthetic limb, continuous movement sequence.
(b) Biofeedback training: limb load devices to facilitate prosthetic weight acceptance.
(c) Training with use of least restrictive assistive device; parallel bars may interfere with learning and independent ambulation in some patients.
(5) Functional activities training: including transfers, stairs, curbs, ramps, down and up from floor, recreational activities, etc.
(6) Regular inspection and maintenance of the prosthesis.
(7) Hygiene: care of stump socks, interior of the socket.
(8) Facilitate prosthetic acceptance.

3. Selected prosthetic gait deviations.

a. Transfemoral amputation.
(1) Circumduction: the prosthesis swings out to the side in an arc. Possible causes: a long prosthesis, locked knee, small or loose socket, inadequate suspension, foot plantar flexed, abduction contracture, poor knee control.
(2) Abducted gait: prosthesis is laterally displaced to the side. Possible causes: crotch or medial wall discomfort, long prosthesis, low lateral wall or malalignment, tight hip abductors.
(3) Vaulting: the patient rises up on the sound limb to swing the prosthesis through. Possible causes: prosthesis too long, inadequate suspension, socket too small, prosthetic foot set in too much plantarflexion, too little knee flexion.
(4) Lateral trunk bending during stance: the trunk bends toward the prosthetic side. Possible causes: low lateral wall, short prosthesis, high medial wall; weak abductors, abductor contracture, hip pain, short amputation limb.
(5) Forward flexion during stance: the trunk bends forward. Possible causes: unstable knee unit, short ambulatory aids, hip flexion contracture.
(6) Lumbar lordosis during stance: exaggeration of the lumbar curve. Possible causes: insufficient support from anterior or posterior walls, painful ischial weight-bearing, hip flexion contracture, weak hip extensors or abdominals.
(7) High heel rise: during early swing, the heel rises excessively. Possible causes: inadequate knee friction, too little tension in the extension aid.
(8) Terminal swing impact: the prosthesis comes to a sudden stop as the knee extends during late swing. Possible causes: insufficient knee friction or too much tension in the extension aid; patient fears that the knee will buckle; forceful hip flexion.

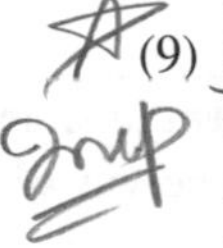

(9) Swing phase whips: at toe-off, the heel moves either medially or laterally. Possible causes: socket is rotated, knee bolt is rotated, foot is malaligned.
(10) Foot rotation at heel strike: as the heel contacts the ground, the foot rotates laterally, sometimes with vibratory motion. Possible causes: foot is malaligned, stiff heel cushion, or plantar flexion bumper.
(11) Foot slap: excessive plantar flexion at heel strike. Possible cause: heel cushion or plantar flexion bumper is too soft.
(12) Uneven step length: patient favors sound limb and limits weight-bearing time on the prosthetic limb. Possible causes: socket discomfort or poor alignment; hip flexion contracture or hip instability.

b. Transtibial amputation.
(1) Excessive knee flexion during stance. Possible causes: socket may be aligned too far forward or tilted anteriorly; plantar flexion bumper is too hard and limits plantar flexion, high heel shoes; knee flexion contracture or weak quadriceps.
(2) Inadequate knee flexion during stance. Possible causes: socket may be aligned too far back or tilted posteriorly; plantar flexion bumper or heel cushion too soft; low heel shoe; anterodistal discomfort, weak quadriceps.

(3) Lateral thrust at midstance. Possible causes: foot is inset too much.
(4) Medial thrust at midstance. Possible causes: foot is outset too much.
(5) Drop off or premature knee flexion in late stance. Possible causes: socket is set too far forward or excessively flexed; dorsiflexion bumper is too soft resulting in excess dorsiflexion of the foot; prosthetic foot keel too short; knee flexion contracture.
(6) Delayed knee flexion during late stance: patient feels as though walking "uphill." Possible causes: socket is set too far back or lacks sufficient flexion; dorsiflexion bumper is too stiff causing excess plantar flexion; prosthetic foot keel too long.

Wheelchairs

Components

1. Postural support system.

a. Seating.
(1) Sling seat: standard on wheelchairs. Hips tend to slide forward, thighs tend to adduct and internally rotate. Reinforces poor pelvic position (posterior pelvic tilt).
(2) Insert or contour seats creates a stable, firm sitting surface; made of wood or plastic, padded with foam.
(a) Improves pelvic position (neutral pelvic position).
(b) Reduces the tendency for the patient to slide forward or sit with a posterior pelvic tilt (sacral sitting).
(3) Seat cushion: distributes weight-bearing pressures. Assists in preventing decubitus ulcers in patients with decreased sensation, prolongs wheelchair sitting times.
(a) Pressure-relieving, contoured foam cushion: uses dense, layered foam; accommodates moderate to severe postural deformity. Easy for caregivers to reposition patients, low maintenance. May interfere with slide transfers.
(b) Pressure-relieving fluid/gel or combination cushion (fluid/gel plus foam). Can be custom-molded. Accommodates moderate to severe postural deformity. Easy for caregivers to reposition patients. Requires some maintenance, heavier, more expensive.
(c) Pressure-relieving air cushion. Accommodates moderate to severe postural deformity. Lightweight, improved pressure distribution. Expensive, base may be unstable for some patients. Requires continuous maintenance.
(4) Adds to measurements to determine back height.
(5) Pressure relief push-ups are required, typically every 15–20 minutes (e.g., the patient with SCI).

b. Back: support to the midscapular region is provided by most standard sling-back wheelchairs.
(1) Lower back height may increase functional mobility, i.e., sports chairs; may also increase back strain.
(2) High back height may be necessary for patients with poor trunk stability or with extensor spasms.
(3) Insert or contour backs: improve trunk extension and overall upright alignment.
(4) Lateral trunk supports: improve trunk alignment for patients with scoliosis, poor stability.

c. Armrests.
(1) Full-length or desk length; desk length facilitates use, proximity to a desk or table.
(2) Fixed-height or adjustable height; adjustable-height arm rests can be raised to facilitate sit-to-stand transfers.
(3) Removable armrests: facilitate transfers.
(4) Wraparound (space saver) armrests: reduce the overall width of the chair by $1^1/_2$ inches.
(5) Upper extremity support surface (trays or troughs) can be secured to the armrests; provides additional postural assistance for patients with decreased use of upper extremities.

d. Leg rests.
(1) Fixed.
(2) Swing-away, detachable: facilitates ease in transfers, front approach to wheelchair when ambulating.
(3) Elevating: indicated for LE edema control, postural support; contraindicated for patients with knee flexor (hamstring) hypertonicity or tightness.

e. Footrests.
(1) Footplates: provide a resting base for feet, feet are neutral with knees flexed to 90 degrees; footplates can be raised or removed to facilitate transfers.
(2) Heel loops: help maintain foot position, prevent posterior sliding of the foot.

(3) Straps (ankle, calf): can be added to stabilize the feet on the foot plates.

2. Wheeled mobility base.

a. Frame.

(1) Fixed or folding.

(a) Folding facilitates mobility in the community, ease of storage.

(b) Rigid frame facilitates stroke efficiency; increases distance per stroke.

(2) Available in heavy-duty, standard, lightweight, active-duty lightweight, ultra-lightweight construction.

(a) In general, the lighter the weight of the frame, the greater the ease of use.

(b) Level of expected activity and environment should be taken into account when deciding on frame construction.

b. Wheels, handrims.

(1) Casters: small front wheels, typically 8 inches in diameter; caster locks can be added to facilitate wheelchair stability during transfers.

(2) Drive wheels: large rear wheels used for propulsion; outer rims allow for hand grip and propulsion.

(a) Projections may be attached to the rims (vertical, oblique, or horizontal) to facilitate propulsion in patients with poor handgrip, e.g., quadriplegia; horizontal or oblique projections widen the chair and may limit maneuvering in the home.

(b) Friction rims/leather gloves: increase handgrip friction, ease of propulsion in patients with poor handgrip.

(c) Construction of drive wheels: standard spokes or spokeless wheels.

c. Tires.

(1) Standard hard rubber tires: durable, low maintenance.

(2) Pneumatic (air-filled) tires: provide a smoother ride, increased shock absorption; require more maintenance.

d. Brakes.

(1) Most brakes consist of a lever system with a cam.

(2) Brakes must be engaged for all transfers in and out of chair.

(3) Extensions may be added to increase ease in both locking and unlocking; e.g., for upper extremity weakness, arthritis.

e. Additional attachments.

(1) Seat belts (pelvic positioner): belt should grasp over the pelvis at a 45-degree angle to the seat.

(2) Seat positioners: can add lateral positioners at hip and knee or medial positioner at knee (adductor pommel) to maintain alignment of the lower extremities, control for spasticity; a seat wedge or a tilt-in-space seat can be used for extensor spasms or thrusting.

(3) Seat back positioners: can add lateral trunk positioners to maintain alignment, control for scoliosis.

(4) Antitipping device: a posterior extension attached to the lower horizontal supports, prevent tipping backward in the chair; also limits going up curbs or over door sills.

(5) Hill-holder device: a mechanical brake that allows the chair to go forward, but automatically brakes when the chair goes in reverse; useful for patients who are not able to ascend a long ramp or hill without a rest.

3. Specialized wheelchairs.

a. Reclining back: indicated for patients who are unable to independently maintain upright sitting position.

(1) Reclining wheelchairs include an extended back and typically elevating leg rests; head and trunk supports may also be added.

(2) Electric reclining back helps to redistribute weight-bearing if patient cannot do active pushups or pressure-relief maneuvers.

b. Tilt-in-space: motorized; entire seat and back may be tipped backwards (normal seat to back angle is maintained); indicated for patients with extensor spasms that may throw the patient out of the chair, or for pressure relief.

c. One-arm drive: drive mechanisms are located on one wheel, usually with two outer rims (or by push lever); patient propels the wheelchair by pushing on both rims (or lever with one hand); difficult for some patients to use, e.g., patients with left hemiplegia, cognitive/ perceptual impairments.

d. Hemiplegic chair (Hemi chair): designed to be low to the ground, allowing propulsion with the noninvolved upper and lower extremities.

e. Amputee chair: wheelchair is modified by placing the drive wheels posterior to the vertical back supports (2 inches backward); increases the length of the base of support and posterior stability; prescribed for patients with bilateral lower-extremity amputations, whose center of gravity is now located more posterior when seated in the wheelchair.

f. Powered wheelchair: utilizes a power source (battery) to propel the wheelchair; prescribed for patients who are not capable of self-propulsion or who have very low endurance.

(1) Microprocessors allow the control of the wheelchair to be adapted to various controls; i.e., joystick, head controls.

(2) Proportional drives: changes in pressure on the control result in directly corresponding changes in speeds.

(3) Microswitching systems: speed is preset; controls turn system on and off; i.e., puff-n-sip tubes for individuals with quadriplegia.

g. Bariatric wheelchair: heavy-duty, extra-wide wheelchair designed to assist mobility in individuals who are obese.
   (1) Selection based on patient characteristics, safety, and function.
   (2) The bariatric client has a center of body mass that is positioned several inches forward compared to the normal-sized person.
      (a) In order to ensure wheelchair stability, the rear axle is displaced forward compared to the standard wheelchair.
      (b) This forward position allows for a more efficient arm push (full-arm stroke with less wrist extension).
   (3) Bariatric wheelchair can be ordered with special adaptations:
      (a) Hard tires versus pneumatic tires for increased durability.
      (b) Adjustable backrest to accommodate excessive posterior bulk.
      (c) Reclining wheelchair to accommodate excessive anterior bulk, cardiorespiratory compromise (e.g., orthostatic hypotension).
      (d) Power application attached to a heavy duty wheelchair to accommodate excessive fatigue.

h. Sports wheelchair: variable; generally include lightweight, solid frame, low seat, low back, seat that accommodates a tucked position, leg straps, slanted drive wheels, small push rims.

Wheelchair Measurements

1. General concepts.

a. Overall the size of the wheelchair must be proportional to the size of the patient and take into account the demands of expected use and the environment in which the chair will be used.

b. Assessments should be taken with the patient on a firm surface (seated or supine).

2. Six key measurements.

a. Seat width.
   (1) Measurement on the patient: width of the hips at the widest part.
   (2) Chair measurement: add 2 inches to the patient's measurement.
   (3) Potential problems.
      (a) Excessive width of the wheelchair will result in added difficulties in reaching the drive wheels and propelling the chair.
      (b) Wheelchair width should accommodate width of doorways; can use a narrowing device; requires coordination to turn the cranking device.
      (c) A wheelchair that is too narrow will result in pressure/discomfort on the lateral pelvis and thighs; lateral space should allow for changes in the thickness of clothing.
   (4) The bariatric client with a pear shape will have increased gluteal femoral weight distribution. Measurement should consider the widest portion of the seated position (e.g., at the forward edge of the seated position). Also consider room for weight-shifting maneuvers for pressure relief, and possible use of lift devices.

b. Seat depth.
   (1) Measurement on the patient: posterior buttock to the posterior aspect of the lower leg in the popliteal fossa.
   (2) Chair measurement: subtract 2–3 inches from the patient's measurement.
   (3) Potential problems.
      (a) Seat depth that is too short fails to support the thigh adequately.
      (b) Seat depth that is too long may compromise posterior knee circulation or result in a kyphotic posture, posterior tilting of pelvis and sacral sitting.

c. Leg length/seat to footplate length.
   (1) Measurement on the patient: from the bottom of the shoe (customary footwear) to just below the thigh in the popliteal fossa; when a seat cushion is used, the height must be subtracted from the patient's measurement.
   (2) Potential problems.
      (a) Excessive leg length will encourage sacral sitting and sliding forward in the chair.
      (b) Length that is too short will create uneven weight distribution on thigh and excessive weight on the ischial seat.

d. Seat height.
   (1) No patient measurement.
   (2) Chair measurement: minimum clearance between the floor and the footplate is 2 inches, measured from the lowest point on the bottom of the footplate.
   (3) Add 2 inches to the patient's leg length measurement.

e. Arm rest height (hanging elbow height).
   (1) Measurement on the patient: from the seat platform to just below the elbow held at 90 degrees with the shoulder in neutral position.
   (2) Chair measurement: add 1 inch to the patient's hanging elbow measurement.
   (3) Potential problems.
      (a) Armrests that are too high will cause shoulder elevation.
      (b) Armrests that are too low will encourage leaning forward.

f. Back height: Height will vary depending upon the amount of support the patient needs.

(1) Measurement on the patient: from the seat platform to the lower angle of the scapula, mid-scapula, top of shoulder, based on the degree of support desired.

(2) If the patient plans to use a seat cushion, the height of the cushion must be added to the patient's measurement.

(3) Potential problems.

(a) Added back height may increase difficulty in getting the chair into a car or van.

(b) Added back height may also prevent the patient from hooking onto the push handle for stabilization and weight relief; e.g., the patient with quadriplegia.

3. **Standard dimensions.** (See Table 11-1).

a. Custom-made wheelchairs add significantly to the cost of a wheelchair.

b. Whenever possible, patients should be matched to standardized chairs.

Wheelchair Training

Many first-time users require instruction in use and care of the wheelchair.

1. **Instruct in good sitting posture and pressure relief.**

a. Instruct in use of wheelchair cushion: care and maintenance, schedule of use (whenever sitting); limitations of cushion.

b. Instruct in periodic pressure reliefs: arm push-ups; weight shifts—leaning to one side, then other.

2. **Wheelchair propulsion.**

a. Instruct in manual wheelchair propulsion.

(1) Both arms on drive (push) wheels, one arm on drive wheel/one foot pulls diagonally across floor under chair (e.g., the patient with hemiplegia), or one arm (one-arm drive, both outer rims located on one side).

(2) Propulsion: forward/backward, flat surfaces, uneven surfaces.

Table 11-1 ➤ STANDARD WHEELCHAIR DIMENSIONS (IN INCHES)

CHAIR STYLE	SEAT WIDTH	SEAT DEPTH	SEAT HEIGHT
Adult	18	16	20
Narrow adult	16	16	20
Slim adult	14	16	20
Hemi/low seat			17.5
Junior	16	16	18.5
Child	14	11.5	18.75
Tiny tot	12	11.5	19.5

(3) Turning: pushing harder with one hand than other; sharp turning: pull one wheel backward while pushing other wheel forward.

(4) Negotiation of obstacles.

b. Power chair training: focus on driving skill and safety; instruct in use of switches (on/off, turns), joystick; maneuverability, safe stopping.

3. **Wheelchair management.**

a. Instruct in use of wheel locks (brakes), foot supports (foot plate, leg rest), elevation of leg rests, and arm rests.

b. Instruct in routine maintenance of wheelchair; normal cleaning and maintenance, power chair (battery) maintenance.

4. **Community mobility.**

a. Ramps.

(1) Ascending: forward lean of head and trunk, use shorter strokes; move hands quickly for propulsion.

(2) Descending ramps: grip hand rims loosely, control chair's descent; or descend in wheelie position (steep ramp).

b. Wheelies: instruct in how to "pop a wheelie" in order to negotiate curbs; the patient learns how to come up onto and balance on the rear wheels with the front casters off the ground (e.g., the patient with paraplegia).

(1) Practice maintaining balance point in wheelie position (therapist tips chair back into position).

(2) Practice moving into wheelie position: patient places hands well back on hand rims; then pulls (moves) them forward abruptly and forcefully. The head and trunk are moved forward to keep from going over backward. Use lightweight wheelchair to facilitate training.

(3) Balancing in wheelie position: chair tips further back when wheels are pushed forward; chair tips toward upright when wheels are pulled back.

(4) Practice curb ascent: place the front casters up on the curb, the patient then pushes rear wheels up curb; momentum used to assist.

(5) Practice curb descent: descending backwards with forward head and trunk lean; descending forwards in wheelie position.

c. Practice ascending/descending stairs: in wheelchair, on buttocks.

d. Instruct in how to fall safely, return to wheelchair.

e. Instruct in how to transfer into a car, place wheelchair inside car by pulling wheelchair behind the car seat, or to use a wheelchair lift (van-equipped).

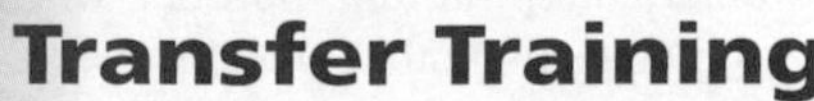

Transfer Training

Dependent Transfers

1. **General concepts:** Minimal or no active participation by patient.
2. **Dependent lift transfer (football transfer).**
   a. Wheelchair is positioned parallel to surface.
   b. Patient is flexed forward at hips in tucked position with hips and knees flexed.
   c. Therapist locks patient's tucked knees between legs; places one hand underbuttocks and one hand on transfer belt.
   d. Patient is rocked forward and lifted using a backward weight shift with therapist in a semisquat position.
   e. Therapist then pivots using small steps and gently lowers patient to support surface.
3. **Dependent stand-pivot transfer.** Similar to above, but patient's lower extremities are extended and in contact with floor.
4. **Hydraulic lift transfer.** Positioning and widening of base of device is critical to stability.

Assisted Transfers

1. **General Concepts.**
   a. Requires some participation by patient; levels of assistance include stand-by, minimal, moderate, or maximal assistance.
   b. Includes verbal cueing or manual assistance for lift, support, or balance control.
   c. Transfer belts, trapeze bars, overhead loops can be used to provide additional control.
2. **Assisted stand-pivot transfer.**
   a. Used for patients who are unable to stand independently and can bear some weight on lower extremities (e.g., patients with CVA, incomplete SCI, hip fracture/replacement).
   b. Wheelchair is placed parallel to surface (on the patient's sound or stronger side).
   c. Therapist can block out one or both of the patient's knees to provide stability; support can be added by placing both hands on the patient (on both buttocks, both on upper back, or one on buttock/one on upper back).
   d. Patient rocks forward and pushes up into standing.
   e. Therapist assists patient with forward weight shift and standing, pivoting toward chair, and controlled lowering toward the support surface.
   f. Variation: assisted squat-pivot transfer for patients who are unable to stand fully; e.g., with marked weakness both lower extremities.
3. **Assisted transfer using a transfer (sliding) board.**
   a. Used for patients with good sitting balance who can lift most but not all of weight of buttocks; e.g., patients with complete level C5 spinal cord injury (SCI).
   b. Wheelchair is placed parallel to surface.
   c. Patient moves forward in chair and board is placed well under buttocks.
   d. Patient performs transfer by doing a series of push-ups and lifts along board.
   e. Therapist assists in lift (hands on buttocks, on transfer belt, or one on buttock/one on belt).
   f. Care must be taken not to pinch fingers under board or drag/traumatize skin.
   g. Feet can remain on foot pedals or be positioned on the floor.
   h. Patients with complete level C6 SCI can be independent with transfer board on level surfaces.
4. **Push-up transfer (pop-over transfer).**
   a. Used for patients with good sitting balance who can lift buttocks clear of sitting surface; can be a progression in transfer training from using a transfer board.
   b. The patient with complete C7 SCI can be independent in transfers without a sliding board.
   c. The patient utilizes the head-hips relationship to successfully complete the transfer (movement of head in one direction results in movement of hips in the opposite direction/towards the support surface being transferred to).

Training

1. **Practice.**
   a. In and out of bed.
   b. In and out of wheelchair.
      (1) Level surfaces.
      (2) Unlevel surfaces: to floor.
   c. On and off toilet, tub seat.
   d. In and out of car.
2. **Instructions.**
   a. Inform patient about the transfer, as well as expectations for the patient.
   b. Synchronize actions using commands and counts.
   c. Reduce assistance as appropriate.

Environmental Considerations

Environmental Modification

1. **Purpose.**
   a. Assess degree of safety, function, and comfort of the patient in the home, community, and work environments.
   b. Provide recommendations to ensure a barrier-free environment, greatest level of functional independence.

2. **Standard adult wheelchair dimensions for environmental access.**
   a. Width: 24–26 inches from rim to rim.
   b. Length: 42–43 inches.
   c. Height (push handles to floor): 36 inches.
   d. Height (armrest to floor): 29–30 inches.
   e. Footrests may extend for very large people.
   f. 360 degrees turning space = 60 inches × 60 inches.
   g. 90 degrees turning space = minimum of 36 inches.
   h. Minimum clear width for doorways and halls = 32 inches; ideal is 36 inches.
   i. High forward reach = maximum of 48 inches from floor; low forward reach = a minimum of 15 inches from the floor.
   j. Side reach = maximum of 24 inches.

3. **Home.**
   a. Entrance: accessible; stairs with handrail, ramp, platform to allow for ease of door opening.
   b. Floors: nonskid surface, carpeting securely fastened; no scatter rugs.
   c. Furniture arrangement: should allow sufficient room to maneuver easily; e.g., with wheelchair, or ambulation with assistive device.
   d. Doors: thresholds should be flush or level (no doorsills); standard door width is 32 inches; outside door swing area requires a minimum of 18 inches for walkers and 26 inches for wheelchairs.
   e. Stairs: uniform riser heights (7 inches high) with a tread depth (a minimum of 11 inches); handrails, recommended height is 32 inches, $^1/_2$ to 2 inches in diameter; nonslip surface; well lighted; color code with warm colors (red, orange, yellow) if visual impairments exist.
   f. Bedroom: furniture arrangement for easy maneuverability; a minimum of 3 feet on side of bed for wheelchair transfers; firm mattress, stable bed, sufficient height to facilitate sit-to-stand transfers; phone accessibility; appropriate height for wall switches is 36–48 inches; outlets a minimum of 18 inches above the floorboard.
   g. Bathroom: optimal toilet seat height is 17–19 inches; tub seat, nonskid tub surface or mat; grab bars securely fastened; optimal height of horizontal grab bars is 33–36 inches.
   h. Kitchen: appropriate height of countertops, for wheelchair users no higher than 31 inches; counter depth of at least 24 inches; accessible equipment and storage areas.

4. **Community/workplace.**
   a. Steps: recommended height is 7–9 inches.
   b. Ramps: recommended ratio of slope to rise is 1:12 (for every inch of vertical rise, 12 inches of ramp is required); minimum of 36 inches wide, with nonslip surface; handrail waist high for ambulators (34–38 inches) and should extend 12 inches beyond the top and bottom of runs; ramp should have level landing at top and bottom.
   c. Parking (handicapped parking): parking space with adjacent 4-foot aisle for wheelchair maneuverability; accessible within a short distance of buildings; curb cutouts.
   d. Building entrance: accessible; accessible elevator.
   e. Access to public telephones, drinking fountains, bathrooms.
   f. Ergonomic assessment of immediate work area: appropriate lighting, temperature, seating surface, height and size of work counter.
   g. Public transportation: accessible.

Appendix A

Gerard Dybel

Ergonomics

1. **General concepts.**
   a. Refers to the relationships among the worker. The work that is done; the tasks and activities inherent in that work; the environment in which the work is performed; ergonomics uses scientific and engineering principles to improve the safety, efficiency, and quality of movement involved in work.
   b. Purpose: maintain the health and productivity of workers at an optimally safe level.
   c. Model of injury/illness prevention: worker behaviors attempt to balance the demands of work with the worker's capacity. Worker behavior in this balance is affected by administrative controls.
   d. Work demands: processes and tools, production levels, work schedules.
   e. Worker capacity: objective assessment of worker's current level of ability to perform the physical demands of a specific identified job.
   f. Administrative controls: changes in the way that work in a job is assigned or scheduled to reduce the magnitude, frequency, or duration of exposure to ergonomic risk factors.
2. **Hazard prevention and control.**
   a. Preferably controlled by the use of engineering interventions.
   b. The ergonomic program should focus on making the job fit the person.
   c. Engineering controls accomplish this by the design or modification of the work station, work methods, and tools to reduce exposure to awkward postures, repetitive motion, and excessive exertion.
3. **Personal Protective Equipment (PPE).**
   a. Can be used to address specific ergonomic stressors.
   b. These devices may include:
      (1) Gloves.
      (2) Protective guards.
      (3) Clothing for protection from the cold or exposure to chemicals.
   c. Braces, splints, and back support belts are considered to be part of the medical management program and are not PPE.
4. **Management Model:** (from APTA [2001] Guide to Physical Therapy Practice, 2nd ed. and Occupational Health Physical Therapy Guidelines
   a. Prevention of Work-Related Injury/Illness. Initial BOD11-99-25-71).
   b. Examination.
      (1) Complete history of the client company's injury/illness experience.
      (2) Ergonomic tests and measures examine:
         - Environment.
         - Site.
         - Tools.
         - Equipment.
         - Materials.
         - Machinery.
         - Physical demands.
         - Physical stressors.
         - Environmental conditions.
      (3) Individual worker tests and measures include:
         - Anthropometrics.
         - Worker's physical capacity.
         - Work and health habits.
   c. Evaluation.
      (1) Injury or illness data analysis.
      (2) Work analysis.
      (3) Evaluation of worker/workforce safety, behavior, and compliance.
   d. Diagnosis.
      (1) Identification of at-risk employees.
      (2) Identification of at-risk work processes/workstations.
      (3) Identification of solutions.
   e. Prognosis is related to preventing injury/illness and should include:
      (1) An estimate of anticipated goals for all interventions.
      (2) An estimate of expected outcomes for all interventions.
   f. Interventions.
      (1) Procedural interventions include:
         - Monitoring at-risk employees and work processes.
         - Ergonomics.
         - Education and training.
         - Health promotion.
         - Return-to-work case management.
         - Occupational health committee/team development.
      (2) Participatory interventions include:
         - Team involvement in work assignment.
         - Human resources management.
         - Labor relations.
         - Design and production standards.

5. Outcomes: generation, analysis, and interpretation of data related to injury/illness prevention and ergonomics.

Role of the Physical Therapist in Occupational Health

1. Examination of individuals.
   a. Work-related impairment.
   b. Functional limitation.
   c. Disability.
   d. Other health-related conditions which prevent individuals from performing their occupational pursuits in order to determine a diagnosis, prognosis, and intervention.

2. Integrate prevention and wellness programs in the workplace, consultation, screening, and education.

3. Physical therapist management of the acutely injured Worker. (From APTA. Occupational Health Physical Therapy Guidelines: Physical Therapist Management of the Acutely Injured Worker. BOD 03-01-17-56).
   a. Management of lost time and minimization of disability.
      (1) Optimize work performance and minimize the development of work-related occupational disability.
      (2) Effective and timely management of the injured worker is enhanced by participation in some form of productive duty and access to on-site or convenient off-site physical therapy services.
      (3) Based on physical work capacity assessment, employers are encouraged to make accommodations to normal duty or provide alternative or transitional duty work.
   b. Management of neuromusculoskeletal injury.
      (1) Diagnosis of the neuromusculoskeletal condition and application of interventions to specific systems and tissue affected by the injury.
      (2) Determination of safe work activity that will not compromise medical stability.
      (3) The design of safe, progressive rehabilitation programs based on the workers' job demands and within the functional and medical limitations.
      (4) Minimization of lost work time by means of aggressive clinical management and promotion of productive work.
   c. Facilitation of timely and appropriate referrals.
      (1) Referrals for necessary interventions are facilitated through constant monitoring of neuromusculoskeletal signs, symptoms, medical stability, and progress.
      (2) Injured workers are processed through the employer's health system working interdependently with physicians and other health-care providers.
   d. Minimization of injury/reinjury incident rate.
      (1) The physical therapist's role in minimizing injury recurrence is to make ergonomic recommendations for:
         • Work station design.
         • Work performance and worker training that may be specific to the worker's neuromusculoskeletal condition.
         • Providing early intervention to workers with potentially disabling neuromusculoskeletal signs or symptoms.
         • Participating in a comprehensive team for the timely dissemination of information, including physician, physical therapist, employer representative, safety management and injured worker.

4. Phases of physical therapy intervention.
   a. Admission to a specific phase of care is based on the physical therapy examination, evaluation, diagnosis, and prognosis of the worker's functional and neuromusculoskeletal status.
   b. Progression from one phase to the next is based on objective, functional tests and measurements. Duration of treatment is influenced by the level of physical activity required by the job if a reasonable accommodation for the job is not available.
      (1) Acute phase: immediate posttrauma, focuses on the control and reduction of localized inflammation, joint or soft tissue restriction, and stabilization and containment of the injury.
      (2) Postacute phase: involvement of the injured worker in more active/functional activities. Functional training to increase ability to perform physical tasks related to community and work reintegration.
      (3) Reconditioning phase: more vigorous therapeutic exercise that emphasizes daily functional and work activities and increased endurance.
      (4) Return-to-work phase: this phase is indicated for workers who have progressed satisfactorily through the reconditioning phase but are not ready to return to work because of physical, functional, behavioral, or vocational deficits. An objective functional capacity evaluation (FCE) may used as a criterion for entry into this phase.

Functional Capacity Evaluation (FCE)

(From APTA. Occupational Health Physical Therapy Guidelines: Evaluating Functional Capacity. BOD 11-01-07-11).

1. Purpose.
   a. Provide an objective measure of a patient's/client's safe functional abilities compared to the physical demands of work.

2. Uses of the FCE.
   a. Return-to-work and job placement decisions.
   b. Disability evaluation.
   c. Determination of work function with nonwork-related illness and injuries.
   d. Determination of function in nonoccupational settings.
   e. Intervention and treatment planning.
   f. Case management and case closure.

3. Definition.
   a. A detailed examination and evaluation that objectively measures the patient's/client's current level of function, primarily within the context of the demands on competitive employment.
   b. Measurements of the FCE are compared to the physical demands of a job or other functional activities, and are used to make return to work/activity decisions, disability determination, or to generate a rehabilitation plan.

4. Specific physical demand characteristics.
   a. Categories of work demands.
      (1) Sedentary.
      (2) Light.
      (3) Medium.
      (4) Heavy.
      (5) Very heavy.
   b. Frequency of work demands.
      (1) Never.
      (2) Occasional.
      (3) Frequent.
      (4) Constant.

5. Physical demands in the workplace.
   a. Physical abilities required to perform work tasks successfully.
   b. Physical demands include:
      (1) Work postures/positions.
      (2) Body movements.
      (3) Forces applied to the worker.
      (4) Repetition of the work tasks.

6. FCE protocols.
   a. A standard protocol includes tests and measures applied consistently to all patients/clients undergoing a functional capacity evaluation.
   b. A job-specific protocol includes tests and measures applied consistently to patient/client undergoing a functional capacity evaluation with reference to a specific, identified job.

Work Conditioning and Work Hardening Programs

(From APTA. Occupational Health Physical Therapy Guidelines: Work Conditioning and Work Hardening Programs. BOD 03-01-17-58)

1. Definitions.
   a. Work conditioning programs.
      (1) Intensive, work-related, goal-oriented conditioning programs.
      (2) Designed specifically to restore systemic neuromusculoskeletal functions, muscle performance, motor function, ROM, and cardiovascular/pulmonary functions.
   b. Work hardening programs.
      (1) Highly structured, goal-oriented, individualized intervention programs designed to return the patient/client to work.
      (2) Multidisciplinary programs that use real and simulated work activities designed to restore physical, behavioral, and vocational functions.

2. Program content.
   a. Work conditioning.
      (1) Requires work conditioning examination and evaluation.
      (2) Utilizes work conditioning and functional activities related to work.
      (3) Provide multihour sessions of up to 4 hours/day, 5 days/week, 8 weeks.
      (4) Addresses physical and functional needs provided by one discipline.
   b. Work hardening.
      (1) Requires work hardening examination and evaluation.
      (2) Utilizes real or simulated work activities.
      (3) Provided in multihour sessions of up to 8 hours/day, 5 days/week, 8 weeks.
      (4) Addresses physical, functional, behavioral, and vocational needs within a multidisciplinary model.

Manual Material Handling and Lifting Limits

1. Factors affecting "safe" load lifting.
   a. Biomechanical factors.
      (1) Greatest biomechanical stressors and the largest moments during lifting occur in the lumbar spine, specifically the L5-S1 disc.
      (2) Disc compressive forces, shear forces, and torsional forces are believed to be largely responsible for vertebral end-plate fractures, disc herniations, and nerve root irritation.
      (3) The weight of the load and the distance from the load to the base of the spine are significant contributors to lumbosacral compressive and shear forces when using either a squat or stooped lifting posture.
   b. Physiological factors.
      (1) The worker's ability to perform dynamic, repetitive lifting is limited by his or her maximal aerobic capacity.

(2) Repetitive lifting tasks could exceed the worker's normal energy capacities, which decrease strength and increase the risk of injury.
(3) Age, gender, and physical conditioning may affect a worker's ability to perform repetitive lifting.
(4) Lifting from floor to knuckle height requires greater whole-body work, although performing lifts above waist height requires greater shoulder and arm muscle work.

c. Psychophysical factors.
(1) The maximal acceptable weight of lift defines what a person can lift repeatedly for an extended period of time without excessive fatigue.
(2) The psychophysical approach provides a means of estimating the combined effects of biomechanical and physiological stressors on manual lifting.

d. Chair dimensions for seated work.
(1) Chair height: sufficient to allow the feet to be placed firmly on the floor or a foot support.
(2) Knee flexion angle is 90 degrees with the popliteal fold about 2–3 cm above the seat surface. If too low, there is excessive knee flexion, the spine is flexed, and the pelvis is posteriorly rotated. If too high, the feet do not reach the floor and there is excessive pressure on the back of the thighs.
(3) Chair length/depth: the seat pan should provide 10 cm clearance from the popliteal fossa to allow for leg movement and prevent pressure on the back of the knees.
(4) Seat pan slope: a backward slope of 5 degrees is suggested for normal, upright sitting.
(5) Arm rest height: the elbow should be flexed to 90 degrees and the shoulder should be in neutral position.

Guidelines for Seated Work

1. **Definition.**
   a. Sitting transfers body weight to supporting areas.
   (1) Seat pan through ischial tuberosities.
   (2) Backrest through soft tissues.
   (3) Armrests through forearms.
   (4) Floor.

   b. Sitting posture varies with the design of the chair and the task being performed.
   (1) Lumbar spine posture during sitting.
   (2) Pelvis rotates posteriorly and lumbar spine flattens when moving from standing to unsupported sitting.
   (3) Knee and hip angles control spinal posture during sitting, caused by the insertion of various muscles on the pelvis and legs.

   c. Lumbar disc pressure during sitting.
   (1) Compression forces measured at L3 disc: pressures measured with the subject standing are about 35% lower than the pressure measured when the subject is sitting without support.
   (2) Use of a lumbar support decreases lumbar disc pressure.
   (3) Backward inclination of the backrest from 90 degrees to 110 degrees results in decreased lumbar disc pressure.
   (4) Decreased disc pressure when arm rests were used.

Upper Extremity Work-Related Musculoskeletal Disorders (WRMSD)

1. **WRMSD Definition.**
   a. Disorders of the muscles, tendons, ligaments, joint cartilage, blood vessels, or spinal discs.
   b. Associated with exposure to known risk factors.
   (1) Excess force.
   (2) Repetition.
   (3) Awkward postures.
   (4) Vibration.
   (5) Temperatures.
   (6) Contact stresses.

   c. Possible relationship between onset and severity of WRMSD and performance of highly repetitive of forceful tasks.

2. **Common Upper Extremity WRMSD.**
   a. Carpal tunnel syndrome.
   b. Tendinitis.
   c. Tenosynovitis.
   d. Ganglion cysts.
   e. Bursitis.
   f. Myositis.
   g. Synovitis.
   h. Fibromyalgia.
   i. Osteoarthritis.
   j. Raynaud's syndrome.
   k. Complex regional pain syndrome (CRPS)/reflex sympathetic dystrophy (RSD).

chapter 12

Professional Roles & Management

WILLIAM FARINA

Institutional Types

Practice Environments

1. **Acute care (short-term hospital).**
   a. Treatment for a short-term illness or health problem.
   b. Average patient length of stay is <30 days. Usual length of stay is <7 days.
   c. Provider may be physician, physician assistant (PA), nurse, physical therapist (PT), etc.
   d. Rapid discharge for next level of care makes the PT's role in patient and family education and in discharge planning increasingly important.

2. **Primary care.**
   a. Basic or first-level health care.
   b. Provided by primary care physicians (PCPs), including family practice physicians, pediatricians, internists, and sometimes obstetric/gynecologic (OB/GYN) physician specialists.
   c. Provided on an outpatient basis.
   d. PTs support primary care teams through examination, evaluation, diagnosis, prognosis, and prevention of musculoskeletal and neuromuscular disorders.
   e. Often the PCP is the "gatekeeper" to other subspecialists, including physical therapy.

3. **Secondary care (specialized care).**
   a. Second-level medical services.
   b. Provided by medical specialists, such as cardiologists, urologists, and dermatologists, who do not have first contact with patients.
   c. This care often requires inpatient hospitalization or ambulatory same-day surgery such as hernia repair.

4. **Tertiary care (tertiary health care).**
   a. Highly specialized, technologically based medical services; e.g., heart, liver, or lung transplants, and other major surgical procedures.
   b. Provided by highly specialized physicians in a hospital setting.
   c. PTs respond to requests for consultation made by other health-care practitioners.

5. **Subacute care.**
   a. An intermediate level of health care for medically fragile patients too ill to be cared for at home.
   b. Provided by medical and nursing services as well as rehabilitative services; e.g., PT, occupational therapy (OT), and speech therapy (ST) at a higher level than is offered in a skilled nursing facility (SNF) on a regular basis.
   c. Provided within the hospital or SNF setting.

6. **Transitional care unit.**
   a. Hospital-based SNF.
   b. Care provided by medical, nursing, and rehabilitation services, including PT, OT, and ST on a daily basis.
   c. Patients are often discharged home, to assisted living facilities, or SNFs.

7. **Ambulatory care (outpatient care).**
   a. Includes outpatient preventative, diagnostic, and treatment services.
   b. Provided at medical offices, surgery centers, or outpatient clinics.
   c. Providers may be physicians, physician assistants (PAs), nurse practitioners, PTs, or others.

d. Less costly than inpatient care. Favored by managed-care plans.
e. Outpatient rehabilitation centers, PT clinics, outpatient satellites of institutions, or privately owned outpatient clinics.

8. Skilled nursing facility (extended care facility).
a. Free-standing or part of a hospital.
b. Care provided by continuous nursing, rehabilitation, and other health-care services on a daily basis.
c. Medicare defines "daily" as 7 days a week of skilled nursing and 5 days a week of skilled therapy.
d. Patients are not in an acute phase of illness, but require skilled care on an inpatient basis.
e. SNFs must be certified by Medicare and meet qualifications, including 24-hour nursing coverage, availability of PT, OT, and ST.

9. Acute rehabilitation hospital.
a. Facility that provides rehabilitation, social, and vocational services to disabled individuals to facilitate their return to maximal functional capacity.
b. Rehabilitation involves the coordinated services of medical, rehabilitative, social, educational, and vocational services for training or retraining.

10. Chronic care facility (long-term care facility).
a. Long-term care facility provides services to patients for 60 days or more.
b. Medical services provided to patients with permanent or residual disability caused by a nonreversible pathological health condition.
c. May require specialized care/rehabilitation.

11. Custodial care facility.
a. Patient care that is not medically required but necessary for the patient who is unable to care for him/herself.
b. Custodial care may involve medical or nonmedical services that do not seek a cure.
c. This type of care is usually not covered under managed-care plans.
d. Daily care is delivered by nonmedical support staff.

12. Hospice care.
a. Care available for dying patients and their families at home or inpatient settings.
b. Hospice team includes: nurses, social workers, chaplains, volunteers, and physicians. PT and OT services are optional.
c. Eligibility for reimbursement includes:
(1) Medicare eligibility.
(2) Certification by physician of terminal illness ($\leq$6 months of life).

13. Home health care.
a. Health care provided to individuals and their families in their homes.
b. Provided by a home health agency (HHA), which may be governmental, voluntary, or private; non-profit or for-profit.
c. Eligible patients include those who:
(1) Are homebound or have great difficulty leaving the home without assistance or an assistive device.
(2) Would experience a health risk leaving the home.
(3) Require skilled care from one of the following services: nursing, PT, OT, or ST.
(4) Have physician certification.
(5) Show potential for progress.
(6) Have more than housekeeping deficits.
d. Environmental safety is consideration of PT; e.g., proper lighting, securing of scatter rugs, handrails, wheelchair ramps.
e. Supplemental equipment may be necessary; e.g., raised toilet seats, grab bars, long-handled utensils, if delivered by a licensed durable medical equipment vendor to the home at the time of hospital discharge.
f. Adaptive equipment ordered in the home is not reimbursable, except for items such as wheelchairs, commodes, and hospital beds.
g. Substance abuse should be reported immediately to the physician.
h. Physical abuse should be communicated immediately and directly to the proper authorities; e.g., department of social service should be notified if child abuse is suspected.
i. The laws that mandate reporting of abuse of an elder, disabled individual, or minor may vary from state to state.

14. School system.
a. The PT serves as a consultant to teachers who work with students with disabilities in the classroom.
b. Major goal of PT treatment is the child's functioning in the school setting.
c. Recommendations are made for adaptive equipment to facilitate improved posture, head control, and function; e.g., using a computer, viewing a blackboard, improving mobility from class to class.

15. Private practice.
a. Entrepreneurial PTs who work for or own a free-standing, independent PT practice.
b. May accept all insurances with provider numbers.
c. Settings vary from sports physical therapy and orthopedic clinics, rehabilitation agencies, occupational health.
d. Must document every visit and complete reevaluations at least every 30 days for reimbursement purposes.

The United States Health-Care System

Organization

1. **Overview.**
   a. A group of decentralized subsystems that serve different populations.
   b. Overwhelmingly private ownership of health-care delivery.
   c. Relatively small federal and state governmental programs that work in conjunction with a large private sector, although the government pays for a large portion of these private sector services through Medicare and Medicaid reimbursement.
   d. Decentralization results in overlap in some areas and competition in others; therefore, health care is primarily a business that is market-driven, especially for patients covered by managed-care insurance.
      (1) Patients are viewed as consumers because of this economic focus.
      (2) Cost containment while maintaining quality of service is a delicate balancing act that is not always achieved.
   e. PCPs have increased significance as the first line for evaluation and intervention, and as the referral source for specialized and/or ancillary services.

2. **Health-care regulations.**
   a. Health care is a highly regulated industry, with most regulations mandated by law, both at the state and federal levels.
   b. Legally mandated regulations are set forth by the Center for Medicare and Medicaid Services (CMS), a division of U.S. Department of Health and Human Services.
      (1) CMS is the federal agency which develops rules and regulations pertaining to federal laws, specifically the Medicare and Medicaid programs.
      (2) Facilities that participate in Medicare and/or Medicaid programs are monitored regularly for compliance with CMS guidelines by federal and state surveyors.
      (3) Often, State Departments of Public Health monitor Medicare/Medicaid compliance of inpatient institutions, and "fiscal intermediaries" are contracted to monitor compliance of Medicare Part B regulations.
      (4) Facilities that repeatedly fail to meet CMS guidelines may lose their Medicare and/or Medicaid certification (e.g., "provider status").
   c. Standards related to safety are set forth and enforced by the Occupational Safety and Health Administration (OSHA), a division of the U.S. Department of Labor.
      (1) Structural standards and building codes are established and enforced by OSHA to ensure the safety of structures.
      (2) The safety of employees and consumers is regulated by OSHA standards for handling infectious materials and blood products, controlling blood-borne pathogens, operating machinery, and handling hazardous substances.
      (3) Material Safety Data Sheets are mandated by OSHA. These sheets give employees information about potentially hazardous materials in the workplace and how to protect themselves.
      (4) The blood-borne pathogen standard requires institutions to have processes in place to reduce the risk of exposure to blood-borne pathogens. This includes a written safety plan, employee training, and proper disposal practices.
      (5) Other OSHA standards cover x-ray safety, electrical and fire safety, and provide for the provision of personal protective equipment (PPE).
   d. Individual states develop their own requirements with state agencies to enforce these regulations. State accreditation to obtain licensure for a health-care facility is mandatory.
   e. Local or county entities also develop regulations pertaining to health-care institutions, (i.e., physical plant safety features such as fire, elevator, and boiler regulations).

3. **Voluntary accreditation.**
   a. Voluntary accreditation and self-imposed compliance with established standards is sought by most health-care organizations.
   b. Accreditation is a status awarded for compliance with standards and regulations, promulgated by the specific accrediting agency.
   c. Accreditation ensures the public that a health-care facility is adequately equipped, meets high standards for patient care, and has qualified professionals and competent staff.
   d. Accreditation affirms the competence of practitioners and the quality of health-care facilities and organizations.
   e. Although national accreditation through an accrediting agency is voluntary, it is mandatory for most

third-party reimbursement to meet eligibility requirements for federal government grants and contracts.
f. CMS and many states accept certain national accreditations as meeting their respective requirements for participation in the Medicare and Medicaid programs and for a license to operate.

4. Voluntary accrediting agencies.
a. Joint Commission on the Accreditation of Health Care Organizations (JCAHO).
(1) The voluntary agency that accredits health-care facilities according to JCAHO established standards and conditions.
(2) JCAHO accredits hospitals, SNFs, home health agencies, preferred provider organizations (PPOs), rehabilitation facilities, health maintenance organizations (HMOs), behavioral health (including mental health and chemical dependency facilities, ambulatory clinics, physician's networks, hospice care, long-term care facilities, and others).
b. Commission on Accreditation of Rehabilitation Facilities (CARF): the voluntary agency that accredits free-standing rehabilitation facilities and the rehabilitative programs of larger hospital systems in the areas of behavioral health, employment (work hardening) and community support services, and medical rehabilitation (spinal cord injury, chronic pain).
c. Accreditation Council for Services for Mentally Retarded and Other Developmentally Disabled Persons (AC-MRDD): a voluntary agency that accredits programs or agencies serving persons with developmental disabilities.
d. Outpatient centers for comprehensive rehabilitation can be accredited by JCAHO, CARF, and/or AC-MRDD.
e. National League for Nursing/American Public Health Association (NLN/APHA): a voluntary agency that accredits home health and community nursing agencies offering nursing and other health services outside hospitals, extended-care facilities, and nursing homes.
f. Some accreditation bodies may perform unannounced or unscheduled site surveys to ensure ongoing compliance.

5. Accreditation process.
a. Accreditation is initiated by the organization that submits an application for review, followed by a survey conducted by the accrediting agency.
b. A self-study or self-assessment is conducted to examine the organization based on the accrediting agency's standards.
c. An onsite review is conducted with an individual reviewer or surveyor, or a team that visits the organization.
d. The accreditation and reaccreditation processes involve all staff. Tasks include document preparation, hosting on site-visit teams, and interviews with accreditors.
e. Once accredited, the organization undergoes periodic review, typically every 3 years.
f. Some accrediting bodies may perform unannounced or unscheduled site surveys to ensure ongoing compliance.

Reimbursement/Third-Party Payers for Health-Care Services

1. Medicare.
a. Administered by federal government CMS, through the extension of Title XVIII of the Social Security Act, 1965.
b. Provides medical coverage and health-care services to individuals:
(1) ≥65 years.
(2) With permanent kidney failure or other long-term disabilities at <65 years.
c. Social Security Amendment of 1983.
(1) Established Medicare's prospective payment system.
(a) Based on diagnostic-related groups (DRGs).
(1) Classification system that places patients into disease categories or groups.
(2) Basis for Medicare's prospective payment system.
(b) Hospital paid a specific amount per diagnosis, regardless of the length of stay, number of services provided, or tests performed.
d. Medicare Part A benefits.
(1) Hospital insurance, that covers:
(a) Inpatient hospital care.
(1) Limits number of hospital days.
(b) Skilled nursing facilities—first 100 days.
(c) HHA.
(d) Hospice care.
(2) Provides basic protection against the cost of health care.
(3) Does not cover all medical expenses or the cost of long-term care.
(4) Provides coverage for patients who have been on Social Security disability for 24 months.
(5) Annual deductible fees paid by the patient.
e. Medicare Part B.
(1) Medical insurance that covers:
(a) Physician visits.
(b) Outpatient laboratory tests and x-rays.
(c) Ambulance transportation.
(d) Outpatient physical and occupational therapy services (hospital and private practice).
(e) Home health care provided by a PT in independent practice (PTIP).

(f) Durable medical equipment (e.g., wheelchairs, canes, walkers) determined to be "medically necessary."
(g) Medical supplies not covered by hospital insurance.
(h) Residents of long-term care facilities.
(2) Each patient must pay a monthly premium.
(3) PT treatment does not need to be given on a daily basis.
(4) The physician responsible for the care of the patient referred for PT must "certify" the plan of care.
(5) Only PT care that is considered to be "skilled," "necessary" and "certified" by the referring physician will be reimbursed by Medicare.

2. Medicaid.
a. A joint state and federal program mandated by Title XIX of the Social Security Act.
b. Provides health-care services to the poor, elderly, and disabled who do not receive Medicare, regardless of age.
c. Benefits vary from state to state.
d. Preauthorization is needed by a physician before treatment can begin.
e. Individual states can determine the scope, duration, and amount of services provided.

3. Worker's compensation.
a. Regulated by state statutes and administered by private insurers, self-insured employers, or other agencies in some states.
b. Provides health care for individuals injured on the job.
c. Some states limit the number of visits per diagnosis, and/or require a preapproval process for reimbursement.
d. Other states require that the total number of visits, total number of weeks (duration), and number of treatments per week (frequency) to be usual, customary, and reasonable.
e. Employers only contribute to the fund.
(1) All large employers (≥10 employees) or high-risk employers must contribute to Worker's Compensation.

4. Private health insurance.
a. Includes commercial insurance, fee-for-service or traditional indemnity plans, or employers who are self-insured.
b. Patient has freedom to choose his/her providers.
c. Preauthorization may not be needed.
d. The number of PT visits should be usual, customary, and reasonable, which are often defined contractually in the insurance policy.

5. Managed health-care systems.
a. Third-party payers direct patients to certain providers and monitor services in order to avoid excessive and inappropriate treatment and limit access.
(1) Third-party payers frequently use gatekeepers (usually the PCP) to manage access to certain providers, including PT.
(2) Use techniques as preadmission certification, concurrent reviews, financial incentives, or penalties.
(3) Goal is to contain costs and ensure favorable patient outcomes.
b. HMO.
(1) A form of managed care that provides a broad spectrum of health services to individuals and families for a preset amount of money.
(2) Employers contract for these services as a benefit to their employees.
(3) Employees may pay a small fee per visit (copay); e.g., $20/visit.
(4) Patients are locked into use of the system of member health-care providers and affiliating facilities.
(5) Some HMOs allow patients to seek care "out of network," but at a higher or additional cost to the patient.
(6) PCPs chosen by individuals act as gate-keepers for medical care beyond their scope of practice.
(a) Must authorize PT services before they can be provided.
(7) Total number of visits per diagnosis is limited.
(8) Types of HMOs:
(a) Individual Practice Associations (IPAs).
(1) Physician groups contract independently with the HMO.
(2) Physicians work out of their own offices instead of a central facility.
(b) Prepaid Group Plan (PGP).
(a) Physicians practice out of a central location.
c. PPO.
(1) A group of providers, usually physicians or hospitals, which offer health-care services as an entity to employers.
(2) Providers discount their fees to attract patients.
(3) Patients are not locked into PPO providers, but receive financial incentives to use services through the PPO network.
(4) An employer can offer its employees a traditional health-care plan, HMO, or PPO.
(5) Preauthorization is needed before services can be provided.
d. Both HMOs and PPOs contain one or more of the following elements:
(1) Capitation: a system whereby providers are paid a certain amount per case, no matter how many visits are rendered.
(2) Copayment: insured's charge for the covered service.
(a) Made at the time of service.
(b) Predetermined amount.

(3) Coinsurance: insured's share of the cost of the covered service.
   (a) Expressed as a percentage; e.g., 80% paid by insurance company and 20% paid by insured.
(4) The provider is at financial risk if services are overutilized. This is called "shared-risk."

6. Health savings accounts.

a. Tax-free savings account that can be used to pay for health-related expenses and retiree health expenses.
b. Must have a High Deductible Health Plan, which is an insurance product that covers catastrophic health occurrences.

7. Personal payment and free care.

a. Individuals without health insurance must personally pay for all medical care.
b. Individuals who cannot pay for health care can receive pro bono, or free, care through philanthropic donations and services.
c. Many states have programs that offset some of the expense of providing free care by relying on other not-for-profit organizations.

8. Restructuring the health-care system.

a. Cost containment created incentives for health-care providers and hospitals to control both cost and utilization of inpatient services by:
   (1) Reducing average length of hospital stay.
   (2) Reducing routine and/or unnecessary diagnostic testing and treatment.
   (3) Increasing of use of outpatient diagnostic testing and treatment.
   (4) Increasing of utilization of home care and skilled long-term care.

9. Health insurance and portability accountability act (HIPAA).

a. Elements of the act.
   (1) Standards and safeguards to assure an individual's right to continuity in health care.
   (2) Privacy and security of health-care records.
   (3) Portability of health insurance.
b. HIPAA privacy rule.
   (1) Patient confidentiality is maintained in all oral, written, and electronic forms.
   (2) Technical, administrative, and physical safeguards for privacy.
   (3) All individuals must be informed of a facility's privacy policies.
   (4) Written consent must be obtained before any personal health information is disclosed or used for other purposes.
      (a) Exemptions to written consent may be made in emergencies or if delay will prevent timely care.
      (b) If language barriers preclude signed consent in emergent or crucial situations, treatment may commence if the physician believes that consent is implied.
   (5) Prior to discussion of a person's status with a family member or other providers, the person may grant permission or object.
      (a) Providers can use clinical judgment to decide whether to discuss a case if the person cannot give permission, or even if there is an objection.
         (1) Documentation for this decision is essential.
   (6) All information disclosed must be the minimum needed for the immediate purpose.
c. Practice implications.
   (1) Physical identifiability of patients must be reduced.
   (2) Charts and other documentation must be stored out of public view and secured.
   (3) Any information stored or transmitted by computers must be safeguarded.
   (4) Faxes must be sent with cover sheets on dedicated lines to secure locations.
   (5) All e-mails should be password-protected.
   (6) All conversations regarding a person's health status must occur in private areas with minimal disclosure.
   (7) Cover sheets should be used on clipboards that contain patient paperwork.
   (8) Treatment may be provided in groups or open clinics. Discussions about these treatments should be done quietly and in a private space.
   (9) There is no guarantee of 100% confidentiality. Reasonable and vigilant safeguards are required.
   (10) HIPAA does not override state laws with more restrictive privacy policies, and defers to state laws regarding minors.
d. Patient rights.
   (1) An individual can access all of their medical records.
      (a) Providers have 30–60 days to respond.
      (b) A reasonable charge can be imposed for copying.
   (2) An individual has the right to request that information in their record be amended.
      (a) The provider may refuse, but must provide a rationale.
      (b) The provider may comply and provide a reason for amending the record. Original documentation is not removed.

Defensible Documentation

1. The International Classification of Functioning, Disability, and Health Resources (ICF) Model.

a. Developed by the World Health Organization (WHO) and endorsed by the American Physical

Therapy Association (APTA), the World Confederation for Physical Therapy, and other international organizations.

b. The ICF model identifies dimensions of functioning (Body Functions and Body Structures, Activities, Participation) and dimensions of disability (impairments, activity limitations, participation restrictions). See Box 12-1 for complete definitions.

c. The ICF model serves as a platform for communication among medical personnel, patients, and their family/caregivers.

d. The ICF model serves as a platform for choosing and comparing interventions.

e. The ICF model uses a unified, standard language and framework and permits documentation of functioning and disability as a multidimensional phenomena experienced at the level of the body, the person, and society.

f. The ICF model represents a shift away from the medical model that focuses on the condition or the disease affecting the individual.

Box 12-1 ➤ TERMINOLOGY: FUNCTIONING, DISABILITY, AND HEALTH

Health condition is an umbrella term for disease, disorder, injury, or trauma, and may also include other circumstances, such as aging, stress, congenital anomaly, or genetic predisposition. It may also include information about pathogeneses and/or etiology.

Body Functions are physiological functions of body systems (including psychological functions).

Body Structures are anatomical parts of the body such as organs, limbs, and their components.

Impairments are the problems in body function or structure, such as a significant deviation or loss.

Activity is the execution of a task or action by an individual.

Participation is involvement in a life situation.

Activity Limitations are difficulties an individual may have in executing activities.

Participation Restrictions are problems an individual may experience in involvement in life situations.

Contextual Factors represent the entire background of an individual's life and living situation.

- **Environmental Factors** make up the physical, social, and attitudinal environment in which people live and conduct their lives, including social attitudes, architectural characteristics, legal, and social structures.
- **Personal Factors** are the particular background of an individual's life, including gender, age, coping styles, social background, education, profession, past and current experience, overall behavior pattern, character, and other factors that influence how disability is experienced by an individual.

Performance describes what an individual does in his or her current environment.

Capacity describes an individual's ability to execute a task or an action (highest probable level of functioning in a given domain at a given moment).

From: The World Health Organization. International Classification of Functioning, Disability, and Health Resources (ICF). World Health Organization, Geneva, 2002. http://www.who.int/classifications/en/

2. Outcome measures organized by the International Classification of Functioning, Disability, and Health (ICF) categories.

a. Physical therapists select tests and measures as a means to:
   (1) Identify and characterize signs and symptoms of pathology/pathophysiology, impairments, functioning and disability.
   (2) Establish a diagnosis and prognosis, select interventions and to document changes in patient/client status.
   (3) Monitor outcomes, document end points of care, and ensure appropriate and timely discharge.

b. Documentation is enhanced by using measurements with demonstrated reliability and validity.

c. Appendix E presents outcome measures which meet these requirements, organized by ICF categories.

3. Medical records.

a. Complete, timely, and accurate documentation is essential for:
   (1) Patient safety.
   (2) Accurate communication between health-care providers.
   (3) Compliance with federal and state regulations.
   (4) Appropriate utilization for third-party payers.
   (5) Historical record for potential legal situations.

b. General guidelines for documentation.
   (1) All documentation must comply with all applicable state, federal, and regulatory agency laws and regulations.
   (2) Compliance with Medicare guidelines and any other guidelines required by the local insurance carrier to ensure reimbursement.
   (3) Patient's right to privacy must always be respected and protected.
   (4) Release of any medical information must be authorized by the patient.
   (5) Records must be kept in a safe and secure place for a certain number of years (varies from state to state; usually 7 years).

c. Basic principles of documentation (see Guide to Physical Therapist Practice, APTA).
   (1) Documentation should be consistent with Guidelines for Physical Therapy Documentation, APTA.
   (2) All documents must be legible.
   (3) Only medically approved abbreviations or symbols can be used.
   (4) Mistakes should be crossed out with a single line through the error, and then initialed and dated by the therapist.
   (5) White-out material should never be used to correct text in a medical record.
   (6) Informed consent for treatment must only be given by a competent adult.

CHAPTER 12

(7) Noncompetent adults or minors must have a parent or legal guardian give written consent/proxy.
(8) Document each episode of treatment.
(9) Patient name and some other unique identifier should be on each page.
(10) Date each entry (some payers require length of time per visit), particularly Medicare and Medicaid.
(11) Sign each entry with first and last names and professional designation.
(12) Record significant events; e.g., phone conversations with the physician or nurse.
(13) Document treatment rendered in objective, measurable, and functional terms.
(14) Document patient's response to treatment.
(15) When goals and outcomes are reached, complete a discharge plan.

d. Progress notes.
(1) Document specific treatment, equipment provided; include signature of therapist who provides care.
(2) Document patient response to treatment, functional progress, goals achieved, revision of goals, and treatment plan modifications.
(3) Interim progress notes can be written by:
(a) PT.
(b) Physical therapist assistant (PTA).
(c) Student (PT or PTA) notes must be cosigned by supervising therapist.

e. Reevaluation/summary progress report.
(1) Completed minimally every 30 days for all Medicare patients; includes:
(a) Restatement of initial problem.
(b) Length of time patient has been treated.
(c) Progress or regression since last summary or initial evaluation.
(d) Rationale for continued care.
(e) Revision of goals and outcomes.
(f) Revision of plan of care.
(g) Changes documented are stated in behavioral, objective, measurable, and (ROM) functional terms; e.g., range of motion, strength, sitting tolerance.
(2) Must be written by a PT.
(a) PT students can complete if cosigned by supervising therapist.

f. Discharge summary includes:
(1) Restatement of initial problem.
(2) Length of time the patient has been treated.
(3) Progress since initial evaluation.
(4) Patient progress toward goal and outcome achievement.
(5) Reason for discharge.
(6) Must be written by a PT.
(a) PT students can complete if cosigned by supervising therapist.

g. Discharge plan.
(1) Referrals, written or verbal, related to patient's continued care.
(a) Additional services.
(b) Type of supervision the patient will require.
(c) Home care.
(d) Family intervention.
(e) Patient and family education requirements.
(f) Written home exercise program (HEP).
(g) List of equipment ordered, vendor's name, and delivery date.
(h) Social and community needs of the patient.
(i) Date of discharge.
(j) A PT should discharge a patient from PT treatment when maximum benefit is reached.
(k) Identifies needs of patient after discharge from a facility.
(1) Preferable setting for discharge.
(2) Must be written by a PT.
(a) PT students can complete if cosigned by supervising therapist.

h. Advance directives.
(1) A legal document which delineates a patient's wishes for future medical care or no medical care.
(2) Are implemented if the patient is cognitively impaired.
(3) Can include living wills and durable power of attorney.

4. Common reasons for payment denials.

a. Incomplete/insufficient documentation. Documentation that is submitted without required documentation elements may cause a denial of payment.
b. Medically unnecessary. Poor documentation which does not fully explain the reasons for therapeutic interventions may result in denial of payment.
c. Incorrect coding: Failure to document the proper CPT, World Health Organization's International Classification of Diseases, 9th Revision, Clinical Modification (ICD-9-CM 2001) or other diagnosis or treatment codes can result in denial of payment.
d. Pay for performance. As pay for performance programs (payment based on improved functional outcomes) grow, poor documentation may result in reduced payments for services.

Elements of Patient/Client Management

1. Initial examination/evaluation/diagnosis/prognosis.

a. The PT performs an initial examination and evaluation to establish a diagnosis and prognosis prior to intervention.
b. The PT examination:
(1) Identifies the PT needs of the patient or client.
(2) Incorporates appropriate tests and measures to facilitate outcome measurement.

(3) Produces data that are sufficient to allow evaluation, diagnosis, prognosis, and the establishment of a plan of care.
(4) May result in recommendations for additional services to meet the needs of the patient or client.
(5) Used to determine proper diagnosis and treatment coding.

2. Examination.
a. History.
(1) Patient's name, age, race, and sex.
(2) Chief complaint and risk factors, relevance for PT intervention, if applicable.
(3) Referral source.
(4) Pertinent diagnosis and medical history.
(5) Demographic characteristics, including pertinent psychological, social, cultural, and environmental factors.
(6) Concurrent medical services provided.
(7) Pertinent problems.
(8) Statement describing patient's understanding of problem.
(9) Goals of the patient and/or patient's family.
b. Objective findings/systems review.
(1) Physiologic and anatomic status.
(a) Cognitive status, alertness, judgment, communication.
(b) Neurological status: pain, sensation, reflexes, balance, motor function, etc.
(c) Musculoskeletal: joint range of motion, strength, posture, etc.
(d) Cardiovascular: vital signs, endurance, etc.
(e) Integumentary.
(2) Functional status: mobility, transfers, activities of daily living (ADLs), work, school, or athletic performance, etc.
(3) Communication ability, affect, cognition, language, and learning style.

3. Evaluation.
a. Analysis of current impairments and effect on function.
b. Analysis of prolonged impairment, functional limitation, and disability.
c. Analysis of living environment, potential discharge destination, and social supports.

4. Diagnosis.
a. Encompasses a cluster of signs, symptoms, syndromes, or categories.
b. Guides therapist in determining appropriate interventions strategy.
c. Guides therapist in referring patient/client to an appropriate practitioner for services outside the scope of PT.

5. Prognosis.
a. Includes predicted optimal level of improvement in function and amount of time needed to reach that level.
b. Can also predict levels of improvement at various intervals during the course of therapy.

6. Plan of care.
a. The PT establishes a plan of care for the patient/client based on the examination, evaluation, diagnosis, prognosis, anticipated goals, and expected outcomes of the planned interventions for identified impairments, functional limitations, and disabilities.
b. The PT, in consultation with appropriate disciplines, plans for discharge of the patient/client, taking into consideration achievement of anticipated goals and expected outcomes, and provides for appropriate follow-up or referral.
c. The PT also addresses risk reduction, prevention, impact on societal resources, and patient/client satisfaction.
d. Identifies realistic long-term and short-term goals and expected functional outcomes.
(1) Goals address impairment, functional limitations, and/or the prevention of additional problems.
(2) Goals should address:
(a) Who will participate in the activity?
(b) A detailed description of the activity.
(c) The connection of the activity to a specific function.
(d) A specific measure for success.
(e) A time measure.

7. Intervention.
a. The PT provides, or directs, and supervises the PT intervention consistent with the results of the examination, evaluation, diagnosis, prognosis, and plan of care.
b. The intervention is:
(1) Provided under the ongoing direct care or supervision of the PT.
(2) Provided in such a way that delegated responsibilities are commensurate with the qualifications and the legal limitations of the PT support and professional personnel involved in the intervention.
(3) Altered in accordance with changes in response or status.
(4) Provided at a level that is consistent with current PT practice.
(5) Interdisciplinary when necessary to meet the needs of the patient or client.
c. Documentation of the intervention is:
(1) Dated and appropriately authenticated by the PT or, when permissible by law, by the PTA, or both.

8. Reexamination.
a. The PT reexamines the patient/client as necessary during an episode of care to evaluate progress or change in patient/client status, and modifies the plan of care accordingly or discontinues PT services.

b. The PT reexamination:
   (1) Identifies ongoing patient/client needs.
   (2) May result in recommendations for additional services, discharge, or discontinuation of PT needs.

9. **Discharge/discontinuation of intervention.**
   a. The PT discharges the patient/client from PT services when the anticipated goals or expected outcomes for the patient/client have been achieved.
   b. The PT discontinues intervention when the patient/client is unable to continue to progress toward goals or when the PT determines that the patient/ client will no longer benefit from PT.
   c. Discharge:
      (1) Occurs at the end of an episode of care, and is the end of PT services provided during that episode.
   d. Discontinuation:
      (1) Also occurs when the patient/client, caregiver, or legal guardian declines to continue intervention.

10. **Successful documentation practices.**
   a. Incorporate evidence-based practice principles. Use standard tests and measures that are valid and reliable, and select interventions based on research and practice.
   b. Demonstrate progress in specific and functional terms.
   c. Document medical necessity and reasons for skilled care.
   d. Document to stand up in a court of law. Document fully, and limit the use of jargon and obscure abbreviations. Sign and date all entries. Be factual and objective.

Management & Legal Issues

Human Resources

1. Interview.
   a. Performed by supervisor, director, and also possibly a member of the human resources department.
   b. Purpose is to meet with prospective employee.
      (1) Exchange questions and answers to obtain enough information to make an informed decision.
      (2) Questions asked are informational to encourage discussion rather than questions that require "yes or no" answers.
      (3) No questions may be asked about a person's age, religion, race, marital status, politics, national origin, or number of children.
      (4) Information regarding academic record, educational program, or references cannot be obtained without consent.
      (5) Many employers will require a criminal background check that requires the consent of the applicant to pursue.
      (6) Interviewer provides information about:
         (a) Advantages and disadvantages of the organization.
         (b) Benefits available.
         (c) Work hours.
         (d) Vacation, sick, and personal time.
         (e) Salary range.
         (f) Job description.
   c. Employers look for the following information in an interview.
      (1) Decision-making style.
      (2) Communications skills.
      (3) Interpersonal skills: poise, tact, ability to work in groups.
      (4) Leadership.
      (5) Achievement record, and relevant employment experience.
      (6) Sense of personal direction.
   d. Documents reviewed for employment:
      (1) Job application: completeness, attention to detail.
      (2) Previous employment experience.
      (3) Transcript from educational institution (especially for new graduates): grade point average and courses taken may be important in interview process.
      (4) Résumé: a brief written summary that highlights personal, educational, and professional qualifications and experience.
      (5) References.
         (a) Professional: former employers, clinical supervisors, faculty.
         (b) Character: family, friend, clergy.

2. **Job descriptions.**
   a. General summary of responsibilities.
      (1) Provides overview of position including supervisor relationships.

b. Specific job responsibilities.
   (1) Identifies the specific responsibilities of the position.
   (2) Establishes performance standards.
   (3) Establishes skilled and nonskilled requirements of job.
   (4) Formalizes basic performance expectations by describing duties in detail.
   (5) Establishes degree of decision-making authority and autonomy.
   (6) Organizational and supervisory relationships of position.
      (a) Position title.
      (b) Department division.
      (c) Title of position's supervisor.
c. Job specifications.
   (1) Educational requirements; e.g., graduate from accredited PT program.
   (2) State licensure.
   (3) Previous experience requirements.
   (4) Essential job functions or specific physical and mental demands of position.
      (a) Lifting requirements.
      (b) Transferring requirements.
      (c) Ambulatory or positioning requirements.
      (d) Proficiency in reading/writing/comprehension.
      (e) Maintaining static postures: performing therapeutic procedures for several minutes.
   (5) Ability to plan and organize time, and other work habits.
   (6) Problem-solving skills.

3. Performance appraisal.

a. Assesses an employee's performance in relation to performance expectations established with objective criteria.
b. Written report and discussed verbally.
c. Frequency can be 3–6 months or annually.
d. Correlates to job description and goals of the organization.
e. Improves communication between the employee and employer.
f. Feedback should be immediate, specific, and communicated directly.
g. Outcomes of performance appraisals can be motivational and used as a reward system; e.g., raises, bonuses, promotions. May also identify performance issues and areas for improvement.
h. Examples of methods of review:
   (1) Essay appraisal: short paragraph on strengths and weaknesses.
   (2) Performance criteria-based method: based on functional job description using a weighted rating scale (most important task gets highest rating); e.g., patient evaluation, weighted average of 5, and personal appearance 2.

4. Unions.

a. Organized group of workers with the same goals and objectives.
b. Provides collective bargaining when negotiating work contracts.
   (1) Salaries.
   (2) Fringe benefits.
   (3) Hours of work.
   (4) Conditions of work site.
c. Mediates grievances due to labor disputes, disciplinary problems, etc.

5. Policy and procedure manual.

a. Provides extensive information on what shall be done and how it shall be done in a PT department.
b. Required by JCAHO, Commission on Accreditation of Rehabilitation Facilities (CARF), and other accrediting agencies. Often required by other state regulatory bodies, such as state boards of public health.
c. Policies are broad statements that guide in decision making. They may include:
   (1) Scope of service.
      (a) Mission and philosophy statement.
      (b) Identifies the types of services provided, hours available, referral requirements (if applicable), staffing, and other general information about the service.
   (2) Operational policies.
      (a) Billing policies.
      (b) Referral policies (if appropriate).
      (c) Medical record management.
      (d) Quality assurance and improvement activities.
      (e) Other applicable clinical policies.
   (3) Human resources policies.
      (a) Vacation: paid time off; varies according to length of employment, seniority, or other criteria.
      (b) Introductory period (also called probationary period).
      (c) Job descriptions and performance appraisal policies.
      (d) Time off, leave of absence, sabbaticals.
         (1) Military service.
         (2) Maternity leave.
         (3) Medical leave.
         (4) Jury duty.
      (e) Dress code.
d. Procedures: specific guides to job behaviors for all departmental personnel, visitors, and patients that standardize activities with a high level of risk.
   (1) Safety and emergency procedures.
   (2) Equipment management, cleaning, maintaining, training requirements, safety inspections.
   (3) Hazardous waste management.
   (4) Disciplinary procedures.

(a) Manager presents problem in clear and concise terms, and specifically references the problem to the job description and expectations.
(b) Discussion is on performance discrepancy.
(c) Employee is given chance to respond.
(d) Manager presents action to be taken and why.
(e) Follow-up date for reevaluation is set.
(f) Consequences of noncompliance are established.
(g) Documentation of meeting is objective.

6. Staff motivation.

a. Sustains individual behavior toward attainment of an objective or goal by providing:
  (1) Challenging work, varied treatment assignments with opportunity to receive feedback regarding performance.
  (2) Good working conditions.
    (a) Essential equipment should be available for proper patient care.
  (3) Recognition of performance (praise or positive feedback, salary, bonuses, raises, and/or promotions).
  (4) Enhanced opportunity to achieve job-related goals.
    (a) Outline of policies.
    (b) Development of a clear job description.
    (c) Outline job responsibilities.
  (5) Concern as a supervisor, in resolving work-related problems.
  (6) Acknowledgment of the contributions of the staff toward realization of the mission, and scope of the service and/or institution.
  (7) Fair compensation based on market factors and required qualifications, while ensuring equity among the staff of the department/service.
  (8) Consultation with supervisor and involved staff member regarding problems that affect his or her employment.
  (9) Realistic job expectations.
    (a) Supervisor should avoid promising more than can be delivered; e.g., promising a promotion to a senior position when no budget has been approved.

7. Continuing education.

a. Ongoing educational program activities.
  (1) Enhances clinical knowledge.
  (2) Exposes therapist to new techniques and technology.
b. Educational programs may be one day, a weekend, or one week.
c. Employer should support and may subsidize a staff member's attendance, promoting professional and educational development.

8. Meetings.

a. Staff meeting.
  (1) Regularly held departmental meetings with a specific agenda set in advance.
  (2) Purpose is to discuss department or hospital/management business, state or national PT issues, and educate staff members.
  (3) Agendas are predetermined to ensure that the objectives and purpose of the meeting are clear.
b. Supervisory meeting.
  (1) Supervisor and staff meet regularly.
    (a) To discuss patient-care issues.
  (2) One-on-one meeting designed to meet the needs of the staff member.
c. Team meeting.
  (1) Usually scheduled at least weekly.
  (2) Interdisciplinary (MDs, nurses, PTs, OTs, social services, etc.) to improve communication between all staff.
  (3) Purpose is to:
    (a) Discuss and coordinate patient care services.
    (b) Set goals and outcomes for individual patients.
    (c) Discuss goal/outcome achievement necessary for discharge.
    (d) Discuss discharge plans including destination, equipment needs, home-care services, etc.
d. Strategic planning.
  (1) Organizational planning process for goal achievement and future goals.
    (a) Based on the organization's mission and philosophy statement.
    (b) Used for developing plans for implementation to achieve identified goals.
  (2) Results of strategic planning process summarized in strategic plan.
    (a) Provides focused direction so goals of organization are achieved.
    (b) Identifies individuals responsible to develop and carry out the plan; e.g., staff members, department director sets the timeline, and the expected outcomes.
    (c) Informs external parties about organization.
    (d) Goals are time related; e.g., 1-year, 3-year, or 5-year plans.
    (e) Methodology for evaluating the progress of the plan should be developed as part of the plan.
    (f) Analysis of progress toward goals should be done by the director/manager at least quarterly.
  (3) Strategic plans are always driven by and consistent with the organization's mission and philosophy.

9. Incident/occurrence and sentinel event reporting.

a. Incident/occurrence report is used to document incidents that involve patients and/or staff and which

result in harm and/or the potential for harm to the patient and/or staff.
   (1) Incident reports are not part of the medical record, nor are they referenced in the medical record.
   (2) Used to document additional information, circumstances, contributing factors that would not be appropriate to include in the medical record.
   (3) Used to evaluate systems and processes that may have contributed to the cause for the purpose of correcting and/or improving underlying causes or contributing factors.
   (4) Are part of an internal quality improvement program.
   (5) Can be used as a component of individual employee performance appraisal and improvement.

b. Sentinel event: a specific, patient-related occurrence in which an unexpected finding or outcome can be analyzed to improve processes, systems, or therapist performance and reduce the likelihood of reoccurrence.
   (1) Part of a comprehensive quality assurance and improvement program.
   (2) When a sentinel event occurs, a "root cause" analysis is done to identify underlying problems with processes, systems, or performance that can be improved to reduce the likelihood of recurrence.
   (3) Many regulatory and accrediting agencies require sentinel event reporting and analysis, particularly on specific types of incidents.

10. Health-care marketing.

a. Assess the true needs and wants of the patient/client (external factors).

b. Analyze the strengths and weaknesses of the organization to meet the needs of the customer (internal factors).

c. A needs assessment should be conducted, before providing a service or planning a new facility to determine:
   (1) Where is the market? (consumer).
   (2) Does a need for the service exist? (environment).
   (3) Who is the competition?
   (4) In-depth analysis of the marketplace, including demographical and epidemiological data.
   (5) Review of the literature.
   (6) Survey of colleagues.

d. Marketing methods may include:
   (1) Brochures, newsletters, educational pamphlets, newspaper articles, Internet, telemarketing.
   (2) Guest appearances on television, radio, and at local organizations.
   (3) Professional referral.
   (4) Word of mouth.
   (5) Yellow pages advertising.
   (6) Direct marketing to managed-care groups; e.g., sport injuries, low back pain.

11. Service management.

a. Management principles, functions, and strategies.
   (1) Management with a positive attitude about change and innovation fosters best practice.
   (2) Successful management supports open communication, team building, decentralization of resources, and the sharing of power.
   (3) Management that utilizes strategic thinking in a systems model can respond proactively to market demands and changes.
   (4) The use of different management styles (i.e., the manager's characteristic way of performing management tasks) has a significant impact on productivity, change, and growth.
   (5) Management's understanding and application of theories of motivation and behavior facilitates appropriate and effective responses to situations, fosters program efficacy, and promotes employee satisfaction.
   (6) Administrative functions of management include program development, fiscal and personnel management, and program evaluation.
   (7) Management by objective (MBO): a complete system of management based on a set of core goals to be accomplished by a program.
      (a) Mission and goals are established.
      (b) Measurable objectives are quantified.
      (c) Specific time frames for accomplishment of objectives are established.
      (d) Staff training needs and deterrents to progress are identified.
      (e) Program evaluation is instituted.

b. Program development.
   (1) Purposes of developing specific programs.
      (a) To directly meet the needs of a specific population(s) or group(s).
      (b) To clearly focus evaluation and intervention efforts and activities.
      (c) To increase visibility and use of available services (e.g., offering an outpatient cardiac rehabilitation program is more visible than individual referrals, resulting in increased recognition and utilization of this service).
      (d) To convert an idea into a practice reality.
   (2) Four basic steps of program development.
      (a) Needs assessment.
         (1) Describe the community, its physical, social, cultural, and economic factors, and populations at risk.
         (2) Describe the target population's demographics, disorder(s), functional level, and presenting problems.
         (3) Identify specific needs of target population.

- Perceived needs of the population as reported by others (e.g., family, physicians, and other professionals).
- Perceived needs as stated by the individual members of the target population.
- Real needs, which are the actual disabilities and functional limitations of the target population.

(4) Determine discrepancy between real and perceived needs.
(5) Determine unmet needs according to priority.
(6) Identify resources available for program implementation.

- Formal or institutional resources such as staff, supplies, money, space.
- Informal resources such as family, friends, cultural or religious figures, self-help/consumer groups.

(7) Needs assessment methods.

- Survey, interview, or self-report of target population. A representative sample is required.
- Key informant involves the surveying of specific individuals who are knowledgeable about the target population's needs.
- Community forums to obtain information through public meetings or panels.
- Service utilization review of records and reports.
- Analysis of social indicators to identify social, cultural, environmental, and/or economic factors that can predict problems.

(b) Program planning.
(1) Define a focus for the program based on needs assessment results.

- Problem areas, functional limitations, and unmet needs that are relevant to the majority of the target population are the priority focus.
- Program level of difficulty as determined by the range of population's functional levels and the level required by the current and expected environment.

(2) Adopt a frame of reference that is most likely to successfully address and meet the needs that are the program's focus.
(3) Establish objectives and goals of the program specifically related to primary focus.

- Set individual goals to be met by the program.
- Determine programmatic goals to establish standards for program evaluation.

(4) Describe integration of program into existing system of care.

- Establish realistic timetable for program implementation.
- Define staff roles, responsibilities, and assignments.
- Identify methods for professional collaboration.
- Determine the physical setting and space requirements.
- Consider potential barriers to program implementation.
- Develop methods to deal effectively with identified obstacles before program implementation.

(5) Develop a referral system for entry into, completion of, and discharge from the program.

- Evaluation protocols standardize information to be obtained from each person referred to the program and assess the type of program services needed.
- Criteria for acceptance into the program and for movement through program levels are set.
- Discharge criteria determine when an individual has achieved maximum gain from the program, usually defined as the achievement of program goals.

(6) Describe the fiscal implications of the program plan.

- Determine projected volume or service demand to estimate revenue.
- Identify resource utilization and projected expenses to estimate costs.
- Directly compare estimated revenue and estimated expenses to determine financial viability of program.

(c) Program implementation.
(1) Initiate program according to time-table and steps set forth in the program plan.
(2) Document program activities, procedures, and use.
(3) Communicate and coordinate with other programs within the system.
(4) Promote program to ensure it reaches target population.

(d) Program evaluation.
(1) Determine if program should continue, change, or be discontinued.

Fiscal Management

1. **Budget.**
   a. A financial plan, for a specific time period, of the amount of funds allotted to cover specific expenses of operating a PT department or private practice.
   b. An integral part of the planning process.
   c. Provides a mechanism of assessing the financial success of the practice, programs, or projects.
   d. Expresses anticipated income and expenditures over specific time periods in terms of:
      (1) Buildings.
      (2) Space.
      (3) Equipment.
      (4) Supplies.
   e. Operating budgets are usually planned for a one-year duration (e.g., the organization's fiscal year), and can be "flexible," changing according to volume and other factors.
   f. A budget is planned for capital expenses, including all major renovation expenses or the purchase of equipment that is reusable and will last a minimum of 3 years. Capital budgeting should be part of the strategic plan.

2. **Expense budgets.**
   a. Represent the amount of money spent by an organization to provide goods and services within a specific period of time.
   b. There are two types of expense budgets:
      (1) Operating expense budgets.
         (a) Related to the day-to-day operation of the organization.
         (b) Include categories relating to: salaries, benefits (sick, vacation, etc.), supplies, utilities (telephone and electric), linen, housekeeping, maintenance, continuing education, etc.
      (2) Capital budgets.
         (a) Deal with the purchase of larger items which will be utilized for >3–5 years, such as new equipment or new buildings.
         (b) Capital expense is equipment which is depreciable, and usually costs >$1000.

3. **Costs.**
   a. There are direct and indirect, fixed and variable, and discretionary costs associated with providing a PT service.
      (1) Direct costs are directly associated with the production of a service, including:
         (a) The cost of salaries for professional staff.
         (b) Treatment supplies (ultrasound gel, massage lotion).
         (c) Treatment equipment.
         (d) Continuing education.
      (2) Indirect costs are necessary to produce a service, but are indirectly associated with that service.
         (a) Utilities (telephone and electric).
         (b) Housekeeping, laundry.
         (c) Marketing services, etc.
      (3) Fixed costs remain unchanged, even with changes in volume.
         (a) Air conditioning.
         (b) Rent.
      (4) Variable costs increase and decrease in direct proportion to the volume of activity.
         (a) Linen and labor costs increase as volume increases.
      (5) Discretionary expenses are those costs that are not essential for providing PT services. They may include budgeting for continuing education, or recognition activities.

4. **Accounts payable.**
   a. Money owed to a creditor (individual who provides a service or equipment) for services rendered.
   b. A part of the budget where debts are listed.

5. **Accounts receivable.**
   a. Money owed to a company (hospital, PT practice) for providing a service; e.g., PT treatment on credit.
   b. An asset expected to benefit future operations.

Quality Assurance and Quality Improvement

1. **Quality assurance (QA).**
   a. Monitor quality.
   b. Monitor appropriateness of care.
   c. Resolve identified problems.

2. **Continuous quality improvement.**
   a. A systematic process that involves ongoing, deliberate, and continuous monitoring of the systems and processes which affect patient care to assure for the highest quality outcomes possible.

3. **Utilization review (UR).**
   a. Written plan to determine:
      (1) Appropriate use of resources.
      (2) Medical necessity of services provided.
      (3) Cost efficiency.
   b. Methods for UR.
      (1) Prospective review.
         (a) Evaluation of proposed treatment plan that specifies how care will be provided.
         (b) Used by third-party payers to approve proposed PT treatment program.
      (2) Concurrent review.
         (a) Evaluation of ongoing treatment program during hospitalization or treatment.

(b) Method to ensure appropriate that care is being delivered.

(3) Retrospective review.

(a) Audits of medical records after treatment was rendered.

(b) Method to ensure appropriate care was given.

(c) Time-consuming, expensive method for third-party payers.

(4) Statistical utilization review (SUR).

(a) Claims data, such as pricing and utilization, are analyzed.

(b) Determines which providers offer the most efficient and cost-effective care.

(5) Peer review.

(a) Performed by peer groups of health professionals.

(b) Retrospective and concurrent review of clients records to determine if services provided are necessary, appropriate, and comprehensive in relation to the patient's needs.

(1) Educational, not punitive.

(2) Aim is improvement of quality of care.

(3) Focuses on how well services are performed in the delivery of care under review.

(4) Determines if the patient's needs have been met.

(c) May also be performed by peer review organization (PRO).

(1) Reviews services provided to Medicare and Medicaid beneficiaries and some managed care plans.

(2) Determines appropriateness of services delivered to patients.

(6) Audit or program evaluation.

(a) Assessment of the management of patients with a specific diagnosis.

(1) Objectives are established for patients; e.g., total hip replacements.

(2) Outcomes are evaluated in terms of range of motion, strength, pain, function, gait level, ability to climb stairs, etc.

(3) Comparisons made between treating therapists, other facilities, etc.

(4) Programs can be modified or improved when indicated.

Professional Standards

1. (See also Appendices A, B, C, and D).

2. Standards are developed by professional associations and are binding only on association members.

a. Code of Ethics helps PTs and PTAs understand how to act morally and professionally (see Appendices A and C).

(1) Code of Ethics (APTA) has been codified as law in many state practice/licensure law and regulations. It is often adopted by many institutions as the standard of behavior for PTs.

b. Guide for Professional Conduct assists in the interpretation of the Code of Ethics (Appendix B).

c. Guide for Conduct of PTAs determines the propriety of their conduct (Appendix C).

Caregiver Definitions and Roles

1. Physical Therapist (PT).

a. A skilled health professional with a minimum of a baccalaureate degree; current accreditation standards mandate postbaccalaureate degree (master's or doctorate).

b. Licensed by each state or jurisdiction following successful performance on National Physical Therapy Examination.

c. Examines patient, evaluates data, establishes diagnosis, prognosis, and plan of care, administers or supervises treatment.

d. Delegates portions of plan of care to supportive personnel; e.g., PTA.

e. Supervises and directs supportive staff (PTA, PT aide) in designated tasks.

f. Reevaluates and adjusts plan of care as appropriate.

g. Performs and documents final evaluation and establishes discharge and follow-up plans.

h. Consultation by giving professional opinions to others to identify problems, recommend solutions, or produce a specific outcome.

(1) May be patient-related consultation to evaluate the quality of PT services.

(2) May be client-related consultation to a business, school, organization, or government agency.

(a) Expert witness.

(b) ADA compliance.

(c) Work-related injury prevention.

(d) Request for a second opinion.

2. Physical Therapy Director.

a. Oversees function, responsibilities, and relationships of all personnel.

b. Establishes, revises, and ensures that policies and procedures are carried out according to established policy and procedures.

c. Acts as liaison with facility administration.

d. Sets department goals and strategic plan.

3. Physical Therapy Supervisor.

a. Qualified experienced PT with a variety of skills including:

(1) Professional knowledge and skill of tasks performed.

(2) Ability to motivate subordinates.

(3) Ability to evaluate staff and give oral and written feedback.
(4) Ability to interview new staff and help develop their skills.
(5) Delegate tasks to appropriate staff.

b. Patient care may or may not be primary responsibility of the supervisor.

4. Physical Therapist Assistant (PTA).

a. Skilled physical therapy technologist, usually with a 2-year associate degree.

b. Must work under the direction and supervision of a PT in all practice settings.
(1) When the PT and PTA are not within the same physical setting, delegated functions by the PTA must be safe and legal physical therapy practice based on:
(a) Complexity and acuity of the patient's needs.
(b) Proximity and accessibility to the PT.
(c) Supervision available in the event of emergencies.
(d) Type of setting in which the service is provided.
(2) In home health, regularly scheduled and documented supervisory meetings are established between the PT and PTA; the frequency is determined by the needs of the patient and the needs of the PTA, and include:
(a) On-site reassessment of the patient.
(b) On-site review of the plan of care with appropriate revision or termination.
(c) Assessment and recommendation for utilization of outside resources.

c. Able to adjust treatment procedure in accordance with changes in patient status within the scope of the established plan of care.

d. May not evaluate, develop, or change plan of care, or write discharge plan or summary.

e. May carry out routine operational functions, including supervision of the physical therapy aide and documentation of patient progress.

5. Physical Therapy Aide.

a. A nonlicensed worker, specifically trained under the direction of a PT or PTA.

b. Functions only with continuous onsite supervision by a PT or, where allowable by law or regulation, the PTA.

c. Performs designated routine tasks related to the operation of a physical therapy service.

d. Job responsibilities may include:
(1) Functional and ambulation activities.
(2) Application of specific heat, cold, and whirlpool treatments.
(3) Equipment maintenance.
(4) Patient transportation.
(5) Secretarial or housekeeping duties.

e. Aides are not licensed by the state and some state laws limit or prohibit treatment procedures by aides.

6. Physical Therapy and Physical Therapist Assistant Student.

a. Performs duties commensurate with level of education.

b. PT clinical instructor (CI) is responsible for all actions and duties of affiliating student.

c. PT may supervise both PT and PTA students.

d. PTA may supervise only an assistant student.

7. Physical Therapy Volunteer.

a. Member of the community.
(1) Interested in assisting PTs with departmental activities.
(2) Takes phone messages, does filing and other basic secretarial tasks.
(3) May not provide or set up patient treatment, transfer patients, clean whirlpools, or maintain equipment.

8. Home Health Aide.

a. A nonlicensed worker (e.g., nursing/rehabilitation assistant) specifically trained to:
(1) Provide personal care and home-management services.
(2) Assist patients to remain in the home environment.

b. Supervised by a nurse, PT, or OT.

c. Responsibilities include:
(1) Bathing, grooming, light housework, shopping, or cooking in some circumstances.
(2) Supervision of home exercise program (HEP) as directed by the PT; e.g., ambulation.

9. Occupational Therapist (OTR/L).

a. A skilled health professional who holds a minimum of a baccalaureate degree and has passed a national certification examination. OTs are licensed by some, but not all, states. The OT provides:
(1) Education and training in ADLs.
(2) Fabrication of orthoses (splints).
(3) Guidance in selection and use of adaptive equipment.
(4) Therapeutic activities to enhance functional performance, and cognitive/perceptual function.
(5) Consultation concerning the adaptation of physical environments for the handicapped.
(6) Creative activities in treatment of physically and emotionally disabled patients.

b. Services are provided on an inpatient basis, outpatient basis, and in industrial environments.

10. Certified Occupational Therapist Assistant (COTA).

a. Skilled technician who holds an associate degree and has passed a national certification examination.

b. Works under the direction of an OT to carry out established treatment.

(1) Cannot evaluate, establish, or revise a plan of care.

c. Performs duties in a rehabilitation or home setting.
   (1) Concerned with functional deficits in activities of daily living (ADLs), including dressing, grooming, hygiene, housekeeping, etc.

11. Speech-Language Pathologist (ST).

a. A skilled health professional who holds a master's degree in communication disorders, completed 1 year of field experience, and passed a national examination to obtain the Certificate of Clinical Competence authorized by the American Speech and Hearing Association.
b. Conducts remedial programs to restore or improve communication of patients with language and speech impairments.
   (1) May arise from physiological or neurological disturbances and defective articulation.
c. Works with OT to correct swallowing problems and cognitive processing deficits; and with PT in the area of positioning and mobility.

12. Certified Orthotist (CO).

a. Designs, fabricates, and fits orthoses (braces, splints, collars, corsets) prescribed by physicians.
b. Successfully completed the examination by the American Orthotic and Prosthetic Association.
c. Provides these devices to patients with disabling conditions of limbs and spine.
d. Works directly with physicians and physical and occupational therapists.

13. Certified Prosthetist (CP).

a. Designs, fabricates, and fits prostheses for patients with partial or total absence of a limb (amputation).
b. Successfully completed the examination by the American Orthotic and Prosthetic Association.
c. Works directly with physicians, PTs, and OTs.
d. Individuals may be certified in both orthotics and prosthetics (CPO).

14. Certified Respiratory Therapy Technician (CRRT).

a. A skilled technician holding an associate degree from a 2-year training program accredited by the Committee in Allied Health Education and Accreditation.
   (1) Passes a national exam to become registered.
b. Administers respiratory therapy as prescribed and supervised by a physician.
   (1) Performs pulmonary function tests.
   (2) Treatments consist of oxygen delivery, aerosols, and nebulizers.
   (3) Maintains all respiratory equipment and assists patients in their use; i.e., ventilators, oxygen, pressure machines, etc.
   (4) Coordinates care with pulmonary PT treatments.

15. Primary Care Physician (PCP).

a. A practitioner, usually an internist, general practitioner, or family medicine physician, who provides primary care services and manages routine health-care needs.
b. Acts as the gatekeeper for patients covered by managed health care.
   (1) Authorizes referrals to other specialty physicians or services, including PT.

16. Physician Assistant (PA).

a. Skilled allied health professional, graduate of an accredited program, usually at the graduate level.
   (1) Required to pass national certification examination.
   (2) One year direct patient contact required.
b. Under the supervision of the supervisory physician, performs routine diagnostic, therapeutic, preventative and health maintenance services in any setting in which the physician renders care.
   (1) Specialties include family medicine, obstetrics, pediatrics, orthopedics, emergency medicine, and others.
c. Able to write PT orders under some circumstances.

17. Physiatrist.

a. A physician specializing in physical medicine and rehabilitation.
   (1) Certified by the American Board of Physical Medicine and Rehabilitation.
   (2) Diagnoses and treats patients with disabilities involving musculoskeletal, neurological, cardiovascular, or other body systems.
b. Primary focus on maximal restoration of physical, psychological, social, and vocational function, and alleviation of pain.
c. May lead the rehabilitation team in coordination of patient care.
   (1) Works directly with PTs, OTs, and STs.

18. Chiropractor (DC).

a. An alternative medical practitioner, usually licensed by a state board.
   (1) Deals with relationship of the nervous system and the spinal column in the restoration and maintenance of health.
b. Services are covered for individuals in most group health plans.
c. Patients may see a chiropractor and PT at the same time.
   (1) PT, with patient's permission, should contact chiropractor to coordinate care.

19. Registered Nurse (RN).

a. A skilled health professional who is a graduate of an accredited nursing program, and licensed by the state board following successful performance on licensure exam.

b. Primary liaison between the patient and the physician.
   (1) Communicates to physician changes in patient's medical or social condition.
   (2) Educates the patient and family to facilitate recovery.
   (3) Makes referrals to other services under physician's direction.
   (4) Supervises other levels of nursing care (licensed practical nurse [LPN], home health aide).
   (5) Administers medication, but cannot change drug dosages.
   (6) Carries out range of motion, bed exercises, transfers, and ambulation as instructed by the PT.

20. Rehabilitation Counselor (Vocational Rehabilitation Counselor).

a. Counsels physically and mentally handicapped individuals.
   (1) Helps patients improve their ability to function optimally in society.
   (2) Administers vocational tests, procures vocational training, and provides occupational information for job placement.

21. Audiologist.

a. A health professional with a graduate degree in audiology.
b. A specialist in hearing disorders and evaluation who works to rehabilitate individuals with hearing loss.
   (1) Uses audiometric tests to assess sensitivity of sense of hearing.
   (2) Uses speech audiometric tests to assess ability to understand selected words.
   (3) Audiometrist is a technician trained to administer audiometric tests selected and evaluated by the audiologist.

22. Consultant.

a. A person who, by training and experience, has acquired a special knowledge in a subject area which has been recognized by a peer group.
b. A person who analyzes situations, offers advice, and solutions to problems.
   (1) For example: physician referral for consultation or advice regarding diagnosis or treatment of a patient.
   (2) Consultant reviews history, examines patient, and writes opinion.
   (3) Responsibility of patient care not delegated to consultant.

23. Athletic Trainer (ATC).

a. A health professional with a minimum of a baccalaureate degree who is an integral part of the health-care system associated with sports.
   (1) Usually works under supervision of a physician.
   (2) Provides injury prevention, recognition, treatment, and rehabilitation after athletic trauma.
b. Settings for delivery of care:
   (1) Secondary schools, colleges and universities, professional athletic organizations, and private or hospital-based clinics.

24. Social Worker (MSW).

a. Usually completed a master's degree from a school of social work accredited by the Council on Social Work Education. After one year of practical field work, they are licensed or registered by the state.
b. Acts as a resource director assisting patients and families with necessary applications for financial resources, appropriate discharge destinations (e.g., skilled nursing facility, custodial care facility), rental and loaner equipment, and support groups, etc.
c. Acts as a personal or family counselor.
d. Educates the patient and family about their medical problems. Also educates home health staff, helping them understand patient and family interaction and crisis management.
e. Acts as an advocate for the patient in dealing with outside agencies and procuring support services.
f. Mediates between the patient and family by alleviating fears, developing realistic expectations of the patient to the family, and interpreting the patient and families' situation to outside relatives and the home health-care team.

25. Alternative support staff: (e.g., massage therapists, exercise therapists, acupuncturists).

a. May work within the supervision of a PT.
b. Employed under their appropriate titles.
c. Involvement in patient care activities should be within the limits of their education and in accordance with applicable laws and regulations and the discretion of the PT.

26. Team roles and principles of collaboration.

a. Overview.
   (1) A team is a group of equally important individuals with common interests who collaborate to develop shared goals and build trusting relationships to achieve these shared goals.
   (2) Members of the team include the patient/client/consumer; his/her family, significant others, and/or caregivers, health-care professionals; and the reimburser's gatekeepers.
   (3) Professional members on the team will vary according to practice setting.
   (4) The consumer, family, significant other, and/or caregiver role on the team has become increasing important. Collaboration with these individuals is even mandated by law (e.g., Omnibus Budget Reconciliation Act of 1990 [OBRA '90], Individuals with Disabilities Education Act [IDEA]).

b. Principles of collaboration.
   (1) Factors that influence effective team functioning.
      (a) Member skill and knowledge.
      (b) Membership stability.
      (c) Commitment to team goals.
      (d) Good communication.
      (e) Membership composition.
      (f) Common language and goals.
      (g) Effective leadership.
c. Types of teams.
   (1) Multidisciplinary.
      (a) A number of professionals from different disciplines conduct assessments and interventions independent from one another.
      (b) Member's primary allegiance is to his/her discipline. Some formal communications occur between team members.
      (c) Limited communications may result in lack of understanding of different perspectives.
      (d) Resources and responsibilities are individually allocated between disciplines; therefore, competition among team members may develop.
   (2) Interdisciplinary.
      (a) All disciplines relevant to the case agree to collaborate for decision-making.
      (b) Evaluation and intervention is still conducted independently within defined areas of each profession's expertise. However, there is a greater understanding of each discipline's perspective.
      (c) Outcomes and goals are team-directed and not bound to discipline specific roles and functions.
      (d) Members tend to use group process skills effectively (e.g., during team planning meetings).
      (e) The exchange of information, prioritization of needs, allocation of resources, and responsibilities are based on members' expertise and skills, not on "turf" issues.
      (f) Ongoing training, support, supervision, cooperation, and consultation among disciplines are important to this model to ensure that professional integrity and quality of care is maintained.
   (3) Intradisciplinary.
      (a) One or more members of one discipline evaluate, plan, and implement treatment of the individual; e.g., PT, PTA, PT consultant.
      (b) Other disciplines are not involved; communication is limited, thereby limiting perspectives on the case.
      (c) This "team" is at risk due to potential narrowness of perspective.
      (d) Comprehensive, holistic care can be questionable.
   (4) Team efficacy.
      (a) Interdisciplinary teams are the most common and considered to be the most effective in today's health-care system.

Patients Rights, Safety, and Malpractice

1. Statutory laws.
   a. Passed by the legislature and impact physical therapy
   b. Licensure laws.
   c. Workers' Compensation Acts.
   d. Medicare/Medicaid.
   e. Americans with Disabilities Act.

2. Goals of statutory laws impacting physical therapy.
   a. Professional licensing laws are enacted by all states.
      (1) Protect the consumer against professional incompetence and exploitation by opportunists.
      (2) Determine the minimal standards of education
         (a) Graduation from an accredited program or its equivalent in PT.
         (b) Successful completion of a national licensing examination.
         (c) Ethical and legal standards relating to continuing practice of PT.
         (d) All PTs must have a license to practice.
         (e) Each state determines criteria to practice and issue a license.
         (f) Licensure examination and related activities are the responsibility of the Federation of State Boards of Physical Therapy.
            (1) All states belong to this association.

3. Nondiscrimination laws.
   a. Prevent a facility from discrimination against employees regarding race, color, religion, gender, or national origin.
   b. Title VII of the Civil Rights Act of 1964 prohibits employment discrimination based on:
      (1) Race.
      (2) Color.
      (3) Sex.
      (4) Religion.
      (5) National origin.
      (6) Sexual harassment.
         (a) Unwanted advancements.
         (b) Creation of a sexually hostile or intimidating work environment.
         (c) Inappropriate conversations, joking, touching, or interference with job performance.
         (d) Victim or harasser can be either a man or woman.

(e) Victim does not have to be the one harassed, only someone adversely affected by the offensive behavior.

c. The Age Discrimination and Employment Act of 1967.

(1) Prohibits employers from discriminating against persons from 40–70 years of age in any area of employment.

d. 1973 Rehabilitation Act.

(1) Prohibits employment discrimination based on disability in:

(a) Federal executive agencies.

(b) All institutions receiving Medicare, Medicaid, and other federal support.

e. The Americans with Disability Act (ADA), 1990.

(1) Prevents discrimination against people with disabilities.

(2) Ensures their integration into mainstream American life.

(3) The definition of "disabilities" encompasses a wide range of physical and mental conditions.

(4) Requires businesses of ≥15 employees to accommodate needs of people with disabilities to facilitate their economic independence in both the public and private sectors.

(5) Equal Employment Opportunity Commission (EEOC) oversees issues and interprets regulations.

(6) Requires reasonable accommodation to the workplace by removing barriers unless this would cause "undue hardship" (an action requiring significant difficulty or expense).

(a) Installing an elevator so the individual could access upper floors might be considered an undue hardship.

(7) PTs serve as consultants to:

(a) Employers helping them meet their responsibilities.

(b) Disabled helping them achieve their rehabilitation potential and rights under law.

f. Individuals with Disabilities Education Act (IDEA).

(1) Enacted in 1975 with the most recent revision in 2004. Ensures that children with disabilities receive appropriate, free public education.

(2) IDEA provides statutes and guidelines for states and school districts regarding the provision of special education and related services.

(3) Establishes Early Intervention Programs [EIP] including PT, OT, ST, and other services as needed.

(a) Services are provided to children with developmental delays (physical, emotional, cognitive or communicative).

(b) Services provided to infants or toddlers "at risk" for developing delays.

(c) Provision for necessary adaptive equipment.

(4) Requires creation of Individualized Education Plans [IEPs].

(a) Guides the team; however, child has the option of not attending planning meetings for the IEP.

(b) Considers evaluation results and child's concerns.

(1) Functional needs, strength, ROM.

(2) Factors such as English proficiency, behavioral issues, vision, hearing and communication needs.

(3) Need for assistive devices.

4. Assuring patient safety.

a. Risk management programs.

(1) Identify, evaluate, and take corrective action against risk.

(a) Potential patient, employee, and/or visitor injury.

(b) Property loss or damage with resulting financial loss or legal liability.

(2) Efforts taken to decrease risk in PT.

(a) Equipment maintenance; e.g., biannual maintenance of electrical equipment.

(b) Staff education; e.g., safety training for staff in use of equipment.

(c) Regular check of essential safety equipment.

(d) Policies to clean equipment and reduce the potential for spreading infection.

(3) Patient and staff safety.

(a) PTs must follow strict federal standards when using any form of patient restraint.

(1) Restraint must be used for a specific reason, i.e. patient safety.

(2) Restraints are considered temporary and may not be used for an indefinite amount of time.

(3) A patient in restraints must be checked on every 30 minutes.

(4) Restraints are not for punishment or to substitute proper staff supervision.

(5) Use proper patient identifiers, such as wrist bands, with patient date of birth, first and last names, or other unique patient identifiers.

(4) Identify risk factors in patient care or patient and therapist safety; e.g., more than three incidents of patient falls on the rehabilitation floor may require an in-service in transfer training.

(5) Proper and timely reporting of adverse patient occurrence or reactions as required by federal or state statute. These may include:

(a) Adverse reactions to regulated medicines.

(b) Incidents involving abuse or neglect of patients.

(c) Outbreaks of disease that may affect public safety (i.e., influenza).

(4) "Reportable" occurrences such as violence against patients where significant harm is caused to the patient (i.e., nursing home patient with a fall resulting in severe fracture or death).

(6) Annual certification/recertification of staff in cardiopulmonary resuscitation (CPR).

b. Malpractice: PTs are personally responsible for negligence and other acts that result in harm to a patient through professional/patient relationships.

(1) Negligence.
  (a) Failure to do what reasonably competent practitioners would have done under similar circumstances.
  (b) To find a practitioner negligent, harm must have occurred to the patient.
  (c) Each individual (PT, PTA, student PT, or student PTA) is liable for his/her own negligence.

(2) Supervisors or superiors may also be found negligent due to the actions of their workers if they provided faulty supervision or inappropriate delegation of responsibilities.

(3) PT fails to perform a duty, thus causing harm.

(4) Ethical principles are violated in caring for patients; e.g., acting without consent, breaking of confidentiality, lack of respect for patients.

(5) Patients may also contribute to negligence if they do not follow directions of the therapist.

(6) The institution is usually found negligent if a patient was harmed as a result of an environmental problem.
  (a) Slippery floor.
  (b) Fall in a poorly lit hall.

(7) The institution is also liable if an employee was incompetent or not properly licensed.

(8) PTs, PTAs, or students may be liable for:
  (a) Adverse reactions to treatment, such as burns (e.g., leaving a hot pack on too long), falls during gait training, injuries from therapeutic exercise, or harm caused by defective equipment.
  (b) Any action or inaction that is inconsistent with the Code of Ethics or the Standards of Practice that results in harm to a patient.

(9) Patients, parents, or legal guardians can refuse treatment by a student practitioner.

(10) PT may be asked to be an expert witness or testify in a malpractice case for:
  (a) The plaintiff (victim).
  (b) The defendant (accused).

(11) PT's role in emergency preparedness and disaster management.
  (a) PTs are taking on a larger role in an organization's emergency preparedness plan (EPP) and a more active role when an organization is faced with a disaster.
  (b) Internal disaster.
    (1) Power or utility failures.
    (2) Telecom or equipment failure.
    (3) Fire/bomb scare.
    (4) Internal environmental conditions.
  (c) External disaster.
    (1) Terrorism.
    (2) Weather- related: floods, hurricanes, etc.
    (3) Civil disturbances.
    (4) Hazmat incidents. (Hazardous materials)
    (5) Large community casualty incidents.
    (6) Possible PT roles.
      - Helping to triage casualties. → based upon severity
      - Assessing patients with musculoskeletal injuries, freeing up other providers.
      - Command and control functions/communications.
      - Patient transportation.

(12) Emergency preparedness planning.
  (a) Many state and federal agencies require that health organizations have some form of EPP ready.
  (b) PTs can play key roles in developing EPPs.
    (1) Liaison with other local first responders, such as the fire and police departments.
    (2) Help develop and build the communication infrastructure to be used during a disaster.
    (3) Assist in determining which critical services are to be offered and which are secondary.
    (4) Help coordinate internal resources.
    (5) Participate in disaster drills.

Appendix A

Code of Ethics

Preamble

The Code of Ethics for the Physical Therapist (Code of Ethics) delineates the ethical obligations of all physical therapists as determined by the House of Delegates of the American Physical Therapy Association (APTA). The purposes of this Code of Ethics are to:

Define the ethical principles that form the foundation of physical therapist practice in patient/client management, consultation, education, research, and administration.

Provide standards of behavior and performance that form the basis of professional accountability to the public.

Provide guidance for physical therapists facing ethical challenges, regardless of their professional roles and responsibilities.

Educate physical therapists, students, other health care professionals, regulators, and the public regarding the core values, ethical principles, and standards that guide the professional conduct of the physical therapist.

Establish the standards by which the American Physical Therapy Association can determine if a physical therapist has engaged in unethical conduct.

No code of ethics is exhaustive nor can it address every situation. Physical therapists are encouraged to seek additional advice or consultation in instances where the guidance of the Code of Ethics may not be definitive.

This Code of Ethics is built upon the five roles of the physical therapist (management of patients/clients, consultation, education, research, and administration), the core values of the profession, and the multiple realms of ethical action (individual, organizational, and societal). Physical therapist practice is guided by a set of seven core values: accountability, altruism, compassion/caring, excellence, integrity, professional duty, and social responsibility. Throughout the document the primary core values that support specific principles are indicated in parentheses. Unless a specific role is indicated in the principle, the duties and obligations being delineated pertain to the five roles of the physical therapist. Fundamental to the Code of Ethics is the special obligation of physical therapists to empower, educate, and enable those with impairments, activity limitations, participation restrictions, and disabilities to facilitate greater independence, health, wellness, and enhanced quality of life.

Principle #1

Physical therapists shall respect the inherent dignity and rights of all individuals.

(Core Values: Compassion, Integrity)

1A. Physical therapists shall act in a respectful manner toward each person regardless of age, gender, race, nationality, religion, ethnicity, social or economic status, sexual orientation, health condition, or disability.

1B. Physical therapists shall recognize their personal biases and shall not discriminate against others in physical therapist practice, consultation, education, research, and administration.

Principle #2

Physical therapists shall be trustworthy and compassionate in addressing the rights and needs of patients/clients.

(Core Values: Altruism, Compassion, Professional Duty)

2A. Physical therapists shall adhere to the core values of the profession and shall act in the best interests of patients/clients over the interests of the physical therapist.

2B. Physical therapists shall provide physical therapy services with compassionate and caring behaviors that incorporate the individual and cultural differences of patients/clients.

2C. Physical therapists shall provide the information necessary to allow patients or their surrogates to make informed decisions about physical therapy care or participation in clinical research.

2D. Physical therapists shall collaborate with patients/clients to empower them in decisions about their health care.

2E. Physical therapists shall protect confidential patient/client information and may disclose confidential information to appropriate authorities only when allowed or as required by law.

Principle #3

Physical therapists shall be accountable for making sound professional judgments.

(Core Values: Excellence, Integrity)

3A. Physical therapists shall demonstrate independent and objective professional judgment in the patient's/client's best interest in all practice settings.

3B. Physical therapists shall demonstrate professional judgment informed by professional standards, evidence (including current literature and established best practice), practitioner experience, and patient/client values.

3C. Physical therapists shall make judgments within their scope of practice and level of expertise and shall communicate with, collaborate with, or refer to peers or other health care professionals when necessary.
3D. Physical therapists shall not engage in conflicts of interest that interfere with professional judgment.
3E. Physical therapists shall provide appropriate direction of and communication with physical therapist assistants and support personnel.

Principle #4

Physical therapists shall demonstrate integrity in their relationships with patients/clients, families, colleagues, students, research participants, other healthcare providers, employers, payers, and the public.

(Core Value: Integrity)

4A. Physical therapists shall provide truthful, accurate, and relevant information and shall not make misleading representations.
4B. Physical therapists shall not exploit persons over whom they have supervisory, evaluative or other authority (e.g., patients/clients, students, supervisees, research participants, or employees).
4C. Physical therapists shall discourage misconduct by healthcare professionals and report illegal or unethical acts to the relevant authority, when appropriate.
4D. Physical therapists shall report suspected cases of abuse involving children or vulnerable adults to the appropriate authority, subject to law.
4E. Physical therapists shall not engage in any sexual relationship with any of their patients/clients, supervisees, or students.
4F. Physical therapists shall not harass anyone verbally, physically, emotionally, or sexually.

Principle #5

Physical therapists shall fulfill their legal and professional obligations.

(Core Values: Professional Duty, Accountability)

5A. Physical therapists shall comply with applicable local, state, and federal laws and regulations.
5B. Physical therapists shall have primary responsibility for supervision of physical therapist assistants and support personnel.
5C. Physical therapists involved in research shall abide by accepted standards governing protection of research participants.
5D. Physical therapists shall encourage colleagues with physical, psychological, or substance related impairments that may adversely impact their professional responsibilities to seek assistance or counsel.
5E. Physical therapists who have knowledge that a colleague is unable to perform their professional responsibilities with reasonable skill and safety shall report this information to the appropriate authority.
5F. Physical therapists shall provide notice and information about alternatives for obtaining care in the event the physical therapist terminates the provider relationship while the patient/client continues to need physical therapy services.

Principle #6

Physical therapists shall enhance their expertise through the life-long acquisition and refinement of knowledge, skills, abilities, and professional behaviors.

(Core Value: Excellence)

6A. Physical therapists shall achieve and maintain professional competence.
6B. Physical therapists shall take responsibility for their professional development based on critical self-assessment and reflection on changes in physical therapist practice, education, healthcare delivery, and technology.
6C. Physical therapists shall evaluate the strength of evidence and applicability of content presented during professional development activities before integrating the content or techniques into practice.
6D. Physical therapists shall cultivate practice environments that support professional development, life-long learning, and excellence.

Principle #7

Physical therapists shall promote organizational behaviors and business practices that benefit patients/clients and society.

(Core Values: Integrity, Accountability)

7A. Physical therapists shall promote practice environments that support autonomous and accountable professional judgments.
7B. Physical therapists shall seek remuneration as is deserved and reasonable for physical therapist services.
7C. Physical therapists shall not accept gifts or other considerations that influence or give an appearance of influencing their professional judgment.
7D. Physical therapists shall fully disclose any financial interest they have in products or services that they recommend to patients/clients.
7E. Physical therapists shall be aware of charges and shall ensure that documentation and coding for physical therapy services accurately reflect the nature and extent of the services provided.
7F. Physical therapists shall refrain from employment arrangements, or other arrangements, that prevent physical therapists from fulfilling professional obligations to patients/clients.

Principle #8

Physical therapists shall participate in efforts to meet the health needs of people locally, nationally, or globally.

(Core Values: Social Responsibility)

8A. Physical therapists shall provide *pro bono* physical therapy services or support organizations that meet the health needs of people who are economically disadvantaged, uninsured, and underinsured.

8B. Physical therapists shall advocate to reduce health disparities and health care inequities, improve access to health care services, and address the health, wellness, and preventive health care needs of people.

8C. Physical therapists shall be responsible stewards of health care resources and shall avoid over-utilization or under-utilization of physical therapy services.

8D. Physical therapists shall educate members of the public about the benefits of physical therapy and the unique role of the physical therapist.

Appendix B

Guide for Professional Conduct

Purpose

1. This Guide for Professional Conduct (Guide) is intended to serve physical therapists in interpreting the Code of Ethics (Code) of the American Physical Therapy Association (Association), in matters of professional conduct. The Guide provides guidelines by which physical therapists may determine the propriety of their conduct. It is also intended to guide the professional development of physical therapist students. The Code and the Guide apply to all physical therapists. These guidelines are subject to change as the dynamics of the profession change and as new patterns of health-care delivery are developed and accepted by the professional community and the public. This Guide is subject to monitoring and timely revision by the Ethics and Judicial Committee of the Association.

Interpreting Ethical Principles

1. The interpretations expressed in this Guide reflect the opinions, decisions, and advice of the Ethics and Judicial Committee. These interpretations are intended to assist a physical therapist in applying general ethical principles to specific situations. They should not be considered inclusive of all situations that could evolve.

Principle 1

1. A physical therapist shall respect the rights and dignity of all individuals and shall provide compassionate care.
   a. Attitudes of a physical therapist.
      (1) A physical therapist shall recognize, respect, and respond to individual and cultural differences with compassion and sensitivity.
      (2) A physical therapist shall be guided at all times by concern for the physical, psychological, and socioeconomic welfare of patients/clients.
      (3) A physical therapist shall not harass, abuse, or discriminate against others.

Principle 2

1. A physical therapist shall act in a trustworthy manner towards patients/clients, and in all other aspects of physical therapy practice.
   a. Patient/physical therapist relationship.
      (1) A physical therapist shall place the patient/client's interest(s) above those of the physical therapist. Working in the patient/client's best interest requires knowledge of the patient/client's needs from the patient/client's perspective. Patients/clients often come to the physical therapist in a vulnerable state and normally will rely on the physical therapist's advice, which they perceive to be based on superior knowledge, skill, and experience. The trustworthy physical therapist acts to ameliorate the patient's/ client's vulnerability, not to exploit it.
      (2) A physical therapist shall not exploit any aspect of the physical therapist/patient relationship.
      (3) A physical therapist shall not engage in any sexual relationship or activity, whether consensual or nonconsensual, with any patient while a physical therapist/patient relationship exists. Termination of the physical therapist/patient relationship does not eliminate the possibility that a sexual or intimate relationship may exploit the vulnerability of the former patient/client.
      (4) A physical therapist shall encourage an open and collaborative dialogue with the patient/client.
      (5) In the event the physical therapist or patient terminates the physical therapist/patient relationship while the patient continues to need physical therapy services, the physical therapist should take steps to transfer the care of the patient to another provider.
   b. Truthfulness.
      (1) A physical therapist has an obligation to provide accurate and truthful information. A physical therapist shall not make statements that he/she knows or should know are false, deceptive, fraudulent, or misleading.
   c. Confidential information.
      (1) Information relating to the physical therapist/patient relationship is confidential and may not be communicated to a third party not involved in that patient's care without the prior consent of the patient, subject to applicable law.
      (2) Information derived from peer review shall be held confidential by the reviewer unless the physical therapist who was reviewed consents to the release of the information.
      (3) A physical therapist may disclose information to appropriate authorities when it is necessary to protect the welfare of an individual or the com-

munity or when required by law. Such disclosure shall be in accordance with applicable law.

d. Patient autonomy and consent.
   (1) A physical therapist shall respect the patient's/client's right to make decisions regarding the recommended plan of care, including consent, modification, or refusal.
   (2) A physical therapist shall communicate to the patient/client the findings of his/her examination, evaluation, diagnosis, and prognosis.
   (3) A physical therapist shall collaborate with the patient/client to establish the goals of treatment and the plan of care.
   (4) A physical therapist shall use sound professional judgment in informing the patient/ client of any substantial risks of the recommended examination and intervention.
   (5) A physical therapist shall not restrict patients' freedom to select their provider of physical therapy.

Principle 3

1. A physical therapist shall comply with laws and regulations governing physical therapy and shall strive to effect changes that benefit patients/clients.
   a. Professional practice.
      (1) A physical therapist shall comply with laws governing the qualifications, functions, and duties of a physical therapist.
   b. Just laws and regulations.
      (1) A physical therapist shall advocate the adoption of laws, regulations, and policies by providers, employers, third party payers, legislatures, and regulatory agencies to provide and improve access to necessary health-care services for all individuals.
   c. Unjust laws and regulations.
      (1) A physical therapist shall endeavor to change unjust laws, regulations, and policies that govern the practice of physical therapy.

Principle 4

1. A physical therapist shall exercise sound professional judgment.
   a. Professional responsibility.
      (1) A physical therapist shall make professional judgments that are in the patient/client's best interests.
      (2) Regardless of practice setting, a physical therapist has primary responsibility for the physical therapy care of a patient and shall make independent judgments regarding that care consistent with accepted professional standards.
      (3) A physical therapist shall not provide physical therapy services to a patient/client while his/her ability to do so safely is impaired.
      (4) A physical therapist shall exercise sound professional judgment based upon his/her knowledge, skill, education, training, and experience.
      (5) Upon accepting a patient/client for physical therapy services, a physical therapist shall be responsible for: the examination, evaluation, and diagnosis of that individual; the prognosis and intervention; re-examination and modification of the plan of care; and the maintenance of adequate records, including progress reports. A physical therapist shall establish the plan of care and shall provide and/or supervise and direct the appropriate interventions.
      (6) If the diagnostic process reveals findings that are outside the scope of the physical therapist's knowledge, experience, or expertise, the physical therapist shall so inform the patient/client and refer to an appropriate practitioner.
      (7) When the patient has been referred from another practitioner, the physical therapist shall communicate pertinent findings and/ or information to the referring practitioner.
      (8) A physical therapist shall determine when a patient/client will no longer benefit from physical therapy services.
   b. Direction and supervision.
      (1) The supervising physical therapist has primary responsibility for the physical therapy care rendered to a patient/client.
      (2) A physical therapist shall not delegate to a less qualified person any activity that requires the professional skill, knowledge, and judgment of the physical therapist.
   c. Practice arrangements.
      (1) Participation in a business, partnership, corporation, or other entity does not exempt physical therapists, whether employers, partners, or stockholders, either individually or collectively, from the obligation to promote, maintain or comply with the ethical principles of the Association.
      (2) A physical therapist shall advise his/her employer(s) of any employer practice that causes a physical therapist to be in conflict with the ethical principles of the Association. A physical therapist shall seek to eliminate aspects of his/ her employment that are in conflict with the ethical principles of the Association.
   d. Gifts and other consideration(s).
      (1) A physical therapist shall not invite, accept, or offer gifts, monetary incentives, or other considerations that affect or give an appearance of affecting his/her professional judgment.
      (2) A physical therapist shall not offer or accept kickbacks in exchange for patient referrals.

Principle 5

1. A physical therapist shall achieve and maintain professional competence.
   a. Scope of competence.
      (1) A physical therapist shall practice within the scope of his/her competence and commensurate with his/her level of education, training and experience.
   b. Self-assessment.
      (1) A physical therapist has a lifelong professional responsibility for maintaining competence through on-going self-assessment, education, and enhancement of knowledge and skills.
   c. Professional development.
      (1) A physical therapist shall participate in educational activities that enhance his/her basic knowledge and skills.

Principle 6

1. A physical therapist shall maintain and promote high standards for physical therapy practice, education and research.
   a. Professional standards.
      (1) A physical therapist's practice shall be consistent with accepted professional standards. A physical therapist shall continuously engage in assessment activities to determine compliance with these standards.
   b. Practice.
      (1) A physical therapist shall achieve and maintain professional competence.
      (2) A physical therapist shall demonstrate his/ her commitment to quality improvement by engaging in peer and utilization review and other self-assessment activities.
   c. Professional education.
      (1) A physical therapist shall support high-quality education in academic and clinical settings.
      (2) A physical therapist participating in the educational process is responsible to the students, the academic institutions, and the clinical settings for promoting ethical conduct. A physical therapist shall model ethical behavior and provide the student with information about the Code of Ethics, opportunities to discuss ethical conflicts, and procedures for reporting unresolved ethical conflicts.
   d. Continuing education.
      (1) A physical therapist providing continuing education must be competent in the content area.
      (2) When a physical therapist provides continuing education, he/she shall ensure that course content, objectives, faculty credentials, and responsibilities of the instructional staff are accurately stated in the promotional and instructional course materials.
      (3) A physical therapist shall evaluate the efficacy and effectiveness of information and techniques presented in continuing education programs before integrating them into his or her practice.
   e. Research.
      (1) A physical therapist participating in research shall abide by ethical standards governing protection of human subjects and dissemination of results.
      (2) A physical therapist shall support research activities that contribute knowledge for improved patient care.
      (3) A physical therapist shall report to appropriate authorities any acts in the conduct or presentation of research that appear unethical or illegal.

Principle 7

1. A physical therapist shall seek only such remuneration as is deserved and reasonable for physical therapy services.
   a. Business and employment practices.
      (1) A physical therapist's business/employment practices shall be consistent with the ethical principles of the Association.
      (2) A physical therapist shall never place her/his own financial interest above the welfare of individuals under his/her care.
      (3) A physical therapist shall recognize that third-party payer contracts may limit, in one form or another, the provision of physical therapy services. Third-party limitations do not absolve the physical therapist from making sound professional judgments that are in the patient's best interest. A physical therapist shall avoid underutilization of physical therapy services.
      (4) When a physical therapist's judgment is that a patient will receive negligible benefit from physical therapy services, the physical therapist shall not provide or continue to provide such services if the primary reason for doing so is to further the financial self-interest of the physical therapist or his/her employer. A physical therapist shall avoid over-utilization of physical therapy services.
      (5) Fees for physical therapy services should be reasonable for the service performed, considering the setting in which they are provided, practice costs in the geographic area, judgment of other organizations, and other relevant factors.
      (6) A physical therapist shall not directly or indirectly request, receive, or participate in the dividing, transferring, assigning, or rebating of an unearned fee.
      (7) A physical therapist shall not profit by means of a credit or other valuable consideration, such as an unearned commission, discount, or gratuity,

in connection with the furnishing of physical therapy services.

(8) Unless laws impose restrictions to the contrary, physical therapists that provide physical therapy services within a business entity may pool fees and monies received. Physical therapists may divide or apportion these fees and monies in accordance with the business agreement.

(9) A physical therapist may enter into agreements with organizations to provide physical therapy services if such agreements do not violate the ethical principles of the Association or applicable laws.

b. Endorsement of products or services.

(1) A physical therapist shall not exert influence on individuals under his/her care or their families to use products or services based on the direct or indirect financial interest of the physical therapist in such products or services. Realizing that these individuals will normally rely on the physical therapist's advice, their best interest must always be maintained, as must their right of free choice relating to the use of any product or service. Although it cannot be considered unethical for physical therapists to own or have a financial interest in the production, sale, or distribution of products/services, they must act in accordance with law and make full disclosure of their interest whenever individuals under their care use such products/services.

(2) A physical therapist may receive remuneration for endorsement or advertisement of products or services to the public, physical therapists, or other health professionals provided he/she discloses any financial interest in the production, sale, or distribution of said products or services.

(3) When endorsing or advertising products or services, a physical therapist shall use sound professional judgment and shall not give the appearance of Association endorsement unless the Association has formally endorsed the products or services.

c. Disclosure.

(1) A physical therapist shall disclose to the patient if the referring practitioner derives compensation from the provision of physical therapy.

Principle 8

1. A physical therapist shall provide and make available accurate and relevant information to patients/ clients about their care and to the public about physical therapy services.

a. Accurate and relevant information to the patient.

(1) A physical therapist shall provide the patient/client accurate and relevant information about his/her condition and plan of care.

(2) Upon the request of the patient, the physical therapist shall provide, or make available, the medical record to the patient or a patient-designated third party.

(3) A physical therapist shall inform patients of any known financial limitations that may affect their care.

(4) A physical therapist shall inform the patient when, in his/her judgment, the patient will receive negligible benefit from further care.

b. Accurate and relevant information to the public.

(1) A physical therapist shall inform the public about the societal benefits of the profession and who is qualified to provide physical therapy services.

(2) Information given to the public shall emphasize that individual problems cannot be treated without individualized examination and plans/programs of care.

(3) A physical therapist may advertise his/her services to the public.

(4) A physical therapist shall not use, or participate in the use of, any form of communication containing a false, plagiarized, fraudulent, deceptive, unfair, or sensational statement or claim.

(5) A physical therapist that places a paid advertisement shall identify it as such unless it is apparent from the context that it is a paid advertisement.

Principle 9

1. A physical therapist shall protect the public and the profession from unethical, incompetent, and illegal acts.

a. Consumer protection.

(1) A physical therapist shall provide care that is within the scope of practice as defined by the state practice act.

(2) A physical therapist shall not engage in any conduct that is unethical, incompetent or illegal.

(3) A physical therapist shall report any conduct that appears to be unethical, incompetent, or illegal.

(4) A physical therapist may not participate in any arrangements in which patients are exploited due to the referring sources' enhancing their personal incomes as a result of referring for, prescribing, or recommending physical therapy.

Principle 10

1. A physical therapist shall endeavor to address the health needs of society.

a. Pro bono service.

(1) A physical therapist shall render pro bono publico (reduced or no fee) services to patients lacking the ability to pay for services, as each physical therapist's practice permits.

b. Individual and community health.
   (1) A physical therapist shall be aware of the patient's health-related needs and act in a manner that facilitates meeting those needs.
   (2) A physical therapist shall endeavor to support activities that benefit the health status of the community.

Principle 11

1. A physical therapist shall respect the rights, knowledge, and skills of colleagues and other health-care professionals.
   a. Consultation.
      (1) A physical therapist shall seek consultation whenever the welfare of the patient will be safeguarded or advanced by consulting those who have special skills, knowledge, and experience.
   b. Patient/provider relationships.
      (1) A physical therapist shall not undermine the relationship(s) between his/her patient and other health-care professionals.
   c. Disparagement.
      (1) Physical therapists shall not disparage colleagues and other health-care professionals.

From American Physical Therapy Association, JAPTA, 2004, with permission.

Appendix C

Guide for Conduct of the Physical Therapist Assistant

Preamble

The Standards of Ethical Conduct for the Physical Therapist Assistant (Standards of Ethical Conduct) delineate the ethical obligations of all physical therapist assistants as determined by the House of Delegates of the American Physical Therapy Association (APTA). The Standards of Ethical Conduct provide a foundation for conduct to which all physical therapist assistants shall adhere. Fundamental to the Standards of Ethical Conduct is the special obligation of physical therapist assistants to enable patients/clients to achieve greater independence, health and wellness, and enhanced quality of life.

No document that delineates ethical standards can address every situation. Physical therapist assistants are encouraged to seek additional advice or consultation in instances where the guidance of the Standards of Ethical Conduct may not be definitive.

Standards:

Standard #1

Physical therapist assistants shall respect the inherent dignity, and rights, of all individuals.

1A. Physical therapist assistants shall act in a respectful manner toward each person regardless of age, gender, race, nationality, religion, ethnicity, social or economic status, sexual orientation, health condition, or disability.

1B. Physical therapist assistants shall recognize their personal biases and shall not discriminate against others in the provision of physical therapy services.

Standard #2

Physical therapist assistants shall be trustworthy and compassionate in addressing the rights and needs of patients/clients.

2A. Physical therapist assistants shall act in the best interests of patients/clients over the interests of the physical therapist assistant.

2B. Physical therapist assistants shall provide physical therapy interventions with compassionate and caring behaviors that incorporate the individual and cultural differences of patients/clients.

2C. Physical therapist assistants shall provide patients/clients with information regarding the interventions they provide.

2D. Physical therapist assistants shall protect confidential patient/client information and, in collaboration with the physical therapist, may disclose confidential information to appropriate authorities only when allowed or as required by law.

Standard #3

Physical therapist assistants shall make sound decisions in collaboration with the physical therapist and within the boundaries established by laws and regulations.

3A. Physical therapist assistants shall make objective decisions in the patient's/client's best interest in all practice settings.

3B. Physical therapist assistants shall be guided by information about best practice regarding physical therapy interventions.

3C. Physical therapist assistants shall make decisions based upon their level of competence and consistent with patient/client values.

3D. Physical therapist assistants shall not engage in conflicts of interest that interfere with making sound decisions.

3E. Physical therapist assistants shall provide physical therapy services under the direction and supervision of a physical therapist and shall communicate with the physical therapist when patient/client status requires modifications to the established plan of care.

Standard #4

Physical therapist assistants shall demonstrate integrity in their relationships with patients/clients, families, colleagues, students, other healthcare providers, employers, payers, and the public.

4A. Physical therapist assistants shall provide truthful, accurate, and relevant information and shall not make misleading representations.

4B. Physical therapist assistants shall not exploit persons over whom they have supervisory, evaluative or other authority (eg, patients/clients, students, supervisees, research participants, or employees).

4C. Physical therapist assistants shall discourage misconduct by healthcare professionals and report illegal or unethical acts to the relevant authority, when appropriate.

4D. Physical therapist assistants shall report suspected cases of abuse involving children or vulnerable adults to the supervising physical therapist and the appropriate authority, subject to law.

4E. Physical therapist assistants shall not engage in any sexual relationship with any of their patients/clients, supervisees, or students.
4F. Physical therapist assistants shall not harass anyone verbally, physically, emotionally, or sexually.

Standard #5

Physical therapist assistants shall fulfill their legal and ethical obligations.

5A. Physical therapist assistants shall comply with applicable local, state, and federal laws and regulations.
5B. Physical therapist assistants shall support the supervisory role of the physical therapist to ensure quality care and promote patient/client safety.
5C. Physical therapist assistants involved in research shall abide by accepted standards governing protection of research participants.
5D. Physical therapist assistants shall encourage colleagues with physical, psychological, or substance related impairments that may adversely impact their professional responsibilities to seek assistance or counsel.
5E. Physical therapist assistants who have knowledge that a colleague is unable to perform their professional responsibilities with reasonable skill and safety shall report this information to the appropriate authority.

Standard #6

Physical therapist assistants shall enhance their competence through the lifelong acquisition and refinement of knowledge, skills, and abilities.

6A. Physical therapist assistants shall achieve and maintain clinical competence.
6B. Physical therapist assistants shall engage in life-long learning consistent with changes in their roles and responsibilities and advances in the practice of physical therapy.
6C. Physical therapist assistants shall support practice environments that support career development and lifelong learning.

Standard #7

Physical therapist assistants shall support organizational behaviors and business practices that benefit patients/clients and society.

7A. Physical therapist assistants shall promote work environments that support ethical and accountable decision-making.
7B. Physical therapist assistants shall not accept gifts or other considerations that influence or give an appearance of influencing their decisions.
7C. Physical therapist assistants shall fully disclose any financial interest they have in products or services that they recommend to patients/clients.
7D. Physical therapist assistants shall ensure that documentation for their interventions accurately reflects the nature and extent of the services provided.
7E. Physical therapist assistants shall refrain from employment arrangements, or other arrangements, that prevent physical therapist assistants from fulfilling ethical obligations to patients/clients.

Standard #8

Physical therapist assistants shall participate in efforts to meet the health needs of people locally, nationally, or globally.

8A. Physical therapist assistants shall support organizations that meet the health needs of people who are economically disadvantaged, uninsured, and underinsured.
8B. Physical therapist assistants shall advocate for people with impairments, activity limitations, participation restrictions, and disabilities in order to promote their participation in community and society.
8C. Physical therapist assistants shall be responsible stewards of healthcare resources by collaborating with physical therapists in order to avoid over-utilization or under-utilization of physical therapy services.
8D. Physical therapist assistants shall educate members of the public about the benefits of physical therapy.

From American Physical Therapy Association, with permission.

Appendix D

Standards of Practice for Physical Therapy

1. Preamble.

a. The physical therapy profession's commitment to society is to promote optimal health and function in individuals by pursuing excellence in practice. The American Physical Therapy Association attests to this commitment by adopting and promoting the following Standards of Practice for Physical Therapy. These Standards are the profession's statement of conditions and performances that are essential for provision of high-quality professional service to society and provide a foundation for assessment of physical therapy practice.

2. Legal/Ethical Considerations.

a. Legal considerations.
   (1) The physical therapist complies with all the legal requirements of jurisdictions regulating the practice of physical therapy.
   (2) The physical therapist assistant complies with all the legal requirements of jurisdictions regulating the work of the assistant.

b. Ethical considerations.
   (1) The physical therapist practices according to the Code of Ethics of the American Physical Therapy Association.
   (2) The physical therapist assistant complies with the Standards of Ethical Conduct for the Physical Therapist Assistant of the American Physical Therapy Association.

3. Administration of the Physical Therapy Service.

a. Statement of mission, purposes, and goals.
   (1) The physical therapy service has a statement of mission, purposes, and goals that reflects the needs and interests of the patients and clients served, the physical therapy personnel affiliated with the service, and the community.

b. Organizational plan.
   (1) The physical therapy service has a written organizational plan.

c. Policies and procedures.
   (1) The physical therapy service has written policies and procedures that reflect the operation of the service and that are consistent with the Association's standards, mission, policies, positions, guidelines, and Code of Ethics.

d. Administration.
   (1) A physical therapist is responsible for the direction of the physical therapy service.

e. Fiscal management.
   (1) The director of the physical therapy service, in consultation with physical therapy staff and appropriate administrative personnel, participates in planning for, and allocation of, resources. Fiscal planning and management of the service is based on sound accounting principles.

f. Improvement of quality of care and performance.
   (1) The physical therapy service has a written plan for continuous improvement of quality of care and performance of services.

g. Staffing.
   (1) The physical therapy personnel affiliated with the physical therapy service have demonstrated competence and are sufficient to achieve the mission, purposes, and goals of the services.
   (2) The physical therapy service has a written plan that provides for appropriate and ongoing staff development.

h. Physical setting.
   (1) The physical setting is designed to provide a safe and accessible environment that facilitates fulfillment of the mission, purposes, and goals of the physical therapy service. The equipment is safe and sufficient to achieve the purposes and goals of the service.

i. Collaboration.
   (1) The physical therapy service collaborates with all appropriate disciplines.

4. Patient Client Management.

a. Patient client collaboration.
   (1) Within the patient client management process, the physical therapist and the patient client establish and maintain an ongoing collaborative process of decision making that exists throughout the provision of services.

b. Initial examination/evaluation/diagnosis/prognosis.
   (1) The physical therapist performs an initial examination and evaluation to establish a diagnosis and prognosis prior to intervention.

c. Plan of care.
   (1) The physical therapist establishes a plan of care and manages the needs of the patient/client based on the examination, evaluation, diagnosis,

prognosis, goals, and outcomes of the planned interventions for identified impairments, functional limitations, and disabilities.

(2) The physical therapist involves the patient client and appropriate others in the planning, implementation, and assessment of the plan of care.

(3) The physical therapist, in consultation with appropriate disciplines, plans the discharge of the patient client taking into consideration achievement of anticipated goals and expected outcomes, and provides for appropriate follow-up or referral.

d. Intervention.

(1) The physical therapist provides, or directs and supervises, the physical therapy intervention consistent with the results of the examination, evaluation, diagnosis, prognosis, and plan of care.

e. Reexamination.

(1) The physical therapist reexamines the patient/client as necessary during an episode of care to evaluate progress or change in patient/client status and modifies the plan of care accordingly or discontinues physical therapy services.

(2) The physical therapist reexamination.

(a) Identifies ongoing patient/client needs.

(b) May result in recommendations for additional services, discharge, or discontinuation of physical therapy needs.

f. Discharge/discontinuation of intervention.

(1) The physical therapist discharges the patient/client from physical therapy services when the anticipated goals or expected outcomes for the patient/client have been achieved.

(2) The physical therapist discontinues intervention when the patient/client is unable to continue to progress toward goals or when the physical therapist determines that the patient/client will no longer benefit from physical therapy.

g. Communication/coordination/documentation.

(1) The physical therapist communicates, coordinates and documents all aspects of patient/ client management including the results of the initial examination and evaluation, diagnosis, prognosis, plan of care, interventions, response to interventions, changes in patient/client status relative to the interventions, reexamination, and discharge/discontinuation of intervention and other patient client management activities.

h. Education.

(1) The physical therapist is responsible for individual professional development. The physical therapist assistant is responsible for individual career development.

(2) The physical therapist and the physical therapist assistant, under the direction and supervision of the physical therapist, participate in the education of the students.

(3) The physical therapist educates and provides consultation to consumers and the general public regarding the purposes and benefits of physical therapy.

(4) The physical therapist educates and provides consultation to consumers and the general public regarding the roles of the physical therapist, the physical therapist assistant, and other support personnel.

i. Research.

(1) The physical therapist applies research findings to practice and encourages, participates in, and promotes activities that establish the outcomes of patient/client management provided by the physical therapist.

j. Community responsibility.

(1) The physical therapist demonstrates community responsibility by participating in community and community agency activities, educating the public, formulating public policy, or providing pro bono physical therapy services.

k. Glossary.

(1) Client. An individual who is not necessarily sick or injured but who can benefit from a physical therapist's consultation, professional advice, or services. A client also is a business, a school system, or other entity that may benefit from specific recommendations from a physical therapist.

(2) Diagnosis. Both the process and the end result of the evaluation of information obtained from the patient examination. The physical therapist organizes the evaluation information into defined clusters, syndromes, or categories to determine the most appropriate intervention strategies for each patient.

(3) Evaluation. A dynamic process in which the physical therapist makes clinical judgments based on data gathered during the examination.

(4) Examination. The process of obtaining a history, performing relevant systems reviews, and selecting and administering specific tests and measures.

(5) Intervention. The purposeful and skilled interaction of the physical therapist with the patient or client. Intervention has three components: direct intervention; instruction of the patient or client and of the family; and coordination, communication, and documentation.

(6) Patient. An individual who is receiving direct intervention for an impairment, functional limitation, disability, or change in physical function and health status resulting from injury, disease, or other causes; an individual receiving healthcare services.

(7) Physical. therapist patient management model The model on which physical therapists base management of the patient throughout the

episode of care, including the following elements: examination, evaluation and reevaluation, diagnosis, prognosis, and intervention leading to the outcome.

(8) Plan of care. A plan that specifies the long-term and short-term outcomes/goals, the predicted level of maximal improvement, the specific interventions to be used, the duration and frequency of the intervention required to reach the outcomes/goals, and the criteria for discharge.

(9) Prognosis. The determination of the level of maximal improvement that might be attained by the patient and the amount of time needed to reach that level.

(10) Treatment. One or more interventions used to ameliorate impairments, functional limitations or disability or otherwise produce changes in the health status of the patient; the sum of all interventions provided by the physical therapist to a patient during an episode of care.

Acknowledgement to Judith D. Hershberg, PT, DPT, MS; Catherine S. Lane, PT, DPT, MS; Linda Arslanian, PT, DPT, MS; and Rita P. Fleming-Castaldy, PhD, OTL, FAOTA for their original contributions in formulating this chapter.

Appendix E

Table 12-1 ➤ OUTCOME MEASURES ORGANIZED BY THE INTERNATIONAL CLASSIFICATION OF FUNCTIONING, DISABILITY, AND HEALTH (ICF) CATEGORIES

BODY STRUCTURE AND FUNCTION MEASURES	REFERENCES
Manual Muscle Test (MMT)	Hislop HJ, Montgomery J. Daniels and Worthingham's Muscle Testing: Techniques of Manual Examination, 8th ed. Saunders (Elsevier), Philadelphia, 2007. Kendall, F, McCreary E, Provance P, et al. Muscles Testing and Function with Posture and Pain, 5th ed. Lippincott Williams & Wilkins, Baltimore, 2005.
Joint Motion	Norkin C, White, J. Measurement of Joint Motion, 4th ed. FA Davis, Philadelphia, 2009.
Modified Ashworth Scale	Bohannon RW, Smith, MB. Interrater reliability of a modified Ashworth scale of muscle spasticity. Phys Ther 67:206–207, 1987. Blackburn M, van Vliet P, Mockett SP. Reliability of measurements obtained with the Modified Ashworth Scale in the lower extremities of people with stroke. Phys Ther 82:25–34, 2002. Haas BM, Bergstrom E, Jamous A, et al. The interrater reliability of the original and the modified Ashworth scale for the assessment of spasticity in patients with spinal cord injury. Spinal Cord 34:560–564, 1996.
Glasgow Coma Scale (GCS)	Jennett B, Teasdale G. Management of Head Injuries. FA Davis, Philadelphia, 1981.
Rancho Levels of Cognitive Function (LOCF) [TBI]	Hagen C, Malkmus D, Durham P. Levels of cognitive functioning. In: Rehabilitation of the Head Injured Adult: Comprehensive Physical Management. Downey, CA: Professional Staff Association of Ranchos Los Amigos Hospital, 1979.
ASIA Impairment Scale – Standard Neurological Classification of Spinal Cord Injury	American Spinal Injury Association: International Standards for Neurological Classification of Spinal Cord Injury. American Spinal Injury Association, Chicago, 2006.
Mini Mental State Exam (MMSE)	Folstein MF, Folstein SE, McHugh PR. "Mini-mental state." A practical method for grading the cognitive state of patients for the clinician. J Psychiatr Res 12(3):189, 1975.
Fugl-Meyer [CVA]	Fugl-Meyer AR, Jaasko L, Leyman I, et al. The post-stroke hemiplegic patient: a method for evaluation and performance. Scand J Rehabil Med 7:13–31, 1975. Fugl-Meyer AR. Post-stroke hemiplegia assessment of physical properties. Scand J Rehabil Med 63:85–93, 1980. Gladstone DJ, Danells CJ, Black S. The Fugl-Myer assessment of motor recovery after stroke: a critical review of its measurement properties. Neurorehabil Neural Repair 16:232, 2002.
National Institutes of Health (NIH) Stroke Scale [CVA]	Brott T, Adams HP, Olinger CP, et al. Measurements of acute cerebral infarction: a clinical examination scale. Stroke 20:864–70, 1989.

BODY STRUCTURE AND FUNCTION MEASURES	REFERENCES
	Goldstein LB, Bertels C, Davis JN. Interrater reliability of the NIH stroke scale. Arch Neurol 46:660–662, 1989. Heinemann A, Harvey R, McGuire JR, et al. Measurement properties of the NIH stroke scale during acute rehabilitation. Stroke 28:1174–1180, 1997. The NIH Stroke Scale is available online at: *http://www.ninds.nih.gov/doctors/NIH_Stroke_Scale.pdf*
Postural Assessment Scale for Stroke Patients (PASS) [CVA]	Benaim C, Pérennou DA, Villy J, et al. Validation of a standardized assessment of postural control in stroke patients: the Postural Assessment Scale for Stroke Patients (PASS). Stroke 30:1862–1868, 1999. Pyoria O, TaLvitie U, Nyrkko H, et al. Validity of the Postural Control and Balance for Stroke Test. Physiother Res Int 12(3):162–174, 2007.
Unified Parkinson's Disease Rating Scale (UPDRS)	Fahn S, Elton R. Unified Parkinson's Disease Rating Scale. In: Fahn S, et al (eds): Recent Developments in Parkinson's Disease, Vol 2. Macmillan Health Care Information, Florham Park, NJ, 1987:153–167. Unified Parkinson's Disease Rating Scale available online at: *http://www.mdvu.org/library/ratingscales/pd/updrs.pdf*
Functional Independence Measure (FIM)	Guide for the Uniform Data Set for Medical Rehabilitation (Adult FIM) version 4.0, State University of New York at Buffalo, 1993. Dodds TA, Martin DP, Stolov WC, et al. A validation of the functional independence measurement and its performance among rehabilitation in-patients. Arch Phys Med Rehabil 74:531–536, 1993. Linacre JM, Heinemann AW, Wright BD, et al. The structure and stability of the Functional Independence Measure. Arch Phys Med Rehabil 75:127–132, 1994. Long WB, Sacco MJ, Coombes SS, et al. Determining normative standards for Functional Independence Measure transitions in rehabilitation. Arch Phys Med Rehabil 75:144–148, 1994. Hamilton BB, Laughlin JA, Fielder RC, et al. Interrater reliability of the 7-level Functional Independence Measure (FIM). Scand J Rehabil Med 26:115–119, 1994. The FIM is available online at: email: info@udsmr.org *web site: http://www.udsmr.org*
Functional Assessment Measure (FIM + FAM)	Linn RT, et al. Does the Functional Assessment Measure (FAM) extend the Functional Independence Measure (FIM ™) Instrument? A Rasch analysis of stroke patients. J Outcome Measure 3:339, 1999. Hall KM. The Functional Assessment Measure (FAM). J Rehabil Outcomes 1(3):63–65, 1997. Hall KM, Mann N, High WM, et al. Functional measures after traumatic brain injury: Ceiling effects of FIM, FIM+FAM, DRS, and CIQ. J Head Trauma Rehabil 11(5):27–39, 1996. The FIM + FAM is available online at: *http://www.birf.info/pdf/tools/famform.pdf*
Barthel Index (BI)	Granger CV, Devis LS, Peters MC, et al. Stroke rehabilitation analysis of repeated Barthel Index measures. Arch Phys Med Rehabil 60:14–17, 1979.

(Continued on following page)

ACTIVITY MEASURES	REFERENCES
	Mahoney FI, Barthel DW. Functional evaluation: The Barthel Index. Maryland State Med J 14:61–65, 1965.
Physical Performance Test	Reuben DB, Siu AL. An objective measure of physical function of elderly populations: The Physical Performance Test. J Am Geriatr Soc 38:1105, 1990.
Disabilities of the Arm, Shoulder, and Hand Outcome Measure (DASH)	Beaton DE, Davis AM, Hudak P, McConnell S. The DASH (Disabilities of the Arm, Shoulder and Hand) Outcome Measure: What do we know about it now? Br J Hand Ther 6(4):109–118, 2001. Beaton DE, Katz JN, Fossel AH, et al. Measuring the whole or the parts? validity, reliability & responsiveness of the disabilities of the arm, shoulder, and hand outcome measure in different regions of the upper extremity. J Hand Ther 14(2):128, 2001. Bot SDM, Terwee CB, van der Windt DAWM, et al. Clinimetric evaluation of shoulder disability questionnaires: A systematic review of the literature. Ann Rheum Dis 63(4):335, 2004. Available online at: *http://www.dash.iwh.on.ca/*
Lower Extremity Functional Scale (LEFS)	WangY-C, Hart DL, Stratford PW, Mioduski JE. Clinical Interpretation of a Lower-Extremity Functional Scale–derived computerized adaptive test. Phys Ther 89(9):957 2009. Lin CW, Moseley AM, Refshauge KM, Bundy AC. The Lower Extremity Functional Scale has good clinimetric properties in people with ankle fracture. Phys Ther 89(6):580, 2009. Binkley JM, Stratford PW, Lott SA, Riddle DL. The Lower Extremity Functional Scale (LEFS): Scale development, measurement properties, and clinical application. Phys Ther 79(4):371, 1999. Available online at: *http://www.tac.vic.gov.au/upload/LE.pdf*
High Level Mobility Assessment Tool (HiMat) [TBI]	Williams GP, Robertson V, Greenwood KM, et al. The high-level mobility assessment tool (HiMAT) for traumatic brain injury. Part 1: Item generation. Brain Injury19(11):925–932, 2005. Williams GP, Robertson V, Greenwood, KM et al. The high-level mobility assessment tool (HiMAT) for traumatic brain injury. Part 2: Content validity and discriminability. Brain Injury 19(10): 833–843, 2005. Williams GP, Greenwood KM, Robertson VJ, et al. High-Level Mobility Assessment Tool (Hi-MAT): Inter-rater reliability, retest reliability, and internal consistency. Phys Ther 86:395–400, 2006. The HiMat is available online at: *http://www.tbims.org/combi/himat/index.html*
Wheelchair Skills Test (WST) [SCI]	Kirby RL, Dupuis DJ, MacPhee AH, et al. The Wheelchair Skills Test (version 2.4): measurement properties. Arch Phys Med Rehabil 85:794, 2004 Videotapes for Wheelchair Users and Wheelchair Skills Program (WSP) Version 4.1 Manual available online at: *http://www.wheelchairskillsprogram.ca/eng/overview.htm* Additional online resources The Powered Wheelchair Training Guide *http://www.wheelchairnet.org/WCN_Prodserv/Docs/PWTG/WCN_PWTG.html* The Manual Wheelchair Training Guide

ACTIVITY MEASURES	REFERENCES
	http://www.wheelchairnet.org/wcn_prodserv/Docs/WCN_MWTG.html A Guide to Wheelchair Selection *http://www.wheelchairnet.org/WCN_Prodserv/Docs/WCN_PVAguide.html*
Wolf Motor Function Test (WMFT) [CVA]	Wolf SL, Catlin PA, Ellis M, et al. Assessing Wolf Motor Function Test as outcome measure for research in patients after stroke. Stroke 32:1635, 2001. Morris DM, Uswatte G, Crago JE, et al. The reliability of the Wolf Motor Function Test for assessing upper extremity function after stroke. Arch Phys Med Rehabil 82:750, 2001.
Motor Activity Log (MAL) [CVA]	Wolf SL, Thompson PA, Morris DM, et al. The EXCITE trial: Attributes of the Wolf Motor Function Test in patients with subacute stroke. Neurorehabil Neural Repair 19:194, 2005. Uswatte G, Taub E, Morris D, et al. The Motor Activity Log-28: Assessing daily use of the hemiparetic arm after stroke. Neurology 67:1189, 2006. Van der Lee JH, Beckerman H, Knol DL, et al. Clinimetric properties of the motor activity log for the assessment of arm use in hemiparetic patients. Stroke 35:1410, 2004.
Berg Balance Scale (BBS)	Berg K, Wood-Dauphinee S, Williams J, et al. Measuring balance in the elderly: preliminary development of an instrument. Physiother Can 41:304–311, 1989. Berg KO, Maki B, Williams JI, et al. Clinical and laboratory measures of postural balance in an elderly population. Arch Phys Med Rehabil 73:1073–1080, 1992. Berg KO, Wood-Dauphince SL, Williams JI, et al. Measuring balance in the elderly: Validation of an instrument. Can J Public Health 83:S7–11, 1992. Berg KO, Wood-Dauphinee S, Williams JI. The balance scale: reliability assessment with elderly residents and patients with an acute stroke. Scand J Rehabil Med 27:27–36, 1995.
Functional Reach (FR)	Duncan P, et al. Functional Reach: A new clinical measure of balance. J Gerontol 45:M192, 1990. Duncan PW, Studenski S, Chandler J, Prescott B. Functional reach: Predictive validity in a sample of elderly male veterans. J Gerontol 47: M93, 1992. Weiner DK, Duncan PW, Chandler J, Studenski SA. Functional Reach: A marker of physical frailty. J Am Geriatr Soc 40:2–3, 1992.
Multidirectional Reach	Newton R. Validity of the multi-directional reach test: A practical measure for limits of stability in older adults. J Gerontol Med Sci 56(4):M248–52, 2001. Newton R. Validity of MDRT. J Gerontol 56A.4:M248, 2001.
Modified Functional Reach (seated)	Lynch SM, Leahy P, Barker S. Reliability of measurements obtained with a modified functional reach test in subjects with spinal cord injury. Phys Ther 78(2):128, 1998.
Stops Walking When Talking (SWWT)	Lundin-Olsson L, Nyberg L, Gustafson Y. Stops walking when talking as a predictor of falls in elderly people. Lancet 348:617, 1997.
Timed Up & Go (TUG)	Ng SS, Hui-Chan CW. The Timed Up & Go test: Its reliability and association with lower-limb impairments and locomotor capabilities in people with chronic stroke. Arch Phys Med Rehabil 86:1641–1647, 2005.

(Continued on following page)

ACTIVITY MEASURES	REFERENCES
	Podsiadlo D, Richardson S. The Timed "Up & Go": A test of basic functional mobility for frail elderly persons. J Am Geriatr Soc 39:142–148, 1992.
Performance Oriented Mobility Assessment (POMA) (Tinetti)	Tinetti M. Performance-oriented assessment of mobility problems in elderly patients. J Am Geriatr Soc 34:119–126, 1986.
Clinical Test for Sensory Integration in Balance (CTSIB)	Shumway-Cook A, Horak F. Assessing the influence of sensory interaction on balance. Phys Ther 1986;66(10): 1548–1550.
Modified Clinical Test for Sensory Integration in Balance (mCTSIB)	Rose DJ. Fallproof! A Comprehensive Balance and Mobility Training Program. Human Kinetics, Champaign, IL, 2003.
Functional Gait Assessment (FGA)	Wrisley DM, Marchetti GF, Kuharsky DK, Whitney SL. Reliability, internal consistency, and validity of data obtained with the functional gait assessment. Phys Ther 84:906–918, 2004.
Modified Emory Functional Ambulation Profile (mEFAP)	Baer HR, Wolf SL. Modified Emory Functional Ambulation Profile: An outcome measure for rehabilitation for post stroke gait dysfunction. Stroke 32:973, 2001. Wolf SL, Catlin PA, Gage K. Establishing the reliability and validity of measurements using the Emory Functional Ambulation Profile. Phys Ther 79:1122, 1999. Nelson, AJ: Functional ambulation profile. Phys Ther 54:1059, 1974.
10 Minute Walk Test	Collen FM, Wade DT, Bradshaw CM. Mobility after stroke: reliability of measures of impairment and disability. Int Disabil Studies 12:6–9, 1990. Bohannon RW, Andrews AW, Thomas MW. Walking speed: Reference values and correlates for older adults. J Orthop Sports Phys Ther 77:86, 1996.
6 Minute Walk Test	Enright, PL, Sherrill, DL. Reference equations for the six-minute walk in healthy adults. Am J Respir Crit Care Med 158:1384–1387, 1998. Liu J, Drutz C, Kumar R, et al. Use of six minute walk test post stroke. Is there a practice effect? Arch Phys Med Rehabil 89:1686–1692, 2008. Fulk GD, Echternach JL, Nof L, O'Sullivan S. Clinometric properties of the six-minute walk test in individuals undergoing rehabilitation poststroke. Physiother Theory and Pract 24:195–204, 2008.
Dynamic Gait Index (DGI)	Shumway-Cook A, Woollacott M. Motor Control—Translating Research into Clinical Practice, 3rd ed. Lippincott Williams & Wilkins, 2007:395–396. Jonsdottir J, Cattaneo D. Reliability and validity of the Dynamic Gait Index in persons with chronic stroke. Arch of Phys Med and Rehabil 88(11):1410–1415, 2007. Walker ML, Austin G, Banke GM, et al. Reference group data for the Functional Gait Assessment. Phys Ther 87(11):1468–1477, 2007 Wrisley D. Functional Gait Assessment Phys Ther 84(10): Appendix, 2007.
Observational Gait Analysis (OGA)	Norkin C: Examination of gait. In: O'Sullivan S, Schmit. T. Physical Rehabilitation, 5th edition. FA Davis, Philadelphia, 2007:320–334. Pathokinesiology Service and Physical Therapy Department: Observational Gait Analysis Handbook. Los Amigos Research and Education Institute, Inc, Downey, CA, 2001. Perry JP. Gait Analysis: Normal and Pathological Function. Thorofare, NJ: Slack, 1992.

PARTICIPATION MEASURES	REFERENCES
The MOS SF-36 Health Survey	Anderson C, Laubscher S, Burns R. Validation of the short-form (SF-36) health survey questionnaire among stroke patients. Stroke 27:1812–1816, 1996. Ware JE, Sherbourne CD. The MOS 36-Item Short-Form Health Survey (SF-36), 1: conceptual framework and item selection. Med Care 30:473–483, 1992. The SF-36 Health Survey is available online at: *http://www.rand.org/health/surveys/sf36item/*
Participation Objective, Participation Subjective (POPS)	Brown M, Dijkers MPJ, Gordon W, et al Participation Objective, Participation Subjective: A measure of participation combining outsider and insider perspectives. J Head Trauma Rehabil 19(6), 459–481, 2004. Mascialino G, Hirshson C, Egan M, et al. Objective and subjective assessment of long-term community integration in minority groups following traumatic brain injury. NeuroRehabilitation 24 (1):29–36, 2009. The POPS is available online at: *http://www.tbims.org/combi/pops/Appendix%20I.doc*
Impact of Participation and Autonomy (IPA)	Cardol M., de Haan RJ, de Jong BA, et al. Psychometric properties of the impact on participation and autonomy questionnaire. Arch Phys Med Rehabil 82(2):210–216, 2001. The IPA is available online at: *http://www.nivel.nl/pdf/INT-IPA-E.pdf*
Activities and Balance Confidence Scales (ABC)	Lajoie Y, Gallagher SP. Predicting falls within the elderly community: Comparison of postural sway, reaction time, the Berg Balance Scale, and the Activity-specific Balance Confidence scale for comparing fallers and non-fallers. Arch Gerontol Geriatr 38:11–26, 2004. Myers AM, Fletcher PC, Myers AN, et al. Discriminative and evaluative properties of the ABC Scale. J Gerontol 53A: M287–M294, 1998. Powell LE, Myers AM. Activities-specific Balance Confidence (ABC) Scale. J Gerontol 50A:M28–34, 1995. The ABC Scale is available online at: *http://www.pacificbalancecenter.com/forms/abc_scale.pdf*
Tinetti Falls Efficacy Scale (FES)	Harada N, Chiu V, Damon-Rodriquez J. Screening balance and mobility impairment in elderly individuals living in a residential care facility. Phys Ther 75:462–469, 1995.
Dizziness Handicap Inventory (DHI)	Jacobson GP, Newman CW. The development of the dizziness handicap inventory. Arch Otolaryngol Head Neck Surg 16:424–427, 1990.
Modified Fatigue Impact Scale (mFIS)	Fisk JD, Pontefract A, Ritvo PG, et al. The impact of fatigue on patients with multiple sclerosis. Can J Neurol Sci 21(1):9, 1994. Fisk JD, Ritvo PG, Ross L, et al. Measuring the functional impact of fatigue: Initial validation of the Fatigue Impact Scale. Clin Infect Dis Suppl 1:S79, 1994.
Outpatient Physical Therapy Improvement in Assessment Log (OPTIMAL)	Guccione AA, Mielenz TJ, Devellis RF, et al. Development and testing of a self-report instrument to measure actions: outpatient physical therapy improvement in movement assessment log (OPTIMAL). Phys Ther 85(6):515–530, 2005. *Optimal is available online at: http://www.apta.org*

(Continued on following page)

PARTICIPATION MEASURES	REFERENCES
Craig Handicap Assessment and Reporting Technique (CHART)	Walker N, Mellick D, Brooks CA, et al. Measuring participation across impairment groups using the Craig Handicap Assessment Reporting Technique. Am J Phys Med Rehabil 82(12):936–941, 2003. Hall KM, Dijkers M, Whiteneck G, et al. The Craig Handicap Assessment and Reporting Technique (CHART): Metric properties and scoring. J Rehabil Outcomes Measure 2(5):39–49, 1998. CHART is available online at: *http://www.tbims.org/combi/chart/index.html*
Stroke Impact Scale (SIS)	Duncan PW, Lai SM, Bode RK, et al. Stroke Impact Scale-16: A brief assessment of physical function. Neurology 60(2):291, 2003. Lai SM, Perera S, Duncan PW, et al. Physical and social functioning after stroke: Comparison of the Stroke Impact Scale and Short Form-36. Stroke 34(2):488, 2003. Duncan PW, Bode R, Lai SM, et al. Rasch analysis of a new stroke-specific outcome scale: The Stroke Impact Scale. Arch Phys Med Rehabil 84(7):950, 2003. Guide for Stroke Impact Scale Administration is available at: *http://www2.kumc.edu/coa/SIS/SIS_admin_guide.doc* The SIS is available online at: *http://www.chrp.org/pdf/HSR082103_SIS_Handout.pdf*

Note: All websites referenced in table accessed September 30, 2009.

Key: TBI: traumatic brain injury; SCI: spinal cord injury; CVA: cerebrovascular accident.

From O'Sullivan S, Schmitz T (2010). Improving Functional Outcomes in Physical Rehabilitation. Philadelphia, FA Davis, with permission.

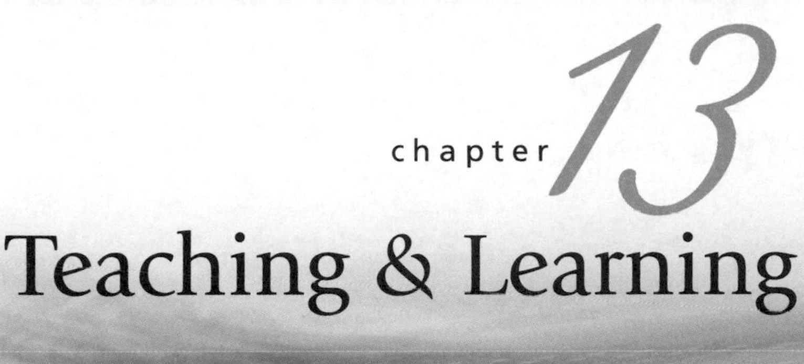

chapter 13 Teaching & Learning

SUSAN B. O'SULLIVAN

Physical Therapist Roles and Responsibilities

Patient/Client-Related Instruction

1. **The process of:** informing, educating, or training patients/clients, families, significant others, and caregivers in order to promote and optimize physical therapy services (APTA Guide To Physical Therapist Practice, 2nd ed. Phys Ther 81: 47, 2001).

2. **Provided across all settings.** For all patients/clients on promoting understanding of:
   a. Current condition, impairments, functional limitations, and disabilities.
   b. Anticipated goals and expected outcomes, the plan of care, specific intervention elements, and self-management strategies.
   c. Elements necessary for the smooth transition to home or an alternate setting, work, and community.
   d. Individualized family service plans (IFSPs) or individualized education plans (IEPs).
   e. Safety awareness, and risk factor reduction and prevention.
   f. Health promotion, wellness, and fitness.

Educational Programs

1. **Instruction and educational programs are provided for:**
   a. Other therapists, health care providers, staff, and/or students in academic and/or clinical settings. Programs can be formal or informal.
   b. Instruction and educational programs are provided for local, state, and federal agencies.
   c. The general public to increase awareness of health issues and roles of the physical therapist.

Clinical Education of Students

1. **Instruction and supervision of physical therapy or physical therapist assistant students.**
   a. Provided by clinical instructors during scheduled clinical education experiences.
   b. Close communication and collaboration with the school and the academic coordinator of clinical education is necessary.

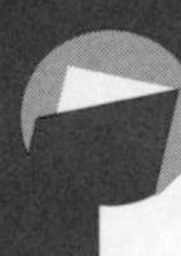

Educational Theory

"Learning is the process whereby knowledge is created through the transformation of experience" (Kolb, 1984).

Learning Styles

1. **Characteristic mode.**
   a. Of gaining, processing, and storing information. Learning styles differ across dimensions.

2. **Analytical versus intuitive learners.**
   a. Analytical/objective learner.
      (1) Processes information in a step-by-step order.
      (2) Perceives information in an objective manner; is able to use facts and easily understand relationships between them.
      (3) Perceives information in an abstract, conceptual manner; information does not need to be related to personal experience.
      (4) Learns best with structure, step by step learning; may have difficulty comprehending the big picture.
   b. Intuitive/global learner.
      (1) Processes information all at once, in a simultaneous manner; not in an ordered sequence.
      (2) Perceives information in a subjective manner: reflects on personal experiences.
      (3) Perceives information in a concrete manner: information assimilated about practical, real-life experiences.
      (4) Learns best if information is connected to personal experiences and presented in a practical, real-life context. If not, knowledge may be disregarded. May have difficulty ordering steps and comprehending details.

3. **Reasoning: inductive versus deductive.**
   a. Inductive reasoner (assimilator): observes similarities, can develop theoretical models to explain relationships.
   b. Deductive reasoner (converger): analyzes problems in depth; applies information, theoretical models to practical situations.

4. **Initiative: active versus passive learner.**
   a. Active/aggressive learner: exhibits initiative, actively seeks information; may reach conclusions quickly before all information is gathered.
   b. Passive learner: often exhibits little initiative; responds best to directed learning.

Learning Theories

1. **Behaviorist (stimulus-response theory).**
   a. Basic premises.
      (1) Behavior is modified in response to a given stimulus.
      (2) Behavior is determined by its consequences; the response of one behavior becomes the stimulus for the next response (chaining).
      (3) Learning occurs because the behavior is reinforced (learned association).
   b. Behavior can be controlled or shaped by operant conditioning (behavior modification techniques).
      (1) Desired or correct behaviors are identified.
      (2) Frequent and scheduled reinforcements are given to reinforce the desired behaviors; e.g., praise, encouragement, candy.
         (a) Accuracy of reinforcement is critical; e.g., use of rewards that are meaningful to the individual.
         (b) Timing of reinforcement is critical: immediate versus distant or delayed; e.g., use of a reinforcement schedule.
      (3) Negative behaviors are ignored; unreinforced behaviors are weakened and eventually extinguished.
      (4) Behavior that has aversive consequences (punishment) is less likely to occur again; aversive conditioning is less powerful as a tool for learning than positive reinforcements.
      (5) The environment is altered to promote correct responses; e.g., a closed environment with reduction of distractors.
      (6) Repetition is a necessary prerequisite for learning.
      (7) Clinical uses: limited; e.g., may be used when working with adults with impaired or limited cognitive abilities (traumatic brain injury, stroke) or young children.
   c. Prominent theorists: B.F. Skinner, G. Watson.

2. **Cognitive theory.**
   a. Basic premises.
      (1) Focus is on cognitive development of intellectual abilities and skills, from:
         (a) Symbolic function (ages 2 to 8).
         (b) Concrete mental operations (ages 8 to 12).
         (c) Conceptual thought (ages 12 and up).
      (2) Thinking emerges with language development.

(3) Perceptual features are important conditions of learning; e.g., figure-ground, directional signs, sequence.

b. Cognitive strategies are used; e.g., repeated challenges to thinking.
   (1) Knowledge is organized by the teacher; the teacher is the expert; a pedagogical approach (the art and science of teaching children).
   (2) Learning is culturally relative.
   (3) Cognitive feedback is used to confirm and correct knowledge.
   (4) Goal-setting by learner is important for motivation.
   (5) Both divergent and convergent theory is nurtured.

c. Prominent theorists: J. Piaget, J.S. Bruner.

3. Humanist.

a. Basic premises.
   (1) Personal freedom and dignity of the individual is emphasized in the learning process.
   (2) Understanding of the learner's needs and feelings is sought.
   (3) The learner experiences unconditional positive regard, acceptance, and understanding.

b. Teaching is student-centered; e.g., self-discovery, self-appropriated learning, experiential learning.
   (1) Promotes active learning (self-initiated) rather than passive; e.g., knowledge is organized by the learner, not for the learner.
   (2) Learning addresses relevant problems and issues.
   (3) A positive learning climate is facilitated.
   (4) The teacher is a facilitator and resource-finder.
   (5) Learning is evaluated by the learner; e.g., self-assessment.

c. Prominent theorists: Carl Rogers, A.H. Maslow.

4. Adult learning (andragogy).

a. Basic characteristics of adult learners.
   (1) The learner is self-directed: goal-oriented, seeks knowledge for own sake.
   (2) Has a rich core of experience that serves as a broad base for learning.
   (3) Demonstrates a readiness to learn.
   (4) Demonstrates a problem-centered orientation to learning.

b. Teaching is learner-centered.
   (1) The teacher interacts with the learner: helps to clarify the learning problem, structure the learning environment to enhance learning, provide resources.
   (2) Learners share the responsibility for planning the learning experience; actively participate in the learning process.
   (3) The learning process makes use of the experiences of the learner.

c. Prominent theorists: M. Knowles, J.R. Kidd.

Behavioral Objectives from the Educational Domains

1. Cognitive: objectives concern mental processes, the acquisition of intellectual skills; e.g., remembering and recalling knowledge, thinking, problem-solving, creating.

a. Level 1.0 Knowledge: involves recall of previously learned information; e.g., knows specific facts, terminology, criteria, methodology; the learner is able to:
   (1) Remember or recall information; e.g., defines, describes.
   (2) Organize and reorganize information; e.g., matches, reproduces.

b. Level 2.0 Comprehension: involves understanding at its lowest level; the learner is able to:
   (1) Translate, interpret, and extrapolate information; e.g., defends, distinguishes, explains.
   (2) Use information; e.g., predicts, infers.

c. Level 3.0 Application: involves use of abstractions; the learner is able to:
   (1) Apply knowledge and concepts to situations; e.g., modifies, changes, relates.
   (2) Formulate and utilize rules or generalize methods; e.g., predicts, manipulates.

d. Level 4.0 Analysis: involves the breakdown of information into component parts to enable clear understanding; the learner is able to:
   (1) Clarify information; e.g., recognizes unstated assumptions, fallacies in reasoning; correctly answers questions on licensure examination.
   (2) Indicate how the information is organized or arranged; e.g., analyze relationships or organizational structure.
   (3) Distinguish facts from inferences, hypotheses; e.g., differentiates, discriminates.

e. Level 5.0 Synthesis: involves putting together of elements to form a whole; the learner is able to:
   (1) Produce unique communications; e.g., write a report, relate a clinical experience effectively.
   (2) Formulate a plan of care or research proposal.

f. Level 6.0 Evaluation: involves making judgments about the value of material or methods; the learner is able to:
   (1) Produce a judgment about the accuracy of information using internal criteria; e.g., judge the accuracy, consistency of a written research report.
   (2) Produce a judgment of material using external criteria; e.g., use major theories to evaluate material, judge the value of a clinical report.

2. Affective: objectives concern feelings and emotions; e.g., interests, attitudes, appreciations, values, emotional sets or biases.

a. Level 1.0 Receiving (attending): objectives involve attending to phenomena and stimuli; the learner demonstrates:

(1) Awareness; e.g., describes the clinical environment (objects and structures around him), people, and situations.
(2) Willingness to receive; e.g., listens to others, demonstrates tolerance and sensitivity to human needs, cultural differences.
(3) Selected attention; e.g., attends closely to discussions of human values or judgments.

b. Level 2.0 Responding: objectives involve responses or actions; the learner demonstrates:
(1) Compliance; e.g., willingness to respond to hospital rules.
(2) Acceptance of responsibility; e.g., protects confidentiality of patients.
(3) Satisfaction in responses; e.g., takes pleasure in communicating effectively with patients and families.

c. Level 3.0 Valuing: objectives involve accepting and internalizing worth or value; the learner demonstrates:
(1) Consistency of response in situations based on holding a value; e.g., respects human dignity of patients through appropriate actions in varying situations.
(2) Preference for and commitment to a value; e.g., actively participates in discussions about viewpoints such as euthanasia.

d. Level 4.0 Organization: objectives involve organization of a value system; the learner demonstrates:
(1) Conceptualization; e.g., recognizes or forms judgments based on a value; accepts responsibility for own behavior.
(2) Ordered relationships; e.g., able to look at health care policies affecting the elderly and formulates a life plan for advocacy.

e. Level 5.0 Characterization by a value or value complex; objectives involve:
(1) Persistent and consistent behaviors influenced by a well-developed value system; e.g., displays safety consciousness, self-reliance in working independently.
(2) Consistent adherence to a professional code of ethics; e.g., displays consistent professional behaviors.

3. **Psychomotor:** objectives concern motor skills; e.g., writing, speaking, performing motor acts or skills; objectives include an aspect of performance; the learner demonstrates ability to:
   a. Write a plan of care smoothly and legibly.
   b. Set up clinical equipment quickly and correctly.
   c. Operate clinical equipment safely and skillfully.
   d. Perform manual therapeutic exercise skills correctly and effectively.
   e. Perform functional mobility skills safely and correctly.
   f. Perform activities of daily living independently and safely.

Instruction

Instructional Process

1. **Learner/needs assessment:** identify relevant characteristics and needs of the learner prior to the educational experience.
   a. Determine what the learner needs to know.
      (1) Current level of knowledge.
      (2) Plans/needs for the future.
   b. Determine what the learner brings to the learning experience.
      (1) Educational background, previous knowledge and experiences.
      (2) All instruction should take into account the influences of age, culture, gender roles, race, sex, sexual orientation, and socioeconomic status.
   c. Determine the learner's readiness to learn.
      (1) Learning style.
      (2) Capabilities, attentiveness, energy level.
   d. Identify impairments that may impact on learning: e.g., perceptual deficits, visual impairments, communication impairments, confusion, memory loss, emotional dysregulation.
   e. Identify available resources; e.g., information about facilities, materials, time available for the instructional process.

2. **Analysis of data, formulation of objectives of instruction.** (See Figure 13-2).
   a. Specify what the learner should learn (goals and behavioral objectives).
      (1) Identify what the learner will do; e.g., describe, discuss, explain.
      (2) Identify what the criteria of performance are; e.g., given a list of risk factors that the learner will correctly identify.
      (3) Specify the conditions of the performance; e.g., 75% of the time.

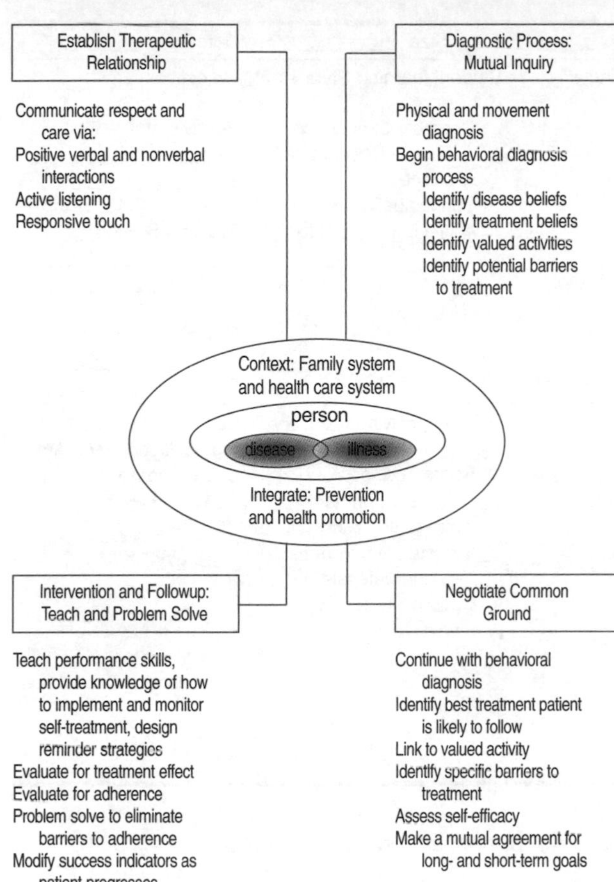
Establish Therapeutic Relationship
Communicate respect and care via:
Positive verbal and nonverbal interactions
Active listening
Responsive touch
Diagnostic Process: Mutual Inquiry
Physical and movement diagnosis
Begin behavioral diagnosis process
Identify disease beliefs
Identify treatment beliefs
Identify valued activities
Identify potential barriers to treatment
Context: Family system and health care system
person
disease
illness
Integrate: Prevention and health promotion
Intervention and Followup: Teach and Problem Solve
Teach performance skills, provide knowledge of how to implement and monitor self-treatment, design reminder strategies
Evaluate for treatment effect
Evaluate for adherence
Problem solve to eliminate barriers to adherence
Modify success indicators as patient progresses
Negotiate Common Ground
Continue with behavioral diagnosis
Identify best treatment patient is likely to follow
Link to valued activity
Identify specific barriers to treatment
Assess self-efficacy
Make a mutual agreement for long- and short-term goals

Figure 13-1 • Patient-Practitioner Collaborative Model. From: Shepard, K and Jensen, G: Handbook of Teaching for Physical Therapists. Boston, Butterworth-Heinemann, 1997, p 252, with permission.

(4) Set goals that are attainable, mutually agreed upon by learner and instructor.

(5) Use clear, unambiguous, and measurable terms; e.g., family/caregiver will demonstrate understanding of safety measures to prevent falls by correctly describing proper use of brakes and transfer sequence 100% of the time within 2 weeks.

b. Set priorities.

(1) Determine which educational goals are most important, what sequence is needed.

(2) Ensure maximum utilization of available teaching time.

(3) Avoid bombardment; e.g., too much, too soon.

(4) Repetition is important for learning; build in experiences that reinforce instruction.

3. Analysis of instruction/planning (what, how, where, when).

a. Select what materials to use; options include print, audiovisual media, computer assisted instruction, models.

b. Select what methods of teaching are appropriate; options include individual instruction, group discussion, organized classes/lecture, demonstration and modeling, tutorials. Also includes written or pictorial instruction; e.g., home exercise program.

(1) Choice of method is dependent on:

(a) The individual learner/unique characteristics; e.g., preferences for rate and style of learning, motivation.

(b) Objectives of instruction.

(2) A variety of teaching methods is typically helpful to reinforce the learning.

c. Select what activities are likely to help the learner achieve the stated objectives.

4. Implementation: strategies to affect mastery of learning.

a. Individuals learn best when:

(1) They are actively involved in goal setting and the learning process; learning is not dictated by the instructor.

(2) Learners need to feel free to freely express their own ideas, beliefs, and concerns.

(3) There is respect and trust between learner and instructor.

(4) The instructor is supportive and nonjudgmental.

b. Therapist/teacher should recognize that:

(1) Individuals learn at different rates.

(2) Trial and error and introspection are an essential part of the learning process.

(3) Experiential learning is more effective than didactic learning.

(4) Reinforcement is necessary to ensure a sense of competence and success.

c. Therapist/teacher roles and responsibilities.

(1) Gain the learner's attention, motivation, and active participation.

(2) Provide an overview of the learning process: objectives, purposes, nature of the task, and procedures to follow.

(3) Stimulate recall of previous learning; relate present learning to past and future learning.

(4) Monitor and control the learning.

(a) Organize learning units over a period of time.

(b) Break down learning into a series of steps or units.

(c) Determine the best sequence(s) of learning units and experiences; e.g., sequence from familiar to unfamiliar, simple to complex, concrete to abstract.

(d) Provide ample opportunity for practice and repetition.

(e) Progress at a comfortable pace for the learner.

(f) Give timely feedback, provide accurate knowledge of results.

(g) Reward successful behaviors.

(5) Monitor and control the environment.

(6) Reduce conditions that have a negative impact on learning; e.g., pain or discomfort, anxiety,

Teacher ____________	Institution ____________	Audience ____________	Class Size ____________	Date/Time ____________
Philosophical Orientation + (%) __ Cognitive Processing-Reasoning __ Academic Rationalism __ Technology __ Social Adaptation __ Social Reconstruction __ Personal Relevance	Learning Theory + (%) __ Behaviorism __ Gestalt/Problem-Solving Experience __ Piaget/Cognitive Structure	Domain of Learning + (%) __ Cognitive __ Affective __ Psychomotor __ Perceptual __ Spiritual	Student learning Style + (%) __ Concrete Experience __ Reflective Observation __ Abstract-Conceptualization __ Active Experimentation	Objectives Behavioral 1. ____________ 2. ____________ Problem Solving 1. ____________ 2. ____________ Outcome 1. ____________ 2. ____________
Teaching Aids + A. Audiovisual __ Computer Generated __ Blackboard __ Overhead Projector __ Slides __ Videotape; film B. Handouts __ Class Objectives __ Small Group Tasks __ Assigned Readings __ Lecture Outline __ Laboratory Exercises	Format of Delivery + (%) __ Lecture __ Laboratory __ Seminar-Discussion __ Independent Study	Student Evaluation + (%) __ Practical Exam __ Written Short Answers __ Written Essay __ Report or Project	Teaching Environment + __ Room Arrangement __ Room Environment: temperature, light, acoustics, cleanliness __ Teacher Materials: podium, chalk/pens, media setup	Subject Background Prep (content, sequence, time, skill, demonstration) The Learning Experience

Figure 13-2 • The Preactive Teaching Grid.
From Shepard, K and Jensen, G: Handbook of Teaching for Physical Therapists. Boston, Butterworth-Heinemann, 1997, p 40, with permission.

fear, frustration, feelings of failure, humiliation or embarrassment, boredom, time pressures.

5. **Evaluation.**
   a. Initial evaluation.
      (1) Determine relevant previous achievement, learning skills.
      (2) Utilize diagnostic tests.
      (3) Determine aptitude/choice of learning approaches.
   b. Formative evaluation (diagnostic-progress assessment).
      (1) Analyze what learning has occurred, what must still be learned.
      (2) Institute appropriate changes/modifications in the teaching plan.
   c. Summative evaluation (outcome assessment).
      (1) Assess attainment of learning objectives and content/skills.
      (2) Determine effectiveness of teaching materials/methods.
   d. Sources: direct observation of behaviors, written and verbal feedback, formal checklists, questionnaires, pre- and post-tests.

6. **Documentation:** provide a complete record of activities and outcomes to assure accountability, continuity of care. Include:
   a. Educational plan: objectives and activities.
   b. Progression and modification of the educational plan; document the need for change.
   c. Outcomes: document the learner's progress and attainment of the learning objectives.

Interventions—Media

The selection of appropriate media can enrich the learning experience, clarify and support a presentation provide for self-instruction or individualized tutorial. Selection should be based on the needs assessment. Cost and availability are factors that may also enter into the decision making process. Media can include, but are not limited to:

1. **Print: written handouts.**
   a. Advantages: low cost.
   b. Disadvantages: can be boring; inappropriate for educational level of individual; culturally biased.
2. **Computer-assisted instruction.**
   a. Advantages: can be individually paced; novel.
   b. Disadvantages: higher cost; limited availability in clinical setting.
3. **Audiovisuals.**
   a. Slides (PowerPoint).
      (1) Advantages: easy to add color, realistic.
      (2) Disadvantages: no motion, cost, availability; lights must be low during presentation.

b. Audiotapes.
   (1) Advantages: self paced.
   (2) Disadvantages: most learners are visually oriented.
c. Film/DVD/Videotapes.
   (1) Advantages: demonstrates movement, 3-dimensional.
   (2) Disadvantages: can be time-consuming.
d. Models.
   (1) Advantages: can provide visual and "hands on" experience.
   (2) Disadvantages: limited choices, cost.

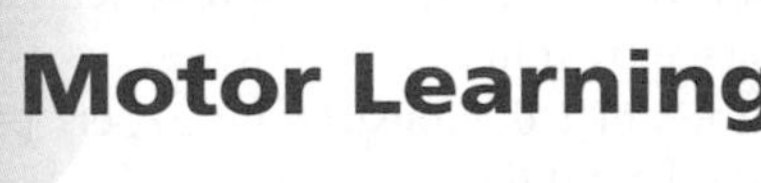

Motor Learning

"Motor learning is a set of internal processes associated with practice or experience leading to relatively permanent changes in the capability for skill" (Schmidt, 1999)

Phases of Motor Learning

1. **Cognitive phase:** the learner develops an understanding of the task; the process of cognitive mapping allows the learner to determine what to do.
2. **Associative phase:** the learner has determined a strategy, practices it, and makes adjustments in how the motor skill is performed.
3. **Autonomous phase:** the learner has practiced the motor skill to the extent that the performance becomes largely automatic; characterized by high-level skilled performance with few adjustments needed.
4. **(See Table 2-13).**

Motor Learning Evaluation

1. **Performance:** there is an acquired capability to perform the motor skill with practice.
   a. Performance may not always present an accurate picture of learning since it can be affected by fatigue, motivation, or stress.
   b. Determine efficiency (spatial and temporal organization or movement), level of effort, automaticity, and speed of decision making.
2. **Retention:** the skill can be demonstrated after a period of no practice, called the retention interval.
   a. Vary the retention interval: minutes, hours, or days.
   b. Determine the capability to retain the skill, perform without decrement.
3. **Generalizability:** an acquired capability to adapt the skill to permit performance of other similar related tasks.
   a. Vary the skill: have the patient perform the same skill in different postures; e.g., lower trunk rotation in sidelying, kneeling, standing.
   b. Modify the skill: e.g., upper extremity PNF patterns with elbow straight, elbow flexing, or elbow extending.
4. **Resistance to contextual change:** there is an acquired capability to perform what is learned in other environments.
   a. Vary the environment: in the clinic, on the nursing unit, at home, in the community.
   b. Determine the capability to retain the skill, perform without decrement.

Motor Learning Strategies

1. **Strategies vary by stage of motor learning.** (See Table 2-10).
2. **Ensure learner readiness.**
   a. Optimal arousal facilitates learning; high arousal and low arousal states interfere with learning (Inverted U theory).
   b. Optimal cognitive function: attention, concentration, memory ensures learning.
      (1) Vary strategies with specific cognitive impairments.
      (2) Avoid mental fatigue: give frequent rests.
   c. Communicate, encourage, and support learner; reduce fear and apprehension.
3. **Identify and describe the skill.**
   a. Identify the reasons why the skill is important to learn; stress links to functional independence, patient goals.
   b. Promote insights into the relationship between parts of the task and the whole task, current learning, and previous learning.
4. **Demonstrate the skill.**
   a. At ideal performance parameters (spatial and temporal organization).

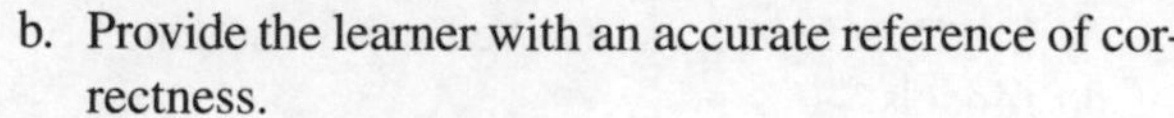

b. Provide the learner with an accurate reference of correctness.

5. Control the environment.
a. A closed environment is important for early motor learning; reduce environmental distractors.
b. Later learning will benefit from a shift toward a more open environment; vary the environment, introduce distractors.

6. Schedule appropriate practice sessions.
a. Promote practice of variations of the task to promote generalizability, improved retention.
b. Promote practice of the task in varying environments to promote resistance to contextual change.
c. Use distributed practice with frequent rest periods for learners who demonstrate poor endurance, cognitive impairments (poor attention, concentration, memory); or when the task is complex, long, and energy-intensive.
d. Vary practice schedules.
(1) Variable practice (random or serial practice order of tasks) improves retention, enhances depth of cognitive processing and active learning.
(2) Constant practice and blocked practice order improve performance, early learning.
e. Use mental practice: to cognitively rehearse task, preview movement, decrease apprehension.
f. Promote practice during off-therapy times.

7. Provide appropriate feedback.
a. Maximize active learning: allow for trial and error learning; don't bombard with feedback. The learner needs to actively process intrinsic information, self-correct responses.
b. Select appropriate (intact) sensory systems: visual, auditory, tactile, proprioceptive feedback.
c. Include both knowledge of results (KR) and knowledge of performance (KP) information.
d. Vary feedback schedules:
(1) Summed, fading, or bandwidth schedules improve retention, enhance depth of cognitive processing and active learning.
(2) Feedback after every trial improves performance, early learning.
e. Provide motivational feedback: reinforce desired skills, behaviors.

8. Demonstration and modeling.
a. Useful to reduce errors, improve learning and performance by imitation.
b. Use therapist demonstration, expert patients with similar disabilities, videotapes.

9. Guided movement (active assisted movement).
a. Useful during early learning, not during associative or autonomous learning.
b. Useful for slow positioning tasks; e.g., the therapist actively assists the patient in moving from supine to sitting or sitting to standing.
c. Useful to reduce anxiety and inspire trust; ensure safety.

10. Transfer training as appropriate.
a. Parts-to-whole transfer: for complex tasks with highly independent parts.
(1) Demonstrate the integrated whole skill.
(2) Break the skill down into component parts.
(3) Practice the individual component parts.
(4) Practice the integrated whole skill (each treatment session); delaying practice of the integrated whole skill may interfere with learning (parts to whole transfer).
b. Bilateral transfer: practice movements with sound limb before practice with involved limb; e.g., the patient with stroke.

11. Evaluate outcomes.
a. Level of independence, safety.
b. Level of function, ease of movement effort.

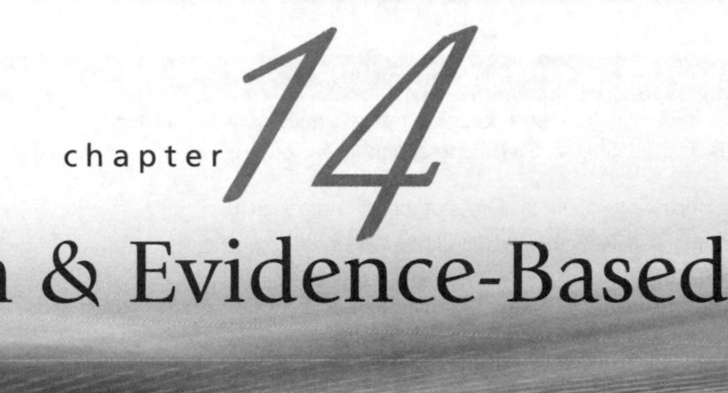

chapter 14 Research & Evidence-Based Practice

SUSAN B. O'SULLIVAN

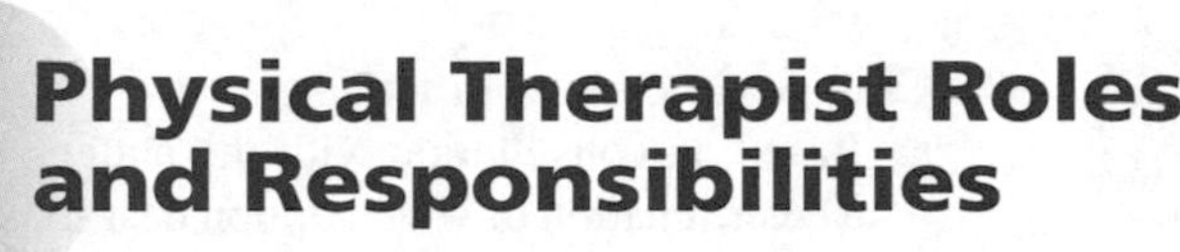

Physical Therapist Roles and Responsibilities

Physical Therapists Use Evidence-Based Practice (EBP)

1. **Definition of EBP:** The "conscientious, explicit and judicious use of current best evidence in making decisions about the care of individual patients" (Sackett et al, 2000).
2. **Clinical decisions are based on:**
   a. Systematic review of research evidence: studies included are rigorous and clinically relevant, "best available external clinical evidence" (i.e., randomized trials and meta-analysis).
   b. Clinical expertise of the therapist; proficiency and judgment acquired through clinical practice, acquisition of clinical skills, and continued educational development. For example, the clinician accurately identifies the patient's health status and needs, the risks and benefits of possible interventions.
   c. Patient values: values and unique qualities (preferences, concerns, expectations) are identified and integrated into clinical decisions.
3. **EBP is a four-step process.** (See Table 14-1).
4. **Electronic Medical Databases.** (See Table 14-2).
5. **Evidence-Based Clinical Practice Guidelines (CPGs):** systematically developed statements to assist the clinician and patient in decisions about appropriate courses of action.
   a. CPGs are developed through a combination of current best scientific evidence (e.g., systematic research and meta-analysis), expert judgment, and analysis of patient preferences combined with outcome-based guidelines.
   b. Guidelines issued by professional groups and governmental agencies are developed by expert consensus.
   c. Focus is on specific conditions or aspects of care. See Chapter 1, Musculoskeletal Physical Therapy for examples of specific clinical practice guidelines on neck pain, hip pain, meniscal and cartilage lesions, and plantar fasciitis (Appendices A–D).
6. **APTA clinical research agenda.**
   a. Support, explain, and enhance physical therapy clinical practice by facilitating research that is primarily useful to clinicians.
   b. Revised agenda (Phys Ther 80:499, 2000).

Physical Therapists Conduct Research in Clinical and Academic Settings

1. **Steps.**
   a. The research question/proposal is developed and submitted for ethical approval and funding (Institutional Review Board).
   b. The research study is conducted.
   c. The research data is analyzed and reported (i.e., presentation and written publication).

Table 14-1 ➤ STEPS IN EVIDENCE BASED PRACTICE

Step 1	A clinical problem is identified and an answerable research question is formulated. • The question is clearly defined and related to a clinical decision (e.g., whether to use a therapeutic, preventive, or diagnostic intervention). • The question is focused to clarify the target of the literature search.
Step 2	A systematic literature review is conducted and best evidence is collected. • Sources of evidence include books, journals, clinical protocols, colleagues. • Stronger sources of evidence include a systematic review using an electronic search of the medical literature; see Electronic Medical Databases (Table 14-2). • Articles are selected that are most likely to provide valid results (e.g., randomized controlled trials [RCTs]).
Step 3	The research evidence is summarized and critically analyzed. • The type (design) of the study is identified. • Study methods are identified (e.g., Were all patients who entered the trial properly accounted for and attributed at the conclusion of the study? Were appropriate samples of patients used? What are the inclusion and exclusion criteria?) • Statistical methods and analysis are identified (e.g., Are results presented clearly? Statistically significant?)
Step 4	The research evidence is synthesized and applied to clinical practice. • Best evidence is available and applied to clinical practice using clinical decision analysis.

Physical Therapists Incorporate Research Evidence Into Practice

1. **Steps.** (See Table 14-1).
2. **Sources:** Evidence presented in publications, websites, discussion groups , presentations (Table 14-2).
3. **Changes in clinical practice.**
   a. Based on consultation with the patient, to arrive at a determination of which option best suits the patient (a client-centered approach).
   b. Physical therapists must exercise good clinical judgment in determining applicability of the research results to the specific patient (i.e., similarity to the research group).

Table 14-2 ➤ ELECTRONIC MEDICAL DATABASES

- PubMed—US National Library of Medicine's search service to Medline and Pre-Medline (database of medical and biomedical research) http://www.ncbi.nlm.nih.gov/ pubmed/
- APTA Open Door-Hooked on Evidence (database of evidence-based physical therapy practice) http://www.apta.org/AM/ Template.cfm?Section=Research &Template=/MembersOnly
- Cochrane Database of Systemic Reviews (Cochrane Reviews) (database of systematic reviews of RCTs; primary source for clinical effectiveness information) http://www. www.cochrane.org/ reviews
- CINAHL (database of nursing and allied health research) http://www.cinahl.com
- Physiotherapy Evidence Database (PEDro) (database of physical therapy RCTs, systematic reviews, and evidence-based clinical practice guidelines) http://www.pedro.fhs.usyd.edu.au/ index.html
- The Sheffield Evidence for Effectiveness and Knowledge http://www.shef.ac.uk/seek/ infosearch.htm#guide
- The Centre for Health Evidence http://www.cche.net/usersguides/ start.asp Tacking
- ERIC (database of education research) http://www.eric.ed.gov/
- Ovid (database of health and lifescience research) http://www.ovid.com
- DARE (database of abstracts of reviews of evidence from medical journals) http://www.york.ac.uk/inst/crd/ crddatabases.htm
- RehabDATA (database of disability and rehabilitation research) http://www.naric.com/research
- Center for International Rehabilitation Research Information and Exchange (database of rehabilitation research) http://www.cirrie.buffalo.edu

Research Design

Methods

Common denominators include statement of the problem, formation of a research question, collection and analysis of data, results, and conclusions.

1. **Historical research:** involves investigation of a variety of data sources.
   a. Uses sources of data already available.
      (1) Primary sources: original documents, eyewitness accounts, direct recordings of events.
      (2) Secondary sources: description of an event by other than an eyewitness, summary information in textbooks, newspaper accounts.
   b. Investigates authenticity of the data (external criticism).
   c. Evaluates worth of the data (internal criticism).
      (1) Ensures that data are accurate (validity).
      (2) Ensures that data are reliable.
   d. Data synthesis: researcher determines relationships based on analyses and inferences; draws conclusions.
2. **Descriptive research:** involves collecting data about conditions, attitudes, or characteristics of subjects or groups of subjects.
   a. Determines and reports existing phenomena.
   b. Data collection: typically done through questionnaire survey, interview, or observation.
      (1) Permits classification, identification.
      (2) Data can be used for prediction, decision-making.
   c. Examples of descriptive research.
      (1) Case studies or clinical reports: in-depth investigation of an individual, group, or institution.
      (2) Developmental research: studies of behaviors that differentiate individuals at different levels of age, growth, or maturation.
      (3) Longitudinal studies: differentiate changes in an individual or group of individuals over time; e.g., developmental sequences.
      (4) Normative research: investigates standards of behavior, standard values for given characteristics of a sample; e.g., gait characteristics.
      (5) Qualitative research: seeks facts or causes of social phenomena, complex human behavior.
         (a) Utilizes people's own written or spoken words, behaviors through interview or observation.
         (b) Develops concepts, insights, and understanding from patterns in the data; uses inductive reasoning.
         (c) Emphasis is on understanding of human experience, e.g., holistic view of people and settings.
3. **Correlational research:** attempts to determine whether a relationship exists between two or more quantifiable variables and to what degree.
   a. Describes relationships, predicts relationships among variables without active manipulation of the variables.
   b. Limitations.
      (1) Cannot establish cause-and-effect relationships; limits interpretation of results. 
      (2) May fail to consider all variables that enter into a relationship.
   c. Degree of relationship is expressed as correlation coefficient, ranging from –1.00 to +1.00.
      (1) If the correlation is near +1.00, the variables are positively correlated.
      (2) If the correlation is near 0.00, the variables are not related.
      (3) If the correlation is near –1.00, the variables are inversely related.
   d. Examples of correlational research.
      (1) Retrospective: investigation of data collected in the past. Prospective: recording and investigation of present data.
      (2) Descriptive: investigation of several variables at once; determines existing relationships among variables.
      (3) Predictive: useful to develop predictive models.
4. **Experimental research:** attempts to define a cause and effect relationship through group comparisons.
   a. Alleged cause or treatment (the independent variable) is manipulated.
   b. Effect or difference (the dependent variable) is determined.
   c. Designs.
      (1) True experimental design: includes random assignment into experimental group (receives treatment) or control group (no treatment). All other experiences are held similar.
      (2) Cohort design: quasi-experimental design, subjects are identified and followed over time for changes/outcomes following exposure to an intervention; lacks randomization, may or may not have a control group.
      (3) Within-subject design (repeated measures): subjects serve as their own controls; randomly assigned to treatment or no treatment blocks.

(4) Between-subject design: comparisons made between groups of subjects.

(5) Single-subject experimental design: involves a sample of one with repeated measurements and design phases.

(a) A-B design: involves two phases, a pretreatment or baseline phase followed by an intervention or treatment phase.

(b) A-B-A design (multiple baseline design): involves three phases—a baseline phase and a treatment phase, followed by a second baseline phase.

(c) A-B-A-B (multiple baseline, multiple treatment): includes baseline, treatment, and additional baseline and treatment phases.

(6) Factorial design: refers to the number of independent variables utilized; e.g., single factor, multifactor.

5. **Causal-comparative research:** attempts to define a cause-and-effect relationship through group comparisons.
   a. Ex post facto research: the cause or independent variable has already occurred; cannot be manipulated (e.g., gender) or should not be manipulated (e.g., type of brain injury).
   b. Groups are compared based on the dependent variable.

6. **Epidemiology:** the study of disease frequency and distribution in a community; the science concerned with examining and determining the specific causes of health problems and interrelationships of factors.

Variables

1. **Independent variable:** the activity or factor believed to bring about a change in the dependent variable; the cause or treatment.
2. **Dependent variable:** the change or difference in behavior that results from the intervention (independent variable); the outcome that is being evaluated.

Hypothesis

1. **Definition:** A tentative and testable explanation of the relationship between variables; the results of an experiment determine if the hypothesis is accepted or rejected.
   a. Directional hypothesis (research hypothesis): a generalization that predicts an expected relationship between variables.
   b. Null hypothesis: states that no relationship exists between variables, a statistical hypothesis; any relationship found is the result of chance or sampling error.
      (1) The null hypothesis is rejected; meaning that a significant difference was observed between groups or treatments.
      (2) The null hypothesis is accepted; meaning that no significant difference was observed between groups or treatments.

Data Types (Table 14-3)

1. **Nominal scale:** classifies variables or scores into two or more mutually exclusive categories based on a common

Table 14-3 ➤ EXAMPLES OF STATISTICAL ANALYSES ACCORDING TO THE STUDY'S PURPOSE AND THE DATA'S LEVEL OF MEASUREMENT

PURPOSES	LEVELS OF MEASUREMENT		STATISTICS
Describe the Variable	Nominal	→	Frequency, Percentage
	Ordinal	→	Median, Mode, Range
	Interval	→	Mean, Median, Mode, Range, Standard Deviation, Skew of the Distribution
Relationship	Nominal	→	Chi Square
	Ordinal	→	Spearman's Rank Order or Kendall's Tau Correlations
	Interval	→	Pearson's Product Moment Correlation, Partial Correlation, Multiple Correlation, Multiple Regression
Difference	Nominal	→	One group: Chi Square Two groups: Independent: Chi Square; Paired: McNemar Test More than two groups: Independent: Chi Square; Paired: Cochran's Q
	Ordinal	→	Two groups: Independent: Mann-Whitney U; Paired: Wilcoxon Signed Rank More than two groups: Independent: Kruskal-Wallis; Paired: Friedman ANOVA
	Interval	→	Two groups: Independent: t-test; Paired: Paired t-test; Statistical Control: ANCOVA More than two groups: Independent: ANOVA; Across time: Repeated ANOVA; Statistical Control: ANCOVA

Nominal: characteristics into categories
Ordinal: rank ordering, no specific intervals between ranks
Interval: values rank ordered on a scale that has equal distances (intervals) between points on that scale
Prepared by Nina Coppens, PhD, RN, University of Massachusetts, Lowell.

set of characteristics; the lowest level of measurement; e.g., subjects are classified as male or female, tall or short, etc.

2. **Ordinal scale:** classifies and ranks variables or scores in terms of the degree to which they possess a common characteristic; intervals between ranks are not equal; e.g., subjects are ranked in a graduating class according to grade point average; manual muscle test grades (normal, good, fair, poor, trace, zero) are ranked as an ordinal scale.

3. **Interval scale:** classifies and ranks variables or scores based on predetermined equal intervals; does not have a true zero point; e.g., an IQ test with scores ranging from 0 to 200; temperature scales (Fahrenheit or Celsius).

4. **Ratio scale:** classifies and ranks variables or scores based on equal intervals and a true zero point; the highest, most precise level of measurement; e.g., goniometry, scales for height, weight, or force allow the use of precise physical measures (ratio data) for research.

Sampling

1. **The selection of individuals (a sample) for a study from a population.** The sample represents the larger group from which they were selected.
   a. Random: all individuals in a population have an equal chance of being chosen for a study.
   b. Systematic: individuals are selected from a population list by taking individuals at specified intervals; e.g., every 10th name.
   c. Stratified: individuals are selected from a population from identified subgroups based on some predetermined characteristic; e.g., by height, weight, or gender.
   d. Double-blind study: an experiment in which the subject and the investigator are not aware of group assignment.
   e. Effect size: the size (quantity, magnitude) of the differences between sample means; allows a statistical test to find a difference when one really does exist.
   f. Generalizability: the degree to which a study's findings based on a sample apply to an entire population.

Instrumentation

1. **Instrument selection:** with established validity and reliability.

2. **Gold standard:** an instrument with established validity can be used as a standard for assessing other instruments.

Informed Consent

1. **A document that includes consent of an individual prior to participation in a study with full disclosure of risks and benefits; ethical disclosure.**

2. **Components.**
   a. Information about the general nature of what is to take place.
   b. Any risks to the individual and what will be done to minimize the risks.
   c. Possible benefits.
   d. An ethical disclosure.

Problems Related to Measurement

1. **Control.**
   a. The researcher attempts to remove the influence of any variable other than the independent variable. In order to evaluate its effect on the dependent variable.
      (1) Control group: the group in a research study that resembles the experimental group but who do not receive the new or different treatment (e.g., treated as usual); provides a baseline for interpretation of results.
      (2) Experimental group: the group in a research study that receives a new or novel treatment that is under investigation.
      (3) Intervening variable: a variable that alters the relationship (intervenes) between the independent and dependent variable; may not be directly observable or easy to control (e.g., anxiety).
2. **Validity.**
   a. The degree to which a test, instrument, or procedure accurately measures what it is supposed to or intended to measure.
   b. Types.
      (1) Internal validity: the degree to which the observed differences on the dependent variable are the direct result of manipulation of the independent variable, and not some other variable.
      (2) External validity: the degree to which the results are generalizable to individuals (general population) or environmental settings outside of the experimental study.
      (3) Face validity: the assumption of validity based on the appearance of an instrument as a reasonable measure of a variable; may be used for initial screening of a test instrument but psychometrically unsound.
      (4) Content validity: the degree to which an instrument measures an intended content area.

a Determined by expert judgment.
b Requires both item validity and sampling validity.

(5) Concurrent validity: the degree to which the scores on one test are related to the scores on another criterion test with both tests being given at relatively similar times; usually involves comparison to the gold standard.
(6) Predictive validity: the degree to which a test is able to predict future performance.
(7) Construct validity: the degree to which a test measures an intended hypothetical abstract concept (nonobservable behaviors or ideas).

3. Threats to validity.

a. Sampling bias (selection bias): the researcher introduces systematic sampling error; e.g., a sample of convenience (the use of volunteers or available groups) instead of random selection of subjects.
b. Failure to exert rigid control over subjects and conditions: intervening variables interact with the dependent variable; e.g., in a longitudinal pediatric study, the outcome is due to the maturation of the child rather than the treatment intervention.
c. The administration of the pretest influences scores on the posttest; e.g., a learning effect occurs as a result of taking a test.
d. The measurement instrument is not accurate, the test does not measure the characteristic it purports to measure; e.g., muscle strength, not motor control.
e. Pretest-treatment interaction: subjects respond differently to the treatment because of the pretest.
f. Multiple treatment interference: more than one treatment is being given to the subjects at the same time; or carry-over effects from an earlier treatment influence the results of a later treatment, e.g., effects of ultrasound following application of a hot pack.
g. Experimenter bias: expectations of the researcher about the expected outcomes of the study influence the results of a study.

h. Hawthorne effect: the subject's knowledge of participation in an experiment influences the results of a study.
i. Placebo effect: subjects respond to a sham treatment with positive effects; e.g., taking a sugar pill instead of an experimental drug results in a change.

4. Reliability.

a. The degree to which a test consistently measures what it is intended to measure.

(1) Interrater (intertester) reliability: the degree to which two or more independent raters can obtain the same rating for a given variable; the consistency of multiple raters.
(2) Intrarater (intratester) reliability: the degree to which one rater can obtain the same rating for a given variable on multiple measurement trials; an individual's consistency of rating.
(3) Test-retest reliability: the degree to which the scores on a test are stable or consistent over time; a measure of instrument stability.
(4) Split-half reliability: the degree of agreement when a test is split in half and the reliability of first half is compared to the second half; a measure of internal consistency of an instrument.

5. Threats to reliability.

a. Errors of measurement: random errors or systematic errors; e.g., repeat measurements of blood pressure may vary as a result of physiological changes (fear, anxiety).

6. Objectivity.

Agreement among expert judges on what is observed or what is done; e.g., scoring of a perceptible sign or symptom is the same, regardless of who is observing the phenomena (e.g., Licensure Exam).

7. Subjectivity.

Refers to a testing format that may differ depending upon the person grading the test (e.g., figure skating judging)

8. Sensitivity and specificity.

a. Sensitivity: a test's ability to correctly identify the proportion of individuals who truly have a disease or condition (a true positive).
b. Specificity: a test's ability to correctly identify the proportion of individuals who do not have a disease or condition (a true negative).
c. Predictive value: a test's ability to estimate the likelihood that a person will test positive (or negative) for a target condition.
d. True positive: individuals are correctly identified as having the target condition.
e. True negative: individuals are correctly identified as not having the target condition.
f. False positive: individuals are identified as having the target condition when they do not.
g. False negative: individuals are identified as not having the target condition when they do.

Evaluating the Evidence: Levels of Evidence and Grades of Recommendation

Definitions

1. **Systematic Review (SR) including meta-analysis:** a review in which the primary studies are summarized, critically appraised, and statistically combined; usually quantitative in nature with specific inclusion/exclusion criteria.
2. **Randomized Controlled Trial (RCT):** an experimental study in which participants are randomly assigned to either an experimental or control group to receive different interventions or a placebo.
3. **Cohort study:** a prospective (forward-in-time) study; a group of participants (cohort) with a similar condition is followed for a defined period of time; comparison is made to a matched group that does not have the condition.
4. **Homogeneity:** SR free of variations (heterogeneity) in the directions and degree of results between individual studies.
5. **Case-control study:** a retrospective (backward-in-time) study. A group of individuals with a similar condition (disease) is compared with a group that does not have the condition to determine factors that may have played a role in the condition.
6. **Case report (study):** type of descriptive research in which only one individual is studied in depth, often retrospectively.

Adapted from Centre for Evidence-based Medicine, Oxford-Centre for Evidence-Based Medicine. (http://www.cebm.net/levels of evidence.asp)

Levels of Evidence

Evidence is evaluated by "best" study design (Table 14-4).

Table 14-4 ➤ LEVELS OF EVIDENCE

LEVEL	DESCRIPTION	GRADE OF RECOMMENDATION
1	Level 1a: SR (with homogeneity) of multiple RCTs; randomization of large numbers of patients; multicenter; substantial agreement of size and direction of treatment effects. Level 1b: Individual RCT with narrow confidence level; treatment effects precisely defined. Level 1c: All-or-none case series. In absence of RCT, overwhelming evidence of substantial treatment effect following introduction of a new treatment (e.g., vaccine).	A
2	Level 2a: SR (with homogeneity) of cohort studies (comparison groups). Prospective: patients are identified for study before outcomes achieved. Level 2b: Individual cohort study or low-quality RCT (small N). Quality study includes more than 80% follow-up of patients enrolled in study.	B
3	Level 3a: SR (with homogeneity) of case-control studies (case comparison). Level 3b: Individual case-control study. Retrospective: patients identified for study after outcomes have been achieved.	B
4	Case-series and poor-quality cohort and case-control studies. Largely descriptive studies.	C
5	Expert opinion without explicit critical appraisal, or based on physiology, bench research, or first principles. Observations not made on patients	D (Lowest scientific rigor; expert opinion without explicit critical appraisal)

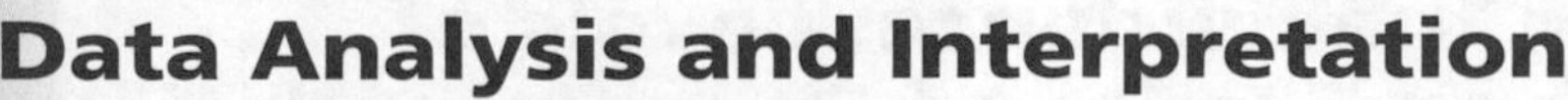

Data Analysis and Interpretation

Descriptive Statistics

1. **Purpose:** Summarize and describe data.
2. **Measures of central tendency:** a determination of average or typical scores.
   a. Mean: the arithmetic average of all scores (X).
      (1) Add all scores together and divide by the number of subjects (N).
      (2) The most frequently used measure of central tendency; appropriate for interval or ratio data.
   b. Median: the midpoint, 50% of scores are above the median and 50% of scores are below; appropriate for ordinal data.
   c. Mode: the most frequently occurring score; appropriate for nominal data.
3. **Measures of variability:** a determination of the spread of a group of scores.
   a. Range: the difference between the highest score and the lowest score.
   b. Standard deviation (SD): a determination of variability of scores (difference) from the mean.

1. If examining for relationships (correlations):

- Are there only two variables?
  - No → Are the data ranked?
    - No → One variable predicted from others?
      - Partial correlation
      - Dependent variable continuous?
        - Discriminant function
        - Multiple correlation
    - Yes → One dependent variable?
      - Kendall's coefficient
      - Kendall's multiple tau
  - Yes → Are the data frequency counts? (nominal or categorical data)
    - No → Are data ranked? (ordinal data)
      - Are both continuous? (interval data)
        - Pearson's r
      - Kendall's tau / Spearman's rho
    - Yes → Contingency coefficient

2. If examining for differences between groups:

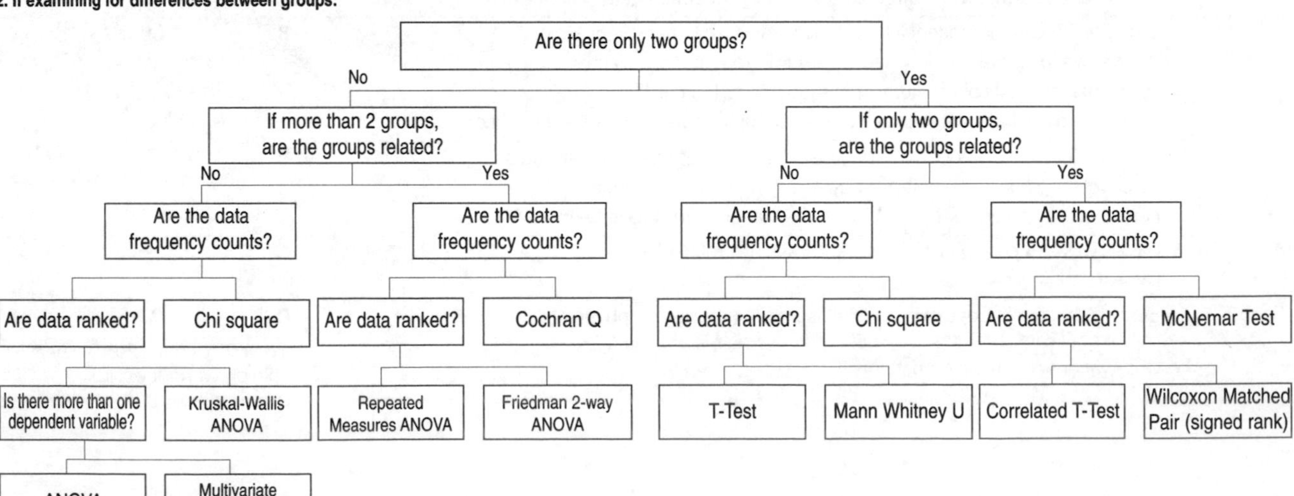

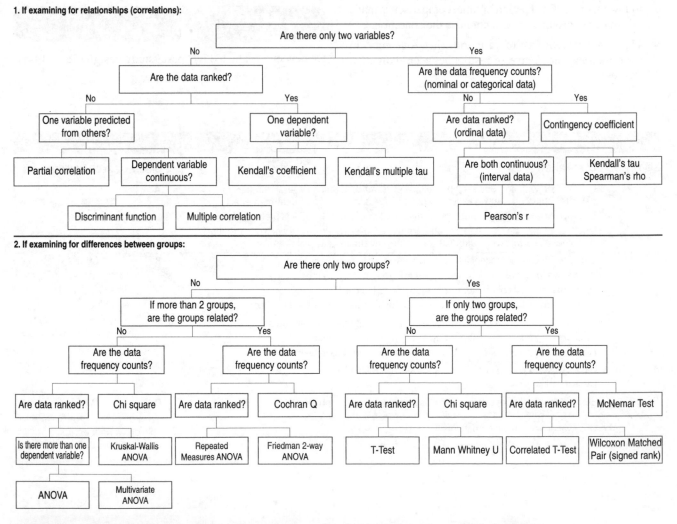

Figure 14-1 • Clinical decision making: Flow diagram for determining appropriate statistics.
Key: follow flow diagram to the right with yes answers; follow flow diagram to left with no answers.
Adapted from materials prepared by Dr. L Zaichkowsky, Boston University.

(1) Subtract each score from the mean, square each difference, add up all the squares, and divide by the number of scores.
(2) The most frequently used measure of variability.
(3) Appropriate with interval or ratio data.

c. Normal distribution: a symmetrical bell-shaped curve indicating the distribution of scores; the mean, median, and mode will be similar.
(1) Half the scores are above the mean and half the scores are below the mean.
(2) Most scores are near the mean, within one standard deviation; approximately 68% of scores fall within –1 or +1 SD of the mean.
(3) Frequency of scores decreases further from the mean.
(a) Approximately 95% of scores fall within –2 or +2 SD of the mean.
(b) Approximately 99% of scores fall within –3 or +3 SD of the mean.
(4) Distribution may be skewed (not symmetrical) rather than normal: scores are extreme, clustered at one end or the other; the mean, median, and mode are different.

d. Percentiles and quartiles: describe a score's position within the distribution, relative to all other scores.
(1) Percentiles: data are divided in 100 equal parts; position of score is determined.
(2) Quartiles: data are divided into 4 equal parts and position of score is placed accordingly.

Inferential Statistics

1. Purpose.

a. Help determine how likely the results of a study of a sample can be generalized to the whole population.

2. Concepts.

a. Standard error of measurement: an estimate of expected errors in an individual's score; a measure of response stability or reliability.

b. Tests of significance: an estimation of true differences, not due to chance; a rejection of the null hypothesis.
(1) Probability levels are associated with inferential analyses. Alpha level: preselected level of statistical significance.
(a) Most commonly set at 0.05 or 0.01; indicates that the expected difference is due to chance; e.g., at 0.05, only 5 times out of every 100 or a 5% chance, often expressed as a value of P.
(b) Allows rejection of the null hypothesis: there are true differences on the measured dependent variable.
(2) Degrees of freedom: based on number of subjects and number of groups; allows determination of level of significance based on consulting appropriate tables for each statistical test.
(3) Errors.
(a) Standard error: expected chance variation among the means, the result of sampling error.
(b) Type I error: the null hypothesis is rejected by the researcher when it is true; e.g., the means of scores are concluded to be truly different when the differences are due to chance.
(c) Type II error: the null hypothesis is not rejected by the researcher when it is false; e.g., the means of scores are concluded to be due to chance when the means are truly different.
(d) By increasing sample size, using random selection, and having valid measures, the chance of both Type I and II errors is decreased.

3. **Parametric statistics:** testing is based on population parameters; includes tests of significance based on interval or ratio data.

a. Assumptions.
(1) A normal distribution exists in the population studied of the variable measured, or distribution is known. In a large, representative sample, the assumption of normal distribution is probably met.
(2) Random sampling is performed.
(3) Variance in the groups is equal.

b. T-test: a parametric test of significance used to compare two independent groups created by random assignment and identify a difference at a selected probability level (e.g., 0.05).
(1) T-test for independent samples: compares the difference between two independent groups; e.g., a test to determine whether an intervention (a new hand splint) improves the function of patients with rheumatoid arthritis.
(2) T-test for paired samples: compares the difference between two matched samples; e.g., Does therapy improve function in siblings with autism?
(a) One-tailed t-test: based on a directional hypothesis; evaluates differences in data on only one end of a distribution, either negative or positive; e.g., patients who receive a certain treatment exhibit better rehabilitation outcomes than those who do not.
(b) Two-tailed t-test: based on a nondirectional hypothesis; evaluates differences in data on both positive and negative ends of a distribution; tests of significance are almost always two-tailed; e.g., either group of patients (treatment or control) may exhibit better rehabilitation outcomes.
(3) Inappropriate use of t-tests: use of a t-test to compare more than two means within a single sample; e.g., three modes of exercise are compared within a single sample.

c. Analysis of variance (ANOVA): a parametric test used to compare three or more independent treatment groups or conditions at a selected probability level.
   (1) Simple (one-way) ANOVA: compares multiple groups on a single independent variable; e.g., three sets of posttest scores (balance scores from a Balance Master) are compared from three different categories of elderly: young elderly (65–74); old elderly (75–84); and old and frail elderly (>85).
   (2) Factorial ANOVA (multifactorial) compares multiple groups on two or more independent variables; e.g., two groups of injured patients (those with severe ankle sprain and moderate ankle sprain) and a control group are compared for muscle activation patterns and sensory perception in each limb.

d. Analysis of covariance (ANCOVA): a parametric test used to compare two or more treatment groups or conditions while also controlling for the effects of intervening variables (covariates), e.g., two groups of subjects are compared on the basis of gait parameters using two different types of assistive devices; subjects in one group are taller than subjects in the second group; height then becomes the covariate that must be controlled during statistical analysis.

4. **Nonparametric statistics:** testing not based on population parameters; includes tests of significance based on ordinal or nominal data.
   a. Used when above parametric assumptions cannot be met.
   b. Less powerful than parametric tests, more difficult to reject the null hypothesis; e.g., can be used with small sample and with ordinal or nominal level data.
   c. Chi square test: a nonparametric test of significance used to compare data in the form of frequency counts occurring in two or more mutually exclusive categories; e.g., subjects are asked to rate treatment preferences.

5. **Correlational statistics:** used to determine the relative strength of a relationship between two variables; e.g., compare progression of radiologically observed joint destruction in rheumatoid arthritis and its relationship to demographic variables (gender, age), disease severity, and exercise frequency.
   a. Pearson product-moment coefficient (r): used to correlate continuous data with underlying normal distribution on interval or ratio scales; e.g., the relationship between proximal and distal development in infants is examined.
   b. Spearman's rank correlation coefficient (r_{ss} or Spearman's rho): a nonparametric test used to correlate ordinal data; e.g., the relationship of verbal and reading comprehension scores is examined.
   c. Point biserial correlation: one variable is dichotomous (nominal) and the other is ratio or interval; e.g., the relationship between elbow flexor spasticity and side of stroke (left or right) in stroke patients is examined.
   d. Rank biserial correlation: one variable is dichotomous (nominal) and the other is ordinal; e.g. the relationship between gender and functional ability is examined.
   e. Intraclass correlation coefficient (ICC): a reliability coefficient based on an analysis of variance.
   f. Strength of relationships.
      (1) Positive correlations range from 0 to +1.00: indicates that as variable X increases, so does variable Y.
         - High correlations: >0.76 to 1.00.
         - Moderate correlations: 0.51 to 0.75.
         - Fair correlations: 0.26 to 0.50
         - Low correlations: 0.00 to 0.25.
         - 0 means no relationship between variables.
      (2) Negative correlations range from –1.0 to 0: indicates that as variable X increases, variable Y decreases; an inverse relationship.
   g. Common variance: a representation of the degree that variation in one variable is attributable to another variable.
      (1) Determined by squaring the correlation coefficient, e.g., a correlation coefficient of 0.70 means that the common variance is 49%, i.e., the variation in one variable can be explained by the other 49% of the time.

6. **Linear regression:** used to establish the relationship between two variables as a basis for prediction.
   a. An examination of two continuous variables that are linearly correlated. The variable designated X is the independent or predictor variable. The variable designated Y is the dependent or criterion variable.
   b. The purpose is to generate an equation which relates X to Y, such that if given values of X, Y can be predicted, e.g., blood pressure (Y) is examined by age (X); answers the question, Can systolic blood pressure be predicted from age?

Computer Simulated Examinations

Examinations are on the enclosed computer disc. Follow the instructions on the CD. After completing each examination, your performance will be analyzed in terms of knowledge of specific systems, content areas, domains, and reasoning skills. The questions that follow are the CD examinations with highlighted correct answer, category and reasoning subtype icon. Separate TEACHING POINTS for each question contain the correct answer and incorrect choices explanations plus the reasoning rationale.

Questions with Teaching Points

DOMAINS

- Cardiac, Vascular, Lymphatic, and Pulmonary
- Musculoskeletal
- Neuromuscular
- Integumentary
- Metabolic/Endocrine, Gastrointestinal, Genitourinary, and Multiple System Involvement
- Devices, Modalities, Administration, etc.

CATEGORIES

- Clinical Applications of Foundational Sciences (Pediatric & Adult)
- Examination of the Patient/Client (Pediatric & Adult)
- Foundations for Evaluation, Differential Diagnosis, and Prognosis (Pediatric & Adult)
- Interventions (Pediatric & Adult)
- Equipment, Devices, and Therapeutic Modalities (Pediatric & Adult)
- Teaching and Learning; Research and Evidence-Based Practice; Safety, Protection, and Emergencies; Healthcare Roles

CRITICAL REASONING STRATEGIES

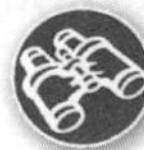 Inductive Reasoning

 Inference

 Analysis

 Deductive Reasoning

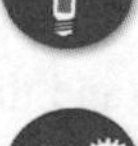 Evaluation

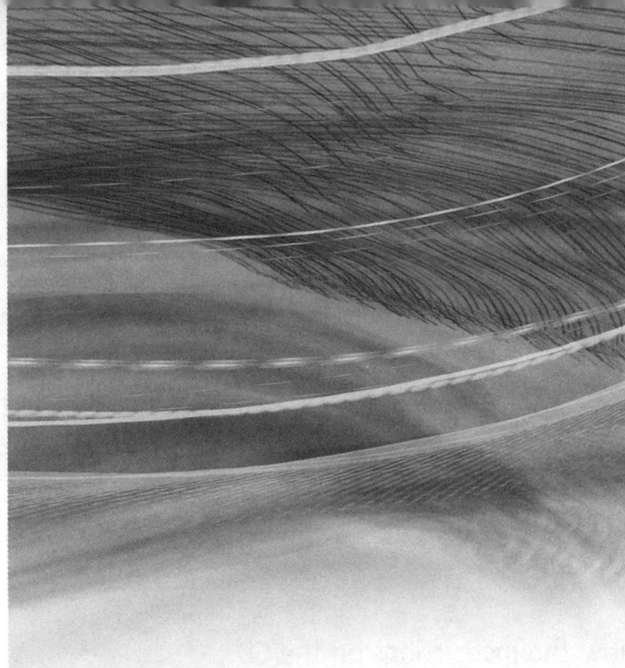

Examination A

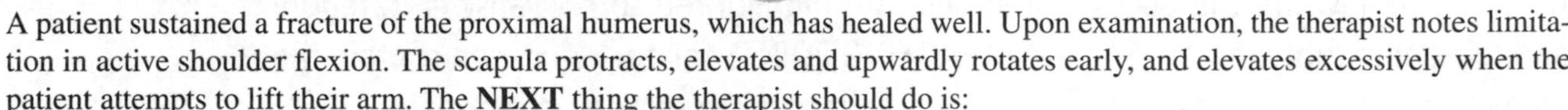

A1 | Musculoskeletal | Patient Examination

A patient sustained a fracture of the proximal humerus, which has healed well. Upon examination, the therapist notes limitation in active shoulder flexion. The scapula protracts, elevates and upwardly rotates early, and elevates excessively when the patient attempts to lift their arm. The **NEXT** thing the therapist should do is:

CHOICES:

1. Passive shoulder flexion and glenohumeral accessory mobility testing.
2. Manual muscle test of serratus anterior and rhomboids.
3. Manual resistance exercises for the supraspinatus and infraspinatus.
4. Large amplitude oscillations performed at the end-range of joint play for the glenohumeral inferior and posterior capsule.

TEACHING POINTS

CORRECT ANSWER: 1

Based on the information given, the **NEXT** thing the therapist should do is determine WHAT is causing the impairments so that the therapist can target treatment to the tissue/s at fault. Limitation of active shoulder flexion can be due to weakness (less than 3/5 strength) of any of the following muscles: deltoid, supraspinatus, serratus anterior, and upper trapezius. However, the loss of active shoulder flexion could also be due to capsular restrictions. A patient who sustained a proximal humerus fracture and resulting immobilization would likely have a capsular restriction as well as muscle atrophy. One must determine the primary impairment in the limitation of active shoulder flexion. Performing passive shoulder flexion and glenohumeral accessory mobility testing will help determine the tissue at fault. If full passive ROM is found, further testing of individual muscles is necessary to determine which muscles to strengthen. If there are restrictions in passive shoulder flexion and capsular restrictions, a program including joint mobilization is appropriate.

INCORRECT CHOICES:

2. Manual muscle test of serratus anterior and rhomboids. Certainly, restricted shoulder flexion could be due to weakness in the serratus anterior. However, a weak serratus anterior would result in retraction of the scapula and possible winging, not protraction and upward rotation of the scapula. In addition, the rhomboids are downward rotators, retractors, and elevators of the scapula. In this scenario, the scapula upwardly rotated and protracted, two actions that are antagonistic to rhomboid action. Therefore, weakness of the rhomboids would not be a concern.
3. Manual resistance exercises for the supraspinatus and infraspinatus. This treatment would be appropriate for weakness of the rotator cuff. This is incorrect, since there is not enough information to begin treatment (no indication that the loss of ROM and excessive scapular motion are due to rotator cuff weakness).
4. Large amplitude oscillations performed at the end-range of joint play for the glenohumeral inferior and posterior capsule. This treatment would be appropriate for capsular restrictions. This is incorrect, as there is not enough information to begin treatment (no indication that the loss of ROM and excessive scapular motion are due to capsular restrictions).

TYPE OF REASONING: INDUCTIVE

This question provides a diagnosis and group of symptoms, and the test taker must reason a next course of action, based on an understanding of the diagnosis. This requires inductive reasoning skill, where clinical judgment is paramount to arriving at a correct conclusion. For this situation, the therapist should perform passive shoulder flexion and glenohumeral accessory mobility testing to determine the cause of the impairments. If you answered incorrectly, review musculoskeletal examination techniques, especially for the shoulder.

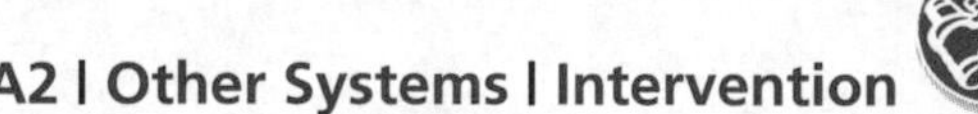

A2 | Other Systems | Intervention

Which of the following exercises should be used for a patient 2 weeks posttransurethral resection of the prostate (TURP) without complications?

CHOICES:

1. Kegel exercises.
2. Trunk stabilization.
3. Hip and leg presses.
4. Proprioception retraining.

TEACHING POINTS

CORRECT ANSWER: 1

Kegel exercises strengthen the pelvic floor muscles and are appropriate in males following prostate procedures.

INCORRECT CHOICES:

To be performed properly, the other choices would require some abdominal or trunk contraction, which could exacerbate urinary incontinence. Proprioception retraining does not address the central problem.

TYPE OF REASONING: INDUCTIVE

This question requires one to use clinical judgment to determine the best course of action according to the diagnosis presented. In this situation, Kegel exercises are ideal, because a TURP can affect pelvic floor strength. Questions that ask about an ideal course of action related to a diagnosis often require inductive reasoning skills. If this question was answered incorrectly, review information on TURP.

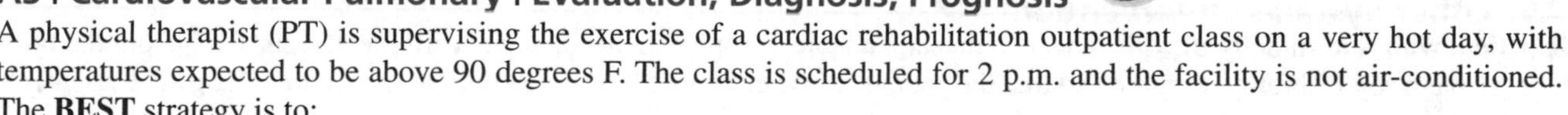

A3 | Cardiovascular-Pulmonary | Evaluation, Diagnosis, Prognosis

A physical therapist (PT) is supervising the exercise of a cardiac rehabilitation outpatient class on a very hot day, with temperatures expected to be above 90 degrees F. The class is scheduled for 2 p.m. and the facility is not air-conditioned. The **BEST** strategy is to:

CHOICES:

1. Decrease the exercise intensity by slowing the pace of exercise.
2. Increase the warm-up period to equal the total aerobic interval in time.
3. Keep the same time of the exercise class because of scheduling requirements.
4. Shift to intermittent exercise but decrease the rest time.

TEACHING POINTS

CORRECT ANSWER: 1

Clinical decisions should focus on reducing the environmental costs of exercising (change the time of day of the exercise class to reduce the heat stress) or reducing the overall metabolic costs of the activity (decrease the pace of exercise, add more rest periods).

INCORRECT CHOICES:

Altering the warm-up period does not lower the overall cost of the aerobic exercise period. Shifting to intermittent exercise is appropriate; rest time should be increased. Keeping the same time of the exercise class because of scheduling requirements is contraindicated.

TYPE OF REASONING: EVALUATION

This question requires one to determine the inherent danger of exercise for a patient with a known cardiac history during hot weather, and to what extent this danger could result in harm to the patient. The test taker who chooses the correct answer realizes that this answer is superior to the others, because it protects the patient from potential or actual harm. If this question was answered incorrectly, review information on exercise of the cardiac patient and environmental conditions.

EXAM A

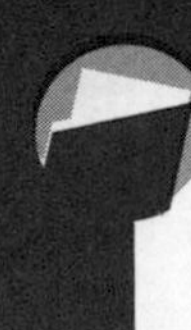

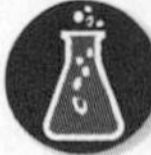

A4 | Devices, Admin., etc. | Equipment, Modalities

A patient has a transtibial amputation and has recently been fitted with a patellar tendon–bearing (PTB) socket. During initial prosthetic checkout, the PT instructs the patient to walk several times in the parallel bars, and then sit down and take the prosthesis off. Upon inspection of the skin, the therapist would expect no redness in the area of the:

CHOICES:

1. Anterior tibia and tibial crest.
2. Patellar tendon and tibial tuberosity.
3. Medial tibial and fibular plateaus.
4. Medial and lateral distal ends of the residual limb.

TEACHING POINTS

CORRECT ANSWER: 1

In a PTB socket, reliefs are provided for pressure-sensitive areas: the anterior tibia and tibial crest, fibular head, and fibular (peroneal) nerve.

INCORRECT CHOICES:

All the other choices are considered pressure-tolerant areas.

TYPE OF REASONING: ANALYSIS

The test taker must consider past knowledge and experiences with lower extremity amputation and use of a PTB socket in order to arrive at the correct conclusion. If the test taker does not recall the pressure-relief properties of a PTB socket, one must draw upon his/her understanding of anatomy and the likelihood of pressure sores in more sensitive skin areas after this type of amputation and ambulation with any prosthetic device.

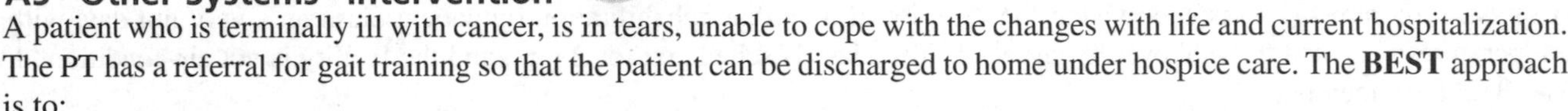

A5 | Other Systems | Intervention

A patient who is terminally ill with cancer, is in tears, unable to cope with the changes with life and current hospitalization. The PT has a referral for gait training so that the patient can be discharged to home under hospice care. The **BEST** approach is to:

CHOICES:

1. Ask the patient questions in order to obtain a detailed history.
2. Ignore the tears and focus on therapy, but in a compassionate manner.
3. Encourage denial so the patient can cope better with life's challenges.
4. Take time now to allow the patient to express fears and frustrations.

TEACHING POINTS

CORRECT ANSWER: 4

It is important to be supportive of a patient who is experiencing losses and resentment. Allow the patient to fully verbalize feelings and frustrations.

INCORRECT CHOICES:

Ignoring the patient's responses or encouraging denial will not allow for healing and acceptance. In an emotional state, the patient may be unable to give an accurate history.

TYPE OF REASONING: EVALUATION

In this situation, the test taker must have a firm understanding of the ethical obligations to the patient and also weigh the fact that the referral is for gait training in preparation for discharge home. In order to arrive at the correct answer, one must find a way to address the patient's needs, while still considering the long-term goal of the patient. Questions such as these are challenging because they require one to consider the emotional value of the patient's situation with the duty of the PT.

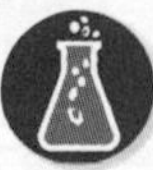

A6 | Devices, Admin., etc. | Equipment, Modalities

The examination reveals muscle spasm of the piriformis, which is compressing the sciatic nerve and producing pain in the posterior hip region. The pain has been worsening over the past 3 months. What is the correct ultrasound (US) setting for this case?

CHOICES:

1. 1 MHz pulsed at 1.0 W/cm^2.
2. 3 MHz continuous at 1.0 W/cm^2.
3. 3 MHz pulsed at 1.0 W/cm^2.
4. 1 MHz continuous at 1.0 W/cm^2.

TEACHING POINTS

CORRECT ANSWER: 4

Continuous US is applied to achieve thermal effects (i.e., chronic pain). 1 MHz of continuous US provides deep heating to a depth of 3–5 cm. At this frequency, attenuation (absorption) is less in superficial tissues. This allows more energy to be absorbed, thus producing more heat in deeper tissue layers.

INCORRECT CHOICES:

Pulsed US is used when nonthermal effects are desired (i.e., acute soft tissue injuries). A 3-MHz frequency is used for the treatment of superficial structures 1–2 cm deep, while a 1-MHz frequency can reach tissue 3–5 cm deep, such as the piriformis.

TYPE OF REASONING: ANALYSIS

Here, the test taker must consider the symptomatology plus the specific treatment parameters given for US treatment and determine what will most likely improve the symptomatology. The test taker must have sound knowledge of US properties, including thermal vs. nonthermal applications. If this question was answered incorrectly, review guidelines on US treatment.

A7 | Neuromuscular | Foundational Sciences

An injury classified as American Spinal Injury Association (ASIA A) is a complete injury. This lesion is below L1, making it a cauda equina injury (injury is to peripheral roots and nerves, a lower motor neuron injury). Because regeneration is possible, some recovery of function can be expected.

CHOICES:

1. A spastic or reflex bladder.
2. Some recovery of function, because damage is to peripheral nerve roots.
3. Loss of motor function and pain and temperature sensation below the level of the lesion with light touch, proprioception, and position sense preserved.
4. Greater loss of upper extremity function than lower extremity function with early loss of pain and temperature sensation.

TEACHING POINTS

CORRECT ANSWER: 2

A spinal cord lesion below L1 is a cauda equina lesion (injury to peripheral roots and nerves, lower motor neuron injury). Because regeneration is possible, some recovery in function can be expected.

INCORRECT CHOICES:

A spastic or reflex bladder is associated with upper motor neuron injury. Other choices describe the deficits associated with anterior cord syndrome (choice 3) or central cord syndrome (choice 4).

TYPE OF REASONING: ANALYSIS

This question requires recall of neuroanatomy, including where the spinal cord ends in the column to become the cauda equina. Also, the test taker must understand the difference between upper and lower motor neuron injuries in order to determine that damage to the cauda equina level results in lower motor neuron symptomatology.

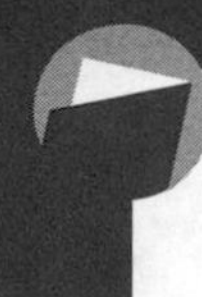

A8 | Devices, Admin., etc. | Teaching, Research, Roles

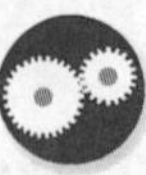

A patient with left hemiplegia receives a new ankle-foot orthosis (AFO). The PT is overwhelmed with too many patients and asks the physical therapy student to take over. This is the student's first affiliation (second day) and he/she has never performed an orthotic checkout for a patient with an AFO. The supervising therapist will be in the same vicinity treating other patients. This task should be:

CHOICES:

1. Delegated to the student who could call out to the supervisor if problems arise.
2. Delegated to another PT.
3. Delegated to the physical therapy assistant (PTA) who is working nearby.
4. Not completed now and the patient sent back to his/her room.

TEACHING POINTS

CORRECT ANSWER: 2

This might be unsafe for the patient. The task of orthotic checkout should be delegated to another PT.

INCORRECT CHOICES:

The PT student or PTA should not perform advanced tasks for the first time without instruction or direct supervision. Postponing the task would be an option only if another PT were unavailable.

TYPE OF REASONING: EVALUATION

This question requires test takers to draw upon their professional principles to deduce what is ethically appropriate for the PT. The test taker must consider ethical guidelines, proper supervision of students, and patient safety.

A9 | Musculoskeletal | Intervention

A patient has been diagnosed with acute synovitis of the temporomandibular joint. Early intervention should focus on:

CHOICES:

1. Application of an intraoral appliance and phonophoresis.
2. Joint mobilization and postural awareness.
3. Instruction to eat a soft food diet and phonophoresis.
4. Temporalis stretching and joint mobilization.

TEACHING POINTS

CORRECT ANSWER: 3

Phonophoresis and education regarding consumption of only soft food should help resolve the acute inflammatory process in the temporomandibular joint.

INCORRECT CHOICES:

Application of an intraoral appliance occurs only when the acute inflammation is not resolved or bruxism continues. Joint mobilization should not be attempted with an acute inflammation.

TYPE OF REASONING: INFERENCE

This case requires one to infer the best course of action for a patient with temporomandibular joint disorder. The potential choices for this patient require the test taker to determine what would result in the best possible outcome for the patient and to consider how each approach and modality will likely provide such a positive result.

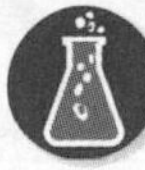

A10 | Musculoskeletal | Intervention

During a cervical spine examination, the PT observes restricted left rotation of the C7–T1 spinal level. After stabilizing the thoracic spine, the therapist's hand placement for mobilization to improve left rotation should be at the:

CHOICES:

1. Posterior right C7 articular pillar.
2. Posterior left C7 articular pillar.
3. Tip of T1 spinous process.
4. Posterior left C6 articular pillar.

TEACHING POINTS

CORRECT ANSWER: 1

The most effective hand placement for mobilization into greater left rotation is at the posterior aspect of the right C7 articular pillar because it rotates the C7 vertebra to the left.

INCORRECT CHOICES:

Hand placement on the left of C6 or C7 articular pillars will promote right rotation. Hand placement on the T1 spinous process will create a posteroanterior glide, which will promote flexion at the T1–2 segment and extension at the C7–T1 segment.

TYPE OF REASONING: ANALYSIS

The test taker must have a solid understanding of anatomy and joint mobilization techniques in order to reason out the best way to facilitate left rotation of the C7 vertebra and provide manual therapy for the cervical vertebrae in general. If this question was answered incorrectly, review joint mobilization guidelines for the cervical spine.

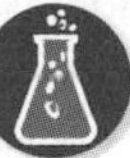

A11 | Neuromuscular | Foundational Sciences

An appropriate fine motor behavior that should be established by 9 months of age is the ability to:

CHOICES:

1. Pick up a raisin with a fine pincer grasp.
2. Build a tower of four blocks.
3. Hold a cup by the handle while drinking.
4. Transfer objects from one hand to another.

TEACHING POINTS

CORRECT ANSWER: 4

Transferring objects from one hand to another is a task developmentally appropriate for an 8 or 9 month-old.

INCORRECT CHOICES:

Using a fine pincer grasp and building a tower of four blocks are skills that develop later. Holding a cup by the handle while drinking usually occurs by 12 months of age.

TYPE OF REASONING: ANALYSIS

In this question, the test taker must understand the fine motor developmental milestones of infants in order to reason which answer is most age-appropriate. If this question was answered incorrectly, review the fine motor developmental milestones of infants up to 1 year.

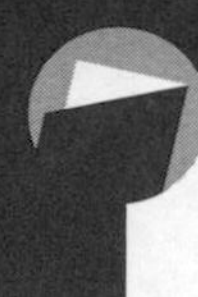

A12 | Neuromuscular | Evaluation, Diagnosis, Prognosis

A patient with a 10-year history of Parkinson's disease (PD) has been taking levodopa (Sinemet) for the last 5 years. The patient presents with deteriorating function and is no longer able to walk independently due to constant and uncontrolled involuntary movements. During the examination, the PT observes the patient is restless, with constant dancing, athetoid-like movements of his legs. The therapist's **BEST** course of action is to:

CHOICES:

1. Complete the treatment session, focusing specifically on documenting the effects of rigidity.
2. Document the observations and refer the patient back to the physician for possible medication adjustment.
3. Talk to the spouse to see if the patient is taking any drugs with hallucinogenic effects, such as selegiline.
4. Examine for additional signs of chronic levodopa therapy, such as dizziness and headache.

TEACHING POINTS

CORRECT ANSWER: 2

Dyskinesias (involuntary movements) are caused by an adverse effect of prolonged use of dopamine. Other changes include gastrointestinal disturbances (nausea, vomiting) and mental disturbances (restlessness, general overactivity, anxiety, or depression). Medication adjustment may reduce some of these effects and improve function.

INCORRECT CHOICES:

Although the symptoms described in the other choices may also occur with pharmacological management of PD, they do not adequately explain the presence of adventitious or involuntary movements. Selegiline is used in early PD; its main adverse effects include nausea, dry mouth, dizziness, anxiety, and hallucinations. Failure to notify the physician of these documented adverse effects can jeopardize the patient's functional outcomes and safety.

TYPE OF REASONING: EVALUATION

One must understand the common symptomatology of PD, as well as the benefits and side effects of levodopa therapy. Questions such as this are challenging, because determining the basis for new or unexpected symptomatology requires one to rely on facts and also judgment to arrive at the best possible conclusion.

A13 | Devices, Admin., etc. | Teaching, Research, Roles

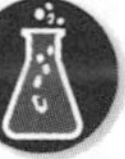

A patient who is to undergo surgery for a chronic shoulder dislocation asks the PT to explain the rehabilitation following a scheduled surgical reconstructive procedure. The therapist's **BEST** response is to:

CHOICES:

1. Explain in detail about the surgical procedure.
2. Tell the patient to ask the surgeon for information about the procedure and appropriate rehabilitation.
3. Explain how patients typically respond to the surgery and outline the progression of exercises.
4. Refer the patient to a physical therapy clinical specialist who is an expert on shoulder reconstructive rehabilitation.

TEACHING POINTS

CORRECT ANSWER: 3

Assess the needs of the patient and provide appropriate information. The PT is well qualified to provide information on the expected rehabilitation process.

INCORRECT CHOICES:

Do not "pass the buck" unless the information is outside of the scope of the therapist's expertise.

TYPE OF REASONING: ANALYSIS

In this scenario, the test taker must understand physical therapy scope of practice and the typical needs of a patient about to undergo surgery. One must be careful not to overburden the patient with detailed information, instead providing factual information that is beneficial and common-sense.

A14 | Cardiovascular-Pulmonary | Patient Examination

Which of the following is a correct reason to terminate a maximum exercise tolerance test for a patient with pulmonary dysfunction?

CHOICES:

1. Electrocardiogram (ECG) monitoring reveals heart rate (HR) increase and normal rhythm.
2. Patient exhibits dyspnea and a drop of 20 mm Hg in arterial oxygen pressure (PaO_2).
3. ECG monitoring reveals flat ST segment.
4. Patient reaches age-predicted maximal HR.

TEACHING POINTS

CORRECT ANSWER: 2

A maximum exercise tolerance test is a sign- or symptom-limited test. Dyspnea with a drop of 20 mm Hg in PaO_2 is an indication for stopping the test.

INCORRECT CHOICES:

Achieving age-adjusted predicted maximum HR is not a sign or symptom, and therefore does not stop the test. HR is expected to increase with normal rhythm. ST segment depression, not a flat ST segment, reveals ischemia and would be a reason to stop the test.

TYPE OF REASONING: DEDUCTIVE

One must have a solid understanding of pulmonary rehabilitation, including the typical and atypical responses of the patient. One would expect to see age-predicted maximal HR, which should not cause alarm. However, a therapist would not want to see symptomatology that indicates the patient is not tolerating the test and may be displaying signs of distress.

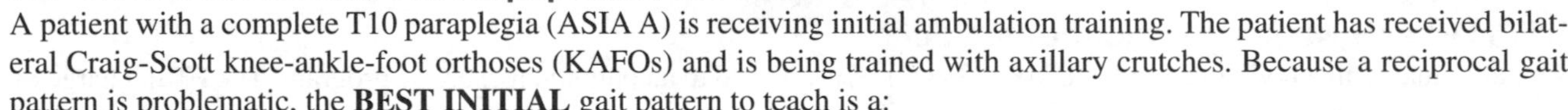

A15 | Devices, Admin., etc. | Equipment, Modalities

A patient with a complete T10 paraplegia (ASIA A) is receiving initial ambulation training. The patient has received bilateral Craig-Scott knee-ankle-foot orthoses (KAFOs) and is being trained with axillary crutches. Because a reciprocal gait pattern is problematic, the **BEST INITIAL** gait pattern to teach is a:

CHOICES:

1. Four-point.
2. Swing-to.
3. Two-point.
4. Swing-through.

TEACHING POINTS

CORRECT ANSWER: 2

An injury classified as American Spinal Injury Association (ASIA) A is a complete injury. A swing-to gait pattern is indicated initially for individuals with limited use of both lower extremities, bilateral KAFOs, and trunk instability.

INCORRECT CHOICES:

A swing-through gait pattern is faster but less stable. This patient can be progressed to this gait pattern after his initial training. This patient is unable to perform a four-point or two-point reciprocal gait with a T10 lesion.

TYPE OF REASONING: INFERENCE

The test taker must understand the requirements for gait for patients with complete SCI, including a progression of gait patterns from least to most challenging and most to least stabilizing. If this question was answered incorrectly, review information on gait patterns and mobility for patients with complete T10 paraplegia and, by extension, all levels of SCI.

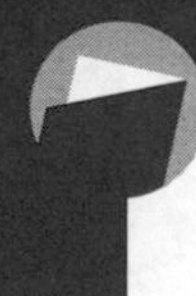

A16 | Other Systems | Evaluation, Diagnosis, Prognosis

After mastectomy, a patient receiving home care cannot accept the loss of her breast. She reports being weepy all the time with loss of sleep. She is constantly tired and has no energy to do anything. The **BEST** action the PT can take is to:

CHOICES:

1. Contact her primary physician and request a psychological consult.
2. Tell the nurse case manager to monitor the patient closely.
3. Tell her depression is common at first, but will resolve with time.
4. Have her spouse observe her closely for possible suicidal tendencies.

TEACHING POINTS

CORRECT ANSWER: 1

The patient is experiencing depression and grief over her loss. Significant, persistent symptoms are an indication for referral to a qualified professional (psychologist).

INCORRECT CHOICES:

She is no longer an inpatient; thus, a nurse case manager would not be able to regularly monitor her behavior. Major depression does not necessarily resolve with time, and is not an expected consequence of mastectomy. The patient has not expressed any suicidal tendencies. If so, the therapist would need to contact the physician immediately.

TYPE OF REASONING: EVALUATION

The test taker must understand the scope of practice of physical therapy to arrive at a correct conclusion. While a PT can provide support for a patient who is adjusting to a loss, the test taker must understand that the degree of symptomatology is beyond the scope of the therapist, and requires referral to a mental health professional for appropriate support and follow-through. Evaluation-type questions are challenging because they require one to go beyond facts and exercise judgment to make the best decision for the patient.

A17 | Other Systems | Foundational Sciences

An individual with a body mass index BMI of 33 $kg.m^{-2}$ is referred to an outpatient exercise program. The PT in charge of the program recognizes this patient is at increased risk for:

CHOICES:

1. Hyperthermia during exercise.
2. Hypothermia during exercise.
3. Rapid weight loss during the initial weeks.
4. Increased anxiety and depression.

TEACHING POINTS

CORRECT ANSWER: 1

A patient with a BMI of 33 $kg.m^{-2}$ is obese (BMI > 30 $kg.m^{-2}$) and is at increased risk for hyperthermia during exercise (as well as orthopedic injury).

INCORRECT CHOICES:

Weight loss is the result of a complex interplay between diet and exercise, and not the result of exercise alone. A balanced program of exercise and diet will produce effects over time, not just in the initial weeks. An appropriately prescribed exercise program should decrease anxiety and depression. Hypothermia is not typical with obesity.

TYPE OF REASONING: INFERENCE

This question requires one to infer a patient's risk factors based on the diagnosis provided. This is an inferential reasoning skill, because one must determine what may be true of a patient, although one cannot be 100% certain. In this case, the patient is likely to have hyperthermia during exercise. If this question was answered incorrectly, review risk factors for patients with obesity, especially exercise risk factors.

A18 | Other Systems | Evaluation, Diagnosis, Prognosis

A middle-aged patient is 10 days postoperative left total knee arthroplasty and is being seen by a home care PT. The patient has been taking hydrocodone with ibuprofen for pain since the surgery. The patient has progressed to walking using standby assistance and a standard walker and active assisted lower extremity exercises. Today, the patient is complaining of back and groin pain of 7/10 when lying in bed or sitting. The pain is 5/10 when standing. A recent International Normalized Ratio (INR) clotting time is within therapeutic levels. Which of the following screening questions is the **BEST** choice for the therapist to ask in consideration of these new symptoms?

CHOICES:

1. When was your last pain medication?
2. Have you been screened for colon cancer?
3. When was your last bowel movement?
4. Do you have any pain or tenderness in your left calf?

TEACHING POINTS

CORRECT ANSWER: 3

Postoperative constipation is common in patients taking opioids. The lack of laxatives in the medication profile would indicate a possible problem with constipation and symptoms of groin pain that is relieved on standing.

INCORRECT CHOICES:

The pain medication timing would not be significant with the change in pain level on positional change. The normal INR, a measure of clotting time, would make screening for deep venous thrombosis (DVT) less of a priority. Screening for colon cancer most likely would have been done as part of the general medical examination for surgery.

TYPE OF REASONING: INFERENCE

Inferential reasoning requires one to draw conclusions based on facts, beliefs, and assumptions. In order to arrive at a correct conclusion, the test taker must understand the side effects of taking opioids. In this situation, the patient presents with the common side effect of constipation from opioid use. If this question was answered incorrectly, review common side effects of opioid use.

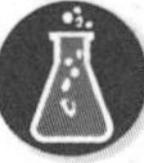

A19 | Musculoskeletal | Evaluation, Diagnosis, Prognosis

During an examination of a patient who complains of back pain, the PT notes pain with end range active range of motion (AROM) into left hip flexion, abduction, and external rotation. The origin of the pain is **MOST LIKELY** the:

CHOICES:

1. Sartorius muscle.
2. Sacroiliac (SI) joint.
3. Left kidney.
4. Capsule of the hip joint.

TEACHING POINTS

CORRECT ANSWER: 2

Pain at end range of flexion, abduction, and external rotation, and extension (FABERE test) is diagnostic for SI joint dysfunction because it both gaps and compresses the joint.

INCORRECT CHOICES:

Pain at the mid range into hip flexion, abduction, and external/lateral rotation suggests hip joint pathology. Patient reported low back pain, and if the sartorius or the hip were involved, the complaint of pain would have been reported in the anterior and medial thigh. Renal pain is often referred to the costovertebral region, flank, or lower abdominal quadrant.

TYPE OF REASONING: ANALYSIS

To arrive at a correct answer, the test taker must understand typical pain patterns associated with different disorders and dysfunctions. Here, the pain pattern is directly associated with SI joint dysfunction. If this question was answered incorrectly, review information on SI joint dysfunction.

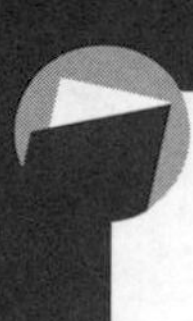

A20 | Devices, Admin., etc. | Teaching, Research, Roles

A PT wants to compare frequencies of carpal tunnel syndrome (CTS) occurring in different groups of individuals: assembly line workers and computer programmers. The appropriate statistical tool to use for analysis of the data is:

CHOICES:

1. Simple one-way analysis of variance (ANOVA).
2. t-test.
3. Normal distribution curve.
4. Chi square test.

TEACHING POINTS

CORRECT ANSWER: 4

Chi square is a nonparametric statistical test used to compare relationships using nominal data. In this example, frequencies of CTS occurring in two different groups of workers are compared.

INCORRECT CHOICES:

The other choices are parametric tests (t-test, ANOVA) that explore differences at a selected probability level. The normal distribution curve is not relevant.

TYPE OF REASONING: DEDUCTIVE

This question is very factual in nature and requires one to understand the properties of each statistical test listed. One must understand that the research study described is comparing frequency of CTS in two different groups of workers. The ANOVA would be best when comparing different variables, and the t-test is best for comparing two groups that are statistically different from each other. The normal distribution curve is not detailed enough for this level of analysis.

A21 | Devices, Admin., etc. | Teaching, Research, Roles

In a research study in which there is a skewed distribution with extreme scores on a balance measure that deviate from the performance of the total group, the **MOST** accurate representation of central tendency is:

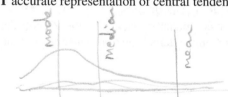

CHOICES:

1. Mean.
2. Mode.
3. Median.
4. Standard deviation.

TEACHING POINTS

CORRECT ANSWER: 3

The median is the middle value with equal scores above and below. It is the most accurate measure of performance in skewed distribution with extreme scores.

INCORRECT CHOICES:

The mean is the average score; it is calculated by dividing the sum of the scores by the number of scores. The mode is the most frequently occurring score in a distribution. Standard deviation is a measure of variance, not central tendency.

TYPE OF REASONING: DEDUCTIVE

This question is very factual, and requires one to recall the definitions of mean, mode, median, and standard deviation. These terms are important for any quantitative research project, and should be reviewed if the question was answered incorrectly.

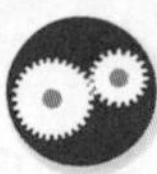

A22 | Neuromuscular | Evaluation, Diagnosis, Prognosis

A factory worker injured the right arm in a factory press with damage to the ulnar nerve at the elbow. A diagnostic electromyogram (EMG) was performed 3 weeks after the injury, with evidence of spontaneous fibrillation potentials. In this case, the PT recognizes that:

CHOICES:

1. Denervation has occurred.
2. Reinnervation is complete.
3. Neurapraxia has occurred.
4. Reinnervation is in process.

TEACHING POINTS

CORRECT ANSWER: 1

Spontaneous fibrillation potentials and positive sharp waves present on EMG 2 to 3 weeks after injury are evidence of denervation. This occurs with axonotmesis, a class 2 peripheral nerve injury (PNI) with axonal damage and Wallerian degeneration distal to the lesion.

INCORRECT CHOICES:

Polyphasic motor units of low amplitude and short duration are evidence of reinnervation. Neurapraxia is a class 1 PNI with local compression or blockage. EMG typically reveals no spontaneous activity.

TYPE OF REASONING: EVALUATION

One must understand the meaning behind spontaneous fibrillation potentials as an indication of either atrophy or healing. In this case, the symptoms indicate atrophy, not healing, but a test taker may mistakenly believe that fibrillation indicates early healing and recovery in the future. If answered incorrectly, review information on EMG testing and diagnostic indicators.

A23 | Devices, Admin., etc. | Equipment, Modalities

A patient is recovering from a right cerebrovascular accident (CVA), resulting in severe left hemiplegia and visuospatial deficits. In addition, there is a large diabetic ulcer on the left foot with pitting edema. The **BEST** choice for wheelchair prescription for this patient is:

CHOICES:

1. Hemiplegic chair with elevating legrest on the left.
2. Powered wheelchair with joystick and elevating legrests.
3. Lightweight active duty wheelchair with elevating legrests.
4. One-arm drive chair with elevating legrest on the left.

TEACHING POINTS

CORRECT ANSWER: 1

A hemiplegic chair has a low seat height (17$^1/_2$ inches as compared with the standard seat height of 19$^1/_2$ inches) and is the best choice for this patient. The patient propels it with the sound right hand and leg. An elevating legrest on the left is indicated for edema.

INCORRECT CHOICES:

A one-arm drive wheelchair has both drive mechanisms located on one wheel. The patient can propel the wheelchair by using one hand. It is contraindicated in patients with cognitive or perceptual deficits (as in this case). The electric wheelchair with joystick might also work but is significantly more expensive and less transportable and would also require increased maintenance. The seat height of a standard height wheelchair (lightweight active duty wheelchair) would be too high to allow propulsion using the sound foot and hand.

TYPE OF REASONING: ANALYSIS

A number of important symptoms are described in this question, and the test taker must analyze all of the symptoms (not just some) in order to make the best choice in wheelchair prescription. When balancing the diabetic issues, hemiplegia, and visuospatial deficits, one must conclude that a hemiplegic chair with elevating legrest provides the safest, most effective means of mobility.

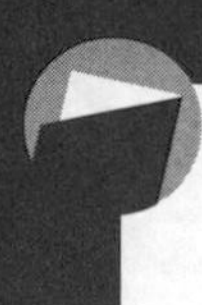

A24 | Other Systems | Evaluation, Diagnosis, Prognosis

A 14 year-old boy with advanced Duchenne's muscular dystrophy is administered a pulmonary function test. The value that is **UNLIKELY** to show any deviation from normal is:

CHOICES:

1. Vital capacity.
2. Forced expiratory volume in 1 second (FEV_1).
3. Functional residual capacity.
4. Total lung capacity.

TEACHING POINTS

CORRECT ANSWER: 3

Becuase muscular dystrophy does not change the lung parenchyma, resting end-expiratory pressure (REEP) will occur at the same point of equilibrium between lung recoil and thoracic outward pull. Therefore, functional residual capacity will not change.

INCORRECT CHOICES:

Muscular dystrophy will alter the respiratory muscles' ability to pull in air and blow out air; therefore, vital capacity, total lung capacity, and FEV_1 will be decreased.

TYPE OF REASONING: INFERENCE

One must understand typical pulmonary symptomatology associated with Duchenne's muscular dystrophy to choose the correct answer. Not only does the test taker reason symptomatology, but he/she also relies on recall of pulmonary terminology and what they directly relate to in terms of function. If this question was answered incorrectly, refer to pulmonary symptomatology of Duchenne's muscular dystrophy and definitions of lung volumes and capacities.

A25 | Devices, Admin., etc. | Equipment, Modalities

A patient fractured the right mid tibia in a skiing accident 3 months ago. After cast removal, a severe foot drop was noted. The patient wants to try electrical stimulation orthotic substitution. The PT would set up the functional electrical stimulation to contract the appropriate muscles during:

CHOICES:

1. Late stance at push-off.
2. Mid swing.
3. Early stance at foot-flat.
4. Late stance at toe-off.

TEACHING POINTS

CORRECT ANSWER: 2

Foot drop is a swing phase deficit. Stimulation of the dorsiflexor muscles during the swing phase places the foot in a more neutral position and prevents the toes from contacting the ground and interfering with the gait pattern.

INCORRECT CHOICES:

Plantarflexors are active from heel strike to foot-flat, and from heel-off to toe-off.

TYPE OF REASONING: ANALYSIS

One must understand the nature of foot drop and the action of dorsiflexors during ambulation in order to choose the correct answer. The test taker who chooses the correct answer understands through analysis that dorsiflexion is needed during swing phase, because the toes may drag on the ground and interfere with the swing. If this question was answered incorrectly, refer to information related to ambulation with foot drop.

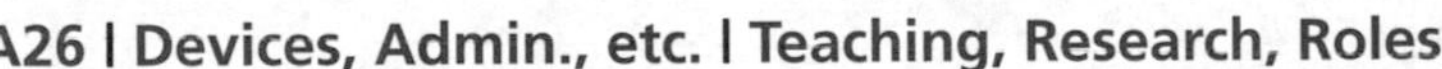

A26 | Devices, Admin., etc. | Teaching, Research, Roles

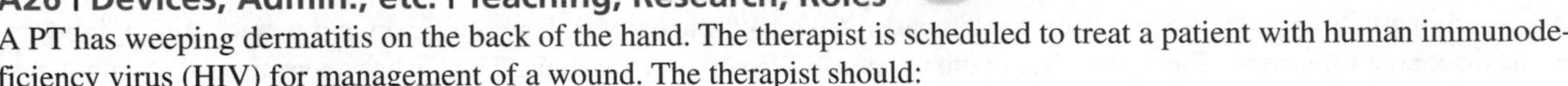

A PT has weeping dermatitis on the back of the hand. The therapist is scheduled to treat a patient with human immunodeficiency virus (HIV) for management of a wound. The therapist should:

CHOICES:

1. Double glove and treat as scheduled.
2. Use sterile precautions with mask and gloves.
3. Continue with treatment as scheduled, but wash hands thoroughly before and after.
4. Refuse to treat that patient.

TEACHING POINTS

CORRECT ANSWER: 4

Blood and Body Fluid Precautionary Guidelines from the Centers for Disease Control and Prevention (CDC) state that a healthcare worker with exudative lesions or weeping dermatitis should refrain from all direct patient care and from handling patient care equipment until the condition resolves.

INCORRECT CHOICES:

The other choices do not offer adequate protection to the patient.

TYPE OF REASONING: EVALUATION

Evaluation questions require one to go beyond facts and make sound judgments that result in the best possible outcome for those who are involved. In this situation, the test taker must reason what would best protect the therapist, as well as the patient, from harm. Because of the nature of the wound, the therapist should decide against direct patient care. Knowledge of CDC Guidelines is crucial.

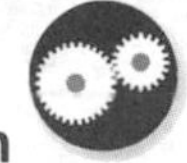

A27 | Musculoskeletal | Patient Examination

As a PT progresses through his/her examination, it is becoming evident that a current patient is anterior cruciate ligament (ACL) deficient in the right knee. Which of the following tests would be **UNNECESSARY** for determining whether the ACL was ruptured?

CHOICES:

1. Lachman's test.
2. Anterior drawer test.
3. Slocum's test.
4. Lateral pivot shift test.

TEACHING POINTS

CORRECT ANSWER: 2

The anterior drawer test places the knee in 90 degrees of flexion. In this position, the knee joint capsule is the primary constraint to movement, so performing this test may result in a false-negative determination.

INCORRECT CHOICES:

The other tests are all appropriate tests to assess the integrity of the ACL.

TYPE OF REASONING: EVALUATION

In order to draw a correct conclusion, one must understand the findings resulting from each of the listed tests, especially as it applies to ACL integrity. In this situation, the anterior drawer test is unnecessary because of the possibility of a false negative. If this question was answered incorrectly, review information on the anterior drawer test.

EXAM A

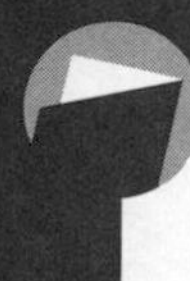

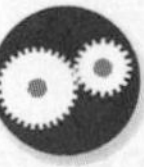

A28 | Devices, Admin., etc. | Teaching, Research, Roles

An elderly patient has been hospitalized for the past 3 days with pneumonia. The physician and patient are hoping for a home discharge tomorrow. The patient lives with a sister in a first floor apartment. The PT has determined that ambulation status is independent with rolling walker and endurance is only up to 15 feet, not enough to allow the patient to get from the bed to the bathroom (a distance of 20 feet). The therapist should recommend:

CHOICES:

1. Postponing her discharge until the patient can walk 20 feet.
2. A skilled nursing facility placement until endurance increases.
3. A bedside commode and referral for home health services.
4. Outpatient physical therapy until the patient's condition improves.

TEACHING POINTS

CORRECT ANSWER: 3

Clinical decision making in this case should focus on the patient's ability to manage in the home. Environmental modifications (the addition of a commode) and assistance of a home care aide should allow the patient to safely return home. Home physical therapy should focus on improving endurance to regain independence in the home. Treatment in the home is the most cost-effective in this case.

INCORRECT CHOICES:

Postponing discharge or placing the patient in a skilled nursing facility is not necessary. Patient does not have the mobility and endurance to attend outpatient therapy.

TYPE OF REASONING: EVALUATION

One must consider multiple factors to arrive at a correct conclusion. One must first consider the physician's constraints with the patient's home environment and her current abilities. Questions that require evaluation require you to make judgments based on professional opinions and experience, which can be challenging for test takers.

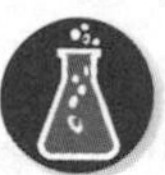

A29 | Neuromuscular | Intervention

A PT examines a patient with a right CVA and determines that the patient has a profound deficit of homonymous hemianopsia. The **BEST INITIAL** strategy to assist the patient in compensating for this deficit is to:

CHOICES:

1. Teach the patient to turn the head to the affected left side.
2. Provide constant reminders, printed notes on the left side, telling the patient to look to the left.
3. Place items, eating utensils on the left side.
4. Rearrange the room so that while the patient is in bed, the left side is facing the doorway.

TEACHING POINTS

CORRECT ANSWER: 1

A patient with homonymous hemianopsia needs to be made aware of the deficit and instructed to turn the head to the affected left side (a compensatory training strategy).

INCORRECT CHOICES:

Initial strategies include placing items on the right (unaffected side), not the left side, so that the patient can successfully interact with the environment. Later, as there is ability to compensate, items can be moved to midline, and finally to the affected left side.

TYPE OF REASONING: ANALYSIS

The test taker must consider what the **BEST INITIAL** strategy is, which is key to answering this analysis-type question. Although all of the choices are possibilities and relevant, focusing on these key words helps one to arrive at the correct conclusion that teaching the patient to turn his/her head needs to occur first.

A30 | Neuromuscular | Intervention

A patient with multiple sclerosis (MS) exhibits moderate fatigue during a 30-minute exercise session. When the patient returns for the next regularly scheduled session 2 days later, the patient reports going right to bed after the last session. Exhaustion was so severe, the patient was unable to get out of bed until late afternoon of the next day. The PT's **BEST** strategy is to:

CHOICES:

1. Treat the patient in a warm, relaxing environment.
2. Utilize a massed practice schedule.
3. Utilize a distributed practice schedule.
4. Switch the patient to exercising in a warm pool.

TEACHING POINTS

CORRECT ANSWER: 3

Common problems in MS include fatigue and heat intolerance. Exercise intensity should be reduced, and a distributed practice schedule should be used, in which rest times equal or exceed exercise times.

INCORRECT CHOICES:

A massed practice schedule in which the exercise time exceeds the rest time is contraindicated as is a warm environment or warm pool, which can increase fatigue.

TYPE OF REASONING: INFERENCE

In this question, one must form a hypothesis about why the symptoms have occurred and what will best remedy them. Having a firm understanding of the nature of MS and heat intolerance that often accompanies MS helps one to arrive at the correct answer.

A31 | Other Systems | Foundational Sciences

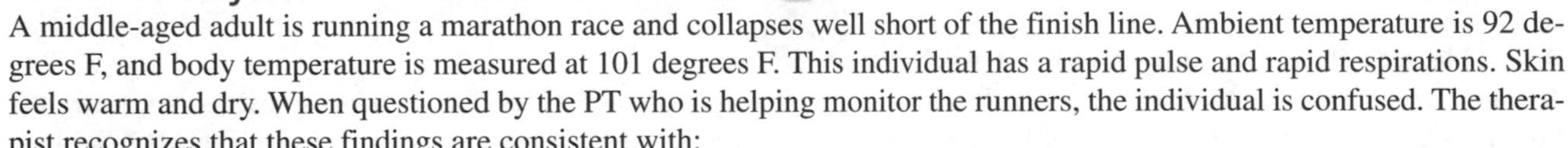

A middle-aged adult is running a marathon race and collapses well short of the finish line. Ambient temperature is 92 degrees F, and body temperature is measured at 101 degrees F. This individual has a rapid pulse and rapid respirations. Skin feels warm and dry. When questioned by the PT who is helping monitor the runners, the individual is confused. The therapist recognizes that these findings are consistent with:

CHOICES:

1. Hypervolemic shock.
2. Hypovolemic shock.
3. Anaphylactic shock.
4. Septic shock.

TEACHING POINTS

CORRECT ANSWER: 2

This individual is demonstrating signs and symptoms of dehydration (inadequate fluid intake) and hypovolemic shock. Pulse and respirations are increased; BP (BP) may decline. Restlessness, anxiety, and confusion may all be present.

INCORRECT CHOICES:

Hypervolemia is an abnormal increase in the volume of circulating blood. Anaphylactic shock is a severe hypersensitivity (allergic reaction) to a substance with symptoms of local allergen-antibody interaction (hives, edema, warmth, erythema) as well as systematic symptoms of flushing, wheezing, dyspnea, and anxiety. Septic shock (sepsis) is a systematic inflammatory response to infection characterized by fever, tachycardia, tachypnea, and organ failure.

TYPE OF REASONING: ANALYSIS

This question requires one to analyze the symptoms presented and determine the most likely diagnosis. This requires analytical reasoning skill. In this situation, the runner's symptoms indicate hypovolemic shock. If this question was answered incorrectly, review signs and symptoms of hypovolemic shock.

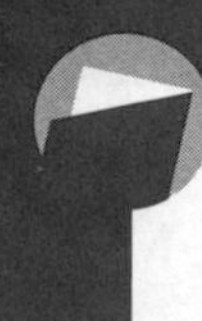

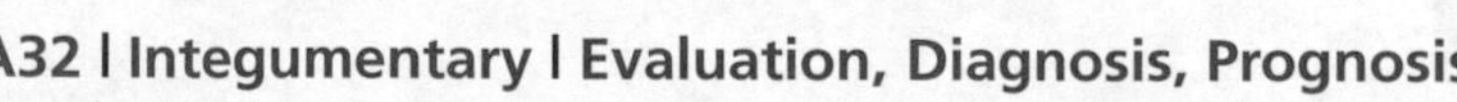

A32 | Integumentary | Evaluation, Diagnosis, Prognosis

A patient with a venous stasis ulcer near the left medial malleolus is referred for physical therapy. Skin changes consistent with stasis dermatitis are evident in the lower leg. Physical examination reveals patent femoral, popliteal, and pedal pulses. An enlarged and dilated greater saphenous vein is evident in the standing position. The **MOST** important physical therapy intervention to consider for this patient is:

CHOICES:

1. Daily walking for 30–60 minutes.
2. Elastic wraps and daily exercises.
3. Daily warm water baths and exercise.
4. Compression therapy with exercise.

TEACHING POINTS

CORRECT ANSWER: 4

Compression therapy is the mainstay of nonoperative treatment of venous stasis ulcers, and works with exercise to facilitate movement of excess fluid from the lower leg. Dressings are applied before compression bandages. Pliable, nonstretchable dressing wraps (e.g., Unna boot) or custom-fitted graduated compression stockings can be used to assist in venous circulation.

INCORRECT CHOICES:

Elastic wraps are easy to apply, but provide only light support and do little to assist circulation. Prolonged hydrotherapy is contraindicated for venous ulcers. Exercise alone will not adequately control venous stasis.

TYPE OF REASONING: INDUCTIVE

The test taker must evaluate each treatment approach and determine which one will, most likely, result in improvement of the venous stasis ulcer. One must understand the nature of stasis ulcers and how they respond or do not respond to each of the treatment approaches. In this type of question, knowledge plus clinical judgment is used to arrive at the correct answer.

A33 | Neuromuscular | Patient Examination

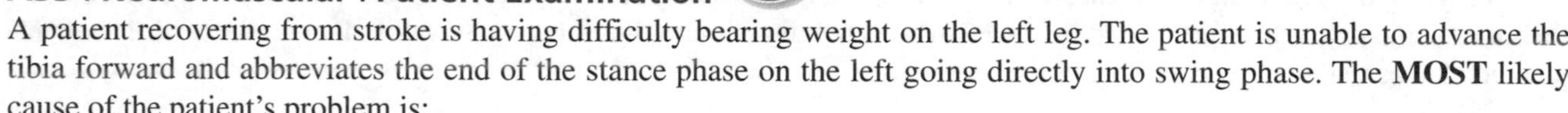

A patient recovering from stroke is having difficulty bearing weight on the left leg. The patient is unable to advance the tibia forward and abbreviates the end of the stance phase on the left going directly into swing phase. The **MOST** likely cause of the patient's problem is:

CHOICES:

1. Weakness or contracture of hip extensors.
2. Spasticity or contracture of the plantar flexors.
3. Spasticity of the anterior tibialis muscle.
4. Weakness or contracture of the dorsiflexors.

TEACHING POINTS

CORRECT ANSWER: 2

Forward advancement of the tibia from midstance to heel-off is controlled by eccentric contraction of the plantar flexors; from heel-off to toe-off, the plantar flexors contract concentrically. Either spasticity or contracture of the plantar flexors would limit this forward progression. Patients compensate by going right into swing, typically with a circumducted gait or with increased hip and knee flexion because there is no push-off.

INCORRECT CHOICES:

Spasticity or contracture of the dorsiflexors is typically not seen, and could not cause this deficit. Weakness of the hip extensors would be evident at heel-strike, with a backward lean of the trunk.

TYPE OF REASONING: INDUCTIVE

In this type of question, one must use mental imagery to "see" the problem in this patient's gait pattern. In choosing the correct answer, the test taker must make a link between the descriptions of the problem and a specific issue in muscle groups. This requires one to utilize clinical judgment, which is an inductive reasoning skill.

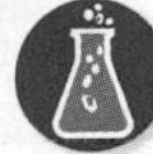

A34 | Musculoskeletal | Foundational Sciences

With a traction injury to the anterior division of the brachial plexus, the PT would expect to see weakness of the elbow flexors, wrist flexors, and forearm pronators. The therapist would also expect to find additional weakness in:

CHOICES:

1. Wrist extension.
2. Forearm supination.
3. Thumb abduction.
4. Lateral rotation of the shoulder.

TEACHING POINTS

CORRECT ANSWER: 3

Thumb abductors are innervated by the median nerve, primarily by the C6 nerve root. The anterior divisions contribute to nerves that primarily serve flexors and, in this case, the thumb.

INCORRECT CHOICES:

All other choices are innervated by nerves off the posterior division. Wrist extensors include the extensor carpi radialis longus (ECRL), entensor carpi radialis brevi (ECRB), innervated by the radial nerve C6–7 and the extensor carpi ulnaris (ECU), innervated by the radial nerve C6–8. Supination results from action of the biceps brachii (musculocutaneous nerve C5–6) and the supinator (radial nerve C6).

TYPE OF REASONING: ANALYSIS

One must have a firm understanding of neuroanatomy to answer the question correctly. The test taker should recognize that the symptoms indicated all correspond to median nerve injury. In this type of question, one is analyzing what the symptoms mean for patient functioning and expected symptomatology, given the exact location of injury.

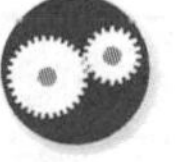

A35 | Other Systems | Interventions

A frail, elderly patient has recently been admitted to a skilled nursing facility following a fall-related injury (fractured hip with open reduction, internal fixation). The patient lived alone on the second floor and was unable to return home. The patient is extremely agitated over being in a nursing facility and demonstrates early signs of dementia, exclaiming to the PT, "Leave me alone, I just want to get out of here!" An important approach to take while working with this patient is to:

CHOICES:

1. State clearly and firmly what is going to happen in therapy.
2. Be calm and supportive, and use only one- or two-level commands.
3. Minimize verbal communication and maximize guided movements.
4. Promise anything to calm the patient down, as long as some walking occurs.

TEACHING POINTS

CORRECT ANSWER: 2

An agitated patient with dementia does not process information easily. A calm and supportive approach with low-level commands (one or two actions) provides the best approach for this patient.

INCORRECT CHOICES:

Establishing rules, confrontation, and making unrealistic promises that cannot be kept may increase agitation. Guided movements may help, but communication should be maintained.

TYPE OF REASONING: EVALUATION

In this type of question, one must assess the value of the four possible choices. In this scenario, the test taker should be able to determine that an agitated patient with dementia will require a calm approach with simple commands to reduce agitation. This type of question requires one to weigh the strength of statements, which is an evaluative skill.

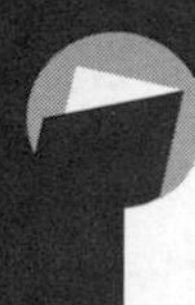

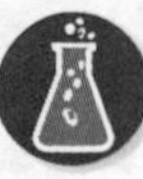

A36 | Other Systems | Foundational Sciences

A elderly patient is being treated for depression following the death of her husband. She is currently taking a tricyclic antidepressant medication (amitriptyline) and has a recent history of a fall. The PT suspects the precipitating cause of the fall is the medication, because it can cause:

CHOICES:

1. Hyperalertness.
2. Hypertension.
3. Dyspnea.
4. Postural hypotension.

TEACHING POINTS

CORRECT ANSWER: 4

Most tricyclic antidepressants have significant anticholinergic and sedative properties and may cause lethargy, sedation, arrhythmias, hypotension, and blurred vision, thus increasing fall risk. The elderly are particularly susceptible to adverse drug effects because of a multitude of factors.

INCORRECT CHOICES:

Hypertension, tachycardia, and convulsions can result when tricyclic antidepressants are used in combination with monoamine oxidase (MAO) inhibitors. Hyperalertness and dyspnea are not expected adverse reactions/side effects of this medication.

TYPE OF REASONING: ANALYSIS

One must understand the common adverse reactions/side effects of medications in order to answer this question correctly. In analysis questions, the test taker weighs all of the information provided in order to determine which response seems to be the most likely to be true.

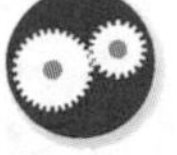

A37 | Cardiovascular-Pulmonary | Foundational Sciences

A patient has class III heart disease and is continually in and out of congestive heart failure (CHF). Digitalis (digoxin) has been prescribed to improve heart function. The patient will demonstrate understanding of the adverse side effects of this medication by recognizing the importance of contacting the primary physician with the appearance of which of the following symptoms?

CHOICES:

1. Confusion and memory loss.
2. Tachycardia.
3. Involuntary movements and shaking.
4. Weakness and arrhythmias.

TEACHING POINTS

CORRECT ANSWER: 4

Class III heart disease is characterized by marked limitation of physical activity; the patient is comfortable at rest, but less than ordinary physical activity causes fatigue, palpitation, dyspnea, or anginal pain. Digitalis (digoxin) is frequently used to treat CHF (it slows HR and increases force of myocardial contraction). Adverse reactions/side effects of digitalis can include fatigue, headache, muscle weakness, bradycardia, and supraventricular or ventricular arrhythmias, including ventricular fibrillation, without premonitory signs.

INCORRECT CHOICES:

The other choices are not expected adverse reactions of this medication.

TYPE OF REASONING: EVALUATION

In this situation, the test taker must determine what constitutes caregiver understanding or competence. This requires the test taker to evaluate the four choices that equate to understanding, which requires judgment and knowledge of class III heart disease. This means that one should have a sound understanding of class III heart disease and typical adverse reactions/side effects of digoxin therapy.

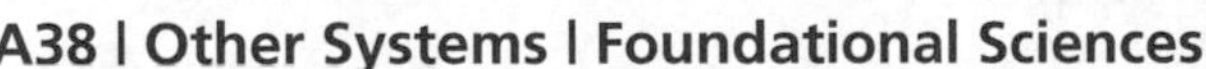

A38 | Other Systems | Foundational Sciences

A patient with HIV is hospitalized with a viral infection, and has a history of four infectious episodes within the past year. The PT recognizes that ongoing systemic effects are likely to include:

CHOICES:

1. Decreased erythrocyte sedimentation rate (ESR).
2. Redness, warmth, swelling, and pain.
3. Fever, tachycardia, and a hypermetabolic state.
4. Low-grade fever, malaise, anemia, and fatigue.

TEACHING POINTS

CORRECT ANSWER: 4

Repeat infections produce a chronic inflammatory state. Systemic effects include low-grade fever, weight loss, malaise, anemia, fatigue, leukocytosis, and lymphocytosis.

INCORRECT CHOICES:

Inflammatory activity can be detected by an elevated ESR. Redness, warmth, swelling, and pain are signs of acute inflammation. Fever, tachycardia, and a hypermetabolic state are signs of the systemic effects of an acute inflammation.

TYPE OF REASONING: INFERENCE

One must infer or draw a reasonable conclusion about the likely ongoing systemic effects of a patient with HIV. This requires inferential reasoning skill. For this case, the patient is likely to exhibit a low-grade fever, malaise, anemia, and fatigue, given the diagnosis and history of multiple infectious episodes. If this question was answered incorrectly, review systemic effects of HIV, especially symptoms of chronic inflammatory state.

A39 | Other Systems | Interventions

A PT is treating a patient with active hepatitis B infection. Transmission of the disease is best minimized if the PT:

CHOICES:

1. Washes hands before and after treatment.
2. Wears gloves during any direct contact with blood or body fluids.
3. Have the patient wear a gown and mask during treatment.
4. Have the patient wear gloves to prevent direct contact with the therapist.

TEACHING POINTS

CORRECT ANSWER: 2

Standard precautions specifiy that health care workers wear personal protective equipment (moisture-resistant gowns, masks) for protection from the splashing of blood, other body fluids, or respiratory droplets resulting from direct body contact with the patient.

INCORRECT CHOICES:

Although hand washing is important, it is not as important as wearing gloves when the health care worker comes in direct contact with blood or body fluids. The patient with risk of transmission of known or suspected infectious agents is typically isolated in a single-patient room and wears protective equipment (masks) only when being transported out of the room. Gowns or gloves are not typically worn.

TYPE OF REASONING: INFERENCE

In this situation, the test taker must weigh all the elements of the scenario to determine what will best protect the PT from exposure. This type of question requires the test taker to consider what the consequences may be for all the choices given. One must have a solid understanding of universal or standard precautions coupled with knowledge of mode of transmission of hepatitis B to come to the correct conclusion.

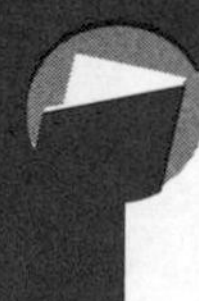

A40 | Devices, Admin., etc. | Equipment, Modalities

A patient complains of pain (7/10) and limited range of motion (ROM) of the right shoulder as a result of chronic overuse. The PT elects to use procaine hydrochloride iontophoresis as part of physical therapy intervention for this patient's problems. To administer this substance, it would be appropriate to use:

CHOICES:

1. Continuous biphasic current, with the medication under the anode.
2. Continuous monophasic current, with the medication under the anode.
3. Continuous monophasic current, with the medication under the cathode.
4. Interrupted biphasic current, with the medication under the cathode.

TEACHING POINTS

CORRECT ANSWER: 2

Because like charges are repelled, the positively charged medication would be forced into the skin under the positive electrode (anode). A continuous, unidirectional current flow is very effective in repelling ions into the skin. Procaine is a positive medicinal ion, and will be repelled from the anode (positive pole).

INCORRECT CHOICES:

A pulsed, interrupted, or bidirectional current generates less propulsive force owing to the discontinuous nature of the current. The cathode is not an appropriate choice to administer this medication.

TYPE OF REASONING: DEDUCTIVE

The test taker must understand the properties of iontophoresis, including positive and negative charges of the electrodes and medication used. Using the skills of deductive reasoning, the test taker reasons out what seems most likely to occur and least likely to occur, given the four possible choices. If this question was answered incorrectly, review information on iontophoresis guidelines and medications.

A41 | Cardiovascular-Pulmonary | Foundational Sciences

A contraindication to initiating extremity joint mobilization on a patient with chronic pulmonary disease may include:

CHOICES:

1. Reflex muscle guarding.
2. Long-term corticosteroid therapy.
3. Concurrent inhalation therapy.
4. Functional chest wall immobility.

TEACHING POINTS

CORRECT ANSWER: 2

Very often, patients with chronic pulmonary disease have been managed using corticosteroid therapy. Long-term steroid use has the catabolic effects of osteoporosis, weakened supporting joint structures, and muscle wasting, making joint mobilization contraindicated.

INCORRECT CHOICES:

There would not be any increase in reflex muscle guarding in a patient with pulmonary disease over that in other patient populations. Inhalation therapy, even with a corticosteroid, has minimal systemic uptake of the drug and, therefore, would not be a contraindication to performing joint mobility. A functionally limited thorax may be considered when deciding on the starting body position for joint mobility, but will not change the ability to perform the task.

TYPE OF REASONING: DEDUCTIVE

This type of question requires the test taker to reason out which negative symptomatology may contraindicate the use of joint mobilization. In order to choose the correct answer, one must understand the effects of joint mobilization and the effects of long-term corticosteroid therapy on soft tissue. The recall of protocols and guidelines is a deductive reasoning skill.

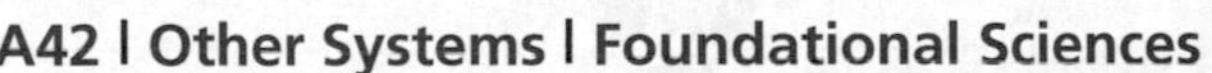

A42 | Other Systems | Foundational Sciences

An elderly and frail individual is receiving physical therapy in the home environment to improve general strengthening and mobility. The patient has a 4-year history of taking nonsteroidal anti-inflammatory drugs (NSAIDs) such as, aspirin for joint pain, and recently began taking a calcium channel blocker (verapamil). The PT examines the patient for possible adverse reactions/side effects that could include:

CHOICES:

1. Increased sweating, fatigue, chest pain.
2. Stomach pain, hypertension, confusion.
3. Weight increase, hyperglycemia, hypotension.
4. Paresthesias, incoordination, bradycardia.

TEACHING POINTS

CORRECT ANSWER: 2

With advanced age, the capacity of the individual to break down and convert drugs diminishes (secondary to decreased liver and kidney function, reduced hepatic and renal blood flow, etc.). Some drugs additionally slow metabolism (e.g., calcium channel blockers like verapamil and diltiazem or antigout drugs like allopurinol). NSAIDs are associated with potential gastrointestinal (GI) effects (stomach pain, peptic ulcers, GI hemorrhage), peripheral edema, and easy bruising and bleeding. NSAIDs can also lessen the effects of antihypertensive drugs. Central nervous system (CNS) effects can include headache, dizziness, lightheadedness, insomnia, tinnitus, confusion, and depression.

INCORRECT CHOICES:

The other choices are not expected adverse reactions.

TYPE OF REASONING: DEDUCTIVE

This question requires the test taker to recall the typical side effects of taking both NSAIDs and calcium channel blockers. This is factual recall of information, which is a deductive reasoning skill. For this scenario, the PT should anticipate potential side effects of stomach pain, hypertension, and confusion. If this question was answered incorrectly, review side effects of NSAIDs and calcium channel blockers.

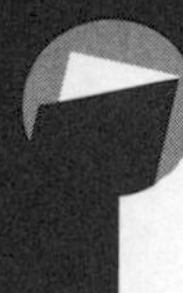

A43 | Cardiovascular-Pulmonary | Evaluation, Diagnosis, Prognosis

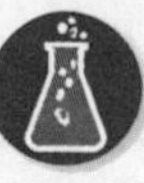

A computer programmer with no significant past medical history presents to the emergency room with complaints of fever, shaking chills, and a worsening productive cough. Complaints of chest pain over the posterior base of the left thorax are made worse on inspiration. An anteroposterior x-ray shows an infiltrate on the lower left thorax at the posterior base. This patient's chest pain is **MOST** likely caused by:

CHOICES:

1. Inflamed tracheobronchial tree.
2. Angina.
3. Trauma to the chest.
4. Infected pleura.

TEACHING POINTS

CORRECT ANSWER: 4

The case is supportive of a pulmonary process as evidenced by radiography and history. Because the radiographic findings and the pain are in the same vicinity and worsen with inspiration, the likelihood is that this pain is pleuritic in origin.

INCORRECT CHOICES:

Angina is not the most likely cause, because the cardiac system is not involved. There is no history of trauma to the chest and no trauma was found radiographically, making it unlikely as the source of pain. An inflamed tracheobronchial tree would not usually reflect pain in the posterior base of the left thorax.

TYPE OF REASONING: ANALYSIS

In this question, the test taker must have a solid foundation of pulmonary disorders in order to recognize the symptoms indicative of pleuritis. The test taker uses analytical skills to match the symptoms presented with the most likely cause of those symptoms. The key to finding the correct answer is in the results of the x-ray and complaints of pain.

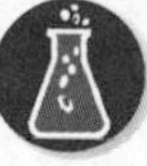

A44 | Cardiovascular-Pulmonary | Evaluation, Diagnosis, Prognosis

An elderly patient is being examined by the PT. The therapist notes a irregular, dark-pigmented ulcer over the medial malleolus. The patient states this is not painful. The **MOST** likely diagnosis is:

CHOICES:

1. Arterial ulcer.
2. Venous ulcer.
3. Diabetic ulcer.
4. Arterial insufficiency.

TEACHING POINTS

CORRECT ANSWER: 2

This patient is demonstrating signs and symptoms of a venous ulcer: irregular, dark pigmentation, usually shallow, and appearing on the distal lower leg (medial malleolus is the most common area). There is little pain associated with venous ulcers.

INCORRECT CHOICES:

Arterial ulcers also have irregular edges, but are not typically dark. They are painful, especially if the legs are elevated, and are common in the distal lower leg (toes, feet lateral malleolus, anterior tibial area). Diabetic ulcers are associated with arterial disease and peripheral neuropathy. They appear in locations where arterial ulcers appear, and are typically not painful. Signs and symptoms of arterial insufficiency include decreased or absent pulses and pale color. Intermittent claudication is common in early disease, whereas in late stages, patients exhibit rest pain and ischemia.

TYPE OF REASONING: ANALYSIS

This question provides a description of symptoms and the test taker must determine the most likely diagnosis. Questions of this nature require analytical reasoning skill, as various symptoms are analyzed in order to draw a reasonable conclusion about the corresponding diagnosis. In this case, the symptoms are indicative of a venous ulcer. If this question was answered incorrectly, review signs and symptoms of venous ulcers.

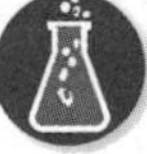

A45 | Integumentary | Evaluation, Diagnosis, Prognosis

A elderly and frail resident of an extended care facility presents with hot, red, and edematous skin over the shins of both lower extremities. The patient also has a mild fever. The **MOST** likely cause of the symptoms is:

CHOICES:

1. Dermatitis.
2. Cellulitis.
3. Herpes simplex infection.
4. Scleroderma.

TEACHING POINTS

CORRECT ANSWER: 2

Cellulitis is an inflammation of the cellular or connective tissue in or close to the skin. It is characterized by skin that is hot, red, and edematous. Fever is a common finding.

INCORRECT CHOICES:

Dermatitis produces red, weeping, crusted skin lesions, but is not commonly accompanied by fever. Location on shins makes herpes an unlikely choice, and there are no skin eruptions or vesicles. Scleroderma is a collagen disease producing tight, drawn skin.

TYPE OF REASONING: ANALYSIS

One must determine the cause of the symptoms in this type of question. This requires the test taker to recall properties of infection and diagnoses that do or do not support the symptoms described. If this question was answered incorrectly, review information on infection, inflammation, and cellulitis.

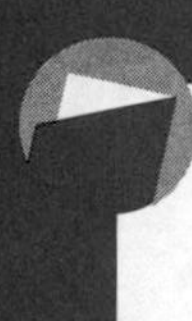

A46 | Devices, Admin., etc. | Equipment, Modalities

A 10 year-old presents with pain (4/10) and limited knee ROM (5–95 degrees) following surgical repair of the medial collateral ligament and ACLs. In this case, the modality that can be used with **PRECAUTION** is:

CHOICES:

1. Premodulated interferential current.
2. Continuous shortwave diathermy.
3. High-rate transcutaneous electrical stimulation.
4. Low-dose US.

TEACHING POINTS

CORRECT ANSWER: 4

Because the epiphyseal plates do not close until the end of puberty, US energy should be applied with caution around the epiphyseal area due to its potential to cause bone growth disturbances. However, there is no documented evidence that US creates any direct untoward effects on the growth plates, especially if applied at low dosage.

INCORRECT CHOICES:

Electrical stimulation or deep thermotherapy would have no deleterious effects on the epiphyseal plates, because no mechanical effects on hard tissue are associated with their use.

TYPE OF REASONING: INFERENCE

In this scenario, the test taker must understand the properties of all the electrical modalities listed, but most importantly recognize that the key to answering the question correctly is the age of the patient. The age of the patient should be the primary consideration when choosing the correct modality. If this question was answered incorrectly, refer to indications, contraindications, and precautions guidelines of electrical modalities.

A47 | Musculoskeletal | Foundational Sciences

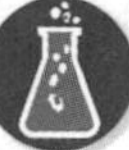

A weight lifter exhibits marked hypertrophy after embarking on a strength training regime. Hypertrophy can be expected to occur following at least:

CHOICES:

1. 1–2 weeks of training.
2. 3–4 weeks of training.
3. 2–3 weeks of training.
4. 6–8 weeks of training.

TEACHING POINTS

CORRECT ANSWER: 4

Hypertrophy is the increase in muscle size as a result of resistance training, and can be observed following at least 6–8 weeks of training. Individual muscle fibers are enlarged, contain more actin and myosin, and have more, larger myofibrils.

INCORRECT CHOICES:

The other choices are too brief a time interval to show demonstrable changes. Some strengthening can occur, but no obvious hypertrophy.

TYPE OF REASONING: ANALYSIS

This question requires knowledge of resistance training and muscle properties in order to answer the question correctly. The test taker uses analysis skills, using knowledge of muscle-building properties to arrive at the correct conclusion.

A48 | Musculoskeletal | Foundational Sciences 

A diagnosis of bicipital tendinitis has been made following an evaluation of a patient with shoulder pain. The **BEST** shoulder position to expose the tendon of the long head of the biceps for application of phonophoresis would be:

CHOICES:

1. Lateral rotation and extension.
2. Medial rotation and abduction.
3. Horizontal adduction.
4. Abduction.

TEACHING POINTS

CORRECT ANSWER: 1

The long head of the biceps is best exposed in shoulder lateral rotation and extension, due to its attachment at the supraglenoid tubercle of the scapula, which is at the medial aspect of the shoulder joint.

INCORRECT CHOICES:

Medial rotation and abduction places the long head of the biceps deep to the anterior deltoid and pectoralis major muscles. The anterior surface of the shoulder, including the long head of the biceps, loses exposure with horizontal adduction.

TYPE OF REASONING: ANALYSIS

This question requires sound knowledge of musculoskeletal anatomy of the shoulder in order to choose the correct answer. One must consider how the position of the shoulder is key to effectively exposing the long head of the biceps, which can be done only through solid knowledge of shoulder anatomy. Some test takers may find it helpful to use mental imagery to picture what happens to the biceps tendon when each of the shoulder positions is assumed.

A49 | Neuromuscular | Intervention 

A patient is unable to bring a foot up on the next step during a training session on stair climbing. The PT's **BEST** course of action to promote learning of this task is to have the patient practice:

CHOICES:

1. Marching in place in the parallel bars.
2. Standing up from half-kneeling.
3. Step-ups onto a low step while in the parallel bars.
4. Balance on the stairs while the therapist passively brings the foot up.

TEACHING POINTS

CORRECT ANSWER: 3

Active task-specific practice of stepping using a low step represents the best choice to ensure motor learning.

INCORRECT CHOICES:

Passively bringing the foot up does not promote active learning. Marching in place and balance on stairs are appropriate lead-up skills to stair climbing, but are not task-specific practice.

TYPE OF REASONING: INFERENCE

In this question, the test taker must consider what choices seem most relevant and most likely to result in future motor performance during stair negotiation. The test taker must ask what seems most likely to result in motor improvement and act as a bridge between where the patient is now and where he/she needs to go to successfully negotiate stairs.

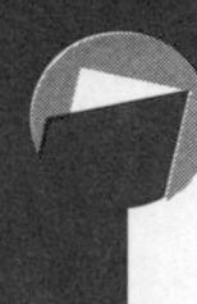

A50 | Integumentary | Foundational Sciences

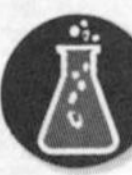

A patient is transferred to a burn clinic with deep, partial-thickness burns over 30% of the body. Healing of this type of burn is characterized by:

CHOICES:

1. Blisters and minimal edema with spontaneous healing.
2. Depressed skin area that heals with grafting and scarring.
3. Moderate edema with spontaneous healing and minimal grafting.
4. Marked edema with slow healing and extensive hypertrophic scarring.

TEACHING POINTS

CORRECT ANSWER: 4

Deep partial-thickness burns involve destruction of the epidermis, with damage of the dermis down into the reticular area. Appearance is mixed red/white color with sluggish capillary refill. Superficial sensation is decreased, while sense of deep pressure is retained. The burn will heal spontaneously in 3–5 weeks if no infection develops (infection can convert the burn to full-thickness). There is marked edema with excessive scarring (hypertrophic).

INCORRECT CHOICES:

Superficial burns heal with minimal edema, whereas superficial partial-thickness burns heal spontaneously with moderate edema and minimal scarring; they do not require grafting. Full-thickness burns require skin grafting; appearance is depressed with significant scarring.

TYPE OF REASONING: ANALYSIS

In this question, the test taker must understand the nature of partial-thickness burns in order to arrive at the correct conclusion. This requires one to analyze the precise meaning of the four choices and determine which answer is most aligned with the characteristics of partial-thickness burns. If this question was answered incorrectly, review information on partial-thickness burns and recovery.

A51 | Devices, Admin., etc. | Equipment, Modalities

A patient with a complete SCI at the T6 level is being discharged home after 2 months of rehabilitation. In preparation for discharge, the rehabilitation team visits the home and finds three standard-height steps going into his home. A ramp will have to be constructed for wheelchair access. The recommended length of his ramp should be:

CHOICES:

1. 60 inches (5 feet).
2. 192 inches (16 feet).
3. 252 inches (21 feet).
4. 120 inches (10 feet).

TEACHING POINTS

CORRECT ANSWER: 3

The architectural standard for rise of a step is 7 inches (steps may vary from 7–9 inches). The recommended ratio of slope to rise is 1:12 (an 8% grade). For every inch of vertical rise, 12 inches of ramp will be required. A straight ramp will have to be 252 inches, or 21 feet, long.

INCORRECT CHOICES:

The other choices do not adequately account for the 1:12 ratio (8% grade).

TYPE OF REASONING: DEDUCTIVE

In this question, one must understand two factors: the architectural standard for rise of a step and guidelines that indicate proper ratio of slope to rise. To arrive at a correct conclusion, one must deduce that the standard rise is 7 inches and the proper ratio is 12 inches of elevation for every 1 inch of rise; therefore, the ramp should be 21 feet. If this question was answered incorrectly, review architectural guidelines for homes.

A52 | Other Systems | Foundational Sciences

A high school wrestler has been taking anabolic-androgenic steroids for the past 6 months to build muscle and improve performance. The PT working with the team suspects illegal drug use and examines the athlete for:

CHOICES:

1. Hypotension, edema, rapid muscular enlargement.
2. Rapid weight loss with disproportionate muscular enlargement.
3. Changes in personality, including passivity and anxiety.
4. Rapid weight gain, marked muscular hypertrophy, mood swings.

TEACHING POINTS

CORRECT ANSWER: 4

Signs and symptoms of anabolic steroid use include rapid weight gain, elevated BP, acne on the face and upper back, changes in body composition with marked muscular hypertrophy, especially in the upper body. Additional signs include frequent bruising, needle marks, male breast enlargement, or in females, secondary male characteristics and menstrual irregularities. With prolonged use, jaundice or changes in personality (mood swings, rages) may develop.

INCORRECT CHOICES:

The other choices are not characteristic of anabolic steroid use.

TYPE OF REASONING: INFERENCE

This question requires the test taker to infer the likely symptoms athletes will exhibit with anabolic steroid use. This requires inferential reasoning skill. In this scenario, the athletes are most likely to demonstrate rapid weight gain, marked muscular hypertrophy, mood swings. If this question was answered incorrectly, review signs and symptoms of anabolic steroid use.

A53 | Cardiovascular-Pulmonary | Evaluation, Diagnosis, Prognosis

A patient with diagnosis of left-sided heart failure (CHF), class II, is referred for physical therapy. During exercise, this patient can be expected to demonstrate:

CHOICES:

1. Severe, uncomfortable chest pain with shortness of breath.
2. Weight gain with dependent edema.
3. Anorexia, nausea with abdominal pain, and distention.
4. Dyspnea with fatigue and muscular weakness.

TEACHING POINTS

CORRECT ANSWER: 4

Left-sided heart failure is the result of the left ventricle failing to pump enough blood through the arterial system to meet the body's demands. It produces pulmonary edema and disturbed respiratory control mechanisms. Patients can be expected to demonstrate progressive dyspnea (exertional at first, then paroxysmal nocturnal dyspnea), fatigue and muscular weakness, pulmonary edema, cerebral hypoxia, and renal changes.

INCORRECT CHOICES:

Severe chest pain and shortness of breath are symptoms of impending myocardial infarction (MI). The other choices describe symptoms associated with right-sided ventricular failure.

TYPE OF REASONING: INFERENCE

In this question, the test taker must understand the difference between left-sided and right-sided CHF, as well as cardiac physiology. Understanding that left-sided failure results in a backup of blood into the lungs helps one to arrive at the correct conclusion of dyspnea, fatigue, and muscular weakness. If this question was answered incorrectly, review information of cardiac physiology and CHF.

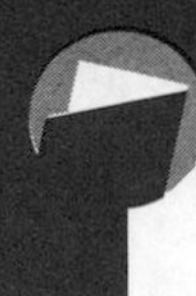

A54 | Musculoskeletal | Intervention

A PT is instructing a student in proper positioning to prevent the typical contractures in the patient with a transfemoral amputation. The therapist stresses positioning the patient in:

CHOICES:

1. Prone-lying with the residual limb in neutral rotation.
2. A wheelchair with a gel cushion and adductor roll.
3. Supine-lying with the residual limb resting on a small pillow.
4. Side-lying on the residual limb.

TEACHING POINTS

CORRECT ANSWER: 1

The typical contractures with a transfemoral amputation are hip flexion (typically from too much sitting in a wheelchair). The residual limb also rolls out into abduction and external rotation. When in bed, hip extension should be emphasized (e.g., prone-lying). When sitting in the wheelchair, neutral hip rotation should be emphasized (e.g., using an abductor roll). Time in extension (prone, supine, or standing) should counterbalance time sitting in a wheelchair.

INCORRECT CHOICES:

Resting in supine with the residual limb resting on a small pillow in a position of hip flexion is contraindicated, as is an adductor roll in wheelchair sitting. Side-lying on the residual limb has no benefit for this patient, and may also position the hip in flexion.

TYPE OF REASONING: INFERENCE

To arrive at a correct conclusion, one must understand the typical contractures associated with a transfemoral amputation. The test taker must infer or draw conclusions about what may occur in the future if the four possible choices are applied. Those who understand that hip flexion, abduction, and external rotation are typical contracture patterns will see that prone lying with the limb in neutral rotation is the only position that discourages the formation of contractures.

A55 | Other Systems | Evaluation, Diagnosis, Prognosis

A PT receives a referral to ambulate a patient who is insulin-dependent. In a review of the patient's medical record, the therapist notices that the blood glucose level for that day is 310 mg/dL. The therapist's **BEST** course of action is to:

CHOICES:

1. Refrain from ambulating the patient; reschedule for tomorrow before other therapies.
2. Ambulate the patient as planned, but monitor closely for signs of exertional intolerance.
3. Postpone therapy and consult with the medical staff as soon as possible.
4. Talk to the nurse about walking the patient later that day after lunch.

TEACHING POINTS

CORRECT ANSWER: 3

Normal fasting plasma glucose is less than 115 mg/dL, while a fasting plasma glucose level greater than 126 mg/dL on more than one occasion is indicative of diabetes. This patient is hyperglycemic with high glucose levels (≥250 mg/dL). Clinical signs that may accompany this condition include ketoacidosis (acetone breath) with dehydration, weak and rapid pulse, nausea/vomiting, deep and rapid respirations (Kussmaul's respirations), weakness, diminished reflexes, and paresthesias. The patient may be lethargic and confused, and may progress to diabetic coma and death if not treated promptly with insulin. Physical therapy intervention is contraindicated; exercise can lead to further impaired glucose uptake. Coordination with the medical staff is crucial, so that the patient's blood glucose levels can be appropriately managed.

INCORRECT CHOICES:

Ambulation is contraindicated. Postponing consultation with the medical staff is potentially dangerous for the patient.

TYPE OF REASONING: EVALUATION

In this scenario, the test taker must recognize the significance of a blood glucose level of 310 mg/dL as being abnormally high and warranting follow-up by nursing personnel. The test taker should also understand what the consequences are of conducting therapy with elevated glucose levels and risk to the patient. Evaluation skills are used because one relies on the knowledge of hyperglycemia to determine what could happen to the patient and, therefore, why therapy must be postponed.

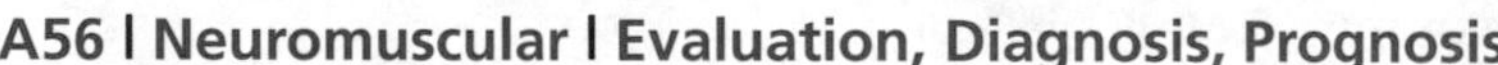

A56 | Neuromuscular | Evaluation, Diagnosis, Prognosis

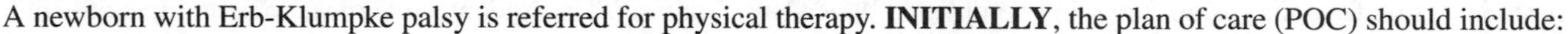

A newborn with Erb-Klumpke palsy is referred for physical therapy. **INITIALLY**, the plan of care (POC) should include:

CHOICES:

1. Partial immobilization of the limb across the abdomen, followed by gentle ROM after immobilization.
2. Passive mobilization of the shoulder in overhead motions.
3. Age-appropriate task training of the upper extremity.
4. Splinting the shoulder in abduction and internal rotation.

TEACHING POINTS

CORRECT ANSWER: 1

Erb's palsy is a paralysis of the upper limb that typically results from a traction injury at birth, causing a brachial plexus injury. Variations include Erb-Duchenne (affecting C5–6 roots), whole arm palsy (affecting C5–T1 roots), and Erb-Klumpke (affecting the lower plexus nerve roots, C8 and T1). Partial immobilization of the limb across the abdomen followed by gentle ROM is the best choice for intial intervention.

INCORRECT CHOICES:

Mobilization in overhead motions is contraindicated. Splinting the shoulder in abduction leads to formation of abduction contractures and later hypermobility of the shoulder. Age-appropriate task training can follow after the initial treatment.

TYPE OF REASONING: EVALUATION

One must understand two factors before arriving at a correct conclusion: the nature of contracture with Erb-Klumpke palsy and the anatomy of the brachial plexus. The test taker who realizes that this condition affects the lower plexus nerve roots understands that splinting in abduction and internal rotation leads to hypermobility and abduction contracture. If this question was answered incorrectly, review brachial plexus injuries in children.

A57 | Musculoskeletal | Intervention

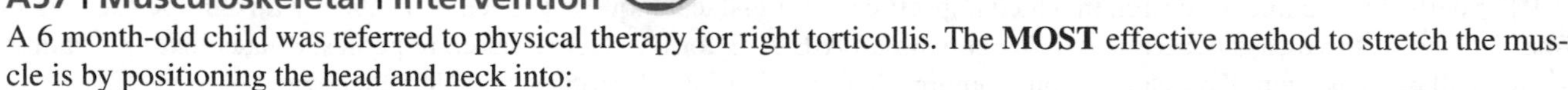

A 6 month-old child was referred to physical therapy for right torticollis. The **MOST** effective method to stretch the muscle is by positioning the head and neck into:

CHOICES:

1. Flexion, left side-bending, and left rotation.
2. Extension, right side-bending, and left rotation.
3. Flexion, right side-bending, and left rotation.
4. Extension, left side-bending, and right rotation.

TEACHING POINTS

CORRECT ANSWER: 4

The right sternocleidomastoid produces left lateral rotation and flexion of the cervical spine. The right sternocleidomastoid is in lengthened position with the head turned to the right and the cervical spine extended.

INCORRECT CHOICES:

The other positions do not effectively stretch the right sternocleidomastoid muscle. Right side-bending and left rotation stretches the left sternocleidomastoid muscle.

TYPE OF REASONING: ANALYSIS

In this question, the test taker must understand the expected symptomatology associated with torticollis, as well as musculoskeletal anatomy of the cervical spine. To arrive at a correct conclusion, one must recall the muscle actions of key musculature affected by right torticollis, as well as which direction of stretch will improve the symptoms.

EXAM A

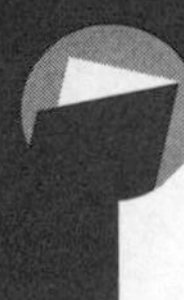

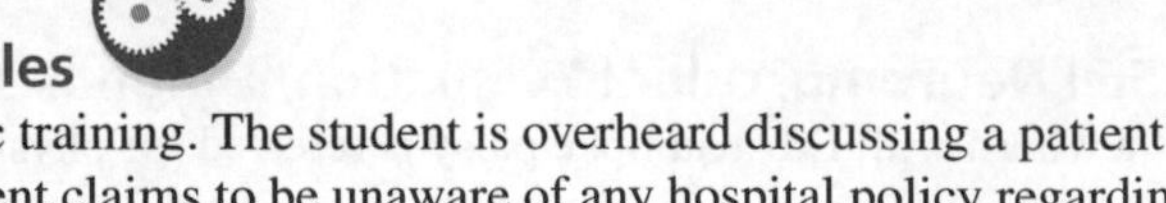

A58 | Devices, Admin., etc. | Teaching, Research, Roles

A student is on final internship following completion of academic training. The student is overheard discussing a patient's history in the elevator. When the PT later points this out, the student claims to be unaware of any hospital policy regarding confidentiality. The therapist's **BEST** analysis of this situation is that:

CHOICES:

1. The student should be expected to value patient confidentiality.
2. Compliance was not a realistic expectation, because the student had recently arrived at this facility.
3. Now that the student is aware of confidentiality restrictions, compliance is expected.
4. Because this is not strictly part of the professional code of ethics, the student should not be expected to demonstrate adherence to this concept.

TEACHING POINTS

CORRECT ANSWER: 1

Valuing and upholding patient confidentiality is an expected behavior for all PTs and physical therapy students, as specified by the American Physical Therapy Association (APTA) Code of Ethics and Health Insurance and Portability Accountability Act (HIPAA) regulations. Because this a final internship, the student should be expected to adhere fully to the APTA's Code of Ethics.

INCORRECT CHOICES:

Ignorance of the APTA's Code of Ethics is no excuse for failure to comply with ethical expectations as well as HIPAA regulations.

TYPE OF REASONING: EVALUATION

The test taker must evaluate the inherent truth in each statement and the ethical duty of a physical therapy student in order to arrive at a correct conclusion. Because all students must adhere to the APTA's Code of Ethics, compliance is realistic and expected in this situation. If this question is answered incorrectly, review the Code of Ethics and HIPAA guidelines on confidentiality.

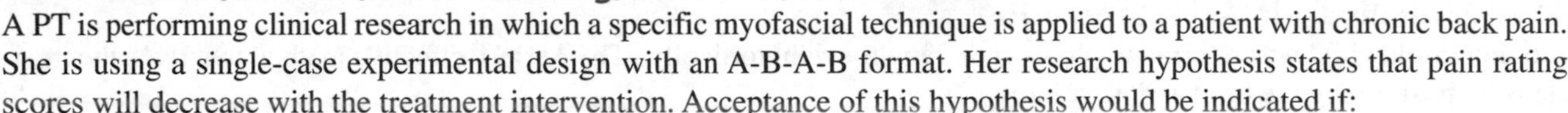

A59 | Devices, Admin., etc. | Teaching, Research, Roles

A PT is performing clinical research in which a specific myofascial technique is applied to a patient with chronic back pain. She is using a single-case experimental design with an A-B-A-B format. Her research hypothesis states that pain rating scores will decrease with the treatment intervention. Acceptance of this hypothesis would be indicated if:

CHOICES:

1. B is equal to A.
2. B is greater than A, at the 1.0 level.
3. B is less than A.
4. B is greater than A, at the 0.05 level.

TEACHING POINTS

CORRECT ANSWER: 3

In an A-B-A-B single-subject design, represents multiple baseline measurements, and represents multiple posttreatment measurements. If the hypothesis is accepted, the pain-rating scores will be lower following treatment compared with the baseline measurements.

INCORRECT CHOICES:

Any choice in which B is equal to or greater than A is incorrect. That would indicate that there was no change in pain or that it increased after treatment.

TYPE OF REASONING: DEDUCTIVE

The test taker must recall the properties of single-subject experimental designs and when to appropriately reject the null hypothesis in order to draw a correct conclusion. Because one is hypothesizing that a given treatment will result in lower pain scores, B must be lower than A to arrive at this conclusion. Questions related to research often require deductive reasoning, because research operates by principles and guidelines, thereby using these guidelines to draw conclusions.

A60 | Neuromuscular | Intervention

A patient is recovering from stroke and demonstrates good recovery in his lower extremity (out-of-synergy movement control). Timing deficits are apparent during walking. Isokinetic training can be used to improve:

CHOICES:

1. Rate control at slow movement speeds.
2. Rate control at varying movement speeds.
3. Reaction time.
4. Initiation of movement.

TEACHING POINTS

CORRECT ANSWER: 2

Patients during recovery from stroke frequently exhibit problems with rate control during walking. They are able to move at slow speeds, but as speed of movement increases, control decreases. An isokinetic device can be an effective training modality to remediate this problem.

INCORRECT CHOICES:

Both initiation of movement and reaction time may be impaired, but are not the likely cause of timing deficits during speed changes while walking.

TYPE OF REASONING: INFERENCE

In this question, the test taker must draw conclusions about the benefits of isokinetic training in later stages of stroke recovery. Also, the test taker must understand the challenges that are often present in rate control with gait speed. If this question was answered incorrectly, review information on gait in stroke recovery and isokinetic training.

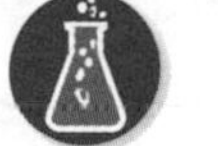

A61 | Musculoskeletal | Intervention

An elderly patient with a transfemoral amputation is having difficulty wrapping the residual limb. The PT's **BEST** course of action is to:

CHOICES:

1. Use a shrinker.
2. Redouble efforts to teach proper Ace bandage wrapping.
3. Apply a temporary prosthesis immediately.
4. Consult with the vascular surgeon about the application of an Unna's paste dressing.

TEACHING POINTS

CORRECT ANSWER: 1

A shrinker is a suitable alternative to elastic wraps. It is important to select the right size shrinker to limit edema and accelerate healing.

INCORRECT CHOICES:

An Unna's paste dressing is applied at the time of initial surgery. Use of a temporary prosthesis should be a prosthetic team decision and is based on additional factors such as age, balance, strength, cognition, and so forth. Continuing to teach elastic bandage wrapping may be inefficient and ultimately fruitless, since the patient is elderly.

TYPE OF REASONING: ANALYSIS

To answer the question correctly, one must analyze the benefits of each approach to remediating the impairment. Because shrinkers are a suitable alternative to elastic wrapping, it is the superior choice. The other possible solutions are not appropriate for the patient at his/her age and stage of recovery, nor are they appropriate to initiate without consultation with the prosthetic team.

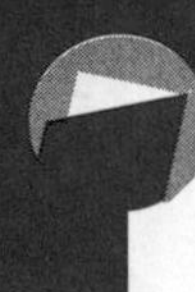

A62 | Cardiovascular-Pulmonary | Intervention

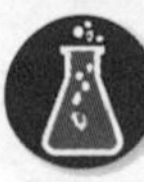

A patient with peripheral vascular disease has been referred for conditioning exercise. The patient demonstrates moderate claudication pain in both legs following a 12-minute walking test. The **MOST** beneficial exercise frequency and duration for this patient is:

CHOICES:

1. 3 times/week, 30 minutes/session.
2. 3 times/week, 60 minutes/session.
3. 2 times/week, BID 20 minutes/session.
4. 5 times/week, BID 10 minutes/session.

TEACHING POINTS

CORRECT ANSWER: 4

Patients with vascular insufficiency and claudication pain should be encouraged to walk daily, 2 to 3 times/day. Duration should be short. The patient should walk to the point of maximum tolerable pain, and be allowed to rest.

INCORRECT CHOICES:

High intensity exercise (30- or 60-minute sessions, 3/week) is contraindicated. Twice-a-week sessions are too infrequent to be beneficial.

TYPE OF REASONING: ANALYSIS

In order to arrive at the correct conclusion, the test taker needs to understand the nature of vascular insufficiency and claudication pain. One must analyze which frequency and duration will not exacerbate the patient's pain, but still provide conditioning exercise. Short, frequent walking intervals to the point of maximum tolerable pain are ideal, and 10-minute sessions provide for this.

A63 | Musculoskeletal | Evaluation, Diagnosis, Prognosis

The radiographic view shown in the diagram that demonstrates the observed spinal defect is:

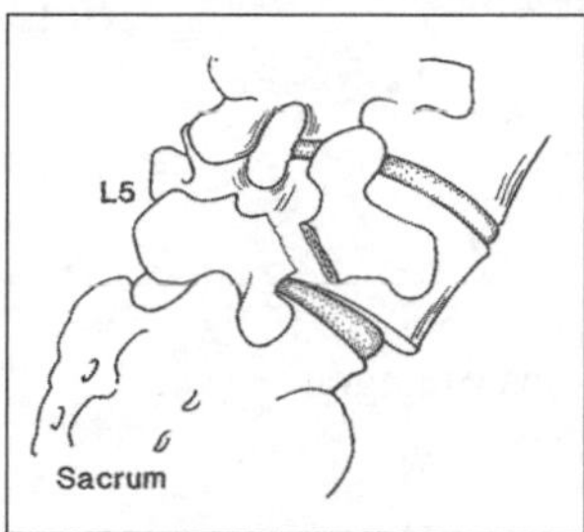

Twomey L, Taylor J (2000) Physical Therapy of the Low Back, 3rd ed. Philadelphia, Churchill Livingstone, Figure 7-1, page 204, with permission.

CHOICES:

1. Lateral.
2. Frontal.
3. Oblique.
4. Posterolateral.

TEACHING POINTS

CORRECT ANSWER: 3

The spinal defect is spondylolisthesis, and the radiographic view that demonstrates the Scotty dog neck fracture is the oblique view.

INCORRECT CHOICES:

A lateral radiographic view will show the degree of anterior or posterior slippage of one vertebra on another, allowing the radiologist to grade the spondylolisthesis. The other choices do not optimally show the defect.

TYPE OF REASONING: EVALUATION

One must rely upon knowledge of the defect displayed on the x-ray, as well as knowledge of which radiographic view will provide the best visualization of this condition. The Scotty dog–shaped fracture is characteristic of spondylolisthesis, which can most ideally be viewed from an oblique view/angle. Knowledge of these two factors helps the test-taker draw the correct conclusion.

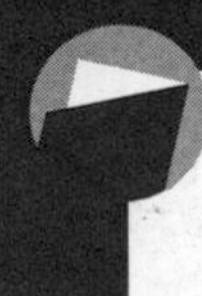

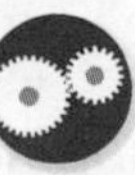

A64 | Other Systems | Evaluation, Diagnosis, Prognosis

A PT is working with a patient with metastatic breast cancer who has been told that she has only months to live. She is quite angry and disruptive during therapy. The PT recognizes that the **MOST** beneficial interaction is:

CHOICES:

1. Forbid all expressions of anger because she is only hurting herself.
2. Provide honest, accurate information about her illness and rehabilitation POC.
3. Allow the patient to express her anger, while refocusing her on effective coping strategies.
4. Provide opportunities for the patient to question her impending death, but limit all expressions of anger.

TEACHING POINTS

CORRECT ANSWER: 3

Anger is a recognized stage in the psychological adaptation to death and dying (Kübler-Ross). Patients should be allowed to express anger, frustration, and resentment. A helpful strategy is to redirect the patient to achieve effective coping strategies (anger management techniques).

INCORRECT CHOICES:

Limiting expressions of anger may only inflame the situation. Whereas honest, accurate information is important, it is not the most useful strategy for this patient at this time.

TYPE OF REASONING: EVALUATION

This type of question requires judgment of a difficult circumstance. The test taker must determine whether anger is a normal expression of what the patient is coping with, and whether the therapist should allow the anger to continue. Understanding the Kübler-Ross stages of grief helps the test taker realize that anger is a normal grief response, and the therapist should help the patient cope effectively with her feelings. If this question was answered incorrectly, review the stages of adjustment to disability, death and dying.

A65 | Musculoskeletal | Evaluation, Diagnosis, Prognosis

While driving the ball during a golf match, a patient felt an immediate sharp pain in the right lower back. The following morning, the patient reported stiffness, with easing of pain after taking a shower. Based on this information, the source of the pain is **MOST** likely:

CHOICES:

1. Nerve root compression.
2. Facet joint impingement.
3. A stress fracture.
4. Diminished blood supply to the spinal cord.

TEACHING POINTS

CORRECT ANSWER: 2

Facet joint dysfunction is exacerbated with sustained positions, and eases with movement. Progressive increase in activity intensifies the pain.

INCORRECT CHOICES:

Stress fracture pain is worse when weight-bearing, and is not necessarily worse in the morning. Nerve root involvement would cause radiating pain to the extremity. The spinal cord has no innervation and is not a source of pain.

TYPE OF REASONING: INFERENCE

The test taker must draw a conclusion for the basis of the patient's symptomatology. A solid understanding of spinal disorders helps one draw the correct conclusion, realizing that the pattern of pain is indicative only of facet joint impingement and not the other conditions. If this question was answered incorrectly, review information on sports medicine and spinal injuries.

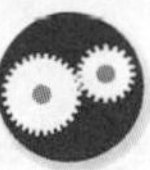

A66 | Devices, Admin., etc. | Teaching, Research, Roles

At 10 a.m., a PT working on an inpatient spinal cord unit is treating a patient with paraplegia. The therapist smells alcohol on the patient's breath. The patient is having difficulty accomplishing a bed-to-chair transfer that was previously done without assistance. In this case, the therapist should:

CHOICES:

1. Confront the patient and ask if alcohol has been consumed.
2. Document and report suspicions of alcoholism to the rehabilitation team at the weekly meeting.
3. Question the patient's family about any history of alcoholism.
4. Document the findings and immediately inform the patient's physician and nurse in charge.

TEACHING POINTS

CORRECT ANSWER: 4

The best response is to discuss a patient problem with the person who is ultimately responsible for the patient. The physician as team leader can effect a change in behavior or seek additional help for the patient. The nurse in charge must also be informed to ensure the safety of the patient.

INCORRECT CHOICES:

Confronting the patient or delaying reporting by asking the family or waiting for a team meeting does not successfully resolve this situation in a timely manner, and may prove harmful to the patient.

TYPE OF REASONING: EVALUATION

This judgment question requires one to determine what will not only address the situation at hand, but also protect the patient from future harm. The test taker must choose the answer that addresses the situation immediately and involves the professionals who hold ultimate responsibility for the patient. Evaluation questions are challenging, in that one must evaluate the merits of each statement and conclude what will result in the best possible outcome.

A67 | Neuromuscular | Intervention

A patient with right hemiparesis has difficulty clearing the more affected foot during the swing phase of gait. An appropriate physical therapy intervention for the right lower extremity might include:

CHOICES:

1. Sitting on a therapy ball, alternating lateral side steps and back to neutral.
2. Pushing backward while sitting on a rolling stool.
3. Forward step-ups in standing, using graduated height steps.
4. Assumption of bridging.

TEACHING POINTS

CORRECT ANSWER: 3

Decreased foot clearance during swing may result from weak hip and knee flexors or from a drop foot (weak dorsiflexors or spastic plantarflexors). Step-ups represent the best choice to functionally strengthen the hip and knee flexors using task-specific training.

INCORRECT CHOICES:

Bridging promotes knee flexion with hip extension. The sitting activities promote hip abduction (therapy ball) and knee extension (pushing backward).

TYPE OF REASONING: INFERENCE

In this question, one must infer which intervention will result in improvement in symptomatology. The test taker must realize that the symptoms presented may be the result of weak hip and knee flexors or drop foot. Regardless, forward step-ups in standing address both of these possibilities.

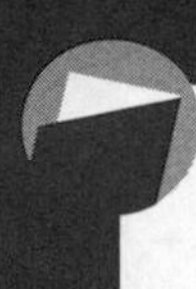

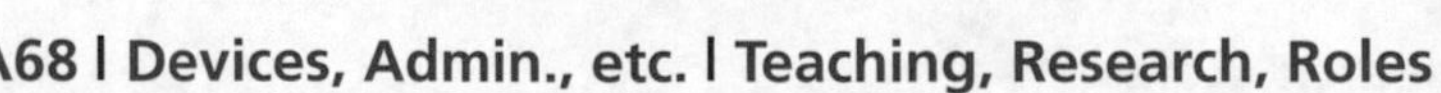

A68 | Devices, Admin., etc. | Teaching, Research, Roles

A researcher reviewed current literature related to moderate exercise for maintaining independence without accelerating disease progression in persons with amyotrophic lateral sclerosis (ALS). The search yielded nine studies: two clinical case reports, two cohort studies, three single randomized controlled trials (RCTs), and two multicenter RCTs. According to levels of evidence (Sackett), which studies provide the best evidence for support of exercise in persons with ALS?

CHOICES:

1. Multicenter RCTs.
2. Cohort/comparison studies.
3. Single-center RCTs.
4. Case series without controls.

TEACHING POINTS

CORRECT ANSWER: 1

According to Sackett's Levels of Evidence, multicenter RCTs (level I RCT) provide the best evidence.

INCORRECT CHOICES:

Level II studies (single randomized clinical trials), are followed by level III (nonrandomized cohort/comparison studies). Level IV includes nonrandomized case control studies, whereas level V includes case series or case reports without controls.

TYPE OF REASONING: DEDUCTIVE

This question requires factual recall of research guidelines, which necessitates deductive reasoning skill. In this question, one must recall that the research studies with the best evidence are the multicenter RCTs. If this question was answered incorrectly, review Sackett's Levels of Evidence, especially RCTs.

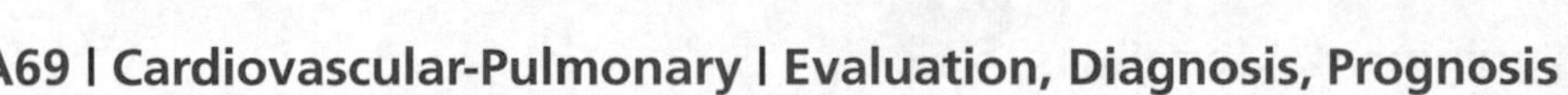

A69 | Cardiovascular-Pulmonary | Evaluation, Diagnosis, Prognosis

A patient is 4 weeks post-MI. Resistive training using weights to improve muscular strength and endurance is appropriate:

CHOICES:

1. If exercise intensities are kept below 85% maximal voluntary contraction.
2. If exercise capacity is greater than 5 METs with no anginal symptoms/ST segment depression.
3. During all phases of rehabilitation, if judicious monitoring of heart rate is used.
4. Only during post–acute phase 3 cardiac rehabilitation.

TEACHING POINTS

CORRECT ANSWER: 2

Resistance training is typically initiated after patients have completed 4–6 weeks of supervised cardiorespiratory endurance exercise. Lower intensities are prescribed. Careful monitoring of BP is necessary, because BP will be higher and HR lower than for aerobic exercise. Patients should demonstrate an exercise capacity greater than 5 METs (metabolic equivalents) without anginal symptoms or ST segment depression. (Source: American College of Sports Medicine: *Guidelines for Exercise Testing and Prescription*, 6th ed.)

INCORRECT CHOICES:

The common use of a percentage of 1 RM (repetition maximum) estimates intensity, and should be used only as a general guideline. Intensity should be assessed using perceived intensity. Exercise should be terminated at a rate of perceived exertion (RPE; Borg Scale 6—20) of 15 to 16. During resistance training, HR response is disproportionate to oxygen consumption and should not be used as a measure of intensity. Resistance training is not restricted to phase 3 programs, as long as proper guidelines are followed.

TYPE OF REASONING: EVALUATION

The test taker must understand the different phases of cardiac rehabilitation and typical guidelines utilized in the recovery process. Also, one must understand MET level activity and impact on cardiac status. This question requires the test-taker's judgment, coupled with knowledge of cardiac rehabilitation guidelines, to arrive at the correct conclusion.

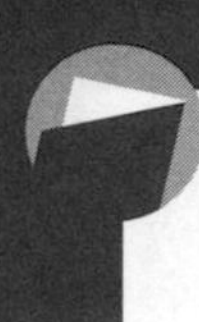

A70 | Devices, Admin., etc. | Equipment, Modalities

A patient diagnosed with lumbar spinal root impingement due to narrowing of the intervertebral foramen has been referred to physical therapy for mechanical traction. What is the lowest percentage of body weight that should be considered for the initial traction force when using a split table?

CHOICES:

1. 15%.
2. 25%.
3. 55%.
4. 85%.

TEACHING POINTS

CORRECT ANSWER: 2

In order to overcome the coefficient of friction of the body moving horizontally over the surface of a table, the traction force should be at least 25% of the body weight when using a split table, or 50% when using a nonsplit table. To achieve joint distraction, a force of 50% body weight is recommended. However, because it is the *initial* traction, a minimum of 25% for the first treatment is recommended to determine patient response. This would provide sufficient force to decrease muscle spasm and stretch the soft tissue, thereby decreasing the compressive force on the spine and allowing for greater ease of joint separation as the force is progressed.

INCORRECT CHOICES:

Forces above 50% are generally not recommended for the lumbar spine.

TYPE OF REASONING: DEDUCTIVE

One must deduce that if the patient is receiving initial mechanical contraction and the guidelines indicate a minimum of 25% body weight, 25% is the only logical conclusion. If this question was answered incorrectly, review mechanical traction guidelines.

A71 | Other Systems | Intervention

A fitness instructor who is 8 months pregnant was recently diagnosed with placenta previa. The PT's most important instructions to her are to continue:

CHOICES:

1. Proper breathing and discontinue pelvic floor exercises.
2. Pelvic floor and discontinue any abdominal exercises.
3. Partial sit-ups and pelvic floor exercises.
4. Abdominal exercises and AROM.

TEACHING POINTS

CORRECT ANSWER: 2

Placenta previa is a condition in which the placenta does not elevate from its original low position (normal in early pregnancy) and assumes a position below the fetus and attached to the lower half of the uterus. It may cover the mouth of the uterus. This is a leading cause of vaginal bleeding and a serious condition that increases morbidity and mortality of both the fetus and the mother. Pelvic floor and breathing exercises are important and should be continued.

INCORRECT CHOICES:

Abdominal exercises can worsen this condition and are contraindicated.

TYPE OF REASONING: INFERENCE

One must infer a couple of issues with this question. First, what is the condition of placenta previa and what may exacerbate the condition? Second, how is the patient's occupation important when recommending modification to her daily routine? The test taker must know the answers to these two questions in order to arrive at a correct conclusion.

A72 | Musculoskeletal | Foundational Sciences

It is important to note the status of the pars interarticularis while reviewing a patient's imaging films. The most appropriate imaging view to identify abnormal anatomy of the pars interarticularis in the lumbar region is:

CHOICES:

1. Anteroposterior view.
2. Lateral view.
3. Oblique view.
4. Lumbosacral view.

TEACHING POINTS

CORRECT ANSWER: 3

For the lumbar region, the oblique view will clearly demonstrate the pars interacrticularis.

INCORRECT CHOICES:

The anteroposterior and lateral views will not demonstrate the pars interarticularis. The lateral view may show anterior displacement of the segment above a pars defect if the condition has progressed to a bilateral displaced fracture of the pars interarticularis (i.e., spondylolisthesis); however, the lateral view will not show the anatomy of the pars interarticularis.

TYPE OF REASONING: INDUCTIVE

One must understand the anatomical nature of a pars interarticularis as a possible indicator of future defects, such as spondylolisthesis or spondylolysis, in order to arrive at the correct conclusion. This requires inductive reasoning as a basis to predict what might happen to this patient based on the findings of the x-ray. If this question was answered incorrectly, review information on imaging of the pars interarticularis.

A73 | Other Systems | Foundational Sciences

A patient with breast cancer had a surgical removal of the mass, followed by 12 weeks of chemotherapy (six treatments) and 8 weeks of radiation therapy (daily). She is referred to physical therapy for mobilization of her upper extremity. The therapist recognizes that in providing postradiation therapy, it is important to:

CHOICES:

1. Observe infection control procedures.
2. Avoid all aerobic exercise for at least 2 months.
3. Avoid stretching exercises that pull on the radiated site.
4. Observe skin care precautions.

TEACHING POINTS

CORRECT ANSWER: 4

Immediate effects of radiation include skin effects (erythema, edema, dryness, itching, hair and fingernail loss, and loose skin). The therapist should observe skin care precautions (avoid topical use of alcohol and drying agents and avoid positioning the patient directly on the radiated area). Exposure to heat modalities is also contraindicated.

INCORRECT CHOICES:

Although postradiation patients are more susceptible to infection due to immunosuppression, there is no evidence of infection in this patient (fever is often the first sign). Stretching exercises are important during and after radiation. Low- to moderate-intensity aerobic exercise is appropriate.

TYPE OF REASONING: INDUCTIVE

This question requires clinical judgment in order to determine the most important procedures and precautions in providing postradiation therapy with a patient. Questions that ask about a best course of action to prevent harm and promote function often require inductive reasoning skill. For this case, the therapist should observe skin care precautions. If this question was answered incorrectly, review therapy guidelines for postradiation patients.

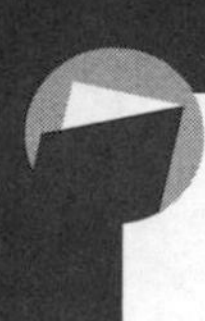

A74 | Neuromuscular | Intervention

A patient with Parkinson's disease (PD) demonstrates a highly stereotyped gait pattern characterized by impoverished movement and a festinating gait. The intervention that would be the **MOST** beneficial to use with this patient is:

CHOICES:

1. Standing and reaching with a body weight support harness.
2. Braiding with light touch-down support of hands.
3. Locomotor training using a rolling walker.
4. Locomotor training using a motorized treadmill and body weight support harness.

TEACHING POINTS

CORRECT ANSWER: 4

The patient with PD typically presents with postural deficits of forward head and trunk, with hip and knee flexion contractures. Gait is narrow-based and shuffling. A festinating gait typically results from persistent forward posturing of the body near the forward limits of stability. Task-specific training using body weight support and treadmill training (BWSTT) is the best choice.

INCORRECT CHOICES:

A rolling walker is contraindicated because it would increase forward postural deformities and festinating gait. Braiding is a complex gait activity that most likely exceeds this patient's abilities. Standing and reaching with body weight support is an important lead-up activity.

TYPE OF REASONING: INFERENCE

Questions such as these are challenging because they are phrased in the manner of most beneficial intervention. One must infer or draw a conclusion as to the most effective method of addressing the impaired gait pattern in order to draw the correct conclusion.

A75 | Neuromuscular | Evaluation, Diagnosis, Prognosis

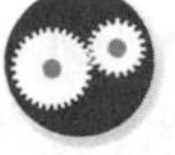

A patient who is recovering from a right CVA reports being thirsty and asks for a can of soda. The PT gives the patient the soda with instructions to open the can. The patient is unable to complete the task. Later, after the treatment session when the patient is alone, the therapist observes the patient drinking from the can, having opened the can on his/her own. The therapist suspects the patient may have a primary deficit in:

CHOICES:

1. Anosognosia.
2. Ideational apraxia.
3. Unilateral neglect.
4. Ideomotor apraxia.

TEACHING POINTS

CORRECT ANSWER: 4

With ideomotor apraxia, a patient cannot perform a task upon command but can do the task when on his/her own.

INCORRECT CHOICES:

With ideational apraxia, a patient cannot perform the task at all. Unilateral neglect might lead the patient to ignore the can completely if positioned on his/her left side. Anosognosia is a more severe form of neglect, with lack of awareness and denial of the severity of one's paralysis.

TYPE OF REASONING: EVALUATION

One must have a firm understanding of the difference between apraxia, neglect, and agnosia in order to arrive at the correct conclusion. Doing so requires one to evaluate the differences between these terms and apply how they fit to the specific circumstances. If this question was answered incorrectly, review the definitions of these terms and other perceptual deficits associated with CVA.

A76 | Other Systems | Patient Examination 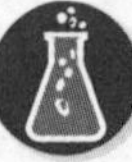

A patient with brittle (uncontrolled) diabetes mellitus is being seen in physical therapy for a prosthetic checkout. The patient begins to experience lethargy, vomiting, and abdominal pain. The therapist notes weakness with some confusion, and suspects:

CHOICES:

1. Ketoacidosis.
2. Respiratory acidosis.
3. Renal acidosis.
4. Llactic acidosis.

TEACHING POINTS

CORRECT ANSWER: 1

An insulin deficiency in a patient with diabetes leads to the release of fatty acids from adipose cells with a production of excess ketones by the liver (diabetic ketoacidosis [DKA]). Signs and symptoms include alterations in GI function (anorexia, nausea and vomiting, abdominal pain), neural function (weakness, lethargy, malaise, confusion, stupor, coma, depression of vital functions), cardiovascular function (peripheral vasodilation, decreased HR, cardiac dysrhythmias), skin (warm and flushed), and increased rate and depth of respiration. The therapist should report these changes immediately; the patient is in need of immediate intravenous insulin, fluid and electrolyte replacement solutions.

INCORRECT CHOICES:

The other choices do not have a similiar pattern of signs and symptoms. Respiratory acidosis is caused by inadequate ventilation and the retention of carbon dioxide. Renal acidosis is the result of kidney failure, with accumulation of phosphoric and sulfuric acids. Lactic acidosis is an accumulation of lactic acid in the blood due to tissue hypoxia, exercise, hyperventilation, or some drugs.

TYPE OF REASONING: ANALYSIS

This question provides a group of signs and symptoms and the test taker must determine the likely diagnosis, which requires analytical reasoning skill. In this situation, the symptoms are most indicative of ketoacidosis. If this question was answered incorrectly, review ketoacidosis signs and symptoms in patients with diabetes.

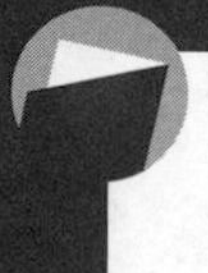

A77 | Cardiovascular-Pulmonary | Patient Examination

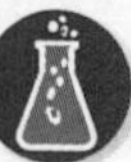

A 62 year-old patient has chronic obstructive pulmonary disease (COPD). Which of these pulmonary test results will be not be increased when compared with those of a 62 year-old healthy individual?

CHOICES:

1. Total lung capacity.
2. FEV_1/FVC (forced vital capacity) ratio.
3. Residual volume.
4. Functional residual capacity.

TEACHING POINTS

CORRECT ANSWER: 2

An obstructive pattern on pulmonary function tests includes increased total lung capacity, caused by destruction of alveolar walls. This same destruction causes an increased residual volume, with a resulting increased functional residual capacity and decreased vital capacity. The GOLD classification (Global Initiative for Obstructive Lung Disease) of an FEV_1/FVC ratio below 70% is indicative of COPD.

INCORRECT CHOICES:

The other choices are all increased with COPD.

TYPE OF REASONING: ANALYSIS

The test taker must understand the physiology and symptomatology of COPD to arrive at a correct conclusion, which is an exception to the expected value. One uses knowledge of physiology of the pulmonary system coupled with expected pulmonary changes in COPD by analyzing the different pulmonary test outcomes. If this question was answered incorrectly, review pulmonary volumes and capacities and COPD symptomatology.

A78 | Devices, Admin., etc. | Equipment, Modalities

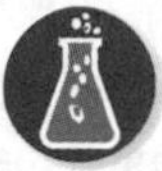

A patient with a transfemoral amputation has been fitted with a prosthesis that utilizes a quadrilateral socket. During prosthetic checkout, the PT should examine pressure tolerance areas of the residual limb with the device off. These include:

CHOICES:

1. Ischial tuberosity and lateral sides of residual limb.
2. Adductor magnus and medial side of residual limb.
3. Distolateral end of femur and ischial seat.
4. Perineal area and medial side of the residual limb.

TEACHING POINTS

CORRECT ANSWER: 1

A quadrilateral socket for a transfemoral amputation is designed to selectively load tissues that are pressure-tolerant. The ischial tuberosity, gluteals, and lateral sides of the residual limb are pressure-tolerant areas.

INCORRECT CHOICES:

The other choices are not pressure-tolerant areas. Reliefs are provided for pressure-sensitive areas (adductor longus tendon, hamstring tendons, sciatic nerve, gluteus maximus, and rectus femoris).

TYPE OF REASONING: ANALYSIS

The test taker must understand the properties of a quadrilateral socket, including typical pressure-tolerant and pressure-sensitive areas. This type of question requires one to analyze the likelihood of each statement to be true given one's knowledge of transfemoral amputation and quadrilateral sockets. If this question was answered incorrectly, review information on transfemoral amputation and design properties of quadrilateral sockets.

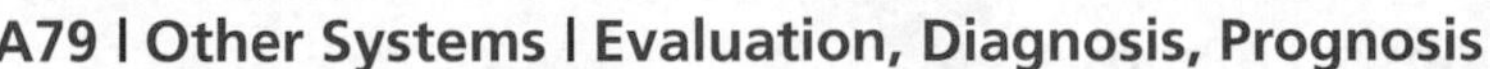
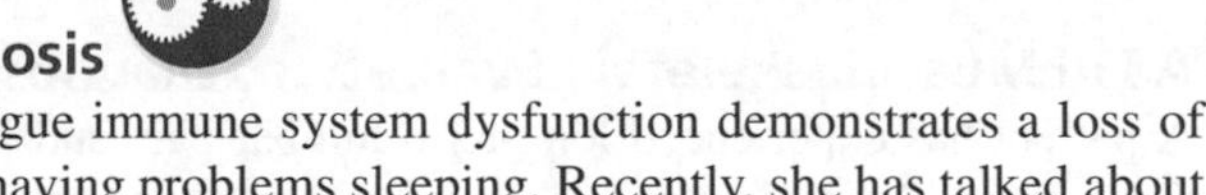

A79 | Other Systems | Evaluation, Diagnosis, Prognosis

A patient recently diagnosed with fibromyalgia and chronic fatigue immune system dysfunction demonstrates a loss of interest in all activities and outlets. She is not eating well and is having problems sleeping. Recently, she has talked about suicide as her only hope. The PT's **BEST** course of action is to:

CHOICES:

1. Present a positive attitude and tell her she will feel better soon.
2. Refer her to a fibromyalgia support group.
3. Refer her to an occupational therapy (OT) intervention group.
4. Immediately contact her primary physician.

TEACHING POINTS

CORRECT ANSWER: 4

This patient is presenting with signs of clinical depression. Her primary physician should be contacted immediately, especially if suicide is mentioned.

INCORRECT CHOICES:

Other choices do not address the need for immediate attention for suicidal tendencies. Do not "pass the buck," relying on OT or support group staff to act in a timely manner.

TYPE OF REASONING: EVALUATION

This judgment question requires consideration of patient safety and which response protects the patient from harm. With any patient who describes suicidal ideation, the PT is required to immediately contact the patient's primary physician, who can provide further instruction/action on what to do. In evaluation questions, one must ask, "What is best for the patient, given the information provided?"

A80 | Musculoskeletal | Intervention

An elderly patient has been confined to bed for 2 months, and now demonstrates limited ROM in both lower extremities. Range in hip flexion is 5–115 degrees, and knee flexion is 10–120 degrees. The **MOST** beneficial intervention to improve flexibility and ready this patient for standing is:

CHOICES:

1. Manual passive stretching, 10 repetitions each joint, two times a day.
2. Tilt-table standing, 20 minutes, daily.
3. Mechanical stretching using traction and 5-lb weights, 2 hours, twice daily.
4. Hold-relax techniques followed by passive range of motion (PROM), 10 repetitions, two times a day.

TEACHING POINTS

CORRECT ANSWER: 3

Prolonged mechanical stretching involves a low-intensity force (generally 5–15 lb) applied over a prolonged period (30 minutes to several hours). It is generally the **MOST** beneficial way to manage long-standing flexion contractures.

INCORRECT CHOICES:

Manual passive stretching and tilt-table standing are shorter-duration stretches that are not likely to be as effective in this case. Hold-relax techniques can be used to improve flexibility in the presence of shortening of muscular elements, but are not likely to be effective in this case, because of the short duration and long-standing contracture affecting connective tissue elements.

TYPE OF REASONING: ANALYSIS

This type of question requires one to have knowledge of two factors: the properties of long-standing contractures and indications for using different types of stretching interventions. One must consider the type of contractures this patient has developed, and what will most effectively impact the contractures over a longer period of time. To arrive at a correct conclusion, one uses reasoning skills to analyze the effectiveness of each approach.

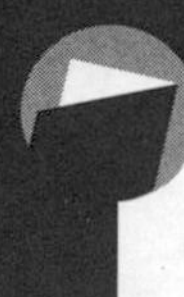

A81 | Musculoskeletal | Evaluation, Diagnosis, Prognosis

A patient has experienced long-term lumbar pain and is diagnosed with degenerative joint disease (DJD) of the lumbar facet joints. The patient complains of numbness, paresthesias, and weakness of the bilateral lower extremities that increase with extended positions or walking greater than 100 feet. Pain persists for hours after assuming a resting position. The patient reports the ability to ride a stationary bike for 30 minutes without any problems. Physical therapy intervention should include:

CHOICES:

1. Increasing cardiovascular endurance with walking for 30 minutes, twice a day.
2. Limiting extended spinal positions and improving the dynamic control of the trunk musculature.
3. Back extension strengthening throughout the entire ROM.
4. Traction and limitation of weight-bearing positions.

TEACHING POINTS

CORRECT ANSWER: 2

Spinal stenosis presents with bilateral dysesthesias and pain in extended positions and/or during walking for distances greater than 100 feet. Physical therapy intervention should emphasize improving dynamic control of the trunk to limit long-term extended spinal positions.

INCORRECT CHOICES:

Improving the cardiovascular status will not change the condition of spinal stenosis. Patients will not tolerate walking 30 minutes without the correct intervention. The signs and symptoms clearly demonstrate that this patient's condition is spinal stenosis. The evidence is clear that patients with spinal stenosis should perform extension exercises, but only in the range of full trunk flexion to neutral. Traction has not been shown to have efficacy to manage patients with spinal stenosis of the lumbar region.

TYPE OF REASONING: INDUCTIVE

Inductive reasoning requires diagnostic thinking, in which the test taker must determine the nature of the diagnosis and intervention. Here, one must understand that the symptoms indicate spinal stenosis, and that the patient requires limitations in long-term extended spinal positions. This type of reasoning also requires one to be a "forward thinker" and determine the best course of action for future functioning.

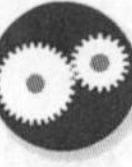

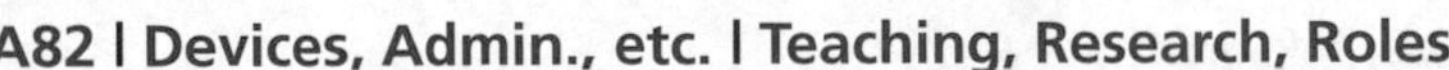

A82 | Devices, Admin., etc. | Teaching, Research, Roles

A PT is instructing a kindergarten teacher in a behavior management program for a child with developmental disabilities who has been mainstreamed into the regular classroom. The therapist requests that the teacher encourage the child to maintain a head-retracted sitting position in the class. The strategy that would be **MOST** beneficial in this situation is to:

CHOICES:

1. Have the teacher give a smile sticker when the child sits with head retracted.
2. Train the teacher in manual handling techniques to assist the child in head retraction.
3. Have the teacher issue a verbal reprimand whenever the child slumps in the chair.
4. Have the teacher encourage the classmates to tell the child to sit up in the chair.

TEACHING POINTS

CORRECT ANSWER: 1

Positive reinforcement (use of the smile sticker) is an effective way to shape behavior by operant conditioning. Positive behaviors are encouraged (hold head in a retracted position).

INCORRECT CHOICES:

Negative behaviors are ignored (slumping in the chair). Manual handling techniques do not promote active control. Classmates should never be involved in reprimands.

TYPE OF REASONING: EVALUATION

One must evaluate the worth of each of these potential approaches to behavioral management of a child. Requiring judgment and knowledge of the effectiveness of positive versus negative reinforcements helps one to arrive at the correct conclusion. In this circumstance, positive reinforcement is most effective, and results in the shaping of positive behaviors.

A83 | Devices, Admin., etc. | Teaching, Research, Roles

A PT has recently attended a professional conference on myofascial release. The therapist has been asked to share this information with PT colleagues during an in-service session. The therapist's **BEST INITIAL** activity is to:

CHOICES:

1. Ask colleagues to select a suitable time and place for the therapist's lecture.
2. Provide a comprehensive packet of handouts in advance of the first in-service session.
3. Organize a PowerPoint presentation and prepare a handout.
4. Survey colleagues about their current level of knowledge using a brief questionnaire.

TEACHING POINTS

CORRECT ANSWER: 4

In order to better share the information, the PT needs to determine what information and skills colleagues currently have. A brief questionnaire is an effective means to achieve this goal.

INCORRECT CHOICES:

The other choices demonstrate planning of the learning experience **WITHOUT** the benefit of a needs assessment.

TYPE OF REASONING: INFERENCE

For the PT to be most effective in delivering information to a group of people, he/she must understand what knowledge the group already has. Otherwise, the presentation is less effective. Therefore, one must infer or draw conclusions of the needs of the group to arrive at a correct answer.

A84 | Other Systems | Evaluation, Diagnosis, Prognosis 

A patient who is 3 months post-CVA is being treated in physical therapy for adhesive capsulitis of the right shoulder. Today, the patient complains of new symptoms, including constant burning pain in the right upper extremity that is increased by the dependent position and touch. The right hand is mildly edematous and stiff. In this case, the intervention that is contraindicated is:

CHOICES:

1. Stress loading using active compression during upper extremity weight-bearing activities.
2. Passive manipulation and ROM of the shoulder.
3. Positional elevation, compression, and gentle massage to reduce edema.
4. AROM exercises of the limb within a pain-free range to regain motion.

TEACHING POINTS

CORRECT ANSWER: 2

This patient is demonstrating early signs of complex regional pain syndrome (CRPS) type I (formerly known as reflex sympathetic dystrophy). These changes typically begin up to 10 days after injury. Passive manipulation and ROM of the shoulder can further aggravate the patient's sympathetically maintained pain.

INCORRECT CHOICES:

In type I CRPS, all of the other treatments listed can be used.

TYPE OF REASONING: INDUCTIVE

Using diagnostic thinking, one must first understand what the symptoms are indicative of and then determine what the best course of action is. The test taker must understand that the symptoms are consistent with CRPS, and that passive manipulation would only heighten the pain response. If this question was answered incorrectly, review information on CRPS and appropriate interventions.

A85 | Neuromuscular | Foundational Sciences 

To prepare a patient with an incomplete T12 paraplegia (ASIA A) for ambulation with crutches, the upper quadrant muscles that would be **MOST** important to strengthen include the:

CHOICES:

1. Upper trapezius, rhomboids, and levator scapulae.
2. Deltoid, triceps, and wrist flexors.
3. Middle trapezius, latissimus dorsi, and triceps.
4. Lower trapezius, latissimus dorsi, and triceps.

TEACHING POINTS

CORRECT ANSWER: 4

The upper quadrant muscles that are most important to strengthen for crutch gaits include the lower trapezius, latissimus dorsi, and triceps. Shoulder depression and elbow extension strength are crucial for successful crutch gait.

INCORRECT CHOICES:

The other choices include muscles not critical to swing-to or swing-through crutch gaits required by a patient with a complete SCI (ASIA A) at T12.

TYPE OF REASONING: INFERENCE

In this question, one must use knowledge of kinesiology coupled with the understanding of T12 paraplegia to arrive at a correct conclusion. One must infer what muscles are most important to strengthen to facilitate ambulation with crutches. The test taker who understands kinesiology well will be able to see that the lower trapezius, latissimus dorsi, and triceps are key muscles in activating scapular depression and elbow extension for crutch use.

A86 | Cardiovascular-Pulmonary | Foundational Sciences

A patient is recovering at home from an MI and percutaneous transluminal coronary angioplasty. The PT decides to use pulse oximetry to monitor the patient's responses to exercise and activity. An acceptable oxygen saturation rate (SaO_2) to maintain throughout the exercise period is:

CHOICES:

1. 82%.
2. 75%.
3. 92%.
4. 85%.

TEACHING POINTS

CORRECT ANSWER: 3

Normal SaO_2 is 95%–98%. A 92% SaO_2 is lower than normal but acceptable.

INCORRECT CHOICES:

Unacceptable oxygen saturation rates during exercise are all other choices (85%, 82%, 75%).

TYPE OF REASONING: DEDUCTIVE

Using recall of factual information, the test taker must deduce what the proper protocol is for oxygen saturation in patients. When using pulse oximetry, the therapist should expect a minimum of less than 88% saturation during exercise. All other saturation levels are below the acceptable standards. Deductive reasoning questions often require one to recall standards and protocols to make proper decisions.

A87 | Devices, Admin., etc. | Equipment, Modalities

Following major surgery of the right hip, a patient ambulates with a Trendelenburg gait. Examination of the right hip reveals abductor weakness (gluteus medius 3/5) and ROM limitations in flexion and external rotation. As part of the intervention, the PT opts to include functional electrical stimulation to help improve the gait pattern. Stimulation should be initiated for the:

CHOICES:

1. Right abductors during swing on the right.
2. Right abductors during stance on the right.
3. Left abductors during stance on the right.
4. Left abductors during swing on the right.

TEACHING POINTS

CORRECT ANSWER: 2

During the stance phase of gait, the hip abductors of the support limb are activated to maintain the pelvis in a relatively horizontal position. This allows the opposite foot to clear the floor during swing.

INCORRECT CHOICES:

Stimulation of the right abductors throughout swing or the left hip abductors during swing or stance would not compensate for the weakness of the right hip abductors during the support period.

TYPE OF REASONING: INFERENCE

The test taker must have a solid understanding of functional electrical stimulation properties coupled with knowledge of kinesiology to arrive at a correct conclusion. One must first consider the limitations of the patient in the right hip, what a Trendelenburg gait pattern is, and then which muscle groups should be targeted to improve the gait pattern. If this question was answered incorrectly, review information on electrical stimulation of the lower extremity for gait improvement.

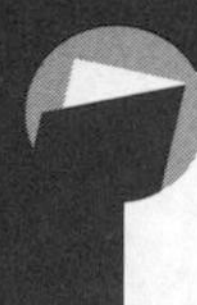

A88 | Musculoskeletal | Foundational Sciences

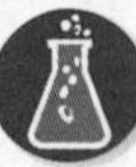

A patient was referred to physical therapy complaining of loss of cervical AROM. X-rays showed DJD at the uncinate processes in the cervical spine. The motion that would be **MOST** restricted would be:

CHOICES:

1. Flexion.
2. Extension.
3. Rotation.
4. Side bending.

TEACHING POINTS

CORRECT ANSWER: 4

The uncinate processes (joints of Luschka) are located at the inferolateral aspect of the lower cervical vertebrae. Side bending is lost with degenerative changes at the joint that the uncinate process makes with the vertebra below.

INCORRECT CHOICES:

Other motion is restricted, but to a lesser degree. Review the joints of Luschka in the Review & Study Guide if necessary.

TYPE OF REASONING: ANALYSIS

Knowledge of cervical anatomy and DJD of the spine is important for arriving at the correct conclusion. The test taker must consider how the degeneration affects functional motion of the cervical spine and to what degree. If this question was answered incorrectly, review information on cervical anatomy and DJD of the spine.

A89 | Musculoskeletal | Evaluation, Diagnosis, Prognosis

A patient is unable to perform overhead activities because of a painless inability to reach past 80 degrees of right shoulder abduction. The "empty can" test was positive. Early subacute physical therapy intervention should focus on:

CHOICES:

1. Active assistive pulley exercises.
2. Modalities to reduce pain and inflammation.
3. Superior translatory mobilizations to increase glenohumeral arthrokinematic motion.
4. Resistance exercises for the affected muscles.

TEACHING POINTS

CORRECT ANSWER: 1

The patient is most likely suffering from a supraspinatus tear or impingement. Acute physical therapy intervention should focus on reduction of pain and inflammation. During the **early subacute phase**, active assistive pulley exercises would be indicated to promote healing of the supraspinatus muscle and maintain AROM of the glenohumeral joint.

INCORRECT CHOICES:

Performing a superior glide of the glenohumeral joint would not be beneficial to improve elevation of the arm. Use of modalities is not the focus at this point of intervention. Resistance exercise would be too difficult, and not beneficial to promote healing of the injured tissues.

TYPE OF REASONING: INFERENCE

One must draw a conclusion based on the evidence presented in order to arrive at the correct answer. In this scenario, the test taker must understand what an empty can test is and what a positive test indicates in order to infer the diagnosis and the best intervention approach. If this question was answered incorrectly, review information on supraspinatus tear/impingement and empty can test.

A90 | Devices, Admin., etc. | Teaching, Research, Roles

Two PTs are asked to perform a test on the same group of patients using the Functional Independence Measure (FIM). The results of both sets of measurements reveal differences in the PTs' scores, but not in the repeat measurements. This is indicative of a problem in:

CHOICES:

1. Concurrent validity.
2. Intrarater reliability.
3. Interrater reliability.
4. Construct validity.

TEACHING POINTS

CORRECT ANSWER: 3

Interrater reliability is the degree to which two or more independent raters can obtain the same rating for a given variable. In this case, two therapists obtained different FIM scores for the same group of patients, indicating a problem in interrater reliability.

INCORRECT CHOICES:

Intrarater reliability is the consistency of an examiner on repeat tests. Issues of validity (Does the test measure what it says it measures?) are not relevant.

TYPE OF REASONING: DEDUCTIVE

This type of question requires one to consider facts and evidence to determine the correct conclusion. This question essentially requires one to recognize the definition of interrater reliability. If this question was answered incorrectly, review information on reliability testing.

A91 | Neuromuscular | Evaluation, Diagnosis, Prognosis

A patient is recovering from a complete SCI (ASIA A) with C5 tetraplegia. The PT is performing PROM exercises on the mat when the patient complains of a sudden, pounding headache and double vision. The therapist notices that the patient is sweating excessively, and determines BP at 240/95. The therapist's **BEST** course of action is to:

CHOICES:

1. Lay the patient down immediately, elevate the legs, and then call for a nurse.
2. Place the patient in a supported sitting position and continue to monitor BP before calling for help.
3. Sit the patient up, check/empty catheter bag, and then call for emergency medical assistance.
4. Lay the patient down, open the shirt, and monitor respiratory rate closely.

TEACHING POINTS

CORRECT ANSWER: 3

The patient is exhibiting autonomic dysreflexia (an emergency situation). The therapist should first sit the patient up and check for irritating or precipitating stimuli (e.g., a blocked catheter). The next step is to call for emergency medical assistance.

INCORRECT CHOICES:

Placing the patient supine can aggravate the situation. Continuing to monitor BP before calling for help causes an unnecessary delay in emergency services.

TYPE OF REASONING: EVALUATION

This question requires one to use clinical judgment to determine the best course of action. The test taker must recognize that these symptoms indicate autonomic dysreflexia, an emergency situation, requiring measures to remedy the situation as quickly as possible.

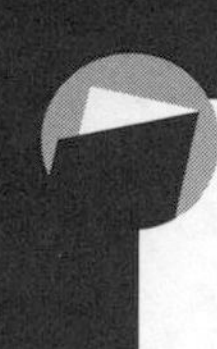

A92 | Devices, Admin., etc. | Equipment, Modalities

A child presents with a flatfoot deformity, with abduction of the forefoot in relation to the weight-bearing line. The forefoot is inverted to the varus position when inspected from the frontal plane. Correct choices for orthotic management of this foot deformity include:

CHOICES:

1. Thomas heel, UCBL insert, or metatarsal bar.
2. Lateral wedge, UCBL insert, or scaphoid pad.
3. Scaphoid pad, metatarsal bar, or Thomas heel.
4. Thomas heel, UCBL insert, or scaphoid pad.

TEACHING POINTS

CORRECT ANSWER: 4

Orthotics can be used to correct a hypermobile flatfoot in children. Correction for a pes planus deformity (support of the longitudinal arch) can be achieved by a University of California Biomechanics Laboratory (UCBL) insert, scaphoid pad, or Thomas heel.

INCORRECT CHOICES:

A metatarsal bar is indicated to take pressure off the metatarsal heads and improve push-off. A lateral wedge (lateral post) is used to support forefoot valgus.

TYPE OF REASONING: INFERENCE

This question requires one to assess the different device choices, have knowledge of their indications, and then apply it to the patient's diagnosis. The test taker must infer which device will not result in functional improvement of the foot deformity. If this correction was answered incorrectly, review information on pes planus deformity and correction.

A93 | Integumentary | Intervention

A child with full-thickness burns to both arms is developing hypertrophic scars. The **BEST** initial intervention to manage these scars is:

CHOICES:

1. Primary excision followed by autografts.
2. Application of custom-made pressure garments.
3. Application of compression wraps.
4. Application of occlusive dressings.

TEACHING POINTS

CORRECT ANSWER: 2

Following burns, edema and hypertrophic scarring can be effectively controlled with custom pressure garments. Pressure should be maintained 23 hours per day, often for 6–12 months.

INCORRECT CHOICES:

Surgery (surgical release) is an option of last resort. Compression wraps (elastic bandages) and occlusive dressings have no impact on hypertrophic scarring.

TYPE OF REASONING: ANALYSIS

One must determine the meaning of hypertrophic scarring and reasonable approaches to resolve the problem. In this question, the patient requires pressure garments because they are effective in controlling hypertrophic scarring, whereas the other methods are not effective or are used as a last resort. If this question was answered incorrectly, review information on full-thickness burns, hypertrophic scarring, and pressure garments.

A94 | Cardiovascular-Pulmonary | Evaluation, Diagnosis, Prognosis

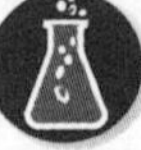

A patient with COPD has developed respiratory acidosis. The PT instructs a PT student participating in the care to monitor the patient closely for:

CHOICES:

1. Disorientation.
2. Tingling or numbness of the extremities.
3. Dizziness or lightheadedness.
4. Hyperreflexia.

TEACHING POINTS

CORRECT ANSWER: 1

A patient with respiratory acidosis may present with many symptoms of increased carbon dioxide levels in the arterial blood. Significant acidosis may lead to disorientation, stupor, or coma.

INCORRECT CHOICES:

The other choices are signs and symptoms of respiratory alkalosis or a decrease of carbon dioxide in the arterial blood.

TYPE OF REASONING: ANALYSIS

One must recall the symptoms of respiratory acidosis in order to arrive at the correct conclusion. In order to do so, the test taker must be knowledgeable of COPD and pulmonary physiology and analyze how the condition matches the symptoms presented. If this question was answered incorrectly, review pulmonary physiology and COPD information.

A95 | Musculoskeletal | Intervention

A computer programmer in her second trimester of pregnancy was referred to physical therapy with complaints of tingling and loss of strength in both of her hands. Her symptoms are exacerbated if she is required to use her keyboard at work for longer than 20 minutes. The **MOST** beneficial physical therapy intervention is:

CHOICES:

1. Dexamethasone phonophoresis to the carpal tunnel.
2. Ice packs to the carpal tunnel.
3. Hydrocortisone iontophoresis to the volar surfaces of both wrists.
4. Placing the wrists in resting splints.

TEACHING POINTS

CORRECT ANSWER: 4

Gestational CTS is not an unusual phenomenon, and results from extra fluid retention. The most effective intervention would be to place the wrists in a neutral position in splints. The carpal tunnel is, therefore, not compromised by poor hand positioning while at work.

INCORRECT CHOICES:

Modalities that use steroids are contraindicated for pregnant women. Although ice packs may relieve discomfort, they do little to correct the source of the problem.

TYPE OF REASONING: INFERENCE

In this question, the test taker must infer the merits of the different potential intervention approaches (what is most appropriate). First, one must recognize that these symptoms are indicative of CTS and then determine what best alleviates the symptoms, given the four choices. One must understand symptomatology and effective treatment approaches for CTS to answer the question correctly.

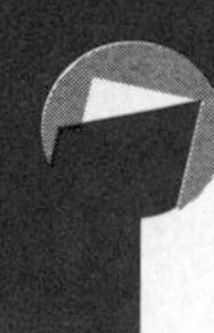

A96 | Devices, Admin., etc. | Equipment, Modalities

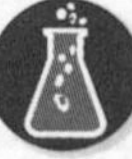

A PT is working in an elementary school system with a child who demonstrates moderate to severe extensor spasticity and limited head control. The **MOST** beneficial positioning device is a:

CHOICES:

1. Wheelchair with adductor pommel.
2. Wheelchair with a back wedge and head supports.
3. Supine stander with abduction wedge.
4. Prone stander with abduction wedge.

TEACHING POINTS

CORRECT ANSWER: 2

A wheelchair wedge and head supports holding one's trunk and head in slight flexion will help decrease the extensor tone, and is the most appropriate positioning in the educational setting.

INCORRECT CHOICES:

An abduction pommel controls scissoring of the legs, but does not control head and upper truck necessary for functioning in the school environment. Standers (prone or supine) maintain the lower extremities in extension, enhancing extensor tone.

TYPE OF REASONING: ANALYSIS

The test taker must determine which of the four possible positioning devices is most effective in addressing the child's issues. This requires knowledge of wheelchair seating and positioning and properties of spasticity in children. If this question was answered incorrectly, review information on seating and positioning for children with spasticity.

A97 | Neuromuscular | Foundational Sciences

A patient with complete C6 tetraplegia (ASIA A) should be instructed to initially transfer with a sliding board using:

CHOICES:

1. Shoulder depressors and triceps, keeping the hands flexed to protect tenodesis grasp.
2. Pectoral muscles to stabilize the elbows in extension and scapular depressors to lift the trunk.
3. Shoulder extensors, external rotators, and anterior deltoid to position and lock the elbow.
4. Serratus anterior to elevate the trunk with elbow extensors stabilizing.

TEACHING POINTS

CORRECT ANSWER: 3

The patient with complete C6 quadriplegia will lack triceps (elbow extensors), and should be taught to lock the elbow for push-up transfers by using shoulder external rotators and extensors to position the arm; the anterior deltoid locks the elbow by reverse actions (all of these muscles are functional).

INCORRECT CHOICES:

Triceps are not functional in this patient. Pectoral muscles cannot be used to stabilize the elbows in extension.

TYPE OF REASONING: INDUCTIVE

This question requires one to understand upper body kinesiology, cervical innervation, and transfers for individuals with SCI. Using skills of diagnostic thinking, coupled with knowledge of SCI and kinesiology, the test taker must match innervation of musculature with functional transfers. If this question was answered incorrectly, review cervical innervation levels and transfer skills for SCI.

A98 | Devices, Admin., etc. | Teaching, Research, Roles

A PT volunteered to teach a stroke education class on positioning techniques for family members and caregivers. At the conclusion of the class, caregivers will be expected to utilize the skills taught. The **BEST** choice of teaching method is to utilize:

CHOICES:

1. Therapist demonstration, caregiver practice, and follow-up individual discussion.
2. Therapist demonstration with caregiver role-playing patient.
3. Multimedia (PowerPoint and handouts) that accompany an oral presentation.
4. Question and answer session that addresses the specific concerns of the caregiver.

TEACHING POINTS

CORRECT ANSWER: 1

A variety of teaching methods including demonstration, practice, and discussion has the best chance of reinforcing learning in a diverse group. Using only one type of teaching methodology is not likely to be as successful in meeting the needs of all the group members. Psychomotor skills are best learned by practice, not lecture or just question and answer. Feedback should include both knowledge of performance and knowledge of results.

INCORRECT CHOICES:

The other choices do not adequately address these educational principles.

TYPE OF REASONING: INFERENCE

One must infer to draw a conclusion about the best approach for educating a group of individuals. Because the group may have differing needs and abilities in learning information, one must provide a variety of approaches to delivering the information. Inference reasoning requires one to use his/her knowledge and beliefs to formulate a correct decision.

A99 | Cardiovascular-Pulmonary | Intervention

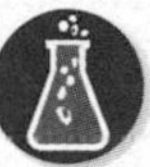

A patient with active tuberculosis (TB) is referred for physical therapy. The patient has been hospitalized and on appropriate antituberculin drugs for three weeks. During treatment, the therapist should observe what precautions?

CHOICES:

1. The patient must wear a tight-fitting mask at all times.
2. The patient must be treated in a private, negative-pressured room.
3. The patient can be treated in the PT gym, without precautions.
4. The therapist must wear personal protective equipment at all times.

TEACHING POINTS

CORRECT ANSWER: 3

Primary disease lasts approximately 10 days to 2 weeks. Two weeks on appropriate antituberculin drugs renders the host noninfectious. The patient can be safely treated in the PT gym without precautions. Medication is taken for prolonged periods (e.g. 9-12 months).

INCORRECT CHOICES:

When the patient is diagnosed with active primary TB, the patient should be in a private, negative-pressured room. The room is considered a potentially infective environment. The therapist should observe all standard precautions (wearing personal protective equipment). The patient need only wear a mask when leaving the room. However this patient is noninfectious.

TYPE OF REASONING: ANALYSIS

One must draw upon their recall of protocols and procedures in TB management in order to make a correct decision about what would be inappropriate in this situation. Standard precautions or universal precautions provide guidelines for this situation, as well as knowledge of the modes of transmission for active TB. Safety of the therapist is of paramount importance in this case.

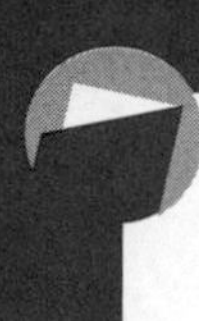

A100 | Musculoskeletal | Evaluation, Diagnosis, Prognosis

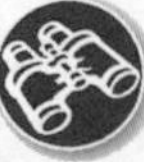

A 12 year-old has been referred to a physical therapy clinic for treatment of patellar tendinitis. The examination reveals that the patient is unable to hop on the affected lower extremity because of pain. The PT decides to refer the patient back to the pediatrician for an x-ray of the knee. The patient returns for therapy with the x-ray shown in the figure. The therapist's initial intervention should focus on:

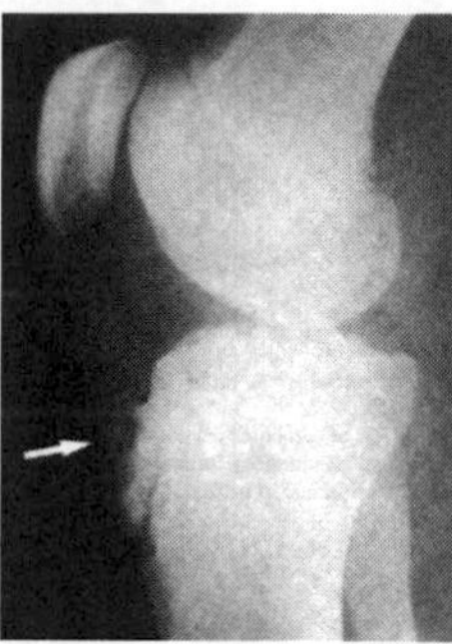

Magee D (2002). Orthopedic Physical Assessment, 4th ed. Philadelphia, W. B. Saunders, Figure 12-149, page 746, with permission.

CHOICES:

1. Aggressive plyometric exercises with focus on endurance training.
2. Iontophoresis using dexamethasone and patient education regarding avoidance of squatting and jumping activities.
3. Fitting the patient with crutches for non–weight-bearing ambulation and initiation of hydrocortisone phonophoresis.
4. Patient education regarding avoiding falls onto the affected knee, and open-chain knee, extension exercises to improve quadriceps strength.

TEACHING POINTS

CORRECT ANSWER: 2

The dysfunction observed on the x-ray is Osgood-Schlatter disease. The radiograph depicts epiphysitis of the tibia at the attachment of the patellar tendon seen in adolescents. It occurs as the result of activities that require continued explosive contractions of the quadriceps muscle complex during pubescent growth spurts. Patient education should focus on controlling knee-loading activities such as squatting and jumping. Iontophoresis using dexamethasone (a corticosteroid) provides a safe mechanism to deliver local anti-inflammatory medication.

INCORRECT CHOICES:

Explosive contractions of the quadriceps complex should be avoided. Ambulation and AROM activities maintain mobility while the structure heals. Phonophoresis would be contraindicated because it may be painful to move the sound head over the affected area. In addition, US should be used with precaution over open epiphyses. Open-chain knee extension exercise may aggravate symptoms due to the increased load at the attachment of the patellar tendon to the tibial tuberosity.

TYPE OF REASONING: INDUCTIVE

One uses skills of diagnostic thinking to make a determination of the condition depicted on the x-ray. Therefore, one must have knowledge of Osgood-Schlatter disease, symptomatology, and treatment of the condition in order to choose the best response for this challenging question. If this question was answered incorrectly, review information on Osgood-Schlatter disease symptomatology and treatment approaches.

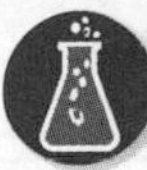

A101 | Musculoskeletal | Foundational Sciences

A patient with a history of low back pain has been receiving physical therapy for 12 weeks. The patient is employed as a loading dockworker. He performs repetitive lifting and carrying of boxes weighing between 15 and 30 lb. An appropriate engineering control to reduce the stresses of lifting and carrying would be to:

CHOICES:

1. Use job rotation.
2. Issue the employee a back support belt.
3. Require the worker to attend a class in using correct body mechanics while performing the job.
4. Provide a two-wheel handcart for use in moving the boxes.

TEACHING POINTS

CORRECT ANSWER: 4

Implementation of an engineering control technique can be accomplished by designing or modifying the workstation, work methods, and tools to eliminate/reduce exposure to excessive exertion, awkward postures, and repetitive motions.

INCORRECT CHOICES:

The other choices do not fit the definition of an engineering control technique.

TYPE OF REASONING: ANALYSIS

In this question, the test taker must analyze which engineering control is most beneficial and most appropriate to recommend for the worker. To arrive at the correct conclusion, one must understand the patient's work environment, and which environmental control remedies the problem at hand, as well as helps to prevent injury in the future.

A102 | Musculoskeletal | Foundational Sciences

Common compensatory postures the PT would expect for a patient diagnosed with fixed severe forefoot varus are:

CHOICES:

1. Subtalar pronation and medial rotation of the tibia.
2. Excessive ankle dorsiflexion and medial rotation of the femur.
3. Excessive midtarsal supination and lateral rotation of the tibia.
4. Toeing-in and lateral rotation of the femur.

TEACHING POINTS

CORRECT ANSWER: 1

In order to maintain the center of gravity over the base of support, the subtalar joint must pronate, and the entire lower quarter must medially rotate.

INCORRECT CHOICES:

Because the expected compensation is pronation of the ankle and medial rotation of the tibia, the responses with dorsiflexion and/or external rotation are incorrect.

TYPE OF REASONING: INFERENCE

The test taker must understand the diagnosis and nature of fixed severe forefoot varus to arrive at the correct conclusion. This requires knowledge of biomechanics of the lower extremity and typical compensatory postures. If this question was answered incorrectly, review information on forefoot varus deformities.

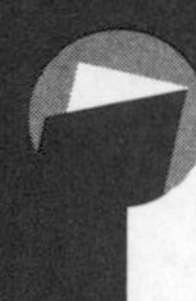

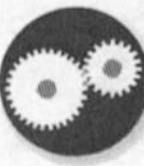

A103 | Musculoskeletal | Intervention

A patient has undergone surgery and subsequent immobilization to stabilize the olecranon process. The patient now exhibits an elbow flexion contracture. In this case, an absolute CONTRAINDICATION for joint mobilization would be:

CHOICES:

1. Soft end-feel.
2. Springy end-feel.
3. Empty end-feel.
4. Firm end-feel.

TEACHING POINTS

CORRECT ANSWER: 3

An empty end-feel (no real end-feel) may be indicative of severe pain and muscle guarding associated with pathological conditions.

INCORRECT CHOICES:

Springy and firm end-feels may be expected after elbow surgery. Soft end-feel is an indication of range limitation because of tissue compression (e.g., in knee flexion, there is contact between the posterior leg and the posterior thigh). None of these is a contraindication for mobilization.

TYPE OF REASONING: EVALUATION

This question requires sound knowledge of joint mobilization strategies, indications, and contraindications. In addition, the test taker must understand what the normal end-feels are for the elbow, especially after immobilization. In this case, the empty end-feel is atypical after immobilization, thereby contraindicating use of joint mobilization techniques.

A104 | Other Systems | Intervention

A middle-aged patient is recovering from surgical repair of an inguinal hernia, and is experiencing some persistent discomfort in the groin area. Patient education should focus on:

CHOICES:

1. Closed-mouth breathing during any lifting.
2. Avoiding straining or turning in bed.
3. Proper lifting techniques and precautions against heavy lifting.
4. Avoiding sitting too long in any one position.

TEACHING POINTS

CORRECT ANSWER: 3

Patients should be educated about proper lifting techniques and precautions against heavy lifting.

INCORRECT CHOICES:

Closed-mouth breathing during lifting is contraindicated, due to increased risk of intra-abdominal pressure with Valsalva's maneuver. Avoiding excessive straining is important. Turning in bed and sitting are part of daily functions.

TYPE OF REASONING: INDUCTIVE

This question requires one to use clinical judgment to determine a best course of action for a patient post–surgical repair of an inguinal hernia. This necessitates inductive reasoning skill. If this question was answered incorrectly, review exercise and education guidelines for patients with inguinal hernia repairs.

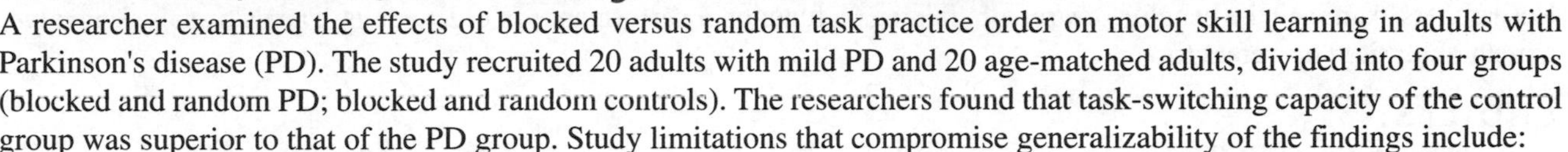

A105 | Devices, Admin., etc. | Teaching, Research, Roles

A researcher examined the effects of blocked versus random task practice order on motor skill learning in adults with Parkinson's disease (PD). The study recruited 20 adults with mild PD and 20 age-matched adults, divided into four groups (blocked and random PD; blocked and random controls). The researchers found that task-switching capacity of the control group was superior to that of the PD group. Study limitations that compromise generalizability of the findings include:

CHOICES:

1. Use of age-matched but not sex-matched controls.
2. Use of only four matched groups.
3. Small sample size and limited number of practice trials.
4. Use of limited outcome measures.

TEACHING POINTS

CORRECT ANSWER: 3

Generalizability refers to the ability to apply these research findings of the PD sample to the larger populations of all patients with mild PD. The small sample size and limited practice duration compromise the generalizability of this study. The researchers correctly refer to this as a pilot study.

INCORRECT CHOICES:

Use of limited outcome measures will impact the validity of the results. The use of four matched groups is an adequate design, as is the use of age-matched controls.

TYPE OF REASONING: DEDUCTIVE

This question requires factual recall of research guidelines in order to arrive at a correct conclusion. In this case, the study limitations that compromise generalizability of the findings include small sample size and limited number of practice trials. If this question was answered incorrectly, review research guidelines and generalizability of research findings.

A106 | Musculoskeletal | Intervention

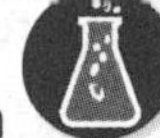

A patient has lumbar spinal stenosis encroaching on the spinal cord. The PT should educate the patient to **AVOID:**

CHOICES:

1. Bicycling using a recumbent cycle ergometer.
2. Use of a rowing machine.
3. Tai chi activities.
4. Swimming using a crawl stroke.

TEACHING POINTS

CORRECT ANSWER: 4

Continuous positioning in spinal extension increases symptoms in patients with spinal stenosis. Activities such as swimming using a crawl stroke place the spine in this position.

INCORRECT CHOICES:

All other activities described do not require the patient to maintain a continuous extended spinal position.

TYPE OF REASONING: ANALYSIS

In this question, the test taker must understand the symptomatology of spinal stenosis and avoidance of certain postures to prevent increases in symptoms. Using the skills of analyzing information presented, one must reason which functional activity most likely encourages continuous spinal extension and should, therefore, be avoided. If this question was answered incorrectly, review information on spinal stenosis.

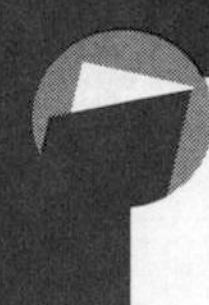

A107 | Devices, Admin., etc. | Teaching, Research, Roles

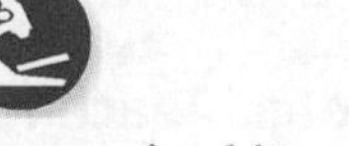

Researchers examined the benefits of strength training on functional performance in older adults. The data analysis involved a meta-analysis. This refers to:

CHOICES:

1. Pooling of data of RCTs to yield a larger sample.
2. A mechanism to critically evaluate studies.
3. Data analysis performed by the Cochrane Collaboration.
4. Pooling of data of all available studies to yield a larger sample.

TEACHING POINTS

CORRECT ANSWER: 1

Meta-analysis refers to pooling of data of RCTs to yield a larger sample. In this example, pooling of data from 121 RCTs yielded a sample of 6,700 people older than age 60. Meta-analysis provides a mechanism for quantitative systematic review.

INCORRECT CHOICES:

Non-RCTs (case-control studies, case reports) are excluded. The Cochrane Collaboration is one source of meta-analysis reviews. Critically evaluating systematic reviews is a separate process.

TYPE OF REASONING: DEDUCTIVE

This question requires one to recall the guidelines for meta-analysis research. This is factual recall of information, which is a deductive reasoning skill. If this question was answered incorrectly, review meta-analysis research guidelines.

A108 | Devices, Admin., etc. | Teaching, Research, Roles

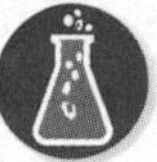

A group of 100 patients who experienced low back pain as a result of a work-related injury were identified and followed over a period of 1 year. Differential outcomes were recorded. Factors were hypothesized that influenced the probability of a good outcome. This study is an example of a:

CHOICES:

1. Case-control study.
2. Case report study.
3. Case series study.
4. Cohort study.

TEACHING POINTS

CORRECT ANSWER: 4

A cohort design involves evaluating the relationship between a potential exposure (risk factors) and an outcome (disease or condition). The cohorts are followed forward in time (prospective study) to determine outcomes.

INCORRECT CHOICES:

A case-control study is a study that identifies a group with common characteristics (a disease or condition) and compares them with a suitable group (age-matched) without the condition. A case report is a detailed description of the management of a patient. Case series involves a description of the management of several patients (multiple case reports).

TYPE OF REASONING: ANALYSIS

This question requires one to analyze the information presented about the research study and then draw a reasonable conclusion about the type of study described. This requires analytical reasoning skill. If this question was answered incorrectly, review research design guidelines, especially cohort studies.

A109 | Integumentary | Patient Examination

During the initial examination of a client with an ulcer superior to the medial malleolus, the PT notes hemosiderosis and liposclerosis. There are no signs of infection, there is minimal drainage, granulation is present, and the wound bed is clean except for a small amount of yellow fibrin deposits. The next action the therapist should take is:

CHOICES:

1. Perform an ankle-brachial index (ABI).
2. Apply a four-layer bandaging system.
3. Apply an Unna boot.
4. Débride the wound with whirlpool irrigation.

TEACHING POINTS

CORRECT ANSWER: 1

The description of the wound is characteristic of a venous stasis ulceration, which is evident by the location (common site is superior to the medial malleolus), hemosiderosis (an accumulation of hemosiderin, a brown-colored pigment), and the liposclerosis (thickening of the tissue). Although this is a venous insufficiency wound, there could be a concomitant arterial disease, and before any type of compression therapy is applied (primary management for venous ulcerations), arterial perfusion must be assessed. The ABI is performed using a Doppler US and comparing the systolic pressure of the tibial or dorsalis pedis artery with that of the brachial artery. An ABI of 1 is normal.

INCORRECT CHOICES:

An ABI of 0.5–0.8 indicates signs of decreased arterial perfusion are present, and any compression therapies will be contraindicated. Applying a four-layer bandage system (e.g., Profore) or an Unna boot is an appropriate compression therapy if arterial disease is absent. Débriding the wound in this case is not necessary (small amounts of fibrin deposits are normal), and whirlpool irrigation is harmful to granulation. In addition, placing the limb in a dependent position may further aggravate the condition.

TYPE OF REASONING: INFERENCE

In this question, the test taker must have knowledge of venous and arterial insufficiency in order to choose the correct answer. In order to do this, one must infer how the symptoms relate to the nature of the patient's ulcer and its type, which requires inferential reasoning skill. If this question was answered incorrectly, review information on symptoms of venous and arterial insufficiency and the typical presentation of venous stasis ulcers.

A110 | Musculoskeletal | Evaluation, Diagnosis, Prognosis

An 11 year-old was referred to physical therapy with complaints of vague pain at his right hip and thigh that radiated to the knee. AROM is restricted in abduction, flexion, and internal rotation. A gluteus medius gait was observed with ambulation for 100 feet. The **BEST** choice for PT intervention is:

CHOICES:

1. Open-chain strengthening of the right hip abductors and internal rotators for avascular necrosis of the hip.
2. Hip joint mobilization to improve the restriction in motion as the result of Legg-Calvé-Perthes disease.
3. Orthoses to control lower extremity position as the result of femoral anteversion.
4. Closed-chain partial weight–bearing lower extremity exercises for slipped capital femoral epiphysis.

TEACHING POINTS

CORRECT ANSWER: 4

This patient is exhibiting signs and symptoms of slipped capital femoral epiphysis, characterized by a gluteus medius gait. Closed-chain exercises with weight-bearing to tolerance will help regain or maintain functional muscular strength and normal motion.

INCORRECT CHOICES:

The signs and symptoms are consistent with slipped capital femoral epiphysis and not any of the other conditions. Avascular necrosis of the femoral head (osteochrondritis dissecans) involves the necrosis and separation of a small segment of the subchondral bone from the femoral head (epiphysis). The hip is painful upon weightbearing. Legg–Calvé–Perthes disease (osteochrondrosis of the femoral head) produces a painful hip with limited motion in abduction and internal rotation. Deformity (flattening) of the femoral head is a complication. Femoral anteversion occurs when the femoral neck is directed anteriorly when the knee is directed anteriorly. Review treatments for each of these conditions if you selected one of these choices.

TYPE OF REASONING: INDUCTIVE

Inductive reasoning is used for diagnostic circumstances, in which one must match symptomatology to the most likely diagnostic indicator. If this question was answered incorrectly, review information on slipped capital femoral epiphysis and the other lower extremity conditions mentioned.

A111 | Devices, Admin., etc. | Teaching, Research, Roles

A researcher states that he expects that there will be no significant difference between 20 and 30 year-olds after a 12-week exercise training program using exercise HRs and myocardial oxygen consumption as measures of performance. The kind of hypothesis that is being used in this study is a(n):

CHOICES:

1. Experimental hypothesis.
2. Research hypothesis.
3. Null hypothesis.
4. Directional hypothesis.

TEACHING POINTS

CORRECT ANSWER: 3

The null hypothesis is a statistical hypothesis that states that there is no relationship (or difference) between variables. Any relationship found will be a chance relationship, not a true one.

INCORRECT CHOICES:

A directional or research (experimental) hypothesis predicts an expected relationship between variables (e.g., 20 year-olds will demonstrate improved measures of performance when compared with 30 year-olds).

TYPE OF REASONING: DEDUCTIVE

Research questions often require the use of deductive reasoning, which requires knowledge of protocols and rules. Here, the test taker must recall the definitions for the different types of hypotheses formulated in research. If this question was answered incorrectly, review information on the different types of hypotheses.

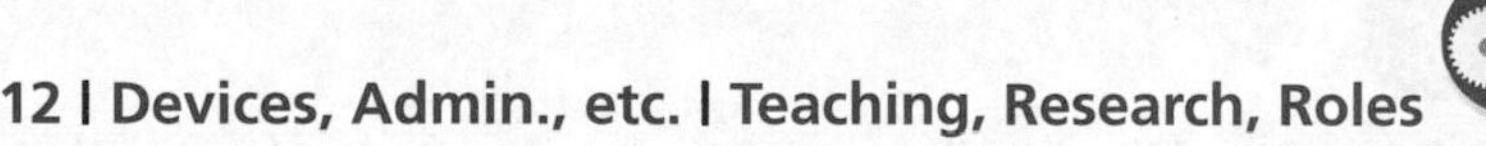

A112 | Devices, Admin., etc. | Teaching, Research, Roles

A PT was treating a patient in a room shared with two other patients. The patient in the next bed was uncomfortable, and asked the therapist to reposition one leg. The therapist placed the leg on two pillows, as requested by the patient. Unknown to the therapist, this patient had a femoral artery graft 2 days prior. As a result, the graft became occluded and the patient was rushed to surgery for a replacement. The patient claimed the therapist placed the leg too high on the pillows, causing the occlusion of the original graft, and sued for malpractice. The hospital administrator and legal team decided that:

CHOICES:

1. The therapist was functioning outside the common protocols of the hospital and, therefore, did not support the actions of the therapist.
2. The therapist was functioning according to common protocols of the institution and, thus, supported the actions of the therapist.
3. It was the patient's fault for requesting the position change and, therefore, supported the actions of the therapist.
4. They would counter-sue, because the patient was responsible for requesting the position change.

TEACHING POINTS

CORRECT ANSWER: 1

The therapist was acting outside of his/her area of responsibility and did something that caused the patient harm. The therapist demonstrated negligence, defined as a failure to do what a reasonably competent practitioner would have done under similar circumstances, and as a result, the patient was harmed.

INCORRECT CHOICES:

The therapist was not operating within standard protocols by changing the position of an unfamiliar patient, no matter how well-meaning. The patient was naïve about the effects of position changes, but may request a change. The therapist is not obligated to fulfill the patient's desires (especially a patient not being treated by the therapist) and, in this case, by doing so, caused harm. Consulting with a nurse, physician's assistant, or other practitioner first would have been the wise course of action.

TYPE OF REASONING: EVALUATION

In this situation, the test taker must evaluate the strength of the statements presented and determine which statement has the most merit. One must rely on the guidelines of physical therapy practice and hospital protocols to determine whether the response of the therapist constituted negligence. If this question was answered incorrectly, review concepts of negligence.

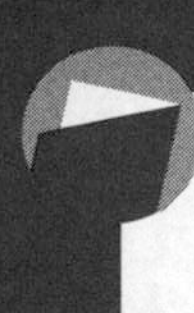

A113 | Neuromuscular | Intervention

A patient has a 3-year history of multiple sclerosis (MS). One of the disabling symptoms is a persistent and severe diplopia, which leaves the patient frequently nauseated and immobile. A beneficial intervention strategy to assist the patient in successfully participating in rehabilitation would be to:

CHOICES:

1. Provide the patient with special glasses that magnify images.
2. Instruct the patient to close both eyes and practice movements without visual guidance.
3. Provide the patient with a soft neck collar to limit head and neck movements.
4. Patch one eye.

TEACHING POINTS

CORRECT ANSWER: 4

Double vision (diplopia) can be managed by patching of one eye. Patients are typically on an eye-patching schedule that alternates the eye that is patched. Loss of depth perception can be expected with eye patching, but is not as disabling as diplopia.

INCORRECT CHOICES:

Having the patient use magnifiying glasses or a soft neck collar does not correct the primary deficit. Although practice with eyes closed may be part of a rehabilitation program, it also does not address the primary deficit. This patient will need eyes open for daily functional activity.

TYPE OF REASONING: INFERENCE

The test taker must infer or draw conclusions about how the four possible treatment options will be the best remedy for diplopia. This requires knowledge of the condition of diplopia and how eye patching is the superior choice for remedying the condition. If this question was answered incorrectly, review information about treatment of diplopia.

A114 | Neuromuscular | Intervention

The **BEST** choice for positioning strategy for a patient recovering from acute stroke who is in bed and demonstrates a flaccid upper extremity is:

CHOICES:

1. Supine with the affected arm flexed, and with the hand resting on the stomach.
2. Side-lying on the sound side, with the affected shoulder protracted, and the arm extended resting on a pillow.
3. Supine with the affected elbow extended, and the arm positioned close to the side of the trunk.
4. Side-lying on the sound side, with the affected upper extremity flexed overhead.

TEACHING POINTS

CORRECT ANSWER: 2

Most patients with stroke recover from flaccidity and develop spasticity. Positioning for the patient with early stroke stresses (1) protection against ligamentous strain and the development of a painful subluxed shoulder and (2) positions counter to the typical spastic posture of flexion and adduction with pronation. Side-lying with the affected upper extremity supported on a pillow, with the shoulder protracted and the elbow extended, accomplishes both of these goals.

INCORRECT CHOICES:

The other positions fail to accomplish these goals. The affected arm should not be flexed (choice 1), as flexion-adduction spasticity typically develops in the affected upper extremity. Supine with arm extended at the side (choice 3) and sidelying on sound side with affected arm flexed overhead (choice 4) do not provide needed support for a painful, subluxed shoulder.

TYPE OF REASONING: INDUCTIVE

One must have a good understanding of the nature of stroke, and the potential for spasticity and subluxation of the shoulder. Therefore, the test taker must reason via clinical judgment (an inductive skill) which bed positioning should discourage development of these conditions and protect the ligaments from undue strain. If this question was answered incorrectly, review information on CVA and bed positioning.

A115 | Integumentary | Evaluation, Diagnosis, Prognosis

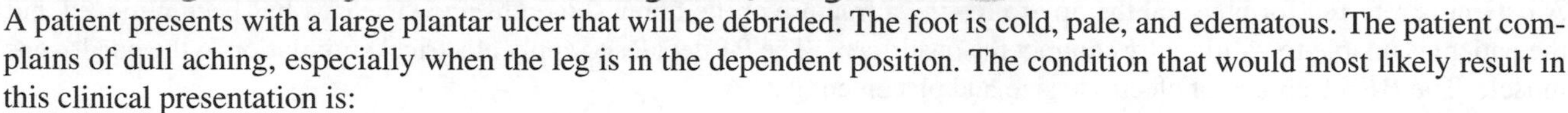

A patient presents with a large plantar ulcer that will be débrided. The foot is cold, pale, and edematous. The patient complains of dull aching, especially when the leg is in the dependent position. The condition that would most likely result in this clinical presentation is:

CHOICES:

1. Chronic arterial insufficiency.
2. Chronic venous insufficiency.
3. Acute arterial insufficiency.
4. DVT.

TEACHING POINTS

CORRECT ANSWER: 2

Venous ulcers typically present with minimal pain (dull aching). Venous congestion and aching are relieved by leg elevation. Chronic venous insufficiency is also characterized by thickening, coarsening, and brownish pigmentation of the skin around the ankles. The skin is usually thin, shiny, and cyanotic.

INCORRECT CHOICES:

Arterial insufficiency typically presents with severe pain (claudication and in severe cases rest pain). The forefoot typically exhibits dependent rubor and pallor with decreased or absent pulses on elevation. Skin is typically cool, pale, and shiny.

TYPE OF REASONING: ANALYSIS

This question requires one to recall the common symptomatology for chronic venous insufficiency and to differentiate the symptoms from other disorders of the lower extremity. In this case, one must recognize that a painless ulcer is usually indicative of chronic venous insufficiency. If this question was answered incorrectly, review common symptoms of chronic venous insufficiency, as well as other common vascular disorders.

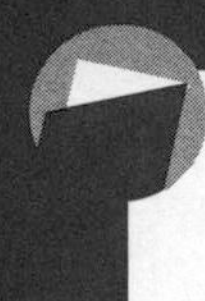

A116 | Devices, Admin., etc. | Equipment, Modalities 

A patient is referred for physical therapy following a fracture of the femur 6 months ago. The cast has been removed, but the patient is unable to volitionally contract the quadriceps. The PT decides to apply electrical stimulation to the quadriceps muscle. The **BEST** choice of electrode size and placement is:

CHOICES:

1. Large electrodes, closely spaced.
2. Small electrodes, closely spaced.
3. Large electrodes, widely spaced.
4. Small electrodes, widely spaced.

TEACHING POINTS

CORRECT ANSWER: 3

Large electrodes are used on large muscles in order to disperse the current (minimize current density under the electrode), enabling a more comfortable delivery of current. Widely spaced electrodes permit the current to travel deeper into the muscle to stimulate a greater number of deeper muscle fibers.

INCORRECT CHOICES:

The other choices do not meet these guidelines. Utilizing small electrodes would cause the current to be concentrated over a smaller surface area, thus increasing the current density under the electrode. Exceeding the current density of an electrode can cause patient discomfort, skin irritation, or a thermal burn. Close spacing of electrodes encourages superficial flow of current, rather than deeper flow.

TYPE OF REASONING: DEDUCTIVE

This type of question requires one to recall protocols and guidelines for electrical stimulation, which is a deductive skill. This question requires one to consider the therapeutic differences between using small versus large and widely versus closely placed electrodes. If this question was answered incorrectly, review information on use of electrical stimulation for large muscles.

A117 | Integumentary | Evaluation, Diagnosis, Prognosis 

While setting a patient up for cervical traction, the PT notices a mole that is brown and black with diffuse edges on the patient's neck. The therapist should:

CHOICES:

1. Discontinue treatment and refer the patient back to the physician.
2. Continue with the traction and report the findings to the physician immediately posttreatment.
3. Continue the treatment; however, document the skin condition.
4. Tell the patient to have the physician inspect the mole.

TEACHING POINTS

CORRECT ANSWER: 2

A mole with irregular edges and multiple colors (black, blue, pale red, or white) is characteristic of a melanoma. It is associated with sun-damaged skin but can appear anywhere on the body. Early recognition before tumor invasion and metastatic spread is critical in improving survival rates. There is no contraindication to treatment, but the physician should be informed by the therapist immediately.

INCORRECT CHOICES:

Delaying reporting of this finding can put this patient at risk for metastatic disease.

TYPE OF REASONING: INFERENCE

In this question, one must draw a conclusion as to whether or not the symptoms described warrant immediate notification of the physician, discontinuation of treatment, or simply notation in the PT's notes. In this instance, the symptoms indicate potential melanoma, and should be reported to the physician immediately, due to the nature of this type of cancer. If this question was answered incorrectly, review information on melanoma.

A118 | Neuromuscular | Evaluation, Diagnosis, Prognosis

A patient suffered a severe traumatic brain injury and multiple fractures after a motor vehicle accident. The patient is recovering in the intensive care unit. The physical therapy referral requests PROM and positioning. On day 1, the patient is semialert, and drifts in and out during physical therapy. On day 2, the patient is less alert with changing status. Signs and symptoms that would require emergency consultation with a physician include:

CHOICES:

1. Developing irritability, with increasing symptoms of photophobia, disorientation, and restlessness.
2. Decreasing function of cranial nerves IV, VI, and VII.
3. Positive Kernig's sign with developing nuchal rigidity.
4. Decreasing consciousness, with slowing of pulse and Cheyne-Stokes respirations.

TEACHING POINTS

CORRECT ANSWER: 4

Signs of increased intracranial pressure secondary to cerebral edema and brain herniation include decreasing consciousness with slowing of pulse and Cheyne-Stokes respirations. Cranial nerve dysfunction is typically noted in CN II (papilledema) and CN III (dilation of pupils).

INCORRECT CHOICES:

The other choices are signs of meningeal irritation and CNS infection. All of the problems listed are serious, and can be life-threatening.

TYPE OF REASONING: INFERENCE

This question requires one to recognize which symptoms are expected after severe brain injury with elevated intracranial pressure, which require immediate physician notification. If this question was answered incorrectly, review information on severe brain injury and typical symptoms.

A119 | Neuromuscular | Foundational Sciences

A PT receives a referral for a patient with neurapraxia involving the ulnar nerve secondary to an elbow fracture. Based on knowledge of this condition, the therapist expects that:

CHOICES:

1. Regeneration is likely in 6–8 months.
2. Nerve dysfunction will be rapidly reversed, generally in 2–3 weeks.
3. Regeneration is likely after 1–1 1/2 years.
4. Regeneration is unlikely, because surgical approximation of the nerve ends was not performed.

TEACHING POINTS

CORRECT ANSWER: 2

Neurapraxia is a mild peripheral nerve injury (conduction block ischemia) that causes transient loss of function. Nerve dysfunction is rapidly reversed, generally within 2–3 weeks. An example is a compression injury to the radial nerve from falling asleep with the arm over the back of a chair (Saturday night palsy).

INCORRECT CHOICES:

If the nerve is cut, the distal part degenerates (Wallerian degeneration). Regeneration (nerve growth and repair) is dependent upon intact Schwann cell and continuity of the nerve pathway. Regrowth is at the rate of 1–4 mm/d. In this case, the nerve injury was not severe enough to initiate regeneration.

TYPE OF REASONING: INDUCTIVE

This question requires one to recall information on peripheral nerve injury and the typical recovery time for this specific type of injury. If this question was answered incorrectly, review information on postfracture peripheral nerve injury.

EXAM A

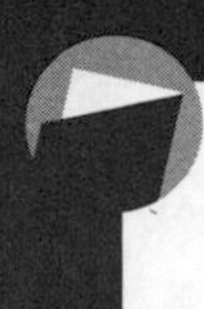

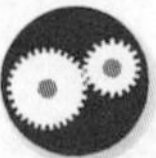

A120 | Devices, Admin., etc. | Teaching, Research, Roles

After 3 weeks of teaching a patient how to ambulate with bilateral crutches and a touch-down gait, the PT determines that the most appropriate kind of feedback to give to the patient is:

CHOICES:

1. Immediate feedback, given after each practice trial.
2. Intermittent feedback, given at scheduled intervals, every other practice trial.
3. Continuous feedback, with ongoing verbal cuing during gait.
4. Occasional feedback, given when consistent errors appear.

TEACHING POINTS

CORRECT ANSWER: 4

In learning a psychomotor skill, the patient must be able to actively process information and self-correct responses. Occasional feedback provides the best means of allowing for introspection, and is appropriate for later practice (associated and autonomous phases of motor learning).

INCORRECT CHOICES:

The other choices emphasize feedback more applicable to very early motor learning (cognitive phase).

TYPE OF REASONING: EVALUATION

In this situation, one must recognize that motor learning strategies vary over the course of training (stages of learning). The test taker must evaluate the value of the different courses of action the therapist could take to assist the patient. In this case, the most value is found in occasional feedback in the presence of errors.

A121 | Other Systems | Evaluation, Diagnosis, Prognosis

A home health PT is treating an elderly patient. On this day, the patient is confused, with shortness of breath and generalized weakness. Given a history of hypertension and hyperlipidemia, the therapist suspects the patient:

CHOICES:

1. Is exhibiting mental changes indicative of early Alzheimer's disease.
2. May be experiencing unstable angina.
3. Forgot to take prescribed hypertension medication.
4. May be presenting with early signs of MI.

TEACHING POINTS

CORRECT ANSWER: 4

An elderly patient with a cardiac history may present with initial symptoms of mental confusion, the result of oxygen deprivation to the brain. The shortness of breath and generalized weakness may be due to generalized circulatory insufficiencies coexisting with the developing MI.

INCORRECT CHOICES:

Early Alzheimer's disease would not produce shortness of breath and generalized weakness. Chest pain would be evident with unstable angina. Hypertension is usually silent (asymptomatic). Occasionally, patients report headache.

TYPE OF REASONING: INFERENCE

One must infer or draw conclusions from the evidence that is presented in this situation. This requires one to recognize that a patient with a cardiac history showing new symptoms of confusion, shortness of breath, and weakness is indicative of MI and not the other choices. If this question was answered incorrectly, review information on symptoms of MI.

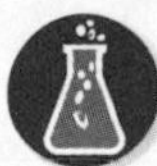

A122 | Musculoskeletal | Foundational Sciences

A baseball pitcher was seen by a PT following surgical repair of a SLAP (superior labral, anterior posterior) lesion of his pitching arm. In follow-up care, the therapist needs to pay attention to the pitching motion. The phase of the throwing motion that puts the greatest stress on the anterior labrum and capsule is:

CHOICES:

1. Wind-up.
2. Cocking.
3. Acceleration.
4. Deceleration.

TEACHING POINTS

CORRECT ANSWER: 2

During the cocking phase, the arm is taken into the end range of humeral external rotation. At that point, the anterior aspects of the capsule and labrum are acting as constraints to prevent excessive anterior glide of the humerus.

INCORRECT CHOICES:

The other phases of the throwing motion do not place the same degree of strain on the anterior labrum and capsule.

TYPE OF REASONING: ANALYSIS

In this question, one must understand what a SLAP lesion is, and the nature of pitching in relation to stresses placed on the anterior capsule and labrum. This requires knowledge of both orthopedics and kinesiology (specifically, throwing mechanics). This type of question requires one to interpret the meaning of the symptoms presented, which is an analysis skill.

A123 | Cardiovascular-Pulmonary | Intervention

A patient is hospitalized in an intensive care unit following a traumatic SCI resulting in C3 tetraplegia (ASIA A). The patient is receiving endotracheal suctioning, following development of significant pulmonary congestion. The recommended time duration for endotracheal suctioning is:

CHOICES:

1. 10–15 seconds.
2. 1–5 seconds.
3. 5–10 seconds.
4. 15–20 seconds.

TEACHING POINTS

CORRECT ANSWER: 1

The recommended time duration for endotracheal suctioning is 10–15 seconds.

INCORRECT CHOICES:

Any longer time (15–20 sec) risks serious hypoxemia, any shorter (1–5 or 5–10 sec) and the risk is ineffective secretion removal.

TYPE OF REASONING: DEDUCTIVE

This type of question requires one to recall protocols and guidelines for endotrachial suctioning, which is a deductive skill. If this question was answered incorrectly, review information about endotracheal suctioning.

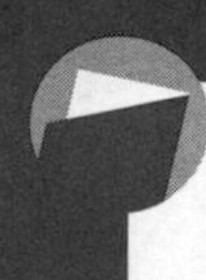

A124 | Integumentary | Intervention

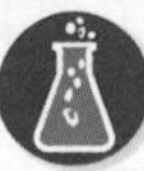

A frail older adult is confined to bed in a nursing facility and has developed a small superficial wound over the sacral area. Because only small amounts of necrotic tissue are present, the physician has decided to use autolytic wound débridement. This is **BEST** achieved with:

CHOICES:

1. Wound irrigation using a syringe.
2. Transparent film dressing.
3. Wet-to-dry gauze dressing with antimicrobial ointment.
4. Sharp débridement.

TEACHING POINTS

CORRECT ANSWER: 2

Autolytic wound débridement allows the body's natural enzymes to promote healing by trapping them under a synthetic, occlusive dressing. Moisture-retentive dressings are applied for short durations (<2 wk). Choices include transparent film dressings or hydrocolloid or hydrogel dressings.

INCORRECT CHOICES:

The other interventions are wound management techniques; however, they are not autolytic.

TYPE OF REASONING: ANALYSIS

One must first understand the nature of autolytic wound débridement in order to arrive at a correct conclusion. This requires one to recall the definition of autolytic, which is the use of the body's natural healing processes. When recalling definitions of words, the skill of analysis is used.

A125 | Devices, Admin., etc. | Equipment, Modalities

A patient was instructed to apply conventional (high-rate) transcutaneous electrical nerve stimulation (TENS) to the low back to modulate a chronic pain condition. The patient now states that the TENS unit is no longer effective in reducing the pain in spite of increasing the intensity to maximum. The PT should now advise the patient to:

CHOICES:

1. Switch to low-rate TENS.
2. Increase the treatment frequency.
3. Switch to modulation mode TENS.
4. Decrease the pulse duration.

TEACHING POINTS

CORRECT ANSWER: 3

Because of the long-term, continuous use of TENS, the sensory receptors accommodated to the continuous current, and no longer responded to the stimuli. Changing to modulation mode (i.e., burst modulation), which periodically interrupts the current flow, does not allow accommodation to occur.

INCORRECT CHOICES:

None of the other choices decreases accommodation. Low-rate TENS is a motor level stimulation, not sensory. Increasing treatment frequency would result in accommodation occurring more quickly. Decreasing the pulse duration would require increasing the intensity to get a response, and the patient has already maximized the intensity.

TYPE OF REASONING: INFERENCE

One must draw a conclusion of why the patient is no longer responding to the TENS therapy, and then what can be clinically done to provide pain relief. In this circumstance, a patient who had previously responded to conventional TENS in the past, but not recently, is indicative of accommodation and requires modification to modulation mode TENS. One uses the skills of inference in this question to draw conclusions about the information presented.

A126 | Neuromuscular | Patient Examination 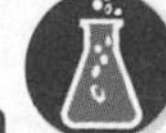

During initial standing, a patient with chronic stroke is pushing strongly backward, displacing the center-of-mass at or near the posterior limits of stability. The most likely cause of this is:

CHOICES:

1. Spasticity of the tibialis anterior.
2. Spasticity of the gastrocnemius-soleus.
3. Contracture of the hamstrings.
4. Contraction of the hip extensors.

TEACHING POINTS

CORRECT ANSWER: 2

The muscles of the foot and ankle move the long lever of the body forward and backward (ankle strategy). The gastrocnemius-soleus moves the body backward, and the anterior tibialis moves the body forward. Poststroke, spasticity of the gastrocnemius-soleus and weakness of the anterior tibialis are common.

INCORRECT CHOICES:

Action of the hip extensors would result in a backward lean, with the center of motion occurring at the hip (hip strategy). Contracture of the hamstrings increases knee flexion and forward trunk lean. Spasticity occurs in lower extremity antigravity extensor muscles, not the anterior tibialis.

TYPE OF REASONING: ANALYSIS

This type of question requires one to analyze the meaning of the information presented and determine the reasons for it. To answer this question correctly, one must have a good understanding of biomechanics to analyze that the backward displacement of the body during standing is indicative of gastrocnemius-soleus spasticity.

A127 | Devices, Admin., etc. | Teaching, Research, Roles 

A patient has been screened using a new test for the presence of a gene (ALG-2) linked to Alzheimer's disease. The physician reports that the patient lacks the gene and should not be at increased risk to develop the disease. Some years later, the same patient develops Alzheimer's, and a repeat test reveals the presence of the gene. The results of the initial test can be interpreted as:

CHOICES:

1. False-negative test result.
2. High-specificity error.
3. Historically inconclusive test result.
4. High-sensitivity error.

TEACHING POINTS

CORRECT ANSWER: 1

In this example, the individual was found not to have the Alzheimer's gene, when years later, he tested positive for the gene and the disease. The original test produced a false-negative result.

INCORRECT CHOICES:

Sensitivity refers to the ability of a test to correctly identify individuals who truly have a disease or condition (a true positive). Specificity refers to a test's ability to correctly identify the proportion of individuals who do not have a disease or condition (a true negative). Findings were reported for the original test, and not as inconclusive.

TYPE OF REASONING: DEDUCTIVE

In this case, the test taker must recognize that the information presented is a definition of false negative. One must recall factual information about the differences between negative versus positive symptoms, as well as the difference between specificity versus sensitivity. If this question was answered incorrectly, review definitions for false negative and positive, specificity, and sensitivity in research.

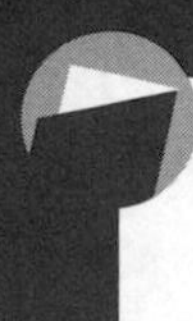

A128 | Other Systems | Evaluation, Diagnosis, Prognosis

A middle-aged adult lives at home with his wife and adult daughter. He has recently been diagnosed with multi-infarct dementia, and is recovering from a fractured hip following a fall injury. In the initial interview with the patient's wife, the PT would expect to find:

CHOICES:

1. History of steady progression of loss of judgment and poor safety awareness.
2. Agitation and sundowning.
3. Perseveration on a thought or activity.
4. History of sudden onset of new cognitive problems and patchy distribution of deficits.

TEACHING POINTS

CORRECT ANSWER: 4

Multi-infarct dementia differs from primary degenerative dementia, Alzheimer's type, in (1) onset: sudden rather than slowly progressive (characteristic of small focal infarcts) and (2) the nature of symptoms: areas of deficits coexist with areas of intact cerebral function.

INCORRECT CHOICES:

Agitation and sundowning (late afternoon wandering) are characteristic of Alzheimer's disease. Perseveration describes getting "stuck" and repeating a thought or activity over and over again, and is sometimes seen following stroke.

TYPE OF REASONING: ANALYSIS

This question asks the test taker to recognize the symptoms of multi-infarct dementia. One must evaluate the information presented and interpret what it means, which is an analysis skill. If this question was answered incorrectly, refer to information on dementia.

A129 | Musculoskeletal | Evaluation, Diagnosis, Prognosis

A 14 year-old girl complains of subpatellar pain after participation in an aerobic exercise program for 2 weeks. The PT's examination shows a large Q angle, pain with palpation at the inferior pole of the patella, and mild swelling at both knees. The **BEST** intervention for this situation is:

CHOICES:

1. Vastus medialis (VM) muscle strengthening.
2. Taping to increase lateral patellar tracking.
3. Vastus lateralis (VL) strengthening.
4. Hamstring strengthening.

TEACHING POINTS

CORRECT ANSWER: 1

Q angles of greater than 15 degrees could be indicative of abnormal lateral patellar tracking. VM muscle strengthening can reduce the tendency for the patella to track laterally.

INCORRECT CHOICES:

VL strengthening can promote greater lateral patellar tracking and further irritation of the patellofemoral joint. VL strengthening may promote an outward pull or dislocation of the patella. Hamstring strengthening does not directly affect tracking of the patella. In the closed chain, problems at the hip or foot can also contribute to patellofemoral pain syndrome. Taping to increase lateral patellar tracking will exacerbate the problem.

TYPE OF REASONING: INDUCTIVE

This question requires one to make a clinical judgment as to the reason for the large Q angle and what can be clinically done to remedy the condition. In this scenario, the test taker should recognize that the abnormal lateral patellar tracking indicates VM weakness. Questions that require one to use diagnostic thinking and clinical judgment use inductive reasoning skills.

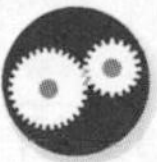

A130 | Neuromuscular | Evaluation, Diagnosis, Prognosis

A PT receives a referral from an acute care therapist to treat a patient with right hemiparesis in the home. The referral indicates that the patient demonstrates good recovery: both involved limbs are categorized as stage 4 (some movements out-of-synergy). The patient is ambulatory with a small-based quad cane. The activity that would be **MOST** beneficial for a patient at this stage of recovery is:

CHOICES:

1. Supine, bending the hip and knee up to the chest with some hip abduction.
2. Sitting, marching in place with alternate hip and flexion.
3. Standing, lifting the foot up behind and slowly lowering it.
4. Standing, small-range knee squats.

TEACHING POINTS

CORRECT ANSWER: 3

Stage 4 recovery is characterized by some movement combinations that do not follow paths of either flexion or extension obligatory synergies. Knee flexion in standing is an out-of-synergy movement.

INCORRECT CHOICES:

All other choices include some degree of in-synergy movements: the supine and sitting options are flexion synergy movements, and the other standing option focuses on knee and hip extension (extension synergy movements).

TYPE OF REASONING: EVALUATION

In this question, one must have a firm understanding of poststroke recovery stages, synergies, and what type of functional activities are ideal for promoting movement appropriate to the stage. Evaluation questions require one to evaluate ideas and determine how valid they are. If this question was answered incorrectly, refer to information on poststroke recovery.

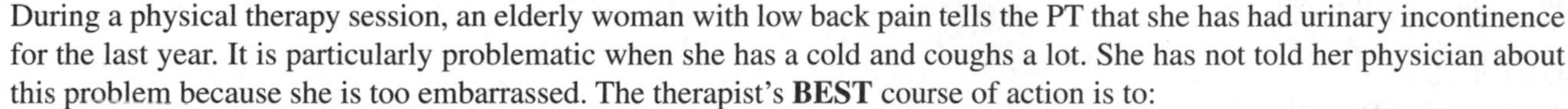

A131 | Other Systems | Evaluation, Diagnosis, Prognosis

During a physical therapy session, an elderly woman with low back pain tells the PT that she has had urinary incontinence for the last year. It is particularly problematic when she has a cold and coughs a lot. She has not told her physician about this problem because she is too embarrassed. The therapist's **BEST** course of action is to:

CHOICES:

1. Examine the patient, document impairments, and discuss findings with the physician.
2. Refer the patient back to the physician.
3. Examine the patient, document impairments, and then refer her back to her physician.
4. Examine the patient and proceed with treatment for low back pain.

TEACHING POINTS

CORRECT ANSWER: 1

The PT should complete the examination of the patient, adequately document the findings, and determine the physical therapy diagnosis. Although many states have direct access laws that permit physical therapy intervention without referral, most insurance companies, including Medicare (affecting the patient in this example), require a physician referral in order for services to be reimbursed. Thus, the therapist needs to consult with the physician to get a referral before initiating any intervention for this problem. This patient demonstrates stress incontinence, a problem that could be successfully treated with physical therapy (e.g., Kegel's exercises and other interventions).

INCORRECT CHOICES:

The other choices do not offer successful resolution for her problems. The therapist is not being an active advocate for the patient in dealing with the incontinence.

TYPE OF REASONING: DEDUCTIVE

In this question, one must recall the appropriate guidelines for physical therapy and treatment in the absence of a physician referral. The patient's age is key in arriving at the correct conclusion. This question requires deductive reasoning, because the test taker must recall protocols and guidelines.

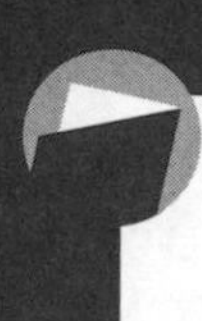

A132 | Neuromuscular | Foundational Sciences

During a sensory examination, a patient complains of a dull, aching pain and is not able to discriminate a stimulus as sharp or dull. Two-point discrimination is absent. Based on these findings, the pathway that is intact is the:

CHOICES:

1. Lateral spinothalamic tract.
2. Dorsal columns/neospinothalamic systems.
3. Fasciculus gracilis/medial lemniscus.
4. Anterior spinothalamic tract.

TEACHING POINTS

CORRECT ANSWER: 4

Sensations interpreted as dull, aching pain travel in the anterior (paleo)spinothalamic tract.

INCORRECT CHOICES:

Discriminative, fast pain is carried in the lateral (neo)spinothalamic tract. Discriminative touch is carried in the proprioceptive pathways (fasciculus gracilis/cuneatus, medial lemniscus).

TYPE OF REASONING: DEDUCTIVE

This question essentially tests one's recall of the various sensory pathways. This information is based on firm guidelines, which is a deductive reasoning skill. If this question was answered incorrectly, review information on the various spinal pathways for sensation.

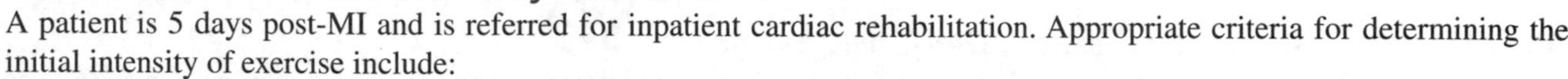

A133 | Cardiovascular-Pulmonary | Intervention

A patient is 5 days post-MI and is referred for inpatient cardiac rehabilitation. Appropriate criteria for determining the initial intensity of exercise include:

CHOICES:

1. Systolic BP < 240 mm Hg or diastolic BP < 110 mm Hg.
2. HR < 120 beats/min and RPE < 13.
3. HR resting plus 30 beats/min and RPE < 14.
4. >1 mm ST segment depression, horizontal or downsloping.

TEACHING POINTS

CORRECT ANSWER: 2

Intensity of exercise is prescribed using HR and RPE and monitored using HR, RPE, and signs of exertional intolerance. For post-MI patients, an RPE < 13 (6–20 scale) and a HR < 120 beats/min (or HR resting plus 20 beats/min) is recommended.

INCORRECT CHOICES:

HR plus 30 beats/min is recommended for postsurgery patients. Signs and symptoms for an upper limit of exercise intensity include choices 1 and 3 along with onset of angina, and ECG disturbances (ventricular arrhythmias, second- or third-degree atrioventricular block, atrial fibrillation, etc). (Source: American College of Sports Medicine, *Guidelines for Exercise Testing and Prescription.*)

TYPE OF REASONING: INFERENCE

One must take the information presented and determine the best course of action that will result in the best outcome, which is an inferential skill. In this situation, one must judge what is the appropriate criterion for exercise for a patient 5 days post-MI, which requires understanding of the nature of MI and guidelines for treatment of it. If this question was answered incorrectly, refer to cardiac rehabilitation guidelines.

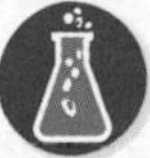

A134 | Other Systems | Evaluation, Diagnosis, Prognosis

A patient is receiving immunosuppressants (cyclosporine) following renal transplantation. Referral to physical therapy is for mobility training using crutches. Initial examination reveals paresthesias in both lower extremities, with peripheral weakness in both hands and feet. The therapist determines the patient is likely experiencing:

CHOICES:

1. Myopathy.
2. Quadriparesis.
3. Peripheral neuropathy.
4. Leukopenia.

TEACHING POINTS

CORRECT ANSWER: 3

This patient is experiencing peripheral neuropathy, as evidenced by the paresthesias and distal weakness in both hands and feet.

INCORRECT CHOICES:

Whereas myopathy may be a potential adverse effect of immunosuppression, it would not present as symmetrical distal weakness with paresthesias. Quadriparesis can also occur with immunosuppression, but would present with spasticity and more widespread paresis. Leukopenia is an abnormal decrease in the number of white blood cells, and can also occur with immunosuppression.

TYPE OF REASONING: ANALYSIS

This question requires one to analyze the symptoms presented in order to determine the most likely diagnosis. This is an analytical reasoning skill. For this case, the patient's symptoms are most likely caused by peripheral neuropathy. If this question was answered incorrectly, review signs and symptoms of peripheral neuropathy.

A135 | Devices, Admin., etc. | Teaching, Research, Roles

A multicenter study was done on the reliability of passive wrist flexion and extension goniometric measurements using volar/dorsal alignment, ulnar alignment, and radial alignment. Significant differences were revealed between the three techniques. An appropriate level for determining significant difference is a *P* value of:

CHOICES:

1. $P = .05$.
2. $P = .015$.
3. $P = .5$.
4. $P = .1$.

TEACHING POINTS

CORRECT ANSWER: 1

A preselected probability level of .05 indicates that the results (in this example, differences in measurements) would be the result of chance only five times of every 100 studies. This level of confidence helps us reject the null hypothesis (there is no difference in goniometric measurement techniques), and is common in most experimental studies (.01 is the other, more stringent level of significance commonly applied).

INCORRECT CHOICES:

The other choices are not the typical *P* value for determining significant differences.

TYPE OF REASONING: DEDUCTIVE

The recall of research guidelines for levels of significance is a deductive skill. If this question was answered incorrectly, refer to research guidelines and determining significance.

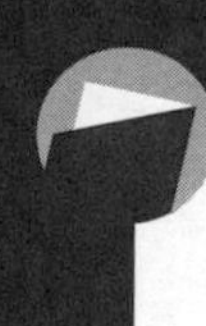

A136 | Musculoskeletal | Intervention

In treating a patient with a diagnosis of right shoulder impingement syndrome, the **FIRST** intervention the PT should consider is to:

CHOICES:

1. Implement a stretching program for the shoulder girdle musculature.
2. Iinstruct the patient in proper postural alignment.
3. Complete AROM in all shoulder motions.
4. Modulate all pain.

TEACHING POINTS

CORRECT ANSWER: 2

Without regaining normal postural alignment and scapular-humeral rhythm, the patient will continue to impinge the supraspinatus and/or biceps tendon at the acromion and never regain normal function of the shoulder.

INCORRECT CHOICES:

It is unlikely that all pain would be controlled. Appropriate AROM exercises and/or stretching could be the focus after posture has been corrected.

TYPE OF REASONING: INDUCTIVE

One must use skills of clinical judgment to determine why instruction in proper postural alignment is a first priority in intervention. Use of clinical judgment and predicting future performance is an inductive skill, an important skill for therapy practice. One must have knowledge of the nature of shoulder impingement syndrome to arrive at the correct conclusion.

A137 | Other Systems | Evaluation, Diagnosis, Prognosis

An elderly and frail patient is being seen for balance instability and frequent falls. The patient arrives for a therapy session complaining of pain and tingling in the forehead, cheek, and jaw on the left side of the face. An inspection of the trunk reveals the eruption of vesicles in the distribution of the T2 dermatome. The PT's **BEST** initial course of action is to:

CHOICES:

1. Refer the patient back to the primary physician immediately.
2. Utilize warm water wraps to relieve the pain and continue with balance training.
3. Have the patient exercise in the pool to promote pain-free movement.
4. Have the patient keep a diary, charting the course and frequency of pain over the next week.

TEACHING POINTS

CORRECT ANSWER: 1

This patient is exhibiting signs and symptoms of a herpes zoster infection (varicella-zoster virus [VZV]). This is also known as shingles; the same virus causes chickenpox in children. VZV affects the sensory ganglia of the spinal cord or cranial nerves (commonly the trigeminal nerve, CN V, and thoracic dermatomes). Early inflammation produces pain and tingling; late symptoms can include postherpetic neuralgia (severe aching or burning pain) that can persist for months or years. The best course of action is to refer the patient back to the physician immediately. Oral antiviral medications (e.g.,acyclovir) and pain meds can be prescribed.

INCORRECT CHOICES:

Other interventions listed can be used to relieve pain but may be contraindicated without a full diagnostic workup and referral. Keeping a diary to chart the course of the pain would unnecessarily delay medical treatment.

TYPE OF REASONING: INDUCTIVE

This question requires clinical judgment to determine a best course of action. One must first understand that the symptoms are indicative of the VZV, and then know the best response to these symptoms. In this case, the therapist must refer the patient back to the physician immediately for follow up. Initial intervention for this entity is outside the scope of physical therapy practice.

A138 | Other Systems | Intervention

An elderly patient is referred to physical therapy following a recent compression fracture at T8. The medical history includes osteoporosis and gastroesophageal reflux disease (GERD). The patient is currently taking antacids. Which of the following is **MOST** important for the therapist to consider in the POC?

CHOICES:

1. Schedule therapy sessions at least 90 minutes after eating.
2. Ensure that the patient eats a small snack before starting exercise.
3. Include sit-ups in supine to strengthen abdominals.
4. Recommend an over-the-counter proton pump inhibitor (PPI) medication.

TEACHING POINTS

CORRECT ANSWER: 1

Gastric contents reflux into the esophagus in GERD. Scheduling therapy at least 90 minutes after eating reduces the possibility of food remaining in the stomach and aggravating the esophagus during therapy.

INCORRECT CHOICES:

Concentric abdominal exercises (sit-ups) are contraindicated in recent thoracic compression fractures. Eating right before a therapy session may aggravate GERD. Recommending a medication change is outside the scope of a PT.

TYPE OF REASONING: INFERENCE

The test taker must infer how each of the possible choices would impact the patient's diagnosis of GERD. Therefore, one must have a solid understanding of the nature of GERD in order to conclude that scheduling therapy sessions at least 90 minutes after eating is the **MOST** important choice. If this question was answered incorrectly, review information on GERD and ideal times for activity and positioning after meals.

A139 | Devices, Admin., etc. | Equipment, Modalities

A patient with spastic hemiplegia is referred to physical therapy for ambulation training. The patient is having difficulty in rising to a standing position due to cocontraction of the hamstrings and quadriceps. The therapist elects to use biofeedback as an adjunct to help break up this pattern. For knee extension, the biofeedback protocol should consist of:

CHOICES:

1. High-detection sensitivity, with electrodes placed close together.
2. Low-detection sensitivity, with electrodes placed far apart.
3. High-detection sensitivity, with electrodes placed far apart.
4. Low-detection sensitivity, with electrodes placed close together.

TEACHING POINTS

CORRECT ANSWER: 4

When the electrodes are close together, the likelihood of detecting undesired motor unit activity from adjacent muscles (crosstalk) decreases. By setting the sensitivity (gain) low, the amplitude of signals generated by the hypertonic muscles would decrease and keep the EMG output from exceeding a visual or auditory range.

INCORRECT CHOICES:

The other choices do not achieve these goals. The wider the spacing of electrodes, the more volume of the muscle is monitored. Thus, when targeting a specific muscle, a narrow spacing should be used. When the focus is not on a specific muscle but instead to encourage a generic motion such as shoulder elevation, then a wider spacing of electrodes can be used. In addition, when working with weakness of a muscle where there is a decreased ability to recruit motor units or a decrease in the size and number of motor units, then a wider spacing and a high sensitivity would be used in order to create an adequate visible signal.

TYPE OF REASONING: DEDUCTIVE

This question requires one to recall the protocols for biofeedback training. One must determine how low-detection versus high-detection will result in different outcomes, as well as differences when the electrodes are placed close together versus far apart.

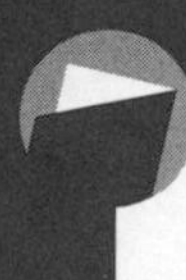

A140 | Integumentary | Intervention

A patient sustained a T10 SCI, (ASIA C), 4 years ago and is now referred for an episode of outpatient physical therapy. During initial examination, the PT observes redness over the ischial seat that persists for 10 minutes when not sitting. The **BEST** intervention in this case would be to:

CHOICES:

1. Switch to a low-density wheelchair foam cushion.
2. Increase the wheelchair armrest height, which is adjustable.
3. Reemphasize the need for sitting push-ups performed every 15 minutes.
4. Switch to a tilt-in-space wheelchair.

TEACHING POINTS

CORRECT ANSWER: 3

Excessive ischial pressure and redness from prolonged sitting require an aggressive approach. Arm push-ups, at least every 15 minutes, are indicated if redness is present.

INCORRECT CHOICES:

Switching to a high-density gel cushion and/or a tilt-in-space chair would also help over the long-term, but does not address the immediate concerns. A foam cushion is generally ineffective. Adjusting the armrest height does not remediate this problem.

TYPE OF REASONING: EVALUATION

One must determine the value in the four possible choices presented as it applies to the patient scenario. In this case, the test taker must determine which approach will provide the most immediate benefit and is effective and appropriate to the diagnosis. This requires knowledge of paraplegia and appropriate pressure relief approaches.

A141 | Musculoskeletal | Foundational Sciences

An adolescent female is referred to physical therapy with a diagnosis of anterior knee pain. Positive findings include pes planus, lateral tibial torsion, and genu valgum. The position that the femur will be in is excessive:

CHOICES:

1. Abduction.
2. Medial rotation.
3. Lateral rotation.
4. Retroversion.

TEACHING POINTS

CORRECT ANSWER: 2

Common abnormal postural findings consistent with anterior knee pain in an adolescent female include pes planus, lateral tibial torsion, and genu valgum. These are compensatory changes that occur when the femur is in excessive medial rotation.

INCORRECT CHOICES:

Abduction is associated with coxa valga (an increase in the angle of the femoral head to the neck), which is not commonly associated with knee pain. Lateral femoral rotation is commonly observed with genu varum. Retroversion of the hip is an abnormally small angle between the femoral neck and the condyles, and is not affected by posture.

TYPE OF REASONING: ANALYSIS

One must analyze the meaning of the symptoms and determine how they affect femoral position in order to arrive at the correct conclusion. This requires knowledge of biomechanics and the meaning of pes planus, tibial torsion, and genu valgum. If this question was answered incorrectly, review information on possible causes of anterior knee pain.

A142 | Neuromuscular | Evaluation, Diagnosis, Prognosis

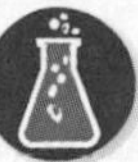

A patient is referred to physical therapy for vestibular rehabilitation. The patient presents with spontaneous nystagmus that can be suppressed with visual fixation, oscillopsia, and loss of gaze stabilization. Additional postural findings include intense disequilibrium, and an ataxic wide-based gait with consistent veering to the left. Based on these findings, the PT determines the patient is most likely exhibiting signs and symptoms of:

CHOICES:

1. Benign paroxysmal positional vertigo (BPPV).
2. Acoustic neuroma.
3. Ménière's disease.
4. Acute unilateral vestibular dysfunction.

TEACHING POINTS

CORRECT ANSWER: 4

This patient is presenting with classic signs and symptoms of unilateral vestibular dysfunction. An abnormal vestibular ocular reflex (VOR) produces nystagmus (involuntary cyclical movements of the eye), loss of gaze stabilization during head movements, and oscillopsia (an illusion that the environment is moving). Abnormal vestibulospinal function produces impairments in balance and gait. Veering to once side is indicative of unilateral vestibular dysfunction (in this case on the left side).

INCORRECT CHOICES:

BPPV is associated with episodic vertigo, nausea, blurred vision, and autonomic changes that occur with head movement, and typically stop within 30 seconds once the head is static. Acoustic neuroma is a benign tumor affecting CN VIII, and is associated with progressive hearing loss, tinnitus, and disequilibrium. Ménière's disease is associated with symptoms of nausea and vomiting, episodic vertigo, and fullness in the ear with low-frequency hearing loss.

TYPE OF REASONING: ANALYSIS

In this question, symptoms are provided, and one must analyze what those symptoms indicate. In this case, the symptoms indicate acute unilateral vestibular dysfunction. One must recall vestibular rehabilitation practice and typical diagnoses seen by PTs, including the symptoms of these disorders. If this question was answered incorrectly, review information on vestibular dysfunction.

A143 | Devices, Admin., etc. | Teaching, Research, Roles

A PT is working with a 10 year-old with cerebral palsy. Part of the exercises in the POC involves using the therapy ball. The choice of educational media that is **BEST** to use when instructing in use of this device is:

CHOICES:

1. Photos of other children using the therapy ball.
2. An oral presentation describing the therapy ball positions.
3. A DVD of another child with cerebral palsy on a therapy ball.
4. Printed handouts with stick figure drawings and instructions.

TEACHING POINTS

CORRECT ANSWER: 3

A DVD of another child with cerebral palsy on the ball represents the best choice to engage this child.

INCORRECT CHOICES:

The other choices, although important educational media, are not likely to adequately present the three-dimensional qualities of performance needed for exercising on the therapy ball.

TYPE OF REASONING: INFERENCE

One must determine which approach to education of a child will provide the best outcome in an exercise program. Inference questions require one to rely on beliefs and assumptions as a basis for decision making, which can be challenging for some test takers. In this case, the DVD is ideal to ensure proper understanding and follow-through of the exercise program.

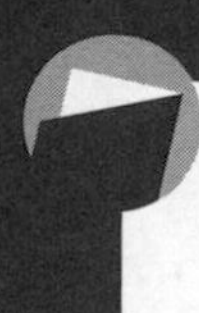

A144 | Devices, Admin., etc. | Teaching, Research, Roles

A sports PT is working with a local high school football team. During the game, a player is tackled violently by two opponents. The therapist determines that the player is unresponsive with normal respirations. The immediate course of action should be to:

CHOICES:

1. Ask for help to log-roll the player on his back, while stabilizing his neck.
2. Summon Emergency Medical Services.
3. Use the chin-lift method to improve the airway.
4. Stabilize the neck, and flip back the helmet face mask.

TEACHING POINTS

CORRECT ANSWER: 2

If the victim is unresponsive, Emergency Medical Services must be activated immediately by calling 911 (or calling a "code," if in a health care facility).

INCORRECT CHOICES:

As long as the patient is breathing, initial stabilization techniques are best left to emergency personnel or experienced first responders. It is most likely that this athlete will have to be placed on a spine board and transported.

TYPE OF REASONING: EVALUATION

One must evaluate the strength of the four possible choices presented and which one will result in the best outcome for the patient. In this question, the symptoms are significant enough that Emergency Medical Services should be summoned immediately, followed by appropriate first aid or cardiopulmonary resuscitation measures. If this question was answered incorrectly, review sports medicine and emergency guidelines and protocols.

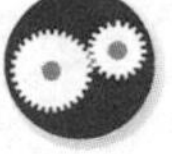

A145 | Neuromuscular | Evaluation, Diagnosis, Prognosis

During a home visit, the mother of an 18 month-old child with developmental delay and an atrioventricular shunt for hydrocephalus tells the PT that her daughter vomited several times, was irritable, and is now lethargic. The therapist's **BEST** course of action is to:

CHOICES:

1. Call for emergency transportation and notify the pediatrician immediately.
2. Give the child a cold bath to try to rouse her.
3. Place the child in a side-lying position and monitor vital signs.
4. Have the mother give the child clear liquids because she vomited.

TEACHING POINTS

CORRECT ANSWER: 1

These signs and symptoms could be the result of increased cerebral edema due to a clogged or infected shunt. Medical attention should be obtained immediately to avoid damage to the brain.

INCORRECT CHOICES:

The other choices do not adequately respond to this emergency situation.

TYPE OF REASONING: EVALUATION

This question requires one to evaluate the symptoms of the child and determine whether or not they constitute an emergency situation. In order to arrive at the correct conclusion, one must understand the nature of hydrocephalus and the use of shunts in children and symptoms that indicate an emergency. Evaluation-type reasoning requires one to make value judgments and determine the value of one's actions.

A146 | Other Systems | Intervention

A woman recently delivered twins. After delivery, she developed a 4-cm diastasis recti abdominis. The **BEST** initial intervention for this problem is to teach:

CHOICES:

1. Pelvic tilts and bilateral straight leg raising.
2. Pelvic floor exercises and sit-ups.
3. Gentle stretching of hamstrings and hip flexors.
4. Protection and splinting of the abdominal musculature.

TEACHING POINTS

CORRECT ANSWER: 4

Diastasis recti abdominis is a condition in which there is a lateral separation, or split, of the rectus abdominis. It is important to teach protection (splinting) of the abdominal musculature.

INCORRECT CHOICES:

Patients should be instructed to avoid full sit-ups or bilateral straight leg raising. Pelvic floor exercises are done, but are not remediation for diastasis recti.

TYPE OF REASONING: INFERENCE

One must understand the diagnosis of diastasis recti abdominis in order to arrive at the correct conclusion. This requires knowledge of possible pre- and postpartum conditions in labor and delivery and kinesiology, especially of the rectus abdominis muscle. If one understand the nature of rectus abdominis tears, the intervention approaches to initiate and activities to avoid are apparent.

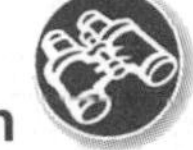

A147 | Cardiovascular-Pulmonary | Intervention

The optimal position for ventilation of a patient with a C5 SCI (ASIA A) is:

CHOICES:

1. Semi-Fowler's.
2. Side-lying, head of bed flat.
3. Supine, head of bed flat.
4. Side-lying, head of bed elevated 45 degrees.

TEACHING POINTS

CORRECT ANSWER: 3

A patient with a C5 ASIA A SCI will not have the abdominal musculature necessary to return the diaphragm to a high-domed position during exhalation. Inspiration will be affected by the change in the diaphragm's resting position. In the supine position, gravity will take the place of abdominals, holding the abdominal contents under the diaphragm, improving the zone of apposition, the height of the diaphragm dome, and therefore, the ability to ventilate.

INCORRECT CHOICES:

The other positions listed negate the positive effects of gravity acting on the abdomen to hold the abdominal contents under the diaphragm.

TYPE OF REASONING: INDUCTIVE

One must utilize clinical judgment coupled with knowledge of ventilation after SCI to arrive at the correct conclusion. The judgment in this situation entails knowledge of the effects of gravity on high–spinal level injury, including the holding of abdominal contents under the diaphragm in a supine position. If this question was answered incorrectly, review information on respiratory capabilities after spinal injury.

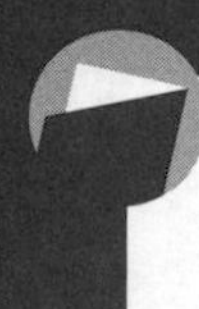

A148 | Devices, Admin., etc. | Teaching, Research, Roles

A 16 year-old patient with osteosarcoma is being seen in physical therapy for crutch training. The parents have decided not to tell their child about the diagnosis. The patient is quite perceptive, and asks the PT directly if it is cancer. The therapist's **BEST** course of action is to:

CHOICES:

1. Discuss the cancer with the patient, gently acknowledging the parents' fears.
2. Change the subject and discuss the plans for that day's treatment.
3. Schedule a conference with the physician and family about these questions.
4. Tell the patient to speak directly with the physician.

TEACHING POINTS

CORRECT ANSWER: 3

The most appropriate strategy is to hold a conference with the physician and family and discuss the patient's questions. Everyone interacting with this patient should be answering questions in the same way. A direct and honest approach is best, but must be consistent with the parents' wishes, because this patient is a minor child.

INCORRECT CHOICES:

The other choices in this scenario do not address the issue at hand effectively or respect the patient's or parents' concerns.

TYPE OF REASONING: EVALUATION

In this situation, one must consider the age of the patient and the wishes of the parents when determining the best course of action. Because the patient is a minor, it is important to schedule a conference with all involved parties to share important information with the patient.

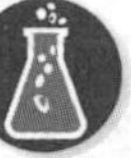

A149 | Neuromuscular | Evaluation, Diagnosis, Prognosis

A patient has a 2-year history of amyotrophic lateral sclerosis (ALS) and exhibits moderate functional deficits. The patient is still ambulatory with bilateral canes, but is limited in endurance. An important goal for the physical therapy plan of care (POC) should be to prevent:

CHOICES:

1. Radicular pain and paresthesias.
2. Overwork damage in weakened, denervated muscle.
3. Further gait deterioration as a result of ataxia.
4. Further functional loss as a result of myalgia.

TEACHING POINTS

CORRECT ANSWER: 2

ALS is a progressive degenerative disease that affects both upper and lower motor neurons. An important early goal of physical therapy is to maintain the patient's level of conditioning, while preventing overwork damage in denervated muscle (lower motor neuron injury).

INCORRECT CHOICES:

Myalgia is common in lower motor neuron lesions. It can be ameliorated but not prevented. Ataxia and radicular pain are not associated with ALS.

TYPE OF REASONING: ANALYSIS

One must have a good understanding of the nature of ALS and typical functional limitations associated with the disease to arrive at the correct conclusion. In this case, it is common knowledge that ALS presents with denervated muscles, and the potential for overwork damage in those muscles exists. This type of question requires one to analyze the meaning of the information presented and interpret the significance of it.

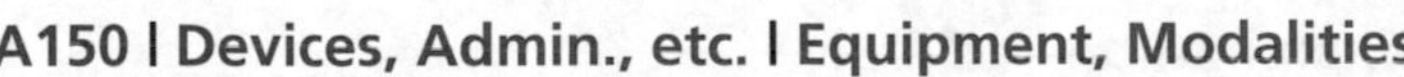
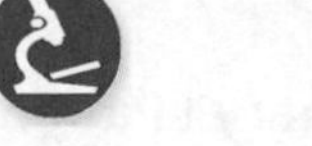

A150 | Devices, Admin., etc. | Equipment, Modalities

A patient has extensive full-thickness burns to the dorsum, of the right hand and forearm, and is being fitted with a resting splint to support the wrists and hands in a functional position. The splint should position the wrist and hand in:

CHOICES:

1. Neutral wrist position, with slight finger flexion and thumb flexion.
2. Slight wrist extension, with fingers supported and thumb in partial opposition and abduction.
3. Slight wrist flexion, with interphalangeal extension and thumb opposition.
4. Neutral wrist position, with interphalangeal extension and thumb flexion.

TEACHING POINTS

CORRECT ANSWER: 2

It is important to recall that functional resting position is slight wrist extension, supported fingers in natural slightly flexed position, and thumb partially opposed to promote proper joint position for recovery and future hand use.

INCORRECT CHOICES:

The other choices do not place the hand in a functional position.

TYPE OF REASONING: DEDUCTIVE

This question requires one to recall the protocol for functional hand position splinting after burns, which is a deductive skill. If this question was answered incorrectly, refer to splinting after burns information.

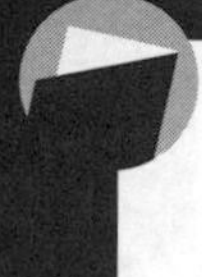

A151 | Cardiovascular-Pulmonary | Patient Examination

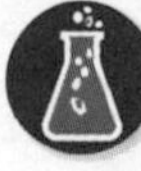

A patient is on the cardiac unit following admission for CHF and a history of an MI. The patient is currently compensated by pharmacological management and is comfortable, alert, and oriented at rest with a normal HR and BP. The telemetric ECG depicts the rhythm in Figure 1. The PT's appropriate interpretation and action is:

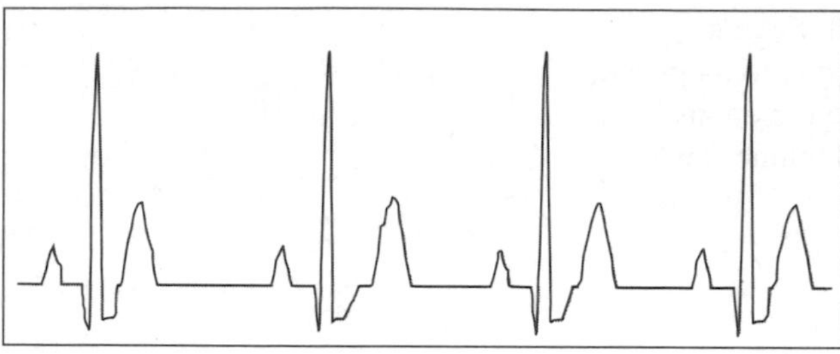

CHOICES:

1. ST segment depression; check medical record for baseline ECG.
2. Normal sinus rhythm; continue to monitor during activity progression.
3. ST segment depression; alert emergency medical personnel.
4. Ventricular tachycardia; alert emergency medical personnel.

TEACHING POINTS

CORRECT ANSWER: 1

The ECG shows ST segment depression. If ST segment depression is present during comfortable, stable rest in a patient with a history of an MI, it likely represents the presence of a nontransmural MI and is the patient's baseline ECG. However, this should be confirmed to rule out silent ischemia.

INCORRECT CHOICES:

This is not normal sinus rhythm, or ventricular tachycardia. ST segment depression alone is not an indication to alert emergency medical personnel.

TYPE OF REASONING: ANALYSIS

This question requires one to make a judgment based on information presented in Figure 1. Questions that require analysis of pictorial information often utilize analytical reasoning skill. To arrive at the correct conclusion, one must recall how ST segment depression appears on an ECG and then make a judgment for an appropriate course of action based on that information. In this case, the best course of action for ST segment depression is to check the medical record for the baseline ECG.

A152 | Devices, Admin., etc. | Teaching, Research, Roles

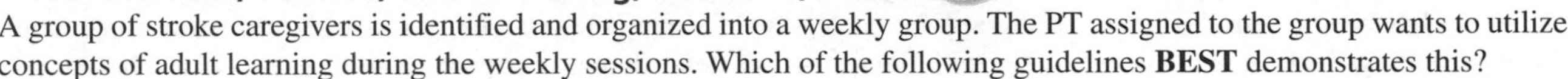

A group of stroke caregivers is identified and organized into a weekly group. The PT assigned to the group wants to utilize concepts of adult learning during the weekly sessions. Which of the following guidelines **BEST** demonstrates this?

CHOICES:

1. The therapist designs the learning experiences based on past classes.
2. The therapist determines the agenda and provides a written schedule.
3. Participants assume an active role in determining the agenda.
4. Participants are guided through their learning using constant feedback.

TEACHING POINTS

CORRECT ANSWER: 3

Guidelines to promote adult learning include allowing participants to assume active control in determining the agenda, building on the participants' past experiences, and allowing adequate time for interaction and learning.

INCORRECT CHOICES:

It is not the philosophy of adult learning for the PT to determine the agenda or the learning experiences without first consulting with the participants. Constant feedback negates active learning.

TYPE OF REASONING: INDUCTIVE

One must understand adult group learning guidelines in order to determine the guideline that is **BEST** for the type of group described. This requires inductive reasoning skill, in which clinical judgment is paramount to arriving at a correct conclusion. If this question was answered incorrectly, review adult group learning guidelines.

A153 | Neuromuscular | Intervention

An 18 month-old child with Down syndrome and moderate developmental delay is being treated at an Early Intervention Program. Daily training activities that should be considered include:

CHOICES:

1. Stimulation to postural extensors in sitting using rhythmic stabilization.
2. Locomotor training using body weight support and a motorized treadmill.
3. Holding and weight shifting in sitting and standing using tactile and verbal cueing.
4. Rolling activities, initiating movement with stretch and tracking resistance.

TEACHING POINTS

CORRECT ANSWER: 3

Children with Down syndrome typically present with generalized hypotonicity. The low tone is best managed by weight-bearing activities in antigravity postures. Typical responses include widened base-of-support and cocontraction to gain stability. Verbal cueing for redirection is generally the best form of feedback to use, along with visually guided postural control.

INCORRECT CHOICES:

Proprioceptors are not in a high state of readiness, and the child may be slow to respond to proprioceptive facilitation techniques (i.e., stretch, resistance, rhythmic stabilization). With developmental delay, this child is not ready for intensive locomotor training.

TYPE OF REASONING: INFERENCE

In this question, the test taker must draw from knowledge of Down syndrome to arrive at the correct conclusion for activities appropriate for an 18-month-old child with this diagnosis. This type of question requires inferential skill, in which the test taker must draw conclusions about the best course of intervention based on the evidence presented.

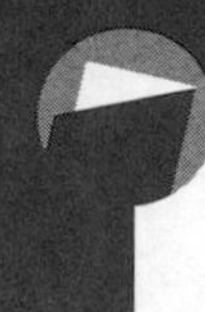

A154 | Musculoskeletal | Evaluation, Diagnosis, Prognosis

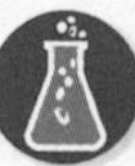

A patient has been referred to physical therapy for acute shoulder pain after shoveling snow in a driveway for 2 hours. Positive findings include pain and weakness with flexion of an extended upper extremity as well as scapular winging with greater than 90 degrees of abduction. The patient's problem is **MOST LIKELY** the result of:

CHOICES:

1. Supraspinatus tendinitis.
2. Compression of the long thoracic nerve.
3. Compression of the suprascapular nerve.
4. Subdeltoid bursitis.

TEACHING POINTS

CORRECT ANSWER: 2

Vigorous upper limb activities can cause inflammation of soft tissues surrounding the shoulder, resulting in compression of the long thoracic nerve and weakness of the serratus anterior. The serratus anterior stabilizes the scapula with greater than 90 degrees of abduction.

INCORRECT CHOICES:

Supraspinatus tendinitis or weakness does not result in scapular winging. The supraspinatus muscle in concert with the deltoids initiates abduction in the upper extremity. Subdeltoid bursitis causes pain with all AROM and does not result in scapular winging.

TYPE OF REASONING: ANALYSIS

This type of question requires the test taker to analyze the symptoms presented and make a determination of the probable diagnosis. The symptoms described indicate compression of the long thoracic nerve, and the key is in the scapular winging. This requires knowledge of shoulder kinesiology and nerve impingement syndromes of this region to arrive at the correct conclusion.

A155 | Neuromuscular | Evaluation, Diagnosis, Prognosis

A patient with multiple sclerosis (MS) demonstrates strong bilateral lower extremity extensor spasticity in the typical distribution of antigravity muscles. This patient would be expected to demonstrate:

CHOICES:

1. Sitting with the pelvis laterally tilted and both lower extremities in windswept position.
2. Sacral sitting with increased extension and adduction of lower extremities.
3. Sitting with both hips abducted and externally rotated.
4. Skin breakdown on the ischial tuberosities and lateral malleoli.

TEACHING POINTS

CORRECT ANSWER: 2

Spasticity is typically strong in antigravity muscles. In the lower extremities, this is usually the hip and knee extensors, adductors, and plantar flexors. Strong extensor tone results in sacral sitting with the pelvis tilted posteriorly. This results in a rounded upper spine (kyphotic) and forward head.

INCORRECT CHOICES:

A laterally tilted pelvis with both lower extremities in a windswept position is likely the result of asymmetrical spasticity. Hips are typically adducted and internally rotated, with extended lower extremities (scissoring position). Skin breakdown can occur on the ischial tuberosities with sacral sitting; breakdown on the lateral malleoli is not likely.

TYPE OF REASONING: INDUCTIVE

In this question, one uses their diagnostic reasoning skills to form links between the symptoms presented and the knowledge of the typical pattern of lower extremity extensor spasticity patterns. Inductive reasoning questions require clinical judgment, coupled with knowledge of the diagnosis to form conclusions. If this question was answered incorrectly, review information on MS and extensor spasticity of the lower extremity.

A156 | Neuromuscular | Foundational Sciences

A patient with multiple sclerosis (MS) has been on prednisolone for the past 4 weeks. The medication is now being tapered off. This is the third time this year that the patient has received this treatment for an MS exacerbation. The PT recognizes possible adverse effects of this medication are:

CHOICES:

1. Weight gain and hyperkinetic behaviors.
2. Hypoglycemia and nausea or vomiting.
3. Muscle wasting, weakness, and osteoporosis.
4. Spontaneous fractures with prolonged healing or malunion.

TEACHING POINTS

CORRECT ANSWER: 3

This patient is receiving systemic corticosteroids to suppress inflammation and the normal immune system response during an MS attack. Chronic treatment leads to adrenal suppression. There are numerous adverse reactions/side effects that can occur. Those affecting the patient's capacity to exercise include muscle wasting and pain, weakness, and osteoporosis, Weight loss is common (anorexia) with nausea and vomiting.

INCORRECT CHOICES:

Adrenal suppression produces hyperglycemia, not hypoglycemia. Spontaneous fractures are not typical. Hyperkinetic behavior is not an expected adverse effect.

TYPE OF REASONING: INFERENCE

This question requires one to draw conclusions about the potential chronic effects of corticosteroid therapy. It requires knowledge of the effects of corticosteroids on multiple body systems. Because of the need to make judgments for what may happen as a result of a therapeutic regimen, the question requires inferential reasoning skill.

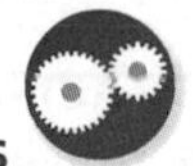

A157 | Other Systems | Evaluation, Diagnosis, Prognosis

A 24 year-old woman, who is 12 weeks pregnant, asks a PT if it is safe to continue with her aerobic exercise. Currently, she jogs 3 miles, three times a week, and has done so for the past 10 years. The therapist's **BEST** answer is:

CHOICES:

1. Jogging is safe as long as the target HR does not exceed 140 beats/min.
2. Jogging is safe at mild to moderate intensities, whereas vigorous exercise is contraindicated.
3. Continue jogging only until the fifth month of pregnancy.
4. Swimming is preferred over walking or jogging for all phases of pregnancy.

TEACHING POINTS

CORRECT ANSWER: 2

According to the American College of Sports Medicine, women can continue to exercise regularly (three times a week) at mild to moderate intensities throughout pregnancy if no additional risk factors are present. After the first trimester, women should avoid exercise in the supine position because this position is associated with decreased cardiac output. Prolonged standing with no motion should also be avoided.

INCORRECT CHOICES:

Non–weight-bearing exercise (swimming) is an acceptable alternative to walking or jogging. However, this patient's interests and skills are with jogging, making it the most appropriate choice. Exercise prescription should be specific to the individual. Using a target HR of 140 or a target date of the fifth month of pregnancy does not allow for this.

TYPE OF REASONING: EVALUATION

In this question, one must determine the benefits and risks of exercise in pregnancy. In order to arrive at the correct conclusion, one must draw upon knowledge of exercise parameters during pregnancy, including appropriate intensities and positions for exercise. This requires the skill of evaluation, or determining the value of statements and making value judgments.

EXAM A

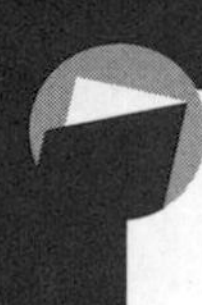

A158 | Musculoskeletal | Intervention

A patient with a grade 2 quadriceps strain returns to physical therapy after the first exercise session, complaining of muscle soreness that developed later in the evening and continued into the next day. The patient is unsure whether to continue with the exercise. The therapist can minimize the possibility of this happening again by using:

CHOICES:

1. Eccentric exercises, 1 set of 10, lifting body weight (sit-to-stand).
2. Eccentric exercises, 3 sets of 10, with gradually increasing intensity.
3. Concentric exercises, 3 sets of 10, at 80% of maximal intensity.
4. Concentric exercises, 3 sets of 10, with gradually increasing intensity.

TEACHING POINTS

CORRECT ANSWER: 4

This patient is experiencing delayed-onset muscle soreness (DOMS) as a result of vigorous exercise or muscular overexertion. It typically begins 12–24 hours after exercise, peaks in 24–48 hours, and can last up to 5–7 days.

INCORRECT CHOICES:

DOMS is usually greater after muscle lengthening or eccentric exercise. It can be lessened by gradually increasing intensity and duration of exercise, and not starting at 80% of maximal intensity.

TYPE OF REASONING: INDUCTIVE

In this question, the test taker must first determine what the cause for the patient's complaints is and then make an appropriate decision for modification of the exercise program to prevent future problems. This requires the skills of inductive reasoning, which is used when making clinical judgments, diagnostic thinking, and decisions that impact future performance.

A159 | Musculoskeletal | Patient Examination

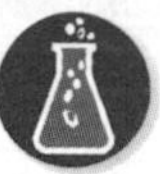

Upon examining a patient with vague hip pain that radiates to the lateral knee, the PT finds a negative FABERE test, negative grind test, and a positive Noble's compression test. The dysfunction is most likely due to:

CHOICES:

1. DJD of the hip.
2. An iliotibial band friction disorder.
3. SI joint dysfunction.
4. irritation of the L5 spinal nerve root.

TEACHING POINTS

CORRECT ANSWER: 2

A positive Noble's compression test is an indication of an iliotibial band friction disorder.

INCORRECT CHOICES:

A negative FABERE test can rule out SI joint dysfunction. A negative grind test eliminates DJD at the hip. There were no findings to implicate the L5 nerve root.

TYPE OF REASONING: ANALYSIS

One must understand the differences between the FABERE test, Noble's compression test, and grind test as well as what these tests are indicative of in order to arrive at the correct conclusion. This requires one to make determinations about the meaning of information, which is an analysis skill. If this question was answered incorrectly, review information on these tests.

A160 | Neuromuscular | Foundational Sciences

A patient suffered carbon monoxide poisoning from a work-related factory accident, and is left with permanent damage to the basal ganglia. Intervention for this patient will need to address expected impairments of:

CHOICES:

1. Motor paralysis with the use of free weights to increase strength.
2. Muscular spasms and hyperreflexia with the use of ice wraps.
3. Impaired sensory organization of balance with the use of standing balance platform training.
4. Motor planning with the use of guided and cued movement.

TEACHING POINTS

CORRECT ANSWER: 4

The basal ganglia functions to convert general motor activity into specific, goal-directed action plans. Dysfunction results in problems with motor planning and scaling of movements and postures. Patients benefit from initial guided movement and task-specific training. Proprioceptive, tactile, and verbal cues can also be used prior to and during a task to enhance movement.

INCORRECT CHOICES:

The other listed deficits (choices) are not seen with basal ganglia disorders. Paralysis, hypertonicity, and hyperreflexia occur with upper motor neuron lesions (corticospinal tract involvement). Problems with sensory organization and selection can occur with traumatic brain injury, and stroke and in children with cerebral palsy, Down syndrome, and learning disabilities.

TYPE OF REASONING: INFERENCE

Questions that ask one to predict the suspected symptomatology of a diagnosis often require the use of inferential reasoning. Here, the test taker must draw conclusions as to how damage to the basal ganglia impacts functional performance. This requires knowledge of neuroanatomy, motor learning, and neurorehabilitation in order to arrive at the correct conclusion.

A161 | Neuromuscular | Patient Examination

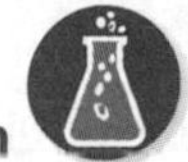

A patient presents with problems with swallowing. When the PT tests for phonation by having the patient say "AH" with the mouth open, there is deviation of the uvula to one side. The therapist then tests for function of the gag reflex and notices decreased response to stimulation. These findings suggest involvement of the:

CHOICES:

1. Vagus nerve.
2. Trigeminal nerve.
3. Facial nerve.
4. Hypoglossal nerve.

TEACHING POINTS

CORRECT ANSWER: 1

These are the tests to examine vagus nerve (CN X) function.

INCORRECT CHOICES:

Incorrect Choices: The trigeminal nerve (CN V) has both sensory and motor components. Sensory tests include pain & light touch to forehead, checks, jaw along with light touch (cotton wisp) to cornea. Motor function involves testing the temporal and masseter muscle (patient clenches teeth and holds against resistance). The facial nerve (CN 7) is tested using motor tests: raise eyebrows, frown, show teeth, smile, close eyes tightly, and puff out both cheeks.
The hypoglossal nerve (CN 12) is testing using motor tests: tongue movements.

TYPE OF REASONING: ANALYSIS

This question requires one to determine how the patient's symptoms relate to a certain diagnosis or impairment. In this scenario, one must recall the functions of the cranial nerves to determine that the symptoms presented indicate damage to CN X.

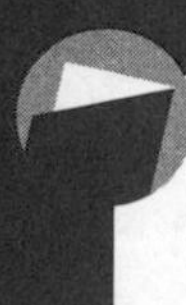

A162 | Cardiovascular-Pulmonary | Foundational Sciences

A patient with COPD is sitting in a bedside chair. The apices of the lungs in this position compared with other areas of the lungs in this position would demonstrate:

CHOICES:

1. Increased perfusion.
2. Increased volume of air at REEP.
3. The lowest oxygenation and highest carbon dioxide content in blood exiting this zone.
4. The highest changes in ventilation during the respiratory cycle.

TEACHING POINTS

CORRECT ANSWER: 2

The gravity-independent area of the lung in the upright sitting position refers to the apices of the lungs, which house the most air at REEP. The gravity-dependent area of the lungs in the upright sitting position refers to the bases of the lungs, which will house the most pulmonary perfusion. The relative increase in blood in the pulmonary capillaries around the alveoli in the bases results in less room for air in those alveoli. Because there is a relative decrease in blood in the pulmonary capillaries around the alveoli in the apices, there is more room for air.

INCORRECT CHOICES:

The apices of the lungs in that position have the least perfusion because of the effects of gravity on blood flow. The apices also have the smallest change in ventilation during the respiratory cycle because they are the most full at rest, and that area has the least ROM of the thorax. The apices of the lung have the highest oxygenation and lowest carbon dioxide content as a result of the small blood volume that passes by these alveoli. Therefore, a relatively small amount of oxygen is extracted from the alveolar air, and a relatively small amount of carbon dioxide is given off into the alveolar air.

TYPE OF REASONING: INFERENCE

One must draw conclusions about the relationship between the upright position of the patient and the apices of the lungs, which is an inferential skill. This requires knowledge of pulmonary physiology and how perfusion changes with changes in position and the effects of gravity. If this question was answered incorrectly, review pulmonary physiology information.

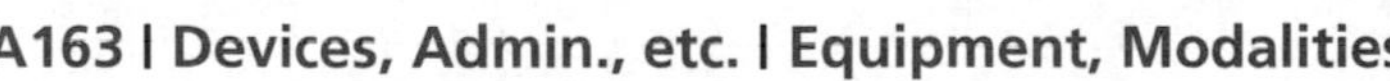

A163 | Devices, Admin., etc. | Equipment, Modalities

Checkout for a lower limb orthosis includes inspection of the alignment of anatomical and orthotic joints. During a sagittal plane checkout, the PT determines that the orthotic hip joint on a hip-knee-ankle-foot orthosis (HKAFO) is malaligned. The correct position is:

CHOICES:

1. Just anterior and superior to the greater trochanter.
2. 3 inches below the anterior superior iliac spine.
3. Just posterior and inferior to the greater trochanter.
4. Lateral to the greater trochanter.

TEACHING POINTS

CORRECT ANSWER: 1

The orthotic hip joint should coincide with a point just anterior and superior to the greater trochanter (the anatomical center of the hip joint).

INCORRECT CHOICES:

The other landmarks are not consistent with the anatomical center of the hip joint.

TYPE OF REASONING: DEDUCTIVE

This question requires one to recall protocols for lower limb orthotic fit and alignment. The recall of facts and guidelines is a deductive skill. In this case, the test taker draws upon knowledge of orthotic inspection to make the proper judgment for what constitutes a proper fit. If this question was answered incorrectly, review anatomical landmarks of the hip joint and orthothic checkout of a HKAFO.

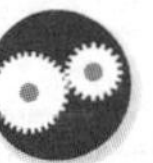

A164 | Devices, Admin., etc. | Teaching, Research, Roles

A PTA is supervising a patient's home exercise program. The patient is 6 weeks poststroke. Part of the POC includes "progressive gait training on level surfaces." The patient falls and sustains a fractured hip. The fall occurred when the PTA took the patient on the stairs for the first time. The responsible party in this case is:

CHOICES:

1. The PT, who is negligent for failing to provide adequate supervision of the PTA.
2. Neither the PT nor the PTA, because patients who have sustained a CVA are always at high risk for falls, and thus, it is a regrettable occurrence only.
3. Both the PT and the PTA, because the PT gave inadequate supervision and the PTA used poor judgment.
4. The PTA, who is completely liable because the POC was altered without communicating with the supervising PT.

TEACHING POINTS

CORRECT ANSWER: 4

Only the supervising PT can alter the established POC. In this case, the treatment plan stipulated progressive ambulation on level surfaces only. Therefore, the PT is not responsible; the PTA is responsible and negligent.

INCORRECT CHOICES:

Ongoing supervision of the PTA in a home setting is not required. Denying negligence because the patient is at high risk for falls is not relevant. The PT is not responsible. The PTA decided to include stair climbing where the fall occurred, and therefore is responsible and negligent. There was nothing in the scenario to suggest that the PTs supervision was inadequate.

TYPE OF REASONING: EVALUATION

Questions that require the test taker to make a decision based on values and judgment calls utilize evaluation skills. In this scenario, the test taker must determine who acted negligently and why. This question demonstrates how the PT was explicit about the POC, but the PTA chose to modify that plan without consent, which constitutes negligence. If this question was answered incorrectly, review roles and responsibilities of the PTA.

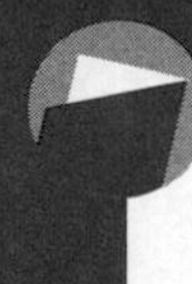

A165 | Musculoskeletal | Intervention

As the result of blunt trauma to the quadriceps femoris muscle, a patient experiences loss of knee function. The **BEST** choice for early physical therapy intervention is:

CHOICES:

1. Aggressive soft tissue stretching to remove blood that has accumulated in soft tissues.
2. Aggressive open-chain strengthening of the quadriceps femoris to regain normal lower extremity strength.
3. Gentle PROM exercises in non–weight-bearing to regain normal knee motion.
4. Gentle AROM exercises in weight-bearing.

TEACHING POINTS

CORRECT ANSWER: 4

Gentle weight-bearing AROM exercises to patient's tolerance will minimize the chance of myositis ossificans and promote improved function.

INCORRECT CHOICES:

Aggressive soft tissue stretching and strengthening can promote myositis ossificans. Gentle PROM exercises in a non–weight-bearing position is not likely to maintain knee function as well as AROM and weight-bearing.

TYPE OF REASONING: INFERENCE

This question requires one to infer or predict what may result from different intervention approaches after blunt trauma to the quadriceps femoris. This requires not only knowledge of risks associated with exercise after this type of trauma, but also awareness of myositis ossificans. If this question was answered incorrectly, review information on myositis ossificans and exercise after blunt muscle trauma of the lower extremity.

A166 | Devices, Admin., etc. | Teaching, Research, Roles

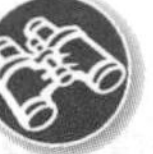

A PT is teaching wheelchair skills to an adolescent with a recent SCI. The **BEST** motivational techniques to ensure full participation are to:

CHOICES:

1. Provide structure and offer frequent feedback to ensure correct responses.
2. Keep sessions short and allow time for frequent discussions.
3. Treat the patient as an adult and incorporate the patient's goals into the POC.
4. Limit anxiety by demonstrating the techniques to the best of the therapist's ability.

TEACHING POINTS

CORRECT ANSWER: 3

Adolescents prefer to be treated as adults. It is important to incorporate the patient's goals into the POC.

INCORRECT CHOICES:

Too much structure limits trial-and-error learning, which is superior for retention of skills. Length of practice sessions should be determined by the difficulty of the skill and ability of the patient. The therapist is often the least successful model to demonstrate motor skills. Use an individual with a similar disability who has mastered the required skill (rehabilitation graduate).

TYPE OF REASONING: INDUCTIVE

This question requires one to utilize clinical judgment to reach a sound conclusion, which is an inductive reasoning skill. For this question, the test taker must consider the age of the individual in order to determine the **BEST** motivational techniques. In this case, treating the patient as an adult and incorporating the patient's goals into the POC is best. If this question was answered incorrectly, review teaching techniques for adolescents.

A167 | Neuromuscular | Patient Examination

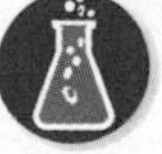

While evaluating the gait of a patient with right hemiplegia, the PT notes foot drop during midswing on the right. The **MOST LIKELY** cause of this deviation is:

CHOICES:

1. Inadequate contraction of the ankle dorsiflexors.
2. Excessive extensor synergy.
3. Decreased proprioception of foot-ankle muscles.
4. Excessive flexor synergy.

TEACHING POINTS

CORRECT ANSWER: 1

Weakness or delayed contraction of the ankle dorsiflexors or spasticity in the ankle plantar flexors may cause foot drop during midswing.

INCORRECT CHOICES:

Excessive extensor synergy would cause plantarflexion during stance. Decreased proprioception of the foot-ankle muscles would cause difficulties with foot placement and balance during stance. A strong flexor synergy can cause dorsiflexion with hip and knee flexion during swing.

TYPE OF REASONING: ANALYSIS

In this question, the test taker must determine the reasons for the foot drop, which requires analytical skills. Analysis is used whenever symptoms are provided, and the test taker must determine what the cause is for them. This question requires knowledge of hemiplegic gait patterns and likely causes for foot drop.

A168 | Devices, Admin., etc. | Teaching, Research, Roles

A patient's daughter wants to look at her father's medical record. He has recently been admitted for an insidious onset of low back pain. The PT should:

CHOICES:

1. Give her the chart and let her read it.
2. Tell her she cannot see the chart because she could misinterpret the information.
3. Tell her that she must have the permission of her father before she can look at the chart.
4. Tell her to ask the physician for permission.

TEACHING POINTS

CORRECT ANSWER: 3

The only times confidentiality can be breached are if the patient agrees, is not competent to make decisions, or is in danger.

INCORRECT CHOICES:

A family member does not have the right to medical information without the patient's permission, unless the patient is a minor child or is incompetent to make decisions. The physician cannot give permission.

TYPE OF REASONING: DEDUCTIVE

This question requires knowledge of protocols and guidelines, which is a deductive reasoning skill. In this scenario, the test taker must understand HIPAA guidelines that stipulate protection of medical information and release of information only with permission of the patient. If this question was answered incorrectly, review information on HIPAA guidelines and confidentiality.

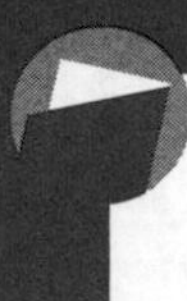

A169 | Devices, Admin., etc. | Equipment, Modalities 

Following a total knee replacement (TKR), continuous passive motion (CPM) is initiated. One of the main objectives in using CPM in this case is to facilitate:

CHOICES:

1. Active knee extension.
2. Active knee flexion.
3. Passive knee flexion.
4. Passive knee extension.

TEACHING POINTS

CORRECT ANSWER: 2

Studies have shown that following a TKR, CPM significantly increases active knee flexion ability as compared with active knee extension or passive motions. The difference is significant 2 weeks postsurgery.

INCORRECT CHOICES:

The other choices are not the focus of, nor do they derive the same benefits of, CPM use.

TYPE OF REASONING: INFERENCE

In this question, one must have a firm understanding of the indications and benefits of CPM after TKRs. It requires the test taker to draw conclusions based on prior knowledge and assumptions, which is an inferential reasoning skill. If this question was answered incorrectly, review information of benefits of CPM after TKR.

A170 | Devices, Admin., etc. | Equipment, Modalities 

The use of ultrasound (US) in the area of a joint arthroplasty is permissible, even if the surrounding area contains:

CHOICES:

1. Plastic implants.
2. Infected tissue.
3. Metal implants.
4. Neoplastic lesions.

TEACHING POINTS

CORRECT ANSWER: 3

Several studies have shown the safe use of US over metal implants. The acoustical energy is dispersed throughout the metal, and is absorbed into the surrounding tissue. There is no significant heating within the implant.

INCORRECT CHOICES:

The other choices are contraindications for the use of US.

TYPE OF REASONING: EVALUATION

One must determine the strength and logic of the statements within this question, which requires the skills of evaluation. Although the test taker must also rely on knowledge of US protocols and contraindications to answer this question, the key is in knowing the potential harm and physiological outcomes when using US over implants, infected tissue, and neoplasms. This type of knowledge goes beyond that of general protocols to facilitate one's judgment of the situation.

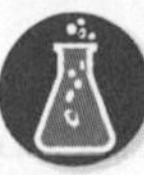

A171 | Neuromuscular | Patient Examination

A PT observes genu recurvatum during ambulation in a patient with hemiplegia. The patient has been using a posterior leaf spring (PLS) orthosis since discharge from subacute rehabilitation 4 weeks ago. The therapist has previously administered Fugl-Meyer Assessment of Physical Performance, and determined the lower extremity score to be 22 (of a possible 34), with strong synergies in the lower extremity and no out-of-synergy movement. The most likely cause of this deviation is:

CHOICES:

1. Extensor spasticity.
2. Hip flexor weakness.
3. Dorsiflexor spasticity.
4. Hamstring weakness.

TEACHING POINTS

CORRECT ANSWER: 1

A hyperextended knee can be caused by extensor spasticity, quadriceps weakness (a compensatory locking of the knee), or by plantarflexion contractures or deformity. The most likely cause in this case is extensor spasticity, which is consistent with strong obligatory synergies (stage 3 recovery).

INCORRECT CHOICES:

Spasticity in dorsiflexors is atypical and would not cause knee hyperextension. Hip flexor and hamstring weakness would result in decreased lower extremity clearance during swing.

TYPE OF REASONING: ANALYSIS

One must understand the various stages and dominant synergy patterns after stroke to arrive at the correct conclusion. In addition, the test taker must understand the Fugl-Meyer Assessment as a basis for understanding the patient's current status and potential reasons for the genu recurvatum. If this question was answered incorrectly, review information on genu recurvatum and stages of stroke recovery.

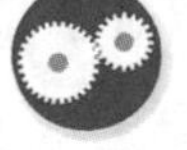

A172 | Cardiovascular-Pulmonary | Evaluation, Diagnosis, Prognosis

During a home visit, a PT is providing postural drainage in the Trendelenburg position to an adolescent with cystic fibrosis. The patient suddenly complains of right-sided chest pain and shortness of breath. On auscultation, there are no breath sounds on the right. The therapist should:

CHOICES:

1. Continue treating as it is possibly a mucous plug.
2. Reposition patient with the head of the bed flat, because the Trendelenburg position is causing shortness of breath.
3. Place the right lung in a gravity-dependent position to improve perfusion.
4. Call Emergency Medical Services, because it may be a pneumothorax.

TEACHING POINTS

CORRECT ANSWER: 4

The combined signs and symptoms of absent breath sounds, sudden onset of chest pain, and shortness of breath indicate a pneumothorax, especially in an adolescent (growth spurt) with pathological changes of lung tissue. This is an emergency situation.

INCORRECT CHOICES:

The other interventions (continuing treating, reposition the patient) do not adequately address the emergency nature of this situation, given the symptoms presented. Potential harm can come to this patient.

TYPE OF REASONING: EVALUATION

This question requires one to make a value judgment and determine the importance of the symptoms described, which is an evaluation skill. In this case, the symptoms indicate a medical emergency, with the key words being "sudden onset" of new symptoms. If this question was answered incorrectly, review information on cystic fibrosis and symptoms of pneumothorax.

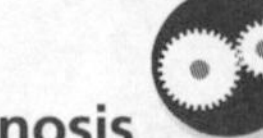

A173 | Musculoskeletal | Evaluation, Diagnosis, Prognosis

A client with rheumatoid arthritis presents at the physical therapy clinic with severe whiplash from a motor vehicle accident 1 week ago. Initial cervical radiograph results revealed osseous structures appeared intact. The client's chief complaints are of cervical pain and sudden falls with loss of consciousness. Examination reveals a positive Romberg sign and hyperreflexia. The PT's **INITIAL** action is to:

CHOICES:

1. Fit this client with a hard cervical collar and contact the referring physician recommending a computed tomography (CT) scan.
2. Immediately inform the referring physician and recommend a magnetic resonance imaging (MRI) scan.
3. Immediately inform the referring physician and recommend another series of radiographs.
4. Perform a test for transverse ligamental laxity.

TEACHING POINTS

CORRECT ANSWER: 1

This patient is exhibiting signs and symptoms of spinal cord compression with upper motor neuron signs (hyperreflexia), a positive Romberg sign, and sudden falls with loss of consciousness. This requires immediate immobilization and contact with the physician for further imaging. Some cervical lesions (nondisplaced dens fracture, rupture of the transverse ligament) require greater imaging detail than radiographs provide. This individual also has rheumatoid arthritis, which is often accompanied by erosion of the dens and facets and ligamental laxity (transverse). Immediately informing the physician is important, and if the client is exhibiting spinal cord compression, immediate stabilization is required.

INCORRECT CHOICES:

Another series of radiographs is inadequate. More detailed imaging is required. An MRI is important, but would likely miss a fracture. Sometimes, MRIs can detect fractures indirectly via imaging bone marrow edema, peripheral edema, or impingement of soft tissue structures. Because there are signs and symptoms of cord compression, it would be unwise to perform ligamentous laxity testing designed to exacerbate the symptoms. Provocation tests are performed only to clear the cervical spine of ligamental laxity, NOT when it is suspected. Upper cord signs require immediate stabilization and contact with the physician.

TYPE OF REASONING: EVALUATION

This question requires the test taker to determine a INITIAL course of action based on an understanding of the severity of the symptoms. This necessitates evaluative reasoning skill. In this case, the PT should fit the patient with a hard cervical collar and contact the referring physician to recommend a CT scan. If this question was answered incorrectly, review signs and symptoms of spinal cord compression, especially upper motor neuron signs, and imaging.

A174 | Neuromuscular | Intervention

A patient with an 8-year history of Parkinson's disease (PD) is referred for physical therapy. During the initial examination, the patient demonstrates significant rigidity, decreased PROM in both upper extremities in the typical distribution, and frequent episodes of akinesia. The exercise intervention that **BEST** deals with these problems is:

CHOICES:

1. Quadruped position, upper extremity PNF D2 flexion and extension.
2. Resistance training, free weights for shoulder flexors at 80% of one repetition maximum.
3. Modified plantigrade, isometric holding, stressing upper extremity shoulder flexion.
4. PNF bilateral symmetrical upper extremity D2 flexion patterns, rhythmic initiation.

TEACHING POINTS

CORRECT ANSWER: 4

The patient with PD typically develops elbow flexion, shoulder adduction contractures of the upper extremities, along with a flexed, stooped posture. Bilateral symmetrical upper extremity PNF D2F patterns encourage shoulder flexion and abduction, with elbow extension and upper trunk extension (all needed motions).

INCORRECT CHOICES:

Both quadruped and modified plantigrade positions encourage postural flexion. The patient needs exercises to improve postural flexibility and AROM, not strength of shoulder flexors.

TYPE OF REASONING: INFERENCE

One must recall the specific patterns of PNF and the ROM that is facilitated with each pattern. In addition, the test taker must use this knowledge of PNF to determine how the patterns will positively impact PD symptomatology, which is an inferential skill. If this question was answered incorrectly, review information on upper extremity PNF patterns and rigidity in PD.

A175 | Devices, Admin., etc. | Teaching, Research, Roles

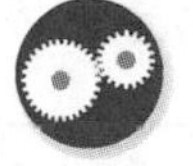

An elderly patient with diabetes is recovering from recent surgery to graft a large decubitus ulcer over the heel of the left foot. The PT is concerned that loss of range at the ankle (−5 degrees to neutral) will limit ambulation and independent status. One afternoon, the therapist is very busy, and requests that one of the physical therapy aides do the ROM exercises. The aide is new to the department but is willing to take this challenge on if the therapist demonstrates the exercises. The therapist's **BEST** course of action is to:

CHOICES:

1. Take 5 minutes to instruct the aide in ROM exercises.
2. Perform the ROM exercises without delegating the task.
3. Reschedule the patient for the next day.
4. Defer the ROM exercises and have the aide ambulate the patient in the parallel bars.

TEACHING POINTS

CORRECT ANSWER: 2

The practice of using supportive personnel falls under the Code of Ethics and under the individual practice acts of the states. Delegated responsibilities should be commensurate with the qualifications (experience, education, and training) of the individual to whom responsibilities are being assigned. In this case, it is not reasonable to assume an aide, newly arrived to the PT department, has the knowledge or skills to do this treatment. The therapist should do the ROM exercises.

INCORRECT CHOICES:

A brief orientation to ROM exercises is not adequate to ensure proper treatment. Deferral of the treatment or rescheduling does not address the concern about loss of ROM.

TYPE OF REASONING: EVALUATION

This question utilizes one's knowledge of the Code of Ethics, as well as prudent measures to take when delegating responsibilities to unskilled personnel. To determine the best course of action, one uses evaluation skills and must consider what will result in the safety and well-being of the patient.

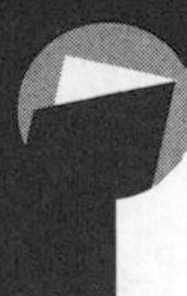

A176 | Musculoskeletal | Evaluation, Diagnosis, Prognosis 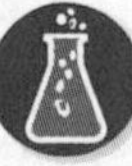

A PT is working with a client who fractured the left fibula 3 months ago. The client is still having pain with exercise. Based on the recent radiograph pictured and the given information, the prognosis for this client is:

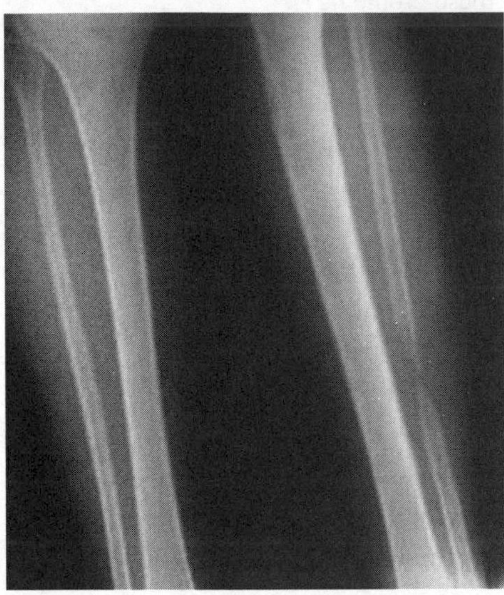

CHOICES:

1. A bone stimulator or surgery will be required.
2. Healing is proceeding normally.
3. Non–weight-bearing is indicated for complete healing.
4. This fracture will require an immobilizer boot for healing.

TEACHING POINTS

CORRECT ANSWER: 1

Normally, radiographic evidence of healing is present within 2–6 weeks (soft callus phase). This radiograph represents a nonunion fracture. A nonunion is a fracture that will not heal, and there are no signs of bone repair over a period of 3 consecutive months (bridging and callus formation are absent). Typical causes of nonunion fractures include infection, inadequate mobilization, poor blood supply, and muscle or some type of tissue interpositioned between the fractured segments. The distal tibia is more frequently the site of nonunion fractures in the long bones of the lower extremity, due to a sometimes inadequate blood supply.

INCORRECT CHOICES:

If there were bridging or a callus formation, but less than expected, then it would be classified as a delayed union fracture. A delayed union is characteristic of a fracture that has not healed within the expected time frame, and there is evidence that it will heal given time and the right environment. In the case of delayed union, a bone stimulator, change in weight-bearing status, and/or the use of an immobilizer boot for the leg may be needed. A fibular fracture typically does not restrict weight-bearing status because this is a non–weight-bearing bone.
Reference image above: http://boneandspine.com/orthopaedic-images/xray-union-shaft-fibula/

TYPE OF REASONING: ANALYSIS

One must analyze the radiograph presented and then make a determination about the prognosis for the patient, given that the patient is 3 months postfracture. This requires analytical reasoning skill, because the test taker must weigh multiple pieces of information for their significance in order to draw a reasonable conclusion. If this question was answered incorrectly, review fracture healing and radiographic evidence.

A177 | Musculoskeletal | Evaluation, Diagnosis, Prognosis

The problems associated with ankylosing spondylitis in its early stages can **BEST** be managed by the PT with:

CHOICES:

1. Postural education.
2. Pain management.
3. Joint mobilization.
4. Stretching of scapular stabilizers.

TEACHING POINTS

CORRECT ANSWER: 1

Postural reeducation will help to prevent further increases in thoracic kyphosis, and costal expansion exercise will improve breathing efficiency.

INCORRECT CHOICES:

Stretching of scapular stabilizers is not indicated because the postural changes may already have overstretched these muscles. Pain management is usually not a factor in the early stages of the condition. Joint mobilization is not a successful intervention in this progressive disorder.

TYPE OF REASONING: INFERENCE

In this question, the test taker must infer or draw conclusions as to which interventions will best meet the needs of a person with an early-onset ankylosing spondylitis. In order to arrive at the correct conclusion, one must understand that the patient's condition is progressive in nature, and that early in the disorder, the patient will benefit the most from postural education. If this question was answered incorrectly, refer to information on management of ankylosing spondylitis.

A178 | Neuromuscular | Evaluation, Diagnosis, Prognosis

A patient is referred for rehabilitation after a middle cerebral artery stroke. Based on this diagnosis, a PT can expect that the patient will present with:

CHOICES:

1. Contralateral hemiplegia with central poststroke pain and involuntary movements.
2. Contralateral hemiparesis and sensory deficits; the arm more involved than the leg.
3. Decreased pain and temperature to the face and ipsilateral ataxia, with contralateral pain and thermal loss of the body.
4. Contralateral hemiparesis and sensory deficits; the leg more involved than the arm.

TEACHING POINTS

CORRECT ANSWER: 2

A CVA affecting the middle cerebral artery will result in symptoms of contralateral hemiparesis and hemisensory deficits with greater involvement of the arm than the leg.

INCORRECT ANSWERS:

The findings presented in choice 1 are characteristic of a CVA affecting the posterior cerebral artery syndrome (central territory). The findings presented in choice 3 are characteristic of a CVA affecting the vertebral artery, and posterior inferior cerebellar artery (lateral medullary syndrome). The findings presented in choice 4 are characteristic of a CVA, affecting the anterior cerebral artery.

TYPE OF REASONING: DEDUCTIVE

This question requires the recall of neuropathology in order to make a determination of which symptoms most closely match damage to the middle cerebral artery. The recall of facts and guidelines is a deductive reasoning skill. If this question was answered incorrectly, review information on CVA and cerebral artery syndromes.

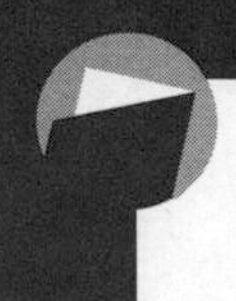

A179 | Cardiovascular-Pulmonary | Foundational Sciences

The cardiac rehabilitation team is conducting education classes for a group of patients. The focus is on risk factor reduction and successful life style modification. A participant asks the PT to help interpret cholesterol findings. Total cholesterol is 220 mg/dL, high-density lipoprotein (HDL) cholesterol is 24 mg/dL, and low-density lipoprotein (LDL) is 160 mg/dL. Analysis of these values reveals:

CHOICES:

1. The levels of HDL, LDL, and total cholesterol are all abnormally high.
2. LDL and HDL cholesterol levels are within normal limits, and total cholesterol should be below 200 mg/dL.
3. The levels of HDL, LDL, and total cholesterol are all abnormally low.
4. The levels of LDL and total cholesterol are abnormally high, and HDL is abnormally low.

TEACHING POINTS

CORRECT ANSWER: 4

Increased total blood cholesterol levels (>200 mg/dL) and levels of LDLs (>130 mg/dL) increase the risk of coronary artery disease (CAD); conversely, low concentrations of HDLs (<40 mg/dL for men and <50 mg/dL for women) are also harmful. The link between CAD and triglycerides is not as clear.

INCORRECT CHOICES:

The other choices are not accurately interpreted. In choice 1, the HDL is abnormally low, not high. In choice 2, neither the LDL nor the HDL is within normal limits. In choice 3, the LDL and total cholesterol are abnormally high, not low.

TYPE OF REASONING: DEDUCTIVE

This question requires the recall of the normal versus abnormal laboratory values for lipoproteins. It is a factual question, which often requires less value judgment but more recall of facts to arrive at the correct conclusion, which is a deductive skill. If the question was answered incorrectly, review information on these laboratory values.

A180 | Devices, Admin., etc. | Teaching, Research, Roles

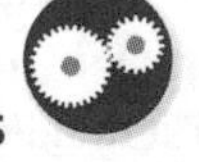

A female PT is treating a football player with an ACL sprain. She is very fond of this patient and enjoys treating him. After a few visits, the football player asks her out to dinner. The therapist's response should be to:

CHOICES:

1. Thank him very much, and invite him for dinner at her apartment with other guests.
2. Transfer the patient care to one of her colleagues, and then go out to dinner with him.
3. Thank him very much, but refuse his invitation while he is receiving treatment as her patient.
4. Thank him very much, and accept his offer for dinner.

TEACHING POINTS

CORRECT ANSWER: 3

Physical therapy departments should have a policy stating that it would be unethical to have sexual contact or dating between staff and patients. The Code of Ethics of the APTA, Principle 4 (Appendix B, Professional Roles and Management Chapter) alludes to this. Some authorities suggest a waiting period of 6 months after discharge from treatment before commencing an intimate relationship.

INCORRECT CHOICES:

Accepting his offer for dinner is not acceptable conduct. Transferring the patient to another PT does not negate the fact that the patient is still receiving active treatment by the clinic staff.

TYPE OF REASONING: EVALUATION

In this question, the test taker must make a value judgment of ethical conduct when working with a patient who makes a request such as this. Evaluation-type questions can be challenging to answer when ethical decisions must be weighed. The Code of Ethics from the APTA is the guiding force behind making the correct decision in this circumstance.

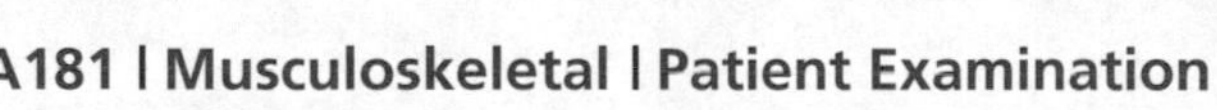

A181 | Musculoskeletal | Patient Examination

A PT is performing the maximal cervical quadrant test to the right with a patient with right C5–6 facet syndrome. The patient would most likely complain of:

CHOICES:

1. Pain in the right cervical region.
2. Tightness in the right upper trapezius.
3. Radicular pain into the right upper limb.
4. Referred pain to the left midscapular region.

TEACHING POINTS

CORRECT ANSWER: 1

The test position would consist of right cervical side-bending with extension. This shortens the upper trapezius and stresses the right cervical facets. When a pathological cervical facet is provoked, the result will cause pain in the ipsilateral cervical region, with referred pain to the ipsilateral scapular region. The test might also compress the nerve root, creating radicular signs, but only on the right side.

INCORRECT CHOICES:

This test would shorten the upper trapezius so it will not cause tightness in the muscle. Radicular pain would be consistent with dysfunction of a spinal nerve, not a facet joint syndrome. Referred pain to the left midscapular region would be caused by a test that was applied to the structures on the left side.

TYPE OF REASONING: ANALYSIS

The test taker must analyze the nature of cervical facet syndrome according to the four choices, and then determine likely patterns of pain during provocative testing to arrive at the correct conclusion. This requires knowledge of cervical anatomy and pathophysiology, as well as understanding of the maximal cervical quadrant test. If this question was answered incorrectly, review information on cervical facet syndrome.

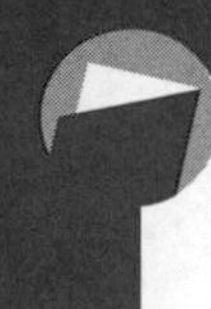

A182 | Neuromuscular | Intervention

A 62 year-old patient developed polio at the age of 6, with significant lower extremity paralysis. The patient initially wore bilateral long leg braces for a period of 2 years and then recovered enough to stop using the braces, but still required bilateral Lofstrand crutches, then a cane to ambulate. Recently, the patient has been complaining of new difficulties, and has had to start using crutches again. The PT suspects postpolio syndrome. The **BEST INITIAL** intervention for this patient based on current findings is to:

CHOICES:

1. Initiate a lower extremity resistance training program utilizing 80% one repetition maximum.
2. Initiate a moderate conditioning program consisting of cycle ergometry 3 times a week of 60 minutes at 75% maximal HR.
3. Instruct in activity pacing and energy conservation techniques.
4. Implement an aquatic therapy program consisting of daily 1-hour aerobics.

TEACHING POINTS

CORRECT ANSWER: 3

The therapist should initially teach this patient activity pacing and energy conservation techniques. It is important to balance rest with activity in order to not further weaken muscles affected by progressive postpolio muscular atrophy.

INCORRECT CHOICES:

Resistance training, conditioning, and aquatic therapy may be helpful in improving activity tolerance if kept at low to moderate intensities (not evident in the incorrect choices). They should not be the therapist's initial priority.

TYPE OF REASONING: INDUCTIVE

In this question, the test taker must have a solid understanding of the nature of postpolio syndrome in order to choose the best answer. In this scenario, because the patient is showing signs that indicate postpolio syndrome, the priority should be pacing oneself during tasks and conserving energy in order to preserve muscle function. If this question was answered incorrectly, review information on postpolio syndrome and appropriate interventions.

A183 | Musculoskeletal | Foundational Sciences

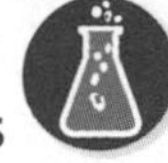

A patient diagnosed with lumbar spondylosis without discal herniation or bulging has a left L5 neural compression. The most likely structure compressing the nerve root is the:

CHOICES:

1. Supraspinous ligament.
2. Ligamentum flavum.
3. Anterior longitudinal ligament.
4. Aosterior longitudinal ligament.

TEACHING POINTS

CORRECT ANSWER: 2

The ligamentum flavum becomes hypertrophied with lumbar spondylosis and may invade the intervertebral foramen, compressing the left L5 spinal nerve root.

INCORRECT CHOICES:

The supraspinous ligament and anterior longitudinal ligaments are unlikely to compress any neurological structures based on their anatomical locations. The posterior longitudinal ligament is so small and centrally located in the lower lumbar region that it is not able to compress a spinal nerve (actually more likely to compress the spinal cord [i.e., cauda equina]).

TYPE OF REASONING: ANALYSIS

The test taker must weigh the information presented in the question and then utilize knowledge of lumbar anatomy in order to arrive at the correct conclusion. One must also rely on knowledge of the nature of lumbar spondylosis to determine what structures are most likely to compress the L5 nerve root when discal herniation is absent. If this question was answered incorrectly, review information on lumbar anatomy and lumbar spondylosis.

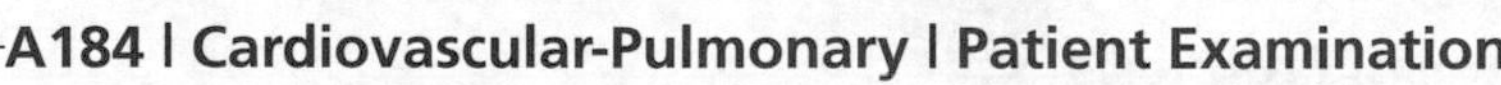
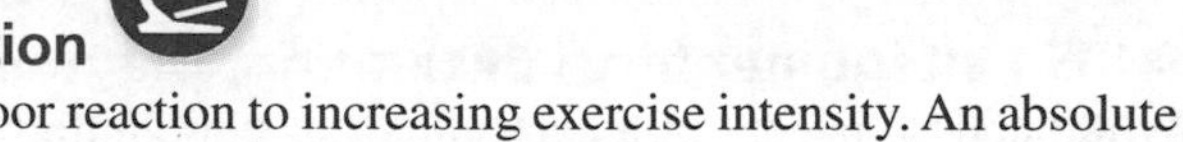

A184 | Cardiovascular-Pulmonary | Patient Examination

During an exercise tolerance test (ETT), a patient demonstrates a poor reaction to increasing exercise intensity. An absolute indication for terminating this test is:

CHOICES:

1. 1.5 mm of downsloping ST segment depression.
2. Onset of moderate to severe angina.
3. Fatigue and shortness of breath.
4. Supraventricular tachycardia.

TEACHING POINTS

CORRECT ANSWER: 2

According to the American College of Sports Medicine, an absolute indication for terminating an exercise bout is the onset of moderate to severe angina. Other absolute indications include acute MI, a drop in systolic BP with increasing workload, serious arrhythmias (second- or third-degree heart blocks, sustained ventricular tachycardia or premature ventricular contractions, atrial fibrillation with fast ventricular response), unusual or severe shortness of breath, CNS symptoms (ataxia, vertigo, confusion), or patient's request.

INCORRECT CHOICES:

The other choices (fatigue, 1.5 mm downsloping ST segment and supraventricular tachycardia) are considered relative indications and would require close monitoring.

TYPE OF REASONING: DEDUCTIVE

This question does necessitate some use of judgment. The key to arriving at the correct conclusion is in the recall of the American College of Sports Medicine guidelines that indicate when exercise should be terminated. The recall of guidelines is a deductive skill, and helps shape our clinical judgment in situations such as this scenario.

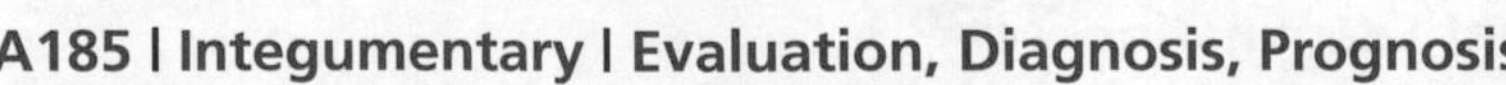

A185 | Integumentary | Evaluation, Diagnosis, Prognosis

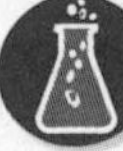

While under the care of a babysitter, this child unfortunately sat down in spilled pool chemicals, and when the child's diaper was later removed, chemical burns were present. The **BEST** terms to characterize the burn depicted in the figure is:

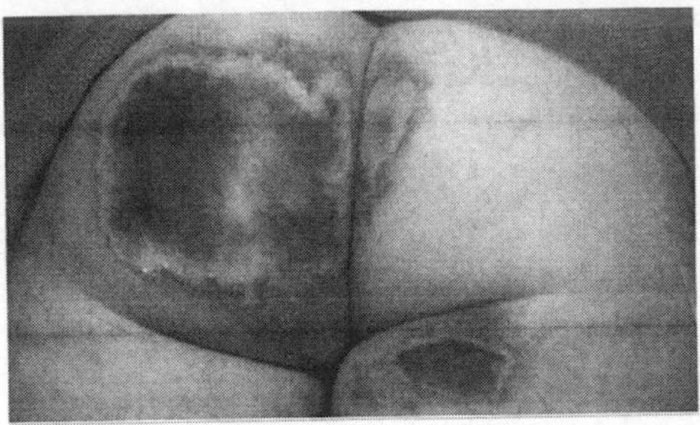

CHOICES:

1. Superficial partial-thickness burn wound with scar formation.
2. Deep, partial-thickness burn wound extending into fascia, muscle, and bone.
3. Superficial burn wound.
4. Full-thickness burn wound.

TEACHING POINTS

CORRECT ANSWER: 4

This is a full-thickness burn wound. It is characterized by white (ischemic) and black (charred) areas. Skin is parchment-like, leathery, and dry. Full-thickness burns heal with skin grafting and scarring.

INCORRECT CHOICES:

Partial-thickness burns are bright pink or red with a wet surface and blisters. This injury extends beyond the superficial skin (pink or red burn with no blisters). Superficial burns heal with minimal to no scarring. There is no indication that this burn extends down to the bone.

TYPE OF REASONING: ANALYSIS

This question requires one to analyze information in a picture, which is an analytical reasoning skill. The test taker must recall the typical presentation of full-thickness burns in order to arrive at a correct conclusion. If this question was answered incorrectly, review information on burn wound classification—differential diagnosis and pictures of full-thickness burns.

A186 | Devices, Admin., etc. | Equipment, Modalities

A patient with a T4 SCI is being measured for a wheelchair. In determining the correct seat height, the PT can use as a measure:

CHOICES:

1. Clearance between the floor and the foot plate of at least 2 inches.
2. Clearance between the floor and the foot plate of at least 4 inches.
3. The patient's leg length measurement plus 4 inches.
4. The distance from the bottom of the shoe to just under the thigh at the popliteal fossa.

TEACHING POINTS

CORRECT ANSWER: 1

The correct measure for seat height in a wheelchair is 2 inches clearance between the floor and the foot plate, measured from the lowest point on the bottom of the footplate.

INCORRECT CHOICES:

Leg measurement from the popliteal fossa to heel with customary footwear in place is used to determine footrest length on the wheelchair, not correct seat height. Clearance of 4 inches is too high.

TYPE OF REASONING: DEDUCTIVE

The measure for seat height in wheelchair prescription is a deductive skill, because the test taker must recall the guidelines for proper wheelchair fit. In this circumstance, the proper guideline is 2 inches of clearance between the floor and the foot plate at its lowest point. If this question was answered incorrectly, review information on seated examination for wheelchair prescription.

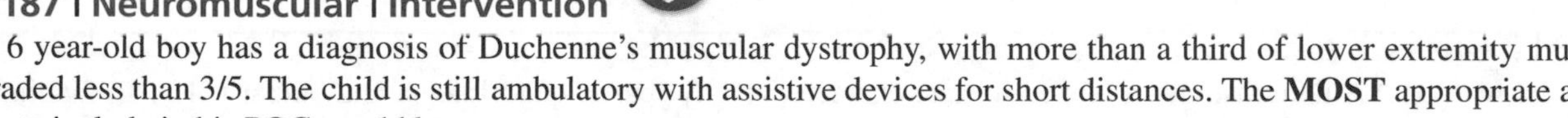

A187 | Neuromuscular | Intervention

A 6 year-old boy has a diagnosis of Duchenne's muscular dystrophy, with more than a third of lower extremity muscles graded less than 3/5. The child is still ambulatory with assistive devices for short distances. The **MOST** appropriate activity to include in his POC would be:

CHOICES:

1. Progressive resistance strength training at 80% maximum vital capacity.
2. 30 minutes of circuit training using resistance training and conditioning exercises.
3. Recreational physical activities such as swimming.
4. Wheelchair sports.

TEACHING POINTS

CORRECT ANSWER: 3

Exercise at low to moderate intensities is the general rule for patients with muscular dystrophy. Because of the young age of this child, exercise should be fun. Recreational exercise (swimming) satisfies this requirement and should be helpful in maintaining functional level as long as possible. At 6 years of age, wheelchair confinement is not usual.

INCORRECT CHOICES:

Muscles with grades of 3 or less will not benefit from active or resistive exercise. Progressive resistance strength training (choice 1) and circuit training (choice 2) can be harmful at high intensities, producing overwork injury. Wheelchair sports (choice 4) is not applicable for a 6 year-old child.

TYPE OF REASONING: INFERENCE

In this question, one must make a link between the diagnosis, the age of the child, and the appropriate interventions. Here, recreational activities such as swimming are appropriate, because the child is ambulatory and encourages maintenance of function for as long as possible. Questions such as these require one to draw conclusions based on evidence presented, which is an inferential skill.

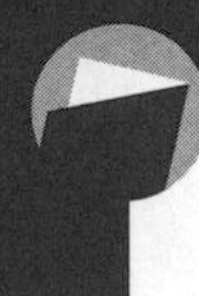

A188 | Devices, Admin., etc. | Teaching, Research, Roles

A PT works in a private outpatient clinic and sells custommade orthotic shoe inserts at a reasonable price to patients. This practice can be viewed as unethical if the:

CHOICES:

1. Therapist realizes all of the profits from the sale of the inserts.
2. Patient's ability to pay is in doubt.
3. Need for the inserts is exaggerated.
4. Inserts are provided as part of pro bono services.

TEACHING POINTS

CORRECT ANSWER: 3

PTs can provide devices (custom-made orthotic shoe inserts) at a reasonable and fair market price. The need for the device must be genuine and not exaggerated for the purposes of increasing revenues to the therapist.

INCORRECT CHOICES:

Pro bono services (from Latin "for the public good") are provided either at a reduced fee or for no fee. The therapist can provide devices pro bono if the patient's ability to pay is in doubt and the need for the device is warranted. A therapist can realize a profit from the sales if not unreasonable.

TYPE OF REASONING: EVALUATION

This question requires one to evaluate the ideas stated in the question and then determine the value of each statement. In this circumstance, the therapist is acting unethically if he/she exaggerates the need for the shoe inserts. Ethical questions can be challenging at times, because one's ethical principles are weighed against the needs of the patient.

A189 | Devices, Admin., etc. | Teaching, Research, Roles

A patient with a CVA demonstrates a locked-in state characterized by spastic quadriplegia and bulbar palsy. To facilitate communication with this patient, the PT should instruct the family to:

CHOICES:

1. Encourage use of eye movements to signal letters.
2. Give the patient a chance to mouth responses, even though vocalization is poor.
3. Look closely at facial expression to detect signs of communication.
4. Use a communication board with minimal hand movements.

TEACHING POINTS

CORRECT ANSWER: 1

Pontine lesions that result in locked-in syndrome leave the patient with an inability to move or speak, but with full cognitive function. By taping one eye open, the patient's ability to receive sensory inputs is increased (sensory deprivation is lessened) and eye movements can be used for communication.

INCORRECT CHOICES:

The family should not expect any other active motor responses from the patient.

TYPE OF REASONING: INDUCTIVE

The test taker must understand how locked-in syndrome affects functioning in order to arrive at the correct conclusion. In this circumstance, communication is best facilitated by eye movements, not other motor movements. If this question was answered incorrectly, review information on locked-in syndrome and communication.

A190 | Musculoskeletal | Intervention 

After performing an ergonomic examination of a computer programmer and workstation, the most appropriate recommendation for achieving ideal wrist and elbow positioning would be to:

CHOICES:

1. Elevate the keyboard to increase wrist flexion.
2. Maintain the keyboard in a position that allows a neutral wrist position.
3. Lower the keyboard to increase wrist extension.
4. Add armrests.

TEACHING POINTS

CORRECT ANSWER: 2

Work involving increased wrist deviation from a neutral posture in either flexion/extension or radial/ulnar deviation has been associated with increased reports of CTS and other wrist and hand problems.

INCORRECT CHOICES:

Increasing wrist flexion or extension can be harmful. Adding armrests does not solve the wrist position problem.

TYPE OF REASONING: DEDUCTIVE

This question requires one to recall the proper ergonomic guidelines for workstation function. In this scenario, it is important to prevent wrist and elbow dysfunction by facilitating neutral wrist positioning when using a keyboard. If this question was answered incorrectly, review ergonomic workstation evaluation guidelines.

A191 | Cardiovascular-Pulmonary | Foundational Sciences 

A patient with congestive heart failure (CHF) is on digitalis to improve myocardial contraction. The patient is a new participant in a phase 2 outpatient cardiac rehabilitation program. The PT expects the effects of this medication to include:

CHOICES:

1. Depressed ST segment on ECG with QT and T wave changes.
2. Increased resting HR.
3. Decreased BP.
4. Reduced exercise capacity.

TEACHING POINTS

CORRECT ANSWER: 1

Digitalis produces characteristic changes on the ECG: gradual downward sloping of ST segment with a flat T wave and shortened QT interval.

INCORRECT CHOICES:

HR is decreased (not increased). BP is unchanged (not decreased). Exercise capacity is increased (not reduced).

TYPE OF REASONING: ANALYSIS

The test taker utilizes analysis skill by determining the meaning of the information presented and then using recall of knowledge of digitalis therapy. If this question was answered incorrectly, review cardiac pharmacology and interpretation information, especially therapeutic uses and effects of digitalis.

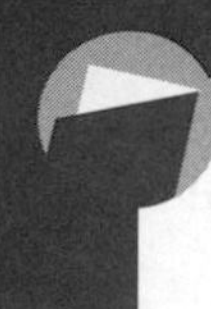

A192 | Cardiovascular-Pulmonary | Intervention

A patient is being treated for secondary lymphedema of the right arm as a result of a radical mastectomy and radiation therapy. The resulting edema (stage 1) can **BEST** be managed in physical therapy by:

CHOICES:

1. Isokinetics, extremity positioning in elevation, and massage.
2. AROM and extremity positioning in a functional arm/hand position.
3. Isometric exercises, extremity positioning in elevation, and compression bandaging.
4. Intermittent pneumatic compression, extremity elevation, and massage.

TEACHING POINTS

CORRECT ANSWER: 4

Lymphedema after surgery and radiation is classified as secondary lymphedema. Stage 1 means that there is pitting edema that is reversible with elevation. The arm may be normal size first thing in the morning, with edema developing as the day goes on. It can be effectively managed by external compression and extremity elevation. Manual lymph drainage (massage and PROM) are also appropriate interventions.

INCORRECT CHOICES:

Exercise and positioning alone would not provide the needed lymph drainage; isometric exercise is contraindicated.

TYPE OF REASONING: INDUCTIVE

The test taker must understand the nature of postmastectomy lymphedema and then recall appropriate interventions to remedy lymphedema to choose the best answer. Questions that require one to use clinical judgment to determine the best course of action in treatment utilize inductive reasoning skill. If this question was answered incorrectly, review lymphedema management guidelines.

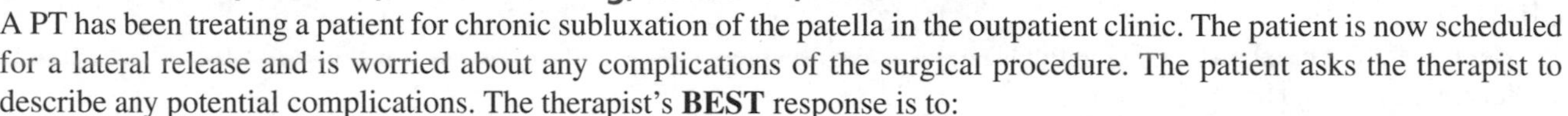

A193 | Devices, Admin., etc. | Teaching, Research, Roles

A PT has been treating a patient for chronic subluxation of the patella in the outpatient clinic. The patient is now scheduled for a lateral release and is worried about any complications of the surgical procedure. The patient asks the therapist to describe any potential complications. The therapist's **BEST** response is to:

CHOICES:

1. Refer the patient to a physical therapy colleague who specializes in knee problems.
2. Suggest that the patient speak with his/her surgeon.
3. Explain how previous patients that the therapist treated responded to the surgery.
4. Do an internet search and print out the information desired by the patient.

TEACHING POINTS

CORRECT ANSWER: 2

It is within the surgeon's scope of practice to discuss the indications and problems that could arise from this surgical procedure.

INCORRECT CHOICES:

It is not within the PT's scope of practice to be the expert that discusses problems associated with surgery. Referral should be made to the physician, not another therapist.

TYPE OF REASONING: EVALUATION

One must have a firm understanding of the scope of practice of the PT to choose the best answer. In this circumstance, if the patient queries about surgical complications, the test taker should understand that this information falls outside the PT's scope of practice and needs to refer to the person who can deliver this information, which is the surgeon.

A194 | Musculoskeletal | Intervention

A patient was referred for physical therapy after a right breast lumpectomy with axillary lymph node dissection. Scapular control is poor when upper extremity flexion or abduction is attempted. Early PT intervention should focus on:

CHOICES:

1. Active assistive pulley exercises to assist rotator cuff muscles following damage to the suprascapular nerve.
2. Strengthening of the right rhomboid to promote normal function of the scapula as a result of damage to the dorsal scapular nerve.
3. Gravity-assisted right upper extremity exercises to promote scapular control following damage to the long thoracic nerve.
4. Strengthening of the right deltoids to help stabilize the shoulder, which compensates for damage to the dorsal scapular nerve.

TEACHING POINTS

CORRECT ANSWER: 3

With axillary dissection, the long thoracic nerve may be damaged. This leads to serratus anterior weakness and loss of scapular control. Gravity-assisted exercises to promote scapular control should be emphasized early in rehabilitation to help restore proper scapular humeral rhythm.

INCORRECT CHOICES:

Because the dysfunction is associated with scapular control, the rotator cuff and deltoid muscles would not be involved. The rhomboids are important for scapular control, but they are innervated by the dorsal scapular nerve, which is not typically injured during the surgical procedure stated.

TYPE OF REASONING: INFERENCE

In this question, the test taker must recognize that the symptoms presented likely indicate long thoracic nerve damage and that gravity-assisted exercise to facilitate proper scapular humeral rhythm is required. This type of question requires one to infer or draw conclusions from the information presented to make an appropriate intervention choice.

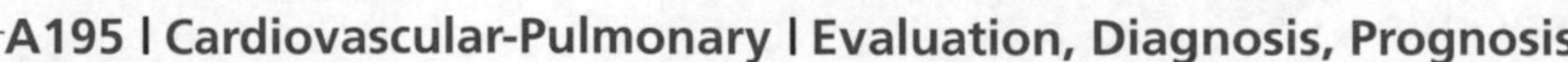

A195 | Cardiovascular-Pulmonary | Evaluation, Diagnosis, Prognosis

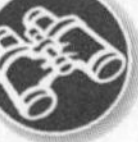

A postsurgical patient is receiving postural drainage, percussion, and shaking to reduce pulmonary congestion. The PT assigned to the case could reduce the frequency of treatment if the:

CHOICES:

1. Color of secretions changes from white to yellow.
2. Patient becomes febrile.
3. Patient experiences an increase in postoperative pain.
4. Amount of productive secretions decreases.

TEACHING POINTS

CORRECT ANSWER: 4

The purpose of postural drainage is to help remove retained secretions. If the amount of secretions diminishes, this might be an indicator that the treatment has been successful and that the frequency of treatment can be reduced.

INCORRECT CHOICES:

The other choices indicate the patient's condition is worsening. Change of secretions from white to yellow (or green) suggests a developing pulmonary infection. An increase in temperature (febrile) also suggests infection (pulmonary, wound, or urinary tract). If the patient reports an increase in postoperative pain, the patient would be unable to handle his/her secretions independent of the PT. All would be an indication to maintain the PT intervention, not decrease it.

TYPE OF REASONING: INDUCTIVE

One must utilize clinical judgment to determine what circumstances warrant a decrease in treatment frequency. In order to arrive at the correct conclusion, one must understand which of the choices indicates pulmonary improvement. In this situation, this is the decrease in productive secretions. If this question was answered incorrectly, review information on postsurgical postural drainage.

A196 | Other Systems | Evaluation, Diagnosis, Prognosis

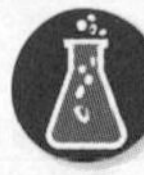

A patient is referred to physical therapy with a complaint of onset of unsteady gait. The past medical history is unremarkable except for a kidney transplant 5 years ago. Medications have included oral steroids and immunosuppression agents without adverse effects. No history of cardiopulmonary problems, recent illnesses, or other significant medical problems are admitted to in the initial interview. The patient was last seen 10 months ago by the primary care provider and 18 months ago by the immunologist. Evaluation shows increased skin turgor around the extremity joints, decreased proprioception (3/5 lower extremity, 4/5 upper extremity), flexibility and strength 4/5 lower extremity, 4+/5 upper extremity) with no difference contralaterally. Berg Balance Test was 40. The **MOST** important action for the PT to take in this case is:

CHOICES:

1. Begin progressive balance retraining, focusing on center of gravity control exercises.
2. Referral for follow-up to both physicians.
3. Begin progressive resistive strengthening exercises using a circuit training program.
4. Referral to a neurologist.

TEACHING POINTS

CORRECT ANSWER: 2

Connective tissue changes, myopathies, and neuropathies can indicate rejection in a patient with a solid organ transplant in either the acute or the chronic stage. Given the onset of the symptoms and length of time since seeing the physicians managing the care, reporting the changes and securing medical follow-up are the most important actions for the therapist.

INCORRECT CHOICES:

Although initiating an exercise program would be indicated, the stated balance exercises are at too low a level considering the Berg Balance score. Progressive resistance exercises would not be the exercise of choice due to possible rejection problems. Referral to a neurologist is not indicated.

TYPE OF REASONING: ANALYSIS

In this question, the test taker must analyze all the pieces of information presented and determine what this information means as a whole for the patient and a potential diagnosis. Questions of this nature, in which many pieces are analyzed in order to understand the whole picture, test analytical reasoning skill. In this scenario, the patient's symptoms are indicative of transplant rejection and require referral to both the primary care physician and the immunologist for follow-up.

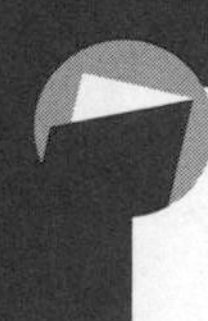

A197 | Devices, Admin., etc. | Teaching, Research, Roles

A PT arrives at work 1 hour before the work day commences, and begins moving treatment tables and rearranging the physical therapy clinic. This operation could have been done during regular hours. The therapist sustained a low back injury as a result of moving the equipment. Payment for the therapist's care relating to this incident would be covered primarily by:

CHOICES:

1. Employee's health insurance.
2. The hospital's insurance company.
3. The PT's own resources.
4. Workers' Compensation.

TEACHING POINTS

CORRECT ANSWER: 4

The employee was injured on the job, even though he or she arrived early. Workers' Compensation covers this injury because it is job-related. Prior approval by the supervisor is not a factor.

INCORRECT CHOICES:

The other choices are not relevant in this example (coverage by the employee's health insurance, the hospital's insurance, or the PT's own resources). The problem is work-related.

TYPE OF REASONING: DEDUCTIVE

Recalling knowledge of Workers' Compensation guidelines is a deductive reasoning skill. One may find it challenging to determine whether or not the PT qualified for these benefits because he/she was moving equipment before the start of the work day. However, the key is in the understanding that the employee was injured while conducting job-related duties. If this question was answered incorrectly, review information on Workers' Compensation.

A198 | Musculoskeletal | Evaluation, Diagnosis, Prognosis

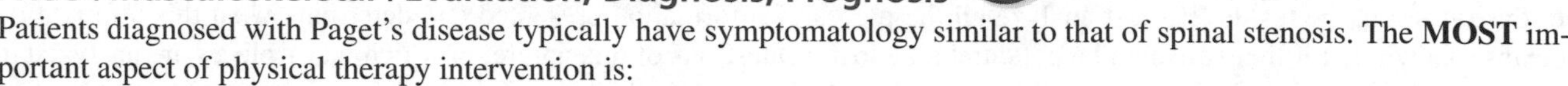

Patients diagnosed with Paget's disease typically have symptomatology similar to that of spinal stenosis. The **MOST** important aspect of physical therapy intervention is:

CHOICES:

1. Postural reeducation to prevent positions that increase symptoms.
2. Strengthening exercises for the abdominals and back muscles.
3. Modalities to decrease pain.
4. Lumbar extension exercises.

TEACHING POINTS

CORRECT ANSWER: 1

Patients should be educated to minimize certain positions for long periods. Symptoms resulting from Paget's disease are aggravated by positions in which the lumbar spine is in extension.

INCORRECT CHOICES:

Because this is a chronic condition, modalities are not the most effective management strategy. Lumbar extension exercises decrease the space within the vertebral foramen, thereby increasing symptoms of pain associated with stenosis and Paget's disease. Strengthening exercises for the abdominal and back muscles do not affect the disease processes of slowly progressive enlargement and deformity of multiple bones.

TYPE OF REASONING: ANALYSIS

It is important to make the link between symptoms of spinal stenosis and Paget's disease when answering this question because the intervention approaches are similar. One utilizes analysis skill by determining the meaning of the information provided and then linking this information to the best intervention approach. If this question was answered incorrectly, refer to information on Paget's disease.

A199 | Devices, Admin., etc. | Equipment, Modalities

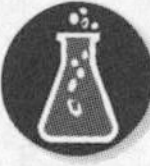

A patient with spastic left hemiplegia experiences severe genu recurvatum during stance phase. The patient is using a double upright metal ankle-foot orthosis (AFO). The cause of the problem might be attributed to the:

CHOICES:

1. Anterior stop, setting the foot in too much plantarflexion.
2. Posterior stop, setting the foot in too much dorsiflexion.
3. AFO, which is not indicated for this patient.
4. Orthosis, allowing for excessive sagittal motion of the foot in stance.

TEACHING POINTS

CORRECT ANSWER: 1

An AFO can be used to assist in knee control for the patient with hemiplegia. An anterior stop that limits dorsiflexion (foot is set in slight plantarflexion) helps create an extension moment at the knee and can thus assist in stabilizing the knee during stance.

INCORRECT CHOICES:

A posterior stop set in about 5 degrees of dorsiflexion imposes a flexion force at the knee at midstance. Thus, it prevents a lax knee from hyperextending. A hinged solid AFO provides slight sagittal motion, aiding in foot-flat position early in stance. An AFO can be indicated in this case.

TYPE OF REASONING: ANALYSIS

One must have a firm understanding of a double upright AFO to arrive at the correct conclusion. If this question was answered incorrectly, review information on uses of double upright AFOs and proper use of anterior/posterior stops settings.

A200 | Cardiovascular-Pulmonary | Evaluation, Diagnosis, Prognosis

A patient complains of difficulty walking. At rest, the skin in the lower leg appears discolored. After walking for about 2 minutes, the patient complains of pain in the leg. A marked pallor is also evident in the skin over the lower third of the extremity. The PT suspects:

CHOICES:

1. Neurogenic claudication.
2. Restless leg syndrome.
3. Vascular claudication.
4. Peripheral neuropathy.

TEACHING POINTS

CORRECT ANSWER: 3

Intermittent claudication (leg pain) occurs with peripheral vascular disease (PVD). Exercising the extremity to the point of claudication results in the development of pain, along with increased pallor of the skin. Pulses may also be decreased or absent because of ischemia. The hallmark of claudication pain is that it is relieved with rest.

INCORRECT CHOICES:

The other choices are all nonvascular causes of leg pain. Neurogenic claudication is associated with burning pain and dysesthesias. Peripheral neuropathy produces aching pain with sensory loss and numbness of the feet. It can progress to involve the hands (stocking and glove distribution). Motor weakness and muscle atrophy can occur (chronic sensorimotor neuropathy) along with autonomic changes (autonomic neuropathy). Restless leg syndrome is associated with "creeping" or "crawling" sensations in the legs that result in involuntary movements.

TYPE OF REASONING: INDUCTIVE

The question requires one to use diagnostic (inductive) thinking. One must recognize the signs and symptoms of each of the choices. If this question was answered incorrectly, review information on PVD and claudication, along with the other conditions mentioned.

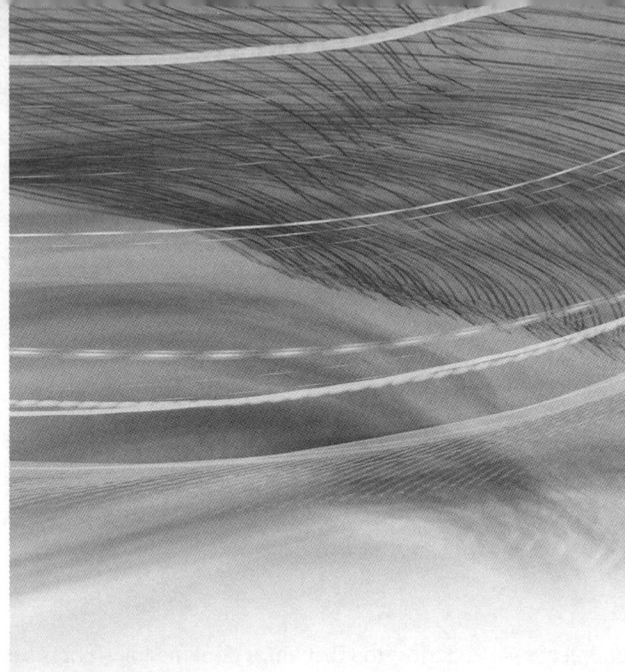

Examination B

B1 | Neuromuscular | Foundational Sciences

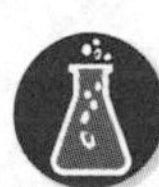

A physical therapy plan of care for a child with spastic cerebral palsy who is 3 years old chronologically and cognitively, but at a 6 month-old gross developmental level would include:

CHOICES:

1. Reaching for a black and white object while in the supine position.
2. Reaching for a multicolored object while in an unsupported standing position.
3. Reaching for a multicolored object while in an unsupported, guarded sitting position.
4. Visually tracking a black and white object held 9 inches from his/her face.

TEACHING POINTS

CORRECT ANSWER: 3

The appropriate task would include the 6 month-old gross developmental level activity of working on unsupported sitting.

INCORRECT CHOICES:

Standing and supine are not appropriate choices (too advanced or not advanced enough). The use of a multicolored object is more appropriate than a black and white object for a 3 year-old cognitive level.

TYPE OF REASONING: ANALYSIS

In this question, the test taker must take into consideration the chronological, cognitive, and gross developmental levels of the child in order to arrive at the correct conclusion. In this scenario, the test taker must provide the appropriate physical challenge for a child developmentally functioning at 6 months in gross development, while providing activities that are appropriate for the 3 year-old cognitive level. If this question was answered incorrectly, review motor and cognitive developmental milestones.

B2 | Musculoskeletal | Intervention

A patient is receiving mobilizations to regain normal mid thoracic extension. After three sessions, the patient complains of localized pain that persists for greater than 24 hours. The therapist's treatment should:

CHOICES:

1. Continue with current mobilizations, followed by a cold pack to the thoracic spine.
2. Place the physical therapy on hold and resume in 1 week.
3. Change mobilizations to gentle, low-amplitude oscillations to reduce the joint and soft tissue irritation.
4. Change to self-stretching activities, because the patient does not tolerate mobilization.

TEACHING POINTS

CORRECT ANSWER: 3

Changing to low-amplitude oscillations will promote a decrease in the pain and tissue irritation. If pain persists for over 24 hours, the soft tissue and joint irritation may progress.

INCORRECT CHOICES:

Pain beyond 24 hours indicates possible tissue damage, so modification would be indicated. Placing the patient on hold would not be indicated or appropriate based on the patient's response. Self-stretching will improve the osteokinematic motion, but not the arthrokinematic motion, so this would not be an appropriate modification.

TYPE OF REASONING: INFERENCE

This question requires one to understand joint mobilization techniques, coupled with recognition of possible results that may occur when utilizing the techniques. In this scenario, the patient's symptoms indicate that the joint mobilization techniques resulted in soft tissue and joint irritation. Therefore, the therapist should consider less irritating mobilization for improved tolerance. If this question was answered incorrectly, refer to joint mobilization information.

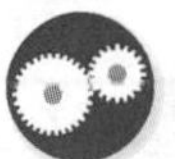

B3 | Neuromuscular | Intervention

A therapist wishes to use behavior modification techniques as part of a plan of care to help shape the behavioral responses of a patient recovering from traumatic brain injury (TBI). The **BEST** form of intervention is to:

CHOICES:

1. Reprimand the patient every time an undesirable behavior occurs.
2. Use frequent reinforcements for all desired behaviors.
3. Allow the patient enough time for self-correction of the behavior.
4. Encourage the staff to tell the patient which behaviors are correct and which are not.

TEACHING POINTS

CORRECT ANSWER: 2

Behavioral modification is best achieved through use of positive reinforcements for all desired behaviors.

INCORRECT CHOICES:

Negative behaviors should be ignored, not reprimanded. Self-correction is not a form of behavior modification.

TYPE OF REASONING: EVALUATION

The test taker utilizes knowledge of behavioral modification techniques to choose the correct answer in this scenario. Using evaluative skills, one determines the value of each of the four choices, and which choice is most aligned with behavioral modification guidelines to promote positive behaviors via positive reinforcement techniques.

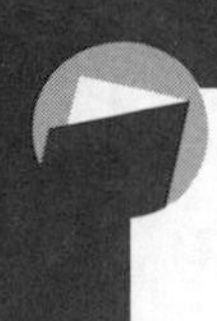

B4 | Neuromuscular | Evaluation, Diagnosis, Prognosis

A patient with multiple sclerosis (MS) presents with dysmetria in both upper extremities. Which of the following interventions is the **BEST** choice to deal with this problem?

CHOICES:

1. 3-lb weight cuffs to wrists during activities of daily living (ADL) training.
2. Pool exercises using water temperatures greater than 85 degrees F.
3. Proprioceptive neuromuscular facilitation (PNF) patterns using dynamic reversals with carefully graded resistance.
4. Isokinetic training using low resistance and fast movement speeds.

TEACHING POINTS

CORRECT ANSWER: 3

Dysmetria is a coordination problem in which the patient is unable to judge the distance or range of movement (overshoots or undershoots a target). Adding manual resistance with PNF can assist the patient in slowing down the movement and achieving better control.

INCORRECT CHOICES:

The patient lacks speed control. Low-resistance, fast-speed isokinetic training is contraindicated. The resistance of water (pool therapy) could help control the speed of movements, but the temperature is too warm (patients with MS demonstrate heat intolerance). Weight cuffs could also help slow the movements down, but would unnecessarily fatigue the patient (patients with MS demonstrate problems with excessive fatigue).

TYPE OF REASONING: INFERENCE

One must understand the deficit of dysmetria in order to arrive at the correct conclusion. Using skills of inference, the test taker uses the knowledge of dysmetria to determine what course of action is useful to promote improved coordination and motor control. If this question was answered incorrectly, review information on dysmetria.

B5 | Devices, Admin., etc. | Equipment, Modalities

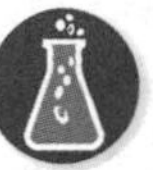

A patient suffered recent fractures of C4 and C5 following trauma received in a motor vehicle accident. Maximum stabilization of his cervical spine can **BEST** be achieved with a:

CHOICES:

1. Four-poster orthosis.
2. Philadelphia collar.
3. Halo orthosis.
4. Milwaukee orthosis.

TEACHING POINTS

CORRECT ANSWER: 3

Maximum stabilization of the cervical spine can be achieved with the use of a halo orthosis. It contains a ring that is attached to the skull by four screws, and two anterior and two posterior uprights that connect the ring to a thoracic orthosis.

INCORRECT CHOICES:

A four-poster orthosis uses a chin and occipital pad, attached to two anterior and two posterior uprights, connected to a thoracic orthosis. It provides moderate control. A Philadelphia collar utilizes a mandibular and occipital extension with a rigid anterior strut. It provides minimal control and is contraindicated. A Milwaukee orthosis is used to stabilize scoliosis. Its frame includes a pelvic girdle, two posterior uprights, and an anterior upright that attaches to a superior upper chest ring.

TYPE OF REASONING: ANALYSIS

In this question, the test taker must be familiar with the four orthoses and their indications for stabilization after cervical fracture. In this case, the halo orthosis provides the most stability. If this question was answered incorrectly, refer to stabilization procedures after cervical fracture.

B6 | Cardiovascular-Pulmonary | Intervention

A patient recovering from cardiac transplantation for end-stage heart failure is referred for exercise training. The patient is receiving immunosuppressive drug therapy (cyclosporine and prednisone). The therapist recognizes that this patient will:

CHOICES:

1. Require longer periods of warm-up and cool-down.
2. Be unable to perform resistance training.
3. Require a frequency of 2–3 times/week.
4. Require short bouts of exercise.

TEACHING POINTS

CORRECT ANSWER: 1

A patient recovering from cardiac transplantation will require longer periods of warm-up and cool-down, because physiological responses to exercise and recovery take longer.

INCORRECT CHOICES:

Low- to moderate-intensity resistance training can be performed. Aerobic exercise should be performed 4–6 times/week, while progressively increasing the duration of training from 15 to 60 minutes per session. (Source: *ACSM Guidelines for Exercise Testing and Prescription*).

TYPE OF REASONING: INFERENCE

This question requires the test taker to infer what may be true of a patient, given the diagnosis of cardiac transplantation. Inferential reasoning skills are utilized whenever one must predict a best course of action or determine what may be true of a person or situation. In this case, the therapist should recognize that the patient will require longer periods of warm-up and cool-down. If this question was answered incorrectly, review exercise guidelines for patients with cardiac transplantation.

B7 | Neuromuscular | Patient Examination

A patient presents with weakness and atrophy of the biceps brachii resulting from an open fracture of the humerus. The therapist's examination includes needle electromyography (EMG) of the biceps. The muscle response anticipated after the needle is inserted and prior to asking the patient to contract the muscle is:

CHOICES:

1. Fibrillation potentials.
2. Electrical silence.
3. Polyphasic potentials.
4. Interference patterns.

TEACHING POINTS

CORRECT ANSWER: 2

Inserting an EMG needle into a normal muscle causes a burst of electrical activity (insertional activity), after which the muscle produces no sound (electrical silence).

INCORRECT CHOICES:

Fibrillation potentials are spontaneous activity seen in relaxed denervated muscle, and polyphasic potentials are produced in the contracted muscle undergoing reorganization.

TYPE OF REASONING: INFERENCE

One must understand the expected responses to EMG needle insertion in order to arrive at the correct conclusion. Inferential skills are used whenever one must determine what may occur based on facts and evidence. In this situation, the test taker must infer what happens after needle insertion and before muscle contraction.

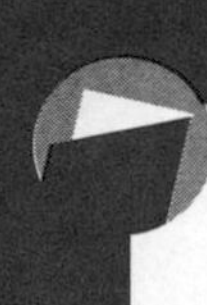

B8 | Other Systems | Evaluation, Diagnosis, Prognosis 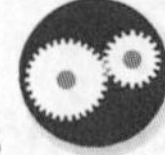

A new staff physical therapist (PT) on the oncology unit of a large medical center receives a referral for strengthening and ambulation for a woman with ovarian cancer. She is undergoing radiation therapy after a surgical hysterectomy. Her current platelet count is 17,000. The treatment of **GREATEST BENEFIT** for this patient at this time is:

CHOICES:

1. Resistance training at 40%, one repetition maximum.
2. Progressive stair climbing using a weighted waist belt.
3. Active range of motion (AROM) exercises.
4. Resistance training at 60%, one repetition maximum.

TEACHING POINTS

CORRECT ANSWER: 3

AROM and ADL exercises are beneficial for this patient.

INCORRECT CHOICES:

Resistive exercise is contraindicated in patients with significant bony metastases, osteoporosis, or low platelet count (<20,000).

TYPE OF REASONING: EVALUATION

One must utilize knowledge of normal platelet counts and contraindications for resistive exercise in patients with cancer. In this situation, the patient's platelet count is low, which should alert the test taker that resistive exercise should be deferred. Questions such as these require one to review the merits of a situation, which is an evaluative skill. Knowledge of normal blood counts is very useful information.

B9 | Other Systems | Intervention 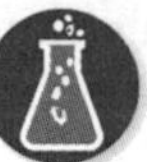

A patient complains of increased pain and tingling in both hands after sitting at a desk for longer than 1 hour. The diagnosis is thoracic outlet syndrome [TOS]. Which treatment would be the **MOST** effective physical therapy intervention?

CHOICES:

1. Strengthening program for the scalenes and sternocleidomastoids.
2. Stretching program for the pectoralis minor and scalenes.
3. Cardiovascular training using cycle ergometry to reduce symptoms of TOS.
4. Desensitization by maintaining the shoulder in abduction, extension, and external rotation with the head turned toward the ipsilateral shoulder.

TEACHING POINTS

CORRECT ANSWER: 2

TOS is described as compression to the neurovascular structures in the scalene triangle, the area defined by the anterior and middle scalenes between the clavicle and the first rib. The compression is a result of a shortened pectoralis minor and scalene muscles. Therefore, a stretching program to these muscles to gain space in the scalene triangle is appropriate.

INCORRECT CHOICES:

Shortening of the scalenes and sternocleidomastoids may be the culprit that caused TOS to develop. Strengthening these muscles would not improve the amount of space in the scalene triangle space. Cardiovascular training, especially performed in the posture using a cycle ergometer, would not improve the disorder. The problem in TOS is too much vascular volume in too small a space. Increasing the vascular volume through that space with cardiovascular exercise will not resolve the symptoms of TOS. Desensitization by putting the shoulder and neck in this position is likely to diminish the space in the scalene triangle and further compress the neurovascular structures that run through that triangle.

TYPE OF REASONING: ANALYSIS

This requires analytical reasoning. If this question was answered incorrectly, review the causes and interventions for TOS.

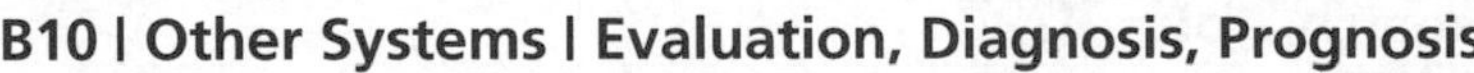

B10 | Other Systems | Evaluation, Diagnosis, Prognosis

A patient with diabetes is exercising. The patient reports feeling weak, dizzy, and somewhat nauseous. The therapist notices that the patient is sweating profusely and is unsteady when standing. The therapist's **BEST** immediate course of action is to:

CHOICES:

1. Call for Emergency Services; the patient is having an insulin reaction.
2. Have a nurse administer an insulin injection for developing hyperglycemia.
3. Insist that the patient sit down until the orthostatic hypotension resolves.
4. Administer orange juice for developing hypoglycemia.

TEACHING POINTS

CORRECT ANSWER: 4

Hypoglycemia, or abnormally low blood glucose, results from too much insulin (insulin reaction). It requires accurate assessment of symptoms and prompt intervention. Have the patient sit down and give an oral sugar (e.g., orange juice).

INCORRECT CHOICES:

Once the patient is stabilized, the physician should be notified. Emergency Services are generally not needed. Profuse sweating does not usually accompany orthostatic hypotension.

TYPE OF REASONING: INDUCTIVE

The test taker must first determine the cause of the patient's symptoms and then the appropriate course of action. Questions such as these utilize one's clinical judgment and diagnostic thinking, which is an inductive reasoning skill. One should recognize that these symptoms are indicative of hypoglycemia and require immediate administration of sugar to relieve symptoms.

B11 | Neuromuscular | Evaluation, Diagnosis, Prognosis

A patient with postpolio syndrome started attending a supervised outpatient exercise program. The patient failed to show up for follow-up sessions. The patient reported increased muscle pain and being too weak to get out of bed for the past 2 days. The patient is afraid to continue with the exercise class. The therapist's **BEST** course of action regarding exercise is to:

CHOICES:

1. Decrease the intensity and duration, but maintain a frequency of 3 times/week.
2. Discharge the patient from the program because exercise is counterproductive in postpolio syndrome.
3. Decrease the frequency to once a week for an hour session, keeping the intensity moderate.
4. Reschedule exercise workouts for early morning when there is less fatigue.

TEACHING POINTS

CORRECT ANSWER: 1

Clinical manifestations of postpolio syndrome include myalgias, new weakness as well as atrophy, and excessive fatigue with minimal activity. Nonexhaustive exercise and general body conditioning are indicated. A change in the exercise prescription (intensity and duration) is warranted.

INCORRECT CHOICES:

The patient should not exercise to the point of fatigue and exhaustion. A frequency of once a week is too little to be beneficial. Rescheduling exercise to early morning does not address the needed change in exercise prescription. Stopping exercise completely will not help this patient.

TYPE OF REASONING: INFERENCE

This question requires the test taker first to understand the nature of postpolio syndrome and then determine the appropriate exercise regimen to prevent further exacerbation of symptoms. Therefore, one must infer, or draw conclusions, from the evidence presented to arrive at the correct decision. If this question was answered incorrectly, review information on postpolio syndrome.

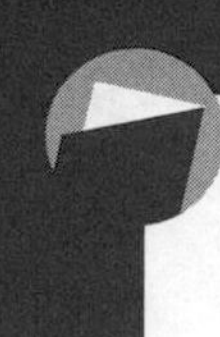

B12 | Devices, Admin., etc. | Teaching, Research, Roles 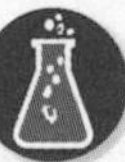

A physical therapy student is on a final clinical rotation. The supervising PT becomes aware that the student tends to process information all at once, not in an ordered step-by-step manner. The therapist's **BEST** strategy to ensure adequate learning for this student is to:

CHOICES:

1. Redirect the student to process information in a step-by-step manner.
2. Focus the student on objective information and interrelationships.
3. Focus the student on learning important relationships and concepts.
4. Provide real-life examples that link learning to personal experiences.

TEACHING POINTS

CORRECT ANSWER: 4

This student learns best using an intuitive or global learning style. The student processes information all at once, and will learn best if information is connected to personal experiences and presented in practical, real-life experiences.

INCORRECT CHOICES:

Sequential learning and focusing on objectives or concepts are better choices for an analytical/objective type of learner.

TYPE OF REASONING: ANALYSIS

One must link how the student's processing of information all at once requires a change in teaching approach to promote improved learning. In this situation, students who learn in this matter require real-life examples and links to personal experience. For this type of question, the test taker must weigh the information presented and analyze which choice best represents the correct answer.

B13 | Cardiovascular-Pulmonary | Intervention 

A patient is recovering from open heart surgery (coronary artery bypass graft [CABG]). The PT supervising the patient's outpatient exercise program at 8 weeks postsurgery recognizes that resistance training with moderate to heavy weights:

CHOICES:

1. Is absolutely contraindicated.
2. Should include upper body exercises only.
3. Should be based on 60–80%, 1 repetition maximum initially.
4. Should be avoided during the first 3 months.

TEACHING POINTS

CORRECT ANSWER: 4

Moderate to heavy resistance exercises should be avoided until the sternum has healed, generally by 3 months. Patients with sternal movement or wound infection should perform lower extremity resistance exercises only.

INCORRECT CHOICES:

Once cleared, initial loads for the upper body should be 30–40%, 1 repetition max, and 50–60% for hips and legs. (Source: *ACSM Guidelines for Exercise Testing and Prescription.*)

TYPE OF REASONING: DEDUCTIVE

One must recall the guidelines for cardiac exercise post-CABG in order to arrive at a correct conclusion. This requires recall of factual guidelines, which is a deductive reasoning skill. For this question, the key words are "8 weeks' postsurgery," which should draw one to conclude that resistance training with moderate to heavy weights should be avoided during the first 3 months. If this question was answered incorrectly, review cardiac exercise guidelines, especially post-CABG.

B14 | Cardiovascular-Pulmonary | Foundational Sciences

A patient is taking a drug from the sympathomimetic group, albuterol (Ventalin). What is the **MOST** important effect of this medication?

CHOICES:

1. Increases airway resistance and decreases secretion production.
2. Reduces airway resistance by reducing bronchospasm.
3. Reduces bronchial constriction and high blood pressure (BP) that accompanies exercise.
4. Increases heart rate (HR) and BP to enhance a training effect during aerobic activity.

TEACHING POINTS

CORRECT ANSWER: 2

Sympathomimetics are a class of drugs that mimic the effects of stimulation of body organs and structures by the sympathetic nervous system. Albuterol (Ventalin) has the primary action of reducing airway resistance by a decrease in bronchospasm.

INCORRECT CHOICES:

Albuterol decreases airway resistance and has no effect on the volume or consistency of airway secretions. The primary effects of albuterol are on β_2 receptors in the bronchiole smooth muscle. It may also have an effect on β_1 receptors, producing cardiovascular adverse reactions of increased BP and tachycardia. These adverse effects can result in a patient monitoring exercise parameters at lower exercise workloads and reducing aerobic training effects.

TYPE OF REASONING: INFERENCE

This question, while requiring knowledge of the effects and side effects of medication (a deductive skill), also requires one to determine the **MOST** important effects (not adverse effects). Therefore, this question utilizes inferential reasoning, in which the test taker must draw conclusions based on the information presented and determine what is most important, which encourages inferential deductive reasoning. If this question was answered incorrectly, refer to information on sympathomimetic medications.

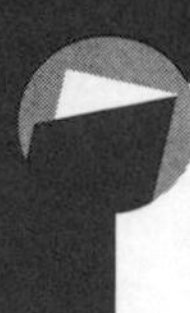

B15 | Other Systems | Foundational Sciences

A PT decides to exercise a patient with lower extremity lymphedema using aquatic therapy. Hydrostatic pressure exerted by the water can be expected to:

CHOICES:

1. Provide joint unloading and enhance ease of active movement.
2. Reduce effusion and assist venous return.
3. Increase resistance as speed of movement increases.
4. Increase cardiovascular demands at rest and with exercise.

TEACHING POINTS

CORRECT ANSWER: 2

The pressure exerted by water on an immersed object is equal on all surfaces (Pascal's law). As the depth of immersion increases, so does hydrostatic pressure. Increased pressure limits effusion, assists venous return, and can induce bradycardia.

INCORRECT CHOICES:

The other choices do not relate directly to hydrostatic pressure. Buoyancy of water provides an environment of relative weightlessness and assists in joint unloading and active movement. Hydromechanics, movement of water molecules, increases the resistance of water as speed of movement increases. Hot water immersion (>35 degrees C) can increase cardiovascular demands at rest and with exercise.

TYPE OF REASONING: DEDUCTIVE

This question primarily requires recall of physics, including hydrostatic pressure and buoyancy. In order to arrive at the correct conclusion, one must apply knowledge of hydrostatic pressure to the patient in this case. This patient has a history of myocardial infarction (MI) and is deconditioned. If this question was answered incorrectly, refer to information on effects of hydrostatic pressure on cardiovascular function.

B16 | Musculoskeletal | Intervention

A therapist determines that a patient is walking with a backward trunk lean with full weight on the right leg. The patient also demonstrates great difficulty going up ramps. The **BEST** intervention to remediate this problem is to:

CHOICES:

1. Stretch hip abductors through side-lying positioning.
2. Stretch hip flexors through prone-lying.
3. Strengthen hip extensors through bridging.
4. Strengthen knee extensors with weights, using 80%, 1 repetition maximum.

TEACHING POINTS

CORRECT ANSWER: 3

Backward trunk lean (gluteus maximus gait) is the result of a weak gluteus maximus. It causes increased difficulty going up stairs or ramps. Functional training exercises such as bridging are indicated.

INCORRECT CHOICES:

The patient is able to perform a backward trunk lean in standing, indicating adequate range in hip flexors. Ability to take full weight on the limb without knee buckling indicates adequate strength of knee extensors. Tightness in hip abductors is rare and would result in the posture (lateral lean) being maintained during all phases of gait.

TYPE OF REASONING: INFERENCE

In this question, the test taker must determine the cause of a backward trunk lean and difficulty ascending ramps, and which muscle groups require strengthening. This type of question requires one to make inferences or draw conclusions from the evidence presented in order to make a clinical decision. If this question was answered incorrectly, review knowledge of gait deviations and their causes.

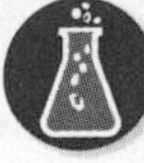

B17 | Integumentary | Patient Examination

If a patient has developed a thick eschar secondary to a full-thickness burn, the antibacterial agent **MOST** effective for infection control is:

CHOICES:

1. Silver nitrate.
2. Sulfamylon.
3. Panafil.
4. Nitrofurazone.

TEACHING POINTS

CORRECT ANSWER: 2

Sulfamylon penetrates through eschar and provides antibacterial control.

INCORRECT CHOICES:

Silver nitrate and nitrofurazone are superficial agents that attack surface organisms. Panafil is a keratolytic enzyme used for selective débridement.

TYPE OF REASONING: ANALYSIS

This question requires recall of the properties of each agent in antibacterial control and then to determine which one would **MOST** effectively promote infection control. Therefore, the test taker must analyze each agent and rely on knowledge of these agents to arrive at the correct conclusion. If this question was answered incorrectly, review information on agents used after burns.

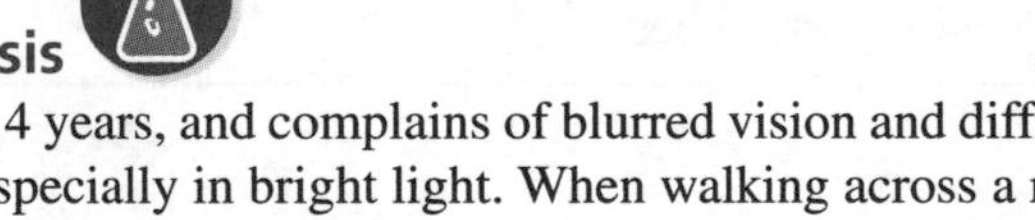

B18 | Neuromuscular | Evaluation, Diagnosis, Prognosis

An elderly person has lost significant functional vision over the last 4 years, and complains of blurred vision and difficulty reading. The patient frequently mistakes images directly in front, especially in bright light. When walking across a room, the patient is able to locate items in the environment using peripheral vision when items are located to both sides. Based on these findings, the therapist suspects:

CHOICES:

1. Glaucoma.
2. Homonymous hemianopsia.
3. Cataracts.
4. Bitemporal hemianopsia.

TEACHING POINTS

CORRECT ANSWER: 3

Cataracts, which cause a clouding of the lens, result in a gradual loss of vision; central vision is lost first, then peripheral.

INCORRECT CHOICES:

Glaucoma produces the reverse symptoms: loss of peripheral vision occurs first, then central vision, progressing to total blindness. Hemianopsia is field defect in both eyes that often occurs following stroke. There was no mention of cerebrovascular accident (CVA) in the question.

TYPE OF REASONING: ANALYSIS

In this question, symptoms are presented and one must make a determination of the most likely diagnosis. These types of questions require analysis of the meaning of information presented that utilizes analytical reasoning skill. If this question was answered incorrectly, refer to information on visual deficits associated with aging.

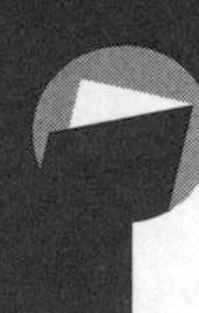

B19 | Devices, Admin., etc. | Teaching, Research, Roles

A therapist publishes a study of a 5 year-old who is injured in a motor vehicle accident with resulting C4 spinal cord injury (ASIA C) (Brown-Sequard syndrome). As part of the patient's comprehensive rehabilitation program, the patient participated in a locomotor training program using a body weight support system 1 month after injury. Training parameters included 3–5 days/wk, 20–30 minutes for 5 months. After training, outcomes included return to walking in the community with assistive devices. This is an example of a:

CHOICES:

1. Cohort study.
2. Case report.
3. Nonrandomized case-control series.
4. Retrospective study.

TEACHING POINTS

CORRECT ANSWER: 2

This is an example of a case report. The therapist provides a detailed description of the management of a patient that may serve as a basis for future research. It is a level V study (Sackett's Levels of Evidence).

INCORRECT CHOICES:

A cohort study and a case-control series involve multiple patients. A retrospective design uses previously collected information in order to answer a research question.

TYPE OF REASONING: DEDUCTIVE

One must recall the guidelines for a case report study in order to arrive at a correct conclusion, which necessitates deductive reasoning skill. For this situation, the study described is an example of a case report, because the study entails an in-depth description of the management of one patient. If this question was answered incorrectly, review research guidelines, especially case report studies.

B20 | Neuromuscular | Intervention

A patient incurred a right CVA 1 month ago and demonstrates moderate spasticity in the left upper extremity (predominantly increased flexor tone). The major problem at this time is a lack of voluntary movement control. There is minimal active movement, with $^{1}/_{4}$ inch subluxation of the shoulder. The initial treatment activity of **GREATEST BENEFIT** is:

CHOICES:

1. Sitting, weight-bearing on extended left upper extremtiy, weight-shifting.
2. PNF D2 flexion pattern, left upper extremity.
3. Quadruped, rocking from side to side.
4. Sitting, left active shoulder protraction with extended elbow, and shoulder flexed to 90 degrees.

TEACHING POINTS

CORRECT ANSWER: 1

Sitting, weight-bearing, and rocking on an extended left upper extremity will help to decrease the flexor tone. It also provides joint compression (approximation) at the shoulder, which will help maintain shoulder position and stimulate stabilizing muscles.

INCORRECT CHOICES:

Quadruped is too strenuous for this patient at this time (maximum weight-bearing on a weak, unstable upper extremity). The other two activities demand more voluntary control than this patient currently demonstrates.

TYPE OF REASONING: INDUCTIVE

The test taker must make a determination of where the patient is currently functioning and match this knowledge to what the patient could most likely tolerate and achieve success in during interventions. In this situation, the patient would benefit the most from weight-bearing activities through the affected extremity with weight-shifting. Questions such as these require clinical judgment, which is an inductive reasoning skill.

B21 | Devices, Admin., etc. | Teaching, Research, Roles

A therapist conducts a study of the effectiveness of hot and cold in treating patients with pain. Two hundred patients are recruited for each treatment group. The pain instrument used has a possible total score of 50, with 50 being the worst pain. Data analysis reveals that group A (heat modalities) has a mean score of 33 with a standard deviation of 1, whereas group B (cold modalities) had a mean of 35 with a standard deviation of 6. Based on these data, the conclusion one should reach is:

CHOICES:

1. Heat has a greater effect on pain relief than cold.
2. The spread of scores with cold treatment demonstrates that variability is greater.
3. Cold has a greater effect on pain relief than heat.
4. The spread of scores with heat treatment demonstrates variability is greater.

TEACHING POINTS

CORRECT ANSWER: 2

The spread of scores with cold treatment (standard deviation of 6) indicates that this treatment produces more variable effects than the heat treatment.

INCORRECT CHOICES:

All other conclusions cannot be determined based on the data presented and the statistical analysis presented.

TYPE OF REASONING: DEDUCTIVE

This question requires recall of research guidelines, especially interpretation of data, which is a deductive reasoning skill. In this scenario, the standard deviation is key to arriving at the correct decision, because it indicates that the cold treatment has produced more variable effects than the heat treatment. If this question was answered incorrectly, refer to information on standard deviation and interpretation of results.

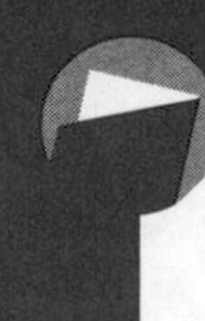

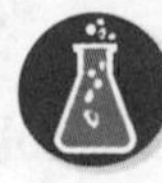

B22 | Musculoskeletal | Patient Examination

The therapist in the photograph is testing which muscle?

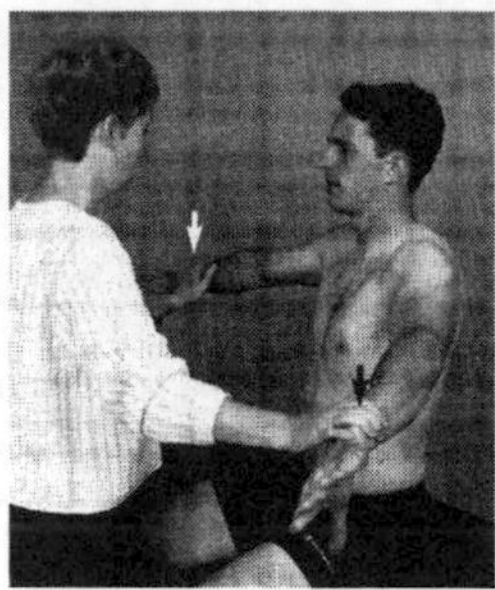

Magee D (2002). Orthopedic Physical Assessment, 4th ed. Philadelphia, W. B. Saunders, Figure 5-94, page 278, with permission.

CHOICES:

1. Supraspinatus.
2. Anterior deltoid.
3. Middle deltoid.
4. Upper trapezius.

TEACHING POINTS

CORRECT ANSWER: 1

The muscle being tested is the supraspinatus. The empty-can position puts the supraspinatus muscle in its most effective position for contraction. Weakness may be a result of inflammation, neuropathy of the suprascapular nerve, or a tendon tear.

INCORRECT CHOICES:

The muscle test for the anterior deltoid would have the humerus and forearm in neutral, rather than internal rotation of the humerus and pronation of the forearm shown in the picture. The muscle test for the middle deltoid would have the shoulder in abduction to 90 degrees. The muscle test for the upper trapezius is the shoulder shrug.

TYPE OF REASONING: ANALYSIS

In this situation, the test taker must recall knowledge of muscle testing of the supraspinatus to arrive at the correct conclusion. Whereas recall of muscle testing positions and procedures can be simple recall, the picture utilizes analysis of information coupled with recall, which becomes an analytical skill. If this question was answered incorrectly, refer to information on special tests of the shoulder complex.

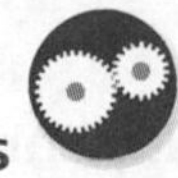

B23 | Devices, Admin., etc. | Equipment, Modalities

A patient presents with pain and instability of the left foot/ankle secondary to poliomyelitis, with more recent development of progressive postpolio muscle atrophy. In this case, a plastic solid ankle-foot orthosis (AFO) is an appropriate prescription in order to:

CHOICES:

1. Provide modest assistance to dorsiflexion while restricting plantar flexion.
2. Control excessive amounts of knee flexion during stance.
3. Maintain dorsiflexion throughout swing.
4. Restrict all movement.

TEACHING POINTS

CORRECT ANSWER: 4

A solid AFO is indicated with severe pain or instability; it limits all foot and ankle movement.

INCORRECT CHOICES:

The other choices do not adequately address these problems. Dorsiflexion assistance during swing can be provided by a posterior leaf spring device. Excessive knee flexion during stance can be controlled using an anterior stop that limits dorsiflexion.

TYPE OF REASONING: EVALUATION

In this question, the test taker must evaluate the merits of the four statements in order to determine which response is most true, given the patient's symptoms and clinical issues. In this situation, a solid AFO is most beneficial with severe pain or instability. If this question was answered incorrectly, review information on indications for AFOs.

B24 | Musculoskeletal | Patient Examination

A patient is referred to physical therapy after an anteroinferior dislocation of the right shoulder. A possible positive examination finding as the result of this trauma would be:

CHOICES:

1. Weak rhomboids.
2. Positive drop arm test.
3. Weak deltoids.
4. Positive Neer's test.

TEACHING POINTS

CORRECT ANSWER: 3

Because of the anatomical position of the axillary nerve, it can be damaged by an anteroinferior dislocation at the glenohumeral joint. This results in weak deltoids.

INCORRECT CHOICES:

A drop arm test evaluates the integrity of the rotator cuff. A Neer test evaluates impingement of the shoulder. The rhomboids are innervated by the dorsal scapular nerve. Anatomically, the dorsal scapular nerve is medial and posterior to the shoulder joint.

TYPE OF REASONING: ANALYSIS

This question requires one to recall musculoskeletal anatomy of the shoulder and the various tests that can be administered to determine dysfunction in the shoulder. For this case, the drop arm test and Neer's test are not administered to determine anterior shoulder dislocation, and rhomboids do not play a role in anterior shoulder stability. Through analysis of the information presented, the test taker should conclude that weak deltoids are the most likely cause.

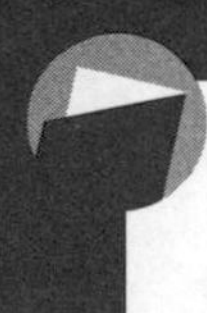

B25 | Devices, Admin., etc. | Teaching, Research, Roles

A team of researchers investigates the use constraint-induced movement therapy on patients with chronic stroke (>1 year poststroke) using a multicenter randomized controlled trial (RCT). This type of design provides the highest level of evidence because it uses:

CHOICES:

1. Alternating experimental and control conditions for a subject.
2. Random assignment to matched cohort groups.
3. A sample of convenience for the intervention group.
4. Random assignment to an experimental or control group.

TEACHING POINTS

CORRECT ANSWER: 4

An RCT uses a randomization process to assign subjects to either an experimental group(s) or a control (comparison) group. Subjects in the experimental group receive the intervention and are then compared with subjects in the control group, who do not receive the intervention.

INCORRECT CHOICES:

Alternating experimental and control conditions for a subject is an A-B-A-B design, typically used in single-subject design studies. A cohort design investigates a group of subjects without a control group (sample of convenience).

TYPE OF REASONING: DEDUCTIVE

One must recall the guidelines for an RCT in order to arrive at a correct conclusion. Questions that require one to recall facts or guidelines often necessitate deductive reasoning skill. For this case, this type of research design provides the highest level of evidence due to the random assignment to an experimental or control group. If this question was answered incorrectly, review research guidelines, especially RCT study designs.

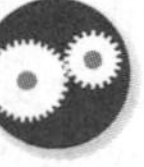

B26 | Devices, Admin., etc. | Teaching, Research, Roles

A therapist has been asked to give an in-service presentation to staff nurses on safe guarding techniques. In order to best prepare for this talk, the therapist should:

CHOICES:

1. Survey the audience a day before the scheduled session.
2. Provide a questionnaire to all participants 2 weeks before the scheduled session.
3. Survey the audience at the scheduled session.
4. Provide a questionnaire to a random sampling of participants 1 week before the scheduled presentation.

TEACHING POINTS

CORRECT ANSWER: 2

A questionnaire to all participants represents the best method of needs assessment in this situation.

INCORRECT CHOICES:

Leaving the survey to the day of or day before the presentation does not allow for adequate advanced planning to meet the group's needs. Using a random sample of participants will not adequately represent the needs of the whole group.

TYPE OF REASONING: EVALUATION

This question requires one to evaluate the merits of the statements presented, and the test taker must determine which course of action best meets the needs of the group. In a situation in which a therapist is preparing for an in-service, it is ideal to perform a needs assessment of the group as a basis for planning the manner in which to deliver information to the group. Evaluation questions can be challenging, because they require one to make a judgment call based on knowledge and experience.

B27 | Neuromuscular | Intervention

The patient with left hemiplegia would be **LEAST** likely to respond in therapy if the motor learning strategies emphasized:

CHOICES:

1. Maximum use of verbal cues.
2. Encouraging the patient to slow down.
3. Simplification/restructuring of the environment, including removal of all clutter.
4. Maximum use of demonstration and gesture.

TEACHING POINTS

CORRECT ANSWER: 4

The patient with left hemiplegia typically demonstrates visuospatial perceptual deficits. Maximum use of demonstration and gesture would be inappropriate to assist this patient in the relearning of motor tasks.

INCORRECT CHOICES:

The other choices are all valid motor learning strategies that can be used to assist the patient with left hemiplegia.

TYPE OF REASONING: INFERENCE

One must utilize knowledge of deficits related to right CVA (and, therefore, left hemiplegia) in order to arrive at the correct conclusion. Because of expected visuospatial deficits, it would be least beneficial to maximize use of demonstration and gestures. The test taker must account for the key information in this question (patient with left hemiplegia) in order to infer the least effective intervention approach.

B28 | Cardiovascular-Pulmonary | Evaluation, Diagnosis, Prognosis

A 2 week-old infant born at 27 weeks gestation with hyaline membrane disease is referred for a physical therapy consult. Nursing reports that the child "desaturates to 84% with handling" and has minimal secretions at present. The PT should:

CHOICES:

1. Provide suggestions to nursing for positioning for optimal motor development.
2. Perform manual techniques for secretion clearance, 2–4 hours daily, to maintain airway patency.
3. Put the PT consult on hold, because the child is too ill to tolerate exercise.
4. Delegate to a physical therapy assistant (PTA) a maintenance program of manual techniques for secretion clearance.

TEACHING POINTS

CORRECT ANSWER: 1

Excessive handling of a premature infant can cause oxygen desaturation. It is in the best interests of the infant to limit the number of handlers. The PT's role should be to assist nursing in developing positioning schedules, positions for feeding, infant stimulation activities, etc.

INCORRECT CHOICES:

At present, there is little information provided that would necessitate the PT or PTA to be a direct caregiver to this child.

TYPE OF REASONING: INDUCTIVE

The test taker must utilize clinical judgment coupled with knowledge of neonatology physical therapy practice to arrive at the correct conclusion. One uses inductive reasoning skills whenever diagnostic thinking or clinical judgment is utilized. If this question was answered incorrectly, refer to information on neonatology practice.

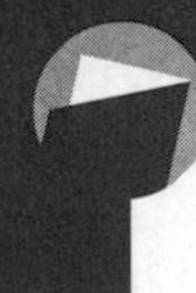
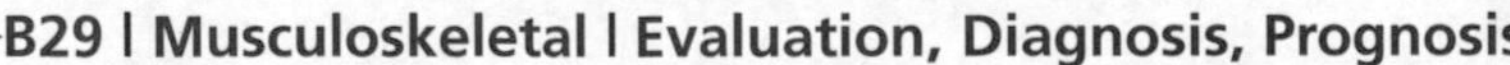

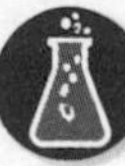

B29 | Musculoskeletal | Evaluation, Diagnosis, Prognosis

A patient sustained a valgus stress to the left knee while skiing. The orthopedist found a positive McMurray's test and a positive Lachman's stress test. The patient has been referred to physical therapy for conservative management of this problem. The **BEST** intervention for the subacute phase of physical therapy is:

CHOICES:

1. Open-chain strengthening of the quadriceps femoris and hip adductors to inhibit anterior translation of the tibia on the femur.
2. Closed-chain functional strengthening of the quadriceps femoris and hip abductors to promote regaining terminal knee extension.
3. Closed-chain functional strengthening of the quadriceps femoris and hamstrings, emphasizing regaining terminal knee extension.
4. Open-chain exercises of the hip extensors and hamstrings to inhibit anterior translation of the femur on the tibia.

TEACHING POINTS

CORRECT ANSWER: 3

The evaluation is suggestive of an unhappy triad injury. Closed-chain exercises are emphasized during the **subacute phase** to enhance functional control of the muscles surrounding the knee. Terminal extension must be achieved during this stage if normal function is to occur.

INCORRECT CHOICES:

Open-chain exercise does not promote regaining functional control for the muscle surrounding the knee. Focus on the hip abductors (rather than the hamstrings) will not promote regaining functional control of the knee joint.

TYPE OF REASONING: ANALYSIS

The test taker must have knowledge of the patient's exact deficits and appropriate interventions in order to make the correct decision in this case. This requires knowledge of McMurray's test, Lachman's test, and rehabilitation strategies after an unhappy triad injury. In this type of question, the meaning of the information presented is analyzed to make the appropriate decision.

B30 | Other Systems | Evaluation, Diagnosis, Prognosis

The patient's chief complaint is increasing difficulty completing ADLs and instrumental activities of daily living (IADLs). The chart review reveals that the patient is being treated for chronic immunosuppression due to a kidney transplant 20 years ago. No other medical history is remarkable. The PT hypothesizes that the impairments **MOST** involved in limiting function are likely related to:

CHOICES:

1. Decreased cardiovascular endurance.
2. Distal somatosensory losses for balance.
3. Impaired joint mobility.
4. Loss of muscle strength.

TEACHING POINTS

CORRECT ANSWER: 4

Long-term therapy with immunosuppression agents including corticosteroids can lead to myopathies and skin changes.

INCORRECT CHOICES:

Although neurotoxicities (peripheral neuropathy) can occur, they are not the most common. Cardiovascular involvement post–kidney transplant is most commonly seen as hypertension, which would not be expected to affect cardiovascular endurance. Joint mobility is unaffected.

TYPE OF REASONING: INFERENCE

This question requires the test taker to use critical reasoning skill to determine the most likely reason for the patient's difficulty in completing ADLs/IADLs. In order to arrive at a correct conclusion, one must consider the patient's diagnosis and results of long-term immunosuppression therapy. In this case, muscle strength is most likely involved in limiting function.

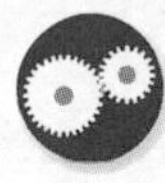

B31 | Devices, Admin., etc. | Teaching, Research, Roles

A patient with TBI has a convulsive seizure during a therapy session. The patient has lost consciousness and presents with tonic-clonic convulsions of all extremities. The therapist's **BEST** response is to:

CHOICES:

1. Initiate rescue breathing immediately and call for help to restrain the patient.
2. Position in side-lying, check for an open airway, and immediately call for emergency assistance.
3. Position in supine with head supported with a pillow, and wait out the seizure.
4. Wrap the limbs with a sheet to prevent self-harm, position in supine, and call for emergency assistance.

TEACHING POINTS

CORRECT ANSWER: 2

This is an emergency situation. In order to prevent aspiration, turn the head to the side or position in side-lying. Check to see whether the airway is open, and wait for tonic-clonic activity to subside before initiating artificial ventilation, if needed.

INCORRECT CHOICES:

Supine positioning can be life-threatening if the tongue falls backward to restrict the airway. Rescue breathing and restraining the patient are not indicated.

TYPE OF REASONING: EVALUATION

This question requires one to make a value judgment of the most appropriate course of action in a treatment situation. In this case, the symptoms of the patient constitute an emergency, and the therapist should undertake first aid actions and call for emergency assistance. If this question was answered incorrectly, refer to first aid guidelines for patients with seizure disorders.

B32 | Devices, Admin., etc. | Teaching, Research, Roles

A therapist wants to know whether neurodevelopmental treatment (NDT) handling techniques produce an improvement in independent rolling that lasts longer than 30 minutes. In this study, rolling is the:

CHOICES:

1. Independent variable.
2. Dependent variable.
3. Intervening variable.
4. Control variable.

TEACHING POINTS

CORRECT ANSWER: 2

The dependent variable is the change or difference in behavior (in this example, rolling) that results from the intervention.

INCORRECT CHOICES:

NDT handling is the independent variable. The terms *intervening* and *control* are not used to correctly define the study.

TYPE OF REASONING: DEDUCTIVE

Information related to research protocols and guidelines are often deductive reasoning–type questions. Here, the test taker must recall factual knowledge to make the correct decision. If this question was answered incorrectly, refer to terminology related to quantitative research, especially for types of variables.

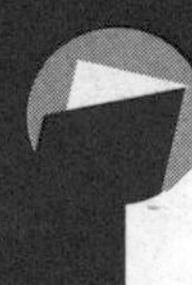

B33 | Cardiovascular-Pulmonary | Evaluation, Diagnosis, Prognosis

An adult with no significant past medical history presents to the emergency room with complaints of fever, shaking chills, and a worsening productive cough. The patient has chest pains over the posterior base of the left thorax, which are made worse on inspiration. What would be an expected physical finding for this patient?

CHOICES:

1. Crackles over the left thorax.
2. Slowed respiratory rate.
3. Symmetrical breathing.
4. Increased chest excursion.

TEACHING POINTS

CORRECT ANSWER: 1

Crackles are a typical finding over the area correlating with an infiltrate.

INCORRECT CHOICES:

With a lower than normal tidal volume, a respiratory rate would have to be elevated, not slowed, to maintain an adequate minute ventilation (respiratory rate times tidal volume = minute ventilation). Because the patient is having pain, thoracic expansion would likely be limited and asymmetrical.

TYPE OF REASONING: INFERENCE

In this question, one must draw conclusions from the evidence presented about the patient. In this situation, the patient's symptoms would **NOT** indicate the possibility of a slowed respiratory rate or symmetrical breathing. Therefore, to arrive at the correct conclusion, one must infer or make conclusions based on the evidence presented.

B34 | Devices, Admin., etc. | Equipment, Modalities

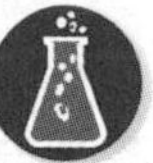

A patient with postpolio syndrome is demonstrating severe genu valgum during standing and walking. This problem can be effectively controlled by prescribing a knee-ankle-foot orthosis (KAFO) with:

CHOICES:

1. A posterior plastic shell.
2. A quadrilateral brim.
3. An anterior knee cap strap.
4. Pretibial and suprapatellar anterior bands.

TEACHING POINTS

CORRECT ANSWER: 1

Genu valgum can be controlled in a KAFO with a properly fitted posterior plastic shell.

INCORRECT CHOICES:

Older braces used a valgus correction strap, which wraps around the medial knee and buckles around the lateral upright. The correction is not as effective as a posterior plastic shell. A quadrilateral brim is used to take some weight-bearing off the limb. Pretibial and suprapatellar anterior bands are used in the KAFO to maintain sagittal stability (three-point pressure system).

TYPE OF REASONING: ANALYSIS

One must utilize their knowledge of KAFOs to make the correct decision in this case. Also, one must understand and analyze the nature of genu valgum according to the patient information presented. If this question was answered incorrectly, review information on indications for KAFOs and genu valgum.

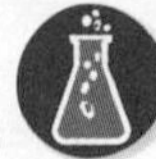

B35 | Other Systems | Evaluation, Diagnosis, Prognosis

An elderly patient is confined to bed after a severe stroke. The patient has a 25-year history of diabetes and diabetic neuropathy in both lower extremities. During an examination of sensory and integumentary integrity, the therapist identifies an ischemic necrosis on the lateral side of the right foot in the region of the fifth metatarsal head. Hypoesthesia is found in both feet, and the patient is not able to sense a 5.07 Semmes-Weinstein monofilament in the right forefoot. The therapist's interpretation is that:

CHOICES:

1. The patient still has normal protective sensation in the right foot.
2. Protective sensation of the foot is lost at the 10-g force level.
3. The foot is insensate with protective sensation loss at the 75-g force level.
4. The patient in unable to perceive sharp/dull sensation.

TEACHING POINTS

CORRECT ANSWER: 2

The neuropathic limb is prone to the development of neuropathic ulcers. Examination is facilitated by the use of Semmes-Weinstein monofilaments. Three sizes of monofilaments are typically used: (1) the 4.17 monofilament provides 1 g of force, and is indicative of normal sensation, (2) the 5.07 monofilament provides 10 g of force, and is indicative of protective sensation loss, and (3) the 6.10 monofilament provides 75 g of force, and reveals a severely insensate foot.

INCORRECT CHOICES:

This patient does not have normal protective sensation. Monofilaments are used to examine pressure sensation (a single-point perception test), and do not reveal any information about sharp/dull sensation.

TYPE OF REASONING: ANALYSIS

One must understand the indications for and administration of the Semmes-Weinstein monofilament test in order to choose the correct answer. The test taker must analyze the information about the patient and make a determination of how this relates to guidelines for interpretation of the monofilament test when administered with this patient. If this question was answered incorrectly, refer to guidelines for monofilament testing and interpretation.

B36 | Devices, Admin., etc. | Equipment, Modalities

A patient strained the lower back muscles 3 weeks ago, and now complains of pain (6/10). Upon examination, the therapist identifies bilateral muscle spasm from T10–L4. The therapist elects to apply interferential current to help reduce pain and spasm. The **BEST** electrode configuration to choose in this case would be:

CHOICES:

1. Two electrodes, with current flow parallel to the spinal column.
2. Two electrodes, with current flow perpendicular to the spinal column.
3. Four electrodes, with current flow diagonal to the spinal column.
4. Four electrodes, with current flow perpendicular to the spinal column.

TEACHING POINTS

CORRECT ANSWER: 3

The crisscrossed electrode configuration allows: (1) a greater area to be treated and (2) current interference to occur between the frequencies of the two circuits because of the diagonal pattern.

INCORRECT CHOICES:

A crisscrossed electrode configuration is needed to create interferential current. None of the other electrode configurations facilitates the flow of current diagonal to the spinal column, which would cause the frequencies to intersect.

TYPE OF REASONING: DEDUCTIVE

This question requires recall of factual information related to the protocol for electrode placement when using interferential current. The test taker must refer to this knowledge to understand that four electrodes with current flowing diagonal to the spinal column are best for treating the patient's symptoms.

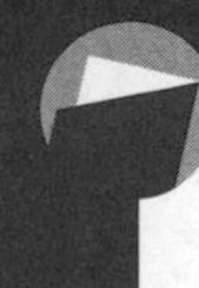

B37 | Neuromuscular | Foundational Sciences

An infant is independent in sitting, including all protective extension reactions and can pull-to-stand through kneeling, cruise sideways, and stand alone. The infant still demonstrates plantar grasp in standing. This infant's chronological age is approximately:

CHOICES:

1. 5 months.
2. 6 months.
3. 8–9 months.
4. 10–15 months.

TEACHING POINTS

CORRECT ANSWER: 3

The 8 to 9 month-old will be able to pull-to-stand, stand alone, and cruise sideways, but because he/she is not yet walking, may still exhibit plantar grasp in the standing position.

INCORRECT CHOICES:

At 5 months, the infant can roll prone to supine and demonstrates head control in supported sitting. At 6 months, the infant can sit independently and pull-to-stand. At 10–15 months, the infant typically begins to walk unassisted.

TYPE OF REASONING: DEDUCTIVE

In this question, one must recall the developmental milestones of an infant in order to arrive at the correct conclusion. This type of recall is factual and based on guidelines, which is a deductive reasoning skill. If this question was answered incorrectly, refer to the developmental milestones and reflexes of infants.

B38 | Musculoskeletal | Evaluation, Diagnosis, Prognosis

A retired bus driver has experienced increasing frequency of low back pain over the last 10 years. The patient states that nonsteroidal anti-inflammatory drugs (NSAIDs) help to relieve the symptoms, but there is always a nagging-type pain. The patient reports significant stiffness in the morning that dissipates by noon after exercising and walking. Pain is exacerbated with frequent lifting and bending activities, as well as sitting for long periods. Physical therapy intervention should emphasize:

CHOICES:

1. Modalities to reduce pain, joint mobilization, and lumbar extension exercises.
2. Joint mobilization, soft tissue mobilization, and flexion exercises.
3. Postural reeducation, soft tissue mobilization, and dynamic stabilization.
4. Modalities to reduce pain, postural reeducation, and dynamic stabilization exercises.

TEACHING POINTS

CORRECT ANSWER: 3

This is a long-term degenerative and postural dysfunction that is manageable with medication and proper physical activity. Therefore, the most effective use of treatment time should emphasize regaining normal postural alignment and functional ADLs.

INCORRECT CHOICES:

Whereas modalities and mobilization can relieve acute pain, this is a chronic problem that demands choices appropriate for long-term management of the problem.

TYPE OF REASONING: INFERENCE

One must consider all of the patient's symptoms and determine what the likely cause(s) of the symptoms is in order to make an appropriate decision for intervention. This requires the use of inferential reasoning, in which decisions are made after drawing conclusions from the evidence presented.

B39 | Devices, Admin., etc. | Teaching, Research, Roles

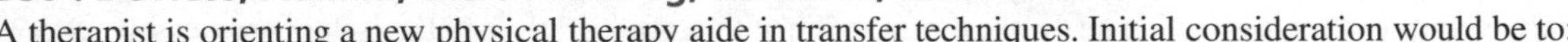

A therapist is orienting a new physical therapy aide in transfer techniques. Initial consideration would be to:

CHOICES:

1. Provide an organized series of talks dealing with patient safety during transfers.
2. Determine specific goals for teaching the techniques.
3. Give a computer-simulated instructional program before actual "hands-on" training takes place.
4. Ask about previous work and other experiences related to transferring individuals.

TEACHING POINTS

CORRECT ANSWER: 4

The therapist's initial analysis of the learner should identify the current level of knowledge and skills about transfer techniques. The therapist can then build on this information to plan appropriate educational goals and teaching methods.

INCORRECT CHOICES:

Determining specific goals or strategies without an adequate needs asssessment is counterproductive.

TYPE OF REASONING: EVALUATION

This question couples knowledge of training staff members with a value judgment, in which the test taker must determine the best way to initiate training to an aide. In this situation, it is best to determine the aide's previous knowledge and experience prior to initiating transfer training. If this question was answered incorrectly, refer to training guidelines for physical therapy personnel.

B40 | Other Systems | Evaluation, Diagnosis, Prognosis

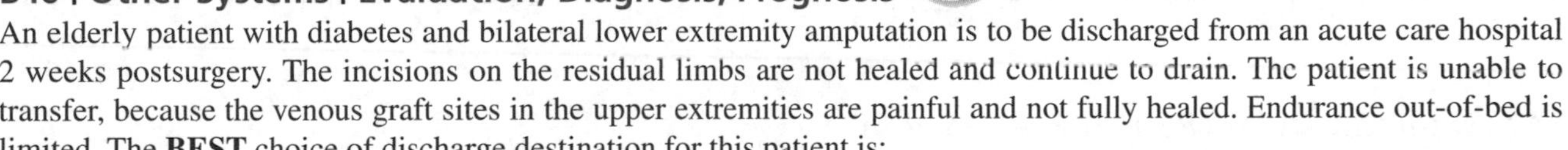

An elderly patient with diabetes and bilateral lower extremity amputation is to be discharged from an acute care hospital 2 weeks postsurgery. The incisions on the residual limbs are not healed and continue to drain. The patient is unable to transfer, because the venous graft sites in the upper extremities are painful and not fully healed. Endurance out-of-bed is limited. The **BEST** choice of discharge destination for this patient is:

CHOICES:

1. Skilled nursing facility.
2. Home.
3. Custodial care facility.
4. Rehabilitation hospital.

TEACHING POINTS

CORRECT ANSWER: 1

A skilled nursing facility is the best facility, because the patient continues to require nursing care for the open wounds. Initiation of physical therapy when this patient is able is also available.

INCORRECT CHOICES:

Discharge to home would be premature, because the patient is unable to transfer. Custodial care involves medical or nonmedical care that does not seek a cure. A rehabilitation hospital is not appropriate at this time, because the patient cannot actively participate in rehabilitation 3 hours/day.

TYPE OF REASONING: INDUCTIVE

One must utilize clinical judgment in this situation to make an appropriate determination for the best discharge situation for this patient. The key is that the patient's current medical status requires continued nursing care, which can be managed at a skilled nursing facility. In addition, the patient can continue to receive rehabilitation at a duration that is most appropriate for the patient's current tolerance for functional activity. Questions that require clinical judgment often utilize inductive reasoning skill.

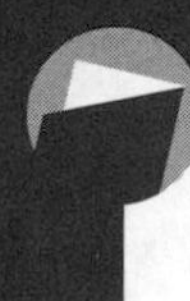

B41 | Neuromuscular | Patient Examination

A patient currently being seen for low back pain awoke one morning with drooping left facial muscles and excessive drooling. The patient was recovering from a cold and had experienced an earache in the left ear during the previous 2 days. The therapist suspects Bell's palsy, which can be confirmed by examining:

CHOICES:

1. Trigger points for pain, especially over the temporomandibular joint (TMJ).
2. Taste over the anterior tongue, and having the patient raise the eyebrows and puff the cheeks.
3. Taste over the posterior tongue, and having the patient protrude the tongue.
4. Corneal reflex and stretch reflexes of facial muscles.

TEACHING POINTS

CORRECT ANSWER: 2

Bell's palsy is a lower motor neuron lesion affecting the branches of the facial nerve, CN VII. Examination of the motor function of the muscles of facial expression (i.e., raise eyebrows, show teeth, smile, close eyes tightly, puff cheeks) and taste over the anterior tongue will reveal deficits of CN VII function.

INCORRECT CHOICES:

Taste over the posterior tongue is a function of CN IX (glossopharyngeal). Strength of tongue protrusion is a function of CN XII (hypoglossal). Pupillary reflexes are a function of CN II (optic).

TYPE OF REASONING: INFERENCE

In this question, the suspected diagnosis and symptoms are provided, but the test taker must determine how to best confirm this diagnosis through testing of the cranial nerves. This question requires inferential critical reasoning, which uses clinical decision-making based on facts and evidence. If this question was answered incorrectly, refer to information on Bell's palsy.

B42 | Neuromuscular | Patient Examination

A PTA is assigned to ambulate a patient with a 10-year history of Parkinson's disease (PD). The PT instructs the PTA to watch for:

CHOICES:

1. Decreased trunk rotation with shorter steps.
2. Wider steps and increased double support time.
3. Unsteady, uneven gait with veering to one side.
4. An abnormally wide base of support.

TEACHING POINTS

CORRECT ANSWER: 1

Gait changes characteristic of PD include loss of arm swing and reciprocal trunk movements, shuffling gait, and festinating gait (an abnormal and involuntary increase in the speed of walking).

INCORRECT CHOICES:

Patients with PD take shorter steps (not longer). Veering to one side only is indicative of a unilateral peripheral vestibular deficiency (the patient veers to the side with the dysfunction). An abnormally wide base of support is indicative of gait unsteadiness, but is not typical in the patient with PD.

TYPE OF REASONING: DEDUCTIVE

This question essentially requires one to recall the typical gait pattern of patients with PD. This type of recall is factual and based on guidelines, thus utilizing deductive reasoning skills. If this question was answered incorrectly, refer to information of gait patterns in PD.

B43 | Cardiovascular-Pulmonary | Foundational Sciences

A patient with congestive heart failure (CHF) is on a regimen of diuretics (chlorothiazide). The potential side effects of this medication that the PT should be alert for include:

CHOICES:

1. Orthostatic hypotension and dizziness.
2. Reflex tachycardia and unstable BP.
3. Myalgia and joint pains.
4. Hyperkalemia and premature ventricular contractions (PVCs).

TEACHING POINTS

CORRECT ANSWER: 1

Thiazide diuretics are used to manage mild to moderate hypertension. Adverse side effects include orthostatic hypotension and dizziness, along with drowsiness, lethargy, and weakness. These represent a safety risk during functional training and gait.

INCORRECT CHOICES:

BP is lowered and is more stable, not less. Hypokalemia (not hyperkalemia) can occur, resulting in increased PVCs. Muscle cramps and weakness can occur. Joint pains are likely caused by a comorbid condition.

TYPE OF REASONING: INFERENCE

The test taker utilizes factual knowledge of side effects of medications, coupled with knowledge of CHF to make the correct decision in this case, using inferential reasoning skills.

B44 | Musculoskeletal | Evaluation, Diagnosis, Prognosis

A patient with a traumatic injury to the right hand had a flexor tendon repair to the fingers. Physical therapy intervention after this type of repair would begin:

CHOICES:

1. After the splint is removed in 2–3 weeks, to allow full AROM of all affected joints.
2. After the splint is removed in 4–6 weeks, to allow ample healing time for the repaired tendon.
3. Within a few days after surgery, to preserve tendon gliding.
4. Within a few days after surgery, to allow for early initiation of strengthening exercises.

TEACHING POINTS

CORRECT ANSWER: 3

Early passive and active assistive exercises promote collagen remodeling to allow free tendon gliding.

INCORRECT CHOICES:

When rehabilitation is delayed by several weeks, adhesions form, which restrict free tendon gliding. Early initiation of strengthening exercises is contraindicated.

TYPE OF REASONING: INDUCTIVE

This question requires one to use clinical judgment to make a determination of the best intervention for a patient who has had a recent flexor tendon repair of the hand. One utilizes knowledge of hand therapy and early tendon repair protocols to arrive at the correct conclusion. If this question was answered incorrectly, review flexor tendon repair information and therapy protocols.

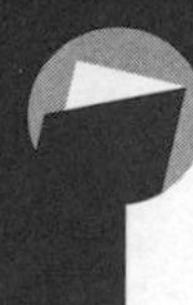

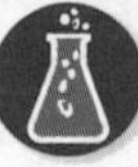

B45 | Musculoskeletal | Evaluation, Diagnosis, Prognosis

A community-dwelling elder fell at home and suffered multiple fractures of the right arm including Colles' fracture of the right wrist and humeral fracture of the right shoulder. The patient is hospitalized for open reduction, internal fixation (ORIF) of the right radius. What is an expected finding with this elderly patient when compared with a younger patient?

CHOICES:

1. Decreased pain and tenderness at the fracture sites.
2. Slower fracture healing time with prolonged rehabilitation.
3. Decreased risk of disorientation after surgery.
4. Malunion at the fracture sites.

TEACHING POINTS

CORRECT ANSWER: 2

Fracture healing in elderly clients is slower and typically results in longer rehabilitation times than for younger clients.

INCORRECT CHOICES:

Hospitalization and surgery frequently cause disorientation and mental confusion as well as complications from prolonged inactivity (e.g., pneumonia). Pain and tenderness are **NOT** decreased at the fracture site. Although fracture healing is slower, malunion (fracture healing within a normally expected time but in an unsatisfactory position) is **NOT** more likely.

TYPE OF REASONING: ANALYSIS

In this situation, one must make a determination of expected findings after this type of injury in an elderly patient. This requires analysis of the information presented and the meaning of this information to determine the correct conclusion.

B46 | Neuromuscular | Patient Examination

The therapist suspects that a patient recovering from a middle cerebral artery stroke is exhibiting a pure hemianopsia. This can be examined using a:

CHOICES:

1. Distance acuity chart placed on a well-lighted wall at patient's eye level 20 feet away.
2. Penlight held approximately 12 inches from the eyes and moved to the extremes of gaze right and left.
3. Penlight held 6 inches from the eyes and moved inward toward the face.
4. Visual confrontation test with a moving finger.

TEACHING POINTS

CORRECT ANSWER: 4

Visual field is examined using the confrontation test. The patient sits opposite the therapist and is instructed to maintain his/her gaze on the therapist's nose. The therapist slowly brings a target (moving finger or pen) in the patient's field of view alternately from the right or left sides. The patient indicates when and where he/she first sees the target.

INCORRECT CHOICES:

Distance acuity vision is tested using a Snellen eye chart at a distance of 20 feet. Ocular pursuit is tested using a penlight moved in an H pattern to the extremes of gaze. Convergence is tested using a penlight and ruler; the patient keeps the penlight in focus as it moves inward from a distance of 4 or 6 inches.

TYPE OF REASONING: INFERENCE

This question basically asks the test taker to recall the appropriate examination approach for hemianopsia. Questions such as these do require recall of factual knowledge (knowledge of the different tests), but then must be applied to the specific patient presented in the question, which moves beyond factual recall to drawing a conclusion, which is an inferential reasoning skill.

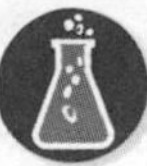

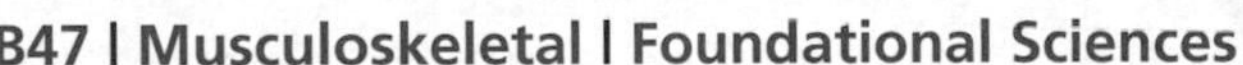

B47 | Musculoskeletal | Foundational Sciences

A patient is recovering from a left tibial amputation and complains of numbness and tingling affecting the dorsal foot and big toe. The patient knows the limb is gone and can't understand why this is happening. The therapist suspects the source of discomfort is most likely pressure from residual limb wrapping affecting the:

CHOICES:

1. Sural nerve.
2. Medial calcaneal nerve.
3. Tibial nerve.
4. Common peroneal (fibular) nerve.

TEACHING POINTS

CORRECT ANSWER: 4

Sensation to the dorsum of the foot and big toe is supplied by the superficial peroneal (fibular) nerve, a branch off of the common peroneal (fibular) nerve. Phantom limb sensation (sensation of a limb that is no longer there) usually occurs in the immediate postoperative phase and can be stimulated by external pressure (residual limb wrapping or rigid dressing). It typically dissipates over time, although some patients may experience the sensation for the rest of their lives. This is a common finding and should not interfere with prosthetic rehabilitation.

INCORRECT CHOICES:

The sural nerve is a distal branch of the tibial nerve that supplies the back of the leg and the lateral side of the foot and little toe. The medial calcaneal nerve is also a branch of the tibial nerve that supplies the heel and medial sole of the foot.

TYPE OF REASONING: ANALYSIS

In this question, the test taker utilizes knowledge of neuroanatomy to arrive at a correct conclusion. Although the patient's phantom limb sensations are typical of postamputation, the challenge in choosing the correct answer is in knowing which nerve would most likely cause the sensation when the amputation is transtibial. If this question was answered incorrectly, refer to information on lower extremity neuroanatomy.

B48 | Devices, Admin., etc. | Teaching, Research, Roles

A therapist investigated the accuracy of pulse oximeter estimates during exercise. Correlational analysis measured the strength of the relationship between two types of ear probe—equipped pulse oximeters during heavy cycle exercise under hypoxic conditions. The investigator found measured arterial oxyhemoglobin saturation (%HbO_2) levels to have a correlation of 0.89 at high saturation, but only 0.68 at low saturation levels. The results of this study suggest:

CHOICES:

1. Both devices are highly accurate at all saturation levels.
2. Accuracy of the measurements increases at higher saturation levels.
3. During heavy exercise, oxygen saturation levels should be interpreted cautiously.
4. Both devices are only moderately accurate.

TEACHING POINTS

CORRECT ANSWER: 2

The result of the study indicates that the correlation between the two types of oximeters was high when oxygen saturation levels were high (0.89), but only moderate (0.68) at low oxygen saturation levels.

INCORRECT CHOICES:

Accuracy was not the same at all saturation levels, and the high correlation during high saturation suggests that the devices are accurate during heavy exercise.

TYPE OF REASONING: DEDUCTIVE

This type of question requires knowledge of guidelines in correlational research and parameters for high versus moderate correlation. This type of knowledge is factual recall, using deductive reasoning skills. If this question was answered incorrectly, refer to correlational research guidelines.

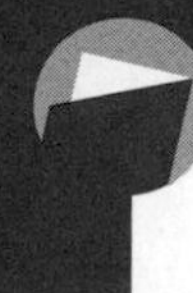

B49 | Musculoskeletal | Patient Examination

A college soccer player sustained a hyperextension knee injury when kicking the ball. The patient was taken to the emergency room of a local hospital and was diagnosed with "knee sprain." The player was sent to physical therapy the next day for rehabilitation. As part of the examination to determine the type of treatment plan to implement, the therapist conducted the test shown in the figure. Based on the test picture, the therapist is examining the integrity of the:

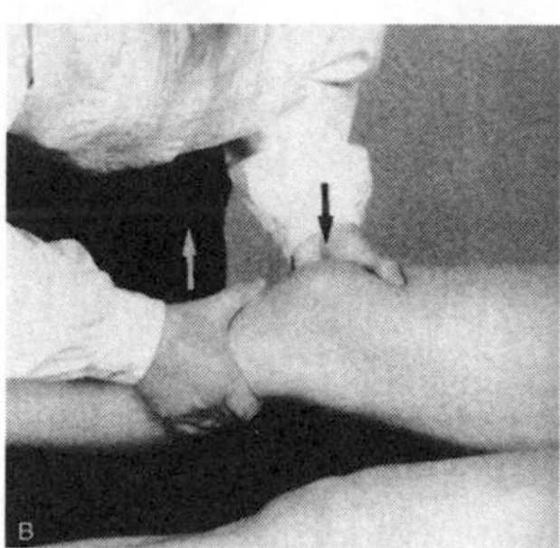

Magee D (2002). Orthopedic Physical Assessment, 4th ed. Philadelphia, W. B. Saunders, Figure 12-27B, page 700, with permission.

CHOICES:

1. Anterior cruciate ligament.
2. Posterior cruciate ligament.
3. Medial meniscus.
4. Iliotibial band.

TEACHING POINTS

CORRECT ANSWER: 1

The test shown in the figure is the Lachman test to determine the integrity of the anterior cruciate ligament.

INCORRECT CHOICES:

The posterior cruciate is examined using the posterior drawer and the reverse Lachman test. The medial meniscus is examined using the McMurray and the Apley tests. The iliotibial band is tested using the Noble compression test.

TYPE OF REASONING: INFERENCE

The question requires the test taker to recall the visual information depicted as a test of integrity of the anterior cruciate ligament. This is factual recall of visual information, but also requires one to sort out other tests that may appear similar in order to arrive at the correct conclusion. This skill is therefore inferential, requiring one to draw conclusions based on visual information.

B50 | Musculoskeletal | Evaluation, Diagnosis, Prognosis

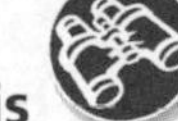

A patient is seen in physical therapy 2 days after a motor vehicle accident. The chief complaints are headaches, dizziness, neck pain with guarding, and a "sensation of a lump in the throat." Plain film x-rays were read as negative. The therapist should refer this patient for a:

CHOICES:

1. Second series of plain film x-rays.
2. Myelogram.
3. T2 magnetic resonance imaging (MRI).
4. Computed tomography (CT) scan.

TEACHING POINTS

CORRECT ANSWER: 4

The primary concern of the therapist is to rule out strong suspicions of an upper cervical spine fracture. CT scan is still preferred for assessing cortical bone, especially spinal fractures.

INCORRECT CHOICES:

Plain films, already taken, did not show any fracture, which is not uncommon. A second series would not be expected to reveal any new information. The T2 MRI and myelogram are not as specific for assessing bony anatomy as the CT scan.

TYPE OF REASONING: INDUCTIVE

One must consider the symptoms of the patient and a possible cause to arrive at the conclusion that a CT would be the most appropriate next step in determining the cause for the symptoms. Inductive reasoning skills are utilized when one must use knowledge of symptoms plus diagnostic skills to make an appropriate decision. If this question was answered incorrectly, refer to information on indications for CT scans.

B51 | Integumentary | Equipment, Modalities

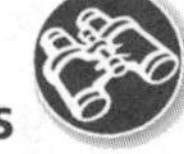

A patient with an acutely sprained ankle will be treated by immersion into an ice water bath. The therapist should tell the patient to expect in order:

CHOICES:

1. Aching, numbness, and burning, followed by intense cold.
2. Burning, intense cold, and aching, followed by numbness.
3. Intense cold, burning, and aching, followed by numbness.
4. Numbness, aching, and intense cold, followed by burning.

TEACHING POINTS

CORRECT ANSWER: 3

Stimulation of the cold receptors produces the perception of intense cold as the cold modality is applied to the skin. The burning and aching sensations are due to the intensity perceived as the tissue temperature decreases. As the transmission of the signals from the skin receptors slows and finally ceases, numbness is produced.

INCORRECT CHOICES:

The other choices do not portray this sequence of expected sensations. Numbness occurs last in the sequence, not first. Intense cold is perceived first, before burning and aching.

TYPE OF REASONING: INDUCTIVE

One must rely on knowledge of applications of cold modalities and expected sensations when applied to arrive at the correct conclusion. Inductive reasoning is utilized via diagnostic thinking and prediction of what may occur, given a set of circumstances. If this question was answered incorrectly, review information on cryotherapy.

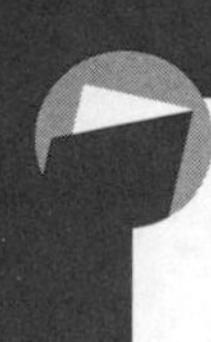

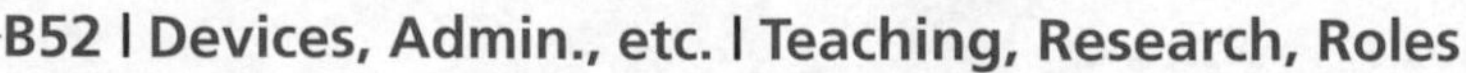

B52 | Devices, Admin., etc. | Teaching, Research, Roles

A patient with cancer is admitted to a local hospital. The patient is given an Advanced Care Medical Directive to review and sign. Guidelines for this document include specifying the rights of individual patients to:

CHOICES:

1. Be informed of a facility's right to modify the format and implementation schedule of the document.
2. Establish mental competence for decision making, with signing witnessed by two adults.
3. Insist on contraindicated palliative treatment, even if the ultimate outcome is death.
4. Be informed of the right to make decisions regarding their medical care upon admission.

TEACHING POINTS

CORRECT ANSWER: 4

Advanced Care Medical Directives are mandated by federal law, the Patient Self-Determination Act of 1990. Patients receiving care from hospitals, nursing facilities, hospices, home health care agencies, and health maintenance organizations that receive federal Medicare or federal-state Medicaid funds must be informed on admission of their right to make decisions regarding their medical care. The facility cannot alter these guidelines.

INCORRECT CHOICES:

Establishing mental competence is not routinely required. Physicians cannot be mandated to give a contraindicated treatment; the patient can, however, refuse a recommended treatment, even if it leads to death.

TYPE OF REASONING: DEDUCTIVE

One utilizes their knowledge of protocols and guidelines to answer questions of deductive reasoning skill. In this question, one must refer to knowledge of Advanced Directives to make the best determination of what it specifies. If this question was answered incorrectly, refer to information related to Advanced Care Medical Directives.

B53 | Neuromuscular | Evaluation, Diagnosis, Prognosis

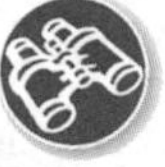

A patient is recovering from stroke, and at 4 months, is ambulating with a straight cane for household distances. During outpatient physical therapy, the therapist has the patient practice walking with no assistive device. Recurvatum is observed that worsens with continued walking. The therapist's **BEST** strategy is to:

CHOICES:

1. Practice isolated small-range quadriceps eccentric control work in standing, and continue with the straight cane.
2. Give the patient a small-based quad cane (SBQC) to improve stability, and have him/her practice AROM in supine.
3. Put the patient on a Cybex and work on increasing quadriceps torque output at higher loads and increasing speeds.
4. Give the patient a KAFO to control the hyperextension and a hemi walker.

TEACHING POINTS

CORRECT ANSWER: 1

Eccentric quadriceps control work (closed-chain exercises) is indicated in order to reduce recurvatum. The patient should continue with the straight cane until able to walk without the device and recurvatum.

INCORRECT CHOICES:

Open-chain exercises (Cybex, AROM) do not adequately address the functional demands of gait. The use of SBQC or hemi walker will not correct the problem. A KAFO is inappropriate to stabilize the knee, which can be effectively stabilized using either an AFO or a Swedish knee cage. The use of an orthosis should be considered only as a last resort.

TYPE OF REASONING: INDUCTIVE

One must use clinical judgment and knowledge of recurvatum in ambulation to arrive at the correct conclusion. Inductive reasoning questions require use of knowledge combined with clinical judgment to determine the best course of action in clinical situations. In this situation, the test taker must recognize that the recurvatum indicates eccentric quadriceps control work.

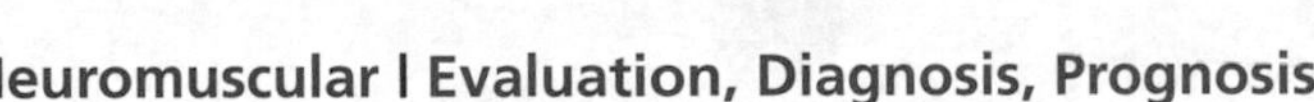

B54 | Neuromuscular | Evaluation, Diagnosis, Prognosis

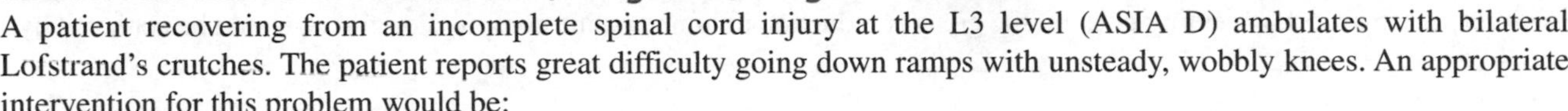

A patient recovering from an incomplete spinal cord injury at the L3 level (ASIA D) ambulates with bilateral Lofstrand's crutches. The patient reports great difficulty going down ramps with unsteady, wobbly knees. An appropriate intervention for this problem would be:

CHOICES:

1. Prolonged icing to reduce hamstring pain.
2. Biofeedback training to reduce knee extensor spasticity.
3. Progressive resistance training for the quadriceps.
4. Stretching using a posterior resting splint for tight plantar flexors.

TEACHING POINTS

CORRECT ANSWER: 3

A spinal cord injury at the level of L3 affects knee extensors. ASIA scale D means the injury is incomplete, with at least half of the key muscles below the neurological level having a muscle grade of 3 or more. A weak knee will wobble or buckle going down stairs or ramps. It is the result of weak quadriceps or knee flexor contracture. Strengthening exercises using progressive resistance training for the quadriceps are indicated.

INCORRECT CHOICES:

Biofeedback training may reduce knee extensor spasticity, but this may only increase knee instability, and is not indicated in this case. There is no indication that hamstring pain or tight plantar flexors are present or precipitating causes of the patient's problem.

TYPE OF REASONING: INFERENCE

In this question, the test taker must understand what impairments result from L3 spinal injury and what clinical interventions can be implemented to improve the patient's deficits. In this situation, the patient's deficits indicate weak knee extensors, which can be strengthened through a progressive resistive exercise program. If this question was answered incorrectly, refer to information on lumbar level spinal cord injury.

B55 | Devices, Admin., etc. | Teaching, Research, Roles

Under HIPPA rules, it is illegal to release protected health information (PHI) without a competent patient's consent to:

CHOICES:

1. The insurance company that is paying for the patient's treatment.
2. The patient's spouse.
3. Another health care provider involved in the care of the patient.
4. Report suspected abuse.

TEACHING POINTS

CORRECT ANSWER: 2

A spouse does not have the legal right to the patient's information without the patient's consent.

INCORRECT CHOICES:

Those individuals involved in the care of the patient, a legal guardian with power of attorney in situations in which the patient is judged mentally incompetant, or the patient's payer have a legal right to information regarding a patient's care without obtaining the patient's consent for releasing information. The therapist has a positive legal obligation to report suspected abuse whether or not consent is granted.

TYPE OF REASONING: EVALUATION

In this question, one must determine the strength of the statements presented as well as which statement adheres to legal guidelines related to HIPPA. Evaluation questions often require test takers to make value judgments and recall certain guidelines in order to make those judgments.

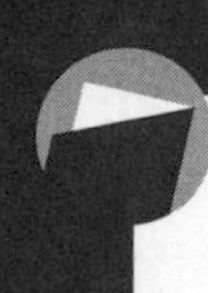

B56 | Musculoskeletal | Evaluation, Diagnosis, Prognosis

With respect to a worker's sitting posture, the greatest reduction in lumbar spine compression forces would be achieved by:

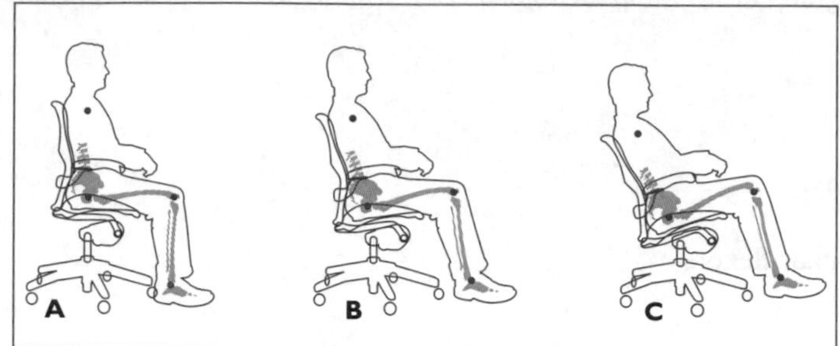

The Kinematics of Sitting. Herman Miller Co., 2002, with permission.

CHOICES:

1. Using a 2-inch gel seat cushion.
2. Increasing the chair backrest–seat angle to between 90 and 110 degrees.
3. Eliminating armrests on the chair.
4. Decreasing the chair backrest–seat angle to 85 degrees.

TEACHING POINTS

CORRECT ANSWER: 2

Maximal reduction of lumbar disc pressures can be achieved by increasing the angle between the seat pan and the chair backrest to between 90 and 110 degrees, using armrests for support, or adding a lumbar support. Combining the effects of all three provides the best solution.

INCORRECT CHOICES:

A gel seat cushion reduces pressures on the ischial seat. Eliminating armrests or decreasing the chair backrest–seat angle would only worsen the problem.

TYPE OF REASONING: INFERENCE

This question requires one to infer visual information from the picture in order to make a clinical determination of the best course of action. Inferential questions require one to make sense of information presented and to draw conclusions from it. Therefore, one must draw conclusions about the sitting posture in the picture in order to determine which solution would most effectively reduce compression forces in the lumbar spine.

B57 | Musculoskeletal | Foundational Sciences 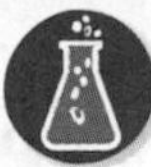

A baseball pitcher has been sent to physical therapy with progressive posterior shoulder pain and weakness of the shoulder abductors and lateral rotators. The therapist notices muscle wasting superior and inferior to the scapular spine. The patient's problem is **MOST LIKELY** attributable to damage involving the:

CHOICES:

1. Spinal accessory nerve.
2. Long head of the biceps brachii.
3. Scalene muscles.
4. Suprascapular nerve.

TEACHING POINTS

CORRECT ANSWER: 4

Microtrauma to the suprascapular nerve can occur with repetitive activities involving shoulder "cocking" and follow-through resulting in inflammation and muscle weakness of the muscles supplied by the suprascapular nerve (the supraspinatus and infraspinatus muscles).

INCORRECT CHOICES:

Damage to the spinal accessory nerve will promote weakness and atrophy of the upper trapezius muscle. Damage to the long head of the biceps brachii or scalene muscles will not present with posterior shoulder pain, weakness with shoulder abduction/external rotation, and/or atrophy of the supraspinatus and infraspinatus muscles.

TYPE OF REASONING: ANALYSIS

This question requires one to rely on knowledge of shoulder neuroanatomy in order to choose the correct solution. This type of recall is factual in nature, with basic analysis or interpretation of the information presented. In this case, the patient's weakness of the shoulder abductors and lateral rotators is indicative of damage to the suprascapular nerve. If this question was answered incorrectly, refer to shoulder neuroanatomy and functional anatomy.

B58 | Devices, Admin., etc. | Teaching, Research, Roles 

Nursing homes that receive Medicare reimbursement for eligible residents are required by law to provide for rehabilitation services, including physical therapy, based on:

CHOICES:

1. Needs assessment performed by a PT.
2. Referral from a physician or physician assistant.
3. Diagnostic categories (Diagnosis-Related Groups [DRGs]).
4. Referral from the nurse case manager or nurse practitioner.

TEACHING POINTS

CORRECT ANSWER: 1

Other professionals (physician, nurse practitioner or case manager, physician assistant) can initiate a referral for physical therapy examination and evaluation of a patient. However, the determination of need for services must be performed by a licensed PT.

INCORRECT CHOICES:

The physician, physician assistant, and nurse case manager can only refer for services. DRGs are a classification system designed to standardize prospective payment for medical care. They are not used to delineate the need for care.

TYPE OF REASONING: DEDUCTIVE

This question requires the test taker to recall Medicare guidelines for reimbursement of physical therapy services and who can most appropriately determine the need for PT services in skilled nursing facilities. This is factual recall of information based on guidelines, which is a deductive reasoning skill. If this question was answered incorrectly, refer to Medicare reimbursement guidelines, especially needs assessments for physical therapy services.

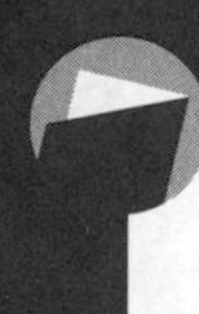

B59 | Neuromuscular | Evaluation, Diagnosis, Prognosis

A patient is recovering from surgical resection of an acoustic neuroma and presents with symptoms of dizziness, vertigo, horizontal nystagmus, and postural instability. To address these problems, physical therapy plan of care should incorporate:

CHOICES:

1. Prolonged bedrest to allow vestibular recovery to occur.
2. Strengthening exercises focusing on spinal extensors.
3. Repetition of movements and positions that provoke dizziness and vertigo.
4. Hallpike's exercises to improve speed in movement transitions.

TEACHING POINTS

CORRECT ANSWER: 3

In patients with unilateral vestibular pathology, habituation training (use of positions and movements that evoke symptoms) will encourage the vestibular system to recalibrate. Good recovery can generally be expected with gradual progression of exercises.

INCORRECT CHOICES:

Prolonged bedrest will delay recovery and may result in incomplete recovery. Strengthening exercises for spinal extensors are not indicated in the case information. Hallpike-Dix maneuver is used for assessment and diagnosis of benign paroxysmal positional vertigo and is not a set of exercises.

TYPE OF REASONING: INFERENCE

One must have knowledge of acoustic neuroma and expected symptomatology in order to choose the correct intervention approach. Inferential reasoning often requires the test taker to draw conclusions based on the evidence presented. Questions that ask what to expect from a diagnosis or a set of symptoms often require use of inferential reasoning. If this question was answered incorrectly, review intervention approaches for vestibular pathology.

B60 | Devices, Admin., etc. | Equipment, Modalities

A patient is beginning ambulation training with a right above-knee prosthesis. The therapist notices that, during early swing, the heel rises excessively. A possible cause is:

CHOICES:

1. Too little tension in the extension aid.
2. Amputee pain.
3. Too much tension in the extension aid.
4. Too much knee friction.

TEACHING POINTS

CORRECT ANSWER: 1

Excessive heel-rise during early swing can be caused by inadequate knee friction or too little tension in an extension aid.

INCORRECT CHOICES:

Too much tension in the extension aid or too much knee friction would cause decreased heel-rise. Amputee pain can cause a variety of problems but is not likely to result in this specific problem.

TYPE OF REASONING: ANALYSIS

When information is presented about a clinical problem and the test taker is called to make a determination of the cause for the problem, analytical reasoning skills are used. One must determine the meaning of the problem in order to choose the correct solution. In this situation, one must understand that excessive heel-rise with an above-knee prosthesis during early swing phase is indicative of too little tension in the extension aid. If this question was answered incorrectly, review prosthetic gait deviations.

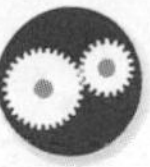

B61 | Other Systems | Evaluation, Diagnosis, Prognosis

A PT is treating an elderly patient in the home. Upon arrival one day, the therapist notices that the patient is confused and skin color and turgor are poor. The patient reports of an "intestinal bug" for the last few days with frequent vomiting and diarrhea. The therapist's **BEST** course of action is to:

CHOICES:

1. Monitor vital signs; if HR is not elevated, get the patient up and walking.
2. Notify the family, and insist that the patient not be alone until the illness is over.
3. Cancel therapy for today, carefully document the findings, and notify the physician.
4. Give the patient water and notify the physician immediately.

TEACHING POINTS

CORRECT ANSWER: 4

This patient is exhibiting signs of dehydration associated with prolonged vomiting and diarrhea. Confusion is a red flag and requires immediate action: administer fluids and notify the physician immediately.

INCORRECT CHOICES:

Giving fluids is the first action the therapist must take. Any other choice jeopardizes the patient's health.

TYPE OF REASONING: EVALUATION

For questions that require one to evaluate a clinical situation and to make a determination of the best course of action (especially if the situation is unexpected), evaluative reasoning is used. Questions such as these are "judgment calls" based on knowledge, experience, and prudence. In this situation, it is most prudent to give the patient water and immediately notify the physician, because the symptoms indicate dehydration.

B62 | Cardiovascular-Pulmonary | Evaluation, Diagnosis, Prognosis

A patient who is 5 weeks post-MI is participating in a cardiac rehabilitation program. The therapist is monitoring responses to increasing exercise intensity. The indicator that exercise should be immediately terminated is:

CHOICES:

1. Systolic BP > 140 mm Hg or diastolic BP > 80 mm Hg.
2. Peak exercise HR > 140.
3. 1.5 mm of downsloping ST segment depression.
4. Appearance of a PVC on the electrocardiogram (ECG).

TEACHING POINTS

CORRECT ANSWER: 3

The upper limit for exercise intensity prescribed for patients post-MI is based on signs and symptoms. Of the choices, only ST segment depression (>1.0 mm of horizontal or downsloping depression) is a significant finding, representative of myocardial ischemia.

INCORRECT CHOICES:

Both HR and BP are expected to rise (the levels of 140 and 140/80 are not significant for most patients). The appearance of a single PVC is also not significant because single PVCs can occur in individuals without a cardiac history.

TYPE OF REASONING: INFERENCE

When questions provide a diagnosis and the test taker must determine the symptoms to watch for, inferential reasoning is used. To answer this question correctly, the test taker must have knowledge of cardiac rehabilitation guidelines and indications for terminating exercise programs. If this question was answered incorrectly, refer to post-MI rehabilitation guidelines.

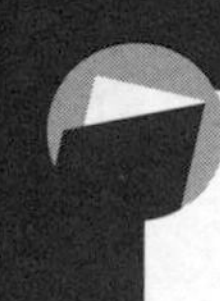

B63 | Other Systems | Intervention

An infant who was 39 weeks gestational age at birth and is now 3 weeks chronological age demonstrates colic. In this case, the **BEST** intervention the PT could teach the mother is:

CHOICES:

1. Stroking and tapping.
2. Fast vestibular stimulation.
3. Neutral warmth.
4. Visual stimulation with a colored object.

TEACHING POINTS

CORRECT ANSWER: 3

Neutral warmth (wrapping) is a calming stimulus.

INCORRECT CHOICES:

All of the other choices would likely increase arousal of the infant. The infant is still too developmentally immature for any of the stimuli other than neutral warmth.

TYPE OF REASONING: INDUCTIVE

One utilizes clinical judgment, with combined knowledge of inhibitory and facilitatory stimuli in infants, in order to choose the best solution. In this scenario, the newborn is too developmentally immature to manage facilitatory stimuli, and requires stimuli that are calming or inhibitory, especially if colic is demonstrated. If this question was answered incorrectly, refer to appropriate stimuli for newborns.

B64 | Neuromuscular | Foundational Sciences

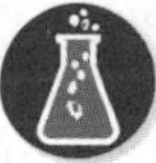

A therapist is treating a patient with Brown-Séquard syndrome that resulted from a gunshot wound. The therapist's examination should reveal:

CHOICES:

1. Loss of motor function and pain and temperature sensation, with preservation of light touch and position sense below the level of the lesion.
2. Loss of upper extremity function (cervical tract involvement), with preservation of lower extremity function (lumbosacral tract involvement).
3. Sparing of tracts to sacral segments, with preservation of perianal sensation and active toe flexion.
4. Ipsilateral weakness and loss of position sense and vibration below the lesion level, with contralateral loss of pain and temperature sensation.

TEACHING POINTS

CORRECT ANSWER: 4

Brown-Séquard syndrome is a hemisection of the spinal cord characterized by ipsilateral weakness and loss of position and vibration sensation below the level of the lesion; there is also contralateral loss of pain and temperature sensation a few segments below the level of the lesion.

INCORRECT CHOICES:

Other choices describe an anterior cord syndrome (choice 1), central cord syndrome (choice 2), or sacral sparing (choice 3).

TYPE OF REASONING: ANALYSIS

This question requires factual recall of neuroanatomy in order to arrive at the correct conclusion. One should recall the nature of Brown-Séquard syndrome as a hemisection of the spinal cord, which results in both ipsilateral and contralateral losses below the level of lesion. One also must separate out the symptoms of other spinal cord syndromes, which are different from this scenario. If this question was answered incorrectly, refer to spinal cord injuries and syndromes.

B65 | Devices, Admin., etc. | Teaching, Research, Roles

A patient is recovering from stroke and presents with moderate impairments of the left upper and lower extremities. The PT's goal today is to instruct the patient in a stand-pivot transfer to the more affected side so the patient can go home on a weekend pass. The wife is attending today's session, and will be assisting the patient on the weekend. The **BEST** choice for teaching this task is to:

CHOICES:

1. Practice the task first with the caregiver, then with the patient.
2. Demonstrate the task, and then practice with the patient.
3. Practice the task first with the patient, then with the caregiver.
4. Demonstrate the task, then have the caregiver practice with the patient.

TEACHING POINTS

CORRECT ANSWER: 2

To ensure optimal motor learning, first demonstrate the task at ideal performance speeds. This provides the patient with an appropriate reference of correction (cognitive map) of the task. Then use guided practice with the patient to ensure safety and successful performance.

INCORRECT CHOICES:

Caregivers should become involved only after initial practice of the task with the patient and after the safety of the patient can be assured.

TYPE OF REASONING: INFERENCE

One must rely upon beliefs and assumptions about the clinical situation above in order to choose the best solution. This is a skill of inferential reasoning, in which the test taker must determine the best course of action to ensure optimal motor learning in educating a caregiver and a patient in transfer skills. Inferential reasoning combines clinical judgment with the need to draw conclusions from evidence presented.

B66 | Integumentary | Foundational Sciences

An elderly and frail individual is referred to physical therapy for mobilization out-of-bed. The therapist performs a skin inspection that reveals a persistent area of redness over the sacrum that is still evident after the patient has been upright for 30 minutes. The therapist recognizes that this is:

CHOICES:

1. A stage II pressure ulcer.
2. Reactive hyperemia.
3. Eczema.
4. A stage I pressure ulcer.

TEACHING POINTS

CORRECT ANSWER: 4

A stage I pressure ulcer is characterized by a defined area of persistent redness (in this example). Additional changes include alterations in skin temperature (warmth or coolness), tissue consistency, and sensation (pain, itching).

INCORRECT CHOICES:

A stage II ulcer involves partial-thickness skin loss with abrasion, blister, or shallow crater. Reactive hyperemia results from temporary occlusion of blood supply to an area, and should reverse within a short time as pressure is reversed. Eczema (dermatitis) is a superficial inflammation of the skin caused by allergic exposure. It may be characterized by extensive erosions, papules, or vesicles with exudate.

TYPE OF REASONING: ANALYSIS

This question provides a description of a condition, and the test taker must determine what the symptoms indicate. This is an analytical reasoning skill. For this case, the symptoms described indicate a stage I pressure ulcer. If this question was answered incorrectly, review pressure ulcer guidelines, especially stage I.

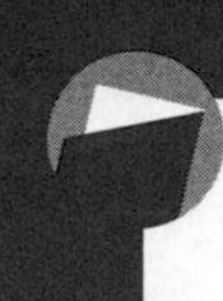

B67 | Devices, Admin., etc. | Equipment, Modalities 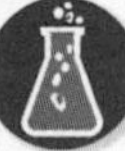

When using a patellar tendon–bearing (PTB) prosthesis, a patient will experience excessive knee flexion in early stance if the:

CHOICES:

1. Socket is aligned too far forward or tilted anteriorly.
2. Socket is aligned too far back or tilted posteriorly.
3. Foot position is outset too much.
4. Foot position is inset too much.

TEACHING POINTS

CORRECT ANSWER: 1

In a PTB prosthesis, the socket is normally aligned in slight flexion to enhance loading on the patellar tendon, prevent genu recurvatum, and resist the tendency of the amputated limb to slide too deeply into the socket. If it is aligned incorrectly (too far anterior or excessively flexed), it will result in excessive knee flexion in early stance.

INCORRECT CHOICES:

A socket aligned too posterior results in insufficient knee flexion. Excessive foot inset results in lateral thrust at midstance. Excessive foot outset results in medial thrust at midstance.

TYPE OF REASONING: ANALYSIS

One must understand and analyze the properties and potential issues in using a PTB prosthesis in order to choose the best response. In this situation, excessive knee flexion in early stance is indicative of the socket aligned too far forward or anteriorly tilted. If this question was answered incorrectly, refer to information on PTB prosthetic alignment.

B68 | Integumentary | Evaluation, Diagnosis, Prognosis 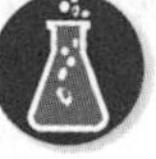

Bluish discoloration of the skin and nailbeds of fingers and toes along with palms that are cold and moist is indicative of:

CHOICES:

1. Liver disease.
2. Carotenemia.
3. Cyanosis.
4. Hypothyroidism.

TEACHING POINTS

CORRECT ANSWER: 3

Bluish discoloration of the skin and nailbeds of fingers and toes, along with palms that are cold and moist are indicative of cyanosis. It is caused by an excess of deoxygenated hemoglobin in the blood. It may be central (due to advanced lung disease, congenital heart disease, abnormal hemoglobin) or peripheral (decreased blood flow, venous obstruction).

INCORRECT CHOICES:

Liver disease produces jaundice (diffusely yellow skin and sclerae). Carotenemia produces a yellow color, especially in the palms, soles, and face (does not affect the sclerae). Hypothyroidism produces dry and cool skin.

TYPE OF REASONING: ANALYSIS

Questions that provide a group of symptoms and the test taker must determine the diagnosis often require analytical reasoning skill. In this situation, the symptoms described indicate the condition of cyanosis. Key words that help one to arrive at a correct conclusion are "bluish discoloration." If this question was answered incorrectly, review signs and symptoms of cyanosis.

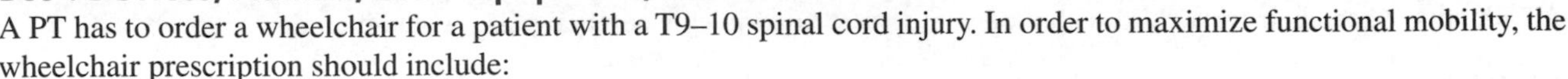

B69 | Devices, Admin., etc. | Equipment, Modalities

A PT has to order a wheelchair for a patient with a T9–10 spinal cord injury. In order to maximize functional mobility, the wheelchair prescription should include:

CHOICES:

1. A low back.
2. Swing-away footrests.
3. Standard height back.
4. Removable armrests.

TEACHING POINTS

CORRECT ANSWER: 3

At T9–10, this patient has partial innervation of the abdominals (innervated T6–12) and full innervation of the upper extremities. A manual wheelchair with a standard back height (mid scapula height) is appropriate for this patient for everyday use.

INCORRECT CHOICES:

If the patient chooses to engage in sports, a low back can improve functional ability. Low wheelchair backs may cause problems with fatigue and back pain over the long-term. Swing-away footrests and removable armrests enhance ease of transfers, not overall functional mobility.

TYPE OF REASONING: INFERENCE

In this question, the test taker must refer to knowledge of thoracic spinal cord injury and intact musculature above the level of injury in order to make the best determination for wheelchair equipment. When one must utilize clinical judgment combined with the ability to draw conclusions based on evidence, inferential reasoning skills are used. If this question was answered incorrectly, refer to thoracic spinal cord injury and wheelchair accessories.

B70 | Musculoskeletal | Patient Examination

A patient complains of persistent wrist pain after painting a house 3 weeks ago. The patient demonstrates signs and symptoms consistent with de Quervain's tenosynovitis. An appropriate special test to confirm the diagnosis is:

CHOICES:

1. Phalen's test.
2. Finkelstein's test.
3. Froment's sign.
4. Craig's test.

TEACHING POINTS

CORRECT ANSWER: 2

Finkelstein's test is specific for reproducing the pain associated with de Quervain's tenosynovitis of the abductor pollicis longus and extensor pollicis brevis.

INCORRECT CHOICES:

Froment's sign is used to identify ulnar nerve dysfunction. Phalen's test identifies median nerve compression in the carpal tunnel. Craig's test identifies an abnormal femoral antetorsion angle, which you hopefully eliminated first.

TYPE OF REASONING: DEDUCTIVE

This question requires factual recall of knowledge of provocative tests for de Quervain's tenosynovitis. In this case, the appropriate test is Finkelstein's test, which reproduces the pain of the abductor pollicic longus and extensor pollicis brevis tendons associated with de Quervain's. If this question was answered incorrectly, refer to provocative testing of the hand or wrist and de Quervain's tenosynovitis.

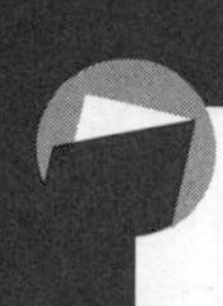

B71 | Devices, Admin., etc. | Equipment, Modalities

An adaptive wheelchair for a child with moderate spastic quadriplegic cerebral palsy would include:

CHOICES:

1. Lateral pads on the seat to keep hips adducted.
2. Movable seat back to allow for extension of the hips and trunk.
3. Movable footrests to allow ankles to plantarflex.
4. A pommel to keep hips abducted.

TEACHING POINTS

CORRECT ANSWER: 4

Hip abduction should be facilitated in sitting with the use of a pommel.

INCORRECT CHOICES:

Hip adduction, extension of the hips, and plantarflexion of ankles should be all controlled for (inhibited), because they are typically strong components of lower extremity spasticity.

TYPE OF REASONING: INFERENCE

In this question, the diagnosis is provided and the test taker must make a determination of how to best manage symptoms associated with the diagnosis. This requires use of inferential reasoning skill, in which one makes clinical assumptions about the diagnosis provided and potential courses of action. In this situation, a child with spastic quadriplegia should have a pommel to maintain hip abduction. If this question was answered incorrectly, refer to information on cerebral palsy and wheelchair positioning.

B72 | Neuromuscular | Patient Examination

An elderly patient with persistent balance difficulty and a history of recent falls (two in the last 3 months) is referred for physical therapy examination and evaluation. During the initial session, it is crucial to examine:

CHOICES:

1. Spinal musculoskeletal changes secondary to degenerative joint disease (DJD).
2. Cardiovascular endurance during a 6-minute walking test.
3. Sensory losses and sensory organization of balance.
4. Level of dyspnea during functional transfers.

TEACHING POINTS

CORRECT ANSWER: 3

A critical component of balance control is sensory input from somatosensory, visual, and vestibular receptors and overall sensory organization of inputs. Initial examination should address these elements before moving on to assess the motor components of balance (e.g., postural synergies). The Clinical Test for Sensory Integration in Balance (CTSIB) or modified CTSIB (Shumway-Cook, Horak) are appropriate instruments.

INCORRECT CHOICES:

Cardiovascular endurance and level of dyspnea during functional transfers are appropriate elements to examine, but should occur after key elements of balance are examined (sensory components and integration; motor and synergistic elements). In this case, DJD changes would not be crucial to examine initially.

TYPE OF REASONING: INDUCTIVE

This case scenario requires the test taker to combine knowledge of the somatosensory system and possible reasons for falls in order to arrive at the correct conclusion. A key facet of this question is in the terms "initial session" and "crucial." These words should cause the test taker to focus on what should come first in a sequence of intervention events and what is most important for the patient. This requires the use of clinical judgment, which is an inductive reasoning skill.

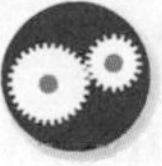

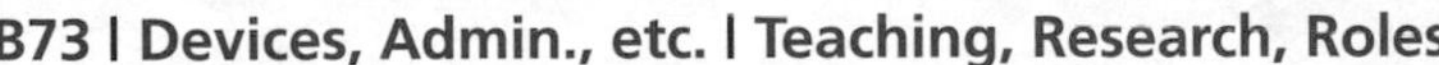

B73 | Devices, Admin., etc. | Teaching, Research, Roles

A patient with adhesive capsulitis of the shoulder sustains a fracture of the shoulder during treatment provided by the PTA. The fracture occurred while the PTA was mobilizing the shoulder joint, which was part of the plan of care established by the PT. The PTA was not familiar with the mobilization techniques to the shoulder. Responsibility in this case falls on:

CHOICES:

1. The PT, who is solely responsible for assessing the competence of the PTA under his/her supervision.
2. The PTA, who is responsible for informing their supervising PT whenever he/she is unfamiliar or uncomfortable with any treatment procedure.
3. Both the PT and the PTA are responsible for establishing effective communication regarding the skills and competencies of the PTA.
4. Neither the PT nor the PTA is responsible for the fracture; it is an accepted risk associated with joint mobilization.

TEACHING POINTS

CORRECT ANSWER: 1

The PT is solely responsible for assessing the competence of all personnel under his/her supervision. Furthermore, it is the responsibility of the supervising PT to exercise sound judgment when delegating responsibility to less skilled personnel.

INCORRECT CHOICES:

The PTA shares responsibility with the PT for good communication and maintaining skills. However, the PT is in the supervisory role and assumes ultimate responsibility ("the buck stops here"). Fractures are not an acceptable risk of joint mobilization.

TYPE OF REASONING: EVALUATION

This question requires some recall of factual guidelines, including supervision and determining competency. However, the question also exposes aspects of judging the value of the statements presented to determine who is responsible for the patient's injury. If this question was answered incorrectly, refer to guidelines related to supervision of personnel.

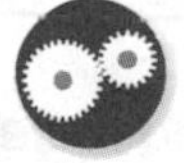

B74 | Devices, Admin., etc. | Teaching, Research, Roles

A patient is referred for physical therapy with a diagnosis of second-degree ankle sprain. The therapist is busy on the telephone when the patient with the ankle sprain arrives for the scheduled appointment. The PTA on staff knows the patient, and has treated the patient previously for a similar injury. The PT should:

CHOICES:

1. Ask the PTA to assess the patient's passive range of motion (PROM) to speed up the process.
2. Complete nonpatient care tasks at another time and examine the patient.
3. Ask the PTA to commence the examination and take over when available.
4. Ask the patient if he/she can wait until the following day for a complete examination.

TEACHING POINTS

CORRECT ANSWER: 2

It is the obligation of the PT to examine this scheduled patient initially in a timely manner and determine the plan of care. This task cannot be delegated.

INCORRECT CHOICES:

The PTA can perform assigned physical therapy tests and interventions under the supervision of a PT. Asking the patient to wait another day is not acceptable.

TYPE OF REASONING: EVALUATION

This question necessitates a value judgment about a clinical situation, which is an evaluative reasoning skill. In this scenario, the PT cannot delegate the task to the PTA and should see the patient first. The discharge summary can be completed at another time. In order to arrive at the correct conclusion, the test taker must have solid understanding of PTA supervision and role delineation.

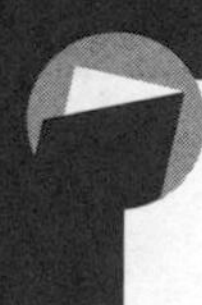

B75 | Musculoskeletal | Patient Examination

During a postural screen for a patient complaining of low back pain, the therapist notices that the knees are in genu recurvatum. Possible contributory postures would include:

CHOICES:

1. Ankle plantarflexion and anterior pelvic tilt.
2. Ankle dorsiflexion and hip abduction.
3. Forefoot varus and posterior pelvic tilt.
4. Lateral tibial torsion and anterior pelvic tilt.

TEACHING POINTS

CORRECT ANSWER: 1

A common contributory problem or correlated motion for genu recurvatum is ankle plantarflexion, due to shortened gastrocnemius muscles. Alterations occurring up the kinetic chain include anterior pelvic tilt to maintain the center of gravity over the feet.

INCORRECT CHOICES:

Ankle dorsiflexion will lead to increased knee flexion. Forefoot varus may lead to tibial internal rotation, but not genu recurvatum. Tibial external rotation will lead to abnormal stresses at the knee joint, but not genu recurvatum.

TYPE OF REASONING: INFERENCE

The test taker must understand the nature of genu recurvatum and contributory postures in order to choose the correct answer. This requires recall of lower extremity musculoskeletal pathology and biomechanics. Questions that require one to draw conclusions based on presented evidence often necessitate the use of inferential reasoning skills. If this question was answered incorrectly, refer to information on postural screening, kinetic chain, and genu recurvatum.

B76 | Musculoskeletal | Foundational Sciences

After treating a patient for trochanteric bursitis for 1 week, the patient has no resolution of pain and is complaining of problems with gait. After reexamination, the therapist finds weakness of the quadriceps femoris and altered sensation at the greater trochanter. This is **MOST** likely due to:

CHOICES:

1. DJD of the hip.
2. Sacroiliac (SI) dysfunction.
3. L4 nerve root compression.
4. L5 nerve root compression.

TEACHING POINTS

CORRECT ANSWER: 3

The positive findings are consistent with an L4 nerve root compression.

INCORRECT CHOICES:

Weakness of only one muscle group is not a common finding for DJD or SI dysfunction. L5 nerve root compression would result in hamstring weakness.

TYPE OF REASONING: ANALYSIS

In this question, the symptoms are provided and the test taker must make a determination of the possible diagnosis. Questions such as these require analytical reasoning skill, using knowledge of neuroanatomy to determine that the most likely cause is L4 nerve root compression. If this question was answered incorrectly, review information on nerve compressions of the lumbar spine.

B77 | Other Systems | Foundational Sciences

A patient in chronic renal failure is being seen in physical therapy for deconditioning and decreased gait endurance. The therapist needs to schedule the patient's sessions around dialysis, which is received 3 mornings a week. The patient is also hypertensive and requires careful monitoring. The therapist's **BEST** approach is to take BP:

CHOICES:

1. Pre- and postactivities, using the nonshunt arm.
2. In sitting when activity has ceased, using the shunt arm.
3. In the supine position, using the shunt arm.
4. Every minute during walking, using the nonshunt arm.

TEACHING POINTS

CORRECT ANSWER: 1

A dialysis shunt would interfere with taking BP. Use the nonshunt arm. Pre- and postexercise measurements are appropriate.

INCORRECT CHOICES:

The shunt arm cannot be used to take BP. Taking BP in the shunt arm or during walking would result in inaccurate measurements.

TYPE OF REASONING: INFERENCE

One must reason the best way to monitor a patient's BP using the appropriate guidelines when the patient has an atrioventricular shunt in the arm for dialysis. Guidelines dictate that you should not take BP on the arm where the shunt is located. Also, monitoring BP is best carried out pre- and postactivity to determine tolerance for activity. This type of reasoning is inferential because one must infer the best approach to patient care, considering the diagnosis and limitations of the patient.

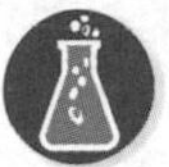

B78 | Integumentary | Evaluation, Diagnosis, Prognosis

A patient who is currently being treated for low back pain arrives for therapy complaining of pain across the middle of the right chest and back. When the therapist inspects the skin, clustered vesicles are apparent in a linear arc. The surrounding skin is hypersensitive. The therapist suspects:

CHOICES:

1. Herpes simplex infection.
2. Psoriasis.
3. Herpes zoster infection.
4. Dermatitis.

TEACHING POINTS

CORRECT ANSWER: 3

Herpes zoster is an acute infection caused by reactivation of the latent varicella-zoster virus (shingles). It is characterized by painful vesicular skin eruptions that follow the underlying route of a spinal (in this case) or cranial nerve. Additional symptoms include fever, gastrointestinal disturbances, malaise, and headache.

INCORRECT CHOICES:

Herpes simplex is an infection caused by the herpes simplex virus. These infections tend to occur on the face (around the mouth and nose). They are sometimes referred to as "cold sores." Psoriasis is a chronic skin condition characterized by red patches covered by dry silvery scales. Dermatitis is an inflammatory condition of the skin characterized by eruptions (not associated with an underlying route of a nerve).

TYPE OF REASONING: ANALYSIS

One must recall the signs and symptoms of herpes zoster infection in order to arrive at a correct conclusion. This requires analytical reasoning skill, because one must weigh the symptoms provided in order to determine the most likely diagnosis. For this question, the key words of "vesicles" and "linear arc" help guide one toward the correct conclusion. If this question was answered incorrectly, review signs and symptoms of herpes zoster infection.

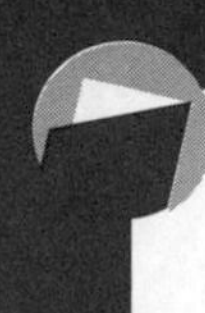

B79 | Devices, Admin., etc. | Teaching, Research, Roles

A therapist wishes to determine the effectiveness of transcutaneous electrical nerve stimulation (TENS) on the relief of pain in a group of 20 patients with phantom limb pain and recruit patients over a 2-year period. All receive a 6-week intervention. The therapist finds that 12 patients with phantom pain had pain relief, whereas 8 had no relief. The **BEST** conclusion that can be reached is that this:

CHOICES:

1. Level 1 RCT provides conclusive evidence of the effectiveness of TENS.
2. Level 3 case-control study provides limited confidence in the effectiveness of TENS.
3. Level 2 cohort design allows small but definitive conclusions to be reached.
4. Level 4 a quasiexperimental study provides only questionable evidence of treatment effectiveness.

TEACHING POINTS

CORRECT ANSWER: 2

Sackett's Levels of Evidence and Grades of Recommendation are used to define the degree of confidence and scientific rigor of the research. Level 3, case-control studies (as in this example), allow some limited confidence in the findings (grade of B).

INCORRECT CHOICES:

True experimental design includes random assignment into experimental group (receives treatment) or control group (no treatment). Level 1 studies require large RCTs and provide maximum confidence in the results (grade of A). Level 2 studies are cohort studies with smaller RCTs and provide good evidence (grade of B). Level 4 studies are poor-quality case series (grade of C), whereas level 5 studies are based on expert opinion only (grade of D).

TYPE OF REASONING: DEDUCTIVE

Questions on protocols and guidelines for research require deductive reasoning skill. Here, no independent judgment is required, but the test taker must recall the guidelines of research, especially case-control studies. An additional skill utilized in this question is interpretation of findings. This does utilize some analytical reasoning skill, but the primary mode of reasoning is factual in nature, which is deductive. If this question was answered incorrectly, review information on Sackett's Levels of Evidence.

B80 | Cardiovascular-Pulmonary | Evaluation, Diagnosis, Prognosis

After an MI, a patient is a new admission to a phase 3 hospital-based cardiac rehabilitation program. During the initial exercise session, the patient's ECG responses are continuously monitored via radio telemetry. The therapist notices three PVCs occurring in a run with no P wave. The therapist should:

CHOICES:

1. Continue the exercise session, but monitor closely.
2. Stop the exercise and notify the physician immediately.
3. Have the patient sit down and rest for a few minutes before resuming exercise.
4. Modify the exercise prescription by decreasing the intensity.

TEACHING POINTS

CORRECT ANSWER: 2

A run of three or more PVCs occurring sequentially is ventricular tachycardia. The rate is very rapid, resulting in seriously compromised cardiac output. This is potentially an emergency situation that can deteriorate rapidly into ventricular fibrillation (no cardiac output) and cardiac arrest.

INCORRECT CHOICES:

The other choices, which involve continuation of exercise, put the patient at serious risk for cardiac arrest.

TYPE OF REASONING: INDUCTIVE

This question requires the test taker to use diagnostic reasoning and clinical judgment to determine whether or not the PVCs and absence of P wave are significant enough to warrant physician notification. This type of reasoning is inductive, and the test taker is called to make a decision for the safety of the patient. In this case, physician notification is warranted, and exercise should be halted immediately. If this question was answered incorrectly, refer to cardiac rehabilitation guidelines and interpretation of ECGs.

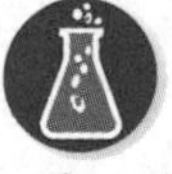

B81 | Neuromuscular | Foundational Sciences

A patient with left hemiplegia is able to recognize his wife after she is with him for a while and talks to him, but is unable to recognize the faces of his children when they come to visit. The children are naturally very upset by their father's behavior. The **BEST** explanation for his problem is:

CHOICES:

1. Ideational apraxia.
2. Anosognosia.
3. Somatognosia.
4. Visual agnosia.

TEACHING POINTS

CORRECT ANSWER: 4

All of the choices are indicative of perceptual dysfunction. This patient is most likely suffering from visual agnosia, which is an inability to recognize familiar objects despite normal function of the eyes and optic tracts. Once the wife talks with him, he is able to recognize her by her voice.

INCORRECT CHOICES:

Ideational apraxia is the inability to perform a purposeful motor act, either automatically or upon command. Anosognosia is the frank denial, neglect, or lack of awareness of the presence or severity of one's paralysis. Somatognosia is an impairment in body scheme.

TYPE OF REASONING: ANALYSIS

In this question, one must recall the meaning of the four choices provided and apply them to the patient's symptoms as described. This requires analytical reasoning, which often requires one to determine the meaning of statements or medical terminology. If this question was answered incorrectly, refer to information on the various perceptual problems after CVA.

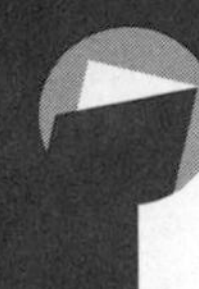

B82 | Cardiovascular-Pulmonary | Foundational Sciences

A home care PT receives a referral to evaluate the fall risk potential of an elderly community-dweller with chronic coronary artery disease (CAD). The patient has fallen three times in the last 4 months, with no history of fall injury except for minor bruising. The patient is currently taking a number of medications. The drug **MOST** likely to contribute to dizziness and increased fall risk is:

CHOICES:

1. Colace.
2. Coumadin sodium.
3. Nitroglycerin.
4. Albuterol.

TEACHING POINTS

CORRECT ANSWER: 3

Of the medications listed, nitroglycerin has greatest risk of causing dizziness or weakness due to postural hypotension. Fall risk is increased even with small doses of nitroglycerin.

INCORRECT CHOICES:

Colace (docusate sodium), an anticonstipation agent, can result in mild abdominal cramps and nausea. Coumadin (warfarin sodium) is an anticlotting medication. Adverse effects can include inceased risk of hemorrhage, which indirectly can result in lightheadedness. Dosages are carefully monitored. Albuterol, a bronchodilator, can cause tremor, anxiety, nervousness, and weakness.

TYPE OF REASONING: INFERENCE

One must infer information from the four medications provided in order to determine the one that is least likely to contribute to increased fall risk. In this circumstance, using inferential reasoning, one recalls the side effects of each medicine and determines that buffered aspirin is least likely to cause increased risk of falls, because this is not one of the common side effects.

B83 | Musculoskeletal | Evaluation, Diagnosis, Prognosis

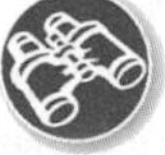

A patient complains of foot pain when first arising that eases with ambulation. The therapist finds that symptoms can be reproduced in weight-bearing and running on a treadmill. Examination reveals pes planus and pain with palpation at the distal aspect of the calcaneus. Early management would include:

CHOICES:

1. Modalities to reduce pain.
2. Use of a resting splint at night.
3. Strengthening of ankle dorsiflexors.
4. Prescription for a customized orthosis.

TEACHING POINTS

CORRECT ANSWER: 2

The symptoms are suggestive of plantar fasciitis. The focus of patient management should be on decreasing the irritation to the plantar fascia. This is most effectively done with a resting night splint.

INCORRECT CHOICES:

Modalities to reduce pain offer some symptomatic relief; however, the pain is not constant. Strengthening the dorsiflexors will not change irritation to the plantar fascia. A customized orthosis may be necessary at a later time if primary symptoms do not resolve after early management.

TYPE OF REASONING: INDUCTIVE

This question requires one to recognize the patient's symptoms as plantar fasciitis and then recall the common treatment strategies for this condition. This requires one to utilize clinical judgment, which is an inductive reasoning skill. If this question was answered incorrectly, refer to guidelines of treatment of plantar fasciitis.

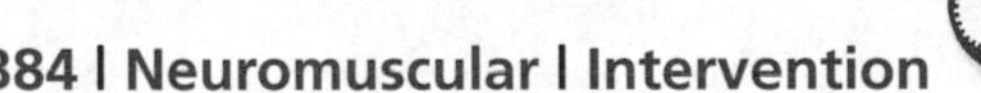

B84 | Neuromuscular | Intervention

A patient with a T10 paraplegia (ASIA A) resulting from a spinal cord injury is ready to begin community wheelchair training. The therapist's goal is to teach the patient how to do a wheelie in order to manage curbs. The **BEST** training strategy is to instruct the patient to:

CHOICES:

1. Throw the head and trunk backward to rise up on the large wheels.
2. Place a hand on the top of the handrims to steady the chair, while throwing the head and trunk forward.
3. Lean backward while moving the hands slowly backward on the rims.
4. Grasp the handrims posteriorly, and pull them forward abruptly and forcefully.

TEACHING POINTS

CORRECT ANSWER: 4

A wheelie can be assumed by having the patient place his/her hands posterior on the handrims and pulling them abruptly and sharply forward. If the patient is unable to lift the casters in this manner, throwing the head back forcefully when pulling the handrims may work. An alternate technique is to grasp the handrims anteriorly, pull backward, then abruptly and forcefully reverse the direction of pull. The therapist can assist by steadying the chair at the patient's balance point until the patient learns to adjust the position through the use of handrim movements forward and backward.

INCORRECT CHOICES:

Throwing the head and trunk backward alone or with moving the hands backward on the rims will not result in a wheelie.

TYPE OF REASONING: EVALUATION

This question requires one to evaluate the merits of each of the four possible solutions and to determine which solution seems most reasonable, which is an evaluative reasoning skill. One must recall knowledge of the strategies and techniques involved in performing a wheelie in order to arrive at the correct conclusion. If this question was answered incorrectly, refer to information on community wheelchair training, especially wheelie techniques.

B85 | Cardiovascular-Pulmonary | Evaluation, Diagnosis, Prognosis

A PT should be alert to recognize the signs and symptoms associated with the onset of aspiration pneumonia. Of the following, the patient **MOST** susceptible to develop this form of pneumonia is one with:

CHOICES:

1. Amyotrophic lateral sclerosis (ALS) with dysphagia and diminished gag reflex.
2. A complete spinal cord lesion at T2, with diminished coughing ability and forced vital capacity (FVC).
3. A circumferential burn of the thorax associated with significant pain.
4. Severe scoliosis with compression of internal organs, including the lungs.

TEACHING POINTS

CORRECT ANSWER: 1

Aspiration pneumonia results from an abnormal entry of fluids or matter (including food) into the airways. A patient with ALS with an inability to swallow (dysphagia) and diminished gag reflex is most susceptible to aspiration pneumonia.

INCORRECT CHOICES:

Others listed may be susceptible to other forms of pneumonia or even, though less likely, aspiration pneumonia.

TYPE OF REASONING: EVALUATION

In this question, the test taker must evaluate the four patient circumstances presented and determine which patient is most at risk for aspiration pneumonia. This requires one to determine the value of the information presented in each patient circumstance, which requires skills in evaluation. To arrive at the correct conclusion, one must understand each diagnosis and risks associated with those diagnoses, which should be reviewed if this question was answered incorrectly.

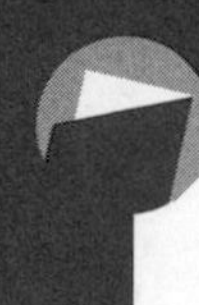

B86 | Musculoskeletal | Intervention 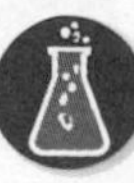

A patient demonstrates quadriceps weakness (4/5) and difficulty descending stairs. The **BEST** intervention to regain functional strength in the quadriceps is:

CHOICES:

1. Isokinetic exercise, at 36 degrees/sec.
2. Progressive resistance exercises, 70% 1 repetition maximum, three sets of 10.
3. Partial squats, progressing to lunges.
4. Maximum isometric exercise, at 45 and 90 degrees of knee extension.

TEACHING POINTS

CORRECT ANSWER: 3

Closed-chain exercises are the most appropriate in this example because of the patient's difficulty descending stairs. Moving the body over a fixed distal segment provides loading to muscles, joints, and noncontractile soft tissues while stimulating the sensory receptors needed for stability and balance.

INCORRECT CHOICES:

Open-chain exercise (all other choices), while improving strength, does not adequately prepare an individual for functional weight-bearing.

TYPE OF REASONING: ANALYSIS

One must analyze the four choices presented in order to determine which activity is best to regain functional quadriceps strength. In this situation, a closed-chain activity is optimal because it is aligned most closely with the patient's functional challenge, which is descending stairs. This requires analytical reasoning skill to determine the precise meaning of the information presented in the four choices. If this question was answered incorrectly, review information on indications for closed-chain exercises.

B87 | Neuromuscular | Foundational Sciences 

Independent community ambulation as the primary means of functional mobility is a realistic functional expectation for a patient with the highest level of complete spinal cord injury at:

CHOICES:

1. Midthoracic (T6–9).
2. High lumbar (T12–L1).
3. Low lumbar (L4–5).
4. Low thoracic (T9–10).

TEACHING POINTS

CORRECT ANSWER: 3

Patients with low lumbar lesions (L4–5) can be independent and functional with bilateral AFOs and canes.

INCORRECT CHOICES:

Patients with complete higher lesions (all other choices) can learn to ambulate with KAFOs and crutches, but exhibit a high rate of orthotic rejection in favor of primary wheelchair mobility. Rejection is due to the high levels of energy expenditure during ambulation.

TYPE OF REASONING: INFERENCE

One must infer the abilities and limitations of each of the spinal injury levels presented in order to make an appropriate determination for the patient who can most realistically perform community ambulation as a primary means of mobility. This requires one to use knowledge of neuroanatomy and spinal innervation levels to determine how the intact musculature can realistically allow for community ambulation. If answered incorrectly, refer to spinal innervation levels and intact musculature for ambulation.

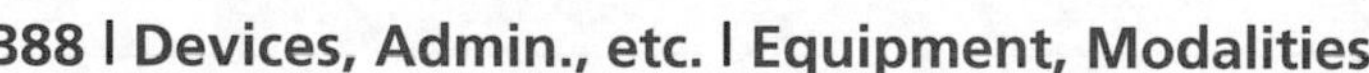

B88 | Devices, Admin., etc. | Equipment, Modalities

A patient presents with multiple fractures of both hands and wrists as a result of a mountain bike accident. Now, 5 weeks later, the patient has vertigo, limited wrist and finger motion, and dry scaly skin over the involved areas. The physical agent of **GREATEST BENEFIT** to select in this case would be:

CHOICES:

1. Paraffin.
2. Hot packs.
3. Functional electrical stimulation.
4. Contact ultrasound (US).

TEACHING POINTS

CORRECT ANSWER: 1

Paraffin bath will provide circumferential heating of the hands and fingers and aid in softening the skin.

INCORRECT CHOICES:

Active exercise, including functional electrical stimulation, would be more effective after the application of paraffin because tissue extensibility and pliability would be increased. Hot packs or US using direct contact would not completely cover the area to be treated.

TYPE OF REASONING: INDUCTIVE

This question requires one to use his/her clinical judgment to make the best determination for a modality to remedy the symptoms of the patient, which is an inductive reasoning skill. In this circumstance, paraffin is ideal for circumferential heating and skin softening. If this question was answered incorrectly, refer to indications for paraffin treatment.

B89 | Devices, Admin., etc. | Equipment, Modalities

An elderly patient demonstrates a history of recent falls (two in the last 2 months) and mild balance instability. The therapist's referral is to examine the patient and recommend an assistive device as needed. Based on the patient's history, it would be **BEST** to select a:

CHOICES:

1. Folding reciprocal walker.
2. Front wheel rolling walker that folds.
3. Standard, fixed-frame walker.
4. Hemi walker.

TEACHING POINTS

CORRECT ANSWER: 2

A rolling walker will provide added stability, while maintaining gait as a continuous movement sequence. The additional benefit of a folding walker facilitates easy transport and mobility in the community.

INCORRECT CHOICES:

A standard fixed-frame walker requires the patient to lift the walker and increases the energy expenditure. A hemi walker decreases the stability offered. A reciprocal walker requires increased motor control to use and also provides less stability.

TYPE OF REASONING: INFERENCE

One must determine how each of the assistive devices will best aid stability for a patient with a history of falls and mild balance instability. Questions that require one to infer information and draw conclusions from that information encourage inferential reasoning skill.

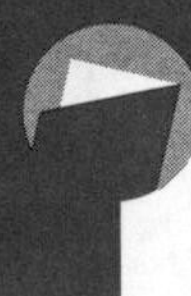

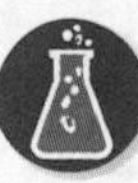

B90 | Musculoskeletal | Intervention

After surgery, a patient develops a stiff pelvis and limited pelvic/lower trunk mobility. The therapist elects to use sitting exercises on a therapy ball to correct these impairments. In order to improve lower abdominal control, the ball would have to move:

CHOICES:

1. Forward, producing posterior tilting of the pelvis.
2. Backward, producing posterior tilting of the pelvis.
3. Forward, producing anterior tilting of the pelvis.
4. Backward, producing anterior tilting of the pelvis.

TEACHING POINTS

CORRECT ANSWER: 1

Contraction of the lower abdominals results in posterior tilting of the pelvis and can be achieved with forward or anterior movement of the therapy ball.

INCORRECT CHOICES:

The other choices incorrectly state the effects of this sitting ball exercise. Backward or posterior motion of the ball produces anterior tilting of the pelvis.

TYPE OF REASONING: ANALYSIS

One must link the motion of the therapy ball to the motion achieved at the pelvis in order to make a correct determination in this scenario. Using analytical reasoning skills, the test taker must determine the meaning of the information presented, and then link this information to improvement in lower abdominal control. In this case, forward motion of the ball will promote posterior pelvic tilt and contraction of the lower abdominals. If this question was answered incorrectly, review principles of therapy ball activities.

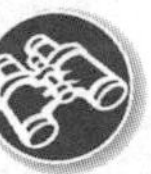

B91 | Neuromuscular | Evaluation, Diagnosis, Prognosis

A patient presents with weakness in the right lower leg 3 weeks after a motor vehicle accident. The patient complains of spontaneous twitching in the muscles of the lower leg. The therapist visually inspects both limbs and determines that muscle bulk is reduced on the involved right limb. Girth measurements confirm a 1-inch difference in the circumference of the right leg measured 4 inches below the patella. Deep tendon reflexes and tone are diminished. Based on these signs and symptoms, the therapist concludes the patient is exhibiting:

CHOICES:

1. Pyramidal tract dysfunction in the medulla.
2. Guillain-Barré syndrome.
3. Brainstem dysfunction affecting extrapyramidal pathways.
4. A peripheral nerve injury.

TEACHING POINTS

CORRECT ANSWER: 4

This patient is exhibiting signs and symptoms of lower motor neuron injury (hypotonia, hyporeflexia, paresis, neurogenic atrophy). The presence of muscle fasciculations is a hallmark sign of lower motor neuron injury.

INCORRECT CHOICES:

Upper motor neuron lesions (cortical or pyramidal tracts) would result in hypertonicity (hypotonicity initially during shock), hyperreflexia, generalized paresis, and variable disuse atrophy. Guillain-Barré syndrome is a lower motor neuron condition that produces symmetrical and ascending signs. Extrapyramidal signs (involuntary movements) are not evident in this case.

TYPE OF REASONING: INDUCTIVE

This question requires one to use diagnostic thinking and clinical judgment, which is an inductive reasoning skill. One should recognize that the hypotonia, hyporeflexia, paresis, and muscle fasciculations are indicative of a lower motor neuron injury and, therefore, a peripheral nerve injury. If this question was answered incorrectly, refer to information regarding lower motor neuron injuries and symptomatology.

B92 | Integumentary | Intervention 

A therapist receives an order for sharp débridement and treatment of a patient with a partial-thickness dermal ulceration. After the second visit, the wound bed is covered with 50% granulation tissue and 50% necrotic tissue that is adherent to the base of the wound bed. Sharp débridement is no longer tolerated. The therapist determines that an enzymatic agent is appropriate, and contacts the patient's physician to discuss this option and obtain a prescription. The **BEST** choice of enzymatic agent to use in this situation is:

CHOICES:

1. Panafil (a keratolytic).
2. Lidocaine spray.
3. Santyl (a collagenase).
4. A wet-to-dry application of Dakin's solution.

TEACHING POINTS

CORRECT ANSWER: 3

Enzymatic agents are useful for débridement, because they are usually selective débriders and cause minimal patient discomfort. Disadvantages include dermatitis and frequent dressing changes. These agents are also slower methods than sharp or mechanical débridement. The referring physician must be contacted in this case, because enzymatic agents are drugs and require a prescription. Necrotic collagen fibers are typically found near the base of the wound, and require an enzymatic agent that is specific for that type of tissue. Santyl is selective for denuded collagen fibers, does not harm granulation, and can be used in combination with antimicrobial powders.

INCORRECT CHOICES:

Panafil (keratolytic) contains papain, urea, and chlorophyllin copper (which often causes the tissue and exudate to turn green) and is most often recommended for more superficial necrotic layers because these layers have more protein. Dakin's (bleach and boric acid) is not an enzymatic débrider, and is cytotoxic and contraindicated in noninfected wounds. Lidocaine spray is a topical anesthetic that can be used to anesthetize a wound.

TYPE OF REASONING: INDUCTIVE

This question requires one to understand the benefits of each of the agents listed in order to determine the best agent to use with the patient's wound. In this situation, Santyl is best because it does not harm granulation tissue and works to débride basilar collagen fibers. Inductive reasoning is utilized in answering this question, because the test taker must use knowledge of the agents, combined with clinical judgment, for a best course of action to arrive at a correct conclusion.

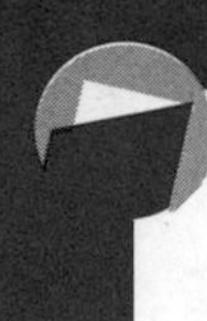

B93 | Cardiovascular-Pulmonary | Evaluation, Diagnosis, Prognosis

A patient with bacterial pneumonia has crackles and wheezes at the left lateral basal segment and decreased breath sounds throughout. The patient is on 4 L of oxygen by nasal cannula with a resulting arterial oxygen saturation (SaO_2) of 90%. Respiratory rate is 28. What is the **MOST BENEFICIAL** intervention for this case?

CHOICES:

1. Postural drainage, percussion, and shaking to the right basilar segments in order to keep the right lung healthy.
2. Postural drainage, percussion, and shaking over the appropriate area on the left lateral thorax for secretion removal.
3. Breathing exercises encouraging expansion of the right lateral basilar thorax, because the left side is not currently participating in gas exchange.
4. Positioning in left side-lying to improve ventilation/perfusion ratios.

TEACHING POINTS

CORRECT ANSWER: 2

A treatment of postural drainage, percussion, and shaking to the appropriate lung segments is advisable. The standard postural drainage position for the lateral basilar segment of the left lower lobe is in side-lying position with the head of bed tipped in full Trendelenburg's position. Given the borderline SaO_2 values on 4 L of oxygen, modification of the position may be necessary for patient tolerance.

INCORRECT CHOICES:

There is nothing that will ensure that the right lung stays healthy or makes it more functional. Therefore, choices 1 and 3 are incorrect answers. Placing the patient in the left side-lying position would increase blood flow to the left lateral base, an area that is getting little ventilation. This position would worsen ventilation/perfusion matching.

TYPE OF REASONING: INDUCTIVE

One must utilize clinical judgment to determine which intervention approach is most beneficial, given the patient's diagnosis and symptoms. This is an inductive reasoning skill, in which clinical judgment and diagnostic thinking are used to arrive at the correct conclusion. If this topic is not well understood, refer to indications for modified postural drainage procedures.

B94 | Other Systems | Evaluation, Diagnosis, Prognosis

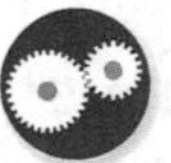

A therapist receives a referral to see an elderly patient in the intensive care unit (ICU) recovering from a severe case of pneumonia. The therapist recognizes that the disorientation is due to delirium rather than dementia because the:

CHOICES:

1. Symptoms are intermittent.
2. Patient demonstrates persistent personality changes.
3. Level of arousal is significantly depressed.
4. Patient has hallucinations throughout the day.

TEACHING POINTS

CORRECT ANSWER: 1

Acutely ill, hospitalized elderly patients frequently exhibit delirium, a fluctuating attention state. Patients demonstrate a fluctuating course with symptoms of confusion that alternate with lucid intervals. Sleep/wake cycles are disrupted and confusion is typically worse at night.

INCORRECT CHOICES:

All other choices are signs of chronic dementia.

TYPE OF REASONING: EVALUATION

One must evaluate the merits of each of the four statements in order to determine which statement most likely seems true for the patient's symptoms and diagnosis. In this case, the disorientation is due to delirium, because the symptoms are intermittent, whereas patients with dementia experience constant, disorientation. Questions that require one to determine the value and merits of statements presented utilize evaluative reasoning skill, which can be challenging because of the need to make a judgment call.

B95 | Devices, Admin., etc. | Teaching, Research, Roles 

A comparison of the effects of exercise in water, on land, or combined on the rehabilitation outcome of patients with intra-articular anterior cruciate ligament reconstructions revealed that less joint effusion was noted after 8 weeks in the water group. An appropriate statistical test to compare the girth measurements of the three groups is:

CHOICES:

1. Spearman rho.
2. Analysis of covariance.
3. ANOVA.
4. Chi square.

TEACHING POINTS

CORRECT ANSWER: 3

ANOVA is a parametric statistical test used to compare three or more treatment groups (in this example, in water, on land, or combined exercise groups) on a measure of the dependent variable (joint effusion girth measurements) at a selected probability level.

INCORRECT CHOICES:

Analysis of covariance compares two or more groups, but also controls for the effects of an intervening variable. Chi square is a nonparametric statistical test used to compare data in the form of frequency counts. Spearman's rho (rank correlation coefficient) is a nonparametric test used to correlate ordinal data.

TYPE OF REASONING: DEDUCTIVE

Questions that require one to recall factual information, especially information related to research protocols, require deductive reasoning skill. One must utilize knowledge of the indications for each statistical test in order to arrive at the correct conclusion. If this question was answered incorrectly, review information on guidelines for the use of ANOVA as well as parametric and nonparametric statistical tests.

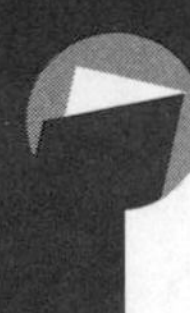

B96 | Neuromuscular | Intervention

A patient has a recent history of strokes (two in the past 4 months) and demonstrates good return in the right lower extremity. The therapist is concentrating on improving balance and independence in gait. Unfortunately, speech recovery is lagging behind motor recovery. The patient demonstrates a severe fluent aphasia. The **BEST** strategy to use during physical therapy is:

CHOICES:

1. Demonstrate and gesture to get the idea of the task across.
2. Utilize verbal cues, emphasizing consistency and repetition.
3. Consult with the speech pathologist to establish a communication board.
4. Have the family present to help interpret during physical therapy sessions.

TEACHING POINTS

CORRECT ANSWER: 1

Fluent aphasia (Wernicke's aphasia) is a central language disorder in which spontaneous speech is preserved and flows smoothly while auditory comprehension is impaired. Demonstration and gesture (visual modalities) offer the best means of communicating with this patient.

INCORRECT CHOICES:

Verbal cues are best for patients with nonfluent aphasia (Broca's aphasia) in which understanding of verbal cues is intact but motor production of speech is not. A communication board is not needed. The family will also have difficulties communicating with the patient.

TYPE OF REASONING: INDUCTIVE

In this question, the patient requires gait training, but has limitations in communication from Wernicke's aphasia. The test taker must determine the best way to communicate with a patient who has this deficit, which is to provide demonstrations and gestures, rather than verbal cues. Questions that elicit clinical judgment to determine a best course of action utilize inductive reasoning skills. If this question was answered incorrectly, refer to information on communication with patients who have Wernicke's aphasia.

B97 | Musculoskeletal | Patient Examination

An individual is walking with a transfemoral prosthesis and demonstrates terminal swing impact. The therapist suspects the:

CHOICES:

1. Prosthesis is externally rotated.
2. Hip flexors are weak.
3. Prosthesis has insufficient knee friction.
4. Prosthesis has too little tension in the extension aid.

TEACHING POINTS

CORRECT ANSWER: 3

Terminal swing impact refers to the sudden stopping of the prosthesis as the knee extends during late swing. Possible causes can include insufficient knee friction or too much tension in the extension aid. In addition, if the patient with an amputation fears the knee will buckle at heel-strike, the patient can use forceful hip flexion to extend the knee.

INCORRECT CHOICES:

Faulty socket contour results in an externally rotated prosthesis. The extension aid has too much tension (not too little). Weak hip flexors would result in decreased force to extend the knee.

TYPE OF REASONING: INFERENCE

One must infer the reason FOR the terminal swing impact when walking with an above-knee prosthesis, which is an inferential reasoning skill (requiring one to draw conclusions based on presented evidence). Using knowledge of above-knee prostheses and proper tension of the extension aid, one can infer that the tension on the extension aid is too high. If this question was answered incorrectly, review information on above-knee prosthesis fit and functions.

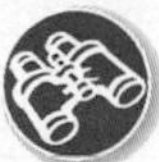

B98 | Integumentary | Intervention

A patient was burned over 40% of the body in an industrial accident, and has full-thickness burns over the anterior trunk and neck and superficial partial-thickness burns over the shoulders. The procedures of **GREATEST BENEFIT** to stabilize this patient out of positions of common deformity include:

CHOICES:

1. Splints utilizing a flexed position for the shoulders and body jacket for the trunk.
2. Plastic cervical orthosis and axillary splints utilizing an airplane position.
3. Soft cervical collar with an intrinsic plus hand splint.
4. A cervical thoracic lumbosacral orthosis (CTLSO) used during all upright activities.

TEACHING POINTS

CORRECT ANSWER: 2

The common deformity for the anterior neck is flexion; the appropriate positioning device is a firm rigid plastic cervical collar that stresses extension. The common deformity of the shoulders is adduction and internal rotation; the appropriate position device is an axillary or airplane splint that stresses abduction, flexion, and external rotation.

INCORRECT CHOICES:

Choices that involve hand splints should be ruled out immediately, because there is no mention of burns to the hands. A CTLSO would prevent neck flexion, but does not deal with the potential shoulder deformities. The CTLSO could also restrict breathing and enhance the risk of pneumonia.

TYPE OF REASONING: INDUCTIVE

This question requires one to recall common positioning techniques after burns to the anterior trunk and neck. Using knowledge of the typical deformity and contracture patterns with burns to this area, one can reason that the solution is to utilize axillary splints and cervical orthosis to bring about abduction, flexion, and external rotation of the shoulders and cervical extension. Questions that require one to make interpretations of clinical guidelines and make judgments from this utilize inductive reasoning skills.

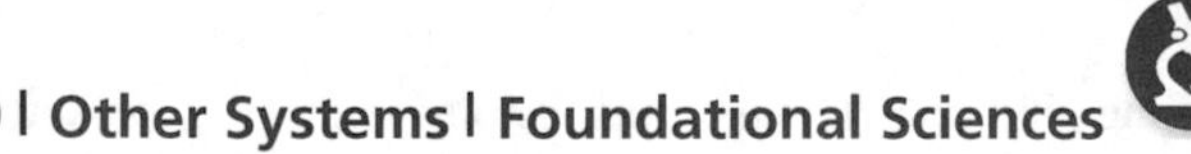

B99 | Other Systems | Foundational Sciences

A patient with type 2 diabetes is referred to physical therapy for exercise conditioning. The therapist recognizes that this patient's diabetes is the result of:

CHOICES:

1. Impaired ability of the tissues to use insulin and insulin deficiency.
2. Pancreatic tumor.
3. Loss of beta-cell function and insulin deficiency.
4. Metabolic syndrome.

TEACHING POINTS

CORRECT ANSWER: 1

Type 2 diabetes results from impaired ability of the tissues to use insulin (insulin resistance), accompanied by a relative lack of insulin or impaired release of insulin.

INCORRECT CHOICES:

Type 1 diabetes results from loss of pancreatic beta-cell function and an absolute insulin deficiency. Metabolic syndrome is a precursor to type 2 diabetes and is evidenced by abdominal obesity, high triglycerides, low high-density lipoprotein (HDL), hypertension, and high fasting plasma glucose (>110 mg/dL). Pancreatic tumor is not a causative factor in type 2 diabetes.

TYPE OF REASONING: DEDUCTIVE

One must recall the factual guidelines of type 2 diabetes in order to arrive at a correct conclusion. This requires deductive reasoning skill. For this situation, type 2 diabetes is the result of an impaired ability of the tissues to use insulin and insulin deficiency. If this question was answered incorrectly, review type 2 diabetes information, especially causes of the condition.

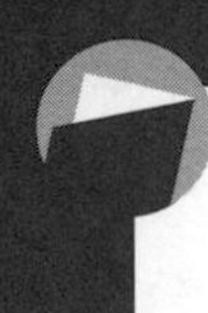

B100 | Neuromuscular | Intervention

Which intervention is **BEST** to improve left-sided neglect in a patient with left hemiplegia?

CHOICES:

1. Hook-lying, holding, light resistance to both hip abductors.
2. Rolling, supine to side-lying on right, using a PNF lift pattern.
3. Bridging with both arms positioned in extension at the sides.
4. Sitting, with both arms extended, hands resting on support surface, active holding.

TEACHING POINTS

CORRECT ANSWER: 2

Incorporating the involved left side into a crossing the midline activity (rolling, using PNF lift) is best.

INCORRECT CHOICES:

All other choices involve symmetrical activity and do little to bring attention to the involved hemiplegic side.

TYPE OF REASONING: INFERENCE

One must link the deficit of the patient (left-sided neglect) to the best treatment approach in order to arrive at the correct conclusion. This requires inferential reasoning skill, as one must infer the course of action that will have the best clinical outcome. In this circumstance, rolling supine to side-lying on the right using a PNF lift pattern is best because it incorporates use of the left side and promotes crossing the midline. If this question was answered incorrectly, review treatment strategies for hemiplegia, especially PNF.

B101 | Devices, Admin., etc. | Teaching, Research, Roles

A patient with TBI receiving physical therapy for the past 2 months has not demonstrated functional improvement. The patient's care is covered by Medicare. The therapist has informed both the physician and the family of this patient's lack of progress. The family insists that the therapist continue to treat the patient, and the physician will continue to certify the patient for more physical therapy. The therapist should:

CHOICES:

1. Continue to provide the care both the family and the referring physician demand; it is the physician's responsibility to determine the appropriateness of physical therapy.
2. Refer the patient to another clinic that is willing to continue treatment despite lack of functional improvement.
3. Modify treatment goals in a manner that will allow the therapist to demonstrate that the treatment is achieving progress toward reasonable goals.
4. Provide the family Medicare "notification of noncoverage" information, and carefully explain it, and their options, which could include paying for the care out-of-pocket.

TEACHING POINTS

CORRECT ANSWER: 4

Medicare requires that physical therapy is skilled and appropriate and demonstrates progress toward reasonable functional goals. Despite the fact that Medicare requires that the physician responsible for the patient "certify" the necessity and appropriateness of physical therapy, this does not absolve the PT from the responsibility of determining whether physical therapy is appropriate. This is the sole responsibility of the PT.

INCORRECT CHOICES:

Neither the physician nor the family can determine the appropriateness of continuing physical therapy. Modifying treatment to ensure progress for continued Medicare coverage or passing the buck with referral to another clinic violates professional ethical codes.

TYPE OF REASONING: DEDUCTIVE

One must understand Medicare coverage guidelines in order to choose the correct solution. Decisions that require one to draw upon knowledge of facts and guidelines require deductive reasoning skill. If this question was answered incorrectly, review Medicare coverage guidelines, especially notification of noncoverage information.

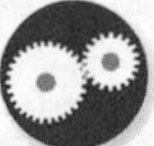

B102 | Cardiovascular-Pulmonary | Evaluation, Diagnosis, Prognosis

A patient with chronic obstructive pulmonary disease (COPD) reports to the fourth outpatient pulmonary rehabilitation session complaining of nausea, gastric upset, and feeling jittery. The patient reports no change in pulmonary symptoms. The PT records the following set of vital signs: temperature 98.6 degrees F, HR 110 beats/min and irregular, BP 150/86, respiratory rate 20. Breath sounds show no change from baseline. The therapist checks the medical record and finds that the patient has no history of gastric disease. The patient is presently taking theophylline, albuterol sulfate (Ventolin), and triamcinolone diacetate (Amcort). The PT should:

CHOICES:

1. Send the patient home and notify the physician of current symptoms.
2. Have the patient increase use of Ventolin to improve respiratory status.
3. Call the patient's physician and report signs of theophylline toxicity.
4. Have the patient stop use of Amcort until he/she schedules an appointment with the physician.

TEACHING POINTS

CORRECT ANSWER: 3

Theophylline is a bronchodilator used to reverse airway obstruction. The combination of symptoms of irregular HR, feeling jittery, and gastric upset is consistent with theophylline toxicity. Because theophylline toxicity can cause arrhythmias and seizures, the patient's physician should be notified by the PT rather than wait for the patient to return home to call the physician. It is also likely that a blood test will be needed to check the theophylline toxicity level and this could be done at the facility.

INCORRECT CHOICES:

Ventolin is a bronchodilator used in the treatment of asthma or COPD. Amcort is an anti-inflammatory agent used to manage bronchial asthma. Neither drug produces the same combination of symptoms described in the case. The therapist should not recommend increasing or stopping a prescribed medication. This is the usually the physician's responsibility.

TYPE OF REASONING: EVALUATION

This question requires one to make a judgment for the well-being of the patient as well as to make a determination of the reason for the patient's symptoms. Value judgments require the use of evaluative reasoning skill in order to determine the best course of action. If this question was answered incorrectly, review information on theophylline toxicity and adverse reactions/side effects of Ventolin and Amcort.

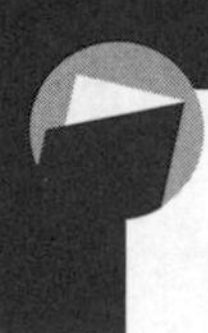

B103 | Neuromuscular | Evaluation, Diagnosis, Prognosis

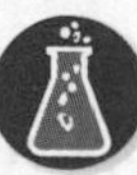

The therapist is treating a 1 year-old child with Down syndrome at home, and notices decreasing strength in the extremities, with neck pain and limited neck motion. Upper extremity deep tendon reflexes (DTRs) are 3+. The therapist suspects:

CHOICES:

1. Upper motor neuron signs consistent with Down syndrome.
2. Atlantoaxial subluxation with spinal cord impingement.
3. Lower motor neuron signs consistent with Down syndrome.
4. Atlantoaxial subluxation with lemniscal impingement.

TEACHING POINTS

CORRECT ANSWER: 2

Ligamentous laxity is a hallmark of Down syndrome, and can lead to atlantoaxial instability (AAI), with spinal cord impingement. This is a medical emergency situation. Decreased muscle strength and increased DTRs are the signs of dislocation from loss of cord function. In this case, the increasing symptomatology (changes in strength, neck pain, limited neck motion, hyperreflexia) is significant for a developing subluxation. Other UMN signs (clonus, positive Babinski response) may also occur.

INCORRECT CHOICES:

Children with Down syndrome often have low tone, not upper motor neuron or lower motor neuron signs. Lemniscal impingement would result primarily in sensory changes.

TYPE OF REASONING: ANALYSIS

In this question, symptoms are provided and the test taker must determine the cause. This type of question requires analytical reasoning, in which the test taker must determine the meaning of the symptoms presented. In this situation, one should determine that the symptoms indicate atlantoaxial subluxation with spinal cord impingement, a medical emergency, which should be reviewed if this question was answered incorrectly.

B104 | Neuromuscular | Evaluation, Diagnosis, Prognosis

Which of the following factors is likely to contribute to subluxation and shoulder pain in hemiplegia?

CHOICES:

1. Spastic paralysis of the biceps.
2. PROM with normal scapulohumeral rhythm.
3. Traction and gravitational forces acting on a depressed, downwardly rotated scapula.
4. Spastic retraction with elevation of scapula.

TEACHING POINTS

CORRECT ANSWER: 3

Shoulder pain and subluxation in hemiplegia may be caused by a number of different factors. One major cause is traction and gravitational forces acting on a depressed, downwardly rotated scapula.

INCORRECT CHOICES:

An appropriate treatment intervention involves PROM with careful attention to maintaining scapulohumeral rhythm. This intervention if performed correctly is **NOT** likely to cause pain. Spastic biceps is likely, but is not a contributing factor to subluxation and pain. Spastic retraction of the scapula is likely but with depression and downward rotation (not elevation).

TYPE OF REASONING: INFERENCE

This question requires the test taker to determine which causative factor is unlikely to result in shoulder pain in hemiplegia. This requires one to draw conclusions from the information presented and to make assumptions about that information, which draws upon inferential reasoning skill. One must have knowledge of the factors that affect subluxation as well as those that do not in order to arrive at the correct conclusion.

B105 | Neuromuscular | Patient Examination

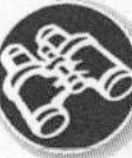

While gait training a patient recovering from a CVA, the therapist observes the knee on the affected side going into recurvatum during stance phase. The **MOST LIKELY** cause of this deviation can be attributed to:

CHOICES:

1. Weakness or severe spasticity of the quadriceps.
2. Weakness of the gastrocnemius-soleus or spasticity of the pretibial muscles.
3. Weakness of both the gastrocnemius-soleus and the pretibial muscles.
4. Severe spasticity of the hamstrings or weakness of the gastrocnemius-soleus.

TEACHING POINTS

CORRECT ANSWER: 1

Severe spasticity of the quadriceps will pull the knee strongly into extension and recurvatum. The patient with a weak quadriceps muscle will compensate by fixing the knee in full extension (recurvatum) during stance, rather than maintaining the knee in a small amount of knee flexion at midstance.

INCORRECT CHOICES:

Weakness of the gastrocnemius-soleus would result in lack of push-off at end of stance. Spasticity of the pretibial muscles or hamstrings is highly unlikely because spasticity typically occurs in antigravity muscles (extensors, adductors, and plantarflexors). Weakness of the pretibial muscles results in drop foot and swing phase difficulties.

TYPE OF REASONING: INDUCTIVE

This question requires one to utilize clinical judgment to arrive at the correct conclusion. Questions that draw upon diagnostic thinking and judgment require inductive reasoning skill. In this case, the test taker uses this judgment to determine the cause for the patient's recurvatum during stance, which is from weakness or severe spasticity of the quadriceps.

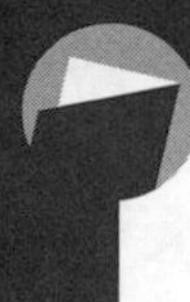

B106 | Integumentary | Evaluation, Diagnosis, Prognosis 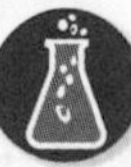

A patient with hemiplegia and a drop foot is referred for physical therapy gait training. Examination reveals a pressure ulcer on the patient's right heel (pictured). The ulcer has dry eschar without edema, erythema, fluctuance, or drainage. The patient is afebrile. The **BEST** choice for intervention for this patient is:

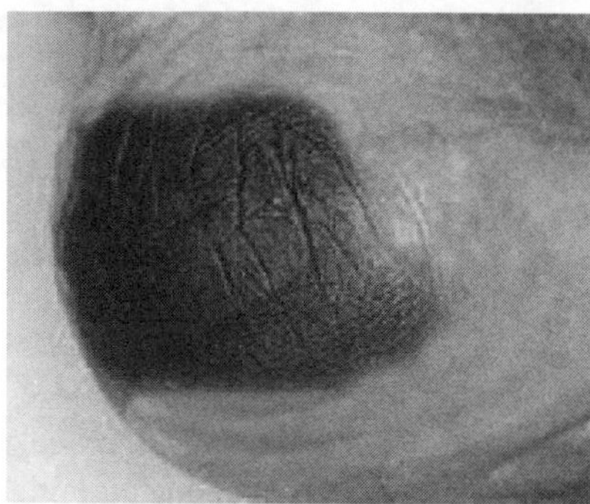

CHOICES:

1. Enzymatic débridement.
2. Refer for an arterial bypass graft.
3. Sharp débridement.
4. Use an AFO with heel pressure relief.

TEACHING POINTS

CORRECT ANSWER: 4

The AFO helps to prevent plantar flexion contractures, while the heel pressure relief prevents further damage to the heel and promotes healing.

INCORRECT CHOICES:

This pressure ulcer, based on the examination findings, is stable and needs to be monitored, not débrided (choices 1 and 3). Arterial bypass grafts are needed if circulation is compromised. There is no indication that this is the case.

TYPE OF REASONING: ANALYSIS

In this question, one must determine the best course of action for the patient with a pressure ulcer on the heel. When one must determine the meaning of visual information presented, such as the picture, analytical reasoning skills are utilized. If this question was answered incorrectly, review information on the treatment of pressure ulcers.

B107 | Devices, Admin., etc. | Teaching, Research, Roles

A therapist has completed a study investigating the relationship between ratings of perceived exertion (RPE) and type of testing modality: arm ergometry versus leg ergometry. The therapist finds a correlation 0.59 with the arm testing, whereas the correlation is 0.79 with the leg testing. Interpretation of these results is that:

CHOICES:

1. Both arm and leg ergometry are only moderately correlated with RPE.
2. Both arm and leg ergometry are highly correlated with RPE.
3. The common variance of both types of testing is only 22%.
4. Leg ergometry is highly correlated with RPE, whereas arm ergometry is only moderately correlated.

TEACHING POINTS

CORRECT ANSWER: 4

In correlational studies, high correlations range from 0.7 to +1.0, and moderate correlations range from 0.35 to 0.69.

INCORRECT CHOICES:

The two types of ergometry do not demonstrate the same degree of correlation (moderate or high). Common variance is a representation of the degree that variation in one variable is attributable to another variable and is determined by squaring the correlation coefficient.

TYPE OF REASONING: DEDUCTIVE

This question requires the test taker to recall information regarding correlation ranges. This information is factual in nature, and requires deductive reasoning skill to choose the correct solution. In this example, a correlation of 0.59 indicates moderate correlation, whereas 0.79 indicates high correlation. If this question was answered incorrectly, refer to information on correlation ranges.

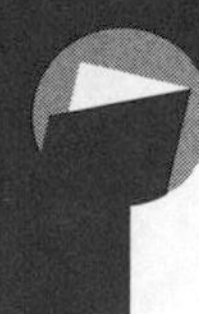

B108 | Musculoskeletal | Evaluation, Diagnosis, Prognosis

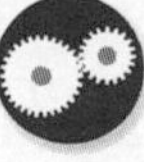

A patient with left knee DJD complains of left-sided knee pain of 2 months' duration. The patient has been followed by outpatient physical therapy for 3 weeks, and feels this condition is worsening. Pain has increased during weight-bearing activities, and the patient can no longer fully extend the left knee. Examination findings include increased swelling, decreased knee AROM into extension, and an antalgic gait. The PT should:

CHOICES:

1. Immediately return the patient to the referring physician with documentation indicating that treatment was ineffective.
2. Continue therapy for another week to ensure that all interventions have been attempted, and then return the patient to the referring physician.
3. Continue physical therapy for another 2 weeks, because there is uncertainty whether the patient understands or is complying with the home exercise program.
4. Tell the patient to see an orthopedic surgeon for possible immediate surgical intervention.

TEACHING POINTS

CORRECT ANSWER: 1

In this case, it would be best to send the patient back to the referring physician with an explanation of what was done, the ineffectiveness of the treatment, and any suggestions for further follow-up.

INCORRECT CHOICES:

The therapist should not continue to treat a patient if the therapist feels no further benefit would be derived by continuing care because it contradicts the American Physical Therapy Association's (APTA's) Code of Ethics. Suggesting the patient needs immediate surgery is outside the scope of the PT's practice.

TYPE OF REASONING: EVALUATION

One must rely on professional conduct principles and apply value judgments to the case situation described in order to arrive at the correct decision. This type of question, in which value judgments are needed to make a decision, necessitates the use of evaluative reasoning skill. In situations in which a patient demonstrates decline in status despite ongoing treatment, it is best to refer the patient back to the physician for follow-up and document the findings regarding this situation.

B109 | Devices, Admin., etc. | Equipment, Modalities

Two months ago, a patient had an inversion sprain affecting the calcaneofibular and anterior talofibular ligaments of the right ankle. The ankle is still painful, very limited in motion, and slightly tender to the touch. As part of physical therapy intervention, US treatment parameters should consist of:

CHOICES:

1. Continuous US at 1 MHz.
2. Pulsed US at 1 MHz.
3. Continuous US at 3 MHz.
4. Pulsed US at 3 MHz.

TEACHING POINTS

CORRECT ANSWER: 3

Because the ankle sprain is chronic in nature, the goal is to decrease pain and increase the range of motion (ROM; tissue extensibility). Increasing the tissue temperature will accomplish these objectives. This will require the heating effects of US produced by continuous US. Because the target structures are close to the skin surface, higher frequencies are used so that the acoustic energy will be absorbed (attenuated) in the superficial layers.

INCORRECT CHOICES:

Pulsed US and continuous US at 1 Hz are NOT the best choices for this patient, because pulsed US does not generate any heat, and a frequency of 1 MHz penetrates too deeply, which would result in periosteal overheating.

TYPE OF REASONING: DEDUCTIVE

The recall of proper US parameters related to chronic ankle sprain utilizes deductive reasoning skill, because knowledge of protocols is required. One must understand the appropriate frequency to use related to the target structures to be treated and the thermal or nonthermal properties achieved with either continuous or pulsed US. In this case, continuous US at 3 MHz is most appropriate to achieve thermal properties over an area of a bony prominence with chronic sprain to the ligaments.

B110 | Neuromuscular | Intervention

In NDT of the patient recovering from stroke, therapy should include:

CHOICES:

1. Reduction of spasticity and abnormal reflex activity through positioning and handling techniques, coupled with movement training.
2. Facilitation of first early movements in synergistic patterns, then out-of-synergy movements.
3. Prolonged positioning out of the typical spastic patterns, followed by PROM.
4. Functional activities emphasizing manual tasks using the less affected side.

TEACHING POINTS

CORRECT ANSWER: 1

The focus of NDT therapy (Bobath's approach) after stroke is to encourage functional return of normal patterns of movement. Movement training utilizes active assisted and active movements with activities designed to break up the abnormal synergies. This is assisted by handling techniques that reduce the influence of spasticity and obligatory reflexes.

INCORRECT CHOICES:

Obligatory synergistic patterns are never encouraged. Prolonged positioning is contraindicated because the patient may stiffen up with excess tone. Activities that utilize only the less affected side are discouraged.

TYPE OF REASONING: INFERENCE

NDT provides guidelines for effective intervention after stroke. This requires one to make assumptions based on facts, which is an inferential reasoning skill. If this question was answered incorrectly, review information on techniques and guidelines of NDT.

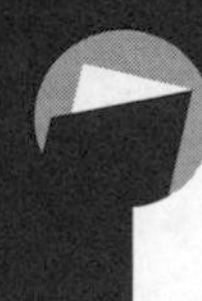

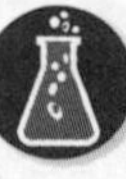

B111 | Devices, Admin., etc. | Equipment, Modalities

A 4 year-old child with moderate spastic diplegia is referred to physical therapy for an adaptive equipment evaluation. Which device/apparatus would be **CONTRAINDICATED**?

CHOICES:

1. Bilateral KAFOs.
2. Prone stander.
3. Tone-reducing AFOs.
4. Posture-control walker (posterior walker).

TEACHING POINTS

CORRECT ANSWER: 1

The knees would not need to be braced using bilateral KAFOs in spastic diplegia because moderate extensor tone can provide antigravity support.

INCORRECT CHOICES:

Tone-reducing AFOs are indicated to stabilize the foot and prevent plantarflexion. A posterior walker and prone stander may both enhance function.

TYPE OF REASONING: ANALYSIS

The test taker must evaluate all of the adaptive devices listed in this question and then determine which device is **contraindicated** given the child's diagnosis. In this situation, bilateral KAFOs are not appropriate. In order to arrive at the correct conclusion, one must analyze each of the devices for their therapeutic value and then determine which device provides the least value.

B112 | Neuromuscular | Intervention

An ambulatory patient recovering from a left CVA is wearing a plastic KAFO to stabilize the right foot. During gait analysis, the therapist observes lateral trunk bending toward the right as the patient bears weight on the right leg at midstance. The **BEST** intervention to correct this problem is:

CHOICES:

1. Provide a lift on the shoe of the involved leg.
2. Strengthen hip flexors on the right side.
3. Strengthen hamstrings on the right side.
4. Strengthen the hip abductors on the right side.

TEACHING POINTS

CORRECT ANSWER: 4

The lateral trunk bending (Trendelenburg's gait) is the result of weak hip abductors on the right (a common problem for patients recovering from stroke). Strengthening of the abductors on the involved right side is indicated.

INCORRECT CHOICES:

The other choices do not address the problem of lateral trunk bending. Weakness of the hip flexors or hamstrings would present as swing phase deficits (inability to shorten the leg so it can clear the floor). The patient is likely to compensate with circumduction. A lift on the left foot might be considered for patients with this problem but is not the intervention of choice.

TYPE OF REASONING: INDUCTIVE

This question requires one to utilize clinical judgment to determine the best choice to correct the Trendelenburg's gait. Questions that encourage diagnostic thinking and clinical judgment utilize inductive reasoning skill. In this situation, the patient's gait pattern indicates weak hip abductors. If this question was answered incorrectly, review information on intervention approaches for Trendelenburg's gait.

B113 | Musculoskeletal | Evaluation, Diagnosis, Prognosis

A 10 year-old boy, who plays catcher on a baseball team, complains of bilateral knee pain that is exacerbated with forceful quadriceps contraction. He has also noticed pain and swelling at the distal attachment of the patellar tendon. The **BEST** early physical therapy intervention is:

CHOICES:

1. Modalities to decrease inflammation.
2. Strengthening exercises for the quadriceps femoris to prevent disuse atrophy.
3. Decreased loading of the knee by the quadriceps femoris muscle.
4. Casting followed by decreased loading of the knee.

TEACHING POINTS

CORRECT ANSWER: 3

Baseball catchers must make forceful contractions of the quadriceps muscles each time they stand up to throw the ball to the pitcher. This may precipitate Osgood-Schlatter disease in the adolescent or preadolescent boy. Early intervention of this condition focuses on reduction of the loading by the quadriceps, but still retaining normal lower extremity function.

INCORRECT CHOICES:

Modalities may provide temporary relief of pain, but it is unlikely that they will alter the inflammation and improve the underlying condition. Strengthening exercise would not be appropriate, because that will lead to continued excessive loading of the structures. Casting is not appropriate, because that may lead to restrictions in normal motion.

TYPE OF REASONING: INDUCTIVE

In this question, the test taker must determine the best intervention approach for a child with bilateral knee pain related to playing catcher. This requires clinical judgment, which is an inductive reasoning skill. One must have an understanding of the nature of this activity on the quadriceps muscles, especially the need for forceful contractions each time the catcher stands up, to arrive at the correct conclusion.

B114 | Integumentary | Intervention

A patient has a decubitus ulcer of 3 months' duration on the lateral ankle. The ankle is swollen, red, and painful, with a moderate to high amount of wound drainage (exudate). The **BEST** dressing for this wound is:

CHOICES:

1. Calcium alginate dressings.
2. Gauze dressings.
3. Semipermeable film dressings.
4. Hydrogel dressings.

TEACHING POINTS

CORRECT ANSWER: 1

Wounds with moderate to high exudate benefit from calcium alginate dressings. The dressings absorb large amounts of exudate (up to 20 times their weight) and form a gel, which maintains the moist wound environment while maintaining good permeability to oxygen.

INCORRECT CHOICES:

Gauze and semipermeable film dressings require a secondary dressing and offer poor conformability to deep wounds. Hydrogel dressings are not recommended for wounds with heavy exudate.

TYPE OF REASONING: INFERENCE

One must infer or draw conclusion based on the information presented in the patient's case, which draws upon inferential reasoning skill. In this situation, calcium alginate dressings are ideal for wounds with moderate to high exudate present. If this question was answered incorrectly, refer to information on wound dressings.

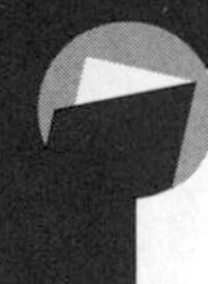

B115 | Musculoskeletal | Patient Examination

A patient was diagnosed with a bulging disc at the right L5–S1 spinal level without nerve root compression. The impairment **MOST LIKELY** to be documented is:

CHOICES:

1. Centralized gnawing pain with loss of postural control during lifting activities.
2. Radicular pain to the right great toe with a compensated gluteus medius gait.
3. Centralized gnawing pain with uncompensated gluteus medius gait.
4. Radicular pain to the right great toe with difficulty sitting for long periods.

TEACHING POINTS

CORRECT ANSWER: 1

Discal degeneration without nerve root compression would likely be exhibited as a centralized gnawing pain with loss of proprioception.

INCORRECT CHOICES:

Because there is no nerve compression, there will not be any type of radicular pain and/or decrease in specific muscle function (beyond the lumbar spine region), so one should not see a decrease in the function of the gluteus medius.

TYPE OF REASONING: INFERENCE

This question provides the diagnosis, and the test taker must determine the most likely symptoms to be present. This type of question in which symptoms must be determined from a diagnosis draws upon inferential reasoning skill. To arrive at the correct answer, the test taker must have a good understanding of the nature of L5–S1 discal degeneration.

B116 | Neuromuscular | Intervention

High-level training for an individual recovering from TBI who demonstrates Rancho Cognitive Function level VII should focus on:

CHOICES:

1. Providing a high degree of environmental structure to ensure correct performance.
2. Providing assistance as needed using guided movements during training.
3. Involving the patient in decision-making and monitoring for safety.
4. Providing maximum supervision as needed to ensure successful performance and safety.

TEACHING POINTS

CORRECT ANSWER: 3

As patients with TBI recover, structure and guidance must be gradually reduced and patient involvement in decision making increased. Safety must be maintained while increasing levels of independence are fostered. Patients at stage VII of recovery often exhibit rote movements (robot syndrome) indicative of the highly structured training utilized for patients during earlier stages of recovery.

INCORRECT CHOICES:

A high degree of structure, assistance, and maximum supervision is not therapeutic at this stage of recovery.

TYPE OF REASONING: DEDUCTIVE

Although this question does require one to utilize clinical judgment, the majority of skill required to answer this question correctly relies upon the recall of the Rancho Cognitive Function Levels and the guidelines for treatment provided within these levels. This is factual information and recall, which ultimately requires deductive reasoning ability to successfully choose the best type of training for the patient. If this question was answered incorrectly, refer to the Rancho Cognitive Function Levels.

B117 | Neuromuscular | Intervention

To correct for the problem of a forward festinating gait in a patient with PD, the therapist should:

CHOICES:

1. Increase cadence using a metronome.
2. Increase stride length using floor markers.
3. Use a toe wedge.
4. Use a heel wedge.

TEACHING POINTS

CORRECT ANSWER: 3

A festinating gait is an abnormal and involuntary increase in the speed of walking in an attempt to catch up with a displaced center of gravity due to the patient's forward lean. The most appropriate intervention would be to use a toe wedge, which would help to displace the patient's center of gravity backward.

INCORRECT CHOICES:

Increasing cadence or stride length would serve only to increase, not decrease, the problem, as will the use of a heel wedge.

TYPE OF REASONING: INDUCTIVE

One must use clinical judgment to determine which approach would best decrease a forward festinating gait pattern in PD. The test taker must understand that forward festination results from forward displacement of center of gravity, which can be improved through the use of a toe wedge to displace the patient's gravity backward. The judgment in this case, utilizing one's knowledge of festinating gait pattern and the intervention approaches proposed, encourages use of inductive reasoning skill.

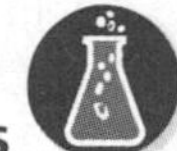

B118 | Musculoskeletal | Foundational Sciences

A patient presents with difficulty with fast movement speeds and fatigues easily. The therapist decides on a strength training program that specifically focuses on improving fast-twitch fiber function. The optimal exercise prescription to achieve this goal is:

CHOICES:

1. Low-intensity workloads for short durations.
2. Low-intensity workloads for long durations.
3. High-intensity workloads for long durations.
4. High-intensity workloads for short durations.

TEACHING POINTS

CORRECT ANSWER: 4

High-intensity exercises at fast contraction speeds for shorter durations (<20 repetitions) are needed to train the highly adaptable fast-twitch IIa fibers.

INCORRECT CHOICES:

Performing workloads at low intensity and slow contraction speeds will challenge slow-twitch (type I) fibers. High-intensity workloads at long durations are contraindicated.

TYPE OF REASONING: ANALYSIS

This question requires one to refer to knowledge of exercise physiology to recall the optimal method of improving fast-twitch fiber function. In order to arrive at the correct solution, one must analyze the information presented and determine its meaning, which is an analytical reasoning skill. If this question was answered incorrectly, refer to information on exercise physiology and fast-twitch fiber exercise.

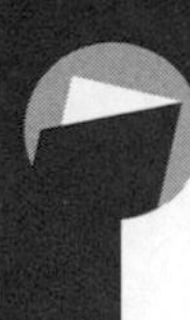

B119 | Musculoskeletal | Patient Examination

A cross-country runner presents with a complaint of pain in the proximal one-third of the right tibia with an insidious onset 4 weeks ago. The pain is present intermittently, and running exacerbates the symptoms. Ligamental testing and soft tissue examination of the knee and leg are unremarkable. Which imaging studies are recommended to be performed **INITIALLY** in order to help establish a diagnosis?

CHOICES:

1. Radiograph and T1 MRI.
2. Bone scan and T2 MRI.
3. Radiograph and bone scan.
4. CT scan and T2 MRI.

TEACHING POINTS

CORRECT ANSWER: 3

This case represents the typical presentation of a stress fracture. Plain radiographs are an inexpensive and quick method to diagnose fractures and healing rates. Stress fractures may take 2–8 weeks before they can be visualized on plain films. If the plain films were negative, then a bone scan is performed (stress fracture, bone bruising).

INCORRECT CHOICES:

If a bone scan is negative, then an MRI (meniscal, bone bruising, soft tissue) or CT scan (small bony irregularities) is ordered. Both MRIs and CT scans are expensive and/or time-consuming. This is most likely a stress fracture, and is best diagnosed by a radiograph and bone scan.

TYPE OF REASONING: INDUCTIVE

One must determine the most likely imaging studies to be initially recommended based on a patient's symptoms. This requires clinical judgment and knowledge of the diagnosis, which necessitate inductive reasoning skill. For this situation, it is likely that a radiograph and bone scan will be recommended, due to the patient's symptoms of stress fracture. If this question was answered incorrectly, review symptoms of stress fractures, especially imaging tests for stress fractures.

B120 | Neuromuscular | Evaluation, Diagnosis, Prognosis

A physical therapy functional goal for a 5 year-old child with a high lumbar lesion (myelomeningocele, L2 level) and minimal cognitive involvement would be:

CHOICES:

1. Community ambulation with HKAFOs and Lofstrand's crutches.
2. Household ambulation with a reciprocating gait orthosis (RGO) and Lofstrand's crutches.
3. Community ambulation with an RGO and Lofstrand's crutches.
4. Household ambulation with KAFOs and rollator walker.

TEACHING POINTS

CORRECT ANSWER: 2

A child with a high-level myelomeningocele will be able to ambulate for limited (household) distances with an RGO and Lofstrand's crutches. Physiological benefits include improved cardiovascular and musculoskeletal functions.

INCORRECT CHOICES:

The child will not be able to be a community ambulator because of the high-energy expenditure necessary with this level of lesion. An RGO is the best choice. The hips are joined by metal cables that prevent inadvertent hip flexion (possible using KAFOs) during a reciprocal two- or four-point gait.

TYPE OF REASONING: INDUCTIVE

This question requires the test taker to assess the value of each of the orthoses and assistive devices presented and then apply their value to the patient's specific diagnosis. This requires one to utilize clinical judgment, in which the test taker uses diagnostic reasoning to determine which solution will be most beneficial for the patient. In this case, an RGO and Lofstrand's crutches are most beneficial for household ambulation.

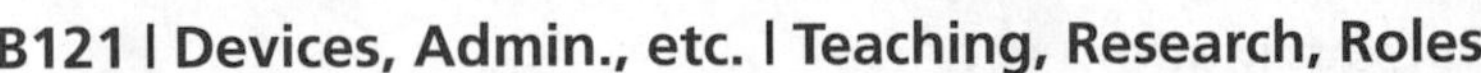

B121 | Devices, Admin., etc. | Teaching, Research, Roles

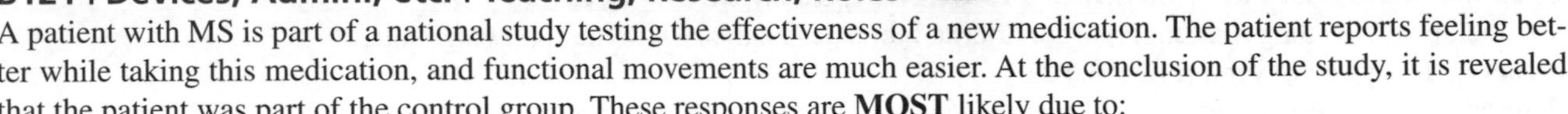

A patient with MS is part of a national study testing the effectiveness of a new medication. The patient reports feeling better while taking this medication, and functional movements are much easier. At the conclusion of the study, it is revealed that the patient was part of the control group. These responses are **MOST** likely due to:

CHOICES:

1. Sampling bias.
2. Hawthorne's effect.
3. Placebo effect.
4. Pretest-treatment interference.

TEACHING POINTS

CORRECT ANSWER: 3

In placebo effect, a subject responds to a sham treatment (in this example, the patient received a pill that did not contain the drug being tested) with positive effects (patient reports she feels much better, moves easier).

INCORRECT CHOICES:

Hawthorne's effect is the subject's knowledge of being part of a study, and that alone might affect the responses. Sampling bias in a national study is unlikely and would not explain the response. Pretest-treatment inference is not a factor in this case; this describes a learning effect that occurs as a result of the pretest.

TYPE OF REASONING: DEDUCTIVE

This question essentially asks one to recall the meaning of a control group in a research study. Patients in control groups receive a sham treatment and do not benefit from any positive effects of the therapeutic regimen under testing. Therefore, the correct answer is placebo effect in this situation, in which the patient believes she has benefited, despite having received no medication. This type of question, while framed within a patient case example, requires direct recall only and encourages deductive reasoning.

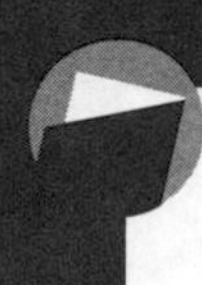

B122 | Cardiovascular-Pulmonary | Patient Examination

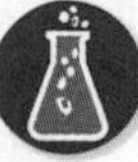

The therapist is reading a recent report of arterial blood gas analysis with the following values:
Fraction of inspired oxygen (FiO_2) = 0.21
Arterial oxygen pressure (PaO_2) = 53 mm Hg
Arterial carbon dioxide pressure ($PaCO_2$) = 30 mm Hg
pH = 7.48
Bicarbonate ion = 24 mEq/L
This would indicate that the patient is in:

CHOICES:

1. Metabolic alkalosis.
2. Respiratory alkalosis.
3. Respiratory acidosis.
4. Metabolic acidosis.

TEACHING POINTS

CORRECT ANSWER: 2

This arterial blood gas shows an increased pH, which is an alkalosis. When looking at arterial blood gas values, carbon dioxide can be viewed essentially as an acid. If the carbon dioxide level is low, then you have less acid, or a resulting alkalosis. This is, therefore, a respiratory alkalosis.

INCORRECT CHOICES:

Because the blood pH is higher than normal (7.35–7.45), the condition is an alkalosis, not an acidosis. If the increased pH was due to a metabolic disorder, a high bicarbonate value would be anticipated. As the HCO_3 is normal (24 mEq/dL), the alkalosis is not from a metabolic cause.

TYPE OF REASONING: ANALYSIS

One must make sense of the information presented in this question and recall the normal laboratory values. This requires analytical reasoning skill, in which one must make an interpretation of information. It is most beneficial to understand the values that indicate respiratory alkalosis to arrive at the correct conclusion. If this question was answered incorrectly, refer to information on arterial blood gas analysis.

B123 | Other Systems | Evaluation, Diagnosis, Prognosis

A retired patient is referred to a cardiac exercise group after a mild MI. From the intake questionnaire, the therapist learns the patient has type 1 insulin-dependent diabetes mellitus (IDDM), controlled with twice-daily insulin injections. In order to minimize the risk of a hypoglycemic event during exercise, the therapist should have the patient:

CHOICES:

1. Avoid exercise during periods of peak insulin activity.
2. Have the patient decrease carbohydrate intake for 2 hours before the exercise session.
3. Monitor blood glucose levels carefully every week during the rehabilitation program.
4. Exercise daily for 40–50 minutes to achieve proper glucose control.

TEACHING POINTS

CORRECT ANSWER: 1

The patient should monitor blood glucose levels frequently when initiating an exercise program and avoid exercise during periods of peak insulin activity (2–4 hours after injection). The therapist should use RPE in addition to HR to monitor exercise intensity.

INCORRECT CHOICES:

A carbohydrate snack should be eaten before and during prolonged exercise bouts. Blood glucose levels should be monitored frequently throughout the day, not weekly. Exercise should begin with daily sessions, 20 minutes twice a day, not 40- to 50-minute sessions. (Source: *ACSM's Guidelines for Exercise Testing and Prescription,* 5th ed.)

TYPE OF REASONING: INFERENCE

This question requires one to understand when peak insulin activity occurs in order to choose the best solution. For patients with IDDM, peak insulin activity occurs between 2 and 4 hours after injection, and therefore, exercise should be avoided during this time frame. One answers this question using inferential reasoning skill by drawing conclusions based on the information presented and making inferences about this information.

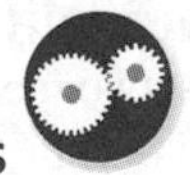

B124 | Neuromuscular | Foundational Sciences

An elderly resident of a community nursing home is diagnosed with Alzheimer's type dementia. In formulating a plan of care, it is important to understand that the patient:

CHOICES:

1. Can usually be trusted to be responsible for own daily care needs.
2. Is more likely to remember current experiences than past ones.
3. Can usually be trusted with transfers with appropriate positioning of the wheelchair.
4. Will likely be resistant to activity training if unfamiliar activities are used.

TEACHING POINTS

CORRECT ANSWER: 4

Activity training is most likely to be successful if done with familiar activities.

INCORRECT CHOICES:

A patient with Alzheimer's disease cannot be trusted to safely perform IADLs or functional mobility skills. Memory for past events may be retained initially, but eventually all memory becomes impaired.

TYPE OF REASONING: EVALUATION

This question requires one to make assumptions about the information presented and then determine the believability of the statements that are made. In this case, it is important to recall that patients with Alzheimer's disease can be resistant to trying unfamiliar activities and should, therefore, have training with familiar activities. When one needs to assess the value of statements made to choose the correct solution, evaluative reasoning skills are utilized.

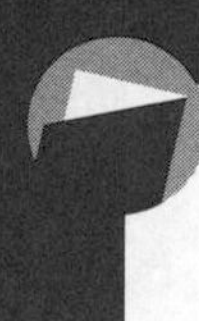

B125 | Devices, Admin., etc. | Teaching, Research, Roles

A patient with a spinal cord injury is having difficulty learning how to transfer from mat to wheelchair. The patient just cannot seem to get the idea of how to coordinate this movement. In this case, the **MOST** effective use of feedback during early motor learning is to:

CHOICES:

1. Provide feedback only after a brief (5-sec) delay.
2. Focus on knowledge of results and visual inputs.
3. Focus on guided movement and proprioceptive inputs.
4. Focus on knowledge of performance and proprioceptive inputs.

TEACHING POINTS

CORRECT ANSWER: 2

During the early stage of motor learning (cognitive stage), learners benefit from seeing the whole task correctly performed. Dependence on visual inputs is high. Developing a reference of correctness (knowledge of results) is critical to ensure early skill acquisition (cognitive mapping).

INCORRECT CHOICES:

Focus on proprioceptive inputs is important during the middle (associative) stage of motor learning. Delayed feedback may be used during later learning.

TYPE OF REASONING: INFERENCE

One must infer information presented in this question, specifically, which approach is most effective during early motor learning. Visual inputs are key during early motor learning with a focus on knowledge of results. To answer this question successfully, one must recall effective teaching principles applied to early learning situations.

B126 | Devices, Admin., etc. | Equipment, Modalities

A patient presents with pain and paresthesia over the first two metatarsal heads of her right foot. Pain is worse after prolonged periods of weight-bearing. She typically wears shoes with 3-inch heels and pointed toes. The **BEST** intervention is a:

CHOICES:

1. Pad placed distal to the metatarsal heads.
2. Scaphoid pad to support the medial longitudinal arch.
3. Thomas' heel to support the medial longitudinal arch.
4. Pad placed proximal to the metatarsal heads.

TEACHING POINTS

CORRECT ANSWER: 4

Compression of the digital nerves in the forefoot results in sensory symptoms of pain and paresthesia (metatarsalgia). It is typically the result of excessively tight shoes. The best intervention is to wear larger shoes, with a metatarsal pad placed proximal to the metatarsal heads to elevate the transverse (anterior) arch and separate the metatarsals. Custom orthotics can also be molded to decrease load. Wearing of high heels should be discouraged. Stretching of plantarflexors may also be helpful.

INCORRECT CHOICES:

A pad placed distal to the metatarsal heads will not provide effective relief of pressure. A scaphoid pad and Thomas' heel are used to support the longitudinal arch and prevent pes valgus, not metatarsalgia.

TYPE OF REASONING: INFERENCE

The test taker must understand and infer what the cause is for the patient's symptoms and then understand the indications for each of the courses of action. In this case, the patient's tight high-heeled shoes are contributing to compression of the digital nerves in the forefoot. Having a thorough understanding of indications for using metatarsal pads, scaphoid pads, and a Thomas' heel is key to arriving at the correct conclusion.

B127 | Musculoskeletal | Evaluation, Diagnosis, Prognosis

A patient developed right throbbing shoulder pain after painting the kitchen. Passive and active glenohumeral motions increase pain. The **BEST INITIAL** intervention for this acute shoulder condition is:

CHOICES:

1. Manual therapy techniques and modalities to reduce pain as the result of subdeltoid bursitis.
2. Correction of muscle imbalances to allow healing of right shoulder supraspinatus tendinitis.
3. Stretching of the pectoralis minor muscle after acromioclavicular joint inflammation.
4. Rotator cuff strengthening exercises to allow ADL function after biceps tendinitis.

TEACHING POINTS

CORRECT ANSWER: 1

Because pain occurs with both AROM and PROM, bursitis is the most likely cause of dysfunction. Initial interventions should focus on reducing pain and inflammation. Modalities and manual therapy are the best choices.

INCORRECT CHOICES:

Supraspinatus and/or bicipital tendonopathy would be most painful with AROM, not both AROM and PROM. An inflammatory condition of the acromioclavicular joint would not be improved by stretching the pectoralis minor muscle.

TYPE OF REASONING: INDUCTIVE

The test taker must determine the best initial intervention for the patient, given one's understanding of the diagnosis and typical intervention approaches. In order to choose the best solution, one must recognize the symptoms as indicative of subdeltoid bursitis and then recognize that modalities and manual therapy techniques to reduce pain and inflammation are the best initial approaches. This decision making process utilizes inductive reasoning skill, in which clinical judgment is paramount to finding the correct solution.

B128 | Other Systems | Evaluation, Diagnosis, Prognosis

A patient has a 5 year history of acquired immunodeficiency syndrome (AIDS). The case worker reports a gradual increase in difficulty with walking. The patient rarely goes out anymore. A referral to PT is initiated. Examination findings reveal typical neuromuscular changes associated with AIDS. These deficits would likely include:

CHOICES:

1. Paraplegia or tetraplegia.
2. Widespread sensory loss resulting in sensory ataxia.
3. Motor ataxia and paresis with pronounced gait disturbances.
4. Progressive rigidity and akinesia with severe balance disturbances.

TEACHING POINTS

CORRECT ANSWER: 3

Alterations in memory, confusion, and disorientation are characteristic of AIDS dementia complex, a common central nervous system (CNS) manifestation of human immunodeficiency virus (HIV) infection. Motor deficits may include ataxia, paresis with gait disturbances, and loss of fine motor coordination. Patients may also develop peripheral neuropathy with distal pain and sensory loss.

INCORRECT CHOICES:

Paraparesis, not paraplegia, might be a finding. Widespread sensory loss, progressive rigidity, and akinesia are not typical findings.

TYPE OF REASONING: EVALUATION

One must evaluate these statements and then recall knowledge of the neuromuscular changes associated with AIDS to arrive at the correct conclusion. This requires determination of the believability of the statements as true of someone with the diagnosis of AIDS, which is an evaluative reasoning skill. If this question was answered incorrectly, refer to information regarding neuromuscular changes associated with AIDS.

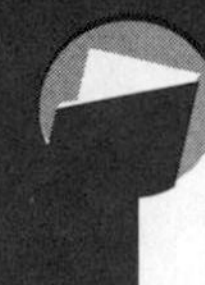

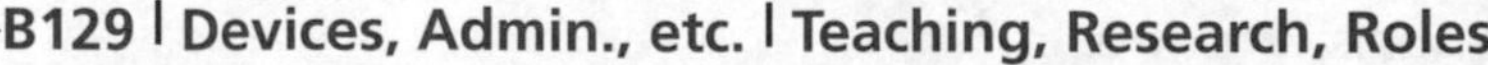

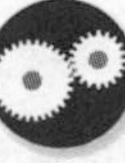

B129 | Devices, Admin., etc. | Teaching, Research, Roles

A new graduate PT has an appointment for a job interview with human resources at a large teaching hospital. The candidate is well dressed, has a professional-looking resume, and is prompt for the 2:00 p.m. appointment. The interviewer is restricted by law from asking about:

CHOICES:

1. Physical ability to perform the job requirements.
2. Malpractice insurance.
3. The applicant's age and marital status.
4. Work hours and sick time.

TEACHING POINTS

CORRECT ANSWER: 3

It is illegal to ask potential applicants their age or marital status. One can ask generically if the candidate is over the age of 18.

INCORRECT CHOICES:

All other items are topics that may be discussed and are not restricted by law.

TYPE OF REASONING: EVALUATION

This question requires one to make a value judgment to determine what is appropriate to discuss in a job interview, which necessitates evaluative reasoning skill. One must recall that information regarding one's specific age or marital status is illegal to inquire from a job applicant, which is factual information, but still requires one to apply his/her beliefs and values in responding to the question. If this question was answered incorrectly, refer to information on interviewing job applicants and questions that are illegal to ask.

B130 | Other Systems | Foundational Sciences

A PT is treating a 2 year-old child with Down syndrome who frequently uses a W sitting position. The main reason to discourage W sitting in this child is that it may cause:

CHOICES:

1. Abnormally low tone because of reflex activity.
2. Femoral antetorsion and medial knee stress.
3. Developmental delay of normal sitting.
4. Hip subluxation and lateral knee stress.

TEACHING POINTS

CORRECT ANSWER: 2

W sitting is a stable and functional position, but may cause later orthopedic problems of femoral antetorsion and knee stress. Children with Down syndrome typically exhibit low tone and hyperextensibility.

INCORRECT CHOICES:

W sitting is not likely to affect low tone or reflex activity. It should also not promote delay of normal sitting. Hip subluxation is unlikely.

TYPE OF REASONING: INFERENCE

One must infer the possible future occurrences from W sitting in order to arrive at the correct answer. First, one must have knowledge of what W sitting is and then understand the stresses that are placed upon the lower extremities, specifically the knees from this sitting position. One infers these stresses, which utilizes inferential reasoning skill, to choose the correct answer. If this question was answered incorrectly, refer to information on W sitting and knee stresses.

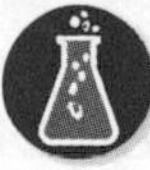

B131 | Neuromuscular | Foundational Sciences

A patient is being examined for impairments after stroke. When tested for two-point discrimination on the right hand, the patient is unable to tell whether the therapist is touching with one or two points. The therapist determines that there is impaired function in the:

CHOICES:

1. Dorsal column/lemniscal pathways and somatosensory cortex.
2. Anterior spinothalamic tract or thalamus.
3. Lateral spinothalamic tract or somatosensory cortex.
4. Spinotectal tract and somatosensory cortex.

TEACHING POINTS

CORRECT ANSWER: 1

Discriminative touch, proprioceptive sensibility, and vibration sense are carried in the posterior white columns (fasciculus cuneatus for the upper extremity and fasciculus gracilis for the lower extremity). The long ascending tracts cross the medulla (sensory decussation) and form the medial lemniscus, which then travels to the thalamus (ventral posterolateral nucleus) and finally to the cortex (postcentral gyrus). Loss of two-point discrimination could result from an insult affecting any of these component parts. Parietal lobe or internal capsule lesions are the most common sites.

INCORRECT CHOICES:

The anterolateral system pathways (spinothalamic tracts) convey pain and temperature. The spinotectal tract conveys information for spinovisual reflexes.

TYPE OF REASONING: ANALYSIS

To answer this question, one must refer to knowledge of applied neuroanatomy, specifically spinal pathways that process discriminative touch of the upper extremity. This requires analysis of the information presented, utilizing analytical reasoning skill to arrive at the conclusion that the dorsal column/lemniscal pathways and somatosensory cortex is impaired. If this question was answered incorrectly, refer to discriminative touch processing of the upper extremity.

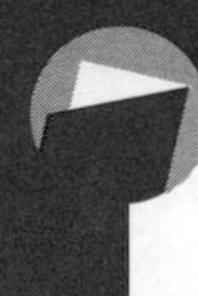

B132 | Cardiovascular-Pulmonary | Evaluation, Diagnosis, Prognosis

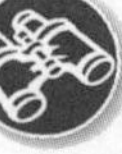

An elderly patient has a history of two MIs and one episode of recent CHF. The patient also has claudication pain in the right calf during an exercise tolerance test. An **INITIAL** exercise prescription that **BEST** deals with these problems is walking:

CHOICES:

1. Five times a week using continuous training for 60 minutes.
2. Three times a week using continuous training for 40-minute sessions.
3. Daily, using interval training for 10- to 15-minute periods.
4. Three times a week using interval training for 30-minute periods.

TEACHING POINTS

CORRECT ANSWER: 3

An appropriate initial exercise prescription for a patient with a history of CHF and claudication pain in the right calf should include low-intensity exercise (walking), low to moderate duration (10–15 min), and higher frequencies (daily). The exercise session should carefully balance activity with rest (interval or discontinuous training).

INCORRECT CHOICES:

All other choices include durations that are too long (60, 40, or 30 min) and do not provide adequate rest periods.

TYPE OF REASONING: INDUCTIVE

One must utilize clinical judgment and diagnostic thinking (an inductive reasoning skill) to choose the best initial exercise prescription for this patient. This requires knowledge of CHF and claudication pain in order to arrive at the best solution. In this case, it is best to balance rest with activity because of the nature of CHF and limited tolerance to exercise.

B133 | Devices, Admin., etc. | Teaching, Research, Roles

After signing a valid informed consent for research experiment, under what circumstances can the subject withdraw from the study?

CHOICES:

1. The subject may withdraw only for safety, comfort, or family emergency reasons.
2. The subject is free to discontinue participation for any reason at any time.
3. The subject has signed an affirmative agreement and must get the researcher's permission to withdraw.
4. The subject may withdraw, but will forfeit any monetary compensation promised for participation.

TEACHING POINTS

CORRECT ANSWER: 2

Subjects may refuse to participate and withdraw from a study at any time. This can occur before or during the experiment. If a patient, quality of care must be maintained. Recognition of this element must be clearly stated in a valid informed consent.

INCORRECT CHOICES:

If promised monetary compensation, it will be paid regardless of withdrawal. The researcher's permission is not required to withdraw. There is no stipulation to state or explain the reason(s) for withdrawal required.

TYPE OF REASONING: DEDUCTIVE

This question requires one to determine what is permissible as an informed consent for participating as a research subject. Recall of information that is placed in consent forms for research is a deductive reasoning skill, which utilizes recall of knowledge and facts. Many questions related to research guidelines and protocols encourage this reasoning. If this question was answered incorrectly, refer to information on informed consent for research.

B134 | Other Systems | Intervention

A patient demonstrates postpartum sacral pain. The patient complains that pain is increased with prolonged walking, ascending or descending stairs, and rising from sit-to-stand. The intervention that is **MOST** beneficial for this problem is:

CHOICES:

1. Cryotherapy and TENS to promote normal healing.
2. Performing mobilization followed by cryotherapy to restore normal motion to the SI joint.
3. Increasing non–weight-bearing with ambulation training and stabilization using a lumbosacral orthosis.
4. Manual therapy techniques of the SI joint to provide relief of symptoms, and therapeutic exercise to restore normal function of the pelvic girdle.

TEACHING POINTS

CORRECT ANSWER: 4

Ligamentous laxity and pain during pregnancy secondary to hormonal influences (relaxin) most commonly affects the SI joint. This ligamentous laxity continues to occur for up to 3 months after pregnancy and leaves the pelvic area vulnerable to injury. SI pain is aggravated by prolonged weight-bearing and stairs. Manual therapy techniques are effective for reducing pain and therapeutic exercise is beneficial to restore normal muscle function.

INCORRECT CHOICES:

Modalities may provide temporary relief of pain, but will not promote any significant impact on healing. Promoting non–weight-bearing does not allow the patient to return to normal function. Mobilization will further stretch joint structures that are already lax.

TYPE OF REASONING: INFERENCE

One must infer the intervention that is most beneficial for a patient with postpartum sacral pain to arrive at the correct conclusion. Questions that encourage one to draw conclusions from evidence utilize inferential reasoning skill. One must understand the nature of postpartum sacral pain from ligamentous laxity and the intervention approach that is most effective in order to arrive at the correct conclusion.

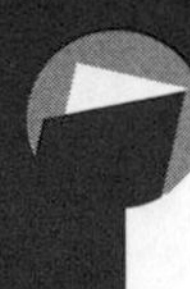

B135 | Devices, Admin., etc. | Equipment, Modalities 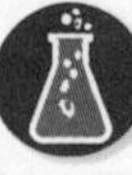

A patient has severe low back pain as a result of chopping wood, and has been receiving US and strengthening exercises to the low back for 2 weeks. The therapist has also been applying TENS, and decides to have the patient use TENS at home. As a safety precaution, it is important to instruct the patient to perform a daily check of the:

CHOICES:

1. Electrodes and leads.
2. Skin and electrodes.
3. Skin and leads.
4. Electrodes and electrode jacks.

TEACHING POINTS

CORRECT ANSWER: 2

Electrodes must be checked regularly for signs of wear or cracking, which would make the delivery of electrical current either ineffective and/or unsafe. Repetitive long-term use of electrodes might produce cracking or uneven wear, which could develop into "hot spots" of increased current density. The increased current density along with continued placement and removal of the electrodes could cause skin irritation and breakdown.

INCORRECT CHOICES:

The leads and electrode jacks are not typically prone to breakdown.

TYPE OF REASONING: ANALYSIS

One must recall the safety guidelines for patients using TENS to choose the correct solution. In this case, it is important to inform the patient to check the skin and electrodes daily to prevent potential injury or irritation. Questions such as these, which require one to determine the meaning of information presented and weigh the information, encourage analytical reasoning skill.

B136 | Integumentary | Evaluation, Diagnosis, Prognosis

A therapist who is working in a burn unit receives a referral to examine a 10 month-old infant who was admitted the previous night. The infant was scalded on the chest. Inspection reveals a large reddened area with thick blisters over one-third of the upper anterior chest. The skin is shiny with a weeping surface. The therapist recognizes that the child has incurred a:

CHOICES:

1. Full-thickness burn.
2. Burn wound infection.
3. Partial-thickness burn.
4. Superficial burn.

TEACHING POINTS

CORRECT ANSWER: 3

This patient has a partial-thickness burn (destruction of the epidermis with damage to the dermis). Skin is red and mottled with intact blisters; broken blisters produce a wet shiny surface.

INCORRECT CHOICES:

A superficial burn (damage to the epidermis) appears red or erythematous. There is no injury to the dermis, and the skin is dry with no blisters. A full-thickness burn (destruction of the epidermal and dermal layers) presents with a white (ischemic) or charred tan color; the surface is parchment-like, leathery, rigid, and dry. Burn wound infection can occur in any patient, but is more common in individuals with extensive burns and open wounds. There is no evidence of infection in this case.

TYPE OF REASONING: ANALYSIS

One must recall the signs and symptoms of a partial-thickness burn and analyze the symptoms in order to arrive at a correct conclusion. This requires analytical reasoning skill. For this case, the symptoms indicate a partial-thickness burn. Key words to help one reach a correct conclusion are "wet and shiny surface" and "reddened area with blisters." If this question was answered incorrectly, review signs and symptoms of burns, especially partial-thickness burns.

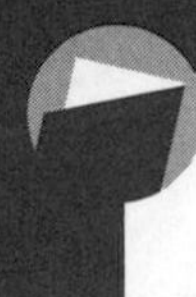

B137 | Other Systems | Evaluation, Diagnosis, Prognosis

An elderly and frail older adult has low vision. The patient recently returned home from a 2-week hospitalization for stabilization of diabetes. The PT's goal is to mobilize the patient and increase ambulation level and safety. The **BEST** intervention strategy for this patient is to:

CHOICES:

1. Keep window shades wide open to let in as much light as possible.
2. Practice walking by having the patient look down at all times.
3. Color-code stairs with pastel shades of blue and green to highlight steps.
4. Practice walking in areas of high illumination and low clutter.

TEACHING POINTS

CORRECT ANSWER: 4

Effective intervention strategies for the elderly patient with low vision include ensuring adequate lighting. Vision and safety decrease dramatically in low lighting. Reducing clutter in the home is also an important strategy to improve safety during ambulation.

INCORRECT CHOICES:

The patient should not continuously look down at the feet, because this poses a safety hazard. This restricts avoidance strategies for environmental objects. Visual acuity decreases dramatically with bright glare from sunlit windows. Color-coded stairs might be of help if they are well lit and if strong colors, not pastels, are used.

TYPE OF REASONING: INFERENCE

This question requires one to recall the guidelines for intervention approaches with people who have low vision. Adequate lighting and low clutter are important to successful and safe navigation in the patient's living spaces. Using the skills of inferential reasoning, the test taker must draw conclusions from the evidence presented and make assumptions about that information.

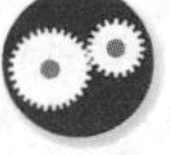

B138 | Cardiovascular-Pulmonary | Evaluation, Diagnosis, Prognosis

The patient has a history of angina pectoris and limited physical activity. As the patient participates in the second exercise class, the PT suspects that angina is unstable and may be indicative of a preinfarction state. The therapist determines this by the presence of:

CHOICES:

1. Angina that responds to rest and interval training but not to continuous training.
2. Arrhythmias of increasing frequency, especially atrial arrhythmias.
3. Angina of increasing intensity that is unresponsive to the nitroglycerin or rest.
4. Prolonged cessation of pain following the administration of nitroglycerin for angina.

TEACHING POINTS

CORRECT ANSWER: 3

Preinfarction or unstable angina pectoris is unrelieved by rest or nitroglycerin (measures that typically reduce most angina). The pain is described as increasing in intensity. Unstable angina is an absolute contraindication to exercise.

INCORRECT CHOICES:

Angina that decreases with rest and interval training along with nitroglycerin is considered stable. Increasing atrial arrhythmias may be a comorbidity, but is not expected with angina.

TYPE OF REASONING: EVALUATION

In this question, the test taker must evaluate the merits of the statements presented and determine which statements seem most indicative of unstable angina. Relying on knowledge of angina pectoris and the indications for unstable angina, the test taker uses evaluative reasoning skill to arrive at the correct conclusion. If this question was answered incorrectly, review information on unstable angina.

B139 | Neuromuscular | Intervention

A patient with a left CVA exhibits right hemiparesis and strong and dominant hemiplegic synergies in the lower extremity. Which activity would be **BEST** to break up these synergies?

CHOICES:

1. Supine-lying, hip extension with adduction.
2. Foot tapping in a sitting position.
3. Bridging, pelvic elevation.
4. Supine, PNF D2F with knee flexing and D2E with knee extending.

TEACHING POINTS

CORRECT ANSWER: 3

The typical lower extremity synergies are effectively broken up using bridging (combines hip extension from the extensor synergy with knee flexion from the flexion synergy).

INCORRECT CHOICES:

Supine hip extension with adduction and foot tapping in the sitting position are in-synergy activities (lower extremity flexion and extension synergies). Supine, lower extremity PNF D2F with knee flexing and D2E with knee extending moves the lower extremity in a pattern closely aligned wih the typical flexion and extension synergies.

TYPE OF REASONING: INFERENCE

This question requires one to determine what will best help a patient to break up a lower extremity synergy pattern after a stroke. Drawing conclusions based on the information presented, the test taker utilizes inferential reasoning to make the determination of which approach will benefit the patient. If this question was answered incorrectly, refer to information on limb synergy patterns and activities that promote this pattern.

B140 | Integumentary | Foundational Sciences

An elderly and frail resident of a nursing home has developed a stage III pressure ulcer. The wound is open with necrosis of the subcutaneous tissue down to the fascia. This elderly patient when compared with a younger patient with the same type of ulcer can be expected to demonstrate:

CHOICES:

1. Increased scarring with healing.
2. Decreased vascular and immune responses resulting in impaired healing.
3. Increased elasticity and eccrine sweating.
4. Increased vascular responses with significant erythema.

TEACHING POINTS

CORRECT ANSWER: 2

Age-associated changes in the integumentary system include decreased vascular and immune responses that result in impaired healing. Rate of healing is considerably slower.

INCORRECT CHOICES:

In the elderly, scarring is typically less than in a younger individual. Both elasticity and eccrine sweating are decreased in the elderly. Vascular responses are typically decreased, not increased.

TYPE OF REASONING: INFERENCE

One must infer or draw a reasonable conclusion about the likely healing abilities of an older adult with a pressure ulcer. This requires inferential reasoning skill. For this case, considering the patient's age as compared with a younger patient, one could expect decreased vascular and immune responses that impair healing. If this question was answered incorrectly, review age changes associated changes in the integumentary system of older adults.

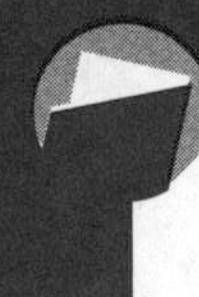

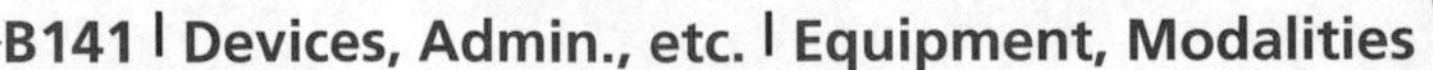

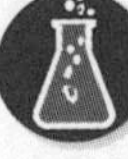

B141 | Devices, Admin., etc. | Equipment, Modalities

A patient with an above-knee prosthesis is walking by swinging the prosthesis out to the side in an arc during swing of the amputated limb. The therapist suspects the prosthesis may have:

CHOICES:

1. An excessively low medial wall.
2. An unstable knee unit.
3. A stiff knee mechanism.
4. Insufficient support from the anterior wall.

TEACHING POINTS

CORRECT ANSWER: 3

A prosthesis that is too long or has a knee mechanism that is too stiff will cause the patient to circumduct or abduct the prosthesis in order to clear the prosthesis and get through swing phase. If it is not compensated, a fall may result.

INCORRECT CHOICES:

The other problems will not result in a circumducted gait pattern. An excessively high (not low) medial wall will produce an abducted gait. An unstable knee unit results in forward flexion of the trunk during stance. Insufficient anterior wall support will result in slippage and an uncomfortable socket. The resulting pain produces an uneven step length.

TYPE OF REASONING: ANALYSIS

In this question, one must determine what the cause is for the circumducted gait pattern. Relying on knowledge of lower extremity prosthetics and gait patterns, one must analyze the meaning of the information presented in order to draw a proper conclusion for the cause, which utilizes analytical reasoning skill. In this case, the likely cause is a stiff knee mechanism.

B142 | Other Systems | Evaluation, Diagnosis, Prognosis

An elderly patient has been hospitalized for 3 weeks after a surgical resection of carcinoma of the colon. The patient is very weak and is currently receiving physical therapy to improve functional ambulation. During the initial sessions, the patient complains of pain in the left shoulder that is aggravated by weight-bearing when using the walker. The therapist decides to:

CHOICES:

1. Notify the physician immediately.
2. Apply pulsed US to decrease pain.
3. Apply heat in the form of a hot pack before ambulation.
4. Ambulate the patient in the parallel bars considering age and diagnosis.

TEACHING POINTS

CORRECT ANSWER: 1

The risk of metastatic disease is present; the therapist should notify the physician immediately.

INCORRECT CHOICES:

Monitoring or modifying the plan of care to reduce pain should be considered only after consultation with the physician. If metastatic disease is present, the US would be contraindicated. Ambulating in the parallel bars exerts the same weight-bearing forces through the upper extremities as a walker.

TYPE OF REASONING: INDUCTIVE

This question requires one to use clinical judgment and diagnostic thinking to make a determination of the cause for the patient's shoulder pain and then what is the best course of action based on this knowledge. In this situation, based on the patient's medical history, it is important to notify the physician immediately because of the risk of metastatic disease. Questions that require clinical judgment to make a determination of a best course of action utilize inductive reasoning skill.

B143 | Devices, Admin., etc. | Equipment, Modalities

A patient sprained the left ankle 4 days ago. The patient complains of pain (4/10), and there is moderate swelling that is getting worse. At this time, which intervention would be **BEST** to use?

CHOICES:

1. Intermittent compression followed by elevation.
2. Contrast baths followed by limb elevation.
3. Cold whirlpool followed by massage.
4. Cold/intermittent compression combination with the limb elevated.

TEACHING POINTS

CORRECT ANSWER: 4

The combination of RICE (rest, elevation, compression, elevation) is best. Cold to decrease pain along with intermittent compression and elevation to facilitate fluid drainage provides the best intervention. Rest is required.

INCORRECT CHOICES:

Contrast baths and whirlpool place the ankle in a dependent position, which might tend to increase edema. The interventions of intermittent compression and elevation should be combined, not sequential.

TYPE OF REASONING: INFERENCE

In this question, the test taker must draw conclusions based on the information presented in the patient's case, which utilizes inferential reasoning skill. The patient's symptoms in this case indicate that cold and intermittent compression with limb elevation are best to relieve pain and facilitate fluid drainage. If this question was answered incorrectly, refer to information on intervention for acute ankle sprain.

B144 | Musculoskeletal | Patient Examination

A patient diagnosed with left lateral epicondylitis has no resolution of symptoms after 2 weeks of treatment. The PT begins a reexamination and finds the left biceps reflex is 1+. The therapist should **NEXT** perform a complete examination of the:

CHOICES:

1. Mid cervical region.
2. Cervicothoracic region.
3. Upper cervical region.
4. Cervicocranial region.

TEACHING POINTS

CORRECT ANSWER: 1

The patient has symptoms (diminished reflex) of a possible left C5 nerve root compression in the mid cervical spine. Any reflex change suggests nerve root irritation or compression. Lateral epicondylitis frequently involves the extensor carpi radialis brevis, which is innervated by spinal nerves emanating from the mid cervical region.

INCORRECT CHOICES:

The presenting symptoms cannot be linked to involvement of the regions listed in the other choices.

TYPE OF REASONING: ANALYSIS

This question provides the symptoms, and the test taker must determine the diagnosis or root cause, which relies primarily on analytical reasoning skill. The test taker must recall knowledge of neuroanatomy to recognize that a 1+ reflex in the left biceps is indicative of possible nerve root compression at the C5 level. If this question was answered incorrectly, refer to information on nerve root compressions of the cervical spine.

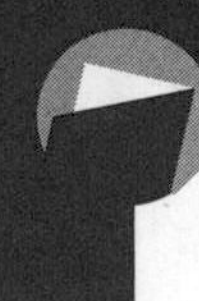

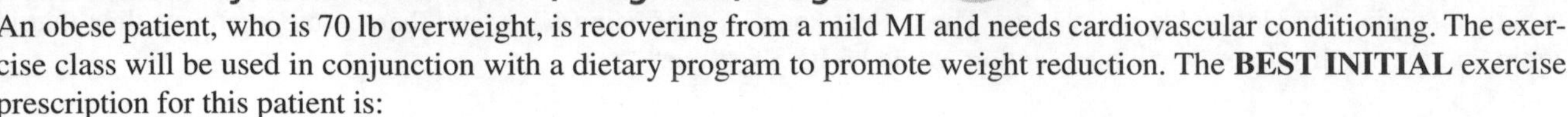

B145 | Other Systems | Evaluation, Diagnosis, Prognosis

An obese patient, who is 70 lb overweight, is recovering from a mild MI and needs cardiovascular conditioning. The exercise class will be used in conjunction with a dietary program to promote weight reduction. The **BEST INITIAL** exercise prescription for this patient is:

CHOICES:

1. Jogging, for 10 minutes at 4 mph.
2. Walking, intensity set at 50% target HR.
3. Walking, intensity set at 75% of HR reserve.
4. Swimming, intensity set at 75% age-adjusted HR.

TEACHING POINTS

CORRECT ANSWER: 2

Obese individuals are typically sedentary, with lower initial levels of physical conditioning. The initial exercise prescription should focus on a lower intensity exercise progressing to longer durations.

INCORRECT CHOICES:

Higher intensity exercise (75% or 85% of HR maximum) should be avoided initially. Jogging is also too intense, and may yield additional orthopedic problems.

TYPE OF REASONING: INDUCTIVE

One must utilize clinical judgment in order to make a determination for the best exercise program for this patient, which is an inductive reasoning skill. This requires diagnostic thinking coupled with knowledge of cardiac exercise prescription for obese individuals. If this question was answered incorrectly, refer to information on appropriate cardiac conditioning exercises for obese individuals.

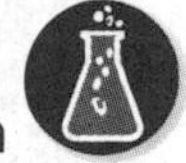

B146 | Musculoskeletal | Patient Examination

A patient underwent a right total hip replacement (THR) 4 months ago. The patient is now referred to physical therapy for gait evaluation. The patient demonstrates shortened stride length on the right. This patient **MOST LIKELY** has:

CHOICES:

1. Contracted hip flexors.
2. Contracted hamstrings.
3. Weakened hip flexors.
4. Weakened quadriceps.

TEACHING POINTS

CORRECT ANSWER: 1

Patients are less active after surgery and spend less time in standing and more time in sitting. The iliopsoas muscles become shortened with increased time in sitting. The contracted iliopsoas limits the patient's ability to extend the hip, which effectively shortens the stride length on the affected side.

INCORRECT CHOICES:

Contracted hamstrings or weak quadriceps result in decreased knee extension during stance and an unstable knee. Weak hip flexors produce decreased limb shortening during swing, typically compensated by circumduction.

TYPE OF REASONING: ANALYSIS

This question provides the symptoms and the test taker must determine the cause for the symptoms, which encourages analytical reasoning skill. In this case, the patient most likely has a contracted iliopsoas muscle, which will shorten the stride length on the right. One must recall reasons for decreased stride length, especially after THR surgery, in order to arrive at the correct conclusion.

B147 | Neuromuscular | Intervention

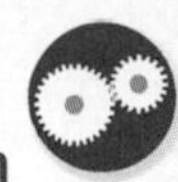

A child with spastic cerebral palsy is having difficulty releasing food from the hand to the mouth. Once the child has brought the food to the mouth, it would be helpful for the caregiver to:

CHOICES:

1. Slowly stroke the finger flexors in a distal-to-proximal direction.
2. Apply a quick stretch to the finger flexors.
3. Slowly stroke the finger extensors in a proximal-to-distal direction.
4. Passively extend the fingers.

TEACHING POINTS

CORRECT ANSWER: 3

Slowly stroking the finger extensors will help to facilitate opening of the hand and allow the child to release the food into the mouth.

INCORRECT CHOICES:

Stimulation of spastic finger flexors (slow stroking, quick stretch) is contraindicated. Passive extension of the fingers will not enhance the activity of feeding.

TYPE OF REASONING: EVALUATION

One must evaluate the merits of the four statements presented to make a determination of the best approach to facilitate finger extension. Using knowledge of neurorehabilitation techniques, the test taker should conclude that stroking the fingers proximal to distal will be most effective in encouraging finger extension. Evaluative reasoning skill is used in this question because the test taker must evaluate the value of statements made to make a judgment for the best course of action.

B148 | Integumentary | Patient Examination

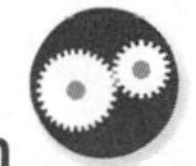

During the examination of the cervical spine of a client for C5 radiculopathy, small groupings of nevi are noted near the superior angle of the left scapula. The **NEXT** action the therapist should take is:

CHOICES:

1. Contact the physician immediately.
2. Ask the patient about any history of moles and examine them closely.
3. Photograph the area in order to provide baseline documentation for the patient's record.
4. Perform a vertebral artery because the nevi are obviously benign growths.

TEACHING POINTS

CORRECT ANSWER: 2

Nevi (moles) should be examined for asymmetry, border irregularities, color, and diameter (>6 mm). It is not uncommon to have a group of moles and they are usually benign, but if there is a transformation of a nevus (plural nevi), then the primary care physician should be contacted. In this situation, the therapist needs to establish a baseline (history and physical examination) of the moles, and then determine whether there is an indication to contact the physician.

INCORRECT CHOICES:

A photograph can be part of the examination, but this does not replace a thorough history and visual inspection. There are no indications for a vertebral artery examination. A vertebral artery examination is performed before manual or mechanical techniques of the cervical spine or if the client exhibits signs or symptoms of vertebral artery compromise.

TYPE OF REASONING: EVALUATION

This question requires the test taker to determine the significance of nevi. In order to determine how significant they are (if at all), the next course of action (setting priorities) would be to ask the patient about any history of moles and then examine them closely. In order to arrive at a correct conclusion, one must evaluate the merits of each of the four possible courses of action presented and decide which action most adequately addresses patient well-being, while being prudent in approach.

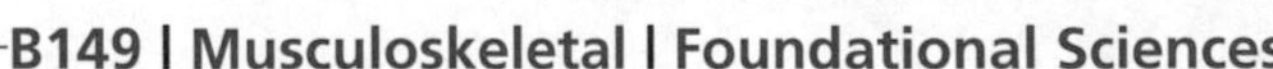

B149 | Musculoskeletal | Foundational Sciences

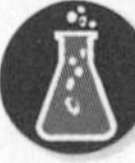

In reference to the figure, when lifting a constant load using either a stoop lift or a squat lift posture, the **MOST** significant contributing factor for increasing lumbar spine compression forces in addition to the weight of the load is:

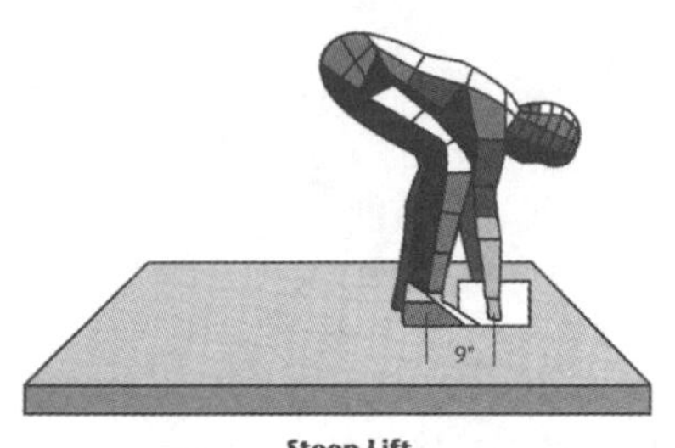

Stoop Lift

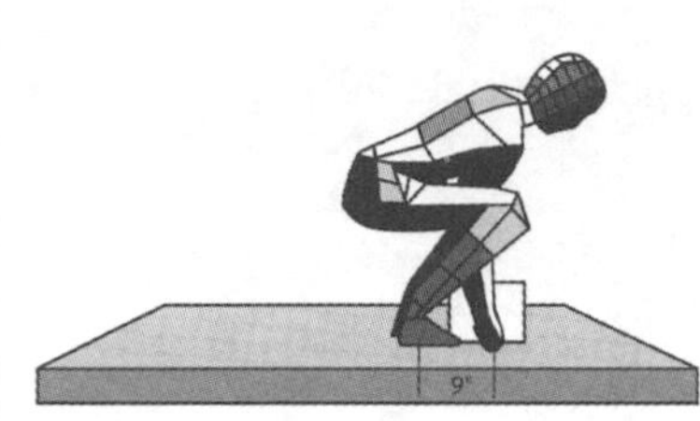

Deep Squat Lift

Musculoskeletal Disorders in the Workplace: Principles and Practice. Nordin M, Andersson G, Pope M (1997). St Louis, Inc., page 122, Figure 10-1, with permission.

CHOICES:

1. The height of the load from the ground.
2. Performing the lift with the lumbar spine in a neutral position rather than in a lordotic posture.
3. The distance of the load from the base of the spine.
4. Performing the lift with the lumbar spine in a kyphotic posture.

TEACHING POINTS

CORRECT ANSWER: 3

Manual lifting biomechanical models have demonstrated high lumbar spine moments, especially when the load is not held close to the body.

INCORRECT CHOICES:

The height of the load from the ground may decrease the overall work but is not the key factor in reducing lumbar compressive forces. The spine should be held in its normal position. A lumbar neutral position may change the biomechanics slightly but will not reduce lumbar compressive forces. Kyphosis occurs in the thoracic region, not lumbar.

TYPE OF REASONING: ANALYSIS

Questions that require one to analyze information presented in pictures often encourage the use of analytical reasoning skill. In this question, one must analyze how the information presented in the picture best depicts how the distance of the load from the base of the spine is the most significant contributing factor for increasing lumbar spine compression forces. If this question was answered incorrectly, review information on biomechanics of lifting.

B150 | Musculoskeletal | Intervention

Nearly 2 months ago, a patient noticed left shoulder pain after walking the dog. This pain has progressively worsened. The patient now is unable to move the left upper extremity overhead while performing ADLs. An orthopedic surgeon diagnosed the problem as adhesive capsulitis. The **MOST** effective direction for glenohumeral mobilization for this patient would be:

CHOICES:

1. Posteroinferior translatory glides.
2. Posterosuperior translatory glides.
3. Anterosuperior translatory glides.
4. Anteroinferior translatory glides.

TEACHING POINTS

CORRECT ANSWER: 1

The diagnosis is left shoulder adhesive capsulitis. Inferior glides will improve the abduction and flexion (overhead motion). Posterior glides have been shown to be the most effective glide to increase glenohumeral external rotation.

INCORRECT CHOICES:

Superior glides will improve extension, not elevation. Based on the concave-convex rule, it seems that anterior glides would be best to promote external rotation at the glenhohumeral joint.

TYPE OF REASONING: INFERENCE

This question requires one to determine the most effective treatment approach in glenohumeral mobilization techniques for adhesive capsulitis. This requires one to have a firm understanding of the nature of adhesive capsulitis, capsular patterns, and joint mobilization techniques of the shoulder to arrive at the correct conclusion. This question utilizes inferential reasoning skill because the test taker must draw conclusion based on the evidence presented for a best course of action.

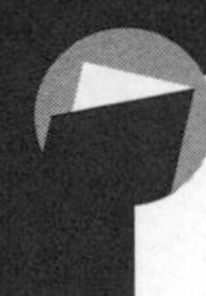

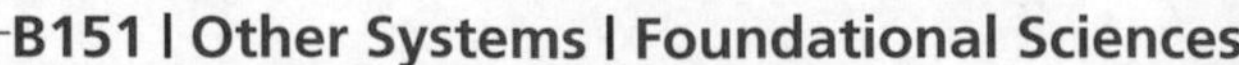

B151 | Other Systems | Foundational Sciences

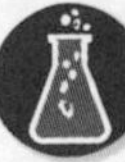

A elderly patient is referred to physical therapy for an examination of functional mobility skills and safety in the home environment. The family reports that the patient is demonstrating increasing forgetfulness and some memory deficits. From the examination, the therapist would expect to find:

CHOICES:

1. Impairments in short-term memory.
2. Periods of fluctuating confusion.
3. Significant impairments in long-term memory.
4. Periods of agitation and wandering, especially in the late afternoon.

TEACHING POINTS

CORRECT ANSWER: 1

Elderly patients with memory impairments typically demonstrate intact immediate recall (e.g., can repeat words); impairments are often noted in memory for recent events (e.g., Why did I come into this room? Who came to see me yesterday?). Long-term memory is usually intact.

INCORRECT CHOICES:

Periods of fluctuating confusion are typically found in delirium, an acute state of disorientation and confusion. Hallucinations or delusions are common (not present in this case). Periods of agitation and wandering (sundowning) are seen in patients with Alzheimer's disease. Whereas the disease begins with mild memory loss (stage I), agitation and wandering typically do not occur until stage II.

TYPE OF REASONING: ANALYSIS

In this situation, the test taker must analyze the patient's symptoms and make a determination of the root cause for them in order to decide what the therapist's findings may be. Analytical questions require one to interpret information and determine the precise meaning of that information. If this question was answered incorrectly, review information regarding age-related memory deficits.

B152 | Neuromuscular | Patient Examination 

A therapist is examining a patient with vestibular dysfunction. The patient is asked to assume a long sitting position with the head turned to the left side. The therapist then quickly moves the patient backward so that the head is extended over the end of the table approximately 30 degrees below horizontal. This maneuver causes severe dizziness and vertigo. A repeat test with the head turned to the right produces no symptoms. The therapist reports these findings as a:

CHOICES:

1. Positive right Hallpike-Dix test.
2. Positive sharpened Romberg's test.
3. Positive left Hallpike-Dix test.
4. Positive positional test.

TEACHING POINTS

CORRECT ANSWER: 3

The test described is the Hallpike-Dix. It is a left positive test because, with the head turned to the left, the change in position produces the patient's symptoms.

INCORRECT CHOICES:

The right Hallpike-Dix test with head turned to the right is negative. The sharpened Romberg's test is used to assess standing balance (dysequilibrium) with the eyes closed and feet in a tandem (heel-toe) position. The Hallpike-Dix test is a positional test; a positive positional test does not delineate or document the side of deficit.

TYPE OF REASONING: DEDUCTIVE

This question requires one to determine which clinical test is represented by the information in the scenario. This requires factual recall of information related to protocols, which is a deductive reasoning skill. In this situation, the scenario describes administration of the Hallpike-Dix maneuver. If this question was answered incorrectly, review information on the Hallpike-Dix maneuver.

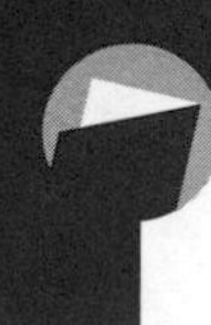

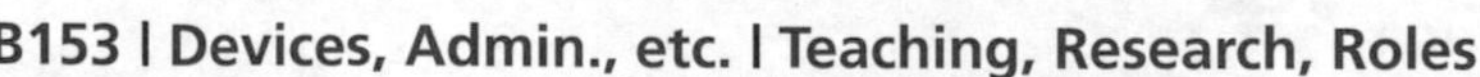

B153 | Devices, Admin., etc. | Teaching, Research, Roles 

A therapist is instructing a patient with a transfemoral lower extremity amputation in prosthetic gait training. The therapist determines that learning is going well because the patient's errors are decreasing and overall endurance is improving. The **BEST** strategy to promote continued motor learning at this point in the patient's rehabilitation is to:

CHOICES:

1. Provide continuous feedback after every walking trial.
2. Have the patient practice walking in varying environments.
3. Have the patient continue to practice in the parallel bars until all errors are extinguished.
4. Intervene early whenever errors appear before bad habits become firmly entrenched.

TEACHING POINTS

CORRECT ANSWER: 2

This patient demonstrates the associative stage of motor learning (errors are decreasing and movements are becoming organized). It is appropriate to gradually progress this patient toward ambulating in a more open (varied) environment.

INCORRECT CHOICES:

Continuous feedback may improve performance, but delays motor learning in the long run. Practicing until errors are extinguished or intervening early whenever errors appear is also an inappropriate strategy for the associative stage of learning. Some trial and error learning is the goal.

TYPE OF REASONING: INDUCTIVE

One must utilize clinical judgment to determine the best strategy to promote continued motor learning with the patient. Use of clinical judgment to make a determination of a best course of action is an inductive reasoning skill. It is important to know the stages of motor learning in order to arrive at the correct conclusion, which should be reviewed if this question was answered incorrectly.

B154 | Cardiovascular-Pulmonary | Intervention 

A young child with newly diagnosed cystic fibrosis is being seen by a PT in the home. Which intervention should be considered for this patient?

CHOICES:

1. Teach the parents secretion removal techniques to all segments of all lobes of both lungs once or twice a day.
2. Teach the child active cycle of breathing technique (ACBT) to be done once or twice a day to clear retained secretions.
3. Teach the child use of the acapella device in postural drainage positions to be performed once or twice a day.
4. Teach the child autogenic drainage for secretion removal to be performed once or twice daily.

TEACHING POINTS

CORRECT ANSWER: 1

For a child this age, proper at-home interventions include secretion removal techniques including manual techniques performed by an adult once or twice a day.

INCORRECT CHOICES:

The use of an acapella device, ACBT, and/or autogenic drainage can be helpful in clearing secretions in patients with cystic fibrosis; however, these three techniques are not appropriate for a child this young, because they rely on independent use and an ability to self-monitor secretion clearance to know how long and how often to perform the techniques.

TYPE OF REASONING: INFERENCE

The test taker must understand the nature of cystic fibrosis and home interventions for the condition to determine what is an acceptable intervention for a **YOUNG** child. Arriving at the correct conclusion requires inferential reasoning, which requires one to draw conclusions from information and form assumptions about the information. If this question was answered incorrectly, review home therapy interventions for young children with cystic fibrosis.

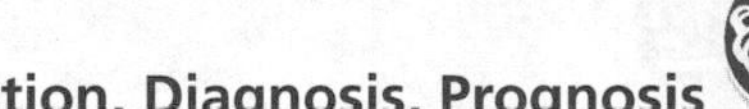

B155 | Other Systems | Evaluation, Diagnosis, Prognosis

A middle-aged woman is referred to a womens' clinic with problems of stress incontinence. She reports loss of control that began with coughing or laughing, but now reports problems even when she exercises (aerobics 3 times/w/k). The **BEST** intervention for this patient is:

CHOICES:

1. Kegel's exercises several times a day.
2. Biofeedback 1 hour/wk to achieve appropriate sphincter control.
3. Functional electrical stimulation 3 times/wk.
4. Behavioral modification techniques to reward proper voiding on schedule.

TEACHING POINTS

CORRECT ANSWER: 1

Symptoms of stress incontinence can be successfully managed through a variety of techniques. Pelvic floor exercises (Kegel's exercises) are the mainstay of treatment and must be performed daily, several times a day, in order to be effective.

INCORRECT CHOICES:

Biofeedback and E-Stim offered weekly or 3 times/wk are not likely to be effective because of insufficient frequency. A voiding schedule does not address the primary impairment.

TYPE OF REASONING: INDUCTIVE

This question requires one to understand the nature of stress incontinence and the appropriate interventions for this condition in order to choose the best intervention approach. Using clinical judgment (an inductive reasoning skill), the test taker determines the best course of action for the patient. If this question was answered incorrectly, review intervention strategies for stress incontinence.

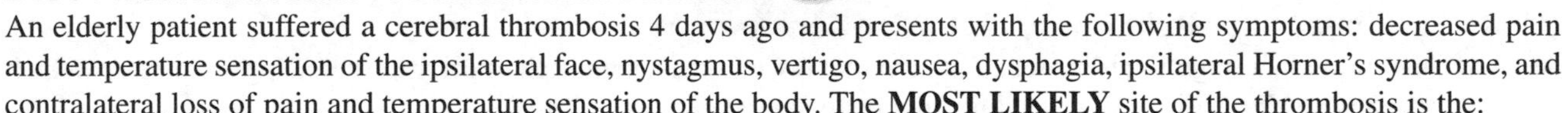

B156 | Neuromuscular | Foundational Sciences

An elderly patient suffered a cerebral thrombosis 4 days ago and presents with the following symptoms: decreased pain and temperature sensation of the ipsilateral face, nystagmus, vertigo, nausea, dysphagia, ipsilateral Horner's syndrome, and contralateral loss of pain and temperature sensation of the body. The **MOST LIKELY** site of the thrombosis is the:

CHOICES:

1. Posterior cerebral artery.
2. Anterior cerebral artery.
3. Posterior inferior cerebellar artery (PICA).
4. Internal carotid artery.

TEACHING POINTS

CORRECT ANSWER: 3

This patient presents with lateral medullary (Wallenberg's) syndrome, which can result from occlusion of the PICA, which is usually a branch of the vertebral artery. It involves the descending tract and nucleus of CN V, the vestibular nucleus and its connections, CN IX and CN X nuclei or nerve fibers, cuneate and gracile nuclei, and spinothalamic tract.

INCORRECT CHOICES:

The symptoms in this case clearly indicate brainstem (cranial nerve) involvement, not cortical involvement (anterior or posterior cerebral artery). An internal carotid artery stroke produces symptoms of combined middle cerebral and anterior cerebral artery strokes.

TYPE OF REASONING: ANALYSIS

This question requires one to recall the symptoms that indicate involvement of the PICA. This requires the test taker to analyze the information presented and interpret it in order to determine that the symptoms are directly indicative of PICA thrombosis. It is important for one to recall applied neuroanatomy related to strokes in order to choose the best answer.

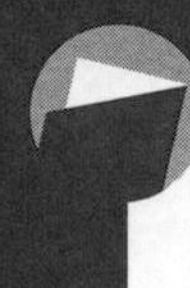

B157 | Integumentary | Intervention

A patient with a 2-inch stage II decubitus ulcer over the left lateral malleolus is referred for physical therapy. The therapist notes a greenish, pungent exudate at the wound site. The therapist decides to use electrical stimulation. The **BEST** choice of polarity and electrode placement is:

CHOICES:

1. Anode placed in the wound.
2. Cathode placed in the wound.
3. Anode placed proximal to wound.
4. Cathode placed proximal to wound.

TEACHING POINTS

CORRECT ANSWER: 2

It is purported that the bactericidal effect produced by negative current is a result of substrate depletion or alteration of the internal processes of the microorganisms. Neutrophils are also attracted to the wound area by chemotaxis to purge the bacteria. The cathode should be placed directly in contact with the wound to cover as much treatment area as possible.

INCORRECT CHOICES:

The anode is used to promote healing in clean noninfected wounds, and placement of an electrode in the wound ensures current will be delivered throughout the wound.

TYPE OF REASONING: DEDUCTIVE

This question requires one to recall the protocol for electrical stimulation in treatment of infected decubitus ulcers. Questions that require one to recall protocols and guidelines require deductive reasoning skill. For this clinical situation, the cathode should be placed in the wound to promote healing. If this question was answered incorrectly, review protocols for electrical stimulation for wound healing.

B158 | Cardiovascular-Pulmonary | Intervention

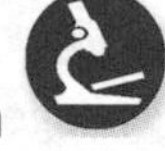

A therapist working in a stage 1 cardiac rehabilitation unit reviews the patient's chart prior to exercising the patient. Which reported laboratory value indicates the need for supplemental oxygen during exercise?

CHOICES:

1. $PaCO_2$ is 45 mm Hg.
2. SaO_2 indicates 84% saturation.
3. PaO_2 is 80 mm Hg.
4. pH is 7.35.

TEACHING POINTS

CORRECT ANSWER: 2

Supplemental oxygen to decrease arterial hypoxemia during exercise becomes warranted when the SaO_2 drops below 88% saturation.

INCORRECT CHOICES:

A PaO_2 between 80 and 100 mm Hg and a $PaCO_2$ between 35 and 45 mm Hg indicates adequate ventilation (normal values). Normal range for pH is 7.35–7.45; pH is an indicator of acidosis (pH $<$ 7.40) or alkalosis (pH $>$ 7.40).

TYPE OF REASONING: DEDUCTIVE

This question requires factual recall of information laboratory values regarding below normal saturation of the need for supplemental oxygen during exercise. This is factual information, which is a deductive reasoning skill. In this situation, supplemental oxygen is needed during exercise if oxygen saturation falls below 88%. The SaO_2 indicates 84% saturation. If this question was answered incorrectly, review oxygen saturation guidelines, especially in patients with cardiac diagnoses.

B159 | Other Systems | Evaluation, Diagnosis, Prognosis

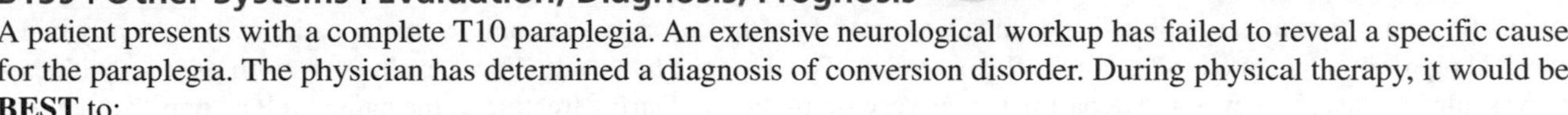

A patient presents with a complete T10 paraplegia. An extensive neurological workup has failed to reveal a specific cause for the paraplegia. The physician has determined a diagnosis of conversion disorder. During physical therapy, it would be **BEST** to:

CHOICES:

1. Initiate ROM and strength training after the patient receives psychological counseling.
2. Discuss possible underlying causes for the paralysis with the patient in an empathetic manner.
3. Initiate functional training consistent with the level of injury.
4. Use functional electrical stimulation as a means of demonstrating to the patient that the muscles are functional.

TEACHING POINTS

CORRECT ANSWER: 3

A conversion disorder (hysterical paralysis) represents a real loss of function for the patient. The therapist should treat this patient the same as any patient with spinal cord injury with similar functional deficits. Early intervention is crucial.

INCORRECT CHOICES:

A psychologist or psychiatrist is best able to help the patient understand the cause of the patient's paralysis. The therapist should be empathetic; however, counseling should not be the main focus of intervention in PT. Confrontation (using E stim to prove the patient has functioning muscles) is contraindicated.

TYPE OF REASONING: EVALUATION

This question requires one to make a value judgment about the best course of action for this patient who has a conversion disorder. It is beneficial to understand what a conversion disorder is and the appropriate role for the PT in order to choose the best response. These types of questions, which require evaluative reasoning, are challenging because of the need to evaluate the believability of statements and make decisions based on values.

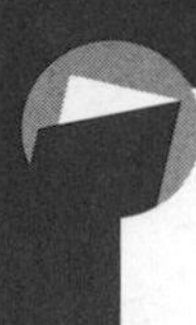

B160 | Devices, Admin., etc. | Teaching, Research, Roles

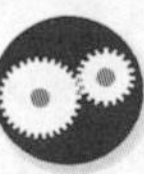

A certified cardiopulmonary clinical specialist was moved off the coronary care unit to treat a patient who recently had a surgical repair of a lacerated index finger flexor tendon. The therapist had dealt almost exclusively with patients with cardiovascular disease; however, the department was very short-staffed. During treatment, the patient felt a "pop," which was the result of a rupture of the newly repaired tendon. The PT in this case should have:

CHOICES:

1. Taken a medical history and asked another therapist to develop the treatment plan.
2. Treated the patient as requested, because the diagnosis was straightforward.
3. Used heat prior to the treatment to increase tendon extensibility.
4. Refused to treat this patient.

TEACHING POINTS

CORRECT ANSWER: 4

Malpractice is considered professional negligence as a result of wrongs or injuries that may occur through professional/patient relationships. Negligence is the failure to do what a reasonable practitioner would have done or not done in a similar circumstance. A supervisor's request to treat a patient can be refused if the therapist feels it is outside the scope of his/her expertise.

INCORRECT CHOICES:

It is inappropriate to ask another therapist to develop a treatment plan or to treat the patient if the therapist does not feel competent to deal with the problem.

TYPE OF REASONING: EVALUATION

This question requires the test taker to rely on his/her value system to determine what would have been the best course of action for this therapist to take. Using one's knowledge, experience, and ethical guidelines, it would have been best for this therapist to refuse to treat the patient because of limitations in knowledge of this area. As a result, negligence has occurred, because the patient has sustained an injury.

B161 | Neuromuscular | Patient Examination

Which is **NOT** considered a normal finding during an examination of a newborn infant?

CHOICES:

1. Symmetry in ROM.
2. Response decrement to repetitive stimuli.
3. Continuous tremulousness.
4. Dramatic skin color changes with change of state.

TEACHING POINTS

CORRECT ANSWER: 3

Continuous tremulousness is an abnormal finding, but occasional tremulousness is not.

INCORRECT CHOICES:

All the other choices are normal findings in a newborn infant.

TYPE OF REASONING: INFERENCE

This question requires one to understand normal activity and responses of infants in order to determine what is **NOT** a normal finding. The test taker must use inferential reasoning, which requires one to draw conclusions and make assumptions from the information presented. If this question was answered incorrectly, review information on abnormal findings in examinations of newborns.

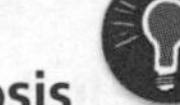

B162 | Neuromuscular | Evaluation, Diagnosis, Prognosis

A patient with long-standing TBI comes into an outpatient clinic using a standard wheelchair. The patient demonstrates sacral sitting with a rounded, kyphotic upper back. The therapist suspects the cause of this posture is:

CHOICES:

1. Uneven weight distribution on the thighs and ischial seat.
2. Decreased floor to seat height.
3. Excessive leg length from seat to the foot plate.
4. Excessive seat width.

TEACHING POINTS

CORRECT ANSWER: 3

Excessive leg length on a wheelchair can result in sliding forward in the wheelchair to reach the foot plate. This results in a posterior tilt of the pelvis and sacral sitting.

INCORRECT CHOICES:

All other choices are not likely to produce these postural deficits.

TYPE OF REASONING: INFERENCE

One must determine the most likely result of excessive leg length from the seat to the foot plate when sitting in a wheelchair. This requires inferential reasoning, in which the test taker must draw conclusions from the information presented. In this situation, the most likely result is sacral sitting and sliding forward in the chair.

B163 | Integumentary | Patient Examination

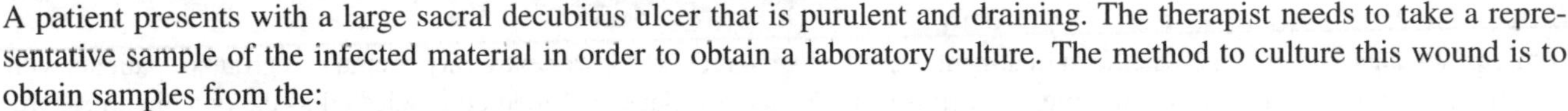

A patient presents with a large sacral decubitus ulcer that is purulent and draining. The therapist needs to take a representative sample of the infected material in order to obtain a laboratory culture. The method to culture this wound is to obtain samples from the:

CHOICES:

1. Exudate in the wound.
2. Dressing, exudate, and surrounding bed linen.
3. Dressing and exudate in the wound.
4. Exudate in the wound and the surrounding tissues.

TEACHING POINTS

CORRECT ANSWER: 1

The specimens must be collected from the wound site with a minimum of contamination by material from adjacent tissues. The exudate provides the best culture.

INCORRECT CHOICES:

The margins of cutaneous lesions or pressure ulcers are usually contaminated with environmental bacteria. Using the dressing for a specimen sample would also contain contaminated tissues.

TYPE OF REASONING: INDUCTIVE

The test taker must use clinical judgment applied to a patient circumstance (an inductive reasoning skill) to determine the best method to obtain a sample culture of a wound. In this situation, it is best to minimize contamination by sampling the exudate in the wound. If this question was answered incorrectly, refer to information on methods for obtaining laboratory cultures.

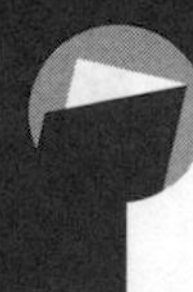

B164 | Cardiovascular-Pulmonary | Foundational Sciences

A phase 2 outpatient cardiac rehabilitation program uses circuit training with different exercise stations for the 50-minute program. One station uses arm ergometry. For arm exercise as compared with leg exercise, at a given workload, the PT can expect:

CHOICES:

1. Higher systolic and diastolic BP.
2. Higher HR and systolic/diastolic BP.
3. Reduced exercise capacity owing to higher stroke volumes.
4. Higher HR and lower systolic BP.

TEACHING POINTS

CORRECT ANSWER: 2

Arm ergometry uses a smaller muscle mass than leg ergometry, with resulting in a lower maximal oxygen uptake. In upper extremity exercise, both HR and BP will be higher than for the same level of work in the lower extremities.

INCORRECT CHOICES:

The other choices do not correctly identify the expected changes with arm exercise.

TYPE OF REASONING: INFERENCE

This question requires one to draw conclusions about arm ergometry and its impact on HR and BP, especially as it relates to leg ergometry. For this scenario, HR and systolic/diastolic BP will be higher with arm ergometry. To arrive at the correct conclusion, one must rely on knowledge of the impact of ergometry on cardiovascular activity, which should be reviewed if this question was answered incorrectly.

B165 | Devices, Admin., etc. | Teaching, Research, Roles

A therapist wants to determine whether a treatment was effective in reducing lower extremity edema in a group of patients with peripheral vascular edema. Volumetric measurements using a water displacement method is selected as the outcome measure. The data were compared to a control group receiving no treatment. Analysis of this data is **BEST** done by employing:

CHOICES:

1. t-test.
2. Chi square.
3. ANOVA.
4. Pearson's product moment.

TEACHING POINTS

CORRECT ANSWER: 1

The data in this study are interval data (values rank ordered on a scale that has equal distances between points on the scale). An appropriate statistic to determine the differences between groups (experimental versus control) is a t-test.

INCORRECT CHOICES:

An ANOVA is also appropriate for interval data and is used for more than two groups. Chi square is appropriate to determine differences between groups if nominal data (rank ordering with no specific intervals between ranks) is used. Pearson's product moment is indicated to determine correlational relationships.

TYPE OF REASONING: DEDUCTIVE

This question requires recall of research guidelines, especially the appropriate statistical test to use with interval data, which is a deductive reasoning skill. In this scenario, the recall of the different types of data and the appropriate statistical tests to use for them are keys to arriving at the correct decision. If this question was answered incorrectly, refer to information on statistical tests for interval data.

B166 | Other Systems | Intervention 

Before liver transplantation, a patient had a body mass index (BMI) of 17 and generalized muscle atrophy, and completed the 6-minute walk with 65% of age-predicted distance. Surgery was 10 days ago, and the patient is able to complete bed mobility with an overhead trapeze, walk independently for short distances with a rolling walker, and complete deep breathing and lower extremity AROM exercises for two sets of 10 repetitions. The patient is being discharged home with family assistance today. Home care physical therapy is scheduled to begin in 1 week. The **BEST** choice for discharge home exercise program is:

CHOICES:

1. Independent ambulation, elastic resistance lower extremity exercise, and active abdominal strengthening.
2. Breathing exercises, ambulation with walker, and AROM lower extremity exercises.
3. Stationary cycling and lower extremity resistance exercises using a 5-lb weight cuff.
4. Independent bed mobility exercises, elastic resistance extremity exercise, and partial sit-ups.

TEACHING POINTS

CORRECT ANSWER: 2

The in-hospital program should be continued until the home care therapist can make his/her own assessment and plan of care. The postoperative goals of improved ventilation, assisted mobility, and AROM are appropriate for the 3-week postoperative time period, considering the debilitation before surgery and the abdominal surgery.

INCORRECT CHOICES:

The other choices essentially change the exercise prescription and introduce unsupervised resistance exercises, which can be harmful to this debilitated patient.

TYPE OF REASONING: INDUCTIVE

This question requires one to consider the benefits of a home exercise program after liver transplantation. Given the patient's current status, the test taker must determine which exercise program will best address the patient's symptoms and result in functional improvement. This requires clinical judgment and prediction of what results will be yielded in the future, which is an inductive reasoning skill.

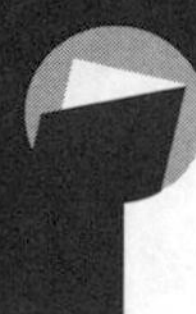

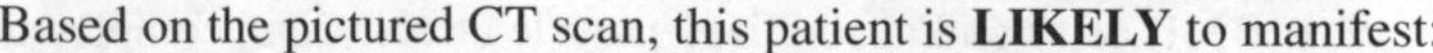

B167 | Neuromuscular | Patient Examination

Based on the pictured CT scan, this patient is **LIKELY** to manifest:

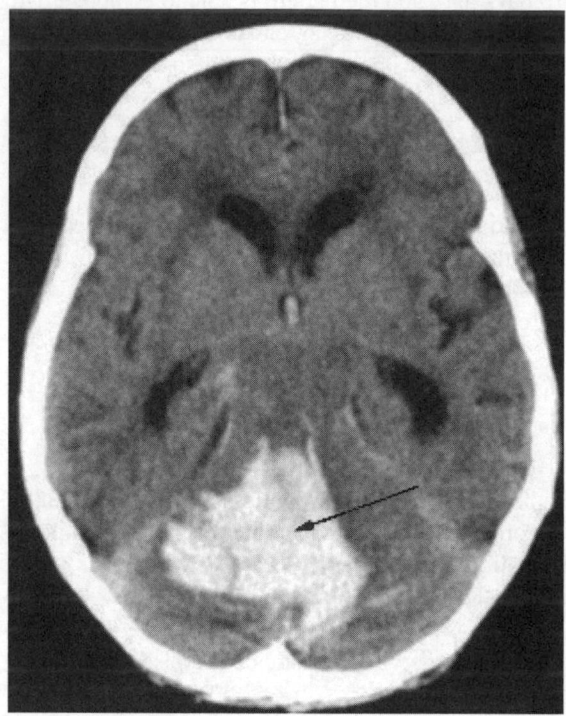

Image from: http://www.med-ed.virginia.edu/courses/rad/headct/index.html

CHOICES:

1. Broca's aphasia.
2. Ataxia.
3. Left-sided unilateral neglect.
4. Wernicke's aphasia.

TEACHING POINTS

CORRECT ANSWER: 2

The arrow is pointing to a hemorrhage in the cerebellum. Damage to this area results in difficulty with movement, postural control, eye-movement disorders, and muscle tone. Ataxia is a common finding.

INCORRECT CHOICES:

Aphasia is more typical of a left cerebral infarct, and left-sided unilateral neglect is typically due to a right cerebral injury. CT scans and MRIs can help the therapist predict clinical manifestations based on the area of injury.

TYPE OF REASONING: ANALYSIS

This question requires the test taker to determine the most likely presentation of symptoms based on the CT image. Questions that require analysis of pictures and graphs often necessitate analytical reasoning skill. In this case, the patient has experienced a hemorrhage in the cerebellum and will most likely display ataxia. If this question was answered incorrectly, review signs and symptoms of cerebellar hemorrhages.

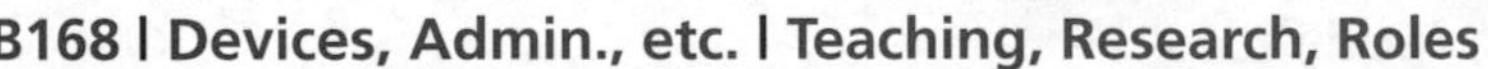

B168 | Devices, Admin., etc. | Teaching, Research, Roles

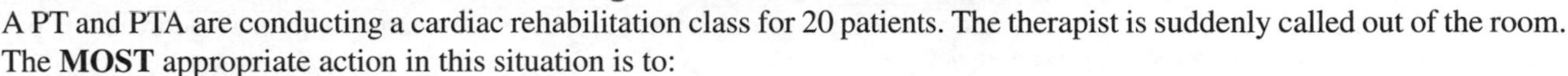

A PT and PTA are conducting a cardiac rehabilitation class for 20 patients. The therapist is suddenly called out of the room. The **MOST** appropriate action in this situation is to:

CHOICES:

1. Terminate the exercises and have the patients monitor their pulses until the therapist returns.
2. Have the PTA supervise the class using the outlined exercise protocol until the therapist returns.
3. Have the patients switch to less intense exercise until the therapist returns.
4. Have the PTA take over the class and teach modified activities.

TEACHING POINTS

CORRECT ANSWER: 2

The PTA can supervise the class using the outlined exercise protocol approved by the PT.

INCORRECT CHOICES:

The class should not be terminated, leaving the patients on their own to monitor their pulses. The PTA or patient should not change the plan of care.

TYPE OF REASONING: EVALUATION

This question requires the test taker to determine the appropriate supervision of PTAs when conducting a group session. This requires recall of supervisory guidelines for personnel, as well as prudence in delegating duties to such personnel, which is an evaluative reasoning skill. In this situation, it is appropriate for the PTA to supervise the class until the therapist returns. If this question was answered incorrectly, review information on supervision of PTAs.

B169 | Musculoskeletal | Intervention

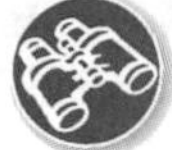

The most efficient intervention to regain biceps brachii strength if the muscle is chronically inflamed and has a painful arc of motion is:

CHOICES:

1. Isometric exercises at the end range of movement only.
2. Active concentric contractions through partial ROM.
3. Active eccentric contractions in the pain-free range.
4. Isokinetic exercises through the full ROM.

TEACHING POINTS

CORRECT ANSWER: 3

For a muscle that is chronically inflamed, focus should be placed on eccentric contractions, because there is less effort and stress placed on the contractile units than with concentric contractions at the same level of work. The exercise should be performed in the pain-free portion of the range.

INCORRECT CHOICES:

Isokinetic, isometric, and isotonic exercises do not allow for pain-free muscle contractions and can cause further inflammation of the muscle.

TYPE OF REASONING: INDUCTIVE

For this question, it is important to have knowledge of kinesiology, exercise physiology, and appropriate exercise for chronically inflamed muscles in order to choose the best exercise approach. This requires diagnostic thinking and clinical judgment, which is an inductive reasoning skill. For this situation, the most appropriate exercise is active eccentric contractions in the pain-free range to avoid further inflammation of the muscle. If this question was answered incorrectly, refer to information on appropriate exercises for various forms of muscle pathology.

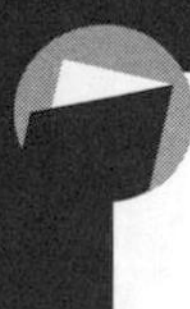

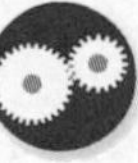

B170 | Devices, Admin., etc. | Equipment, Modalities

During a US treatment, the patient flinches and states that a strong ache was felt in the treatment area. To address this patient's concern, it would be **BEST** to:

CHOICES:

1. Increase the size of the treatment area.
2. Add more transmission medium.
3. Decrease the US intensity.
4. Decrease the US frequency.

TEACHING POINTS

CORRECT ANSWER: 3

Acoustical energy is reflected from the bone into the bone-tissue interface, resulting in rapid tissue temperature elevation and stimulation of the highly sensitive periosteum of the bone. A reduction in intensity is indicated if a strong ache is felt.

INCORRECT CHOICES:

The question assumes that the treatment size of the area is correct. Increasing the size of the treatment area would minimize the ability to elevate the tissue temperature. Thus, the patient would not experience a strong ache from rapid tissue temperature elevation. Adding more transmission medium would encourage transmission of acoustical energy, and thus potentiate the rapid tissue temperature elevation, contributing to the patient's symptom. The frequency has to do with the depth of penetration of the US energy, not the rate/speed at which the tissue temperature is being elevated.

TYPE OF REASONING: EVALUATION

This question requires one to determine the cause for the patient's discomfort during US treatment, and then determine an appropriate course of action, which is an evaluative reasoning skill. For this patient, it is best to decrease the US intensity because the strong ache indicates it is a result of too high an intensity. If this question was answered incorrectly, review information on US guidelines and symptoms warranting change of protocol.

B171 | Devices, Admin., etc. | Teaching, Research, Roles

The Back to Work Center, which specializes in work conditioning, is scheduled for an accrediting site survey. The appropriate agency to conduct this program is the:

CHOICES:

1. Commission on Accreditation of Rehabilitation Facilities (CARF).
2. Joint Commission on Accreditation of Health Care Organizations (JCAHO).
3. Occupational Safety & Health Administration (OSHA).
4. Health & Human Services (HHS).

TEACHING POINTS

CORRECT ANSWER: 1

CARF accredits all rehabilitation facilities, including free-standing work-conditioning centers.

INCORRECT CHOICES:

OSHA and HHS are not accrediting agencies. OSHA is the United States government's principal regulatory agency concerned with the health and safety of workers. HHS is the United States government's principal agency for protecting the *health* of all Americans and providing essential *human services*. JCAHO primarily accredits hospitals, hospices, and home care agencies.

TYPE OF REASONING: DEDUCTIVE

In order to determine the correct solution, one must recall the agency that is responsible for accrediting rehabilitation facilities. This requires factual recall of guidelines and protocols, which is a deductive reasoning skill. For this question, CARF is the appropriate agency to conduct this site survey. If this question was answered incorrectly, refer to information on accreditation agencies, especially CARF.

B172 | Integumentary | Intervention

A patient is recovering from deep partial-thickness burns over the posterior thigh and calf that are now healed. The therapist's examination reveals local tenderness with swelling and pain on movement in the hip area. While palpating the tissues, the therapist detects a mass. The therapist's **BEST** course of action is to:

CHOICES:

1. Continue with ROM exercises but proceed gently.
2. Report these findings promptly to the physician.
3. Use RICE to quiet down the inflammatory response.
4. Use petrissage to work on this area of focal tenderness.

TEACHING POINTS

CORRECT ANSWER: 2

These signs and symptoms are characteristic of heterotopic ossification (HO), an abnormal bone growth typically around a joint. While the etiology is unknown, its presence can lead to serious ROM limitations. These findings should be reported promptly to the physician.

INCORRECT CHOICES:

Petrissage and aggressive ROM exercises could exacerbate the condition. Ice does decrease metabolic activity; however, more in-depth medical management is required.

TYPE OF REASONING: INDUCTIVE

This question requires one to utilize clinical judgment to determine the reason for the patient's symptoms and then determine the best course of action, which is an inductive reasoning skill. In this situation, the findings indicate HO and the therapist should notify the physician promptly. If this question was answered incorrectly, review information on HO.

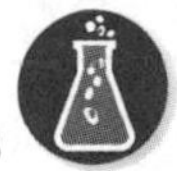

B173 | Other Systems | Foundational Sciences

The PT is reviewing the medical history of a new patient being seen for balance deficits and general deconditioning. The chief finding by the physician before admission 3 days ago was a positive fecal blood test. Which of the following laboratory values would confirm that the patient is safe for balance retraining activities?

CHOICES:

1. Leukocyte count 7,000.
2. Hematocrit 42%.
3. Platelet count 70,000.
4. Erythrocyte sedimentation rate (ESR) 7 mm/1 h.

TEACHING POINTS

CORRECT ANSWER: 2

The stated hematocrit value is within the normal range for both males and females, and indicates the fecal blood loss is not significant at treatment time.

INCORRECT CHOICES:

The leukocyte, platelet, and ESR rate are not significant for implementation of balance retraining.

TYPE OF REASONING: ANALYSIS

This question requires the test taker to determine the value of the information presented and its precise meaning, which is an analytical reasoning skill. One must determine which laboratory value best provides information about the patient's safety in conducting balance retraining activities. In this situation, the hematocrit level is the indicator of a patient's safety to engage in the activity.

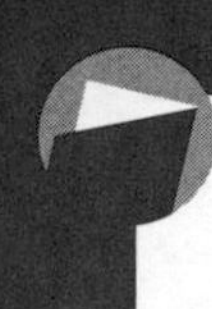

B174 | Cardiovascular-Pulmonary | Patient Examination

ECG changes that may occur with exercise in an individual with CAD and prior MI include:

CHOICES:

1. Bradycardia with ST segment elevation.
2. Significant arrhythmias early on in exercise with a shortened QRS.
3. Bradycardia with ST segment depression > 3 mm below baseline.
4. Tachycardia at a relatively low intensity of exercise with ST segment depression.

TEACHING POINTS

CORRECT ANSWER: 4

The typical exercise ECG changes in the patient with CAD include tachycardia at low levels of exercise intensity. The ST segment becomes depressed (>1 mm is significant). In addition, complex ventricular arrhythmias (multifocal or runs of PVCs) may appear, and are associated with significant CAD and/or a poor prognosis.

INCORRECT CHOICES:

The other choices do not accurately describe the expected ECG changes with exercise. Chronotropic incompetence is indicated by a HR that fails to rise; bradycardia (slowing of HR) is not expected. ST segment elevation with significant Q waves can occur and is indicative of aneurysm or wall motion abnormality.

TYPE OF REASONING: INFERENCE

In order to answer the question correctly, the test taker must recall typical ECG changes for patients who have myocardial ischemia and CAD. Therefore, the test taker must draw conclusions about the patient's diagnosis, which is an inferential reasoning skill. For this patient, one would expect tachycardia and ST segment depression, which should be reviewed if this question was answered incorrectly.

B175 | Musculoskeletal | Intervention

A patient with long-term postural changes exhibits an excessive forward head, and complains of pain and dizziness when looking upward. The **MOST** effective physical therapy intervention is:

CHOICES:

1. Manual therapy techniques to provide pain relief, as well as the incorporation of postural reeducation.
2. Anterior cervical muscle stretching and postural reeducation to relieve vertebral artery compression.
3. Strengthening exercises to the posterior cervical musculature.
4. Postural reeducation to reduce compression of the cervical sympathetic ganglia.

TEACHING POINTS

CORRECT ANSWER: 1

Long-term postural changes with forward head posture include shortening of the posterior muscles, potential joint restrictions, with possible vertebral artery compromise at the occiput. Restoration of normal movement throughout the cervical region and postural reeducation is the best choice for this condition.

INCORRECT CHOICES:

The anterior cervical muscles are most likely already lengthened. Strengthening the posterior muscles will not provide full restoration to the movement restrictions. In addition, the anterior muscle will also benefit from the reconditioning exercises. Postural reeducation by itself will not promote restoration of normal function.

TYPE OF REASONING: INFERENCE

This question provides symptoms and the test taker must determine first what the diagnosis is in order to determine the most effective intervention to remedy the symptoms. Questions that require one to determine a most effective approach in therapy often utilize inferential reasoning skill. If this question was answered incorrectly, refer to information on treatment for vertebral artery compression.

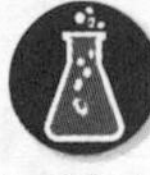

B176 | Cardiovascular-Pulmonary | Patient Examination

A patient with idiopathic dilated cardiomyopathy is on the cardiac unit with telemetry ECG monitoring after a recent admission for decompensated heart failure. Figure 1 depicts this patient's resting telemetric ECG recording, and Figure 2 depicts the patient's exercise (ambulating 2.5 mph on a flat surface in the hallway) telemetric ECG recording. The appropriate interpretation of the change between recordings is:

Figure 1

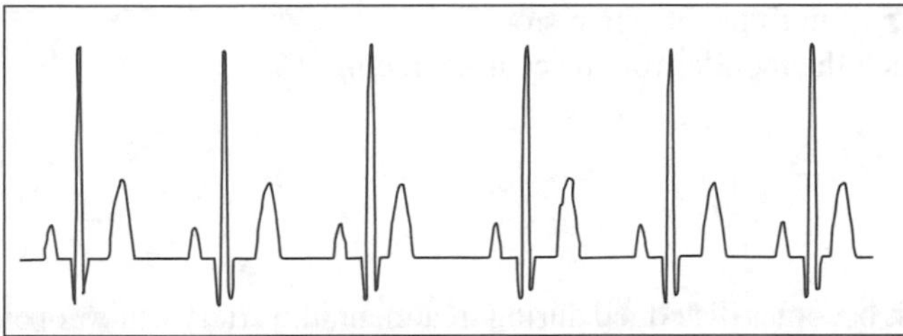

Figure 2

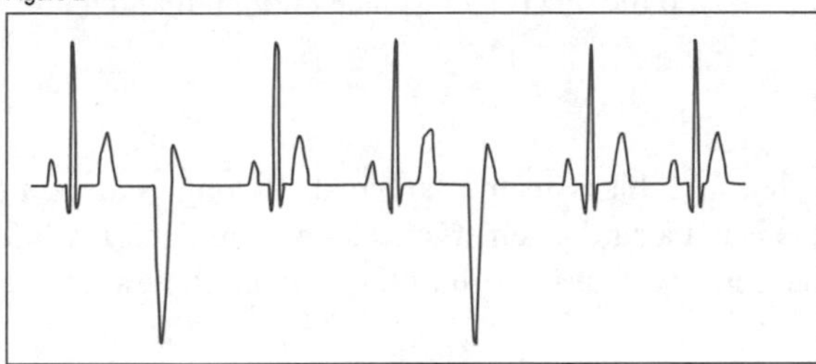

CHOICES:

1. Bradycardia, indicating abnormal response to increasing work demands and high risk.
2. Preventricular contractions, indicating abnormal response to increasing work demands and high risk.
3. Ventricular tachycardia, indicating abnormal response to increasing work demands and moderate risk.
4. Tachycardia, indicating normal response to increasing work demands and normal risk.

TEACHING POINTS

CORRECT ANSWER: 2

New onset of preventricular contractions (wide complex, lack of a P or T wave) indicates an abnormal response to increasing work demands, and indicates high risk for cardiac patients based on American College of Physicians and American Association of Cardiovascular and Pulmonary Rehabilitation risk stratification.

INCORRECT CHOICES:

The rhythm in Figure 2 is not indicative of bradycardia, ventricular tachycardia, or tachycardia.

TYPE OF REASONING: ANALYSIS

Questions that require the test taker to interpret information presented in the form of graphs or charts test analytical reasoning skill. In this situation, the ECG strip indicates PVCs or preventricular contractions with high risk. If this question was answered incorrectly, review information on ECG interpretation, especially PVCs.

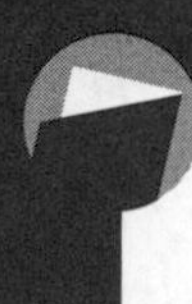

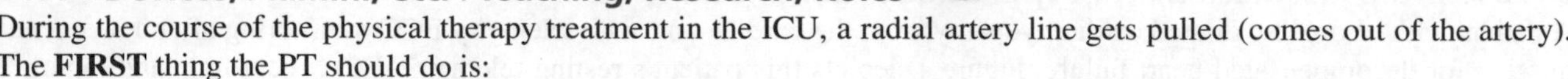

B177 | Devices, Admin., etc. | Teaching, Research, Roles

During the course of the physical therapy treatment in the ICU, a radial artery line gets pulled (comes out of the artery). The **FIRST** thing the PT should do is:

CHOICES:

1. Elevate the arm above heart level to stop the bleeding.
2. Push the code button in the patient's room, because this is a cardiac emergency.
3. Place a BP cuff on the involved extremity and inflate the cuff until the bleeding stops.
4. Reinsert the arterial catheter into the radial artery and check the monitor for an accurate tracing.

TEACHING POINTS

CORRECT ANSWER: 3

A radial arterial line is a catheter placed in the artery itself. If it becomes dislodged during treatment, the artery is now open to bleeding. This arterial bleeding needs to be stopped immediately, although it is not considered a cardiac emergency. Place a BP cuff above the site of bleeding and inflate the cuff to above systole to stop the bleeding or place enough manual pressure on the site to stop the bleeding. Then call for help.

INCORRECT CHOICES:

Elevating the site of bleeding above heart level will not be as effective, because this is an arterial bleed. As long as the heart is pumping with adequate pressure, the site will continue to bleed. This is not a cardiac emergency. Never replace any line that has become disconnected. The line is no longer sterile, and should not be reinserted into the patient. A new, sterile catheter will need to be used if the radial line is to be replaced.

TYPE OF REASONING: EVALUATION

This question requires one to use judgment to evaluate the strength of the statements made in order to arrive at a decision for the first course of action with this patient. In this situation, it is important to stop the bleeding in the most effective manner possible, which is to inflate a BP cuff on the involved extremity until the bleeding stops. Questions such as these can be challenging because one must use a value judgment to make the best decision.

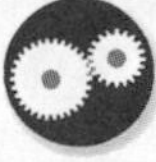

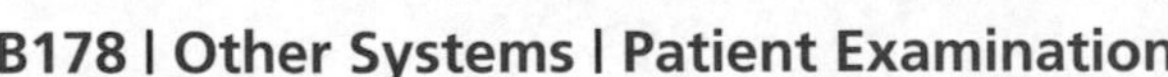

B178 | Other Systems | Patient Examination

A therapist working in an outpatient clinic examines a patient referred for exercise conditioning. During the initial examination, the therapist finds unusual swelling and enlargement in the anterior neck with mild tenderness. The patient does not have any hoarseness or difficulty swallowing. The therapist's **BEST** course of action to:

CHOICES:

1. Document the findings in the medical record.
2. Take girth measurements of the neck.
3. Notify the referring physician.
4. Initiate the plan of care.

TEACHING POINTS

CORRECT ANSWER: 3

This patient is likely exhibiting hyperthyroidism (Graves' disease) and should be referred to the physician of record. Additional manifestations of hyperthyroidism include cardiopulmonary changes (increased HR and respiratory rate, palpitations, dysrhythmias, breathlessness), CNS changes (tremors, hyperkinesias, nervousness, increased DTRs), musculoskeletal changes (weakness, fatigue, atrophy), and integumentary effects (heat intolerance).

INCORRECT CHOICES:

Documenting the findings in the medical record without notifying the physician delays medical intervention. Taking girth measurements at this time is not useful information. This disorder should be treated before beginning an exercise program. The patient will exhibit exercise intolerance and reduced exercise capacity.

TYPE OF REASONING: EVALUATION

This question requires the test taker to determine a best course of action based on the patient's symptoms. Questions such as these necessitate weighing of information to determine its significance and ultimately the best response. In this case, given the significance of the symptoms, the therapist should notify the patient's physician for follow-up. If this question was answered incorrectly, review symptoms of Graves' disease.

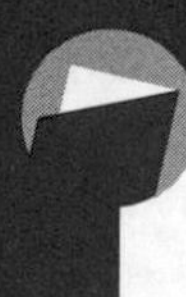

B179 | Integumentary | Intervention 

A patient with a methicillin-resistant *Staphylococcus aureus* (MRSA) infection has been discharged from an isolation setting with an open wound of the buttocks. The patient is now returning to physical therapy as an outpatient. The precaution that needs to be adhered to is:

CHOICES:

1. Treatment can be performed in the therapy gym if contact surfaces are covered.
2. An open wound must be contained within a dressing.
3. Direct contact with the patient should be avoided.
4. Gloves are needed only with dressing changes.

TEACHING POINTS

CORRECT ANSWER: 2

Staphylococcal organisms are spread by contact. Open wounds must be well-contained with a dressing. Standard germicidal cleaning measures (hand washing) should be followed. The therapist should be gloved for any direct contact with the patient's intact skin or surfaces or articles in close proximity to the patient. All equipment should be cleaned with an approved germicidal agent before and after use.

INCORRECT CHOICES:

Isolation in a private room is not required; in ambulatory settings, the patient should be placed in an examination room or cubicle as soon as possible. Treatment in an open gym is inappropriate for patients with MRSA.

TYPE OF REASONING: DEDUCTIVE

The test taker must recall standard precautions for MRSA infection in order to choose the best response. This type of recall is factual and dependent upon knowledge of protocols and guidelines, which is a deductive reasoning skill. If this question was answered incorrectly, review standard precaution guidelines for MRSA.

B180 | Other Systems | Foundational Sciences 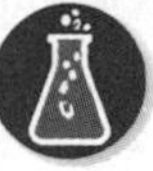

After examining a patient who was referred to physical therapy for posterior thoracic pain, the therapist finds no musculoskeletal causes for the patient's symptoms. Pain may be referred to this thoracic region from the:

CHOICES:

1. Appendix.
2. Ovary.
3. Gallbladder.
4. Heart.

TEACHING POINTS

CORRECT ANSWER: 3

Dysfunction of the gallbladder often refers pain to the thorax.

INCORRECT CHOICES:

The commonly observed referral pattern of the heart is to the chest and upper extremity, the ovaries to the low back, and the appendix to the right lower quadrant.

TYPE OF REASONING: ANALYSIS

This question requires one to refer to knowledge of physiology and of common referred patterns of pain. The test taker must recognize that pain referred to the posterior thoracic region is typical of problems with the gallbladder. To arrive at the correct conclusion, the test taker must analyze the information presented and determine the meaning of that information, which is an analytical reasoning skill.

B181 | Devices, Admin., etc. | Equipment, Modalities

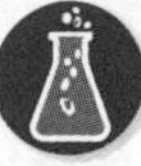

An elderly patient with a transfemoral amputation is being fitted with a temporary prosthesis containing an SACH (solid ankle cushion heel) prosthetic foot. This prosthetic foot:

CHOICES:

1. Absorbs energy through a series of bumpers, permitting sagittal plane motion only.
2. Allows limited sagittal plane motion with a small amount of mediolateral motion.
3. Is an articulated foot with multiplanar motion.
4. Allows full sagittal and frontal plane motion.

TEACHING POINTS

CORRECT ANSWER: 2

The SACH foot is the most commonly prescribed type of prosthetic foot. It provides for sagittal plane motion (primarily plantarflexion) and very limited frontal plane motion (mediolateral motion).

INCORRECT CHOICES:

Articulated feet (joined by a metal bolt or cable to the lower shank section) have rubber bumpers that absorb shock and control plantarflexion excursion. An anterior stop resists dorsiflexion. Full sagittal and frontal plane motions are not allowed.

TYPE OF REASONING: ANALYSIS

One must recall the properties of a SACH foot in order to choose the correct solution. This requires knowledge of prostheses and their indications. The test taker must analyze the information presented and determine the meaning of that information, which is an analytical reasoning skill. If this question was answered incorrectly, refer to information on properties of prosthetic feet.

B182 | Neuromuscular | Intervention

An elderly patient demonstrates significant proprioceptive losses in both lower extremities, distal greater than proximal. The **BEST** strategy to assist in compensatory gait training is to have the patient:

CHOICES:

1. Use light touch-down support on available furniture.
2. Look at the feet for placement while walking.
3. Practice walking on smooth tile floors.
4. Count out loud during each step.

TEACHING POINTS

CORRECT ANSWER: 2

Selection of compensatory strategies for sensory losses is dependent upon careful assessment of the sensory systems contributing to balance (somatosensory, visual, and vestibular). Control should be refocused to use available intact sensory systems. In this case, proprioception is impaired while vision is intact.

INCORRECT CHOICES:

Use of counting can aid gait rhythm, but not foot placement. Light touch-down support can aid balance, but training using available furniture is a bad idea. Walking on smooth tile floors does not address the need for compensatory training.

TYPE OF REASONING: INFERENCE

One must draw conclusions or infer information presented in this question in order to make the determination for the best course of action for this patient. In this case, it is best to have the patient look at his/her feet while walking. Knowledge of compensatory strategies for sensory loss is important for arriving at the correct conclusion, and should be reviewed if this question was answered incorrectly.

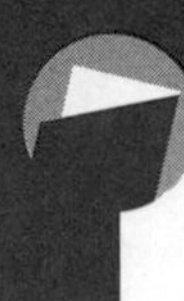

B183 | Cardiovascular-Pulmonary | Patient Examination

A patient in the ICU is referred to physical therapy and presents with significant shortness of breath. Notable on physical examination is a deviated trachea to the left. Which of the following processes would account for such a finding?

CHOICES:

1. Right hemothorax.
2. Left pneumothorax.
3. Left pleural effusion.
4. Right lung collapse.

TEACHING POINTS

CORRECT ANSWER: 1

A right hemothorax (blood was in the pleural space) takes up space in the right hemithorax, shifting the trachea to the left.

INCORRECT CHOICES:

A left pneumothorax and a left pleural effusion take up space in the left thorax. The air (pneumothorax) or the sterile fluid (effusion) in the pleural space would push contents of the left hemithorax, including the trachea, to the right. A lung collapse, or a volume loss phenomenon, on the right would pull the trachea over toward the right.

TYPE OF REASONING: INFERENCE

This question requires the test taker to make a determination for the patient's symptoms, which necessitates use of inferential reasoning. In this situation, the deviated trachea to the left is due to a right hemothorax. One must rely on knowledge of pulmonary pathology to arrive at a correct conclusion, which should be reviewed if this question was answered incorrectly.

B184 | Neuromuscular | Foundational Sciences

A patient complains of pain (7/10) in the shoulder region secondary to acute subdeltoid bursitis. As part of the plan of care during the acute phase, the therapist elects to use conventional TENS, which will modulate the pain primarily through:

CHOICES:

1. Ascending inhibition.
2. Descending inhibition.
3. Stimulation of endorphins.
4. Gate control mechanisms.

TEACHING POINTS

CORRECT ANSWER: 4

The gate control mechanism is activated by the application of conventional (high-rate) TENS at the spinal cord level.

INCORRECT CHOICES:

Ascending inhibition occurs after the gate control mechanism has been activated. Low-rate TENS, having a stronger stimulus and a longer pulse duration, activates the descending inhibition, stimulating endorphin production mechanisms.

TYPE OF REASONING: DEDUCTIVE

This question requires one to recall the properties of conventional TENS and how pain is modulated. This primarily requires recall of the properties of conventional TENS, which is factual knowledge and encourages deductive reasoning skills. Review information on TENS properties and neurophysiological effects if this question was answered incorrectly.

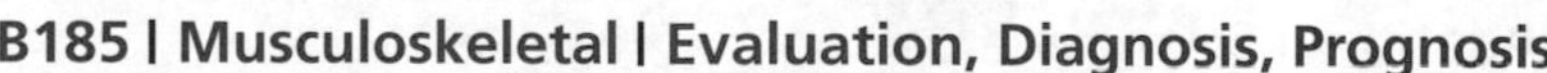

B185 | Musculoskeletal | Evaluation, Diagnosis, Prognosis

A patient described a sudden onset of back pain while trying to lift a heavy barrel. The patient described this pain as constant, unremitting at an intensity of 10/10 over the last 3 days, and unresponsive to pain medications. The patient is unable to work, but is able to drive to the clinic for treatment unaided. There is no history of other back-related symptoms in the past. The symptomatology is **MOST LIKELY** related to:

CHOICES:

1. Discal dysfunction.
2. Neoplastic disease.
3. Early degenerative osteoarthritis.
4. Secondary gain.

TEACHING POINTS

CORRECT ANSWER: 4

A patient who is able to drive to the clinic for treatment and relates a pain level of 10/10 is not providing consistent subjective data. Secondary gain in this case, and not working, is a likely factor.

INCORRECT CHOICES:

Pain from a disc pathology is typically worse in the morning and will decrease (at least slightly) when the patient gets out of bed and begins to walk around. The diagnosis is unlikely to be a neoplastic condition secondary to the acute, traumatic onset. Degenerative oseteoarthritis is described as stiffness in the morning with worsening pain as the activity level increases throughout the day.

TYPE OF REASONING: INDUCTIVE

The test taker must utilize diagnostic thinking and clinical judgment to determine the most likely cause for the patient's symptoms, which is an inductive reasoning skill. In this case, the patient's inconsistency in engagement in activities (driving but not being able to work) most likely has secondary gain involved. If this question was answered incorrectly, review information on secondary gain in patient care.

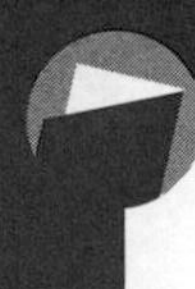

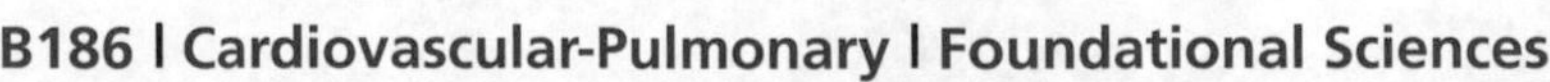

B186 | Cardiovascular-Pulmonary | Foundational Sciences

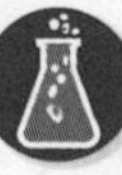

After myocardial infraction (MI), a patient was placed on medications that included a beta-adrenergic blocking agent. When monitoring this patient's response to exercise, the therapist expects this drug will cause HR to:

CHOICES:

1. Be low at rest and rise very little with exercise.
2. Be low at rest and rise linearly as a function of increasing workload.
3. Increase proportionally to changes in systolic BP.
4. Increase proportionally to changes in diastolic BP.

TEACHING POINTS

CORRECT ANSWER: 1

Beta-adrenergic blocking agents (e.g., propranolol [Inderal]) are used to treat hypertension, prevent angina pectoris, and prevent certain arrhythmias. In individuals taking these drugs, HR is low at rest and rises very little with exercise (blunted response). These changes, therefore, invalidate the use of HR to monitor exercise responses. A more sensitive measure would be RPE.

INCORRECT CHOICES:

HR does not rise linearly with exercise in patients on propranolol. The medication is used for treatment of hypertension. Both resting and exercise BP are suppressed.

TYPE OF REASONING: ANALYSIS

This question requires one to recall the indications for beta-adrenergic agents and effects on cardiovascular function. This requires one to interpret information and determine the meaning of that information, which necessitates analytical reasoning skill. If this question was answered incorrectly, review information on effects of beta-blockers on cardiovascular function.

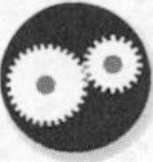

B187 | Devices, Admin., etc. | Teaching, Research, Roles

A male patient, who is from a foreign country, is referred to physical therapy in an acute care setting after a total knee replacement. This patient's faith prevents him from having any physical contact with any female other than his wife. The female PT has spent considerable time reviewing the medical record to prepare for the initial examination. The therapist enters the patient's room and introduces herself to the patient and his wife. The wife explains that the patient cannot be treated by a female. The PT should:

CHOICES:

1. Apologize; proceed with the examination, given his priority post-operative status.
2. Proceed with the examination and instruct the wife to perform the hands-on components of the examination under the therapist's direction.
3. Explain that she will contact her male colleague and he will perform the examination shortly.
4. Document in the patient's chart that the patient refused treatment, and try to have a male colleague see him later that day or the next day.

TEACHING POINTS

CORRECT ANSWER: 3

PTs are obligated to provide services with compassion and caring behaviors that are sensitive to individual and cultural differences. Providing patient-centered care is also required and the patient's beliefs need to be honored. Given the patient's postoperative status, receiving physical therapy is a priority, and the male colleague will need to do so.

INCORRECT CHOICES:

Proceeding with the evaluation, even though valuable time has been spent, would be in violation of the patient's rights and wishes, which is in violation of the Code of Ethics and theories of informed consent. Having the patient's wife perform the hands-on aspects of the examination does not allow for the skilled intervention required by a PT. The patient did not refuse treatment. The methodology of what was offered was against the patient's religious beliefs.

TYPE OF REASONING: EVALUATION

The question requires one to identify that a patient's cultural beliefs and differences need to be honored and patient-centered care needs to be provided. This requires evaluative reasoning skill. In order to answer the question correctly, the test taker must first identify the conflict in providing care as first planned and then formulate an alternative plan that respects the patient's beliefs. If this question was answered incorrectly, review the Code of Ethics Principle 2 (B).

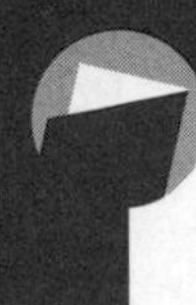

B188 | Other Systems | Evaluation, Diagnosis, Prognosis

A patient has a 20-year history of diabetes. Notable on the examination are the following: vascular insufficiency and diminished sensation of both feet with poor healing of a superficial skin lesion. It is important that the patient understand the precautions and guidelines on foot care for people with diabetes. Which recommendation is **CONTRAINDICATED** to include in patient care instructions?

CHOICES:

1. Wash the feet daily and hydrate with moisturizing lotion.
2. Inspect the skin daily for inflammation, swelling, redness, blisters, or wounds.
3. Use daily hot soaks and moisturize the skin.
4. Wear flexible shoes that allow adequate room and change shoes frequently.

TEACHING POINTS

CORRECT ANSWER: 3

Daily hot soaks are contraindicated because of the increased risk of thermal injury. The patient with diabetes typically has loss of protective sensations.

INCORRECT CHOICES:

All other instructions are correct and important to include in a well-balanced program of foot care.

TYPE OF REASONING: INFERENCE

This question requires one to determine the recommendation to a patient with diabetes that is contraindicated. In this circumstance, one should **NOT** recommend hot soaks because of the risk of thermal injury from loss of protective sensations in the feet. Questions that require one to draw conclusions and formulate opinions based on information presented encourage use of inferential reasoning. If this question was answered incorrectly, refer to guidelines for diabetic foot care.

B189 | Musculoskeletal | Evaluation, Diagnosis, Prognosis

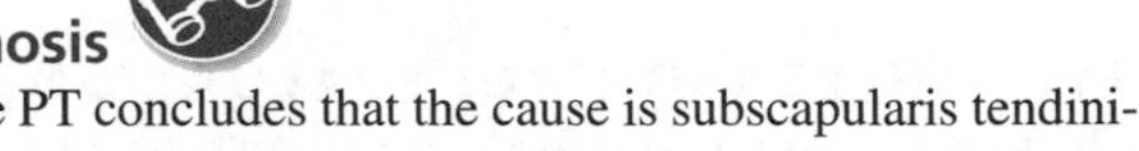

After completing an examination of a patient with shoulder pain, the PT concludes that the cause is subscapularis tendinitis. This clinical finding supportive of this conclusion is:

CHOICES:

1. Pain provoked with active glenohumeral external rotation.
2. Pain provoked with passive glenohumeral external rotation.
3. Tenderness at the greater tubercle of the humerus.
4. Painful resisted shoulder adduction.

TEACHING POINTS

CORRECT ANSWER: 2

The subscapularis is an internal rotator of the humerus. It will be painful if passively stretched into external rotation and irritated when contracting or being resisted when the shoulder internally rotates. The muscle inserts onto the lesser tubercle of the humerus and plays no role in shoulder adduction.

INCORRECT CHOICES:

Active glenohumeral external rotation does not require activation of the subscapularis muscle. The subscapularis attaches to the lesser tuberosity. The subscapularis is not the primary mover for shoulder adduction, so is not likely to be painful with resisted shoulder adduction.

TYPE OF REASONING: INDUCTIVE

This question requires diagnostic reasoning and clinical judgment, which is an inductive reasoning skill. Knowledge of upper extremity orthopedics, especially rotator cuff impairments, is needed to answer this question. One must recall the typical positions and motions that will evoke pain for patients with subscapularis tendinitis in order to arrive at the correct conclusion, which should be reviewed if this question was answered incorrectly.

B190 | Musculoskeletal | Intervention

A soccer player sustained a grade II inversion ankle sprain 2 weeks ago. The **BEST** intervention in the early subacute phase of rehabilitation would most likely include:

CHOICES:

1. Plyometric-based exercise program.
2. Closed-chain strengthening and proprioceptive exercises.
3. Functional soccer-related drills.
4. Mobilization at the talocrural and subtalar joints.

TEACHING POINTS

CORRECT ANSWER: 2

The most effective treatment for this athlete would involve closed-chain exercises and proprioceptive training, appropriate interventions for early **subacute phase** management.

INCORRECT CHOICES:

The other choices are not appropriate or timely for early subacute phase management. These approaches may be useful later in the rehabilitation of this athlete.

TYPE OF REASONING: INFERENCE

One must infer or draw conclusions for the best early intervention approach, given the injury and knowledge of rehabilitation techniques for this injury. This requires inferential reasoning skill, in which the test taker applies this knowledge and formulates conclusions about the patient for a best course of action. If this question was answered incorrectly, review information on early treatment for inversion ankle sprain.

B191 | Devices, Admin., etc. | Equipment, Modalities

A patient is referred for outpatient care after a tendon transfer of the extensor carpi radialis longus. The muscle strength tests poor (2/5) in spite of previous intensive therapy. The therapist elects to apply biofeedback to assist in progressively increasing active motor recruitment. Initially, the EMG biofeedback protocol should consist of:

CHOICES:

1. High-detection sensitivity with recording electrodes placed close together.
2. High-detection sensitivity with recording electrodes placed far apart.
3. Low-detection sensitivity with recording electrodes placed close together.
4. Low-detection sensitivity with recording electrodes placed far apart.

TEACHING POINTS

CORRECT ANSWER: 1

High-detection sensitivity is needed to detect low-amplitude signals generated by a small number of motor units such as in a weak extensor carpi radialis longus.

INCORRECT CHOICES:

Wide electrode placement would pick up signals from more than one muscle and might invalidate the procedure. Low-detection sensitivity may not pick up the necessary motor unit signals.

TYPE OF REASONING: DEDUCTIVE

This question requires application of knowledge of EMG biofeedback protocols in order to determine the best approach to early biofeedback intervention. This encourages deductive reasoning skill, which encourages recall of factual knowledge of protocols to apply information to a specific case situation that of extensor carpi radialis longus tendon transfer. If this question was answered incorrectly, review information on EMG biofeedback guidelines.

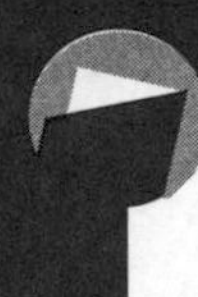

B192 | Other Systems | Evaluation, Diagnosis, Prognosis

A PT receives a home care referral from the nurse case manager. An elderly man has lost functional independence after the recent death of his wife. His past medical history includes stroke with minimal residual disability. Currently, he no longer goes out of his house and rarely even gets out of his chair anymore. During the initial session, the therapist determines that depression may be the cause of his increasing inactivity based on the presence of:

CHOICES:

1. Sleep apnea and weight gain.
2. Complaints of increasing dizziness and palpitations.
3. Low scores on the Geriatric Depression Scale.
4. Weight loss and social withdrawal.

TEACHING POINTS

CORRECT ANSWER: 4

Depression is associated with symptoms of withdrawal, fatigue, and weight loss.

INCORRECT CHOICES:

Sleep apnea is a potentially lethal disorder in which breathing stops for 10 seconds or more, many times a night. It is associated with obesity and anatomical obstruction. Increasing dizziness and palpitations is suggestive of cardiovascular problems. The Geriatric Depression Scale is a valid measure of depression in the elderly. High, not low, scores (>8 of a possible 30) are indicative of depression.

TYPE OF REASONING: INFERENCE

One must recall the typical symptoms associated with depression in the elderly to arrive at the correct conclusion. This requires one to draw conclusions and make assumptions based on the information presented, which is an inferential reasoning skill. If this question was answered incorrectly, review symptoms of depression, especially symptoms in the elderly.

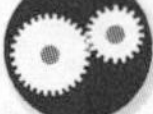

B193 | Devices, Admin., etc. | Teaching, Research, Roles

A PT, practicing in a sports and orthopedic clinic, is scheduled to see a child with bilateral knee pain. The patient arrives for the initial examination, and it is immediately evident that the patient also presents with spastic cerebral palsy and dysarthria. The therapist has no pediatric experience. The PT should:

CHOICES:

1. Complete the initial examination and, before the next visit, search the Internet for appropriate interventions.
2. Inform the parent that he/she will need to find another more specialized PT.
3. Inform the parent of the issue of no pediatric experience, and refer the patient to a PT with appropriate expertise.
4. Complete the initial examination and then advise the parent to see another more specialized PT.

TEACHING POINTS

CORRECT ANSWER: 3

PTs are accountable for making sound professional judgments. The Code of Ethics obligates a PT not only to make judgments within their scope of practice but also to consider their level of expertise. PTs are also obligated to collaborate with or refer to peers when necessary. The treatment of this patient is beyond the therapist's level of expertise; therefore, the PT is obligated to refer to a colleague with the appropriate level of expertise.

INCORRECT CHOICES:

The PT should not perform the initial examination, because this patient's needs exceed the therapist's level of expertise. Although researching interventions is an option to supplement a foundation of interventions, it should not be the resource that determines the plan of care. The PT is obligated to refer the patient to another therapist and not just refuse to see the patient because this may be viewed as abandonment.

TYPE OF REASONING: EVALUATION

The question requires one to identify the limited knowledge of the PT in examining and treating this patient with specific issues and diagnoses. This necessitates evaluative reasoning skill, which is often utilized in ethical situations. In order to answer this question correctly, the test taker needs to identify the limitations in the therapist's scope of practice and level of expertise in relationship to this specific patient, then identify the need for referral when the care required is outside the scope or level of expertise. If this question was answered incorrectly, review the Code of Ethics Principle 3 (C).

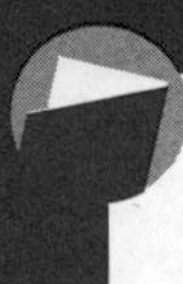

B194 | Cardiovascular-Pulmonary | Patient Examination

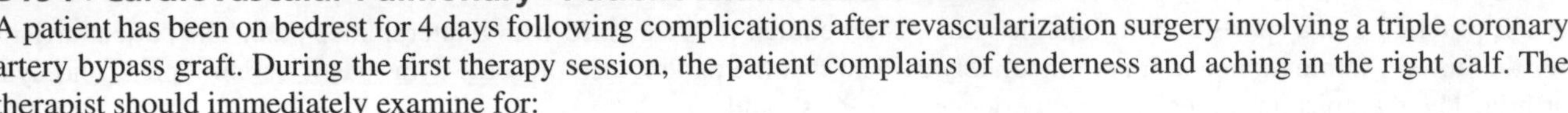

A patient has been on bedrest for 4 days following complications after revascularization surgery involving a triple coronary artery bypass graft. During the first therapy session, the patient complains of tenderness and aching in the right calf. The therapist should immediately examine for:

CHOICES:

1. Bradycardia.
2. Homan's sign.
3. Lowered body temperature.
4. Swelling in the calf or ankle.

TEACHING POINTS

CORRECT ANSWER: 4

Deep vein thrombophlebitis (DVT) is characterized by classic signs of inflammation (tenderness, aching, and swelling), typically in the calf. Rapid screening is possible with Doppler ultrasonography. Color flow venous duplex scanning is the primary diagnostic test for detection of DVT.

INCORRECT CHOICES:

Tachycardia, not bradycardia, may be present. Slight fever can be present, as part of the inflammatory reaction, not lowered temperature. Homan's sign is pain in the calf perceived with squeezing the calf and dorsiflexion; this is not considered reliable and lacks specificity and sensitivity.

TYPE OF REASONING: EVALUATION

This question requires one to evaluate the approaches presented and determine which approach has the most merit, given the patient's current symptoms. This requires evaluative reasoning skill, in which the test taker must weigh arguments and statements made and formulate a conclusion about the strength of these approaches. If this question was answered incorrectly, review symptomatology of DVT.

B195 | Musculoskeletal | Evaluation, Diagnosis, Prognosis

A patient is referred for physical therapy with jaw pain and dysfunction. The patient has experienced three episodes of jaw locking in an open position in the past week. The **MOST LIKELY** cause of this problem is:

CHOICES:

1. Impingement of the temporomandibular ligament.
2. Disc displacement.
3. Lateral pterygoid muscle spasm.
4. Entrapment of the retrodiscal lamina.

TEACHING POINTS

CORRECT ANSWER: 2

This patient is experiencing temperomandibular joint dysfunction (TMJ). The jaw becomes locked in an open position when the disc is displaced. The muscles influence lateral deviation of the jaw with opening.

INCORRECT CHOICES:

The temporomandibular ligament cannot become impinged. The lateral pterygoid muscle would not cause the mouth to be locked open if it experienced a spasm. Entrapment of the retrodiscal lamina is painful, but it is a consequence of a TMJ being locked open secondary to a disc displacement, not a cause.

TYPE OF REASONING: ANALYSIS

This question requires knowledge of TMJ anatomy and typical dysfunction of the joint associated with TMJ disorder. The jaw locking in an open position most likely indicates that the disc has been displaced. Through analytical reasoning, one must interpret or analyze the information presented and determine which problem seems to be the most likely cause. If this question was answered incorrectly, review information on TMJ disorders.

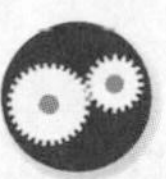

B196 | Other Systems | Evaluation, Diagnosis, Prognosis

An elderly patient is referred to physical therapy after a fall and ORIF for a fracture of the right wrist. During the initial examination, the therapist observes that the patient's skin and eyes have a yellowish hue. The therapist's **BEST** course of action is to:

CHOICES:

1. Continue with the treatment; a yellowish hue is an expected finding 3–4 days post-ORIF.
2. Treat the problem with whirlpool and massage and reevaluate skin color posttreatment.
3. Document the findings and consult with the surgeon immediately after treatment.
4. Send a copy of the examination results to the referring surgeon, emphasizing the skin hue.

TEACHING POINTS

CORRECT ANSWER: 3

This patient is most likely experiencing jaundice as a result of liver dysfunction. The therapist's best course of action is to document the findings and consult with the surgeon immediately, preferably by phone.

INCORRECT CHOICES:

All other choices delay consulting with the primary physican. The symptoms indicate liver dysfunction and jaundice, which warrant immediate contact with the surgeon.

TYPE OF REASONING: EVALUATION

The test taker must determine first what the patient's symptoms are indicative of and then determine what should be the appropriate course of action. Questions such as these, in which value judgments must be made, encourage evaluative reasoning skill.

B197 | Musculoskeletal | Evaluation, Diagnosis, Prognosis

An older adult received a cemented THR 2 days ago. The physical therapy plan of care should have as its **INITIAL** priority:

CHOICES:

1. AROM exercises and early ambulation using a walker, non–weight-bearing.
2. Patient education regarding positions and movements to avoid.
3. PROM exercises and gait training using crutches, weight-bearing to tolerance.
4. Proper technique for transferring to the toilet.

TEACHING POINTS

CORRECT ANSWER: 2

Education regarding positions and movements to avoid is the number one priority. Standard hip precautions stress avoiding excessive flexion, internal rotation, and adduction.

INCORRECT CHOICES:

Patients with cemented THRs should initially be weight-bearing to tolerance using a walker. Transfer training should occur, but it is not the first initial priority.

TYPE OF REASONING: INDUCTIVE

One must utilize clinical judgment and diagnostic thinking (an inductive reasoning skill) to determine the number one priority for this patient with a recent THR. In this situation, it is important to educate the patient regarding positions and movements to avoid, which if not followed could cause potential dislocation of the hip. If this question was answered incorrectly, refer to guidelines for early care of patients with THR.

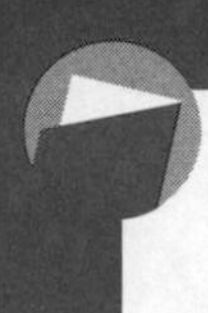

B198 | Devices, Admin., etc. | Teaching, Research, Roles

A patient is referred by an orthopedist with a diagnosis of impingement syndrome of the shoulder. The initial PT examination reveals signs and symptoms that are not consistent with this diagnosis and are more consistent with thoracic spine pain and dysfunction. The therapist treats the patient consistent with PT findings without communicating with the referring physician. Months later, the therapist is sued by the patient's estate. The patient died of undiagnosed metastatic lung cancer. The therapist is:

CHOICES:

1. Not legally licensed to diagnose metastatic cancer, therefore cannot be held responsible for the patient's death.
2. Responsible for making the diagnosis of possible cancer consistent with the PT examination of the patient.
3. Responsible for communicating findings to the referring physician when the findings are inconsistent with the referring physician's diagnosis.
4. Not responsible for the incorrect diagnosis because treatment was appropriate for the PT findings.

TEACHING POINTS

CORRECT ANSWER: 3

When a referral relationship exists with another health care professional, it is the PT's responsibility to communicate with the referring practitioner regarding the physical therapy examination, treatment plan, and management of the referred patient. This is particularly crucial when the findings are inconsistent with the referrer's diagnosis.

INCORRECT CHOICES:

The therapist cannot diagnose metastatic cancer but can be held responsible for not communicating with the primary physican.

TYPE OF REASONING: EVALUATION

This question encourages one to review the actions of the therapist, determine the value of those actions, and then decide whether they were appropriate, which necessitates evaluative reasoning. In this scenario, the therapist should have communicated the findings to the physician for follow-up, especially when they are inconsistent with the physician's findings. Questions that require value judgments are challenging because they move beyond factual knowledge to promote judgment, prudence, and ethical principles.

B199 | Cardiovascular-Pulmonary | Intervention

A patient with stage II primary lymphedema of the right lower extremity is referred for physical therapy. Examination reveals increased limb girth with skin folds/flaps evident. An important component of lymphedema management is manual lymphatic drainage. This procedure should include:

CHOICES:

1. Decongesting the distal portions of the limb first and working proximally.
2. Decongesting the trunk after the limb segments.
3. Decongesting the proximal portions of the limb first and working distally.
4. Deep tissue friction massage for several minutes on fibrotic areas.

TEACHING POINTS

CORRECT ANSWER: 3

Lymphedema is a swelling of the soft tissues that occurs with an accumulation of protein-rich fluid in the extracellular spaces. Causes of primary lymphedema include developmental abnormalities, heredity, surgery, or unknown etiology. Stage II lymphedema is characterized by nonpitting edema with connective scar tissue and clinical fibrosis. Lymphatic drainage is assisted by manual stroking (e.g., Vodder's, Leduc's, Foldi's, Casley-Smith pressure techniques). All techniques use cardinal principles: proximal limb segments before distal, trunk segments before limb segments, and directing the flow of the lymphatics centrally toward the lymphatic ducts.

INCORRECT CHOICES:

The other choices do not adhere to the cardinal principles of lymphatic drainage as explained.

TYPE OF REASONING: DEDUCTIVE

This question requires one to recall factual knowledge—that of manual lymphatic drainage techniques for patients with primary lymphedema. This encourages deductive reasoning skill, in which the test taker must recall the protocols and guidelines for this technique. If this question was answered incorrectly, review information on manual lymphatic drainage techniques.

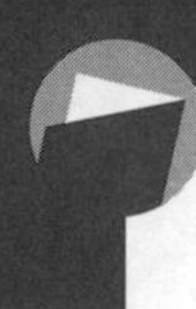

B200 | Devices, Admin., etc. | Equipment, Modalities

A patient with a 10 year history of multiple sclerosis (MS) demonstrates 3+ extensor tone in both lower extremities. The therapist needs to order a wheelchair. It would be **BEST** to recommend a(n):

CHOICES:

1. Standard wheelchair with a 30-degree reclining back.
2. Tilt-in-space wheelchair with a pelvic belt.
3. Electric wheelchair with toe loops.
4. Standard wheelchair with elevating legrests.

TEACHING POINTS

CORRECT ANSWER: 2

A patient with strong extensor tone needs controls over the hips (pelvic belt) to maintain the hips in flexion. The tilt-in-space design best assists in keeping the patient from coming out of the chair when extensor spasms are active.

INCORRECT CHOICES:

The other choices do not adequately address these problems. A reclining back would only increase extensor tone and extensor spasms. Elevating legrests assist circulatory flow in the lower extremities but may increase, not decrease, extensor tone. Toe loops function to keep the feet on the foot pedals. In the event of an extensor spasm, they would not control for proximal tone.

TYPE OF REASONING: INDUCTIVE

The test taker must utilize clinical judgment to determine the best recommendation for this patient, given the diagnosis and symptoms. For this patient, a tilt-in-space wheelchair with a pelvic belt would best address the patient's extensor tone in the lower extremities. If this question was answered incorrectly, review wheelchair prescription for patients with the presence of extensor tone.

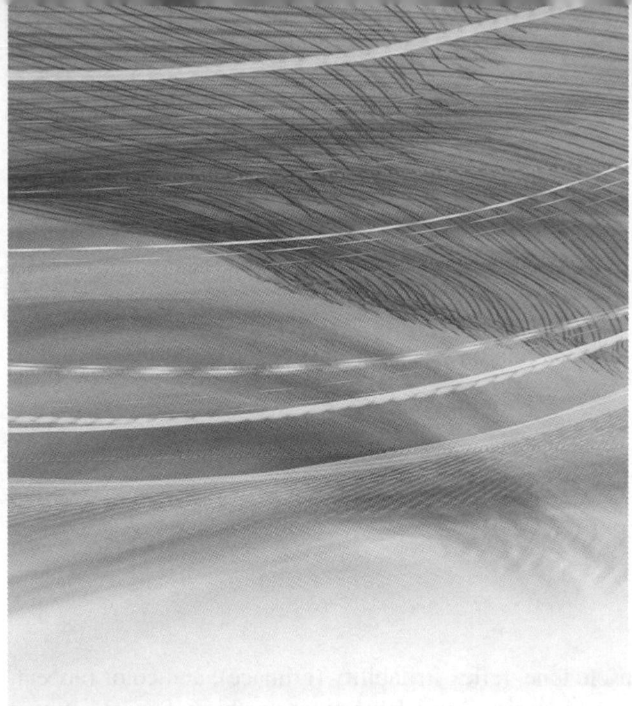

Examination C

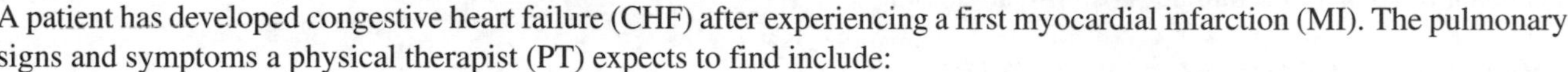

C1 | Cardiovascular-Pulmonary | Evaluation, Diagnosis, Prognosis

A patient has developed congestive heart failure (CHF) after experiencing a first myocardial infarction (MI). The pulmonary signs and symptoms a physical therapist (PT) expects to find include:

CHOICES:

1. Inspiratory wheezing and shortness of breath.
2. Crackles and cough.
3. Cough productive of thick yellow secretions.
4. Crackles and clubbing of the digits.

TEACHING POINTS

CORRECT ANSWER: 2

Patients who present with an MI and CHF have changes in their pulmonary examination, the most common being crackles and dry cough.

INCORRECT CHOICES:

Inspiratory wheezing occurs with extreme airway narrowing, which is not a hallmark of CHF. The cough associated with CHF is most likely nonproductive. Clubbing of the digits is a sign of chronic hypoxia. In this case scenario, this patient presents with his first MI. It is not possible for any chronic changes to have taken place at this point.

TYPE OF REASONING: INFERENCE

This question provides the diagnosis, and the test taker must determine the expected symptoms for this diagnosis. Questions of this nature necessitate inferential reasoning, in which one must draw conclusions based on the information presented. If this question was answered incorrectly, refer to information on symptoms for MI and CHF.

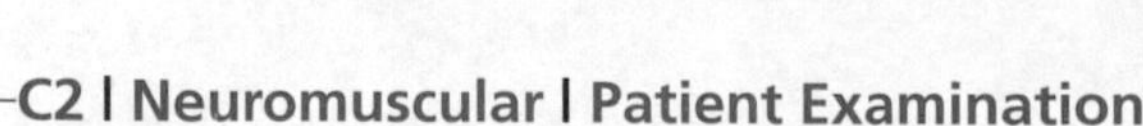

C2 | Neuromuscular | Patient Examination

A newborn is examined at birth using the APGAR test. Based on the following results, the neonatal therapist suspects that neurological complications are likely with an APGAR of:

CHOICES:

1. 3 at 10 minutes.
2. 8 at 5 minutes.
3. 9 at 1 minute.
4. 8 at 1 minute.

TEACHING POINTS

CORRECT ANSWER: 1

The APGAR score is based on heart rate (HR), respiration, muscle tone, reflex irritability (grimace), and color (appearance). APGAR scores are routinely assigned at 1 and 5 minutes and occasionally at 10 minutes postbirth. Scores between 0 and 3 at 1 and 5 minutes are extremely low and indicative of the need for resuscitation. Neurological complications are likely with extremely low APGAR scores, particularly at 10 minutes.

INCORRECT CHOICES:

Scores of 8–10 at 1 or 5 minutes postbirth are normal.

TYPE OF REASONING: INDUCTIVE

The test taker must make a determination of the meaning of the APGAR score as likely to result in neurological complications. This requires one to rely on knowledge of what the scale measures and of score ranges that indicate possible neurological complications. This requires clinical judgment coupled with recall of the properties of the scale, which is an inductive reasoning skill. If this question was answered incorrectly, refer to information on the APGAR Scale.

C3 | Devices, Admin., etc. | Teaching, Research, Roles

A PT requested that a physical therapy assistant (PTA) perform ultrasound (US) to the shoulder of a patient. During the treatment session, the patient experienced an electrical shock. The PT would be responsible for any injury to the patient if it was the result of:

CHOICES:

1. The patient touching the US device during treatment.
2. The PTA failing to use a ground fault interrupter (GFI).
3. The PT having instructed the PTA to use a device that had malfunctioned on the previous day.
4. Faulty circuitry.

TEACHING POINTS

CORRECT ANSWER: 3

The PT, in this case, correctly delegated the US treatment to the PTA. Every individual (PT, PTA) is liable for their own negligence; however, supervisors may assume liability of workers if they provide faulty supervision or inappropriate delegation of responsibilities (not evident in this case). Malfunctioning machine is the correct answer. PTs are liable for use of defective equipment if they contributed to its malfunction or continued to have it used in treatment without having it checked.

INCORRECT CHOICES:

The institution may assume liability if the patient was harmed as a result of an environmental problem such as faulty circuitry or leakage current that would cause the patient to be shocked if they touched the US unit. The standard of practice is such that a GFI is used during administration of US, which would make the PTA primarily liable if a GFI was not used. The patient assumes no liability in this scenario.

TYPE OF REASONING: EVALUATION

This question requires one to determine the value of the statements made in the question and then to determine the believability of these statements as applied to who should be assigned responsibility for the injury. This requires evaluative reasoning skill, in which beliefs and values must be weighed to arrive at a correct conclusion. In this situation, the PT should have taken the malfunctioning unit out of circulation to prevent anyone else from using it, thus making the PT primarily responsible.

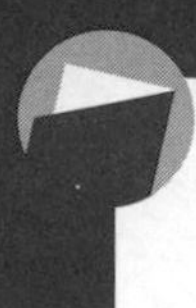

C4 | Cardiovascular-Pulmonary | Intervention

A patient with coronary artery disease received inpatient cardiac rehabilitation after a mild MI. The patient is now enrolled in an outpatient exercise class that utilizes intermittent training. The **BEST** initial spacing of exercise/rest intervals to safely stress the aerobic system is:

CHOICES:

1. 1:1
2. 5:1
3. 2:1
4. 10:1

TEACHING POINTS

CORRECT ANSWER: 3

Presuming that the exercise goals for inpatient cardiac rehabilitation are met, an exercise/rest ratio of 2:1 can be used with this patient to begin exercise in an **outpatient setting** in a safe manner.

INCORRECT CHOICES:

An exercise/rest ratio of 1:1 is appropriate for an initial prescription for inpatient rehabilitation programs with a goal of achieving a 2:1 ratio. Ratios of 5:1 or 10:1 are too stressful to begin outpatient rehabilitation. A 5:1 ratio may be a goal for later exercise programming.

TYPE OF REASONING: INDUCTIVE

One must determine through clinical judgment which exercise/rest interval is **BEST,** given the patient's diagnosis and status. Questions that encourage clinical judgment to determine a best course of action require inductive reasoning skill. If this question was answered incorrectly, review information related to appropriate aerobic exercise and exercise/rest ratios for patients with coronary artery disease.

C5 | Musculoskeletal | Evaluation, Diagnosis, Prognosis

The **BEST INITIAL** intervention to improve functional mobility in an individual with a stable humeral neck fracture is:

CHOICES:

1. Active resistive range of motion (ROM).
2. Isometrics for all shoulder musculature.
3. Pendulum exercises.
4. Heat modalities.

TEACHING POINTS

CORRECT ANSWER: 3

This individual will typically be immobilized with a sling for a period of 6 weeks. After 1 week, the sling should be removed to have the patient perform pendulum exercises to prevent shoulder stiffness.

INCORRECT CHOICES:

Resistive exercises including isometrics are not indicated during this early period. Heat modalities may be effective in reducing pain but do not improve mobility.

TYPE OF REASONING: INFERENCE

One must understand the nature of a stable humeral neck fracture and appropriate interventions in order to arrive at the correct conclusion. One must draw conclusions based on the patient's fracture status, which necessitates inferential reasoning skill. If this question was answered incorrectly, review information on appropriate exercises for stable humeral fractures.

C6 | Musculoskeletal | Intervention

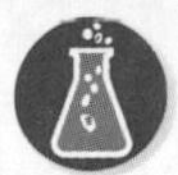

A dancer with unilateral spondylolysis at L4 is referred for physical therapy. The dancer complains of generalized low back pain when standing longer than 1 hour. Interventions for the subacute phase should include strengthening exercise for the:

CHOICES:

1. Abdominals working from neutral to full flexion.
2. Multifidi working from neutral to full extension.
3. Abdominals working from full extension to full flexion.
4. Multifidi working from full flexion back to neutral.

TEACHING POINTS

CORRECT ANSWER: 4

Performing strengthening exercises to the multifidi from flexion to neutral will not stress the pars defect.

INCORRECT CHOICES:

Abdominal strengthening will not provide the segmental stability needed with this condition. Lumbar extension beyond neutral and rotation will tend to aggravate the condition in the early stages of rehabilitation.

TYPE OF REASONING: ANALYSIS

One must understand the nature of unilateral spondylolysis, including symptomatology, in order to choose the best intervention approach. One must analyze the information presented and determine which intervention approach will provide the most benefit, while not stressing the pars defect. This requires analytical reasoning skill, in which the test taker weighs the information presented to choose the best solution.

C7 | Musculoskeletal | Foundational Sciences

A patient has fixed forefoot varus malalignment. Possible compensatory motion(s) or posture(s) might include:

CHOICES:

1. Genu recurvatum.
2. Excessive subtalar pronation.
3. Ipsilateral pelvic external rotation.
4. Hallux varus.

TEACHING POINTS

CORRECT ANSWER: 2

Possible compensatory motions or postures for forefoot varus malalignment include excessive midtarsal or subtalar pronation or prolonged pronation; plantarflexed first ray; hallux valgus; or excessive tibial; tibial and femoral; tibial, femoral, and pelvic internal rotation; and/or all with contralateral lumbar spine rotation.

INCORRECT CHOICES:

The other compensatory motions or deformities are **NOT** typical of this problem.

TYPE OF REASONING: INFERENCE

This question provides the diagnosis and the test taker must determine what compensatory motions or postures are likely to occur. Questions that challenge one to determine possible symptoms from a given diagnosis require inferential reasoning skill. If this question was answered incorrectly, refer to information on forefoot varus malalignment.

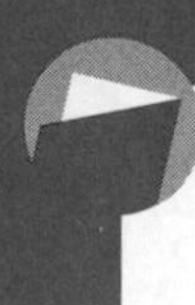

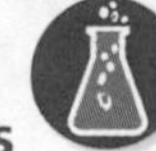

C8 | Integumentary | Foundational Sciences

A PT recently rotated onto a burn unit and is performing débridement techniques using standard precautions. After the session, the therapist experiences itching and skin rash on the hands, watery eyes, and facial swelling. The **MOST** likely cause is:

CHOICES:

1. Atopic dermatitis.
2. Rosacea.
3. Latex allergy.
4. Stasis dermatitis.

TEACHING POINTS

CORRECT ANSWER: 3

The therapist is likely experiencing an immediate hypersensitivity to latex (type I hypersensitivity). Symptoms typically include contact dermatitis, and if severe, swelling and respiratory changes. Whereas gloves are required for sterile débridement, the therapist can switch to nonlatex gloves.

INCORRECT CHOICES:

Atopic dermatitis is a chronic inflammatory skin disease. Rosacea is a chronic form of acne with a vascular component (erythema, telangiectasis). In statis dermatitis, skin is dry and thin with shallow ulcers that develop on the lower legs as a result of venous insufficiency.

TYPE OF REASONING: ANALYSIS

This question provides a group of symptoms and the test taker must determine what the likely cause is for them. This requires analytical reasoning skill. For this situation, the question mentions using standard precautions during the session, from which one should infer that the therapist used latex gloves, especially given the presenting symptoms. Therefore, latex allergy is the correct conclusion in this situation. If this question was answered incorrectly, review signs and symptoms of latex allergies.

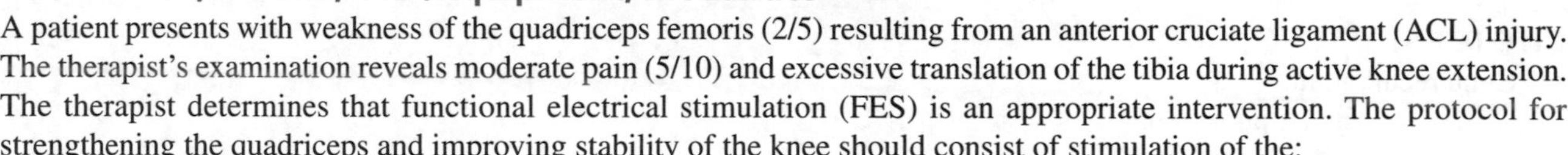

C9 | Devices, Admin., etc. | Equipment, Modalities

A patient presents with weakness of the quadriceps femoris (2/5) resulting from an anterior cruciate ligament (ACL) injury. The therapist's examination reveals moderate pain (5/10) and excessive translation of the tibia during active knee extension. The therapist determines that functional electrical stimulation (FES) is an appropriate intervention. The protocol for strengthening the quadriceps and improving stability of the knee should consist of stimulation of the:

CHOICES:

1. Quadriceps but not the hamstrings.
2. Hamstrings immediately before the quadriceps to produce co-contraction.
3. Hamstrings but not the quadriceps.
4. Quadriceps immediately before the hamstrings to produce co-contraction.

TEACHING POINTS

CORRECT ANSWER: 2

Stimulating the hamstrings just before stimulating the quadriceps will stabilize the tibia and prevent anterior tibial translation during knee extension and during co-contraction of both muscles. This would prevent the moving tibia from placing tension on the injured ACL.

INCORRECT CHOICES:

FES of the quadriceps without setting of the hamstrings first will cause an excessive anterior glide of the tibia. FES of the hamstrings alone will not provide the appropriate treatment because the weakness is in the quadriceps.

TYPE OF REASONING: DEDUCTIVE

One must determine, through the recall of FES protocols, the appropriate method for strengthening the quadriceps and improving knee stability. The recall of protocols and factual information encourages deductive reasoning skill. If this question was answered incorrectly, review information on FES for quadriceps strengthening and improving knee stability.

C10 | Neuromuscular | Evaluation, Diagnosis, Prognosis

A PT is reviewing a medical record prior to examining a patient for the first time. The suspected diagnosis is multiple sclerosis. On the neurologist's note, the therapist finds the following: deep tendon reflex (DTR) right quadriceps is 2+, left quadriceps is 4+. The therapist concludes that:

CHOICES:

1. The right DTR is normal, the left is abnormal.
2. Both DTRs are abnormal and indicative of upper motor neuron (UMN) syndrome.
3. The right DTR is exaggerated, the left is clearly abnormal.
4. Both DTRs are abnormal and indicative of hyporeflexia.

TEACHING POINTS

CORRECT ANSWER: 1

DTRs are graded on a 1–4 scale. Scores include 0 (no response); 1+ (present but depressed); 2+ (normal); 3+ (increased, brisker than average; possibly but not necessarily abnormal); and 4+ (very brisk, hyperactive, with clonus, abnormal). In this case, the right DTR is normal; the left is abnormal, and consistent with strong hypertonicity.

INCORRECT CHOICES:

The other choices do not correctly interpret these findings.

TYPE OF REASONING: INFERENCE

This question requires one to draw conclusions about the information presented, which is an inferential reasoning skill. Here, the test taker must understand the meaning of 2+ and 4+ DTRs of the quadriceps in order to determine that the 2+ is normal and 4+ is abnormal. If this question was answered incorrectly, review information on measurement of DTRs.

C11 | Cardiovascular-Pulmonary | Patient Examination

A patient has an episode of syncope in the physical therapy clinic. The therapist attempts to rule out orthostatic hypotension as the cause of the fainting. This is **BEST** done by:

CHOICES:

1. Checking HR and blood pressure (BP) in supine after 5 minutes' rest, then repeating in semi-Fowler position.
2. Palpating the carotid arteries and taking HR; using the supine position for BP measurements.
3. Checking HR and BP at rest, and after 3 and 5 minutes of cycle ergometry exercise.
4. Checking resting BP and HR in supine and sitting, then repeating measurements after the patient stands for 1 minute.

TEACHING POINTS

CORRECT ANSWER: 4

Orthostatic hypotension is a fall in BP with elevation of position; thus responses to movements (HR and BP) are tested from supine to sitting or sitting to standing. A small increase or no increase in HR upon standing may suggest baroreflex impairment. An exaggerated increase in HR upon standing may indicate volume depletion.

INCORRECT CHOICES:

The other choices do not challenge the system with adequate change of position (supine to semi-Fowler or remaining supine or sitting).

TYPE OF REASONING: INDUCTIVE

One must determine through clinical judgment the **BEST** method to rule out orthostatic hypotension. This requires knowledge of the nature of orthostatic hypotension and how it can be evaluated, which requires inductive reasoning skill. In this case, checking resting BP and HR in sitting and repeating after 1 minute of standing is the **BEST** way to rule the diagnosis out.

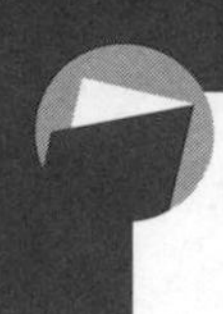

C12 | Integumentary | Evaluation, Diagnosis, Prognosis

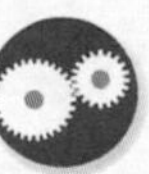

An inpatient with a grade III diabetic foot ulcer is referred for physical therapy. Panafil has been applied to the necrotic tissue BID. The wound has no foul smell; however, the therapist notes a green tinge on the dressing. In this case, the therapist should:

CHOICES:

1. Document the finding and contact the physician immediately.
2. Begin a trial of acetic acid to the wound.
3. Document the finding and continue with treatment.
4. Fit the patient with a total contact cast.

TEACHING POINTS

CORRECT ANSWER: 3

In this case, the therapist should document the findings and continue with treatment. Panafil is a keratolytic enzyme used for selective débridement. A greenish or yellowish exudate can be expected.

INCORRECT CHOICES:

If the exudate was green and had a foul smell, *Pseudomonas aeruginosa* should be suspected. The physician will most likely order a different topical agent. Acetic acid would be the topical agent of choice. A total contact cast can be used only after the wound is free of necrotic tissue.

TYPE OF REASONING: EVALUATION

The test taker must determine the significance of the information presented and evaluate the best course of action, given this information. This requires evaluative reasoning skill, in which one must assign value to the patient's wound status and judge how to proceed.

C13 | Devices, Admin., etc. | Teaching, Research, Roles

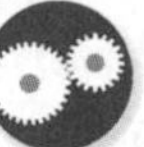

A PT receives a referral to examine the fall risk of an elder who lives alone and has had two recent falls. The activity that represents the **MOST** common risk factor associated with falls in the elderly is:

CHOICES:

1. Climbing on a stepstool to reach overhead objects.
2. Walking with a roller walker with hand brakes.
3. Dressing while sitting on the edge of the bed.
4. Turning around and sitting down in a chair.

TEACHING POINTS

CORRECT ANSWER: 4

Most falls occur during normal daily activity. Getting up or down from a bed or chair, turning, bending, walking, climbing/descending stairs are all high-risk activities.

INCORRECT CHOICES:

Only a small percentage of individuals fall during clearly hazardous activities (e.g., climbing the stepstool). Proper use of an assistive device reduces the risk of falls. Sitting does not typically present a fall risk.

TYPE OF REASONING: EVALUATION

One must reason out the **MOST** common risk factor for an elderly person with a history of falls. This requires the evaluation of the information presented and determining the believability of the statement, which encourages evaluative reasoning skill. In this question, most common risk factors for falls in the elderly are activities that are done during the normal daily mobility activities.

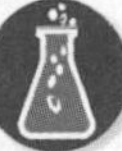

C14 | Devices, Admin., etc. | Equipment, Modalities

A PT is performing a prosthetic checkout on a patient with a transfemoral amputation. The prosthesis has been fitted with a quadrilateral socket. A checkout of the walls of the socket should reveal that the:

CHOICES:

1. Anterior and lateral walls are $2^1/_2$ inches higher than posterior and medial walls.
2. Posterior and lateral walls are 2 inches higher than medial and anterior walls.
3. Height of the posterior wall is 2 inches less than all the other walls.
4. Medial wall is $2^1/_2$ inches higher than posterior wall while anterior and lateral walls are the same height.

TEACHING POINTS

CORRECT ANSWER: 1

The anterior and lateral walls are built $2^1/_2$–3 inches higher than the posterior and medial walls to ensure proper positioning on the ischial seat.

INCORRECT CHOICES:

All other choices would result in improper positioning on the ischial seat with slippage into the socket and improper weight-bearing.

TYPE OF REASONING: ANALYSIS

One must recall the properties of a quadrilateral socket in order to arrive at the correct conclusion. This question requires one to analyze the information presented and determine the most correct information, given one's knowledge of this prosthesis. If this question was answered incorrectly, refer to information on prostheses with quadrilateral sockets.

C15 | Devices, Admin., etc. | Teaching, Research, Roles

A 2 month-old child with bilateral hip dislocations is being discharged home from an acute pediatric facility. The PT has developed a home exercise program and now needs to instruct the parents. The **MOST** important item for the therapist to assess before instructing the parents is:

CHOICES:

1. The financial reimbursement plan.
2. Their degree of anxiety and attention.
3. Their level of formal education.
4. The home environment.

TEACHING POINTS

CORRECT ANSWER: 2

A needs assessment should include a determination of the level of anxiety and ability to attend to the instructions given. If anxiety is high and the parents are unable to attend to the therapist's instructions, risk of failure to perform the home exercises correctly is high.

INCORRECT CHOICES:

Although the other factors may also be considered in the development of a home exercise plan, they do not represent immediate priorities for instruction.

TYPE OF REASONING: INFERENCE

This question requires one to draw conclusions about the diagnosis of the child and the **MOST** important item to assess before instructing the parents. This requires inferential reasoning skill, in which the test taker must make assumptions based on the information presented and determine the most appropriate course of action. In this case, it is most important to determine the parents' degree of anxiety and attention.

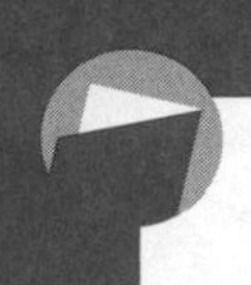

C16 | Devices, Admin., etc. | Teaching, Research, Roles

The grip strength of a group of 50 to 60 year-olds was investigated. A mean score of 40, standard deviation (SD) of 5, and range of 26–57 were reported. The grip strength score for a given patient was determined to be 34. The therapist can safely conclude that in a normal distribution this patient's score fell within:

CHOICES:

1. 99%.
2. 75%.
3. 95%.
4. 34%.

TEACHING POINTS

CORRECT ANSWER: 3

In a normal distribution (bell-shaped curve), 95.45% of scores can be expected to fall within +2 or −2 SD of the mean.

INCORRECT CHOICES:

In a normal distribution, 68% of scores can be expected to fall within +1 or –1 SD of the mean; 99% of scores can be expected to fall within +3 or –3 SDs of the mean.

TYPE OF REASONING: DEDUCTIVE

This question requires factual recall of information related to normal distributions and SDs, which necessitates deductive reasoning skill. One must recall how normal distributions are determined in order to arrive at the correct conclusion. If this question was answered incorrectly, review information related to how to determine normal distributions and SDs.

C17 | Cardiovascular-Pulmonary | Foundational Sciences

Which is **a** typical clinical manifestation of cystic fibrosis (CF)?

CHOICES:

1. Excessive appetite and weight loss.
2. Increased FEV_1 (forced expiratory volume in 1 sec) during pulmonary function testing.
3. Frequent recurrent urinary tract infections.
4. Increase in secretions of the endocrine system.

TEACHING POINTS

CORRECT ANSWER: 1

CF is an inherited disorder affecting the exocrine glands of the hepatic, digestive, and respiratory systems. The patient with CF is prone to chronic bacterial airway infections and progressive loss of pulmonary function from progressive obstructive lung disease. Early clinical manifestations include an inability to gain weight despite excessive appetite and adequate caloric intake.

INCORRECT CHOICES:

The pulmonary function test results in a patients with CF can have a mixed picture of both obstructive and restrictive disease components. It is typical to have a decrease in the FEV_1 value over time, not an increase. There will also be recurrent infections in patients with CF; however, these infections will be in the airways and lung parenchyma. Urinary tract infections, though quite possible, are no different in frequency than in any patient or nonpatient population. Finally, CF is a disorder of the exocrine glands, meaning those glands that excrete secretions. The endocrine system, including the hypothamus, pituitary, thyroid, etc., are not particularly involved in the disease of CF. The pancreas is both an exocrine and an endocrine gland. CF does affect the pancreas by *decreasing* the bicarbonate secretions, reducing the effectiveness of pancreatic enzymes and leading to pancreatic insufficiency.

TYPE OF REASONING: INFERENCE

This question provides the diagnosis, and the test taker must determine the symptomatology that is **expected**. CF is a multisystem disorder, making the possible clinical manifestations quite varied. This questions requires inferential reasoning skill, in which one infers knowledge of CF to arrive at the correct conclusion for what is expected, a gastrointestinal manifestation of poor weight gain despite adequate caloric intake.

C18 | Neuromuscular | Foundational Sciences

An infant demonstrates that the asymmetrical tonic neck reflex (ATNR) is **NOT** obligatory when he/she can turn the head:

CHOICES:

1. To both sides and open the hand.
2. To one side and look at the extended arm on that side.
3. To one side and bring the opposite hand to mouth.
4. And bring the hand to mouth on the same side.

TEACHING POINTS

CORRECT ANSWER: 4

ATNR causes extension of upper extremity on the side the head is turned toward. Bringing the hand to the mouth would not be possible with an obligatory reflex.

INCORRECT CHOICES:

The other choices do not correctly define actions that are limited with an obligatory ATNR. The ATNR is a total upper extremity response and not limited to hand opening or simply looking at the hand.

TYPE OF REASONING: ANALYSIS

In this scenario, if the infant can turn the head and bring the hand to mouth on the same side, the reflex is no longer obligatory. Analytical reasoning skill is used in this question because the test taker must determine the meaning of the information presented and analyze what it means in relation to a correct solution.

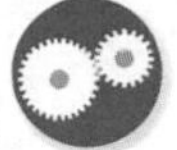

C19 | Devices, Admin., etc. | Teaching, Research, Roles

An elderly patient is referred to physical therapy with back pain. The patient has pancreatic cancer and moderate senile dementia and is unaware of the diagnosis or prognosis, at the family's request. The patient asks the therapist what is the matter and how long will physical therapy take place. The therapist's **BEST** response is:

CHOICES:

1. "I will tell the doctor to answer all of your questions."
2. "Ask the nurse practitioner for this information."
3. "I'll treat the symptoms and see how well you do."
4. To discuss the diagnosis and prognosis with the patient.

TEACHING POINTS

CORRECT ANSWER: 3

The therapist should respond empathetically and use the moment to talk to the patient about the symptoms and physical therapy treatment.

INCORRECT CHOICES:

The diagnosis and prognosis should not be discussed. The family has determined not to tell the patient. Any change would have to be initiated by the family and falls under the domain of the physician. Telling the patient to ask either the physician or the nurse practitioner is not appropriate.

TYPE OF REASONING: EVALUATION

This question requires a value judgment related to a **BEST** course of action for the PT. Value judgments encourage evaluative reasoning skill and are often challenging to answer because they can pose an ethical dilemma. In sensitive situations such as this one, the test taker must determine the responsibility of the therapist. In this scenario, the discussion of the patient's diagnosis and prognosis falls within the domain of the physician.

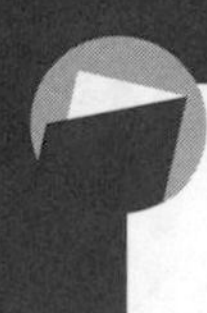

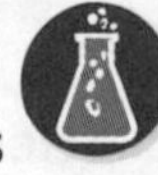

C20 | Other Systems | Evaluation, Diagnosis, Prognosis

During surgery to remove an apical lung tumor, the long thoracic nerve was injured. Muscle testing of the serratus anterior demonstrates its strength to be 3+/5. The **BEST** initial exercises are:

CHOICES:

1. Standing, arm overhead lifts using hand weights.
2. Supine, arm overhead lifts using weights.
3. Sitting, arm overhead lifts using a pulley.
4. Standing, wall push-ups.

TEACHING POINTS

CORRECT ANSWER: 4

The long thoracic nerve supplies the serratus anterior muscle. With a muscle grade of 3+/5, the patient can then begin functional strengthening using standing wall push-ups, with resistance provided by the patient's own body.

INCORRECT CHOICES:

The other exercises would not be optimal or used **INITIALLY** for strengthening a fair plus serratus anterior. Performing overhead exercises with resistance (weights or pulleys) will overload the weakened serratus anterior muscle, causing the patient to compensate and potentially develop inappropriate movement patterns.

TYPE OF REASONING: ANALYSIS

One must recall innervations for the long thoracic nerve in order to arrive at the correct conclusion. This requires analysis of the information presented and interpretation of that information, which requires analytical reasoning skill. Knowledge of neuropathology is helpful to arrive at the correct conclusion. If this question was answered incorrectly, review appropriate exercises for serratus anterior strengthening.

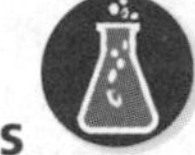

C21 | Musculoskeletal | Evaluation, Diagnosis, Prognosis

A PT examination reveals: posterior superior iliac spine (PSIS) is low on the left; anterior superior iliac spine (ASIS) is high on the left; standing flexion test shows that the left PSIS moves first and farthest superiorly; Gillet's test demonstrates that the left PSIS moves inferiorly and laterally less than right; long sitting test shows that the left malleolus moves short to long; sitting flexion test is negative. In light of these findings, the therapist's diagnosis is:

CHOICES:

1. Left anterior rotated innominate.
2. Left posterior rotated innominate.
3. Left upslip.
4. Iliac inflare on the left.

TEACHING POINTS

CORRECT ANSWER: 2

A posterior rotated innominate is a unilateral iliosacral dysfunction. The question outlines positive physical findings, both static and dynamic, found with this dysfunction. One of these positive findings alone does not confirm the diagnosis of left rotated posterior innominate.

INCORRECT CHOICES:

The findings are opposite to what would be found with a left anterior ilial rotation. If the patient had an upslip, both the PSIS and the ASIS on the left would be elevated. If an inflare was present, the left PSIS would appear more lateral and the ASIS would appear more medial.

TYPE OF REASONING: ANALYSIS

Questions provide the symptoms and the therapist must determine the diagnosis; this requires the use of analytical reasoning skill. This is because of the high need to determine what the cluster of symptoms indicates in terms of deficits and functioning. For this patient, the symptoms indicate a left posterior rotated innominate, which should trigger a review of iliosacral dysfunction if this question was answered incorrectly.

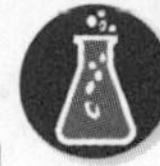

C22 | Integumentary | Patient Examination

A patient recovering from a burn on the back of the hand is referred to physical therapy for mobilization exercises. The therapist observes a 14-cm irregular area that is thick and pink. The therapist documents this finding as:

CHOICES:

1. Atrophic scarring.
2. Hypertrophic scarring.
3. An excoriation.
4. A scale.

TEACHING POINTS

CORRECT ANSWER: 2

Hypertrophic scars are thick (raised) and pink (or red).

INCORRECT CHOICES:

Atrophic scars are thin and white. Excoriation is an abrasion or scratch mark. A scale is a flake of exfoliated epidermis (e.g., dandruff, psoriasis, dry skin).

TYPE OF REASONING: ANALYSIS

This question requires one to determine the clinical findings based on the observation of the patient's skin. This necessitates analytical reasoning skill, because one must analyze the signs presented in order to determine the likely clinical finding. In this case, the therapist's observations are consistent with hypertrophic scarring. If this question was answered incorrectly, review signs and symptoms of hypertrophic scarring, especially in burns.

C23 | Devices, Admin., etc. | Equipment, Modalities

A patient presents with partial- and full-thickness burns on the chest and neck regions. The therapist decides to apply transcutaneous electrical nerve stimulation (TENS) before débridement to modulate pain. Which TENS mode should provide the **BEST** relief?

CHOICES:

1. Conventional (high-rate) TENS.
2. Acupuncture-like (low-rate) TENS.
3. Modulated TENS.
4. Brief intense TENS.

TEACHING POINTS

CORRECT ANSWER: 4

Brief intense TENS is used to provide rapid-onset, short-term relief during painful procedures. The pulse rate and pulse duration are similar to conventional TENS; however, the current intensity is increased to the patient's tolerance.

INCORRECT CHOICES:

In this situation, intensity is the primary determinant of pain relief. Conventional TENS does not use as high of an intensity as brief intense TENS and the application time is longer. Acupuncture-like TENS does not give immediate relief of pain, because it has a long onset. Modulation is used to prevent accommodation, not to provide relief of pain.

TYPE OF REASONING: DEDUCTIVE

One must recall the protocols for TENS use in order to determine the mode that would provide the **BEST** relief of pain for this patient. This requires factual recall of information, which necessitates deductive reasoning skill. In this case, brief intense TENS is **BEST** because it provides rapid-onset, short-term relief during painful procedures.

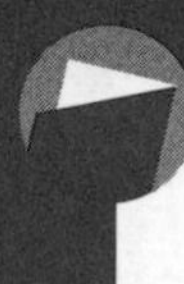

C24 | Neuromuscular | Intervention

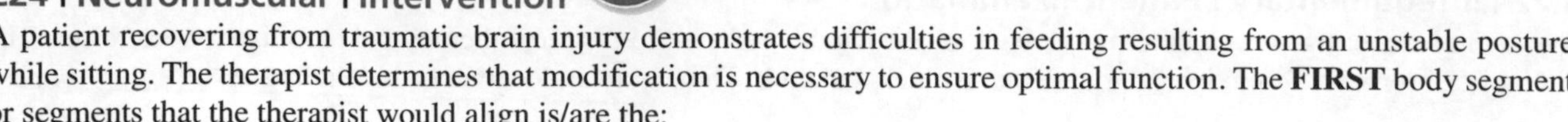

A patient recovering from traumatic brain injury demonstrates difficulties in feeding resulting from an unstable posture while sitting. The therapist determines that modification is necessary to ensure optimal function. The **FIRST** body segment or segments that the therapist would align is/are the:

CHOICES:

1. Pelvis.
2. Head.
3. Lower extremities.
4. Trunk.

TEACHING POINTS

CORRECT ANSWER: 1

Modification of the pelvic position in a neutral posture promotes good lumbar and trunk alignment. Many postural problems are correctable by aligning the pelvis first and achieving a stable base.

INCORRECT CHOICES:

Modifiying the position of the head, trunk, or lower extremities may be necessary but only after achieving a stable base.

TYPE OF REASONING: INDUCTIVE

The test taker must determine through clinical judgment the **FIRST** body segment(s) to align in order to promote good trunk alignment. This requires inductive reasoning skill, in which knowledge of biomechanics and neuropathology is beneficial for arriving at the correct conclusion.

C25 | Neuromuscular | Intervention

A patient demonstrates some out-of-synergy movements in the right upper extremity indicative of stage 4 recovery after a left cerebrovascular accident (CVA). The proprioceptive neuromuscular facilitation (PNF) pattern that represents the **BEST** choice to promote continued recovery of the right upper extremity is:

CHOICES:

1. Chop, reverse chop with right arm leading.
2. Bilateral symmetrical D1 thrust and reverse thrust.
3. Lift, reverse lift with right arm leading.
4. Bilateral symmetrical D2F and D2E, elbows straight.

TEACHING POINTS

CORRECT ANSWER: 1

Both chop and reverse chop patterns move the affected arm out-of-synergy.

INCORRECT CHOICES:

Thrust is an out-of-synergy pattern, and reverse thrust is in-synergy. Lift is an out-of-synergy pattern, and reverse lift is in-synergy. The same is true for bilateral symmetrical D2F (out-of-synergy) and D2E (in-synergy).

TYPE OF REASONING: INFERENCE

In order to arrive at the correct conclusion, one must recall the PNF patterns presented and then match these patterns to the stage of recovery of the patient. The chop, reverse chop with right arm leading encourages out-of-synergy movement, which is most beneficial during stage 4 of recovery. If this question was answered incorrectly, refer to PNF patterns and interventions for stage 4 of stroke recovery.

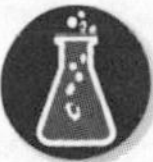

C26 | Cardiovascular-Pulmonary | Intervention

An elderly individual has limited endurance as a result of a sedentary lifestyle. There is no history of cardiorespiratory problems. After an exercise tolerance test, which was negative for coronary heart disease, the **BEST** initial exercise prescription for this individual would be:

CHOICES:

1. 30–50% HR_{max}
2. 60–90% HR_{max}
3. 40–50% HR_{max}
4. 35–50% of VO_{2max}

TEACHING POINTS

CORRECT ANSWER: 2

An appropriate **initial** exercise prescription for an asymptomatic elderly individual with general deconditioning is 60–90% of HR_{max}, which is equivalent to 50–85% of VO_{2max}, or 50–85% of HR reserve (Karvonen's formula). This is within the established intensity guidelines for adults for aerobic exercise training. Duration should be discontinuous and exercise performed most days of the week (*ACSM Guidelines for Exercise Testing and Prescription,* 7th ed).

INCORRECT CHOICES:

All other choices are too conservative. The exercise tolerance test has ruled out coronary heart disease.

TYPE OF REASONING: ANALYSIS

One must analyze the information presented and then determine, given the patient's health status, the **MOST** beneficial initial exercise prescription parameters. Analytical reasoning skill is utilized because the test taker must weigh the information presented and recall the typical prescription parameters for an asymptomatic individual.

C27 | Cardiovascular-Pulmonary | Intervention

A patient is admitted to a coronary care unit with a mild MI. After 2 days, the patient is referred to physical therapy for inpatient cardiac rehabilitation. During an initial exercise session on the unit, the patient reports chest pain, appears anxious, and wants to go back to bed to rest. The therapist's **BEST** initial course of action is to terminate the exercise and:

CHOICES:

1. Sit the patient down and monitor vital signs carefully during the rest period.
2. Contact the attending physician immediately and continue to monitor vital signs.
3. Assist the patient back to bed and contact the charge nurse on the floor.
4. Assign the PTA to assist the patient back to bed and monitor vital signs carefully.

TEACHING POINTS

CORRECT ANSWER: 1

If the chest pain (angina) is exercise-induced, this is an indication to terminate the exercise session (myocardial demand is exceeding myocardial oxygen supply). Recovery is expected after a period of rest.

INCORRECT CHOICES:

If the patient is still anxious, after the rest, it is reasonable to return the patient to the room and inform the nurse. This should be done by the therapist personally in order to carefully monitor the patient's status. The PTA should not be expected to evaluate chest pain or reach a determination about its significance. This is not an emergency situation.

TYPE OF REASONING: EVALUATION

One must make a judgment call for the **BEST** course of action for this patient, given the symptoms presented. Questions that require one to make value judgments necessitate evaluative reasoning skill and can be challenging to answer, because the key to finding the correct solution goes beyond factual knowledge. For this patient, it is best to have the patient sit down and monitor vital signs.

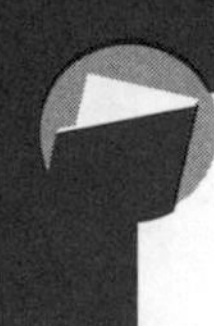

C28 | Integumentary | Evaluation, Diagnosis, Prognosis

A patient with a 10-year history of scleroderma is referred for physical therapy to improve functional status and endurance. The patient was recently treated with corticosteroids for a bout of myositis. Examination findings reveal limited ROM and fibrotic soft tissue along with hyperesthesia. The **BEST** choice for initial intervention is:

CHOICES:

1. Soft tissue mobilization and stretching.
2. Closed-chain and modified aerobic step exercises.
3. Treadmill walking using body weight support at an intensity of 40% HR_{max}.
4. Active range of motion (AROM) exercises and walking in a therapeutic pool.

TEACHING POINTS

CORRECT ANSWER: 4

Scleroderma (progressive systemic sclerosis) is a chronic, diffuse disease of connective tissues causing fibrosis of skin, joints, blood vessels, and internal organs. Patients typically demonstrate symmetrical skin thickening and visceral involvement of the gastrointestinal tract, lungs, heart, and kidneys along with hypersensitivity to touch. The **BEST** choice for initial intervention is to exercise in the pool. The warmth and buoyancy of the water will enhance the patient's movements and decrease pain.

INCORRECT CHOICES:

The other choices are too aggressive at this time and risk increasing the patient's pain, thereby limiting any benefits in flexibility and endurance.

TYPE OF REASONING: INDUCTIVE

One must determine through clinical judgment the **BEST** initial intervention approach for this patient. Knowledge of the nature of scleroderma and expected symptomatology is key to arriving at the correct conclusion, which in this case is AROM exercises and walking in a therapeutic pool. If this question was answered incorrectly, refer to information on intervention approaches for patients with scleroderma.

C29 | Other Systems | Foundational Sciences

A patient is referred to physical therapy after a fall injury (fractured left hip with operative reduction, internal fixation [ORIF]). Medical history reveals a diagnosis of stage 1 Alzheimer's disease. At this stage, the behaviors the therapist would **NOT** expect to find are:

CHOICES:

1. Anxiety and irritability.
2. Profound communication deficits.
3. Memory loss.
4. Difficulty concentrating.

TEACHING POINTS

CORRECT ANSWER: 2

Profound communication deficits (inability to speak), global deterioration of mental functions (delusions, hallucinations, fragmented memory), agitation, and pacing (sundowning) are all characteristic of late stages of this disease.

INCORRECT CHOICES:

Early stage 1 Alzheimer's disease is characterized by memory loss, absentmindedness, anxiety and irritability, difficulty concentrating, and occasional word-finding problems.

TYPE OF REASONING: INFERENCE

One must infer information from the diagnosis presented and the stage of the disease provided. This necessitates inferential reasoning skill, in which one must draw conclusions from the information presented to choose the best solution of what is **NOT** expected in early stage 1.

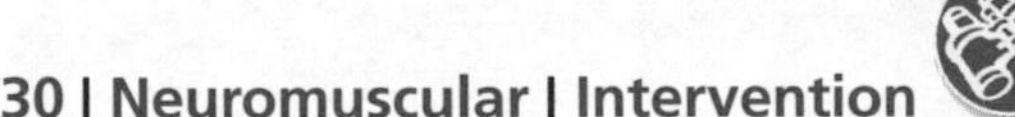

C30 | Neuromuscular | Intervention

A patient recovering from stroke with minimal lower extremity weakness and spasticity is able to walk without an assistive device. The therapist observes that, as the patient walks, there is noticeable hip hiking on the affected side during swing phase. The **BEST** initial intervention is:

CHOICES:

1. Partial wall squats using a small ball held between the knees.
2. Standing, marching with manual pressure applied downward on the pelvis.
3. Marching while sitting on a therapy ball.
4. Bridging exercises progressing to sit-to-stand training.

TEACHING POINTS

CORRECT ANSWER: 3

Hip hiking is a compensatory response for weak hip and knee flexors or extensor spasticity. Active exercises for the hip and knee flexors (marching) is the most appropriate intervention.

INCORRECT CHOICES:

Downward manual pressure on the pelvis strengthens hip hikers. The other choices focus on strengthening hip and knee extensors.

TYPE OF REASONING: INDUCTIVE

The test taker must utilize clinical judgment to determine first what the patient's deficits are (related to the therapist's observation of the patient's gait) and then the **BEST** initial intervention for this patient. One must evaluate the four possible intervention choices given to determine which intervention is **BEST** for addressing the patient's deficits, which requires inductive reasoning skill. In this scenario, marching while sitting on a ball will **BEST** address the patient's weak hip and knee flexors or extensor spasticity.

C31 | Devices, Admin., etc. | Teaching, Research, Roles

The therapist is instructing a patient with traumatic brain injury how to lock the brakes on a wheelchair. The patient is right-handed, and the right upper extremity is more affected than the left. To obtain optimal results, the **BEST** motor learning training strategy is to:

CHOICES:

1. Guide the patient's right hand through the locking motions, then the left.
2. Verbally talk the patient through the locking motions, practicing with both hands simultaneously.
3. Have the patient practice locking the brakes first with the left hand, and then the right.
4. Have the patient practice brake locking using the left hand to assist the right.

TEACHING POINTS

CORRECT ANSWER: 3

Using the motor learning strategy of transfer of training is best to use with this patient. Practice is performed with the less affected extremity first and then progressed to use of the more affected extremity.

INCORRECT CHOICES:

Guided movement (manual or verbal) represents a less active approach than the transfer of training approach. The more passive the performance, the slower the learning will take place. Bilateral tasks are more difficult than performing the task with one limb at a time.

TYPE OF REASONING: INDUCTIVE

The test taker must determine the **BEST** training strategy for a patient with traumatic brain injury, which necessitates inductive reasoning skill and, therefore, clinical judgment. For this patient, it is important to have him/her practice locking the brakes first with his/her left hand and then his/her right in order to encourage effective transfer of training. Knowledge of effective motor learning strategies for patients with brain injury is beneficial for arriving at the correct conclusion.

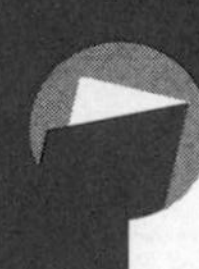

C32 | Devices, Admin., etc. | Teaching, Research, Roles

A PT wants to examine the effects of PNF using the technique of contract-relax on shoulder ROM. A group of 10 patients with adhesive capsulitis were recruited. A matched group of patients were given straight plane active assisted exercise for the same length of time (3 times/wk for 6 wk). In this study, the independent variable is:

CHOICES:

1. Active assisted exercise.
2. PNF contract-relax technique.
3. ROM.
4. Adhesive capsulitis.

TEACHING POINTS

CORRECT ANSWER: 2

The independent variable is the activity or factor believed to bring about a change in the dependent variable. The type of exercise being investigated is PNF contract-relax technique.

INCORRECT CHOICES:

The dependent variable is the difference in behavior that results as a result of the intervention (independent variable); in this case, ROM. The other two choices (active assistive exercise and adhesive capsulitis) are not relevant.

TYPE OF REASONING: DEDUCTIVE

Questions that inquire about research protocols and processes often utilize deductive reasoning skill, which requires logic and factual recall of information. For this question, the test taker must recall the definition of an independent variable and then apply it to the scenario presented. If this question was answered incorrectly, review terminology related to research variables.

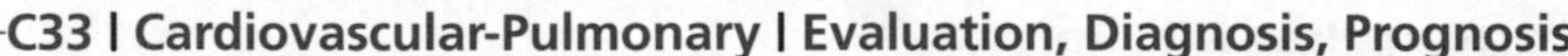

C33 | Cardiovascular-Pulmonary | Evaluation, Diagnosis, Prognosis

A therapist is examining a patient with chronic obstructive pulmonary disease (COPD; GOLD stage III). What would be a clinical finding that the therapist would expect for this patient?

CHOICES:

1. Use of supplemental oxygen.
2. Weight gain.
3. Muscle wasting.
4. Decreased anteroposterior-to-lateral chest ratio.

TEACHING POINTS

CORRECT ANSWER: 3

Muscle wasting is a common manifestation of COPD. The cause of muscle wasting is not clear, but is not simply a malnutrition problem. The results of this muscle wasting is peripheral weakness, impaired functional abilities, poor quality of life and a poor prognostic sign.

INCORRECT CHOICES:

Supplemental oxygen is typically found in patients in stage IV of GOLD, not stage III. Weight loss is a common finding in patients with COPD, especially as the disease progresses. The energy demands of a person with COPD are higher than those of a person without COPD for the same activity. A usual finding is that persons with COPD are less active than their nondiseased counterparts. As the disease progresses, the person with COPD cannot maintain his/her independence with any further decrease his/her activity any lower and weight loss ensues. As lung distruction increases with worsening COPD, there is less elastic recoil properties of the lung to pull the thorax back into what we recognize as a usual thoracic configuration. A barreled chest, or an increased anteroposterior-to-lateral diameter of the chest, is a common finding in advanced, stage III COPD.

TYPE OF REASONING: INFERENCE

One must infer from the symptoms presented what clinical finding would likely be found in a patient with severe (stage III) COPD. This requires knowledge of pulmonary disorders and the typical findings in order to determine, through the process of elimination, what finding is characteristic of that stage of COPD. If this question was answered incorrectly, refer to typical symptoms of COPD.

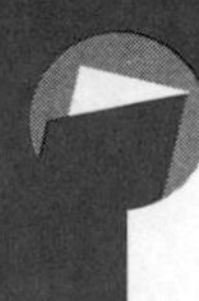

C34 | Devices, Admin., etc. | Teaching, Research, Roles

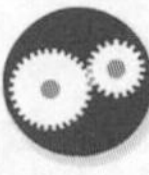

A PT who practices in an outpatient setting has been instructed by the practice manager to always add at 15 minutes to the billing time for every patient encounter in order to account for paperwork time because this is the policy of the center. The PT should:

CHOICES:

1. Follow the directions of the manager.
2. Bill for only the time spent with the patient.
3. Add a modality to the treatment in order to increase billable time.
4. Bill for only the time spent with the patient and report the paperwork billing practice to the proper authorities.

TEACHING POINTS

CORRECT ANSWER: 4

The Code of Ethics obligates a PT to be aware of charges and coding for PT services and obligates the PT to ensure that billing reflects the services provided. The code also obligates the PT to report illegal or unethical acts to the relevant authority. This case demonstrates both illegal and unethical billing, which the PT is obligated to report.

INCORRECT CHOICES:

The manager has directed the PT to practice in an unethical and illegal fashion. It is the PT's responsibility to not bill in this way, but is also obligated to report such practices. Although adding a modality to a patient's treatment may not be harmful if the modality is not indicated, this is unethical practice.

TYPE OF REASONING: EVALUATION

The question requires one to recognize unethical and illegal billing practices and also acknowledge the need to report the situation. This requires evaluative reasoning skill. In order to answer the question correctly, the test taker must first identify the unethical billing practices, and then must know the obligation to report such abuses. If this question was answered incorrectly, review the Code of Ethics Principle 7 (E).

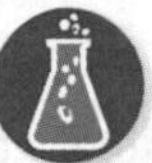

C35 | Musculoskeletal | Intervention

During a postural screen for chronic shoulder pain, the therapist observes excessive internal rotation of the shoulders and winging of the scapula during overhead motion. Intervention should focus on:

CHOICES:

1. Strengthening of pectoral muscles and stretching of upper trapezius.
2. Strengthening of upper trapezius and stretching of pectoral muscles.
3. Strengthening middle and lower trapezius and stretching of pectoral muscles.
4. Strengthening of rhomboids and stretching of upper trapezius.

TEACHING POINTS

CORRECT ANSWER: 3

Abnormal posture that produces excessive internal rotation of the shoulders may result in chronic shoulder impingement syndrome due to a loss of scapular stability with overhead motion. Shoulder pain is likely to continue until a balance between anterior and posterior trunk musculature is achieved. The anterior chest muscles (pectorals) are shortened and need stretching and posterior trunk muscles (middle and lower trapezius) are stretched and need strengthening.

INCORRECT CHOICES:

The pectoralis major and minor need to be stretched not strengthened. Stretching of the upper trapezius will not change this condition.

TYPE OF REASONING: ANALYSIS

Knowledge of shoulder kinesiology and pathology is beneficial to arriving at the correct conclusion for this answer. An understanding that excessive internal rotation of the shoulders and scapular winging could be caused by a weak middle and lower trapezius and shortened pectoral muscles results from a solid understanding of shoulder pathology and kinesiology. Through analytical reasoning, the test taker must determine which muscles are most likely to be affected and, therefore, produce these symptoms.

C36 | Integumentary | Intervention 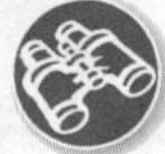

Reexamination of a patient with a dermal ulcer over the coccyx reveals a wound exposing the deep fascia. There is no necrotic tissue, exudate is minimal, and the borders of the ulcer are diffusely covered with granulation tissue. Previous treatment has included daily whirlpool and wet-to-dry dressings with normal saline. Based on the these findings, intervention should consist of:

CHOICES:

1. Continuation of the same treatments.
2. Whirlpool and hydrogel dressings.
3. Calcium alginate dressings.
4. Wound irrigation with pressures below 15 psi.

TEACHING POINTS

CORRECT ANSWER: 4

Low-pressure wound irrigation helps to decrease colonization and prevent infection.

INCORRECT CHOICES:

If the ulcer is clean, whirlpool can damage incipient granulation tissue and should be discontinued. Wet-to-dry dressings help remove necrotic tissue. Calcium alginate is used in the presence of heavy exudates, which is not the case here. Hydrogel would be best because it is nonadherent, keeps wounds moist, and protects granulation buds; however, whirlpool is inappropriate.

TYPE OF REASONING: INDUCTIVE

One must utilize clinical judgment and knowledge of wound care approaches to determine the best intervention approach for this patient, which requires inductive reasoning skill. For this patient, wound irrigation with pressures below 15 psi is most appropriate for the type of wound described. If this question was answered incorrectly, review information on wound care procedures for this type of wound.

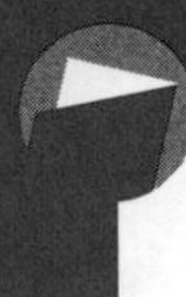

C37 | Musculoskeletal | Evaluation, Diagnosis, Prognosis

The spinal defect shown in the diagram should be managed with avoidance of lumbar spinal:

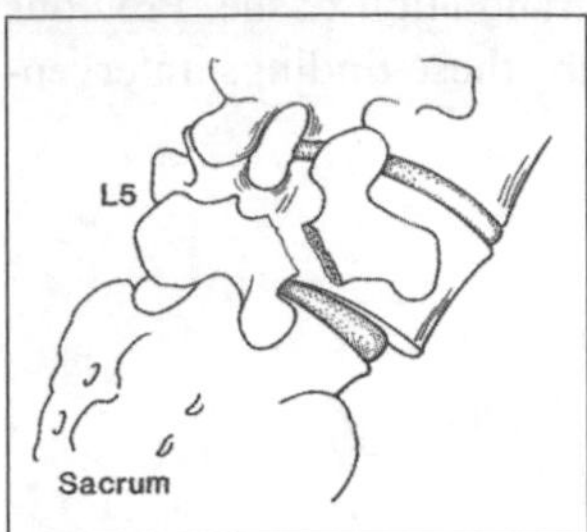

Philadelphia, Churchill Livingstone, Figure 7-1, page 204, with permission. Twomey L, Taylor J (2000) Physical Therapy of the Low Back, 3rd ed.

CHOICES:

1. Flexion.
2. Rotation.
3. Extension.
4. Lateral flexion.

TEACHING POINTS

CORRECT ANSWER: 3

With spondylolisthesis, there is typically an anterior slippage of one vertebra on the vertebra below. Because of the anterior shearing forces acting at the vertebra caused by the wedge shape of the vertebra and gravity, spinal extension positions should be avoided.

INCORRECT CHOICES:

Flexion, rotation, and lateral flexion will cause the bony structures to separate and will not cause any negative compressive loads to the damaged structures.

TYPE OF REASONING: ANALYSIS

One must analyze the spinal defect displayed in the picture and determine the diagnosis in order to determine what lumbar position should be avoided. This requires analytical reasoning skill, in which the precise meaning of the spinal defect must be determined first, before determining the appropriate management of this patient. If this question was answered incorrectly, refer to intervention approaches for spondylolisthesis.

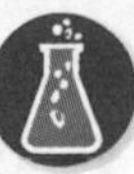

C38 | Neuromuscular | Evaluation, Diagnosis, Prognosis

A computer specialist is unable to work because of weakness and altered sensation in the dominant right hand. The patient complains of pain and tingling of the thumb, index finger, long finger, and radial half of the ring finger. The therapist observes thenar weakness and atrophy. Strength, reflexes, and sensation are within normal limits throughout the remainder of the right upper extremity. The therapist determines these signs and symptoms are characteristic of:

CHOICES:

1. Pronator teres syndrome.
2. Cervical root compression.
3. Ulnar nerve compression.
4. Carpal tunnel syndrome.

TEACHING POINTS

CORRECT ANSWER: 4

The pattern of motor and sensory loss corresponds to the median nerve distribution in the hand. The most likely cause is carpal tunnel syndrome.

INCORRECT CHOICES:

Pronator teres syndrome (also a median nerve problem) produces similar deficits along with involvement of the flexors of the wrist and fingers. Cervical root compression would also produce proximal deficits in strength and sensation. Ulnar nerve compression (ulnar nerve palsy) would produce motor deficits of the flexor carpi ulnaris and medial half of the flexor digitorum profundus, resulting in claw hand. Sensory loss is to the ulnar side of the hand and/or arm.

TYPE OF REASONING: ANALYSIS

This question provides the symptoms, and the test taker must determine the most likely diagnosis. This necessitates analytical reasoning skill, in which one must determine the exact meaning of the symptoms presented to arrive at the correct conclusion. If this question was answered incorrectly, review information on symptoms of carpal tunnel syndrome.

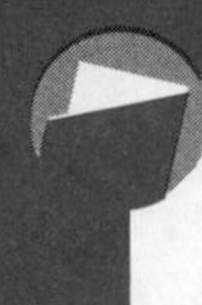

C39 | Neuromuscular | Evaluation, Diagnosis, Prognosis

A patient presents with rapidly progressive symmetrical weakness that started in the distal lower extremity muscles but now has ascended to include proximal trunk and upper extremity muscles. The motor segments of the lower cranial nerves are also showing impairment. The patient complains of abnormal sensations of tingling and burning of the affected extremities. Consciousness, cognition, and communication are all normal. These signs and symptoms are characteristic of:

CHOICES:

1. Postpolio syndrome.
2. Guillain-Barré syndrome.
3. Multiple sclerosis (MS).
4. Amyotrophic lateral sclerosis (ALS).

TEACHING POINTS

CORRECT ANSWER: 2

These signs and symptoms are characteristic of Guillain-Barré syndrome, a peripheral neuropathy in which there is inflammation and demyelination of peripheral motor and sensory nerve fibers. Early in its progression, either upper or lower motor signs may predominate.

INCORRECT CHOICES:

In almost all cases, patients with ALS show features of both UMN and lower motor neuron (LMN) dysfunction. Postpolio syndrome is an LMN syndrome that does not present with sensory paresthesias and is typically asymmetrical. MS will present with UMN signs: spasticity and hyperreflexia.

TYPE OF REASONING: ANALYSIS

This question provides the symptoms, and the test taker must determine what the symptoms most likely indicate. This requires analytical reasoning skill, in which one evaluates the exact meaning of the symptoms presented to arrive at the correct conclusion. If this question was answered incorrectly, review information on symptoms of Guillain-Barré syndrome.

C40 | Cardiovascular-Pulmonary | Foundational Sciences

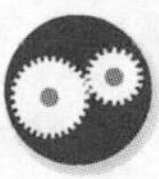

A patient recovering from surgery for triple coronary artery bypass grafts is scheduled to begin a phase III cardiac rehabilitation program. During the resistance training portion of the circuit training program, the therapist instructs the patient to **AVOID** the Valsalva maneuver because:

CHOICES:

1. HR and BP are likely to be elevated.
2. Slowing of pulse and increased venous pressure are possible.
3. A cholinergic or vagal response can occur.
4. The decreased return of blood to the heart can lead to pitting edema.

TEACHING POINTS

CORRECT ANSWER: 2

The Valsalva maneuver results from forcible exhalation with the glottis, nose, and mouth closed. It increases intrathoracic pressures and causes slowing of the pulse, decreased return of blood to the heart, and increased venous pressure. Although Valsalvas occur during normal daily activities (breath holding, straining), they can be dangerous for patients with cardiovascular disease. On relaxation, blood rushes to the heart and can overload the cardiac system, resulting in cardiac arrest.

INCORRECT CHOICES:

HR is not elevated. A cholinergic or vagal response is the result of parasympathetic nervous system (PNS) stimulation providing inhibitory control of the vagus nerve over HR and atrioventricular conduction. Pitting edema is caused by long-term factors such as CHF.

TYPE OF REASONING: EVALUATION

The test taker must determine the value and believability of the reasons presented to **AVOID** the Valsalva maneuver, which encourages evaluative reasoning skill. Having knowledge of the Valsalva maneuver and its effects on HR and venous pressure is important for arriving at the correct conclusion for this question. If this question was answered incorrectly, review information on the Valsalva maneuver.

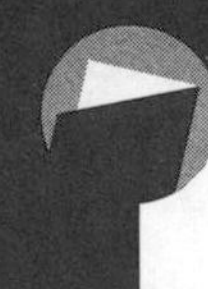

C41 | Cardiovascular-Pulmonary | Evaluation, Diagnosis, Prognosis

A patient experiences color changes in the skin during position changes of the foot. During elevation, pallor develops. When the limb is then positioned in the seated hanging position, hyperemia develops. These changes are indicative of:

CHOICES:

1. Chronic venous insufficiency.
2. Lymphedema.
3. Arterial insufficiency.
4. Deep vein thrombophlebitis.

TEACHING POINTS

CORRECT ANSWER: 3

Arterial insufficiency can be determined by skin color changes during position changes of the foot (termed rubor of dependency test).

INCORRECT CHOICES:

Chronic venous insufficiency can be determined by the history, presence of aching calf pain with prolonged standing, a percussion test in standing, or Trendelenburg's test (retrograde filling test). With chronic venous insufficiency, skin will be dark and cyanotic. Acute deep vein thrombophlebitis (DVT) can be evident with aching calf pain, edema, and muscle tenderness. Lymphedema is evident with visual inspection (i.e., swelling, decreased ROM) and volumetric measurements.

TYPE OF REASONING: INFERENCE

One must infer the exact meaning of the symptoms presented and then draw conclusions about what the diagnosis may be. Questions that inquire about a possible diagnosis for symptoms presented encourage inferential reasoning skill. If this question was answered incorrectly, refer to information on arterial insufficiency of the lower extremity.

C42 | Neuromuscular | Patient Examination

An elderly and frail adult is referred to physical therapy for an examination of balance. The patient has a recent history of falls (two in the last 6 months). Based on knowledge of balance changes in the elderly and scoring of standardized balance measures, the test data that **BEST** indicate increased fall risk is:

CHOICES:

1. Functional Reach of 7 inches.
2. Berg Balance score of 50.
3. Tinetti Performance Oriented Mobility Assessment (POMA) score of 27.
4. Timed Get Up & Go (GUG) test result of 13 seconds.

TEACHING POINTS

CORRECT ANSWER: 1

All of these instruments can be used to examine functional balance and fall risk. A Functional Reach score of < 10 is indicative of increased fall risk.

INCORRECT CHOICES:

A POMA score of 27 out of a possible 28 is an excellent score. (Scores of < 19 indicate a high risk for falls, whereas scores between 19 and 24 indicate moderate risk for falls). A Berg score of 50 out of a possible 56 points also indicates low fall risk. A Timed GUG score of < 20 seconds for the 3-meter walk and turn test indicates low fall risk (scores > 30 sec indicate increased risk).

TYPE OF REASONING: DEDUCTIVE

This question requires one to recall factual information about the various tests described in the question and then determine the meaning of the scores (which also encourages some analytical reasoning). Factual knowledge recall often encourages deductive reasoning skill, in which recall of protocols and guidelines are pivotal to arriving at the correct conclusion. For this scenario, Functional Reach of 7 inches is the **BEST** indicator of increased fall risk. If this question was answered incorrectly, review standardized balance tests.

C43 | Other Systems | Evaluation, Diagnosis, Prognosis

During an examination, a patient complains of right upper quadrant pain and tenderness. The PT percusses over the costal margin at the point where the lateral border of the rectus muscle intersects with the costal margin. The patient complains of acute pain and stops inspiratory effort. This is **MOST** likely indicative of:

CHOICES:

1. Irritation of the psoas muscle by an inflamed appendix.
2. Acute cholecystitis.
3. Peritoneal inflammation.
4. Hernia.

TEACHING POINTS

CORRECT ANSWER: 2

Percussion for costovertebral tenderness that reveals a sharp increase in tenderness with a sudden stop in inspiratory effort is a positive Murphy's sign and is indicative of acute cholecystitis.

INCORRECT CHOICES:

An inflamed appendix results in pain in the right lower quadrant during left-sided pressure (positive Rovsing's sign) or right lower quadrant pain on quick withdrawal (referred rebound tenderness). A hernia produces a bulge in the adominal wall (ventral hernias). Peritoneal inflammation presents with abdominal pain on coughing or with light percussion. Rebound tenderness is also present.

TYPE OF REASONING: INFERENCE

In order to arrive at a correct conclusion, one must have knowledge of the indications for percussion of the costovertebral angle. This requires inferential reasoning skill, in which one draws conclusions based upon evidence and facts. In this situation, percussion is indicated to reveal acute cholecystitis. If this question was answered incorrectly, review indications for Murphy's percussion.

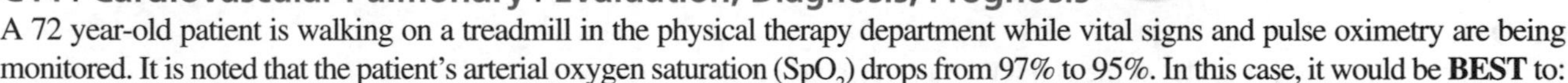

C44 | Cardiovascular-Pulmonary | Evaluation, Diagnosis, Prognosis

A 72 year-old patient is walking on a treadmill in the physical therapy department while vital signs and pulse oximetry are being monitored. It is noted that the patient's arterial oxygen saturation (SpO_2) drops from 97% to 95%. In this case, it would be **BEST** to:

CHOICES:

1. Place a 100% O_2 face mask on the patient for the remainder of the exercise session.
2. Place a 40% O_2 face mask on the patient for the remainder of the exercise session.
3. Place 2 L of O_2 by nasal cannula on the patient for the remainder of the exercise session.
4. Not use supplemental O_2.

TEACHING POINTS

CORRECT ANSWER: 4

A 72-year-old patient would likely have a resting SpO_2 of 95% from the changes associated with aging alone. There is no need to supplement oxygen in this case.

INCORRECT CHOICES:

The guideline for using supplemental oxygen is a $Sp0_2$ of $< 88\%$ or a PaO_2 of < 55 mm Hg. Therefore, the use of oxygen in this scenario is not justified (all other choices). Supplemental O_2 is by prescription only unless it is an emergency.

TYPE OF REASONING: INFERENCE

One must infer the exact meaning of the symptoms presented from this patient in order to make a determination of the **BEST** course of action. For this situation, the patient's response is within normal parameters and does not require supplemental oxygen. Knowledge of oxygen saturation guidelines is key to arriving at the correct conclusion and should be reviewed if this question was answered incorrectly.

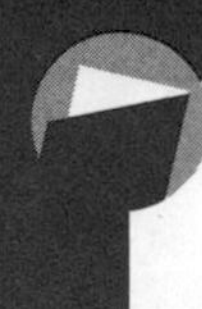

C45 | Devices, Admin., etc. | Equipment, Modalities

The therapist is evaluating the needs of a 6 year-old child who is diagnosed with myelodysplasia at the T10 level. The therapist determines the **MOST** beneficial mobility device for this child to use in the school environment is a:

CHOICES:

1. Bilateral hip-knee-ankle-foot orthosis (HKAFO).
2. Lightweight wheelchair.
3. Bilateral knee-ankle-foot orthosis (KAFO).
4. Parapodium.

TEACHING POINTS

CORRECT ANSWER: 2

The lightweight wheelchair is the **MOST** beneficial choice for this child. It provides effective and efficient mobility.

INCORRECT CHOICES:

Ambulation with orthotic devices at this level lesion requires too much energy and time to be functional. The parapodium permits standing but does not allow for sufficient mobility for the entire school day.

TYPE OF REASONING: INDUCTIVE

One must utilize clinical judgment to determine the **MOST** beneficial mobility device for this child. In order to arrive at the correct conclusion, the test taker must have a thorough understanding of the functional abilities of a child with myelodysplasia at the T10 level. In this case, a lightweight wheelchair is most appropriate, because ambulation requires too much energy and time. If this question was answered incorrectly, review information on thoracic myelodysplasia.

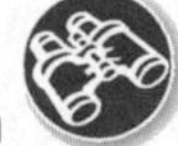

C46 | Musculoskeletal | Intervention

A patient has limited right rotation caused by left thoracic facet joint capsular tightness at T6–7. The arthrokinematic glide that would **MOST** effectively improve right rotation in sitting is:

CHOICES:

1. Superior and anterior glide on the right T6 transverse process.
2. Superior and anterior glide on the left T6 transverse process.
3. Superior and anterior glide on the right T7 transverse process.
4. Superior and anterior glide on the left T7 transverse process.

TEACHING POINTS

CORRECT ANSWER: 2

Because the left thoracic facet joint capsule is restricting movement, motion that would stretch the capsule would facilitate improved right rotation. With right rotation, the left superior facets move upward (opening the joint and stretching the capsule) and the right facets move downward (closing the joint and putting the capsule on relative slack).

INCORRECT CHOICES:

Providing a superior and anterior glide on the right T6 transverse process would improve left rotation. Providing a superior and anterior glide on the left T7 transverse process would improve left rotation at T6–7. Providing a superior and anterior glide on the right T7 transverse process would improve left rotation between T7 and T8.

TYPE OF REASONING: INDUCTIVE

One must utilize clinical judgment to determine the **MOST** effective intervention approach for facilitating improved right rotation. In order to arrive at the correct conclusion, the test taker must have a thorough understanding of normal facet joint capsule motion with rotation. For this patient, a superior and anterior glide to the left T6 transverse process will **MOST** effectively stretch the joint capsule and improve right rotation.

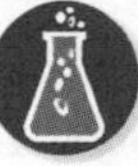

C47 | Musculoskeletal | Foundational Sciences

Electromyogram (EMG) activity in the lower extremities during erect standing is fairly continuous in the:

CHOICES:

1. Anterior tibialis and peroneals.
2. Posterior tibialis and intrinsic foot muscles.
3. Quadriceps femoris and anterior tibialis.
4. Soleus and gastrocnemius.

TEACHING POINTS

CORRECT ANSWER: 4

The soleus and gastrocnemius muscles oppose the dorsiflexion moment that exists at the ankle as a result of the line of gravity, which falls slightly anterior to the lateral malleolus. This fairly continuous activity is crucial for maintaining balance during quiet standing.

INCORRECT CHOICES:

The anterior tibialis, peroneals, and tibialis posterior muscles are inconsistently active and provide transverse stability in the foot during postural sway. The quadriceps femoris and anterior tibialis are active during posterior sway.

TYPE OF REASONING: ANALYSIS

One must recall the muscles that are active in the lower extremity during erect standing in order to arrive at the correct conclusion. This requires one to analyze the various muscles presented and make a determination of the correct solution, which encourages analytical reasoning skill. Knowledge of lower extremity kinesiology is beneficial to choosing the best solution.

C48 | Devices, Admin., etc. | Teaching, Research, Roles

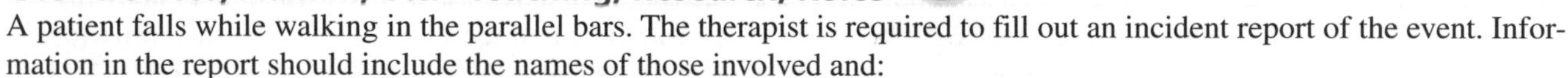

A patient falls while walking in the parallel bars. The therapist is required to fill out an incident report of the event. Information in the report should include the names of those involved and:

CHOICES:

1. The cause of this fall and crossreferences to others who have fallen in the parallel bars.
2. A description of the event, where the patient was injured, and the corrective actions to be taken.
3. What occurred, when and where it occurred, and witness statements.
4. Witness reports and therapist's opinion as to the cause.

TEACHING POINTS

CORRECT ANSWER: 3

The typical information included on an incident report are the names of those involved, inclusive of witnesses, what occurred, when it occurred, and where it occurred.

INCORRECT CHOICES:

An incident report should avoid interpretive information such as cause of the occurrence or corrective actions that were taken. There is no presumption that someone was injured.

TYPE OF REASONING: EVALUATION

One must weigh the information presented and determine which statement is most representative of the information that should appear in an incident report. This requires evaluative reasoning skill, in which one uses judgment to determine the most likely correct solution. If this question was answered incorrectly, review information on components of an incident report.

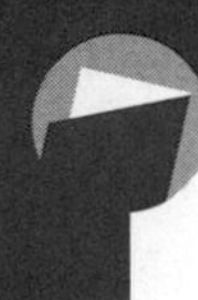

C49 | Devices, Admin., etc. | Equipment, Modalities 

Four days ago, a patient sustained a deep contusion of the lateral thigh as a result of a blow on the leg. After several cryotherapy treatments, the therapist decides to apply US. The parameters that should be used this case are:

CHOICES:

1. Pulsed US at 1 MHz.
2. Continuous US at 1 MHz.
3. Continuous US at 3 MHz.
4. Pulsed US at 3 MHz.

TEACHING POINTS

CORRECT ANSWER: 1

Pulsed US produces nonthermal effects (acoustic steaming, cavitation, microstreaming) which promote tissue repair during the early stages of the inflammation process. The therapist would select 1 MHz for a deep therapeutic effect.

INCORRECT CHOICES:

Continuous US produces thermal effects which are not desired at this stage of healing. Also, 3 MHz is used for superficial structures and would not penetrate to the desired depth to reach the target tissue.

TYPE OF REASONING: DEDUCTIVE

One must recall the appropriate US parameters to treat the patient's condition, which requires deductive reasoning skill. One must also remember the differences between pulsed versus continuous US, 1 MHz frequency versus 3 MHz, and the therapeutic effects on damaged tissue. For this patient, pulsed US at 1 MHz should be used.

C50 | Neuromuscular | Foundational Sciences 

An elderly individual was found unconscious at home and hospitalized with a diagnosis of CVA. Examination by the PT reveals normal sensation and movement on the right side of the body with impaired sensation (touch, pressure, proprioception) and paralysis on the left side of the body. The left side of the lower face and trunk are similarly impaired. The **MOST LIKELY** location of the CVA is the:

CHOICES:

1. Left side of brainstem.
2. Left parietal lobe.
3. Spinal cord.
4. Right parietal lobe.

TEACHING POINTS

CORRECT ANSWER: 4

This patient demonstrates involvement of the long tracts (sensory and motor) indicative of involvement of the contralateral cerebral cortex, parietal lobe.

INCORRECT CHOICES:

Tracts cross in the medulla so it is the right brain that is involved, not the left. The involvement of the face indicates a lesion above the level of the midbrain. A lesion in the spinal cord would not affect the face. A lesion in the brainstem would produce facial signs contralateral to the limb signs.

TYPE OF REASONING: ANALYSIS

The test taker must determine the precise location of the lesion given the symptoms presented. Questions that require one to draw conclusions based on symptoms often encourage analytical reasoning skill. For this patient, the symptoms indicate right parietal lobe damage, which should be reviewed if this question was answered incorrectly.

C51 | Neuromuscular | Foundational Sciences

The loss of sensory function in peripheral neuropathy is often among the first noticeable symptoms. If more than one nerve is involved, the sensory loss typically appears as:

CHOICES:

1. Bandlike dysesthesias and paresthesias in the hips and thighs.
2. Paresthesias affecting primarily the proximal limb segments and trunk.
3. Stocking and glove distribution of the lower and upper extremities.
4. Allodynia of the feet accompanied by pronounced dorsiflexor weakness.

TEACHING POINTS

CORRECT ANSWER: 3

Symmetrical involvement of sensory fibers, progressing from distal to proximal, is the hallmark of polyneuropathy. It is termed "stocking and glove distribution," and is the result of the dying back of the longest fibers in all the nerves from distal to proximal. Sensory symptoms include decreased sensation and pain, paresthesias, and dysesthesias (abnormal sensations such as numbness, tingling, or prickling).

INCORRECT CHOICES:

Proximal involvement (hips) can occur, but only after long-standing disease and distal involvement first. Involvement of the trunk is not typical. Allodynia refers to the perception of an ordinarily painless stimulus as painful, and is not characteristic of polyneuropathy.

TYPE OF REASONING: INFERENCE

This question requires one to determine the likely symptoms for polyneuropathy. This necessitates one to make inferences about the nature of polyneuropathy, which is an inferential reasoning skill. Through knowledge of neuropathology, the test taker should determine that polyneuropathy characteristically appears as a stocking and glove distribution of the hands and feet.

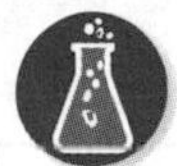

C52 | Cardiovascular-Pulmonary | Intervention

The therapist is supervising a phase II cardiac rehabilitation class of 10 patients. One of the patients, who is being monitored with radiotelemetry, is having difficulty. The therapist decides to terminate the patient's exercise session upon observing:

CHOICES:

1. An increase in HR 20 beats/min above resting.
2. An increase in systolic BP to 150 and diastolic BP to 90.
3. A second-degree atrioventricular (AV) heart block.
4. 1-mm ST segment depression, upsloping.

TEACHING POINTS

CORRECT ANSWER: 3

Criteria for reducing exercise intensity or termination according to the American College of Sports Medicine include (1) onset of angina and other symptoms of exertional intolerance, (2) systolic BP ≥ 240 mm Hg, diastolic BP ≥ 110 mm Hg, (3) >1-mm ST segment depression, horizontal or downsloping, (4) increased frequency of ventricular arrhythmias, (5) second-degree or third-degree AV block or other significant electrocardiogram (ECG) disturbances.

INCORRECT CHOICES:

The other findings do not fall within the criteria listed. HR is expected to rise proportionally to workload intensity unless the patient is on beta-blockers. The rise in BP is not significant enough to stop exercise. 1-mm ST segment depression that is isoelectric or within 1 mm is within normal limits.

TYPE OF REASONING: ANALYSIS

One must determine which symptoms warrant termination of the treatment session and which symptoms merely require monitoring. Through analytical reasoning, the person must interpret the symptoms presented and determine their significance. For this patient, second-degree AV heart block warrants termination of the treatment session. If this question was answered incorrectly, review cardiac rehabilitation guidelines for terminating exercise.

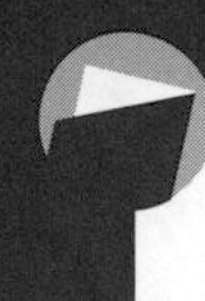

C53 | Cardiovascular-Pulmonary | Intervention

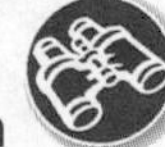

A patient presents with severe claudication that is evident when walking distances greater than 200 feet. The patient also exhibits muscle fatigue and cramping of both calf muscles. Upon examination, the PT finds the skin is pale and shiny with some trophic nail changes. The **BEST** choice for intervention is to:

CHOICES:

1. Begin with an interval walking program, exercising just to the point of pain.
2. Avoid any exercise stress until the patient has been on calcium channel blockers for at least 2 weeks.
3. Utilize a walking program of moderate intensity, instructing the patient that some pain is expected and to be tolerated.
4. Utilize non–weight-bearing exercises such as cycle ergometry.

TEACHING POINTS

CORRECT ANSWER: 1

This patient is exhibiting classic signs of peripheral artery disease (PAD). Rehabilitation guidelines for arterial disease include using an intermittent walking program of moderate intensity and duration, 2–3 times/day, 3–5 days/wk. The patient should be instructed to exercise to the point of claudication pain within 3–5 minutes, not beyond.

INCORRECT CHOICES:

Exhaustive exercise and exercising with persistent pain are contraindicated. Calcium channel blockers may be used in vasospastic disease; exercise is not contraindicated. A cycle ergometry program is less desirable than a walking program (treadmill or track) to reduce claudication. (Source: *American College of Sports Medicine Guidelines for Exercise Testing and Prescription,* ed 7.)

TYPE OF REASONING: INDUCTIVE

One must utilize clinical judgment to determine the **BEST** choice for intervention, which is an inductive reasoning skill. The test taker must understand what the symptoms are indicative of in order to arrive at the correct conclusion. If this question was answered incorrectly, refer to information on exercise for patients with PAD.

C54 | Integumentary | Intervention

A patient is hospitalized with diabetes and a large stage II plantar ulcer located over the right heel. The patient has been non–weight-bearing for the past 2 weeks as a result of the ulcer. The PT determines the **BEST** intervention is:

CHOICES:

1. Clean and bandage with a sterile gauze dressing.
2. A surgical consult because available wound dressings will not promote healing.
3. Clean and débride the wound, and apply a hydrogel dressing.
4. Wash the foot and apply skin lubricants followed by a transparent film dressing.

TEACHING POINTS

CORRECT ANSWER: 3

A stage II ulcer (deep ulcer) involves a partial-thickness skin loss with involvement of epidermis, dermis, or both; it is reversible. Intervention should be directed toward improving perfusion and relieving localized pressure. The wound should be cleaned with an antimicrobial agent, débrided of necrotic tissue, and covered with a sterile dressing. Hydrogel dressings maintain moisture in the wound bed, soften necrotic tissue, and support autolytic débridement. Pressure relief is also an important consideration. Techniques of protective foot care should be taught.

INCORRECT CHOICES:

Application of a dry, sterile gauze dressing is contraindicated, as is the application of skin lubricants. A stage II ulcer has the potential to heal; a surgical consult is not needed at this time.

TYPE OF REASONING: INFERENCE

One must utilize clinical judgment and knowledge of wound care approaches to determine the **BEST** intervention approach for this patient, which requires inductive reasoning skill. For this patient, cleaning and débriding of the wound with application of a hydrogel dressing is most appropriate for the type of wound described. If this question was answered incorrectly, review information on wound care procedures for stage II plantar ulcers.

C55 | Devices, Admin., etc. | Equipment, Modalities

A PT is prescribing a wheelchair for a patient with left hemiplegia who is of average height (5 feet 7 inches). The MOST beneficial feature to include in this prescription is:

CHOICES:

1. Desk armrests.
2. A 17.5-inch seat height.
3. A 20-inch seat height.
4. Elevating legrests.

TEACHING POINTS

CORRECT ANSWER: 2

A hemi- or low-seat wheelchair has a seat height of 17.5 inches. The lower seat height permits the patient to propel and steer the wheelchair using the sound right upper and lower extremities.

INCORRECT CHOICES:

A standard seat height wheelchair (20 inches) is too high to permit efficient use of the sound lower extremity for steering and propulsion. Elevating legrests may be considered if the patient has problems with edema (not indicated in this case). Shorter-length desk armrests are a useful option to allow an individual to get close to tables or work surfaces but they are not a priority in this example.

TYPE OF REASONING: INFERENCE

This question requires one to determine the most beneficial feature in wheelchair prescription for a patient with hemiplegia. This requires knowledge of various wheelchair features and which patient populations derive the most benefit from these features.

C56 | Devices, Admin., etc. | Teaching, Research, Roles

A patient who is participating in a cardiac rehabilitation program suddenly collapses and falls to the floor. The PT is the lone rescuer on site. The therapist checks for a response and finds the patient unresponsive. After activating the emergency response system (phone 911), the therapist, who is a trained health care provider, should:

CHOICES:

1. Give two rescue breaths followed by 15 chest compressions, repeating the cycle for at least 2 minutes.
2. Give 100 chest compressions per minute.
3. Use the automated external defibrillator (AED) to shock the patient after 3 minutes of cardiopulmonary resuscitation (CPR).
4. Begin CPR, and attach and use the AED as soon as it is available.

TEACHING POINTS

CORRECT ANSWER: 4

Guidelines from the American Heart Association (2010) concerning Basic Life Support and CPR specify that the first responder call 911 for unresponsive adults, get an AED (if available), and return to the victim to provide CPR and defibrillation, if needed. Trained HCPs can use ventilations (1 breath every 6-8 seconds) with chest compressions (at least 100/minute).

INCORRECT CHOICES:

The responder should use the AED as soon as possible after beginning CPR, and not wait 3 minutes. The compression rate for adult CPR is about 100/min with a recommended compression-to-ventilation ratio of 30:2. The old ratio was 15:2. Untrained rescuers should use compressions only.

TYPE OF REASONING: DEDUCTIVE

This question requires one to recall the proper and current Basic Life Support for health care provider guidelines. Questions that ask one to recall knowledge of protocols and guidelines necessitates deductive reasoning skill. If this question was answered incorrectly, refer to current guidelines for CPR.

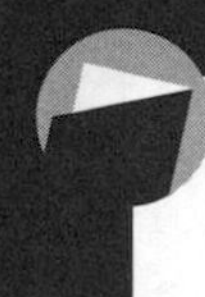

C57 | Musculoskeletal | Evaluation, Diagnosis, Prognosis

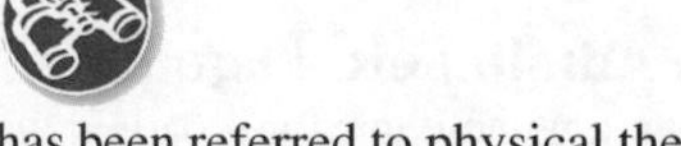

A patient who was casted for 3 weeks after a grade III right ankle sprain has been referred to physical therapy for mobility exercises. Examination shows a loss of 10 degrees of dorsiflexion. The patient will have the **MOST** difficulty in:

CHOICES:

1. Ambulating barefoot.
2. Descending stairs.
3. Descending a ramp.
4. Ambulating over rough surfaces.

TEACHING POINTS

CORRECT ANSWER: 2

Loss of dorsiflexion will make descending stairs most difficult because the ankle must have dorsiflexion during the single-limb support phase during descent.

INCORRECT CHOICES:

Although the activity may be changed, full range in dorsiflexion is not needed for the other choices.

TYPE OF REASONING: INDUCTIVE

The test taker must analyze all of the activities and then utilize clinical judgment to determine which activity requires the most ankle dorsiflexion range. This requires inductive reasoning skill, in which clinical judgment is paramount to finding the correct solution. For this patient, descending stairs would be **MOST** difficult because full-range dorsiflexion is required to complete the task successfully.

C58 | Musculoskeletal | Foundational Sciences

The torque output produced in the sitting position during isokinetic exercise involving the hamstrings is:

CHOICES:

1. Lower than the torque actually generated by the hamstrings.
2. Higher because of eccentric assistance of the quadriceps.
3. Higher than the torque actually generated by the contracting hamstrings.
4. Lower because of resistance of the quadriceps.

TEACHING POINTS

CORRECT ANSWER: 3

Gravity-produced torque adds to the force generated by the hamstrings when they contract, giving a higher torque output than is actually produced by the muscle (gravity-assisted exercise). Testing values may be misleading; software is available to correct for the effects of gravity.

INCORRECT CHOICES:

Hamstring work is lower, not higher, during this activity. Eccentric assistance by the quadricps (effects of reciprocal inhibition) does not lower or significantly raise the work of the hamstrings but rather serves to smooth out contraction.

TYPE OF REASONING: DEDUCTIVE

This question requires one to recall biomechanical guidelines of torque output in exercise. Recall of factual information and guidelines is a deductive reasoning skill. To arrive at the correct conclusion, one must recall that gravity-produced torque adds to the force generated by a contracting muscle, resulting in a higher torque output than what is produced by the muscle itself. If this question was answered incorrectly, review biomechanical guidelines of torque for isokinetic exercises.

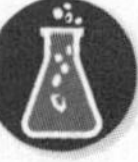

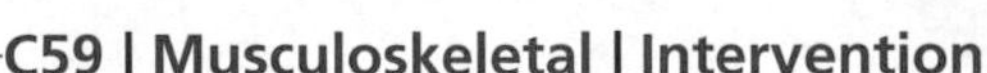

C59 | Musculoskeletal | Intervention

The manual therapy technique appropriate to correct a closing restriction of T5 on T6 is:

CHOICES:

1. Central posteroanterior (PA) pressure at a 60-degree angle on the spinous process of T6 while stabilizing T5.
2. Central PA pressure at a 45-degree angle on the spinous process of T5 while stabilizing T6.
3. Unilateral PA pressure at a 45-degree angle on the right transverse process of T6 while stabilizing T5.
4. Unilateral PA pressure at a 60-degree angle on the left transverse process of T6 while stabilizing T5.

TEACHING POINTS

CORRECT ANSWER: 1

In a closing restriction, the inferior facets of the superior vertebrae will not inferiorly glide on the superior facets of the inferior vertebra. Therefore, T5 inferior facets will not caudally glide on the superior facets of T6. Stabilizing T5 and application of pressure to T6 localizes the cephalad movement of the superior facets T6 on T5 bilaterally. The angle of the thoracic facets is 60 degrees; therefore, the application of force should be at the same plane.

INCORRECT CHOICES:

Providing the force at 45 degrees does not match the anatomical orientation for the facets in that region, so will not be as effective. The force should be a central PA glide because a unilateral glide will promote rotation and/or sidebending rather than extension.

TYPE OF REASONING: ANALYSIS

Knowledge of anatomy and biomechanics is important for choosing the correct solution for this question. The test taker utilizes analytical reasoning skill, determining the meaning of the four choices and deciding which choice most accurately represents the correct manual therapy technique for a closing restriction of T5 on T6. If this question was answered incorrectly, refer to information on manual therapy for closing restriction of thoracic vertebrae.

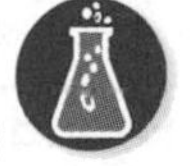

C60 | Neuromuscular | Evaluation, Diagnosis, Prognosis

A patient presents with an acute onset of vertigo overnight. Symptoms worsen with rapid change in head position. If the head is held still, symptoms subside usually within 30–60 seconds. The **MOST** likely cause of these signs and symptoms is:

CHOICES:

1. Benign paroxysmal positional vertigo (BPPV).
2. Bilateral vestibular neuritis.
3. Ménière's disease.
4. Acoustic neuroma.

TEACHING POINTS

CORRECT ANSWER: 1

BPPV is characterized by acute onset of vertigo and is positional, related to the provoking stimulus of head movement.

INCORRECT CHOICES:

Vestibular neuritis is an inflammation of the vestibular nerve caused by a virus and typically produces symptoms of dysequilibrium, nystagmus, nausea, and severe vertigo. Ménière's disease is characterized by a sensation of fullness in the ears associated with abnormal fluid buildup. Additional symptoms include tinnitus, vertigo, nausea, and hearing loss. Acoustic neuroma (vestibular schwannoma) produces unilateral sensorineural hearing loss along with vestibular symptoms.

TYPE OF REASONING: ANALYSIS

One must analyze the symptoms and make a determination of the most likely cause for these symptoms, which requires analytical reasoning skill. For this case, the patient's symptoms **MOST** likely cause is BPPV owing to the nature of an acute onset and being related to changing position of the head. Questions that inquire about a group of symptoms and whereby the test taker must determine the diagnosis often utilize analytical reasoning skill.

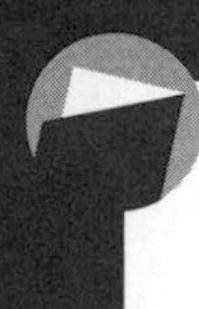

C61 | Cardiovascular-Pulmonary | Foundational Sciences

A patient with a significant history of coronary artery disease is currently taking atropine. Based on knowledge of the effects of this medication, the therapist expects:

CHOICES:

1. Palpitations at rest and with exercise.
2. Orthostatic hypotension.
3. Increased HR and contractility at rest.
4. Increased myocardial ischemia.

TEACHING POINTS

CORRECT ANSWER: 3

Atropine is an anticholinergic agent (it blocks the action of acetylcholine at parasympathetic sites in smooth muscle, secretory glands, and the central nervous system [CNS]). It produces an increase in HR and contractility and is used to treat symptomatic sinus bradycardia and exercise-induced bronchospasm.

INCORRECT CHOICES:

The other choices are not expected effects of this medication but rather adverse cardiovascular reactions (not asked for in this question). These can include tachycardia, orthostatic hypotension, palpitations, ventricular fibrillation, and increased ischemia in patients with MI.

TYPE OF REASONING: INFERENCE

This question requires one to infer the expected effects of atropine, thereby necessitating inferential reasoning skill. For this agent, atropine, one should anticipate possible increased HR and contractility at rest. Knowledge of anticholinergic agents and their effects are beneficial for arriving at the correct conclusion, which should be reviewed if this question was answered incorrectly.

C62 | Cardiovascular-Pulmonary | Foundational Sciences

A patient recovering from stroke is taking warfarin (Coumadin). During rehabilitation, it would be important to watch for potential adverse reactions including:

CHOICES:

1. Edema and dermatitis.
2. Palpitations and edema.
3. Cellulitis and xeroderma.
4. Hematuria and ecchymosis.

TEACHING POINTS

CORRECT ANSWER: 4

Warfarin sodium (Coumadin) is an anticoagulant indicated in the prophylaxis and treatment of venous thrombosis, pulmonary embolism, and thromboembolic disorders. Potential adverse reactions include hematuria and ecchymosis (skin discoloration and hemorrhaging). Serious bleeding is possible with drug toxicity.

INCORRECT CHOICES:

Xeroderma (dry skin), cellulitis (inflammation of tissues), and palpitations (awareness of heart rhythm abnormalities) are not seen as adverse reactions with warfarin.

TYPE OF REASONING: INFERENCE

One must infer the possible effects of warfarin therapy in order to arrive at the correct conclusion. This requires one to understand the common indications for the drug therapy and adverse side effects. For this medication, one should be watchful for hematuria and ecchymosis because of warfarin's properties of blood thinning. If this question was answered incorrectly, review information on warfarin therapy.

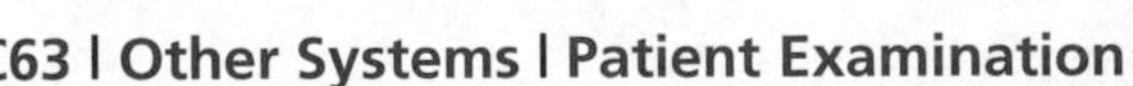

C63 | Other Systems | Patient Examination

The PT reviews the laboratory results of a patient admitted to the acute care hospital yesterday: hematocrit 45%, fasting blood glucose 180 mg/dL, and cholesterol 180 mg/dL. Based on these laboratory results, the patient **MOST** likely has:

CHOICES:

1. Hyperlipidemia.
2. Anemia.
3. Diabetes mellitus.
4. Polycythemia vera.

TEACHING POINTS

CORRECT ANSWER: 3

Fasting blood glucose of 180 mg/dL is abnormal and indicative of diabetes.

INCORRECT CHOICES:

The hematocrit and cholesterol readings are within normal limits. Hyperlipidemia (excessive level of lipids in the blood) and anemia (reduced circulating red blood cells [RBCs]) are not indicated. An elevated hematocrit could be indicative of polycythemia vera (proliferation or hyperplasia of all bone marrow cells with an increase of RBCs and hemoglobin concentration).

TYPE OF REASONING: ANALYSIS

This question requires one to determine the precise meaning of the laboratory values as it relates to a diagnosis for the patient. In this situation, the patient's laboratory values indicate diabetes mellitus. Drawing conclusions based on a group of indicators or symptoms requires analytical reasoning skill. If this question was answered incorrectly, review information on blood glucose laboratory values.

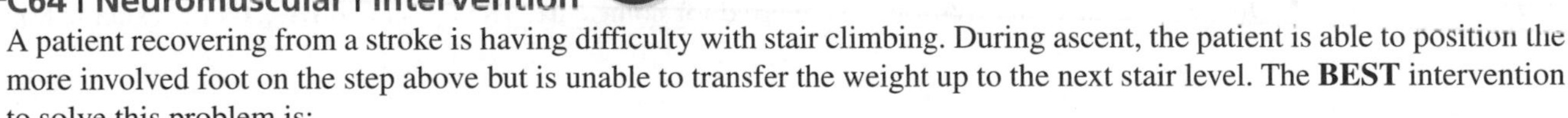

C64 | Neuromuscular | Intervention

A patient recovering from a stroke is having difficulty with stair climbing. During ascent, the patient is able to position the more involved foot on the step above but is unable to transfer the weight up to the next stair level. The **BEST** intervention to solve this problem is:

CHOICES:

1. Bridging, holding.
2. Standing, partial wall squats.
3. Plantigrade, knee flexion with hip extension.
4. Standing, side steps.

TEACHING POINTS

CORRECT ANSWER: 2

The quadriceps muscle is responsible for most of the energy generation needed to transfer up stairs to the next level. Partial wall squats are the **BEST** choice to strengthen these muscles (closed-chain exercise). During forward continuance (corresponding to mid stance), the ankle plantarflexors assist. Hip extensors are also active concentrically, assisting these actions.

INCORRECT CHOICES:

The other choices might be good lead-up activities for gait but would not optimally strengthen the key muscles involved in ascending stairs.

TYPE OF REASONING: ANALYSIS

This question requires one to analyze the described patient challenge and then determine the **BEST** intervention. The test taker must determine what the cause is for the patient who has difficulty transferring weight to ascend stairs, which necessitates analytical reasoning. After analyzing the situation, one should conclude that the quadriceps muscle is weak and partial wall squats in standing would **BEST** address this issue.

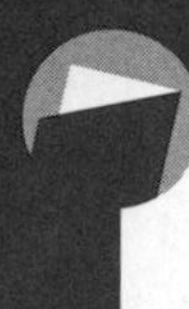

C65 | Cardiovascular-Pulmonary | Evaluation, Diagnosis, Prognosis

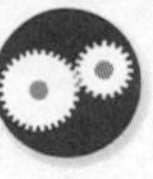

An elderly patient has been hospitalized, on complete bedrest, for 10 days. A physical therapy referral requests mobilization out-of-bed and ambulation. The patient complains of aching in the right calf. The therapist's examination reveals calf tenderness with slight swelling and warmth. The therapist decides to:

CHOICES:

1. Ambulate the patient with support stockings on.
2. Postpone ambulation and report the findings immediately.
3. Begin with ankle pump exercises in bed and then ambulate.
4. Use only AROM exercises with the patient sitting at the edge of the bed.

TEACHING POINTS

CORRECT ANSWER: 2

The patient is exhibiting early signs of acute deep vein thrombophlebitis. These findings should be reported immediately.

INCORRECT CHOICES:

Exercise and ambulation are contraindicated during the acute phase. If DVT is present, the patient will be given anticoagulation medication and will remain on bedrest with elevation of the involved leg until the acute phase subsides.

TYPE OF REASONING: EVALUATION

One must evaluate the patient's symptoms and determine the best course of action, given one's understanding of the symptoms. Here, the patient's symptoms are indicative of a DVT, which necessitates immediate notification and postponement of ambulation. If this question was answered incorrectly, refer to information on DVT and appropriate actions.

C66 | Neuromuscular | Patient Examination

A 9 year-old boy with Duchenne's muscular dystrophy is referred for home care. The PT should **BEGIN** the examination by:

CHOICES:

1. Performing a complete motor examination.
2. Performing a functional examination using the weeFIM.
3. Asking the child and his parents to describe the boy's most serious functional limitations.
4. Asking the parents to outline the boy's past rehabilitation successes.

TEACHING POINTS

CORRECT ANSWER: 3

The child and his parents/caretakers play an important part in determining impairments, functional limitations, disability, and future interventions. Taking a thorough initial history is important in determining what the other components of the examination should be.

INCORRECT CHOICES:

The other choices may indeed be appropriate; however, performing the interview first helps decide which examination tools are needed.

TYPE OF REASONING: INDUCTIVE

Questions such as these are difficult because one must determine what comes first in a process, especially when all the potential choices can be correct in the evaluation of a patient. For this question, the other choices are appropriate when conducting an examination, but the test taker must determine which one most logically should come first. This requires clinical judgment, an inductive reasoning skill.

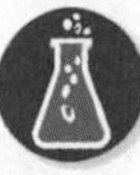

C67 | Musculoskeletal | Evaluation, Diagnosis, Prognosis

During an examination of an adolescent female who complains of anterior knee pain, the PT observes that the lower extremity shows medial femoral torsion and toeing-in position of the feet. The lower extremity position may be indicative of excessive hip:

CHOICES:

1. Anteversion.
2. Medial/internal rotation.
3. Retroversion.
4. Lateral/external rotation.

TEACHING POINTS

CORRECT ANSWER: 1

The pathology commonly associated with medial femoral torsion and toeing-in is hip anteversion due to an increase in the antetorsion angle (>15 degrees) between the femoral condyles and the neck of the femur.

INCORRECT CHOICES:

Excessive internal or external rotation of the hip would not force the patient to stand with toeing-in. Retroversion of the hips would cause the feet to toe-out.

TYPE OF REASONING: ANALYSIS

This question provides the symptoms, and the test taker must determine the likely cause, which requires analytical reasoning skill. Here, the symptoms are analyzed in order to make a determination for the cause of this patient's medial femoral torsion and toeing-in position of the feet. The test taker should conclude that excessive hip anteversion is the cause, which should be reviewed if this question was answered incorrectly.

C68 | Musculoskeletal | Intervention

A patient with osteoporosis and no fractures complains of increased mid and low back pain during breathing and other functional activities. The **MOST** beneficial interventions for this patient include patient education and:

CHOICES:

1. Trunk extension and abdominal stabilization exercises.
2. Trunk rotation and abdominal stabilization exercises.
3. Trunk flexion and extension exercises.
4. Trunk flexion and rotation exercises.

TEACHING POINTS

CORRECT ANSWER: 1

It is important to strengthen from the core to the floor as well as train in proprioception and balance enhancement techniques. Trunk extension and abdominal stabilization exercises are indicated.

INCORRECT CHOICES:

Patients should avoid trunk flexion or rotation exercise because it can cause a compression fracture of the spine.

TYPE OF REASONING: INFERENCE

One must determine first what may be the cause of the patient's pain and then determine the intervention approach that will **BEST** remedy the symptoms. If this question was answered incorrectly, refer to intervention approaches for osteoporosis.

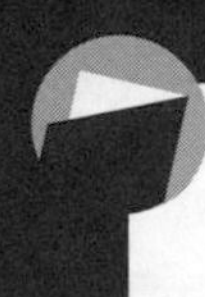

C69 | Devices, Admin., etc. | Teaching, Research, Roles

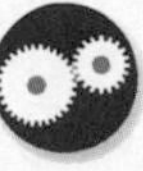

A single 22 year-old woman, who is 3 months pregnant, arrives at a therapist's private practice complaining of shoulder and leg pain. She has a black eye and some bruising at the wrists. The state in which the therapist practices has direct access. The **BEST** course of action for the therapist is:

CHOICES:

1. Administer massage for bruising, TENS, and ice modalities for pain, as indicated by the examination findings.
2. Direct the patient to the nearest ambulatory care center for physician evaluation.
3. Refuse to examine the patient and send her to the nearest emergency room.
4. Examine the patient, and if abuse is suspected, report the findings to the appropriate authorities.

TEACHING POINTS

CORRECT ANSWER: 4

According to the American Physical Therapy Association's (APTA's) Guidelines for Recognizing and Providing Care for Victims of Domestic Violence, this patient falls into a category of high risk. Women between the ages of 17 and 28 years and women who are single, separated, or divorced or who are planning a separation or divorce are at high risk. Battered women usually have more than one injury. Most injuries occur in the head, face, neck, breasts, and abdomen. According to the American Medical Association (AMA), battered women represent 23% of pregnant women who seek prenatal care. The victim may not volunteer information about her situation, but more often than not when asked will reveal it. It is important for the PT to examine the patient, and if abuse is suspected, report the findings to appropriate authorities. The therapist should be familiar with resources available for victims of domestic violence and their own state reporting laws.

INCORRECT CHOICES:

In most state jurisdictions, a PT may be fined or indicted for failure to report (all other choices).

TYPE OF REASONING: EVALUATION

This question requires one to make a judgment call for the **BEST** course of action, given the patient's symptoms. Questions that necessitate professional judgment in ethical situations often utilize evaluative reasoning skill, in which the merits of each potential choice are weighed. For this patient, it is important to do a comprehensive examination and then, if abuse is suspected, report it to the appropriate authorities.

C70 | Devices, Admin., etc. | Equipment, Modalities

An elderly patient presents with a stage III decubitus ulcer on the plantar surface of the right foot. After a series of conservative interventions with limited success, the therapist chooses to apply electrical stimulation for tissue repair. The **BEST** choice for electrical current in this case is:

CHOICES:

1. Low-volt biphasic pulsed current.
2. High-volt monophasic pulsed current.
3. Medium-frequency burst current.
4. Medium-frequency beat current.

TEACHING POINTS

CORRECT ANSWER: 2

Because high-volt pulsed current is a monophasic, unidirectional current, the unidirectional current would produce a therapeutic effect at the active (treatment) electrode. A negative charge (polarity) should be applied for a bactericidal effect or a positive charge given to promote wound healing.

INCORRECT CHOICES:

A biphasic current, which alternates the polarity, would tend to negate the treatment effects. Russian (burst) and interferential (beat) are medium-frequency biphasic currents. Interrupted currents (>0.5-sec interruption) are also not used for tissue healing.

TYPE OF REASONING: DEDUCTIVE

One must recall the appropriate electrical stimulation parameters to treat the patient's condition, which requires deductive reasoning skill. One must recall the differences between currents of differing low-, medium-, and high-volt current, as well as pulsed, burst, and beat current and the therapeutic effects on wound healing. If this question was answered incorrectly, review guidelines for electrical stimulation for wound healing.

C71 | Devices, Admin., etc. | Equipment, Modalities

A patient presents with pain radiating down the posterior hip and thigh as a result of a herniated disc in the lumbar spine. The therapist decides to apply mechanical traction. If the patient can tolerate it, the **PREFERRED** patient position is:

CHOICES:

1. Supine with one knee flexed.
2. Supine with both knees flexed.
3. Prone with no pillow.
4. Prone with pillow under the abdomen.

TEACHING POINTS

CORRECT ANSWER: 3

Placing the patient in the prone position would better align the spine so that the pull of the traction would be along the axis of the vertebral bodies.

INCORRECT CHOICES:

If the prone position is intolerable, then a pillow may be placed under the abdomen. Flexing the spine could exacerbate the disc herniation. A supine, knee-flexed position can be used for spinal stenosis.

TYPE OF REASONING: INDUCTIVE

The test taker must determine which patient position is **PREFERRED** for mechanical traction for a herniated lumbar disc. This requires recall of traction guidelines, but also clinical judgment to determine the correct solution, which necessitates inductive reasoning. Some other positions are acceptable but not preferred. If this question was answered incorrectly, review guidelines for mechanical traction for lumbar disk herniation.

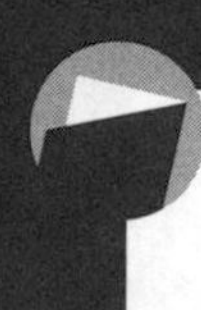

C72 | Neuromuscular | Intervention

A patient recovering from stroke demonstrates hemiparesis of the right upper extremity with moderate flexion and extension synergies (flexion stronger than extension). The therapist's goal is to strengthen the shoulder muscles first to promote elevation of the arm. The **BEST** choice is:

CHOICES:

1. Horizontal adduction with elbow extension.
2. Horizontal adduction with elbow flexion.
3. Abduction with elbow flexion.
4. Abduction with elbow extension.

TEACHING POINTS

CORRECT ANSWER: 4

Obligatory hemiplegic synergies are present and should not be reinforced. Shoulder abduction with elbow extension is the correct choice. It is an out-of-synergy combination that strengthens the shoulder abductors needed to stabilize the shoulder in an elevated position.

INCORRECT CHOICES:

Shoulder abduction with elbow flexion is part of the flexion synergy, whereas adduction with elbow extension is part of the extension synergy. Adduction with elbow flexion is an out-of-synergy combination but does not strengthen muscles needed to elevate and stabilize the upper extremity.

TYPE OF REASONING: INFERENCE

One must evaluate the patient's symptoms and infer the **BEST** method for strengthening the shoulder muscles, thereby requiring inferential reasoning. Given the diagnosis and current status, shoulder abduction with elbow extension is **BEST** because hemiplegic synergies are discouraged using this approach. If this question was answered incorrectly, review limb synergies with stroke and out-of-synergy movement patterns.

C73 | Neuromuscular | Foundational Sciences

A patient recovering from a middle cerebral artery stroke presents with gaze deviation of the eyes. In this type of stroke, the involved eye may deviate:

CHOICES:

1. Toward the hemiplegic side.
2. Upward.
3. Toward the sound side.
4. Down and out.

TEACHING POINTS

CORRECT ANSWER: 3

Unopposed action of the eye muscles causes the eye to deviate in the direction of the intact musculature. Thus, patients with hemispheric lesions involving a large frontal or parital lobe lesion look away from the hemiplegic side and toward the sound side.

INCORRECT CHOICES:

Patients with brainstem pontine lesions cannot look toward the nonparalyzed side. Upward or vertical gaze results from lesions in the upper brainstem. An eye that is deviated downward and out with ptosis is characteristic of a lesion involving CN III.

TYPE OF REASONING: INFERENCE

One must recall the nature of gaze deviation after middle cerebral artery stroke in order to arrive at the correct conclusion. This requires one to utilize inferential reasoning, in which the test taker must draw conclusions from the evidence presented. For this patient, the involved eye may deviate toward the sound side because of the unopposed action of the eye muscles. If this question was answered incorrectly, review information on gaze deviation of the eyes after stroke.

C74 | Cardiovascular-Pulmonary | Patient Examination

A patient is referred for physical therapy after an exercise tolerance test. The physician reports the test was positive and had to be terminated at 7 minutes. Based on the therapist's knowledge of this procedure, the therapist expects the patient may have exhibited:

CHOICES:

1. ST segment depression from baseline of 3-mm horizontal or downsloping depression.
2. A hypertensive response with a BP of at least 170/95.
3. Mild angina and dyspnea with progressive increases in the treadmill speed and grade.
4. ECG changes from baseline of 1-mm ST segment elevation.

TEACHING POINTS

CORRECT ANSWER: 1

A positive exercise tolerance test (graded exercise test) indicates myocardial ischemia with increasing exercise intensities. The optimal test duration is 8–12 minutes but can be terminated if symptoms of exertional intolerance are evident. The American College of Sports Medicine (ACSM) indicates these include ECG changes from baseline (>2 mm horizontal or downsloping; ST segment depression, or > 2-mm ST segment elevation).

INCORRECT CHOICES:

Additional signs of exertional intolerance that indicate the test should be terminated include onset of moderate to severe angina (some angina is expected with increasing work), a drop in systolic BP with increasing workload, serious arrhythmias, signs of exertional intolerance (pallor, cyanosis, cold or clammy skin), unusual or severe shortness of breath (some shortness of breath is expected), CNS signs (ataxia, vertigo, visual or gait problems, confusion), and a hypertensive response equal to or greater than 260/115 (a BP of 170/95 is not a reason for stopping the test. (Source: *ACSM's Guidelines for Exercise Testing and Prescription*, 7th ed. Philadelphia: Lippincott Williams & Wilkins.)

TYPE OF REASONING: INFERENCE

This question requires one to infer information based on the evidence presented. In this case, the test taker must infer what a positive exercise tolerance test indicates and early termination of the test after 7 minutes. If this question was answered incorrectly, refer to information on exercise tolerance testing and ACSM guidelines for terminating the test.

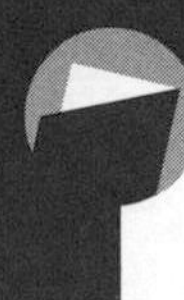

C75 | Musculoskeletal | Evaluation, Diagnosis, Prognosis

A college soccer player sustained a hyperextension knee injury when kicking the ball with the other lower extremity. The patient was taken to the emergency room of a local hospital and was diagnosed with "knee sprain." The patient was sent to physical therapy the next day for rehabilitation. As part of the examination, the therapist conducts the test shown in the figure. The test is positive. The type of exercise that is indicated in the acute phase of treatment is:

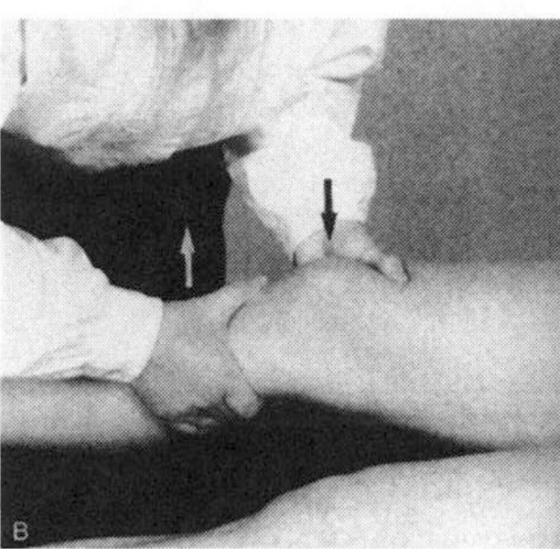

Magee D (2002). Orthopedic Physical Assessment, 4th ed. Philadelphia, W. B. Saunders, Figure 12-27B, page 700, with permission.

CHOICES:

1. Agility exercises.
2. Closed-chain terminal knee extension exercises.
3. Open-chain terminal knee extension exercises.
4. Plyometric functional exercises.

TEACHING POINTS

CORRECT ANSWER: 2

The test that was conducted was a Lachman's test to determine integrity of the ACL. A positive test suggests laxity of the ACL. Closed-chain terminal knee extension exercises are safe and effective secondary to the dynamic stability inherent with this type of exercise.

INCORRECT CHOICES:

Quick cutting/lateral movements that occur in agility training and heavy joint loading that occurs with plyometric exercise should be avoided until the muscular restraints that reduce excessive anterior translation of the affected tibiofemoral joint are strengthened. Open-chain knee extension may place excessive load on the ACL.

TYPE OF REASONING: ANALYSIS

Questions that include analysis of information depicted in pictures often necessitate analytical reasoning skill. This question requires one to determine what type of test is being depicted in the picture and then determine, upon positive result, the best exercise approach. This picture depicts a Lachman's test for determining ACL integrity. The positive test indicates laxity of the ACL and that closed-chain terminal knee extension exercises are best.

C76 | Integumentary | Intervention

A patient with a grade III diabetic ulcer is being treated with a calcium alginate wound dressing. This type of dressing can be expected to:

CHOICES:

1. Absorb exudate and allow rapid moisture evaporation.
2. Facilitate autolytic débridement and absorb exudate.
3. Provide semirigid support for the limb, while maintaining a sterile field.
4. Restrict bacteria from the wound, while supporting the tissues.

TEACHING POINTS

CORRECT ANSWER: 2

Moisture-retentive occlusive wound dressings such as calcium alginate are recommended for use on exudating wounds (grade III ulcer). They maintain a moist wound environment, absorb exudate, provide autolytic débridement, reduce pain at the wound site, or promote faster healing (reepithelialization).

INCORRECT CHOICES:

Calcium alginate dressings do NOT allow rapid evaporation. A disadvantage is that the dressing is very permeable to bacteria, urine, and so forth. Unna's boot is a semirigid dressing that provides limb support.

TYPE OF REASONING: DEDUCTIVE

This question requires one to recall the properties of a calcium alginate wound dressing. Recall of protocols and guidelines and other types of factual information often require deductive reasoning skill. For this question, calcium alginate dressings can be expected to facilitate autolytic débridement and absorption of exudate. If this question was answered incorrectly, review information on calcium alginate and other wound dressings.

C77 | Devices, Admin., etc. | Teaching, Research, Roles

The PT receives a referral to treat a hospitalized patient with adhesive capsulitis and a 5-year history of cirrhosis and hepatitis B. The therapist should:

CHOICES:

1. Use droplet transmission precautions.
2. Use contact precautions.
3. Wear personal protection equipment (PPE) when transporting the patient to therapy.
4. Ask the patient to wear gloves and avoid contact.

TEACHING POINTS

CORRECT ANSWER: 2

Hepatitis B is a viral infection that is transmitted by close contact with the infected patient's body fluids (nasopharyngeal exudate, saliva, sweat, urine, feces, semen, vaginal secretions) and blood and blood products. Health care workers should be vaccinated against the possibility of infection because they are in a high-risk category. Contact precautions should be observed to reduce the risk of microorganism transmission by direct or indirect contact. (refer to Box 6–1, Standard Precautions, Chapter 6).

INCORRECT CHOICES:

Droplet precautions are used when microorganisms can be transmitted by the patient during coughing, sneezing, or talking. The therapist should wear PPE, gloves, and gowns when in direct contact with the patient. The patient does not wear the gloves.

TYPE OF REASONING: DEDUCTIVE

This question causes one to recall the guidelines for standard precautions when working with a patient who has a history of cirrhosis and hepatitis B. The recall of guidelines is factual in nature and necessitates deductive reasoning skill. One must recall how hepatitis B is transmitted to arrive at the correct conclusion. For this patient, the therapist should avoid direct exposure to any blood or body fluids.

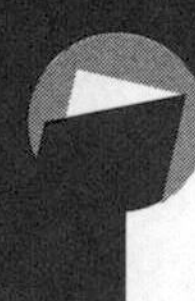

C78 | Musculoskeletal | Foundational Sciences

A patient with a transtibial amputation is learning to walk using a patellar tendon–bearing (PTB) prosthesis and is having difficulty maintaining knee stability from heel-strike to foot-flat. The muscles that are **MOST likely** weak are the:

CHOICES:

1. Knee extensors.
2. Back extensors.
3. Hip flexors.
4. Knee flexors.

TEACHING POINTS

CORRECT ANSWER: 1

The knee extensors (quadriceps) are maximally active at heel-strike (initial contact) to stabilize the knee and counteract the flexion moment.

INCORRECT CHOICES:

Erector spinae, gluteus maximus, and hamstrings contribute to core stability (trunk and pelvis) and assist in counteracting the flexion moment from heel-strike to foot-flat. Hip flexors contribute to initiate swing (acceleration to midswing) whereas knee flexors (hamstrings) decelerate the momentum of the swinging leg (midswing to deceleration).

TYPE OF REASONING: INFERENCE

One must infer the reason for the difficulty in maintaining prosthetic stability in order to choose the correct solution. This requires inferential reasoning, where one must determine the muscles that are **MOST** likely weak.

C79 | Cardiovascular-Pulmonary | Evaluation, Diagnosis, Prognosis

A patient with a history of coronary artery disease and recent MI is exercising in an inpatient cardiac rehabilitation program. Becuase the patient is new, continuous ECG telemetry monitoring is being done. The therapist observes the following. The **BEST** course of action is to:

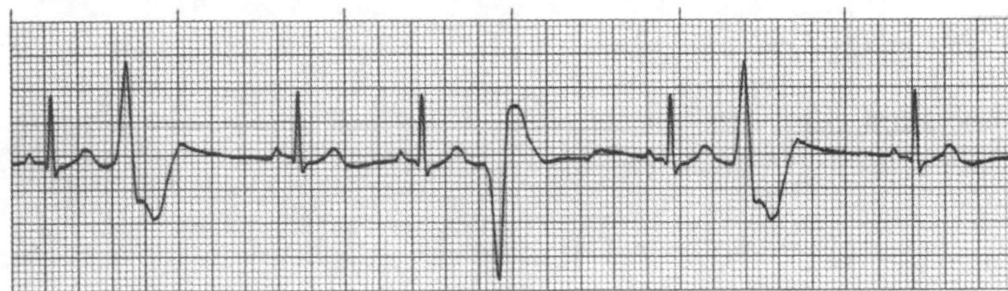

From: Jones, S (2005) ECG Notes. Philadelphia, F.A. Davis, p.51, with permission.

CHOICES:

1. Have the patient sit down and send him/her back to the room after a brief rest period.
2. Activate the emergency medical response team.
3. Have the patient sit down, continue monitoring, and notify the physician immediately.
4. Have the patient sit down, rest, and then resume the exercise at a lower intensity.

TEACHING POINTS

CORRECT ANSWER: 3

This tracing shows premature ventricular contractions (PVCs) that are multifocal (originating from different irritable ventricular focus). These multiform PVCs pose a potential danger of deteriorating into ventricular tachycardia and ventricular fibrillation (cardiac standstill). Because the heart is demonstrating a high degree of irritability, the **BEST** course of action is to stop the exercise, have the patient sit down, continue monitoring carefully, and notify medical staff (attending physician) immediately.

INCORRECT CHOICES:

Failure to report this finding by allowing the patient to rest or return to the room can be life-threatening. The patient has not arrested; therefore, the emergency medical response team should not be activated.

TYPE OF REASONING: EVALUATION

This question actually couples two types of reasoning. First, analytical reasoning is used to evaluate the information depicted in the picture. However, ultimately, evaluative reasoning skill is used to determine the **BEST** course of action, given the information presented. For this patient, the information indicated multifocal PVCs and necessitates termination of exercise with careful monitoring and notification of the physician. If this question was answered incorrectly, refer to information on ECG interpretations and PVCs.

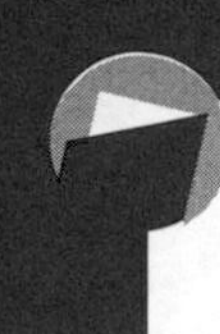

C80 | Neuromuscular | Intervention 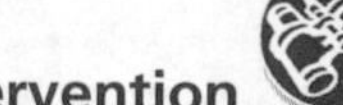

A patient recovering from traumatic brain injury is unable to bring the right foot up on the step during stair climbing training. The **BEST** training activity is to:

CHOICES:

1. Practice stair climbing inside the parallel bars using a 3-inch step.
2. Practice marching in place.
3. Passively bring the foot up and place it on the 7-inch step.
4. Strengthen the hip flexors using an isokinetic training device before attempting stair climbing.

TEACHING POINTS

CORRECT ANSWER: 1

The most appropriate lead-up activity to promote the skill of stair climbing is practice using a 3-inch step in the parallel bars.

INCORRECT CHOICES:

Passive movements do not promote active learning. Marching in place and isokinetic training may improve the strength of the hip flexors but does not promote the same synergistic patterns of muscle activity as the desired skill.

TYPE OF REASONING: INDUCTIVE

One must determine through clinical judgment the **BEST** approach for promoting the skill of stair climbing. This question requires inductive reasoning skill, in which the test taker must first determine the problem and then judge which intervention approach leads up to improving stair climbing ability. If this question was answered incorrectly, review information on exercises to promote stair negotiation.

C81 | Other Systems | Evaluation, Diagnosis, Prognosis

The PT is completing general activity recommendations for a group home of young adults with emotional and behavioral issues. All patients are chemically controlled with either antipsychotic or antidepressant medications. Full-time supervision is available for any activity recommended. Which exercise precautions would be important for the therapist to include?

CHOICES:

1. Promote rhythmic movement to soothing music to avoid agitation.
2. Promote activities with sequential movements to improve memory.
3. Avoid aerobic exercises outdoors when temperature is over 90 degrees F.
4. Avoid games with throwing activities to prevent injuries.

TEACHING POINTS

CORRECT ANSWER: 3

Overheating is detrimental to individuals on antipsychotic or antidepressant medications.

INCORRECT CHOICES:

Assumptions of agitation, memory deficits, or violence in such populations are discriminatory and inaccurate. Although an individual client may demonstrate these, it is inaccurate to suggest these for a group without further individual information.

TYPE OF REASONING: INFERENCE

This question requires one to have knowledge of the adverse/side effects of antipsychotic and antidepressant medications in order to arrive at a correct conclusion. In this situation, the potential adverse effect is overheating; therefore, avoiding aerobic exercise outdoors in temperatures over 90 degrees F is the **MOST** appropriate precaution. If this question was answered incorrectly, review information on adverse effects of antipsychotics and antidepressants.

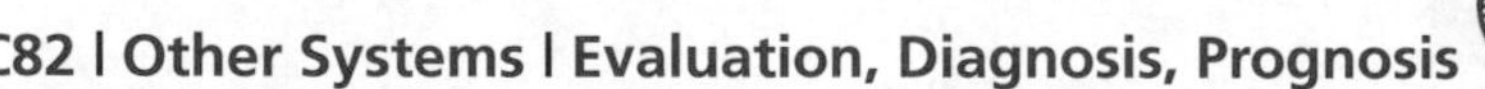

C82 | Other Systems | Evaluation, Diagnosis, Prognosis

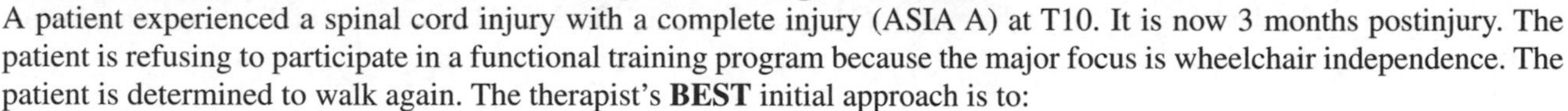

A patient experienced a spinal cord injury with a complete injury (ASIA A) at T10. It is now 3 months postinjury. The patient is refusing to participate in a functional training program because the major focus is wheelchair independence. The patient is determined to walk again. The therapist's **BEST** initial approach is to:

CHOICES:

1. Outline realistic short-term goals to improve independence while maintaining for the possibility of further recovery.
2. Discuss the harmful effects of denial and restrict all discussions to promoting wheelchair independence.
3. Refer the patient for psychological counseling and discharge from physical therapy.
4. Send the patient home for a short time in order to recognize the need for wheelchair training.

TEACHING POINTS

CORRECT ANSWER: 1

This patient is exhibiting denial, the first stage in psychological acceptance (Kübler-Ross). Denial can be protective, particularly in the early phases. However, this patient's denial persists 3 months after injury and is limiting rehabilitation participation and progress. It is important to provide a message of hope tempered with realism. Encouraging realistic short-term goals to improve function is the most appropriate choice.

INCORRECT CHOICES:

The other choices do not satisfy the patient's needs. Restricting discussion, discharging from physical therapy, or sending the patient home for a brief period are confrontational and not the **BEST** initial approach to this problem.

TYPE OF REASONING: EVALUATION

This question necessitates one to determine the merits of the four choices and then determine which seems **BEST**, given the patient's current status and issues. Evaluative reasoning is used for this question because the test taker must weigh the information presented and determine the value of the four approaches. For this patient, it is **BEST** to outline realistic short-term goals to improve function, so goals can be achieved in therapy, while still considering the patient's presence of denial.

C83 | Neuromuscular | Evaluation, Diagnosis, Prognosis

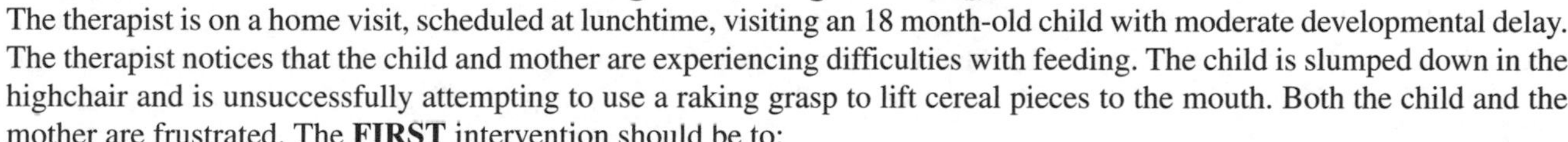

The therapist is on a home visit, scheduled at lunchtime, visiting an 18 month-old child with moderate developmental delay. The therapist notices that the child and mother are experiencing difficulties with feeding. The child is slumped down in the highchair and is unsuccessfully attempting to use a raking grasp to lift cereal pieces to the mouth. Both the child and the mother are frustrated. The **FIRST** intervention should be to:

CHOICES:

1. Work on desensitizing the gag reflex.
2. Recommend that the mother return to breast feeding for a few more months.
3. Recommend that the mother feed the child baby food instead of cereal for a few more months.
4. Reposition the child in a proper sitting position using postural supports.

TEACHING POINTS

CORRECT ANSWER: 4

Feeding can be successful only if the child is positioned in a stable sitting posture: head upright, trunk erect with pelvis neutral and hips flexed to 90 degrees, and feet resting flat. Correct positioning in sitting will facilitate upper extremity function (grasp and release) as well as swallowing.

INCORRECT CHOICES:

The other choices fail to address the central problem in this case, lack of postural support. Changing the child's diet (baby food or breast milk) will not improve the functional skill of feeding.

TYPE OF REASONING: INDUCTIVE

One must determine what should happen **FIRST** when providing interventions for this child. This requires inductive reasoning skill, in which clinical judgment is utilized to determine a best course of action. For this child, the **FIRST** intervention should be to reposition the child in proper sitting and utilize postural supports.

EXAM C

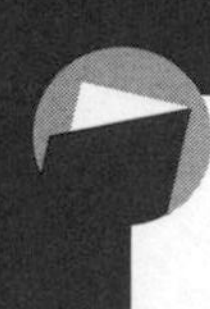

C84 | Musculoskeletal | Intervention

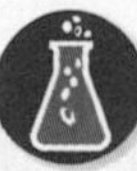

A patient is sent to physical therapy with a diagnosis of "frozen shoulder." The **MOST** effective mobilization technique for restricted shoulder abduction is:

CHOICES:

1. Posterior glide at 10 degrees of abduction.
2. Inferior glide at 55 degrees of abduction.
3. Inferior glide at 95 degrees of abduction.
4. Lateral glide in neutral position.

TEACHING POINTS

CORRECT ANSWER: 2

The convex-concave rule for mobilization applies. The **MOST** effective position to mobilize for improved shoulder abduction is in the resting position (55 degrees). Because the convex humeral head is moving on the concave glenoid, an inferior glide would be **MOST** appropriate to improve shoulder abduction.

INCORRECT CHOICES:

A posterior glide would improve external rotation. An inferior glide at 95 degrees would be outside the normal glenohumeral joints resting position so this technique would not be optimal. A lateral glide (anatomical distraction) is a generic technique that is nonspecific for any one motion and, therefore, not the best choice.

TYPE OF REASONING: ANALYSIS

One must have knowledge of biomechanics and kinesiology in order to arrive at the correct conclusion. In addition, one should understand the diagnosis of frozen shoulder (adhesive capsulitis) and appropriate joint mobilization techniques. This necessitates analytical reasoning skill, in which one must interpret the information presented and determine its precise meaning. If this question was answered incorrectly, review joint mobilization guidelines for treatment of adhesive capsulitis.

C85 | Musculoskeletal | Evaluation, Diagnosis, Prognosis

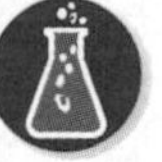

A patient presents with insidious onset of pain in the jaw that is referred to the head and neck regions. As best as the patient can recall, it may be related to biting into something hard. Cervical ROM is limited in flexion by 20 degrees, cervical lateral flexion limited to the left by 10 degrees. Mandibular depression is 10 mm with deviation to the left, protrusion is 4 mm, and lateral deviation is 15 mm to the right and 6 mm to the left. Based on these findings the diagnosis for this patient would be:

CHOICES:

1. Capsule-ligamentous pattern of temporomandibular joint (TMJ) on the left.
2. Weak lateral pterygoids on the left.
3. Weak lateral pterygoids on the right.
4. Cervical spine and TMJ capsular restrictions on the left.

TEACHING POINTS

CORRECT ANSWER: 1

The capsule-ligamentous pattern of the TMJ is limitation on opening, lateral deviation greater to the uninvolved side, and deviation on opening to the involved side. Normal parameters for TMJ measures are 25–35 mm functional, and 35–50 mm normal, normal protrusion is 3–6 mm, and normal lateral deviation is 10–15 mm.

INCORRECT CHOICES:

Weakness of the lateral pterygoids presents as deviation on protrusion to the opposite side of the muscle weakness. A capsular pattern of the cervical spine presents as side flexion and rotation, equally limited, and extension.

TYPE OF REASONING: ANALYSIS

Questions that inquire about a potential diagnosis given a patient's symptoms necessitate analytical reasoning skill. This is because one must weigh the information and analyze the symptoms in order to reach a conclusion that the diagnosis is most likely capsule-ligamentous pattern of TMJ on the left. If this question was answered incorrectly, review information on symptoms of TMJ.

C86 | Devices, Admin., etc. | Teaching, Research, Roles

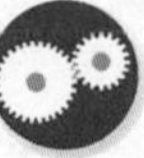

A mother of three is being treated for a Colles' fracture. Her husband wants to look at her medical record. The PT should:

CHOICES:

1. Give him the chart because he is a spouse and has a right to view the information.
2. Not let him look at the chart because he may misinterpret the documentation.
3. Let him look at the chart and be available to answer any questions.
4. Deny access to the chart unless written permission is granted by his wife.

TEACHING POINTS

CORRECT ANSWER: 4

The issue here is patient confidentiality. Spouses do not have access to medical information unless they have consent of their spouse or that of a proxy because of incompetence of the other spouse. In accordance with APTA's Guide for Professional Conduct Principle 1: PTs respect the rights and dignity of all individuals; and 1.2 Confidential Information C: Information derived from the working relationship of PTs shall be held confidential by all parties. HIPAA regulations also limit access to medical record information unless consent is granted.

INCORRECT CHOICES:

The husband should not be allowed to look at the chart. Not letting him look at the chart because of fear he will misinterpret the information is not a valid reason. However, permission must be granted first.

TYPE OF REASONING: EVALUATION

This question provides an ethical situation that requires the test taker to determine the best response, relying on knowledge of the APTA's Guide for Professional Conduct. This follows HIPAA regulations. Questions requiring determination of ethical guidelines and actions often require evaluative reasoning skill.

C87 | Cardiovascular-Pulmonary | Evaluation, Diagnosis, Prognosis

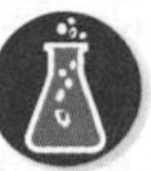

A patient with a recent history of rib fractures suddenly becomes short of breath during a bout of coughing. The patient looks panicked and complains of sharp pain in the left chest. A quick screen shows a deviated trachea to the right, among other signs and symptoms. The **MOST LIKELY** explanation for this is:

CHOICES:

1. Angina.
2. Pulmonary emboli.
3. Pneumothorax.
4. Mucous plugging of an airway.

TEACHING POINTS

CORRECT ANSWER: 3

The deviation of the trachea toward the right, with the chest pain on the left, is a match of symptoms for the occurrence of a pneumothorax on the left. The history of a rib fracture makes pneumothorax all the more likely.

INCORRECT CHOICES:

Whereas all of the pathologies listed would cause panic on the part of the patient, mucous plugging of an airway would not cause pain. The deviation of the trachea would not result from angina or pulmonary emboli, but would happen with a pneumothorax and lung tissue collapse (which could result from mucous plugging).

TYPE OF REASONING: ANALYSIS

This question provides symptoms, and the test taker must determine a cause for them. This necessitates analytical reasoning skill, in which one must produce the correct diagnosis based on the patient's symptoms. If this question was answered incorrectly, review information of symptoms of pneumothorax.

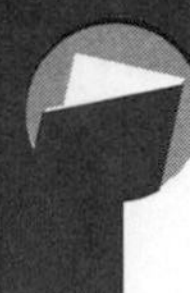

C88 | Musculoskeletal | Foundational Sciences

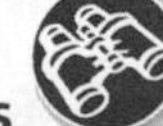

A patient presents with supraspinatus tendinitis. After the initial cryotherapy, the therapist decides to apply US. To effectively treat the supraspinatus tendon, the therapist would place the shoulder joint in:

CHOICES:

1. Slight abduction and external rotation.
2. Slight abduction and internal rotation.
3. Adduction and internal rotation.
4. Adduction and external rotation.

TEACHING POINTS

CORRECT ANSWER: 2

Abduction and internal rotation of the shoulder places the supraspinatus tendon in a good position to apply US by exposing the tendon from under the acromion process.

INCORRECT CHOICES:

The other choices fail to position the supraspinatus tendon in optimal position.

TYPE OF REASONING: INDUCTIVE

One must utilize diagnostic and clinical judgment to determine the best course of action when providing US for supraspinatus tendinitis. Questions that require clinical and diagnostic reasoning utilize inductive reasoning skill.

C89 | Integumentary | Patient Examination

A patient is referred for postmastectomy rehabilitation. During the initial examination, the therapist observes an irregular area of skin on the patient's shoulder about 7 mm in diameter. The patient reports that there has always been a mole there but is more prominent lately and the color has changed, now ranging from black to red to blue. The therapist documents this finding as a:

CHOICES:

1. Benign nevus.
2. Atypical dysplastic nevus.
3. Papule.
4. Wheal.

TEACHING POINTS

CORRECT ANSWER: 2

A nevus is a common mole. A changing nevus (atypical dysplastic nevus) that presents with asymmetry (A), irregular borders (B), variations in color (C), diameter > 6 mm (D), and elevation (E) is indicative of malignant melanoma (the "ABCDEs" from the American Cancer Society).

INCORRECT CHOICES:

A benign nevis does not present with changes and variations in color. A papule is an elevated nevus. A wheal is an irregular, transient superficial area of localized skin edema (e.g., hive, mosquito bite).

TYPE OF REASONING: ANALYSIS

Questions that provide an array of symptoms and the test taker must determine the likely findings often require analytical reasoning skill. For this scenario, the key words including "irregular area" and "variations in color" should assist the test taker in concluding this finding as an atypical dysplastic nevus. If this question was answered incorrectly, review signs and symptoms of skin malignancies from the American Cancer Society.

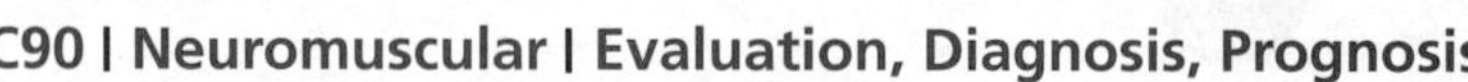

C90 | Neuromuscular | Evaluation, Diagnosis, Prognosis

A patient is 2 days post–left CVA and has just been moved from the intensive care unit to a stroke unit. When beginning the examination, the therapist finds the patient's speech slow and hesitant. The patient is limited to one- and two-word productions, and expressions are awkward and arduous. However, the patient demonstrates good comprehension. These difficulties are consistent with:

CHOICES:

1. Global aphasia.
2. Dysarthria.
3. Wernicke's aphasia.
4. Broca's aphasia.

TEACHING POINTS

CORRECT ANSWER: 4

This patient is demonstrating classic signs of Broca's aphasia (also known as nonfluent, expressive, or motor aphasia). It is the result of a lesion involving the third frontal convolution of the left hemisphere. Broca's aphasia is characterized by slow and hesitant speech with limited vocabulary and labored articulation. There is relative preservation of auditory comprehension.

INCORRECT CHOICES:

Wernicke's aphasia is characterized by impaired auditory comprehension and fluent speech. Global aphasia is a severe aphasia with marked dysfunction across all language modalities. Dysarthria is impairment in the motor production of speech.

TYPE OF REASONING: ANALYSIS

This question provides symptoms and the test taker must determine the diagnosis. This requires analytical reasoning skill, in which one must determine the cause for the symptoms. If this question was answered incorrectly, review symptoms of Broca's aphasia.

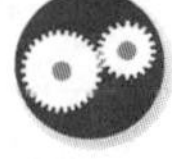

C91 | Neuromuscular | Patient Examination

A patient recovering from traumatic brain injury is functioning at stage IV on the Rancho Los Amigos Levels of Cognitive Functioning Scale. During the therapist's initial examination, the patient becomes agitated and tries to bite the therapist. The **BEST** course of action is to:

CHOICES:

1. Postpone the examination until later in the day when the patient calms down.
2. Postpone the examination for 1 week and then try again.
3. Document the behaviors and engage in a calming activity.
4. Restructure the formal examination so the therapist can complete it in three very short sessions.

TEACHING POINTS

CORRECT ANSWER: 3

Patients in level IV of recovery are confused and agitated. Behavior is bizarre and nonpurposeful relative to the immediate environment. This patient is unable to cooperate directly with formal examination or treatment, lacking both selective attention and memory. The therapist needs to observe and document the behaviors closely and engage the patient in a calming activity such as slow rocking. A quiet, closed environment is critical.

INCORRECT CHOICES:

Because the patient's symptoms are expected for a person in stage IV of Rancho Los Amigos Cognitive Functioning Scale, it is not appropriate to defer treatment or restructure the examination. The patient's immediate needs must be addressed.

TYPE OF REASONING: EVALUATION

One must determine the **BEST** course of action based on evaluating the merits of the four possible choices presented. One must ask, "Are these symptoms expected for this stage of recovery, and if so, what would be **BEST**"? If this question was answered incorrectly, review Rancho stages.

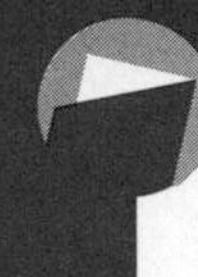

C92 | Cardiovascular-Pulmonary | Intervention

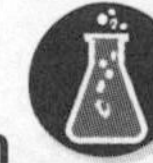

A therapist is working on a cardiac care unit in an acute care facility. After exercising a patient recovering from a ventricular infarct, the therapist notices fatigue and dyspnea after mild activity. Later that day, on a return visit, the therapist notices the patient has a persistent spasmodic cough while lying in bed. HR is rapid (140) and slight edema is evident in both ankles. The patient appears anxious and agitated. The therapist suspects:

CHOICES:

1. Left ventricular failure.
2. Right ventricular failure.
3. Impending MI.
4. Developing pericarditis.

TEACHING POINTS

CORRECT ANSWER: 1

Typical clinical manifestations of left ventricular failure (CHF) include those described in the case example along with an S3 heart gallop, paroxysmal nocturnal dyspnea, orthopnea, and signs and symptoms of pulmonary edema (marked dyspnea, pallor, cyanosis, diaphoresis, tachypnea, anxiety, and agitation).

INCORRECT CHOICES:

Typical clinical manifestations of right ventricular failure include dependent edema of the ankles (usually pitting edema), weight gain, fatigue, right upper quadrant pain, anorexia, nausea, bloating, right-sided S3 or S4, cyanosis of nail beds, and decreased urine output. Impending MI may include anginal pain or discomfort in the chest, neck, jaw, or arms; palpitations; tachycardia; or unusual fatigue or dyspnea. Pericarditis produces substernal pain that may radiate to neck and upper back, difficulty swallowing, pain aggravated by movement or coughing and relieved by leaning forward or sitting upright, and a history of fever, chills, weakness, or heart disease.

TYPE OF REASONING: ANALYSIS

This question provides symptoms of cardiac issues, and the test taker must determine the likely diagnosis. This necessitates analytical reasoning skill, in which one must determine the correct diagnosis based on the patient's symptoms. If this question was answered incorrectly, review symptoms of coronary artery disease.

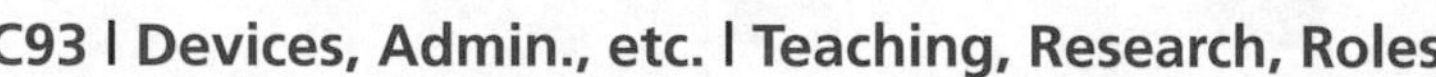

C93 | Devices, Admin., etc. | Teaching, Research, Roles 

A group of researchers conducted a cohort study of patients with chronic stroke to examine the relationship of a new measure of voluntary movement and basic mobility (STREAM) to other measures of impairment and disability. Scores on the STREAM were associated with scores on the Balance Scale and the Barthel Index. The **BEST** choice for data analysis for this study is:

CHOICES:

1. Pearson's product moment correlation.
2. Analysis of variance (ANOVA).
3. Paired t-test.
4. Mann-Whitney U-test

TEACHING POINTS

CORRECT ANSWER: 1

Correlational research attempts to determine whether a relationship exists between two or more quantifiable variables and to what degree. Pearson's product moment correlation is the correct answer.

INCORRECT CHOICES:

The paired t-test, ANOVA, and Mann-Whitney tests measure the difference between two or more groups. Only one group was studied over time in this example.

TYPE OF REASONING: DEDUCTIVE

This question requires factual recall of research guidelines. Any time one must recall guidelines or protocols, deductive reasoning skills are utilized. For this scenario, the **BEST** choice for data analysis for this study is Pearson's product moment correlation, because the study seeks to find a relationship between variables. If this question was answered incorrectly, review correlational research guidelines, especially guidelines for use of Pearson's product moment correlation.

C94 | Other Systems | Foundational Sciences 

A patient has been taking corticosteroids (hydrocortisone) for management of adrenocortical insufficiency and is referred to physical therapy for mobility training after a prolonged hospitalization. Potential adverse effects that one can expect from prolonged use of this medication include:

CHOICES:

1. Confusion and depression.
2. Atrophy and osteoporosis.
3. Decreased appetite and weight loss.
4. Hypotension and myopathy.

TEACHING POINTS

CORRECT ANSWER: 2

Prolonged use of corticosteroids may result in muscle weakness, osteoporosis, fractures, and joint pain. Large doses are associated with cushingoid changes (e.g., moon face, central obesity, hypertension, myopathy, electrolyte and fluid imbalance). Common CNS changes include insomnia and nervousness.

INCORRECT CHOICES:

The other choices are not expected potential adverse effects of corticosteroids.

TYPE OF REASONING: INFERENCE

One must infer or draw conclusions about the expected symptoms of prolonged use of corticosteroids in order to arrive at the correct conclusion. For this patient, one could expect atrophy and osteoporosis to occur. If this question was answered incorrectly, review information on side effects of long-term corticosteroid use.

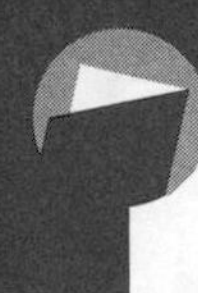

C95 | Integumentary | Foundational Sciences

A PT is treating a patient with deep partial-thickness burns over 35% of the body (chest and arms). Wound cultures reveal a bacterial count in excess of 105/g of tissue on the anterior left arm. The therapist can reasonably expect that:

CHOICES:

1. The risk of hypertrophic and keloid scars is low because there is no viable tissue.
2. The burn area is pain free because all nerve endings in the dermal tissue were destroyed.
3. With antibiotics, spontaneous healing can be expected.
4. The infected wound can convert the area to a full-thickness burn.

TEACHING POINTS

CORRECT ANSWER: 4

A deep partial-thickness burn will heal in about 3–5 weeks if it does not become infected. An infection typically results in conversion of the wound to a full-thickness burn.

INCORRECT CHOICES:

Full-thickness burns (not partial-thickness burns) are without sensation, because the nerve endings are destroyed. However, the area is not pain free, because adjacent areas of partial-thickness burns have intact nerve endings and can be painful. The risk of hypertrophic and keloid scars is high (not low) with deep partial-thickness or full-thickness burns. With wound conversion, grafting will be necessary, because all epithelial cells are destroyed with a full-thickness burn. With an infected wound, spontaneous healing is not expected.

TYPE OF REASONING: INFERENCE

One must determine what a bacterial count of 105/g indicates in order to choose the correct solution. This requires one to draw conclusions about the information presented, which when inferred correctly, indicates that the wound is infected and could convert the burned area to a full-thickness burn. If this question was answered incorrectly, refer to burn care guidelines, especially infected wounds.

C96 | Devices, Admin., etc. | Equipment, Modalities

Recently, a 10 year-old patient has begun walking with supination of the right foot. With the shoe off, the therapist finds a new callus on the lateral side of the metatarsal head of the fifth toe. The **BEST** choice for orthotic prescription is:

CHOICES:

1. Viscoelastic shoe insert with forefoot medial wedge.
2. Scaphoid pad.
3. Thomas' heel.
4. Viscoelastic shoe insert with forefoot lateral wedge.

TEACHING POINTS

CORRECT ANSWER: 4

Supination of the foot (pes cavus) is accompanied by supination of the talocalcaneonavicular (TCN), subtalar, and transversal tarsal joints. It is characterized by an abnormally high arch. The flexible cavus foot generally responds well to orthotic foot control, especially in a child. The best choice is a viscoelastic shoe insert with forefoot lateral wedge.

INCORRECT CHOICES:

The other choices are used to control flexible pes valgus.

TYPE OF REASONING: INDUCTIVE

One must utilize clinical judgment in order to determine the **BEST** choice for orthotic prescription. This requires one to utilize inductive reasoning skill, which also includes diagnostic thinking, in order to determine a best course of action. If this question was answered incorrectly, review orthotic prescription approaches for children with foot supination.

C97 | Musculoskeletal | Intervention

A patient is recovering from a right total hip replacement (posterolateral incision, cementless fixation). The **MOST** appropriate type of bed-to-wheelchair transfer to teach is to have the patient use a:

CHOICES:

1. Stand-pivot transfer to the surgical side.
2. Lateral slide transfer to the surgical side using a transfer board.
3. Stand-pivot transfer to the sound side.
4. Squat-pivot transfer to the surgical side.

TEACHING POINTS

CORRECT ANSWER: 3

During initial healing, it is important to protect the hip from dislocation or subluxation of the prosthesis. With a posterolateral incision, excessive hip flexion and adduction past neutral are contraindicated. This is minimized by transferring to the sound side.

INCORRECT CHOICES:

All other choices emphasize transfer to the surgical side, which can move the hip into adduction. In addition, the stand-pivot transfer with some hip extension is a better choice than transferring with the hip in full flexion.

TYPE OF REASONING: DEDUCTIVE

This question requires one to recall the appropriate guidelines for bed-to-wheelchair transfers of patients with total hip replacements. The recall of guidelines necessitates deductive reasoning, in which factual recall of knowledge is expected. For patients with hip replacements, transfers toward the sound side helps to preserve hip precaution guidelines. If this question was answered incorrectly, review guidelines for transferring patients with hip replacements.

C98 | Devices, Admin., etc. | Equipment, Modalities

A patient with paraplegia at the T10 level wants to participate in wheelchair basketball. An option that should be considered in ordering a wheelchair for this patient is:

CHOICES:

1. A rigid frame.
2. Hard-rubber tires.
3. A mid scapular seat back.
4. A folding frame.

TEACHING POINTS

CORRECT ANSWER: 1

Sports competition wheelchairs are usually made with rigid construction and very strong lightweight materials. The rigid frame allows for better power and distance with each stroke.

INCORRECT CHOICES:

A folding wheelchair does not provide the stability needed for competition sports. Some of the stroke power is distributed through the wheelchair with less distance achieved per stroke. Pneumatic (air-filled) tires provide a smoother ride and improved traction as opposed to hard-rubber tires. A low seat back enhances the user's upper body/arm movements. A higher seat back is indicated for patients with decreased trunk control (not a factor in this example).

TYPE OF REASONING: INDUCTIVE

One must utilize diagnostic reasoning and clinical judgment to determine the best type of wheelchair for a patient with T10 paraplegia who wishes to participate in sports. This requires inductive reasoning skill, in which professional judgment of a best approach is utilized. For this patient, a rigid wheelchair frame is best.

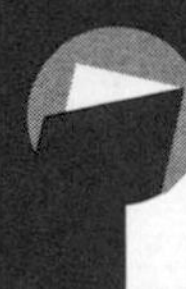

C99 | Neuromuscular | Intervention

The therapist is treating a child with mild developmental delay secondary to 7 weeks prematurity at birth. The child is now 8 months old and is just learning to sit. The **BEST** choice for training activity is:

CHOICES:

1. Standing tilting reactions.
2. Sideward protective extension in sitting.
3. Prone tilting reactions.
4. Supine tilting reactions.

TEACHING POINTS

CORRECT ANSWER: 2

Sideward protective extension in sitting is a functional, protective reaction that normally occurs at about the same time as sitting begins.

INCORRECT CHOICES:

The child who is starting to sit should already have prone and supine tilting reactions. It is too early to begin standing tilting reactions.

TYPE OF REASONING: INFERENCE

One must recall the developmental milestones of infants and infer the **BEST** choice for training in order to choose the correct solution. If this question was answered incorrectly, review the motor developmental milestones of infants.

C100 | Cardiovascular-Pulmonary | Evaluation, Diagnosis, Prognosis

An elderly patient with emphysema and a history of hypertension performs a 12-minute walking exercise tolerance test. Walking distance was 1,106 feet. Vital signs prior to exercise were HR 104, BP 130/76, and SpO_2 93%. At peak exercise, vital signs were HR 137, BP 162/74, and SpO_2 92%. To calculate exercise intensity parameters, the **BEST** method to use is:

CHOICES:

1. 40–85% HR reserve (Karvonen's formula).
2. 70–80% of HR_{max}.
3. 70–85% of age adjusted predicted HR_{max}.
4. 40–50% of maximum metabolic equivalents of the task (METs).

TEACHING POINTS

CORRECT ANSWER: 1

This patient has impaired functional abilities as noted by the low number of feet traveled in 12 minutes. The patient also has a high resting HR, likely the result of pulmonary medications. To correctly prescribe exercise for this patient, high resting HR needs to be taken into consideration. Karvonen's formula, the HR reserve method, uses high resting HR as part of the formula. $[(HR_{max} - HR_{rest}) \times 40 \text{ to } 85\%] + HR_{rest}$ = target HR range.

INCORRECT CHOICES:

If the therapist were to use the formula 70–80% of HR_{max}, the therapist would find that part of the target HR for exercise was lower than the resting HR. Using a predicted number for HR when an actual exercising HR maximum is known is an inaccurate way of prescribing exercise. Finally, because (1) the MET charts are based on a healthy population, (2) the therapist has the actual HR data from the test, and (3) the therapist does not have actual metabolic equivalents during the exercise test, there is no reason to use METs in the calculation of exercise intensity.

TYPE OF REASONING: INDUCTIVE

One must have knowledge of the different methods of calculating exercise intensity in order to choose the **BEST** solution. This requires inductive reasoning skill, in which clinical judgment coupled with knowledge of exercise intensity calculation is utilized to choose the correct answer. If this question was answered incorrectly, review guidelines for calculation using Karvonen's formula.

C101 | Other Systems | Intervention

A patient is recovering from a mild stroke and demonstrates trunk extensor weakness and postural instability. The patient also suffers from severe heartburn and says that previous physical therapy treatments have made it worse. Prior exercises have included holding in side-lying, bridging, and prone on elbows. The **BEST** choice to maximize recovery while minimizing heartburn is to:

CHOICES:

1. Perform trunk stabilization exercises with the patient in Fowler's position.
2. Reduce the number of repetitions of bridging and switch to dynamic reversals.
3. Perform rhythmic stabilization with the patient in sitting.
4. Assure the patient that the heartburn is not aggravated by exercise and suggest taking antacids before physical therapy.

TEACHING POINTS

CORRECT ANSWER: 3

Heartburn is a common symptom of gastrointestinal disorders (gastroesophageal reflux disease [GERD]) and can be aggravated by positioning in supine, prone, or bridging. Modifying the patient's position to upright can alleviate the symptoms and demonstrate to the patient the therapist's concern.

INCORRECT CHOICES:

Changing the position to Fowler's (semi-sitting) improves the stress on the lower esophageal valve (less heartburn) but because it is a supported position does not challenge the patient's postural control. Changing the technique to dynamic reversals does not change the positional deficits of bridging. Recommending medications is outside the scope of practice of the therapist.

TYPE OF REASONING: INFERENCE

This question requires one to understand the circumstances that can aggravate heartburn during exercise in order to arrive at the correct conclusion. Inferential reasoning skills are utilized, because the test taker must weigh the facts and make certain assumptions in order to choose the best solution.

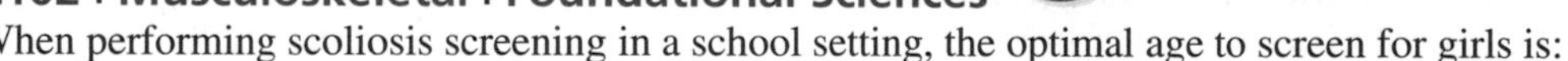

C102 | Musculoskeletal | Foundational Sciences

When performing scoliosis screening in a school setting, the optimal age to screen for girls is:

CHOICES:

1. 6–8.
2. 12–14.
3. 15–17.
4. 9–11.

TEACHING POINTS

CORRECT ANSWER: 4

The most effective age to screen girls for scoliosis is just before the pubescent growth spurt between 9 and 11 years, when the scoliotic curve can increase dramatically. Boys should be screened between 11 and 13 years of age because of differences in the age of onset of puberty between girls and boys.

INCORRECT CHOICES:

Screening can occur at any age, but routine screening should be performed before the pubescent growth spurt. Large changes in abnormal spinal curves can occur during growth spurts.

TYPE OF REASONING: ANALYSIS

One must analyze the merits of performing scoliosis screenings with each of the identified age groups in girls in order to determine the age at which it is optimal to complete the screening. This requires analytical reasoning skill, in which one interprets the various ages and how these ages are relevant to normal development and puberty. If this question was answered incorrectly, review information on scoliosis screening.

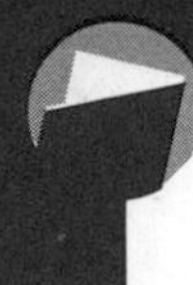

C103 | Neuromuscular | Foundational Sciences

A patient with a confirmed left C6 nerve root compression due to foraminal encroachment complains of pain in the left thumb and index finger. The **MOST** effective cervical position to alleviate this radicular pain in weight-bearing is:

CHOICES:

1. Lower cervical flexion.
2. Left side bending.
3. Lower cervical extension.
4. Right rotation.

TEACHING POINTS

CORRECT ANSWER: 1

Flexion increases the space at the intervertebral foramen, allowing the C6 nerve root to decompress and reduce or alleviate radicular pain.

INCORRECT CHOICES:

Left sidebending, cervical extension, and/or right rotation all close down the foramen on the left hand side, which will increase the compression on the nerve.

TYPE OF REASONING: INFERENCE

This requires the test taker to infer how various cervical positions will result in less pain from C6 nerve root compression. This requires knowledge of anatomy and the cervical position that will increase space at the intervertebral foramen to alleviate pain. Evaluative reasoning skills are utilized whenever one must make a judgment about a best course of action.

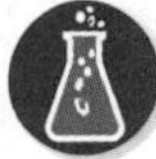

C104 | Musculoskeletal | Foundational Sciences

A patient is standing with excessive subtalar pronation. The therapist examines for possible related motions of:

CHOICES:

1. Tibial and femoral external rotation, with pelvic internal rotation.
2. Tibial, femoral, and pelvic internal rotation.
3. Tibial, femoral, and pelvic external rotation.
4. Tibial and femoral internal rotation with pelvic external rotation.

TEACHING POINTS

CORRECT ANSWER: 2

With the patient standing, the calcaneus is fixed to the ground. Subtalar joint pronation will occur as the talus plantar flexes, adducts, and inverts. In response to subtalar joint pronation, obligatory internal rotation of the tibia, femur, and pelvis occurs.

INCORRECT CHOICES:

External rotation of the tibia, femur, and pelvis would be associated with excessive subtalar supination. The pelvis must follow the rotation present in the lower limb (specifically the femur).

TYPE OF REASONING: ANALYSIS

One must analyze these motions and postures in order to determine which solution is most likely correlated with the excessive subtalar pronation. Through analytical reasoning skill, one should determine that tibial, femoral, and pelvic internal rotation are the possible obligatory motions as a result of the excessive subtalar pronation. If this question was answered incorrectly, tefer to information on postures related to excessive subtalar pronation.

C105 | Devices, Admin., etc. | Teaching, Research, Roles 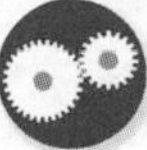

A patient is receiving oupatient physical therapy as a result of a rotator cuff tear has acheived all goals and returned to baseline function. The patient enjoys coming to physical therapy and participates well in treatment. The patient requests to continue with therapy to maintain all achievements because their insurance policy has unlimited physical therapy coverage. The PT should:

CHOICES:

1. Continue to see the patient only if the patient agrees to pay out-of-pocket..
2. Continue to see the patient because physical therapy will be reimbursed by the insurance company.
3. Decrease the frequency of treatment to one time per week.
4. Discharge the patient from physical therapy and do not see the patient under any circumstances.

TEACHING POINTS

CORRECT ANSWER: 1

PTs are obligated to provide therapy services that are indicated according to patient presentation and the examination findings. The Standards of Practice indicate that once the patient's goals are met and the patient has returned to baseline, he/she should be discharged from skilled therapy. The fact that there is unlimited physical therapy coverage should not be a factor in this clinical decision. As long as the PT explains that the therapy is not medically necessary, the patient may still decide that therapy is beneficial to him/her and that he/she must pay out-of-pocket. The Code of Ethics obligates PTs to be responsible stewards of health care resources and avoid both under- and overutilization of services. It would not be considered overutilization of services if the patient was informed of the nature and need of the continued services.

INCORRECT CHOICES:

Even though the insurance would cover continued therapy, it would be unethical for the PT to provide services because this would be overutilization of resources paid by the insurance company. The therapist could continue to see the patient in an ethical manner as long as it was explained that the therapy was not necessary, although the patient chooses to continue treatment. By decreasing the therapy to one time per week, it would still be overutilization because it would be presented to the insurance company as needed services.

TYPE OF REASONING: EVALUATION

The question requires one to recognize the issues of overutilization of services and the unethical behavior in doing so, which is an evaluative reasoning skill. In order to answer the question correctly, the test taker must first identify that skilled physical therapy is no longer indicated and then must know the ethical options for honoring the patient's request for continued therapy. If this question was answered incorrectly, review the Code of Ethics Principle 8 (C).

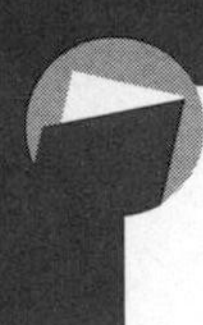

C106 | Devices, Admin., etc. | Equipment, Modalities

A therapist is applying a symmetrical biphasic pulsed current to the vastus medialis to improve patellar tracking during knee extension. The patient complains that the current is uncomfortable. To make the current more tolerable to the patient, yet maintain a good therapeutic effect, the therapist should consider adjusting the:

CHOICES:

1. Pulse rate.
2. Current intensity.
3. Pulse duration.
4. Current polarity.

TEACHING POINTS

CORRECT ANSWER: 3

Decreasing the pulse duration reduces the electrical charge of each pulse, making the current more comfortable by decreasing the total current applied while maintaining the full therapeutic effect.

INCORRECT CHOICES:

The only other parameter that would have a direct effect on comfort would be the intensity. For motor level stimulation, decreasing the intensity would decrease the therapeutic effect by decreasing the quality of the contraction. For sensory level stimulation, decreasing the intensity would decrease the level of sensory input needed for the treatment of pain. The pulse rates used for pain management are typically modulated. For motor level stimulation, decreasing the pulse rate would decrease the quality of the contraction, and increasing the pulse rate could make it more uncomfortable or contribute to muscle fatigue. Changing the polarity would have no effect because a symmetrical biphasic waveform has no net polarity.

TYPE OF REASONING: DEDUCTIVE

This question requires one to factually recall the correct parameters for high-volt pulsed current and how adjustments to the pulse or current results in alterations in therapeutic effect. Factual recall or protocols or guidelines is a deductive reasoning skill. If this question was answered incorrectly, review information on guidelines for high-volt pulsed current.

C107 | Other Systems | Foundational Sciences

Which of the following gastrointestinal sources of pain can refer to the shoulder?

CHOICES:

1. Esophageal pain.
2. Spleen or diaphragmatic pain.
3. Colon or appendix pain.
4. Gallbladder pain.

TEACHING POINTS

CORRECT ANSWER: 2

Spleen or diaphragmatic pain can refer to the shoulder.

INCORRECT CHOICES:

Esophageal pain can refer to the mid back, head, or neck. Colon or appendix pain can refer to the low back, pelvis or sacrum. Gallbladder pain can refer to the mid back and scapular regions.

TYPE OF REASONING: DEDUCTIVE

One must recall the typical referral patterns for gastrointestinal pain in order to determine which refers to the shoulder. This requires deductive reasoning skills, because factual recall of guidelines are used to reach a conclusion. If this question was answered incorrectly, review gastrointestinal pain referral patterns.

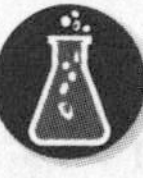

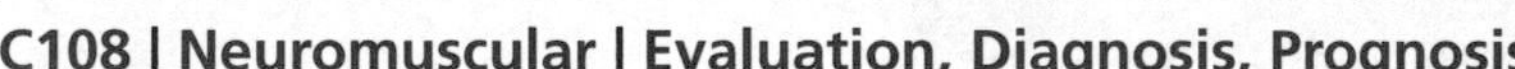

C108 | Neuromuscular | Evaluation, Diagnosis, Prognosis

A patient presents with symptoms of uncoordinated eye movements, profound gait and trunk ataxia, and difficulty with postural orientation to vertical. Balance deficits are pronounced in standing with eyes open and eyes closed. Examination of the extremities reveals little change in tone or coordination. The therapist suspects involvement of the:

CHOICES:

1. Spinocerebellum.
2. Basal ganglia.
3. Premotor cortex.
4. Vestibulocerebellum.

TEACHING POINTS

CORRECT ANSWER: 4

The symptoms are suggestive of cerebellar dysfunction. The vestibulocerebellum (archicerebellum) is concerned with adjustment of muscle tone in response to vestibular stimuli. It coordinates muscle actions to maintain postural coordination and balance control along with eye muscle control (all impaired in this example).

INCORRECT CHOICES:

The spinocerebellum (paleocerebellum) controls muscle tone and synergistic movements of the extremities on the same side of the body. The basal ganglia's functions are complex. It contributes to motor planning and sequencing of voluntary movements. Deficits typically include rigidity, bradykinesia, and tremor along with postural instability. The premotor cortex (precentral area, frontal lobe) stores programs of motor activity assembled as the result of past experience and programs the motor cortex for voluntary movements. It assists the basal ganglia in control of coarse postural movements.

TYPE OF REASONING: ANALYSIS

This question provides the symptoms, and the test taker must determine, through analytical reasoning, the cortical region responsible for the symptoms. If this question was answered incorrectly, review information on cerebellar dysfunction.

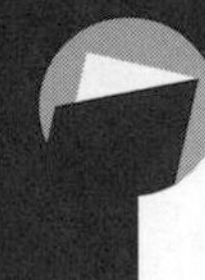

C109 | Other Systems | Evaluation, Diagnosis, Prognosis

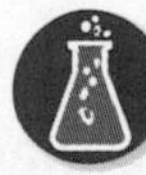

A patient with a 10-year history of diabetes complains of cramping, pain, and fatigue of the right buttock after walking 400 feet or climbing stairs. When the patient stops exercising, the pain goes away immediately. The skin of the involved leg is cool and pale. The therapist checks the record and finds no mention of this problem. The therapist suspects:

CHOICES:

1. Spinal root impingement.
2. Peripheral nerve injury.
3. Peripheral arterial disease (PAD).
4. Raynaud's phenomenon.

TEACHING POINTS

CORRECT ANSWER: 3

Intermittent claudication, often the earliest indication of PAD, is manifested by cramping, pain, or fatigue in the muscles during exercise that is typically relieved by rest. The calf muscle is most commonly affected, but discomfort may also occur in the thigh, hip, or buttock. Cessation of pain immediately upon stopping the exercise is characteristic of intermittent claudication, not other spinal problems. With severe disease, however, pain may be present even at rest.

INCORRECT CHOICES:

The pain associated with spinal root impingement (nerve pain) is often acute and becomes worse or aggravated by extension, side flexion, rotation, standing, walking and exercise in general. It is relieved by lying down. Peripheral nerve injury presents with sensory and motor loss. Raynaud's phenomenon is an intermittent attack of pallor or cyanosis of the small arteries and arterioles of the fingers as a result of inadequate blood flow.

TYPE OF REASONING: ANALYSIS

This is a question that provides the symptoms and one must determine the likely diagnosis. This requires analytical reasoning skill, in which the test taker utilizes knowledge of anatomy, physiology, and pathology to determine the cause. If this question was answered incorrectly, review information on symptoms of PAD.

C110 | Cardiovascular-Pulmonary | Evaluation, Diagnosis, Prognosis

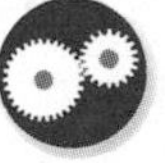

A patient with low back pain has marked elevation of BP and complains of mild to severe mid abdominal pain that increases upon exertion. Palpation reveals a pulsing mass in the lower abdomen. The therapist should:

CHOICES:

1. Instruct in relaxation exercises, because a pulsating mass is not unusual with hypertension.
2. Discontinue treatment and notify the patient's physician immediately.
3. Instruct the patient to contact his/her physician at the conclusion of therapy.
4. Provide hot packs to the abdomen to help relieve the muscle spasm.

TEACHING POINTS

CORRECT ANSWER: 2

This patient is demonstrating signs and symptoms of aortic aneurysm. Pain is intermittent or constant and can be felt in the mid abdominal or low back regions. The pulsating mass is highly significant, and the level of hypertension dramatically increases risk of rupture. This is a serious medical condition; the therapist should notify the physician immediately.

INCORRECT CHOICES:

The therapist should not rely on the patient to contact the physician. All physical therapy intervention should cease.

TYPE OF REASONING: EVALUATION

One must evaluate the significance of the information presented, determine the root cause of the symptoms, and then determine the best course of action. This requires evaluative reasoning skill, in which one evaluates the merits of the four possible choices and determines which approach is most appropriate and safe for the patient. In this case, it is important to discontinue treatment and immediately notify the physician.

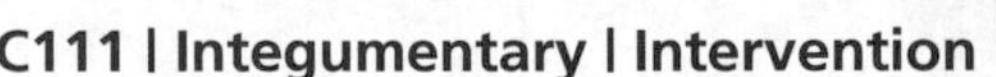
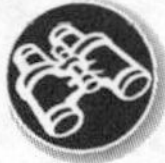

C111 | Integumentary | Intervention

A patient with a 12-year history of diabetes and a small, purulent tunneling wound located on the left heel is referred for wound lavage. The therapist's **BEST** choice is to irrigate the wound using:

CHOICES:

1. Whirlpool with water temperature at 20 degrees C.
2. Hydrogen peroxide spray.
3. A syringe with Dakin's solution while the patient is in the whirlpool.
4. Whirlpool with povidone-iodine.

TEACHING POINTS

CORRECT ANSWER: 4

Wound irrigation (lavage) is an effective way to remove debris and contaminants and reduce bacterial counts on wound surfaces. Whirlpool can be used as a means of wound cleansing and mechanical débridement. Antibacterial agents are typically used (e.g., povidone-iodine [Betadine] or Chloramine-T [Chlorazine]), if the wound is purulent. Limitations of whirlpool include risk of contamination, and use of the dependent position can increase venous congestion and edema.

INCORRECT CHOICES:

Water temperature should be warm (not 20 degrees C) to stimulate peripheral circulation. Hydrogen peroxide is indicated to débride wounds with large amounts of necrotic tissue and is not used for wound lavage. Dakin's solution is an appropriate bactericidal agent; however, it is not administered while the patient is in the whirlpool.

TYPE OF REASONING: INDUCTIVE

This question requires one to utilize clinical judgment and diagnostic thinking to determine the **BEST** choice to irrigate the wound. This necessitates inductive reasoning skill, in which the test taker must refer to knowledge of the various approaches and determine through clinical judgment which approach to wound irrigation will most effectively address the specific wound indicated. If this question was answered incorrectly, refer to information on wound irrigation approaches for purulent wounds.

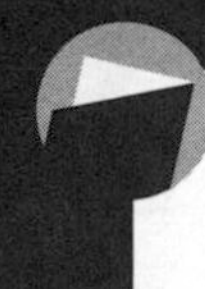

C112 | Other Systems | Evaluation, Diagnosis, Prognosis

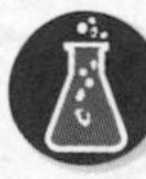

A frail eldery wheelchair-dependent resident of a community nursing home has a diagnosis of organic brain syndrome, Alzheimer's type, stage 2. During the therapist's initial interview, the patient demonstrates limited interaction and mild agitation and keeps trying to wheel the chair down the hall. Because it is late in the day, the therapist decides to resume the examination the next morning. The patient is most likely exhibiting:

CHOICES:

1. Frustration because of an inability to communicate.
2. Disorientation to time and date.
3. Sundowning behavior.
4. Inattention as a result of short-term memory loss.

TEACHING POINTS

CORRECT ANSWER: 3

A patient with stage 2 Alzheimer's disease can be expected to exhibit impaired cognition and abstract thinking, sundowning (defined as extreme restlessness, agitation, and wandering that typically occurs late afternoon), inability to carry out sactivities of daily living, impaired judgment, inappropriate social behavior, lack of insight, repetitive behavior, and a voracious appetite.

INCORRECT CHOICES:

Inability to communicate is characteristic of stage 3. Short-term memory loss and disorientation to time and date are early and persistent signs of the disease.

TYPE OF REASONING: ANALYSIS

This question provides the symptoms, and the test taker must determine, through analytical reasoning, the most likely cause for the patient's behavior. In this situation, the symptoms suggest that the patient with Alzheimer's disease is exhibiting sundowning behavior. If this question was answered incorrectly, review information on Alzheimer's disease and sundowning behavior.

C113 | Musculoskeletal | Intervention

To increase the step length of a patient with a right transfemoral amputation who is taking an inadequate step with the limb, the therapist should:

CHOICES:

1. Provide posterior directed resistance to the right ASIS during stance.
2. Facilitate the gluteals with tapping over the muscle belly.
3. Provide posterior directed resistance to the left ASIS during swing.
4. Provide anterior directed resistance to the right PSIS during swing.

TEACHING POINTS

CORRECT ANSWER: 1

Light resistance and stretch applied to the pelvis (right ASIS) in a posterior direction during mid to late stance will facilitate forward pelvic rotation on that side and enhance forward movement of the limb during swing.

INCORRECT CHOICES:

Anterior directed resistance functions to pull the hip forward but does little to facilitate active forward limb movement. The gluteals function to stabilize the limb during stance (not advance the limb forward). Manual resistance applied to the pelvis during swing may interfere with stepping.

TYPE OF REASONING: INFERENCE

One must infer the best approach to providing directed resistance for the patient with a transfemoral amputation. This requires knowledge of kinesiology and therapeutic exercise in order to arrive at the correct conclusion.

C114 | Other Systems | Evaluation, Diagnosis, Prognosis

An elderly and frail resident of an extended care facility has intractable constipation. During a scheduled visit from the PT, the patient complains of abdominal pain and tenderness. The therapist recognizes the patient may experience pain in the:

CHOICES:

1. Low back and front of the thigh to the knee.
2. Buttock, thigh, and posterior leg.
3. Medial thigh and leg.
4. Anterior hip, groin, or thigh region.

TEACHING POINTS

CORRECT ANSWER: 4

Intractable constipation (obstipation) can cause partial or complete bowel impaction, pain, and tenderness in the lower abdomen. Referred pain is to the anterior hip, groin, or thigh region.

INCORRECT CHOICES:

Pain in the back and front of thigh to knee is characteristic of L2 nerve root compression. Pain in the buttock, thigh, and posterior leg is characteristic of S1 nerve root compression. Pain in the bladder can refer to the medial thigh and leg.

TYPE OF REASONING: INFERENCE

One must infer or draw a reasonable conclusion about the symptoms a client is likely to experience given the diagnosis provided. Inferential reasoning skills are often utilized in cases in which one must determine what may be true of a patient. If this question was answered incorrectly, review signs and symptoms of intractable constipation and pain referral patterns from the viscera.

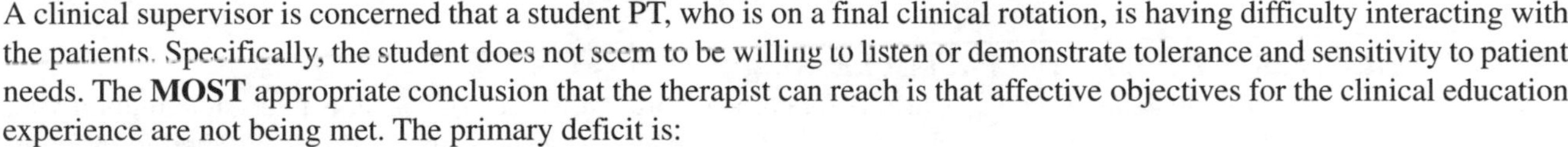

C115 | Devices, Admin., etc. | Teaching, Research, Roles

A clinical supervisor is concerned that a student PT, who is on a final clinical rotation, is having difficulty interacting with the patients. Specifically, the student does not seem to be willing to listen or demonstrate tolerance and sensitivity to patient needs. The **MOST** appropriate conclusion that the therapist can reach is that affective objectives for the clinical education experience are not being met. The primary deficit is:

CHOICES:

1. Level 1.0 Receiving.
2. Level 3.0 Valuing.
3. Level 4.0 Organization.
4. Level 5.0 Adherence to a professional code of ethics.

TEACHING POINTS

CORRECT ANSWER: 1

In the affective domain, level 1.0 deals with attending to phenomena and stimuli. This student lacks these foundation behaviors in the affective domain and is thus functioning at a very low level (failure to be aware of people and situations, willingness to listen to others, and ability to attend closely to discussions).

INCORRECT CHOICES:

The problem is not one of behaviors at the higher levels of the affective domain (all other choices). This student fails to demonstrate the lowest level affective behaviors upon which the higher level skills are built.

TYPE OF REASONING: DEDUCTIVE

This question requires one to recall guidelines and protocols of the clinical education experience, including the affective domain. Knowledge of factual information to determine the correct conclusion is a deductive reasoning skill. If this question was answered incorrectly, review the affective domain and the objectives for the various different levels.

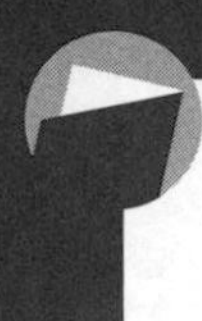

C116 | Devices, Admin., etc. | Teaching, Research, Roles

A therapist wants to investigate the effectiveness of use of the therapeutic pool for decreasing pain in a group of patients with fibromyalgia. Two groups of patients were recruited. One group was assigned to exercises and walking in the pool 3 times/wk for 6 months. The other group was assigned to a gym walking program for the same amount of time. At the end of the study, outcomes were assessed using the McGill Pain Questionnaire and the Health Status Questionnaire. In order to improve reliability, the lead investigator should:

CHOICES:

1. Have the same therapist reassess the patients after 6 months.
2. Have another therapist reassess after 6 months and compare with normalized scores.
3. Utilize a core of four experienced therapists to randomly complete all the assessments.
4. Perform all the final assessments and compare with the initial assessments performed by a core group of therapists.

TEACHING POINTS

CORRECT ANSWER: 1

Reliability is the degree to which a test consistently measures what it is intended to measure. Intrarater reliability is established by having the same rater measure on multiple measurement trials. Interrater reliability can be established if all raters are trained to administer the measurement instruments and demonstrate consistency of rating (there is no evidence of this happening).

INCORRECT CHOICES:

Changing the rater pre- and postintervention or using a group of raters (investigator included) without evidence of measures to train all raters for consistency fails to establish this study's reliability.

TYPE OF REASONING: DEDUCTIVE

Questions that inquire about proper research protocols and improving reliability in conducting studies are questions that require deductive reasoning. This question requires factual recall of reliability and how to improve reliability in studies, which should be reviewed if this question was answered incorrectly.

C117 | Cardiovascular-Pulmonary | Patient Examination

An apparently healthy individual has several risk factors for coronary artery disease. The client is interested in improving overall fitness and cardiac health. After an exercise tolerance test, which was asymptomatic, the client is referred for an exercise class. The **MOST** accurate measure of exercise intensity to monitor during the **FIRST** exercise session is:

CHOICES:

1. Rating of perceived exertion (RPE).
2. MET level.
3. Respiratory rate.
4. HR.

TEACHING POINTS

CORRECT ANSWER: 4

An exercise tolerance test should be performed before commencing an exercise program for all high-risk individuals. The best measurement of exercise intensity in a newly tested and exercising individual is HR.

INCORRECT CHOICES:

RPE will become a valuable measurement tool once the patient becomes adept at using it, but it would not be reliable for the first exercise session. MET level is more of a measurement of workload, not an accurate measurement of an individual's response to exercise. Respiratory rate is not used to prescribe exercise intensity.

TYPE OF REASONING: INDUCTIVE

This question requires the test taker to recall the various measures of exercise intensity and determine, through clinical judgment, which measure will **MOST** accurately monitor the patient's exercise intensity, given his/her diagnosis and symptoms on the **FIRST** visit. Questions that require clinical judgment and diagnostic reasoning require inductive reasoning skill. If this question was answered incorrectly, review measures to monitor exercise intensity for at-risk individuals.

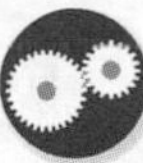

C118 | Neuromuscular | Foundational Sciences

A mother brings her 8 week-old infant to be examined at early intervention because she noticed that the infant was taking steps in supported standing at 2 weeks, but was not able to do it now. The therapist should:

CHOICES:

1. Recommend that a full developmental examination be performed by the early intervention team.
2. Explain that this is normal and that the stepping was a newborn reflex that has gone away.
3. Recommend that the mother bring the infant to a pediatric neurologist.
4. Explain this was due to a stepping reflex that will reemerge around 10 months.

TEACHING POINTS

CORRECT ANSWER: 2

The mother probably saw the neonatal stepping reflex, which is normal in a newborn but is not exhibited in the older infant probably because of anthropomorphic factors and neural maturation. The age that this reflex typically disappears is 2–3 months of age.

INCORRECT CHOICES:

In most infants, pull-to-stand emerges at 8–9 months, whereas unassisted standing and walking occurs at 10 to 15 months. Stepping at this age is not the result of a reflex (does not reemerge later on). A full developmental examination or referral to a neurologist is not indicated, and should be performed only after the child is older and is not walking. It is important to remember that these norms are averages, and that children may be more advanced or slower in reaching these milestones.

TYPE OF REASONING: EVALUATION

One must have firm knowledge of the developmental milestones of infants in order to arrive at the correct conclusion. Using evaluative reasoning, one must evaluate the merits of the four possible choices and determine which solution seems most reasonable, given the infant's symptoms and behaviors. In this case, the behaviors are normal. If this question was answered incorrectly, review the neonatal stepping reflex and developmental milestones for walking.

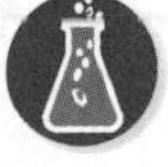

C119 | Musculoskeletal | Patient Examination

A patient complains of pain with mouth opening that makes it difficult to eat foods that require chewing. Examination revealed active mouth opening to be within normal limits of:

CHOICES:

1. 15–24 mm.
2. 35–44 mm.
3. 50–64 mm.
4. 65–74 mm.

TEACHING POINTS

CORRECT ANSWER: 2

Average AROM is approximately 35–50 mm. However, only 25–35 mm of opening between the teeth is required for normal everyday activity.

INCORRECT CHOICES:

The TMJs are considered hypomobile if < 25 mm of opening if achieved. Hypermobility would include values > 50 mm.

TYPE OF REASONING: ANALYSIS

One must recall normal AROM of the TMJ as well as functional AROM ranges in order to arrive at the correct conclusion. Through analytical reasoning, one must review each of the AROM parameters and determine which range seems most reasonable, given one's knowledge of normal ROM guidelines for the TMJ. If this question was answered incorrectly, review AROM guidelines for the TMJ.

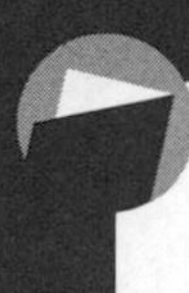

C120 | Other Systems | Foundational Sciences

An elderly and frail individual is receiving physical therapy in the home environment to improve general strengthening and mobility. The patient has a 4-year history of taking nonsteroidal anti-inflammatory drugs (NSAIDs; aspirin) for joint pain, and recently began taking a calcium channel blocker (verapamil). The therapist examines the patient for possible adverse side effects, which could include:

CHOICES:

1. Increased sweating, fatigue, chest pain.
2. Stomach pain, hypertension, dizziness.
3. Weight increase, hyperglycemia, hypotension.
4. Paresthesias, incoordination, bradycardia.

TEACHING POINTS

CORRECT ANSWER: 2

With advanced age, the capacity of the individual to break down and convert drugs diminishes secondary to decreased liver and kidney function, reduced hepatic and renal blood flow, etc. Some drugs additionally slow metabolism (e.g., calcium channel blockers like verapamil and diltiazem or antigout drugs like allopurinol). NSAIDs are associated with potential gastrointestinal effects (stomach pain, peptic ulcers, gastrointestinal hemorrhage), peripheral edema, and easy bruising and bleeding. NSAIDs can also lessen the effects of antihypertensive drugs. CNS effects can include headache, dizziness, lightheadedness, insomnia, tinnitus, confusion, and depression.

INCORRECT CHOICES:

The other choices do not include any of the expected adverse effects listed.

TYPE OF REASONING: DEDUCTIVE

This question requires the test taker to recall the typical side effects of taking both NSAIDs and calcium channel blockers. This is factual recall of information, which is a deductive reasoning skill. For this scenario, the therapist should anticipate potential side effects of stomach pain, hypertension, and dizziness. If this question was answered incorrectly, review side effects of NSAIDs and calcium channel blockers.

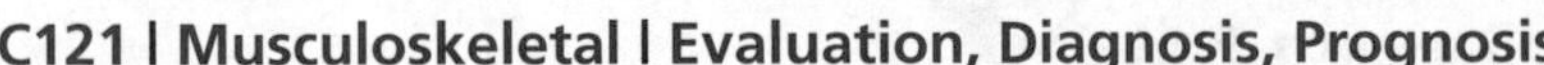

C121 | Musculoskeletal | Evaluation, Diagnosis, Prognosis

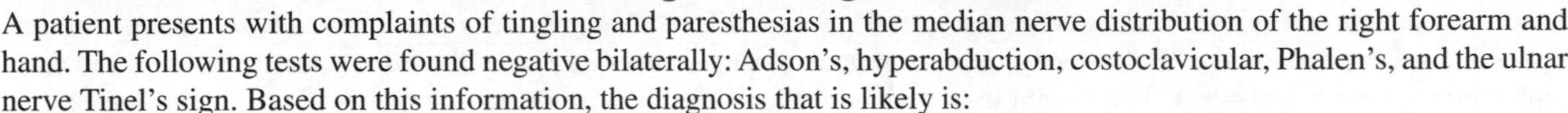

A patient presents with complaints of tingling and paresthesias in the median nerve distribution of the right forearm and hand. The following tests were found negative bilaterally: Adson's, hyperabduction, costoclavicular, Phalen's, and the ulnar nerve Tinel's sign. Based on this information, the diagnosis that is likely is:

CHOICES:

1. Thoracic outlet syndrome (TOS).
2. Pronator teres syndrome.
3. Carpal tunnel syndrome.
4. Ulnar nerve entrapment.

TEACHING POINTS

CORRECT ANSWER: 2

All of these special tests are used to determine neurological compromise of the lower trunk and brachial plexus. Special tests to rule out pronator teres syndrome are (1) passive supination to elongate the pronator, which is tight; this would compress the nerve at that level, and (2) active resistance of pronation, which would compress the nerve as it courses through the pronator muscle belly.

INCORRECT CHOICES:

A negative Adson's test, hyperabduction test, and costoclavicular test will rule out TOS. A negative Phalen's test will rule out carpal tunnel syndrome. A negative ulnar nerve Tinel's sign will rule out ulnar nerve entrapment. By process of elimination, pronator teres syndrome is the only diagnosis remaining.

TYPE OF REASONING: ANALYSIS

One must understand the tests described in the question in order to choose the correct solution. Through analytical reasoning, the test taker must determine what each test indicates (by a negative result) in order to determine the diagnosis that is likely. If this question was answered incorrectly, review information on provocative testing for pronator teres syndrome.

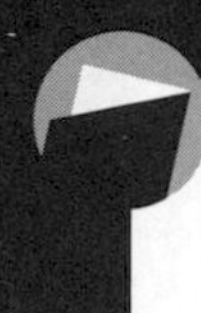

C122 | Devices, Admin., etc. | Teaching, Research, Roles

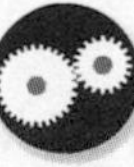

An elderly patient receiving outpatient physical therapy as a result of a CVA presents with a dense left hemiparesis of both upper and lower extremities. The patient requires minimal assistance for transfers and moderate assistance for 50 feet of ambulation with a hemiwalker. The patient lives with and is cared for by a single adult daughter. The patient arrives for a physical therapy session and the therapist notes multiple bruises on the patient's arms and legs. When asked about the bruises, the patient cannot explain how they occurred. Later in the session, the patient reports that her daughter is under a great deal of stress. In this case, the PT should:

CHOICES:

1. Call the police and have the daughter arrested for elder abuse.
2. Contact the Department of Adult Protective Services and file a report for suspected abuse/neglect.
3. Counsel the daughter on how to handle stress and advise her to hire a personal care attendant to help care for the patient.
4. Document the bruises and assess whether the bruises are resolved at the next visit.

TEACHING POINTS

CORRECT ANSWER: 2

PTs are mandated reporters of both child and elder abuse. The Code of Ethics and many state jurisdictions obligate PTs to report suspected cases of abuse involving children and vulnerable adults. Each jurisdiction will have a specific reporting mechanism and procedure that needs to be followed.

INCORRECT CHOICES:

The police should not be called because, at this point, there is no definitive proof of abuse and the patient did not say the daughter was abusing her; therefore, the abuse is not substantiated. Although the therapist may suggest to the daughter that help may be needed in the home, it is beyond the scope of practice to counsel the daughter about stress. Although the therapist should document the bruises, more needs to be done than waiting to the next session to reassess the bruising.

TYPE OF REASONING: EVALUATION

The question requires one to identify the signs of abuse and know the PT's obligation and procedure to report the suspected abuse. This necessitates evaluative reasoning skills. In order to answer this question correctly, the test taker needs to first identify the signs of abuse and then know the rules and regulations regarding mandated reporting and the Code of Ethics obligating the PT to do so. If this question was answered incorrectly, review the Code of Ethics Principle 4 (D).

C123 | Devices, Admin., etc. | Equipment, Modalities

A patient has been referred to the therapist status post fracture of the femur 3 months ago. The patient is unable to volitionally contract the quadriceps. The therapist decides to apply electrical stimulation to stimulate the strengthening of the quadriceps muscle. The **BEST** choice of electrode size and placement is:

CHOICES:

1. Large electrodes, closely spaced.
2. Small electrodes, closely spaced.
3. Small electrodes, widely spaced.
4. Large electrodes, widely spaced.

TEACHING POINTS

CORRECT ANSWER: 4

Two reasons to place a large electrode on a large muscle are to (1) stimulate a large number of muscle fibers and (2) reduce the current density generated under each electrode, making the current more comfortable to the patient. A wide interelectrode spacing will allow the current to stimulate deep muscle fibers.

INCORRECT CHOICES:

Larger amounts of current are used to obtain a contraction out of a muscle. Utilizing small electrodes would cause the current to be concentrated over a smaller surface area, thus increasing the current density under the electrode. Exceeding the current density of an electrode can cause patient discomfort, skin irritation, or a thermal burn. Close spacing of electrodes encourage superficial flow of current rather than deeper flow.

TYPE OF REASONING: DEDUCTIVE

The test taker must determine, through knowledge of electrical stimulation protocols and guidelines, the **BEST** choice of electrode size and placement. The recall of protocols and guidelines is factual in nature and is a deductive reasoning skill. If this question was answered incorrectly, review electrode placement and size guidelines for electrical stimulation.

C124 | Neuromuscular | Intervention

An elderly patient is recovering from a right CVA and demonstrates strong spasticity in the left upper extremity. The therapist wants to reduce the expected negative effects of spasticity in the left upper extremity while the patient is working on sitting control. The **BEST** position for the upper extremity is:

CHOICES:

1. Affected upper extremity extended and internally rotated, with the hand at the side.
2. Left elbow flexed with arm resting on supporting pillow, positioned on the patient's lap.
3. Left shoulder adducted and internal rotation, with arm extended and hand resting on the thigh.
4. Left shoulder abducted and externally rotated, with elbow extended and weight supported on the palm of the hand.

TEACHING POINTS

CORRECT ANSWER: 4

In the upper extremity, spasticity is typically strong in scapular retractors, shoulder adductors, depressors, and internal rotators; elbow flexors and forearm pronators; wrist and finger flexors. The patient should be positioned opposite the expected pattern.

INCORRECT CHOICES:

The other choices all emphasize one or more of the expected spastic muscles/pattern (i.e., internal rotation, elbow flexion, shoulder adduction, and internal rotation).

TYPE OF REASONING: INFERENCE

One must recall the patterns of spasticity in the body after CVA in order to arrive at the correct solution. This requires inferential reasoning skill, in which the test taker must draw conclusions from the evidence presented and determine the possible outcomes from implementing the above positions for this patient. If this question was answered incorrectly, review spasticity after CVA and positioning strategies.

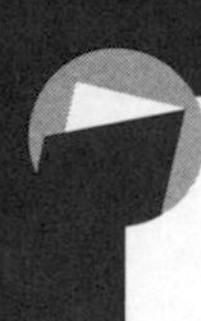

C125 | Neuromuscular | Patient Examination

If the subject's vision is blocked, either by having the subject close the eyes or by placing a barrier between the part being tested and the subject's eyes, the therapist can effectively examine:

CHOICES:

1. Somatosensory integrity.
2. Vestibular/visual/somatosensory integration.
3. Discriminative touch and fast pain, but not proprioception.
4. Conscious proprioception, but not discriminative touch.

TEACHING POINTS

CORRECT ANSWER: 1

The term "somatosensation" refers to conscious relay pathways for discriminative touch, conscious proprioception, fast pain, and discriminative temperature. Sensory examination must rule out vision in order to establish the reliability of sensory testing.

INCORRECT CHOICES:

Vestibular/visual/somatosensory integration can be established only by a series of tests that include both eyes open and eyes closed, and by using flat and compliant (foam) or moving surfaces. The other choices exclude one of the sensory sensations that should be tested with the eyes closed.

TYPE OF REASONING: INFERENCE

One must infer why blocking a subject's vision is important for certain testing protocols in order to arrive at the correct conclusion. Of all the named functions, somatosensory integrity requires the blocking of vision in order to effectively determine that the pathway is intact. Inferential reasoning is utilized, because the test taker must infer why absence of vision is important to determining the functioning of each pathway.

C126 | Musculoskeletal | Patient Examination

An adolescent felt a "clunk" in the lumbar spine 2 weeks ago while lifting weight. There was immediate right lumbar pain and spasm. Posteroanterior and bilateral radiographic views of the lumbar spine were normal except L4 was shifted approximately 1 mm anterior to L5 on the lateral views. Which of the following imaging techniques would give the PT the best information regarding a diagnosis and formulating a plan of care for this individual?

CHOICES:

1. Posteroanterior T1 magnetic resonance imaging (MRI).
2. Posteroanterior computed tomography (CT) scan.
3. Right oblique radiograph.
4. Bilateral oblique radiographs.

TEACHING POINTS

CORRECT ANSWER: 4

The clinician should suspect a spondylolisthesis. A spondylolisthesis is a forward slippage of a vertebra due to a *bilateral* defect in the pars interarticularis. Causes include congenital, acute fracture, or degenerative conditions. The degree of forward slippage is graded on a 1–4 scale (4 being the most severe or a 75–100% slippage) from the lateral view. It is unclear from the description whether there is an actual spondylolisthesis. Bilateral oblique views with a radiograph are needed to see whether there is a fracture at the pars interarticularis bilaterally. This is known as the "Scottie dog" defect (see appendix in Chapter 1 for example).

INCORRECT CHOICES:

A unilateral view would provide information only about one pars interarticularis. Although a CT scan and MRI might add some benefit, the posteroanterior view with these expensive techniques have no added benefit. Depending upon the pathology or presentation of a client, a PT should be able to recommend appropriate medical imaging to ensure accurate and effective patient/client treatment and management decisions.

TYPE OF REASONING: INFERENCE

This question requires one to infer or draw a reasonable conclusion about imaging techniques that would provide the best information about a diagnosis and developing a plan of care. This requires inferential reasoning skill. For this scenario, the best imaging technique would be bilateral oblique radiographs for suspected spondylolisthesis. If this question was answered incorrectly, review symptoms of spondylolisthesis and radiographic imaging.

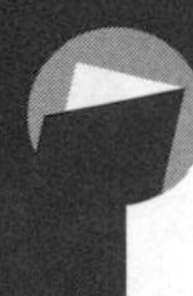

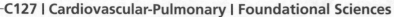

C127 | Cardiovascular-Pulmonary | Foundational Sciences

A therapist is asked to advise a healthy 70 year-old individual who wants to take part in a graduated conditioning program by joining the "Mall Walkers Club." The therapist's **BEST** approach to prescribing the intensity of exercise for this individual is:

CHOICES:

1. Dyspnea scale.
2. Maximal age-related HR.
3. HR reserve formula.
4. 4–8 MET level walking.

TEACHING POINTS

CORRECT ANSWER: 3

Expected changes in the elderly include a lower VO_{2max}, which is evidenced by a lower maximal HR, decreased muscle strength with increased fatigability, and decreased neuromuscular coordination and balance. HR is used as a guide to determine exercise intensity because of the relatively linear relationship between HR and VO_2. The HR reserve method (Karvonen's formula) more accurately depicts the intensity relative to oxygen consumption than HR alone, especially when working with low-fit clients.

INCORRECT CHOICES:

High variability exists for maximal HRs in persons over 65 years of age. Thus, use of this measure is not recommended. MET levels also vary considerably from individual to individual and cannot be relied on; 8 METs represents slow jogging and is not appropriate for this individual. The dyspnea scale measures shorteness of breath and cannot be used to prescribe intensity of exercise.

TYPE OF REASONING: INDUCTIVE

One must determine, given the patient's age and current health status, the **BEST** approach to prescribing the intensity of exercise. This requires clinical judgment and diagnostic reasoning, which is an inductive reasoning skill. If this question was answered incorrectly, review principles of exercise prescription.

C128 | Neuromuscular | Evaluation, Diagnosis, Prognosis

A patient recovering from stroke has been using a bilateral exerciser (UBE) to strengthen muscles in the affected right upper extremity. The patient is now experiencing burning pain in the shoulder that worsens when the limb is touched or moved. Paresthesias and pitting edema in the dorsum of the hand are also present along with painful and diminished ROM of the wrist and fingers. The therapist's **BEST** course of action is to:

CHOICES:

1. Discontinue exercise and use ice for pain relief.
2. Switch to interval exercise and lower the resistance on the UBE.
3. Discontinue UBE exercise, splint the hand and wrist until pain and swelling disappear.
4. Discontinue UBE exercise and initiate elevation, massage, and active assistive ROM.

TEACHING POINTS

CORRECT ANSWER: 4

This patient presents with the classic signs and symptoms of early-stage complex regional pain syndrome (CRPS), type I (reflex sympathetic dystrophy). Interventions are chosen to quiet the sympathetic nervous system and promote pain relief. Edema can be successfully managed with a combination of elevation, massage, and compression bandaging. Restoring ROM (AROM) is also important in the treatment of CRPS.

INCORRECT CHOICES:

Immobilization through splinting is contraindicated because the joints will stiffen with lack of ROM. Thermotherapy is more beneficial than cryotherapy for pain relief because there is no accompanying sympathetic nervous system stimulation as there is with cold. Altering the exercise prescription while continuing with resistive exercise can worsen the problem.

TYPE OF REASONING: INFERENCE

The test taker must first infer the reason for the patient's symptoms and then determine what the **BEST** course of action is to effectively manage those symptoms. If this question was answered incorrectly, review intervention guidelines for CRPS.

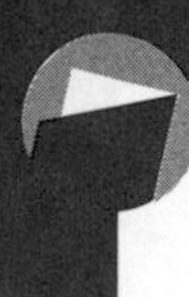

C129 | Other Systems | Evaluation, Diagnosis, Prognosis

The PT has just completed a chart review of a new patient referred for general mobilization after a colon resection with colostomy placement the previous day. At bedside, the therapist observes an intravenous line with clear fluid, a urinary catheter, and oxygen cannula. A second intravenous line is about half way through infusing blood products. All vital signs are stable. Upon taking a history, the patient is found to be alert, oriented, cooperative, and reporting pain at 4/10. The **BEST** plan for the examination is to:

CHOICES:

1. Assess functional abilities monitoring HR, BP, pulmonary status, skin integrity, and tolerance to activity.
2. Request pain medication for this patient because a 4/10 is not consistent with mobilizing a patient.
3. Delay physical assessment due to the infusion of blood products.
4. Postpone examination until postoperative day 3 until patient stabilizes.

TEACHING POINTS

CORRECT ANSWER: 1

A blood transfusion is a type of transplant, meaning transplanting material from one living person to another. Physical therapy tests and measures and interventions need not be withheld while patients are receiving blood products, but the patient should be monitored for signs of acute rejection.

INCORRECT CHOICES:

On postoperative day 1, a pain rating of 4/10 may be the best that is reasonable, even with the best of pharmacological management of pain. Infusion of blood products is not a reason to delay physical therapy examination and intervention; however, adverse reactions to the infusion of blood products would be a reason to abort an examination or intervention. Patients can certainly be seen on postoperative day 1 as long as vital signs are stable and the patient is engaged in the process.

TYPE OF REASONING: INFERENCE

This question requires the test taker to determine a **BEST** course of action, given the information provided, which is an inferential reasoning skill. The key to arriving at a correct conclusion is recognizing that a patient receiving blood products may be at higher risk for symptoms of rejection; therefore, physical assessment should be monitored for these symptoms. If this question was answered incorrectly, review guidelines for physical assessment of patients receiving blood products.

C130 | Devices, Admin., etc. | Teaching, Research, Roles

A group of researchers (the Ottawa Panel) utilized meta-analysis to identify the evidence for aerobic fitness exercises in the management of fibromyalgia. Thirteen randomized, controlled trials (RCTs) and three controlled clinical trials (cohort studies and case-control studies) were selected. The main difference between the two types of trials is the:

CHOICES:

1. Length of the studies.
2. Use of multiple centers versus single-center trials.
3. Duration of the studies.
4. Use of randomization of subjects.

TEACHING POINTS

CORRECT ANSWER: 4

The main difference between the two types of trials is randomization of subjects into experimental and control groups (RCT).

INCORRECT CHOICES:

Meta-analysis involves the combining of a series of independent, previously published studies of similiar purpose to yield a larger target population. RCTs are used and can be either single-center or multiple-center trials. A cohort study is a prospective study involving a group of participants with a similiar condition. Comparison is made with a matched group that does not have the condition. Duration or length of studies are not distinguishing factors between the two types of studies.

TYPE OF REASONING: DEDUCTIVE

One must recall the guidelines for both RCTs and controlled clinical trials in order to arrive at a correct conclusion. Recalling such guidelines is factual information, which requires deductive reasoning skill. If this question was answered incorrectly, review types of research designs, especially RCTs and controlled clinical trials.

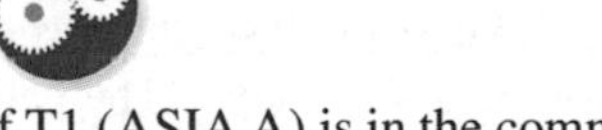

C131 | Neuromuscular | Intervention

A patient with a spinal cord injury at the level of T1 (ASIA A) is in the community phase of mobility training. In order for the patient to navigate a 4-inch-height curb with the wheelchair, the therapist tells the patient to:

CHOICES:

1. Descend backward with the trunk upright and arms hooked around the push handles.
2. Ascend backward with the large wheels first.
3. Lift the front casters and ascend in a wheelie position.
4. Place the front casters down first during descent.

TEACHING POINTS

CORRECT ANSWER: 3

Curbs are ascended in the wheelie position (front casters lifted and moving first). Individuals must learn to use momentum and a strong push to elevate the front casters of the chair (wheelie position) and propel the wheelchair up the curb.

INCORRECT CHOICES:

Patients can descend backward but must use a tucked forward lean position in order to prevent falling backward or they can descend forward using a wheelie position, large wheels landing first. Curbs are not ascended backward or descended with the front casters touching first.

TYPE OF REASONING: EVALUATION

Evaluative reasoning is important to arriving at the correct conclusion for this question, because the test taker must evaluate the merits of the four choices and then determine what is safe and appropriate for this patient. If this question was answered incorrectly, review curb negotiation guidelines for patients with paraplegia.

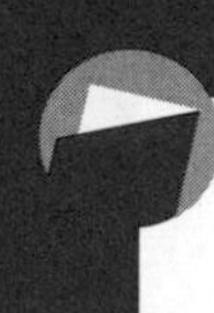

C132 | Cardiovascular-Pulmonary | Foundational Sciences

A patient with a long history of systemic steroid use for asthma control has a contraindication for percussion if there is evidence of:

CHOICES:

1. Decreased bone density.
2. Intercostal muscle wasting.
3. BP > 140/90.
4. Barrel chest.

TEACHING POINTS

CORRECT ANSWER: 1

The only one that is a contraindication to percussion would be decreased bone density, because a rib fracture might be a possible result.

INCORRECT CHOICES:

Although the other choices are sequelae to long-term systemic steroid use, they are not a contraindication for percussion. An increased BP higher than that reported in the scenario might be a contraindication to postural drainage. It is not a contraindication to percussion. Barrel chest is seen in patients with emphysema, not asthma.

TYPE OF REASONING: INFERENCE

One must determine, given an understanding of the nature of long-term systemic steroid use for asthma, which condition would contraindicate percussion. It is beneficial to understand how percussion is performed, because it helps one to reason why decreased bone density would contraindicate the therapy. Inferential reasoning skill is used, because one must infer the effects of long-term steroid use coupled with the nature of percussion therapy when used with patients who have asthma.

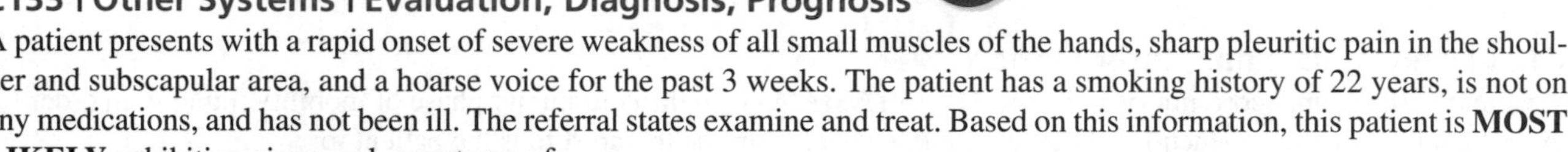

C133 | Other Systems | Evaluation, Diagnosis, Prognosis

A patient presents with a rapid onset of severe weakness of all small muscles of the hands, sharp pleuritic pain in the shoulder and subscapular area, and a hoarse voice for the past 3 weeks. The patient has a smoking history of 22 years, is not on any medications, and has not been ill. The referral states examine and treat. Based on this information, this patient is **MOST LIKELY** exhibiting signs and symptoms of:

CHOICES:

1. A C5–6 bilateral foraminal stenosis.
2. Thoracic outlet syndrome (TOS).
3. Ascending Guillain-Barré syndrome.
4. A Pancoast tumor.

TEACHING POINTS

CORRECT ANSWER: 4

A Pancoast tumor is an apical tumor that is typically found in conjunction with a smoking history. The clinical signs and symptoms can be confused with neurovascular compromise at the level of thoracic outlet. Rapid onset of clinical signs and symptoms and pleuritic pain are highly suspect of an apical tumor. The smoking history and hoarse voice coupled with the other symptoms make this a "red flag" situation that must be reported immediately.

INCORRECT CHOICES:

The pain reported is not typical of Guillain-Barré syndrome (progressive muscle weakness in ascending order and mild sensory symptoms, paresthesias, and hypesthesias). TOS does not typically present bilaterally. Foraminal stenosis in the mid cervical spine will not cause weakness in the hand intrinsics.

TYPE OF REASONING: ANALYSIS

Questions that inquire about a group of symptoms whereby the test taker must determine the diagnosis encourage analytical reasoning skill. One must analyze all of the symptoms presented and determine the precise meaning of that information in order to arrive at the correct conclusion. If this question was answered incorrectly, review Pancoast tumor.

C134 | Devices, Admin., etc. | Teaching, Research, Roles

A group of researchers examined the effects of balance exercises on proprioception. Older adults were randomly assigned to a balance exercise group or a falls prevention group. Twenty-four healthy young adults were used as controls. The researchers found short-term improvements in velocity sense, but not in movement and position sense. In this study, the role of the control group was as:

CHOICES:

1. Matched controls receiving both intervention conditions.
2. Matched controls receiving the balance training intervention.
3. Matched controls receiving the fall prevention education.
4. Comparison with normal proprioception abilities.

TEACHING POINTS

CORRECT ANSWER: 4

The controls were used for comparison to normal proprioception abilities at the ankle joint (the participants were assessed once).

INCORRECT CHOICES:

The controls did not participate in either intervention. Younger adults cannot serve as matched controls to an older age group.

TYPE OF REASONING: DEDUCTIVE

Recall of research guidelines often necessitates deductive reasoning skill. In this case, the test taker must recall the role of a control group as it applies to this specific scenario. If this question was answered incorrectly, review research guidelines and use of control groups in research.

C135 | Devices, Admin., etc. | Equipment, Modalities

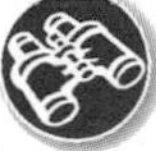

The therapist is applying cervical traction using a cervical harness. The patient complains of pain in the TMJ during the treatment. The therapist should consider:

CHOICES:

1. Reducing the traction poundage and continuing with the treatment.
2. Readjusting the harness and continuing with the treatment.
3. Decreasing the treatment time.
4. Discontinuing traction.

TEACHING POINTS

CORRECT ANSWER: 2

Readjusting the cervical harness angle to increase the force at the back of the skull (occipital protuberance) and lessen the force on the mandible would decrease the pressure on the TMJ and make the treatment more comfortable for the patient.

INCORRECT CHOICES:

When using a cervical harness, there is no way to avoid transmitting the force through the TMJ. Decreasing the force would only decrease the amount, but it would still be concentrated in the TMJ. In addition, decreasing the force may decrease the effectiveness of the treatment. Treatment time does not effect the force being transmitted to the TMJ. Clinically, one would attempt to readjust the harness before discontinuing traction altogether.

TYPE OF REASONING: INDUCTIVE

One must utilize clinical judgment to determine the best course of action for a patient experiencing TMJ pain with cervical traction. Situations that require the test taker to use clinical judgment and diagnostic reasoning encourage inductive reasoning skill. If this question was answered incorrectly, review information on applications of cervical traction and harness adjustments.

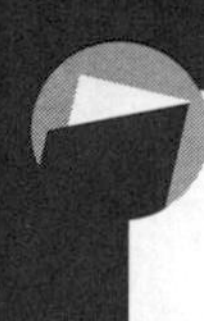

C136 | Musculoskeletal | Intervention 

A therapist is treating a patient with a diagnosis of right shoulder rotator cuff tendinitis. The findings of a work site ergonomic assessment indicate that the worker is required to perform repetitive reaching activities above shoulder height. The most appropriate work site modification would be to:

CHOICES:

1. Allow the worker to take more frequent rests to avoid overuse.
2. Reposition the height of the shelf and items to below shoulder height.
3. Provide the worker with a taller, sit-stand chair.
4. Provide the worker with a standing desk for daily activities.

TEACHING POINTS

CORRECT ANSWER: 2

Work stations should be designed to accommodate the persons who actually work on the job. Work stations should be easily adjustable and designed to be comfortable for the worker. In this case, lowering the height of the shelf for frequent use is best.

INCORRECT CHOICES:

Taking more frequent rests or providing a different chair does not eliminate the essential problem of repetitive overhead reach that is causing the shoulder tendinitis. Using a standing desk would eliminate overhead reach, but is not as practical as lowering the shelf. In the workplace, individuals cannot be expected to stand all day long.

TYPE OF REASONING: INFERENCE

One must infer the best solution to alleviate the patient's right shoulder rotator cuff tendinitis, given the nature of the patient's work environment. In this situation, one should infer that the overhead repetitive reaching is the cause for the diagnosis; therefore, reaching below shoulder height would help to alleviate the symptoms. If this question was answered incorrectly, refer to information on ergonomic workstation assessment.

C137 | Devices, Admin., etc. | Teaching, Research, Roles 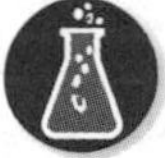

A therapist is conducting a falls prevention workshop for a group of caregivers of individuals with Parkinson's disease. Much of the material is presented at basic introductory level. During the last class, the participants are shown a PowerPoint presentation depicting various home environments and asked to identify hazards. According to the taxonomy of cognitive behavioral objectives, this activity involves:

CHOICES:

1. Analysis.
2. Comprehension.
3. Synthesis.
4. Recall.

TEACHING POINTS

CORRECT ANSWER: 1

The cognitive domain has six levels. This activity involves analysis, the ability to distinguish how an environment is organized or arranged (level 4.0).

INCORRECT CHOICES:

Comprehension involves understanding at its lowest level, the ability to use (translate, interpret) information (level 2.0), synthesis is a high-level activity and involves the putting together of elements to form a whole (formulate a plan of care) (level 5.0). Recall or knowledge is the lowest level and involves the ability to remember information (define or describe) (level 1.0).

TYPE OF REASONING: ANALYSIS

This question provides a description of an educational activity, and the test taker must recall not only cognitive taxonomy guidelines (deductive reasoning skill) but also how those guidelines apply to the educational activity described, which requires analytical reasoning. If this question was answered incorrectly, review the taxonomy of cognitive behavioral objectives.

C138 | Devices, Admin., etc. | Equipment, Modalities

A patient presents with pain of the right Achilles' tendon as well as on the plantar aspect of the right heel. Pain developed insidiously and has now lasted several months. On gait analysis, the therapist observes abnormal supination throughout the stance phase of gait. The **BEST** choice for orthotic intervention is a:

CHOICES:

1. Cushion heel with medial rearfoot and forefoot posts.
2. UCBL (University of California Biomechanics Laboratory).
3. Flexible shoe insert with forefoot varus post.
4. Metatarsal pad.

TEACHING POINTS

CORRECT ANSWER: 1

This patient is presenting with symptoms of plantar fasciitis and heel pain. A cushion heel with an orthotic that provides support to the longitudinal arch (medial rearfoot and forefoot posts) is the best choice for intervention.

INCORRECT CHOICES:

A UCBL insert is prescribed to realign a flexible flatfoot. Forefoot posting is used to correct an abnormal forefoot position (pronation of the subtalar joint) in relationship to the rearfoot. A metatarsal pad is used to transfer stress from painful metatarsal heads in metatarsalgia.

TYPE OF REASONING: INFERENCE

One must first infer what the cause(s) for the symptoms are and then, based on this reasoning, determine the **BEST** choice for orthotic intervention. This necessitates inferential reasoning, in which one must draw conclusions from the information presented in order to make a **BEST** course of action determination. If this question was answered incorrectly, review plantar fasciitis and orthotic shoe inserts.

C139 | Cardiovascular-Pulmonary | Patient Examination

A patient has a 10-year history of peripheral vascular disease (PVD) affecting the right lower extremity. During auscultation of the popliteal artery, the therapist would expect to find:

CHOICES:

1. A bruit.
2. A positive Homan's sign.
3. 4+ pulses.
4. Intense pain and cramping.

TEACHING POINTS

CORRECT ANSWER: 1

A bruit is a swishing sound that occurs in the presence of narrowing of an artery. It is a characteristic finding of PVD present on auscultation.

INCORRECT CHOICES:

All other choices are not revealed on auscultation. Pulse palpation of the extremities will likely reveal a 0 (no pulse) or 1+ (diminished, barely perceptible), not 4+ (bounding, very strong). Homan's sign is pain in the calf when the foot is passively dorsiflexed. It is no longer considered an accurate test to detect DVT. Severe or intense pain with cramping is a likely response when the patient subjectively grades ambulatory ischemic pain. It is not auscultation.

TYPE OF REASONING: INFERENCE

This question requires one to infer what a therapist should find with a patient who has a history of PVD. One must have a solid understanding of the nature of PVD and examination measures in order to choose the correct solution. If this question was answered incorrectly, review PVD examination.

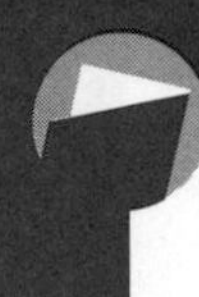

C140 | Other Systems | Foundational Sciences

A therapist is working in a major medical center and is new to the acute care setting. An orientation session for new employees concerns infection control. The therapist recognizes that the most common infection transmitted to health care workers is:

CHOICES:

1. Hepatitis A.
2. Human immunodeficiency virus (HIV).
3. Hepatitis B.
4. Tuberculosis.

TEACHING POINTS

CORRECT ANSWER: 3

Health care workers are most likely to contract hepatitis B (estimated incidence 300,000 new acute cases in United States each year). Transmission is through exposure to blood and blood products and infected body fluids.

INCORRECT CHOICES:

Hepatitis A has a much lower reported incidence (35,000 new cases each year), and is transmitted primarily through the fecal-oral route and contaminated food or water. HIV and tuberculosis also have lower incidences. HIV has a similar route infection as hepatitis B, whereas tuberculosis is an airborne infectious disease. See Box 6–1 Standard Precautions.

TYPE OF REASONING: DEDUCTIVE

Recall of the most common infection transmitted to health care workers is factual information, which necessitates deductive reasoning skill. Through recall of infection control information, one should conclude that hepatitis B is the most common infection to be transmitted. If this question was answered incorrectly, refer to infection control guidelines, especially transmission of hepatitis B.

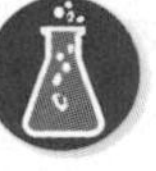

C141 | Musculoskeletal | Evaluation, Diagnosis, Prognosis

A patient presents with pain, joint swelling, subcutaneous olecranon nodules, and increased erythrocyte sedimentation rate (ESR). These findings are characteristic of:

CHOICES:

1. Rheumatoid arthritis (RA).
2. Fibromyalgia.
3. Systemic lupus erythematosus (SLE).
4. Osteoarthritis.

TEACHING POINTS

CORRECT ANSWER: 1

RA is characterized by morning stiffness, pain, and relatively symmetrical joint involvement. Laboratory abnormalities in RA include positive serum rheumatoid factor (RF) and elevated ESR. Articular and extra-articular manifestations include weight loss, malaise, nodulosis, and vasculitis. Synovial fluid analysis reveals elevated white blood cell count and protein count.

INCORRECT CHOICES:

Osteoarthritis (OA), or degenerative joint pain, and fibromyalgia both produce pain but do not produce the laboratory findings reported or nodulosis. SLE is an immunological disorder characterized by inflammatory lesions in multiple organ systems. It is diagnosed by client history (multiple organ involvement, especially of skin, joints, serous membranes), systemic symptoms (e.g., fever, malaise, fatigability), and appearance of skin rash (erythema). ESR is elevated in patients with SLE; however, nodulosis and joint malformations are not expected.

TYPE OF REASONING: ANALYSIS

One must analyze the symptoms presented in order to make a determination of the likely diagnosis. This requires analytical reasoning skill, in which one must determine the meaning of the symptoms in order to determine a diagnosis for the patient. In this case, the symptoms indicate rheumatoid arthritis, which should be reviewed if this question was answered incorrectly.

C142 | Devices, Admin., etc. | Equipment, Modalities 

A patient with a transfemoral amputation and an above-knee prosthesis demonstrates knee instability while standing. The patient's knee buckles easily when performing weight shifts. The therapist suspects the cause of his problem is a:

CHOICES:

1. Prosthetic knee set too far posterior to the trochanter-knee-ankle (TKA) line.
2. Prosthetic knee set too far anterior to the TKA line.
3. Weak gluteus medius.
4. Tight extension aide.

TEACHING POINTS

CORRECT ANSWER: 2

In order to increase stability of the knee, the prosthetic knee is normally aligned posterior to a line extending from the trochanter to the ankle (TKA line). A knee set anterior to the TKA line will buckle easily.

INCORRECT CHOICES:

A prosthetic knee set too far posterior to the TKA would result in excessive knee stability and difficulty flexing the knee. The gluteus medius contributes to stability during stance, primarily lateral stability. Weak abductors can result in trunk lateral bend during stance. An extension aide assists knee extension during the latter part of swing phase. A tight extension aide will result in terminal swing impact during late swing.

TYPE OF REASONING: INDUCTIVE

Clinical judgment and diagnostic reasoning are utilized to determine the likely cause for the patient's knee instability while standing. Through inductive reasoning, the test taker should determine that the prosthetic knee is set too far anterior to the TKA line. If this question was answered incorrectly, review information on prosthetic adjustment/alignment for above-knee prostheses.

C143 | Devices, Admin., etc. | Equipment, Modalities

An adolescent with developmental disabilities is referred to a wheelchair clinic for a new wheelchair. The patient presents with a severe kyphoscoliosis. The therapist determines the **BEST** wheelchair modification to order is a:

CHOICES:

1. Sling seat with dense foam cushion.
2. Firm seat back with lateral posture supports and increased seat depth.
3. Contoured foam seat.
4. Firm seat with lateral knee positioners.

TEACHING POINTS

CORRECT ANSWER: 3

A contoured foam seat that accommodates to the patient's body contours and provides an adequate seat base and lateral support to stabilize the scoliosis provides the **BEST** option.

INCORRECT CHOICES:

A sling seat tends to increase asymmetries. Increasing the seat depth encourages a posterior pelvic tilt and increases kyphosis. A firm seat with lateral knee positioners does not address trunk problems.

TYPE OF REASONING: INDUCTIVE

One must utilize clinical judgment and diagnostic thinking to determine the **BEST** wheelchair modification to order for a patient with severe kyphoscoliosis. This requires knowledge of the various modification devices described in the options and what they address in order to determine that a contoured foam seat is the best solution.

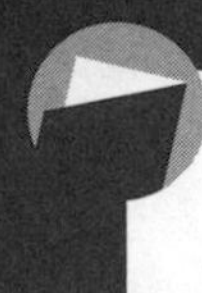

C144 | Devices, Admin., etc. | Teaching, Research, Roles

A group of researchers recruited 19 individuals with multiple sclerosis to participate in a study comparing the effects of an 8-week aerobic training program on exercise capacity. Specifically, walking capacity, maximum exercise tolerance, and fatigue levels were examined. Eleven subjects completed the study. This study is an example of a:

CHOICES:

1. Case series.
2. Case report.
3. Cohort study.
4. Single RCT.

TEACHING POINTS

CORRECT ANSWER: 3

This is a cohort study. It investigates a group of individuals with common characteristics. All subjects receive a common intervention and are examined according to a predetermined set of dependent variables (walking capacity, maximum exercise tolerance, and fatigue levels). It is a quasi-experimental study with limited generalizibility.

INCORRECT CHOICES:

No control group was used, so it is not a RCT. It is also not a case series or case report because all subjects were treated the same.

TYPE OF REASONING: DEDUCTIVE

One must recall the guidelines for a cohort study in order to arrive at a correct conclusion. This necessitates recall of guidelines and principles, which is a deductive reasoning skill. If this question was answered incorrectly, review cohort study guidelines.

C145 | Devices, Admin., etc. | Teaching, Research, Roles

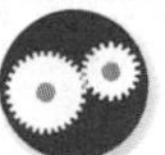

A patient who is undergoing spinal cord rehabilitation is viewed as uncooperative by staff. The patient refuses to complete the training activities outlined to promote independent functional mobility. A review of history reveals that previously the patient was the director of a company with a staff of 20. The **MOST** appropriate strategy the therapist can adopt is to:

CHOICES:

1. Carefully structure the activities and slow down the pace of training.
2. Have the patient work with a supervisor who is a person in authority.
3. Refer the patient to a support group before resuming rehabilitation.
4. Involve the patient in goal setting and structuring the training session.

TEACHING POINTS

CORRECT ANSWER: 4

An andragogical approach is best. The patient is an adult learner who should be allowed to share in the responsibility for planning the learning experience and goal setting. The therapist should help clarify the problem, structure the learning environment, and provide necessary resources.

INCORRECT CHOICES:

Passing the buck or transferring responsibility to a supervisor is not appropriate . Requiring participation in a support group before continuing rehabilitation or slowing down the pace of training would negatively impact rehabilitation and result in increased length of stay.

TYPE OF REASONING: EVALUATION

One must evaluate the merits of each statement in order to make a best course determination for this patient. This question requires a judgment call and a value judgment, which necessitates evaluative reasoning skill. For this patient, it is **MOST** appropriate to involve the patient in goal setting and have him participate in structuring the training session.

C146 | Devices, Admin., etc. | Teaching, Research, Roles

A group of 10 patients is recruited into a study investigating the effects of relaxation training on BP. One group of patients is scheduled to participate in a supervised cardiac rehabilitation program that includes relaxation training 3 times a week for 12 weeks. The other group of patients is instructed to perform activities as usual. At the conclusion of the study, there was no significant difference between the groups; BP decreased significantly in both groups. The investigator can reasonably conclude:

CHOICES:

1. The activities of the nonrehabilitation group were not properly monitored and may account for these results.
2. Cardiac rehabilitation is not effective in reducing BP.
3. Both groups had BPs initially so high that reductions should have been expected.
4. The rehabilitation group was not properly monitored.

TEACHING POINTS

CORRECT ANSWER: 1

To ensure adequate control, the researcher should attempt to remove the influence of any variable other than the independent variable in order to evaluate its effect on the dependent variable. In this study, the investigator did not adequately investigate the usual activities of the control group. The small number of subjects may also have contributed to lack of significance.

INCORRECT CHOICES:

Accepting any statements concerning initial BP or changes in BP is not warranted because data on specific BPs were not provided. The rehabilitation group was closely supervised.

TYPE OF REASONING: INFERENCE

Whereas research-related questions are typically factual in nature, requiring deductive reasoning skill, this question specifically asks for one to draw conclusions based on evidence and infer the reason for the research outcomes, which is an inferential reasoning skill.

C147 | Devices, Admin., etc. | Equipment, Modalities

A patient is using a right KAFO. During orthotic checkout, the therapist discovers that the height of the medial upright is excessive. As weight is transferred onto the orthotic leg during gait, the therapist expects that this patient will demonstrate:

CHOICES:

1. Posterior trunk bending.
2. Lateral lean toward the left.
3. Lateral lean toward the right.
4. Anterior trunk bending.

TEACHING POINTS

CORRECT ANSWER: 3

Lateral trunk bending toward the orthotic stance leg can result from (1) excessive height of the medial upright (in this example), (2) weak gluteus medius (Trendelenburg's gait), (3) abduction contracture, or (4) a short leg.

INCORRECT CHOICES:

Posterior trunk bending is associated with a weak gluteus maximus, whereas anterior trunk bending is associated with a weak quadriceps. Lateral lean to the left is not expected because it would cause pain in the groin region.

TYPE OF REASONING: INFERENCE

This question asks one to infer the likely results of a KAFO that has excessive medial upright height, which requires inferential reasoning. Having knowledge of KAFOs and proper fitting of them, one should conclude that a patient with this issue will demonstrate lateral lean toward the right. If this question was answered incorrectly, review information on orthotic checkout and orthotic gait analysis.

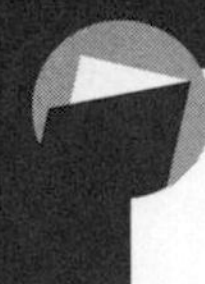

C148 | Devices, Admin., etc. | Equipment, Modalities 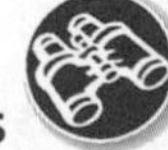

During gait, a patient with hemiparesis drags the toes during swing. Upon further examination, the patient has weak dorsiflexors (able to lift the foot against gravity through half range) and a grade of 2 upon examining tone in the plantarflexors using the Modified Ashworth Scale. An appropriate orthotic modification to correct this problem is an ankle-foot orthosis (AFO) with:

CHOICES:

1. A dorsiflexion assist.
2. Spiral plastic design.
3. A solid ankle.
4. A dorsiflexion stop.

TEACHING POINTS

CORRECT ANSWER: 3

A solid AFO is indicated to control footdrop in the presence of spasticity. A grade of 2 (Modified Ashworth Scale) indicates marked increase in muscle tone throughout the range, but the affected part can be moved.

INCORRECT CHOICES:

A dorsiflexion assist and spiral AFO are contraindicated, because they fail to adequately control spasticity and can actually increase spasticity. An anterior or dorsiflexion stop limits dorsiflexion and can be used with weakness of the plantarflexors (not a problem in this case).

TYPE OF REASONING: INDUCTIVE

This question requires diagnostic reasoning, because the test taker must determine an appropriate orthotic modification to correct the patient's problem. Diagnostic reasoning requires inductive reasoning skill, and one should determine through this skill that a solid ankle AFO will best correct the problem. Knowledge of AFOs is necessary to arrive at the correct conclusion.

C149 | Neuromuscular | Evaluation, Diagnosis, Prognosis 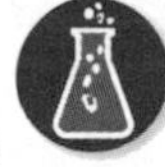

A therapist is examining a 24 month-old child and observes that the child can sit independently, creep in quadruped, pull-to-stand, cruise sideways, but not walk without support. The therapist concludes that this child is exhibiting:

CHOICES:

1. Normal cephalocaudal motor development.
2. Delay in achieving developmental milestones.
3. Normal gross motor development.
4. Slow maturation that is within normal limits.

TEACHING POINTS

CORRECT ANSWER: 2

The 12 to 15 month-old child should be ambulating. At 24 months, lack of ambulation is indicative of developmental delay. Other developmental milestones include sitting at 6 months and creeping, pull-to-stand, and cruise at 8–9 months.

INCORRECT CHOICES:

These findings are not indicative of normal motor milestones (normal cephalocaudal motor development, normal gross motor development, slow maturation within normal limits). In fact, 24 months represents considerable delay in ambulation.

TYPE OF REASONING: ANALYSIS

One must recall the normal developmental milestones of children in order to determine through analytical reasoning that a 24-month-old child who is not ambulating is delayed. Analytical reasoning is utilized whenever one must determine the precise meaning of information and make interpretations from that information. If this question was answered incorrectly, review the developmental milestones of children through the first 2 years.

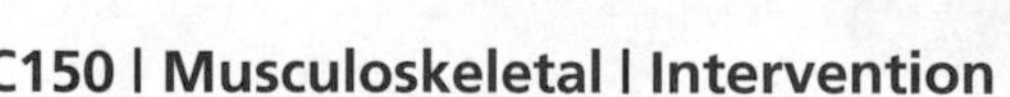

C150 | Musculoskeletal | Intervention

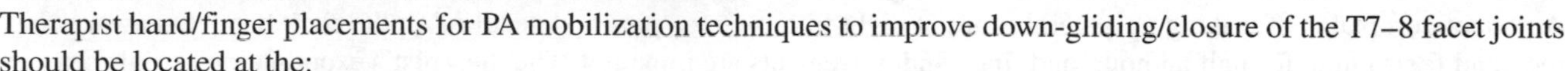

Therapist hand/finger placements for PA mobilization techniques to improve down-gliding/closure of the T7–8 facet joints should be located at the:

CHOICES:

1. Transverse processes of T8.
2. Spinous process of T8.
3. Transverse processes of T7.
4. Spinous process of T6.

TEACHING POINTS

CORRECT ANSWER: 1

The axis of motion for the mid thoracic vertebrae is above the spinous processes and below the transverse processes. Therefore, if down-gliding/closure of T7–8 vertebral segment is required, the therapist's hand placement should be at the transverse process of T8 or the spinous process of T7.

INCORRECT CHOICES:

PA pressures on the spinous process in this region of the thoracic spine will cause the spinous process to glide into and compress the spinous process of the segment below, so no arthrokinematic glide will occur. A PA central glide to the transverse process of T7 will increase extension between T6 and T7.

TYPE OF REASONING: ANALYSIS

One must determine the correct mobilization techniques to improve down-gliding/closure of the T7–8 facct joints in order to arrive at the correct conclusion. This requires knowledge of appropriate mobilization techniques of the thoracic spine, including how to mobilize facet joints. Through analytical reasoning, one should conclude that the correct hand/finger placements should be located at the transverse processes of T8.

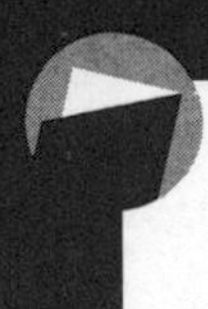

C151 | Musculoskeletal | Evaluation, Diagnosis, Prognosis

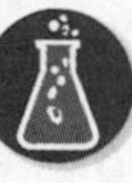

A patient complains of waking up several times at night from severe "pins and needles" in the right hand. On awakening, the hand feels numb for half an hour, and fine hand movements are impaired. The therapist's examination reveals sensory loss and paresthesias in the thumb, index, middle, and lateral half of the ring finger and reduced grip and pinch strength. Some thenar atrophy is present. Based on these examination findings, the **MOST** appropriate diagnosis is:

CHOICES:

1. Thoracic outlet syndrome (TOS).
2. Ulnar nerve entrapment.
3. Carpal tunnel syndrome.
4. Pronator teres syndrome.

TEACHING POINTS

CORRECT ANSWER: 3

Carpal tunnel syndrome is the result of compression of the median nerve under the flexor retinaculum at the wrist. It is characterized by thenar atrophy and sensory loss. Symptoms are worse at night and include burning, tingling, pins and needles, and numbness into the median nerve sensory distribution (palmar and dorsal thumb, index, middle, and lateral half of the ring finger).

INCORRECT CHOICES:

TOS is a neurovascular compression syndrome caused by compression of nerves and/or vessels in the neck. It is characterized by brachial neuritis with or without vascular and vasomotor disturbances in the uper extremity. Electrophysiological studies indicate proximal and not distal compression. Ulnar nerve entrapment typically presents with nocturnal numbness and sensory loss in the little finger and half of the ring finger. The palm is typically not affected. Pronator teres syndrome arises from compression of the median nerve at the elbow with radiation into the radial aspect of the hand. Pronation is possible but weak (not evident in this case). Numbness extends into the median nerve distribution. With passage of time, atrophy of the thenar muscles will occur.

TYPE OF REASONING: ANALYSIS

One must analyze the symptoms presented in order to make a determination of the likely diagnosis. This requires analytical reasoning skill, in which one must determine the meaning of the symptoms in order to determine a diagnosis for the patient. In this case, the symptoms indicate carpal tunnel syndrome, which should be reviewed if this question was answered incorrectly.

C152 | Musculoskeletal | Patient Examination

A patient is referred for physical therapy with a diagnosis of degenerative joint disease affecting C2 and C3. The patient complains of pain and stiffness in the cervical region and transient dizziness with some cervical motions. The **BEST** initial examination procedure is:

CHOICES:

1. Lhermitte's test.
2. Vertebral artery test.
3. Oppenheim's test.
4. Adson's maneuver.

TEACHING POINTS

CORRECT ANSWER: 2

The vertebral artery test checks the integrity of the blood flow through the artery in the cervical region. Because the patient is experiencing symptoms of circulatory disturbance and a unilateral pull could compress the left cervical structures, the vertebral artery test is an appropriate screening test. The test consists of passively placing the patient's head in extension and side flexion. Then the head and neck are slowly rotated to the laterally flexed side and held for 30 seconds. Some of the positive signs may be syncope, lightheadedness, nystagmus, or visual disturbances.

INCORRECT CHOICES:

Lhermitte's sign is pain down the spine and into the upper or lower limbs with passive flexion of the neck. It is used to identify dysfunction of the spinal cord associated with upper motor neuron lesions, and is typically positive in MS. Adson's maneuver is a test for TOS. Oppenheim's test involves running a fingernail along the crest of the tibia; a positive test is the same as a positive Babinski.

TYPE OF REASONING: INFERENCE

One must first determine the meaning of each of the four possible tests and then infer which one is the **BEST** initial test, given the patient's diagnosis and symptoms. If this question was answered incorrectly, review the vertebral artery test.

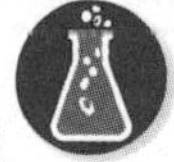

C153 | Neuromuscular | Evaluation, Diagnosis, Prognosis

A young adult otherwise healthy patient is recovering from a complete spinal cord injury (ASIA A) at the level of L4. Functional expectations for this patient include:

CHOICES:

1. Ambulation using bilateral AFOs and canes.
2. Ambulation using bilateral KAFOs and a reciprocating walker.
3. Ambulation using bilateral KAFOs, crutches, and a swing-through gait.
4. Ambulation using reciprocating gait orthoses and a reciprocating walker.

TEACHING POINTS

CORRECT ANSWER: 1

A spinal cord lesion at the level of L4 is considered an LMN injury (cauda equina injury). Intact movements include hip flexion, hip adduction, and knee extension. The quadriceps becomes *fully* innervated at L4. This patient can be expected to be a functional ambulator using bilateral AFOs and crutches or canes.

INCORRECT CHOICES:

All other choices include othotic devices that offer control of joints that is not needed (orthotic bracing of knees and hips). Also crutches or walkers should not be needed.

TYPE OF REASONING: ANALYSIS

One must recall past knowledge of neuroscience related to spinal cord injury in order to determine the functional expectations for the patient with complete L4 injury. In order to arrive at the correct conclusion, one must analyze the four possible choices and determine which choice is most aligned with one's knowledge of injury at this level. If this question was answered incorrectly, review functional expections for patients with lumbar spinal cord injuries.

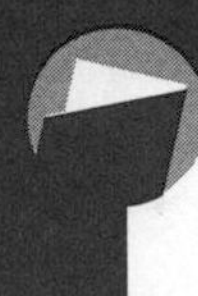

C154 | Neuromuscular | Patient Examination

To examine a patient with a suspected deficit in graphesthesia, the therapist should ask the patient to shut his/her eyes and identify:

CHOICES:

1. Differently weighted, identically shaped cylinders placed in the hand.
2. The vibrations of a tuning fork when placed on a bony prominence.
3. A series of letters traced on the hand.
4. Different objects placed in the hand and manipulated.

TEACHING POINTS

CORRECT ANSWER: 3

Graphesthesia is the ability to recognize numbers, letters, or symbols traced on the skin.

INCORRECT CHOICES:

Barognosis is the ability to recognize different weights placed in the hand using identically shaped objects. Pallesthesia is the ability to recognize vibratory stimuli (i.e., a vibrating tuning fork placed on a bony prominence). Stereognosis is the ability to recognize different objects placed in the hand and manipulated. During testing, vision is occluded.

TYPE OF REASONING: DEDUCTIVE

This question requires factual recall of the definition of graphesthesia, which is a deductive reasoning skill. Using past knowledge of neuroscience is beneficial to arriving at the correct solution. If this question was answered incorrectly, review sensory testing procedures.

C155 | Neuromuscular | Intervention

A patient recovering from stroke is ambulatory without an assistive device and demonstrates a consistent problem with an elevated and retracted pelvis on the affected side. The **BEST** therapeutic exercise strategy is to manually apply:

CHOICES:

1. Anterior-directed pressure during swing.
2. Light resistance to forward pelvic rotation during swing.
3. Downward compression during stance.
4. Light resistance to posterior pelvic elevation during swing.

TEACHING POINTS

CORRECT ANSWER: 2

An elevated and retracted pelvis is a common problem during gait for many patients recovering from stroke. Providing light resistance to forward pelvic rotation actively engages those muscles and reciprocally inhibits the spastic retractors.

INCORRECT CHOICES:

Providing anterior-directed pressure during swing or resistance to pelvic elevation may serve only to increase abnormal tone in those muscles. The problem is a swing phase deficit; downward compression during stance is inappropriate for this problem.

TYPE OF REASONING: INDUCTIVE

One must utilize clinical judgment in order to determine which therapeutic exercise strategy would **BEST** address the patient's problem. Using inductive reasoning skill, the test taker must analyze the four possible choices and then rely on knowledge of mobility challenges in stroke in order to determine the **BEST** course of action for this patient.

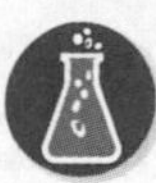

C156 | Neuromuscular | Foundational Sciences

A therapist suspects lower brainstem involvement in a patient with ALS. Examination findings reveal motor impairments of the tongue with ipsilateral wasting and deviation on protrusion. These findings confirm involvement of cranial nerve:

CHOICES:

1. IX.
2. XII.
3. XI.
4. X.

TEACHING POINTS

CORRECT ANSWER: 2

The hypoglossal (CN XII) controls the movements of the tongue. Ipsilateral wasting and the deviation to the ipsilateral side on protrusion are indicative of damage.

INCORRECT CHOICES:

Involvement of the glossopharyngeal (CN IX) results in slight dysphagia, loss of taste in the posterior third of the tongue, and loss of gag reflex. Involvement of the spinal accessory nerve (CN XI) results in minor problems in deglutition and phonation along with weakness in ipsilateral shoulder shrugging. Involvement of the vagus (CN X) results in dysphagia, hoarseness, and paralysis of the soft palate.

TYPE OF REASONING: ANALYSIS

This question requires one to recall the functions of the 12 cranial nerves and then determine which nerve is most likely impaired in this situation. Questions that involve determining an impairment based on a group of symptoms require analytical reasoning skill. If this question was answered incorrectly, review examination of the 12 cranial nerves.

C157 | Musculoskeletal | Evaluation, Diagnosis, Prognosis

A baseball pitcher reports insidious onset of symptoms characteristic of impingement, including catching and popping in the throwing arm. Examination reveals that glenohumeral passive internal rotation is painful and limited to 30 degrees. External rotation is less symptomatic and has 130 degrees of passive range. The PT should first:

CHOICES:

1. Begin elastic resistance exercises for impingement.
2. Mobilize the glenohumeral joint to increase internal rotation ROM.
3. Recommend an anteroposterior radiograph.
4. Recommend an MRI.

TEACHING POINTS

CORRECT ANSWER: 4

The therapist should suspect a labral tear. This is a common finding among pitchers and athletes who do a lot of throwing (especially those who present with abnormal ROM findings and instability symptoms of popping and catching). Although this athlete may present with impingement, an MRI is warranted to fully diagnose the condition and to develop an appropriate treatment plan.

INCORRECT CHOICES:

Beginning treatment without definitive testing is contraindicated. Plain radiographs are inappropriate for suspected soft tissue lesions.

TYPE OF REASONING: INDUCTIVE

This question requires clinical judgment to determine a best course of action for a patient with painful passive internal rotation with limitations in range. Questions that require one to weigh a group of symptoms and determine a best course of action often necessitate inductive reasoning skill. If this question was answered incorrectly, review signs and symptoms of labral tear and diagnostic testing.

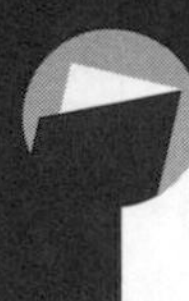

C158 | Other Systems | Foundational Sciences 

A woman is hospitalized in the intensive care unit with extensive trauma after a motor vehicle accident. A review of her medical record reveals the following laboratory values: hematocrit 28%, hemoglobin 10 g/100 mL, and serum white blood cell (WBC) count 12,000/mm³. The **MOST** accurate conclusion the therapist can reach is:

CHOICES:

1. Hematocrit and hemoglobin values are abnormal; WBC is normal.
2. Only hematocrit values are abnormal.
3. Only serum WBC is abnormal.
4. All values are abnormal.

TEACHING POINTS

CORRECT ANSWER: 4

The hematocrit value is abnormally low; women average 42% with a normal range from 37% to 47%. The hemoglobin value is also abnormally low; women average 12–16 g/100 mL of blood. The low values are most likely due to blood loss. The serum WBC (leukocytes) is abnormally high; normal values are 5,000–10,000/mm³. The elevated count (>10,000) indicates acute infection.

INCORRECT CHOICES:

The other choices present findings in which only some, not all, of the values are abnormal.

TYPE OF REASONING: DEDUCTIVE

One must recall the normal laboratory values for female adults in order to arrive at the correct conclusion. This necessitates deductive reasoning, in which recall of factual knowledge and protocols is utilized to determine the correct solution. In this situation, all of the laboratory values are abnormal. If this question was answered incorrectly, review the parameters for these adult laboratory values.

C159 | Integumentary | Evaluation, Diagnosis, Prognosis 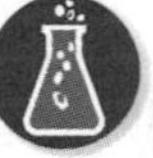

A patient with a transfemoral amputation is unable to wear a total contact prosthesis for the past 4 days. Examination of the residual limb reveals erythema and edema extending over most of the lower anterior limb. The patient tells the therapist that the limb is very itchy and painful. The **MOST LIKELY** cause of these symptoms is:

CHOICES:

1. Cellulitis.
2. Dermatitis.
3. Impetigo.
4. Herpes zoster.

TEACHING POINTS

CORRECT ANSWER: 2

This patient is exhibiting symptoms of contact dermatitis. Primary treatment is removal of the offending agent (in this case, the total contact prosthesis) and treatment of the involved skin with lubricants, topical anesthetics, and/or steroids. The patient may require a thin sock if the problem does not resolve.

INCORRECT CHOICES:

Cellulitis is a suppurative inflammation of the dermis and subcutaneous tissues frequently accompanied by infection. Impetigo is a staphylococcal infection with small macules (unraised spots) or vesicles (small blisters). Herpes zoster is a viral infection with red papules along the course of a nerve or dermatome.

TYPE OF REASONING: ANALYSIS

This question requires the test taker to determine the **MOST LIKELY** cause for the patient's symptoms, which is an analytical reasoning skill. In order to arrive at the correct conclusion, one must analyze the four possible choices and determine which choice is most aligned with one's knowledge of skin irritations, inflammations, and infections. If this question was answered incorrectly, review symptoms and treatment approaches for dermatitis.

C160 | Integumentary | Evaluation, Diagnosis, Prognosis 

A patient is largely confined to bed and has a stage IV sacral pressure ulcer of three months' duration. The **BEST** choice of intervention is:

CHOICES:

1. A 2-inch, convoluted foam mattress.
2. Gentle wound cleansing and wet-to-dry gauze dressings.
3. Surgical repair.
4. Nutritional supplements and pressure relief with a flotation mattress.

TEACHING POINTS

CORRECT ANSWER: 3

A stage IV pressure ulcer is characterized by full-thickness skin loss with extensive destruction, tissue necrosis, or damage to muscle, bone, or supporting structures. Surgical repair is indicated for patients with extensive and chronic ulcers.

INCORRECT CHOICES:

The other interventions are not viable options to resolve this problem. They can be effective in treating ulcers with less extensive damage (stages I–III). After surgery, the use of pressure relieving devices is indicated.

TYPE OF REASONING: INDUCTIVE

This question requires one to determine what the **BEST** intervention approach is for not only the patient in the scenario but also all patients who share a similar diagnosis and current status. Questions that require one to make more global assumptions through clinical judgment necessitate inductive reasoning skill. In this situation, the **BEST** intervention is surgical repair because of the extensive skin loss and tissue destruction. If this question was answered incorrectly, review wound care guidelines for stage IV pressure ulcers.

C161 | Musculoskeletal | Patient Examination 

Following a hip fracture that is now healed, a patient presents with weak hip flexors (2/5). All other muscles are within functional limits. During gait, the therapist expects that the patient may walk with:

CHOICES:

1. Forward trunk lean.
2. A circumducted gait.
3. Excessive hip flexion.
4. Backward trunk lean.

TEACHING POINTS

CORRECT ANSWER: 2

Circumduction is a compensation for weak hip flexors or an inability to shorten the leg (weak knee flexors and ankle dorsiflexors). Hip hiking can also compensate for an abnormally long leg (lack of knee flexion and dorsiflexion).

INCORRECT CHOICES:

Excessive hip flexion is a compensation for footdrop. Forward trunk lean and backward trunk lean are stance phase deviations that compensate for quadriceps weakness and gluteus maximus weakness, respectively.

TYPE OF REASONING: INFERENCE

This question requires the test taker to draw conclusions based on evidence presented, which is an inferential reasoning skill. Questions of this nature often provide a diagnosis, and the test taker must infer the likely symptoms. In this case, the test taker must determine that a patient with weak hip flexors will display a circumducted gait pattern during ambulation. If this question was answered incorrectly, review causes for a circumducted gait pattern.

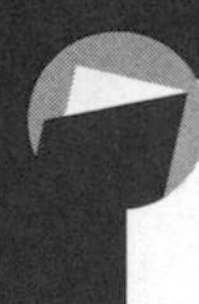

C162 | Musculoskeletal | Intervention

An elderly patient with a left transfemoral amputation complains that, when sitting, the left foot feels cramped and twisted. The therapist's **BEST** choice of intervention is:

CHOICES:

1. Hot packs and continuous US to the residual limb.
2. Iontophoresis to the distal residual limb using hyaluronidase.
3. Appropriate bed positioning with the residual limb in extension.
4. Icing and massage to the residual limb.

TEACHING POINTS

CORRECT ANSWER: 4

This patient is experiencing phantom pain, a common occurrence seen in as many as 70% of patients with lower limb amputations. Treatment interventions can include icing, pulsed US, TENS, or massage. Medical interventions include injections and surgical procedures (rhizotomy, neurectomy).

INCORRECT CHOICES:

Prolonged inactivity and bedrest are contraindicated. Hyaluronidase is indicated for edema reduction. Continuous US is used to achieve thermal effects; heating is not indicated in this case.

TYPE OF REASONING: INDUCTIVE

This question asks the test taker to first consider what the cause for the symptoms is and then determine the **BEST** choice for intervention with this patient. This is an inductive reasoning skill, in which diagnostic reasoning is used to determine best approaches to clinical situations. For this patient, the symptoms clearly indicate phantom pain, and icing and massage to the residual limb are **BEST** to treat the symptoms.

C163 | Devices, Admin., etc. | Teaching, Research, Roles

A researcher uses a group of volunteers (healthy college students) to study the effects of therapy ball exercises on ankle ROM and balance scores. Twenty volunteers participated in the 20-minute ball exercise class 3 times a week for 6 weeks. Measurements were taken at the beginning and end of the sessions. Significant differences were found in both sets of scores and reported at the local physical therapy meeting. Based on this research design, the therapist concludes:

CHOICES:

1. Therapy ball exercises are an effective intervention to improve ankle stability after chronic ankle sprain.
2. The validity of the study was threatened with the introduction of sampling bias.
3. The reliability of the study was threatened with the introduction of systematic error of measurement.
4. The Hawthorne effect may have influenced the outcomes of the study.

TEACHING POINTS

CORRECT ANSWER: 2

The investigator used a sample of convenience and, therefore, introduced systematic sampling error (a threat to validity). Random selection of subjects would improve the validity of this study.

INCORRECT CHOICES:

Generalization to a group of patients with chronic ankle sprain cannot be made. There was no systematic error in measurement in this example. The Hawthorne effect refers to the influence that the subject's knowledge of participation in the experiment had on the results of the study.

TYPE OF REASONING: INFERENCE

The test taker must determine what the most likely conclusion should be to this research study, given the protocol implemented. Questions that require one to draw conclusions based on evidence necessitate inferential reasoning skill to come to the correct conclusion. In this study, the validity has been threatened by convenience sampling. If this question was answered incorrectly, review guidelines to improve validity in research.

C164 | Cardiovascular-Pulmonary | Intervention

A patient has a very large right-sided bacterial pneumonia. Oxygen level is dangerously low. The body position that would **MOST** likely improve the patient's arterial oxygen pressure (PaO_2) is:

CHOICES:

1. Right side-lying with the head of the bed in the flat position.
2. Prone-lying with the head of the bed in the Trendelenburg position.
3. Supine-lying with the head of the bed in the Trendelenburg position.
4. Left side-lying with the head of the bed in the flat position.

TEACHING POINTS

CORRECT ANSWER: 4

In order to match perfusion and ventilation, the therapist needs to place the unaffected side in a gravity-dependent position, or that of left side-lying.

INCORRECT CHOICES:

Although prone and supine with the head of the bed in the flat position might be helpful, these positions would not be as likely to show as much improvement as left side-lying. The use of the Trendelenburg position (head lower than legs) is inappropriate.

TYPE OF REASONING: INFERENCE

The test taker must infer the best body position in order to improve the patient's PaO_2 level. Knowledge of pulmonary rehabilitation guidelines is important in order to arrive at the correct conclusion. If this question was answered incorrectly, refer to pulmonary rehabilitation guidelines for patients with low PaO_2, especially body positions in bed.

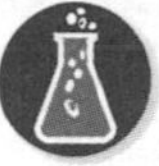

C165 | Musculoskeletal | Evaluation, Diagnosis, Prognosis

An examination of a patient reveals drooping of the shoulder, rotatory winging of the scapula, an inability to shrug the shoulder, and complaints of aching in the shoulder. Based on these findings, the cause of these symptoms would **MOST** likely be due to:

CHOICES:

1. Muscle imbalance.
2. A lesion of the long thoracic nerve.
3. A lesion of the spinal accessory nerve.
4. Strain of the serratus anterior.

TEACHING POINTS

CORRECT ANSWER: 3

Rotary winging occurs when the inferior angle of one scapula is rotated farther from the spine than the inferior angle of the other scapula. The shoulder drooping and inability to shrug the shoulder are secondary to a lesion of the spinal accessory nerve (CN XI), which innervates the trapezius muscle.

INCORRECT CHOICES:

Although this type of winging could be found with all of these answers, the findings of shoulder drooping and inability to shrug the shoulder clearly point to a lesion of CN XI.

TYPE OF REASONING: ANALYSIS

This question requires the test taker to determine the diagnosis based on symptoms presented, which is an analytical reasoning skill. Knowledge of neuroscience and nerve innervations of the cervical spine is beneficial to arriving at the correct conclusion. If this question was answered incorrectly, refer to innervations of the spinal accessory nerve and symptoms of lesions associated with this nerve.

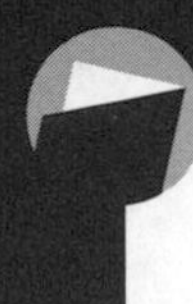

C166 | Devices, Admin., etc. | Equipment, Modalities

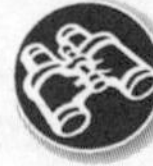

A patient with spastic hemiplegia is referred to the therapist for ambulation training. The patient is having difficulty with standing up from a seated position as the result of co-contraction of the quadriceps and hamstrings during the knee and hip extension phase. The therapist wishes to use biofeedback beginning with simple knee extension exercise in the seated position. The plan is to progress to sit-to-stand training. The initial biofeedback protocol should consist of:

CHOICES:

1. High-detection sensitivity with recording electrodes placed closely together.
2. Low-detection sensitivity with recording electrodes placed closely together.
3. Low-detection sensitivity with recording electrodes placed far apart.
4. High-detection sensitivity with recording electrodes placed far apart.

TEACHING POINTS

CORRECT ANSWER: 2

By initially placing the electrodes close together, the therapist decreases the likelihood of detecting undesired motor units from adjacent active muscles (crosstalk). By setting the biofeedback sensitivity (gain) low, the therapist would decrease the amplitude of the signals generated by the hypertonic muscles and keep the EMG output from exceeding a visual and/or auditory range (scale).

INCORRECT CHOICES:

The other choices fail to use optimal placing of electrodes (electrodes placed far apart) or sensitivity (high-detection) to optimize outcomes. The wider the spacing of electrodes, the more volume of the muscle is monitored. Thus, when targeting a specific muscle, a narrow spacing should be used. When the focus is not on a specific muscle but rather to encourage a general motion such as shoulder elevation, then a wider spacing of electrodes can be used. In addition, when working with weakness of a muscle in which there is a decreased ability to recruit motor units or there is a decrease in the size and number of motor units, then a wider spacing and a high sensitivity would be used in order to create an adequate visible signal.

TYPE OF REASONING: INDUCTIVE

One must utilize clinical judgment and diagnostic reasoning in order to determine the most appropriate initial biofeedback protocol. This requires knowledge of biofeedback guidelines and benefits of using high- versus low-detection sensitivity and electrodes placed either closely together or far apart. If this question was answered incorrectly, review biofeedback guidelines of the lower extremity.

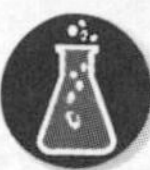

C167 | Neuromuscular | Foundational Sciences

Examination of a patient recovering from stroke reveals a loss of pain and temperature sensation on the left side of the face along with loss of pain and temperature sensation on the right side of the body. All other sensations are normal. The therapist suspects a lesion in the:

CHOICES:

1. Midbrain.
2. Right cerebral cortex or internal capsule.
3. Left posterolateral medulla.
4. Left cerebral cortex or internal capsule.

TEACHING POINTS

CORRECT ANSWER: 3

A lesion in the posterolateral medulla cause mixed sensory loss (described in this case). Pain and temperature are affected whereas discriminative touch and proprioception are not (the medial lemniscus is not involved).

INCORRECT CHOICES:

Sensory loss will be completely contralateral (not mixed) only after the discriminative sensory tracts (fasciculus gracilis and fasciculus cuneatus) cross in the upper medulla. Patients with lesions above the medulla (midbrain, cortex, or internal capsule) will present with contralateral sensory loss.

TYPE OF REASONING: ANALYSIS

This question requires the test taker to determine the location of a lesion based on symptoms presented, which is an analytical reasoning skill. Knowledge of neuroscience and the discriminative sensory tracts is beneficial to arriving at the correct conclusion. If this question was answered incorrectly, refer to information regarding the discriminative sensory tracts and lesions.

C168 | Neuromuscular | Foundational Sciences

A patient is taking the drug baclofen to control spasticity after spinal cord injury. This medication can be expected to decrease muscle tone and pain. Adverse reactions of concern to the PT can include:

CHOICES:

1. Hypertension and palpitations.
2. Drowsiness and muscle weakness.
3. Headache with visual auras.
4. Urinary retention and discomfort.

TEACHING POINTS

CORRECT ANSWER: 2

Baclofen, used in the management of spasticity, can produce CNS depression (drowsiness, fatigue, weakness, confusion, vertigo, dizziness, and insomnia), occurring in less than 10% of patients. Additional adverse effects can include hypotension and palpitations and urinary frequency. Vomiting, seizures, and coma are signs of overdosage.

INCORRECT CHOICES:

Adverse effects include hypotension (not hypertension) and edema. Headache with visual auras is characteristic of migraines. Urinary adverse effects include frequency (not retention).

TYPE OF REASONING: DEDUCTIVE

One must recall the possible adverse effects of taking baclofen in order to arrive at the correct conclusion. This requires knowledge of guidelines and factual information, which is a deductive reasoning skill. If this question was answered incorrectly, refer to therapeutic uses of baclofen, including adverse effects.

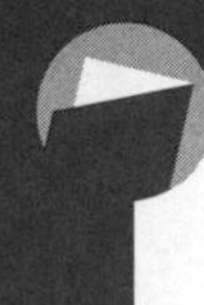

C169 | Other Systems | Evaluation, Diagnosis, Prognosis

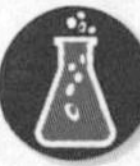

A patient with RA has joined a supervised walking program for remediation of mild heart disease. The patient has been taking NSAIDs regularly for the past 10 years. During an exercise session in week 3, the patient experiences pallor, fatigue, and some dizziness and confusion. The patient denies any musculoskeletal pain. The therapist recognizes the patient may be experiencing:

CHOICES:

1. Enhanced circulation.
2. Anemia.
3. Hypoglycemia.
4. Hyperglycemia.

TEACHING POINTS

CORRECT ANSWER: 2

Regular use of NSAIDs may cause anemia (with symptoms as in this example) because of gastrointestinal bleeding. Musculoskeletal pain is masked.

INCORRECT CHOICES:

Although hypoglycemia can also produce dizziness, fatigue, and confusion, the patient would also likely demonstrate increased sweating, hand tremors, poor coordination, and unsteady gait. Hyperglycemia during exercise would likely result in signs and symptoms of weakness, thirst, dry mouth, nausea, and vomiting. There is no evidence of a glucose disorder in this case.

TYPE OF REASONING: ANALYSIS

This question provides a group of symptoms, and the test taker must determine the likely diagnosis, which requires analytical reasoning skill. The key word that helps the test taker to arrive at a correct conclusion is "NSAIDs," which has the potential to cause anemia. If this question was answered incorrectly, review side effects of taking NSAIDs.

C170 | Cardiovascular-Pulmonary | Foundational Sciences

A patient is exercising in a phase 3 outpatient cardiac rehabilitation program that utilizes circuit training. One of the stations utilizes weights. The patient lifts a 5-lb weight, holds it for 20 seconds, and then lowers it slowly. The therapist corrects the activity and tells the patient to reduce the length of the static hold. Resistance exercise with static holding can be expected to produce:

CHOICES:

1. Abnormal oxygen uptake.
2. Lower HR and arterial BP.
3. Higher HR and arterial BP.
4. Reduced normal venous return to the heart and elevated BP.

TEACHING POINTS

CORRECT ANSWER: 3

Dynamic exercise facilitates circulation, while isometric (static) exercise hinders blood flow, producing higher HRs and arterial BPs. Rise in BP is related to degree of intensity (effort).

INCORRECT CHOICES:

Resistance exercise does little to increase oxygen uptake. HR and BP are higher (not lower). The Valsalva maneuver (forced expiration against a closed glottis) that accompanies breath holding produces increased intrathoracic pressure, which in turn hinders normal venous return to the heart. Breath holding is more likely with isometric exercise, but is not always present.

TYPE OF REASONING: INFERENCE

One must infer the likely outcomes of static exercise on BP and HR in order to arrive at the correct conclusion. This requires one to draw conclusions based on the information presented, which is an inferential reasoning skill. In this case, one should expect an elevated HR and arterial BP as a result of isometric exercise, which should be reviewed if this question was answered incorrectly.

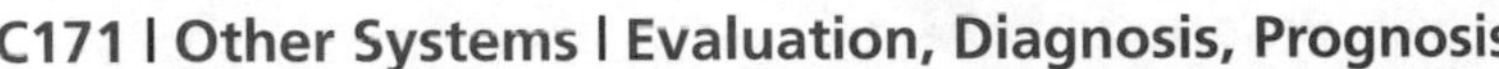

C171 | Other Systems | Evaluation, Diagnosis, Prognosis

A 10 year-old boy with hemophilia fell and injured himself while skateboarding. He was admitted to a pediatric acute care facility with a referral to physical therapy that afternoon. Examination reveals a hemarthrosis in his left knee. The **BEST** initial intervention for this patient is:

CHOICES:

1. Rest, ice, elevation, and non–weight-bearing ambulation with crutches.
2. Rest with pool exercises to maintain ROM and strength.
3. A hot pack for the knee, splint, and instruction in AROM exercises.
4. Mild resistive exercises and partial weight-bearing ambulation using crutches.

TEACHING POINTS

CORRECT ANSWER: 1

Hemarthrosis (bleeding into joint spaces) is associated with swelling, joint pain, and decreased ROM and movement. Optimal treatment involves pain management along with rest, ice, elevation, and functional splinting. The patient should be non–weight-bearing during ambulation.

INCORRECT CHOICES:

Weight-bearing and exercise during an acute bleed are contraindicated (all other choices).

TYPE OF REASONING: INDUCTIVE

One must utilize clinical judgment and diagnostic reasoning to determine the **BEST** initial intervention for this patient. This necessitates inductive reasoning skill, in which the test taker's knowledge of hemarthrosis treatment guidelines helps to guide reasoning for the **BEST** intervention approach. If this question was answered incorrectly, review treatment guidelines for hemarthrosis.

C172 | Other Systems | Evaluation, Diagnosis, Prognosis

An elderly male patient recovering from a fractured hip repaired with ORIF has recently been discharged home. During a home visit, his wife tells the therapist that he woke up yesterday morning and told her he couldn't remember much. Upon examination, the therapist finds some mild motor loss in his right hand and anomia. The therapist affirms the presence of short-term memory loss. The **BEST** course of action is to:

CHOICES:

1. Refer him to his physician, because the therapist suspects Alzheimer's dementia.
2. Refer him to his physician immediately, because the therapist suspects a stroke.
3. Advise the family to document and record any new problems that they notice over the next week, then report back to the therapist.
4. Ignore the findings, because they are expected after surgical anesthesia.

TEACHING POINTS

CORRECT ANSWER: 2

The presence of focal signs (incoordination, anomia) with cognitive signs (memory loss) is indicative of impaired brain function and may be the result of small strokes. This is the most likely choice given the spotty symptoms he presents with as well as their sudden onset.

INCORRECT CHOICES:

Senile dementia, Alzheimer's type, can include some of the same symptoms but the onset is gradual and the course is typically slowly progressive. The reporting of these findings to the primary physician should not be delayed. Further diagnostic workup is indicated. Hospital admission and anesthesia can cause temporary cognitive difficulties (delirium), but these should not persist with discharge home.

TYPE OF REASONING: EVALUATION

In this question, the test taker must determine the **BEST** course of action, given the nature of the patient's new symptoms. This requires evaluative reasoning skill, in which one evaluates the merits of each possible course of action in order to arrive at the correct conclusion. If this question was answered incorrectly, review symptoms of transient ischemic attack and stroke.

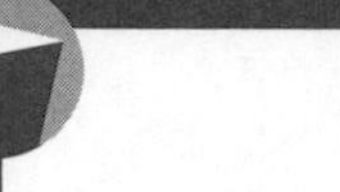

C173 | Other Systems | Evaluation, Diagnosis, Prognosis

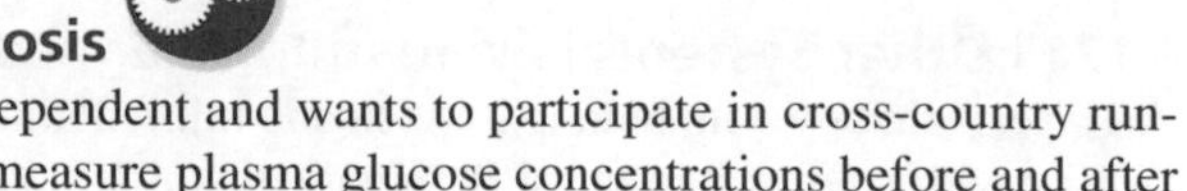

An adolescent with a 4-year history of type 2 diabetes is insulin dependent and wants to participate in cross-country running. The PT working with the school team advises the athlete to measure plasma glucose concentrations before and after running. In addition, the student should:

CHOICES:

1. Consume a carbohydrate after practice to avoid hyperglycemia.
2. Increase insulin dosage immediately before running.
3. Consume a carbohydrate before or during practice to avoid hypoglycemia.
4. Avoid carbohydrate-rich snacks within 12 hours of a race.

TEACHING POINTS

CORRECT ANSWER: 3

During exercise of increasing intensity and duration, plasma concentrations of insulin progressively decrease. Exercise-induced hypoglycemia (abnormally low levels of glucose in the blood) is common for exercising athletes with diabetes. Hypoglycemia associated with exercise can occur up to 48 hours after exercise. To counteract these effects, the individual may need to reduce his insulin dosage or increase carbohydrate intake before or after running. Consuming a carbohydrate product before or during the race will have a preventive modulating effect on hypoglycemia.

INCORRECT CHOICES:

Hyperglycemia (abnormally high levels of glucose in the blood) is more a risk for individuals with uncontrolled type 1 diabetes. These patients should demonstrate glycemic control before starting an exercise program. Consuming carbohydrates will not lessen the likelihood of hyperglycemia.

TYPE OF REASONING: EVALUATION

One must evaluate the merits of each of the four possible courses of action in order to arrive at the correct solution. This requires knowledge of the effects of exercise on glucose concentrations in athletes with diabetes. Through evaluative reasoning, one should conclude that the athlete should consume a carbohydrate snack before or during practice or a race to avoid hypoglycemia. If this question was answered incorrectly, review guidelines for exercise with athletes with diabetes and carbohydrate consumption.

C174 | Other Systems | Foundational Sciences

Why are chronic urinary tract infections more common in adult women than men?

CHOICES:

1. Angiotensin II, antidiuretic hormone (ADH), and endothelin effects are greater.
2. Incidence of urinary tract stones is greater.
3. The urethra is short and close to the vagina and rectum.
4. Sodium reabsorption is increased in the distal tubule and collecting duct.

TEACHING POINTS

CORRECT ANSWER: 3

Chronic urinary tract infections are more common in women due to the shorter length of the urethra in females with closer entrance to the vagina and rectum. Additional risk factors for females include pregnancy and effects of estrogen decline during peri- and postmenopausal years.

INCORRECT CHOICES:

Gender differences are not a factor in the other three choices. Angiotensin II, ADH, and endothelins are humoral substances that cause vasoconstriction of renal vessels. Elimination of sodium and potassium is regulated by the glomerular filtration rate and by humeral agents. Urinary tract infections are associated with stasis of urine flow and obstruction.

TYPE OF REASONING: DEDUCTIVE

This question requires the recall of factual information, which necessitates deductive reasoning. For this situation, the test taker must recall the reason why urinary tract infections are more common in adult women than in men, which relates to the length and location of the urethra in women. If this question was answered incorrectly, review urinary tract infection guidelines in adults.

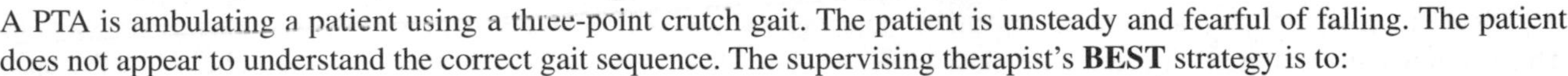

C175 | Devices, Admin., etc. | Teaching, Research, Roles

A PTA is ambulating a patient using a three-point crutch gait. The patient is unsteady and fearful of falling. The patient does not appear to understand the correct gait sequence. The supervising therapist's **BEST** strategy is to:

CHOICES:

1. Instruct the PTA to have the patient sit down and utilize mental practice of the task.
2. Tell the PTA and patient to stop the ambulation and work on dynamic balance activities instead.
3. Instruct the PTA to use a distributed practice schedule to ensure patient success.
4. Intervene and teach the correct sequence because the PTA is apparently unable to deal with this special situation.

TEACHING POINTS

CORRECT ANSWER: 1

Mental rehearsal (mental practice) is the best strategy to have the patient learn the correct sequence. In the non–weight-bearing position, the patient's anxiety is lessened, leaving the patient free to concentrate on the task at hand.

INCORRECT CHOICES:

The PT should provide appropriate guidance to the PTA but not necessarily take over care. Lack of understanding about the gait sequence rather than balance difficulties seems to be the major problem. Distributed practice with long rest times does not address the main difficulty.

TYPE OF REASONING: EVALUATION

This question requires one to evaluate the value of each of the four possible solutions and then determine which solution is the **BEST** strategy, given the patient's challenges. Evaluative reasoning questions often require the test taker to make value judgments, which can be challenging for many test takers.

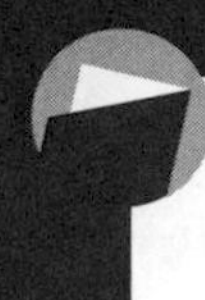

C176 | Musculoskeletal | Patient Examination

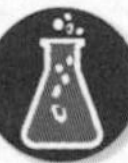

A therapist is reviewing x-rays from a patient with a trimalleolar fracture. The **BEST** radiographic views to visualize this bony anomaly are:

CHOICES:

1. PA and lateral.
2. Lateral and coronal.
3. Anteroposterior and lateral.
4. Oblique and lateral.

TEACHING POINTS

CORRECT ANSWER: 3

A trimalleolar fracture includes fracture of both malleoli and the posterior rim of the tibia. The anteroposterior view of the ankle demonstrates the distal tibia and fibula, including the medial and lateral malleoli and the head of the talus. The fractures of both malleoli will be visable with this view. The lateral view provides evidence of the fracture at the posterior rim of the distal tibia.

INCORRECT CHOICES:

An oblique view of the foot demonstrates the phalanges, the metatarsals, and the intermetatarsal joints. PA view is not routine for the ankle. A coronal view is also not indicated for this type of fracture.

TYPE OF REASONING: ANALYSIS

One must recall the nature of a trimalleolar fracture in order to make a determination of the **BEST** radiographic view for observation of this anomaly. This necessitates analytical reasoning skill, in which one must interpret the information presented in order to make a determination of a **BEST** course of action. If this question was answered incorrectly, review radiographic examination guidelines for trimalleolar fractures.

C177 | Devices, Admin., etc. | Equipment, Modalities

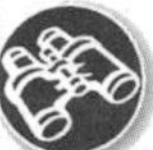

A patient presents with pain and muscle spasm of the upper back (C7–T8) extending to the lateral border of the scapula. This encompasses a 10 × 10-cm area on both sides of the spine. If the US unit only has a 5-cm^2 sound head, the therapist should treat:

CHOICES:

1. The entire area in 5 minutes.
2. The entire area in 10 minutes.
3. Each side, allotting 2.5 minutes for each section.
4. Each side, allotting 5 minutes for each section.

TEACHING POINTS

CORRECT ANSWER: 4

The total treatment area is too large for the 5-cm^2 sound head to produce adequate tissue heating. Sonating the two areas independently will allow more time for the tissue temperature to rise during the treatment time in each area.

INCORRECT CHOICES:

Moving the transducer too fast to cover both sides adequately in the allotted time does not allow sufficient time for the acoustic energy to produce heat because the head is not in a given area long enough. Increasing the treatment time will not affect the rate of heat production. Two minutes is too brief to produce sufficient tissue heating.

TYPE OF REASONING: INDUCTIVE

This question requires clinical judgment and diagnostic reasoning in order to determine the best approach when providing US treatment for this patient. This requires recall of proper US treatment guidelines, including consideration of the size of the sound head and size of the area to be treated. If this question was answered incorrectly, review US treatment guidelines for larger treatment areas.

C178 | Devices, Admin., etc. | Equipment, Modalities 

A patient with chronic cervical pain is referred to an outpatient physical therapy clinic. Past medical history reveals: appendectomy, 12 years ago; chronic heart disease; demand-type pacemaker, 8 years ago; whiplash injury, 2 years ago. At present, the patient complains of pain and muscle spasm in the cervical region. The modality that is **CONTRAINDICATED** in the case is:

CHOICES:

1. Mechanical traction.
2. US.
3. Hot pack.
4. TENS.

TEACHING POINTS

CORRECT ANSWER: 4

All electrical stimulation devices are contraindicated when a patient has a demand-type pacemaker. The electrical signals could interfere with the rhythmic signals of the pacemaker.

INCORRECT CHOICES:

All other modalities could be considered in the management of this patients pain and muscle spasm. The presence of a pacemaker is not contraindicated for the application of traction and hot pack to the cervical region. US is contraindicated only over or in the area of the pacemaker.

TYPE OF REASONING: INFERENCE

One must infer which modality is contraindicated for the patient and why, given the patient's past medical history. This requires inferential reasoning skill, in which one must draw conclusions based on the information presented. If this question was answered incorrectly, review contraindications for TENS therapy.

C179 | Neuromuscular | Patient Examination 

In posturography testing, patients who sway more or fall under conditions with the eyes closed and platform moving (condition 5) or with the visual surround moving and platform moving (condition 6) are likely to demonstrate:

CHOICES:

1. Problems with sensory selection.
2. Vestibular deficiency.
3. Somatosensory dependency.
4. Visual dependency.

TEACHING POINTS

CORRECT ANSWER: 2

The Clinical Test for Sensory Integration in Balance (Sensory Organization Test) using dynamic posturography testing is positive for vestibular deficiency with loss of balance on conditions 5 and 6. Patients who are surface-dependent (somatosensory) have difficulties with conditions 4, 5, and 6.

INCORRECT CHOICES:

Patients who are visually dependent have difficulties with conditions 2, 3, and 6. Sensory selection problems are evident with loss of balance on conditions 3–6. (See Chapter 2 for a complete description of this test.)

TYPE OF REASONING: INFERENCE

One must first determine what conditions 5 and 6 are indicative of in posturography testing in order to arrive at the correct conclusion. This necessitates inferential reasoning, in which one must draw conclusions from the information presented in order to determine what the patient is likely to demonstrate. If this question was answered incorrectly, refer to posturography testing.

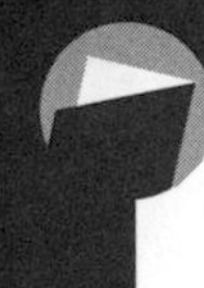

C180 | Neuromuscular | Foundational Sciences

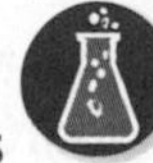

A patient presents with severe, frequent seizures originating in the medial temporal lobes. After bilateral surgical removal of these areas, the patient is unable to remember any new information just prior to the surgery to the present. The patient cannot recall text read minutes ago or remember people previously met. These outcomes are indicative of:

CHOICES:

1. Loss of the hippocampus and declarative memory function.
2. Loss of procedural memory and integration with frontal cortex.
3. A primary deficit from the loss of the amygdala.
4. Loss of integration of the temporal lobe with the basal ganglia and frontal cortex.

TEACHING POINTS

CORRECT ANSWER: 1

Declarative memory refers to conscious, explicit, or cognitive memory. It is a function of the cerebral cortex and the hippocampus.

INCORRECT CHOICES:

Procedural memory (unconscious memory or implicit memory) refers to the recall of skills and habits and emotional responses. It is the result of integrated action of the frontal cortex (neocortex), thalamus, and striatum of the basal ganglia. The amygdala is a collection of nuclei in the anteromedial temporal lobe, forming the core of the limbic circuits. It is important for triggering feelings and drive-related behaviors.

TYPE OF REASONING: ANALYSIS

This question requires the test taker to determine the diagnosis based on symptoms presented, which is an analytical reasoning skill. In this situation, the symptoms are indicative of loss of the hippocampus and declarative memory function. Knowledge of neuroscience and the cortical structures responsible for declarative memory function are beneficial to arriving at the correct conclusion. If this question was answered incorrectly, refer memory functions and structures.

C181 | Other Systems | Evaluation, Diagnosis, Prognosis

A 14 year-old with a body mass index of 33 kg/m^2 and a history of limited participation in physical activities is referred for exercise training. The nutritionist has prescribed a diet limiting his caloric intake. The **BEST** initial exercise prescription is:

CHOICES:

1. 3 weekly sessions of 50 minutes at 70–85% VO_{2max}.
2. 3 weekly sessions of 30 minutes at 60–70% VO_{2max}.
3. 2 weekly sessions of 60 minutes at 50% VO_{2max}.
4. 2 daily sessions of 30 minutes at 40–70% VO_{2max}.

TEACHING POINTS

CORRECT ANSWER: 4

This individual is obese (body mass index $\geq$ 30 kg/m^2) and will benefit from exercise to increase energy expenditure and diet to reduce caloric intake. The initial exercise prescription should utilize low-intensity with longer-duration exercise. Splitting the training into 2 sessions each day is a good choice. The goal is to work toward bringing the target HR into a suitable range. Obese individuals are at increased risk of orthopedic injuries and require close monitoring.

INCORRECT CHOICES:

Weekly sessions at high intensities (70–85% VO_{2max}) and long duration (50 min) are contraindicated. Weekly sessions (2–3 times/wk) are not as beneficial initially as are daily sessions at shorter durations and moderate intensities.

TYPE OF REASONING: INDUCTIVE

One must utilize clinical judgment and diagnostic reasoning to determine the **BEST** initial exercise prescription for this individual. This necessitates inductive reasoning skill, in which one must refer to knowledge of exercise for individuals with obesity to arrive at the correct conclusion. If this question was answered incorrectly, review exercise prescription guidelines for the obese.

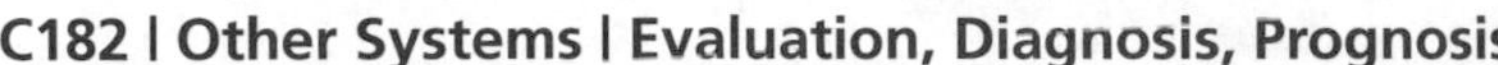
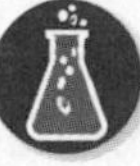

C182 | Other Systems | Evaluation, Diagnosis, Prognosis

A patient is admitted to a hospital after a fall. A review of the patient's medical chart reveals a BP of 160/85, a triglyceride level of 160 mg/dL, and a fasting blood glucose level of 115 mg/dL. Weight is 310 lb. Examination of the patient reveals a rotund man with a 54-inch waistline. These findings are indicative of:

CHOICES:

1. Chronic heart disease.
2. Type 1 diabetes.
3. Metabolic syndrome.
4. Cushing's syndrome.

TEACHING POINTS

CORRECT ANSWER: 3

This patient is exhibiting four of the risk factors of metabolic syndrome (diagnosis is made if three or more are present). Risk factors include (1) abdominal obesity: waist circumference > 40 inches in men or > 35 inches in women; (2) elevated triglycerides: triglyceride level of 150 mg/dL or higher; (3) low high-density lipoprotein (HDL) cholesterol or being on medicine to treat low HDL: HDL level < 40 mg/dL in men or 50 mg/dL in women; (4) elevated BP: systolic BP ≥ 130 mm Hg and/or diastolic BP = 85 mm Hg; and (5) fasting plasma glucose level > 100 mg/dL. The therapist's plan of care should be reflective of the patient's increased risk for heart disease, stroke, and diabetes and assist the patient in lifestyle changes that reduce these risk factors.

INCORRECT CHOICES:

No mention is made of absolute insulin deficiency (type 1 diabetes). Although these are risk factors for heart disease, they do not specifically define or characterize chronic heart disease. Cushing's syndrome (glucocorticoid hormone excess) refers to the manifestations of hypercortisolism from any cause. Patients typically exhibit a round "moon face" with a protruding abdomen or "buffalo hump" on the back along with muscle weakness and wasting.

TYPE OF REASONING: ANALYSIS

This question requires one to analyze all of the signs and symptoms presented and then draw a conclusion about a potential diagnosis. Questions of this nature require analytical reasoning skill. If this question was answered incorrectly, refer to signs and symptoms of metabolic syndrome.

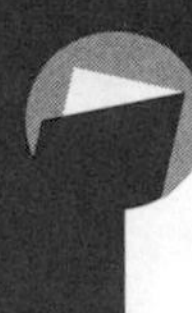

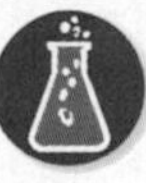

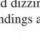

C183 | Other Systems | Evaluation, Diagnosis, Prognosis

A patient in an exercise class develops muscle weakness and fatigue. Examination reveals leg cramps and hyporeflexia. The patient also experiences frequent episodes of postural hypotension and dizziness. Abnormalities on the ECG include a flat T wave, prolonged QT interval, and depressed ST segment. These findings are suggestive of:

CHOICES:

1. Hyperkalemia.
2. Hypocalcemia.
3. Hyponatremia.
4. Hypokalemia.

TEACHING POINTS

CORRECT ANSWER: 4

Hypokalemia, decreased potassium in the blood, is characterized by these signs and symptoms. Other possible symptoms include respiratory distress, irritability, confusion or depression, and gastrointestinal disturbances.

INCORRECT CHOICES:

Hyperkalemia is excess potassium in the blood. Hyponatremia is decreased sodium in the blood, and hypocalcemia is decreased calcium in the blood. These conditions cannot produce this battery of symptoms.

TYPE OF REASONING: ANALYSIS

This question requires the test taker to determine the diagnosis based on the symptoms described, which is an analytical reasoning skill. The test taker must analyze the symptoms in order to determine the most likely cause for them. If this question was answered incorrectly, refer to signs and symptoms of of the conditions listed (Chapter 6).

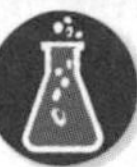

C184 | Other Systems | Evaluation, Diagnosis, Prognosis

An older adult with advanced coronary artery disease and diabetes is receiving functional mobility training in a physical therapy clinic. While walking after lunch, the patient experiences difficulty breathing, starts hyperventilating, and suffers an episode of syncope. The **MOST LIKELY** cause of these symptoms is:

CHOICES:

1. Postprandial hypertension.
2. Coronary artery disease.
3. Hyperglycemia.
4. Seizures.

TEACHING POINTS

CORRECT ANSWER: 2

Lack of oxygen to the brain is the most probable cause of the fainting. Heart failure with dyspnea and hyperventilation can decrease cerebral blood flow by as much as 40%. Postprandial hypotension (a drop in BP after a meal) and hypoglycemia could also cause syncope, but would not likely cause dyspnea and hyperventilation.

INCORRECT CHOICES:

Hypertension or hyperglycemia are not typically seen after a meal (postprandial). Seizures would present with additional clinical features (e.g., an olfactory or visual aura, tongue biting, motor twitching).

TYPE OF REASONING: ANALYSIS

This question requires the test taker to determine the cause for the patient's symptoms, which is an analytical reasoning skill. In this scenario, after considering the patient's past medical history, one should conclude that the symptoms are due to coronary artery disease. If this question was answered incorrectly, refer to symptoms of advanced coronary artery disease.

C185 | Other Systems | Intervention

A patient is referred to a woman's health specialist PT with a diagnosis of pelvic pain and uterine prolapse. Physical therapy intervention should focus on:

CHOICES:

1. Protective splinting of abdominal musculature.
2. External stabilization with a support belt.
3. Gentle abdominal exercises with incisional support.
4. Kegel's exercises to strengthen pubococcygeal muscles.

TEACHING POINTS

CORRECT ANSWER: 4

Intervention should focus on pelvic floor rehabilitation (Kegel's exercises to strengthen pubococcygeal muscles) along with postural education and muscle reeducation.

INCORRECT CHOICES:

Diastasis recti abdominis requires protective splinting of abdominal musculature during initial separation (>2 cm split of the rectus abdominis after pregnancy). External stabilization with a support belt may be required for sacroiliac dysfunction. Postcesarean interventions include gentle abdominal exercises with incisional support. There was no mention of pregnancy or postpregnancy complications.

TYPE OF REASONING: INFERENCE

One must infer or draw a reasonable conclusion about the best intervention approach for a patient with pelvic pain and uterine prolapse. This requires inferential reasoning skill, because one must determine which therapeutic approach will have the most effective outcome of improving function. If this question was answered incorrectly, review exercise guidelines for patients with uterine prolapse.

C186 | Devices, Admin., etc. | Teaching, Research, Roles

A therapist is working with a patient recovering from traumatic brain injury (Rancho Levels of Cognitive Functioning, level IV). This is the patient's first time in the physical therapy gym. While the therapist attempts to work with the patient on sitting control, the patient becomes agitated and combative. Which strategy is the **BEST** choice in this situation?

CHOICES:

1. Enlist the help of a PTA to support the patient while slowly instructing the patient again.
2. Remove the patient to a quiet environment and provide support and calming stimuli.
3. Return the patient to his/her room and try the training activity later in the day.
4. Give the patient a 5-minute rest and resume the training activity.

TEACHING POINTS

CORRECT ANSWER: 2

The best choice is to remove the patient to a quiet room and provide calming stimuli and support. At level IV Rancho Level of Cognitive Function, the therapist can expect the patient to be confused, inappropriate, and highly distractable. The environment should be changed. Memory is severely impaired and the patient is unable to learn new information.

INCORRECT CHOICES:

Enlisting the PTA or resuming training after a 5-minute rest does not change the environment nor calm the patient. Rescheduling for the afternoon similarly does not address the central problem of the patient's level IV behaviors.

TYPE OF REASONING: INFERENCE

Questions that inquire about a **BEST** approach to a therapeutic situation often necessitate inferential reasoning skill. In this situation, the test taker must determine the **BEST** choice for a patient with traumatic brain injury and Rancho level IV behaviors. Review Levels of Cognitive Function after traumatic brain injury and beneficial training strategies for each level.

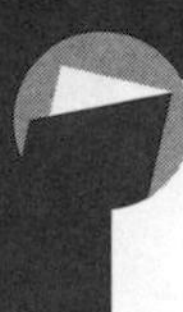

C187 | Neuromuscular | Intervention

A patient has a 10-year history of Parkinson's disease and has been on levodopa (Carbidopa) for the past 6 years. The patient has fallen 3 times in the past month, resulting in a Colles' fracture. The therapist decides to try postural biofeedback training using a platform balance training device. The training sequence should focus on:

CHOICES:

1. Decreasing the limits of stability and improving increasing anterior weight displacement.
2. Increasing the limits of stability and improving increasing anterior weight displacement.
3. Decreasing the limits of stability and improving increasing posterior weight displacement.
4. Increasing the limits of stability and improving center of pressure alignment.

TEACHING POINTS

CORRECT ANSWER: 4

The patient with Parkinson's disease exhibits significant balance impairments including loss of postural reflexes; decreased limits of stability; flexed, stooped posture that alters the center of pressure in an anterior direction; freezing; and orthostatic hypotension. Platform balance training should work toward improving the limits of stability and center of pressure alignment (the patient should focus on reducing anterior displacement).

INCORRECT CHOICES:

The patient is too unstable; decreasing limits of stability is contraindicated, as is promoting anterior weight displacement.

TYPE OF REASONING: INFERENCE

One must infer the most appropriate training sequence for biofeedback postural training in order to arrive at the correct conclusion. This involves inferential reasoning, in which one must consider the patient's diagnosis and current limitations in order to choose the most appropriate training sequence. If this question was answered incorrectly, refer to balance deficits and training strategies for patients with Parkinson's disease.

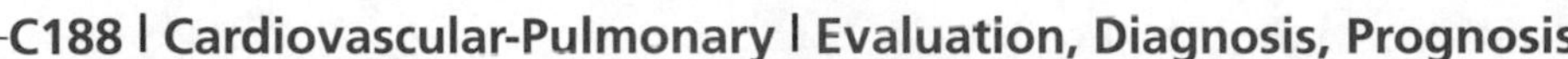

C188 | Cardiovascular-Pulmonary | Evaluation, Diagnosis, Prognosis

A patient is recovering from MI and is referred for supervised exercise training. While working out on a treadmill, the patient begins to develop mild shortness of breath. Upon inspection of the ECG readout, the therapist determines the presence of:

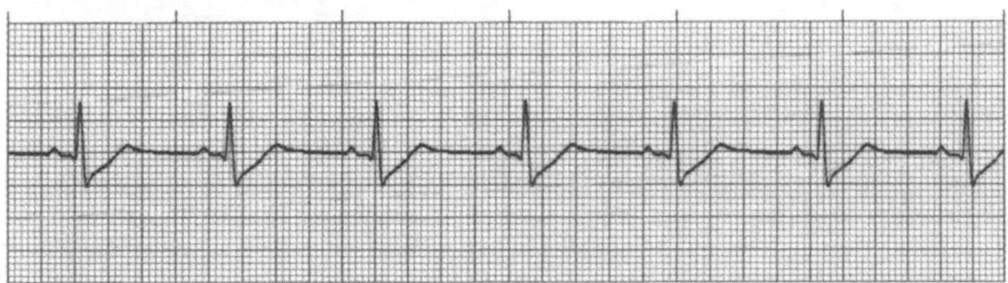

From: Jones, S (2005) ECG Notes. Philadelphia, F.A. Davis, p. 162, with permission.

CHOICES:

1. Sinus rhythm with upsloping ST segment depression.
2. Sinus rhythm with sinoatrial blocks.
3. Sinus rhythm with downsloping ST segment depression.
4. Tachycardia with abnormal P waves.

TEACHING POINTS

CORRECT ANSWER: 1

This patient is exhibiting sinus rhythm with upsloping ST segment depression. An abnormal ECG response is defined as ≥1 mm of horizontal or downsloping depression at 80 msec beyond the J point (Source: American College of Sports Medicine, *ACSM's Guidelines for Exercise Testing and Prescription,* 7th ed). Associated clinical signs suggestive of myocardial ischemia include dyspnea and angina. After a review of this patient's exercise responses coupled with the ECG findings, the therapist correctly determines that the exercise session does not have to be terminated. The therapist should continue to closely monitor the patient's responses.

INCORRECT CHOICES:

This tracing does NOT indicate the other conditions listed (sinoatrial block, downsloping ST segment depression, or tachycardia with abnormal P waves).

TYPE OF REASONING: ANALYSIS

Questions that require one to analyze visual information depicted in pictures, charts, etc., necessitates analytical reasoning skill. This question requires the test taker to appropriately interpret the ECG readout in order to determine the correct diagnosis. If this question was answered incorrectly, review ECG interpretation guidelines.

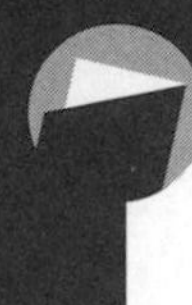

C189 | Musculoskeletal | Evaluation, Diagnosis, Prognosis

A 16 year-old boy with Duchenne's muscular dystrophy has been confined to using a power wheelchair for the past 3 years and is beginning to develop a 10-degree Cobb's angle scoliosis. The **BEST** strategy to help slow this spinal curvature at this time would be to:

CHOICES:

1. Emphasize spinal rotation exercises.
2. Alternate the side of the wheelchair power control.
3. Emphasize spinal extension exercises.
4. Order a new wheelchair with a reclining seat back.

TEACHING POINTS

CORRECT ANSWER: 2

Alternating the side of the power control will help keep upper extremity activity and sitting in the wheelchair more symmetrical.

INCORRECT CHOICES:

Trunk rotation and extension exercises will not reduce scoliosis. Lateral postural supports may be indicated. A reclining seat back is not.

TYPE OF REASONING: INDUCTIVE

One must utilize clinical judgment and diagnostic reasoning to determine the **BEST** strategy to improve the patient's scoliosis. This requires inductive reasoning skill, in which the test taker must analyze the patient's current symptoms and refer to past knowledge of the diagnosis in order to make a best course determination. For this patient, alternating the side of the wheelchair power control will **BEST** help to slow the spinal curvature.

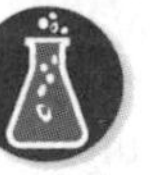

C190 | Musculoskeletal | Evaluation, Diagnosis, Prognosis

A patient presents with a complaint of severe neck and shoulder pain of 2 days' duration. The patient reports falling asleep on the couch watching TV, and has been stiff and sore since. There is tenderness of the cervical muscles on the right, with increased pain upon palpation. Passive ROM is most limited in flexion, then side-bending left, and then rotation left, and active extension. Side-bending right and rotation right arealso painful. Based on these examination findings, the patient's diagnosis is:

CHOICES:

1. Cervical radiculopathy.
2. Facet syndrome.
3. Cervical strain.
4. Herniated disc.

TEACHING POINTS

CORRECT ANSWER: 2

A facet syndrome presents with localized pain.

INCORRECT CHOICES:

Cervical radiculopathy presents with arm pain in the dermatomal distribution and increased pain by extension and rotation or side flexion. Cervical strain presents with pain on activity or when the muscle is on stretch. Cervical disc herniation has a dermatomal pain distribution with an increase of pain on extension, and pain on flexion may either increase or decrease (most common).

TYPE OF REASONING: ANALYSIS

This question requires the test taker to determine the diagnosis based on symptoms presented, which is an analytical reasoning skill. For this patient, the symptoms are indicative of facet syndrome. Knowledge of spinal disorders is required for arriving at the correct conclusion. If this question was answered incorrectly, refer to symptoms of facet syndrome.

C191 | Musculoskeletal | Intervention

A postal worker (mail sorter) complains of numbness and tingling in the right hand. Examination reveals a median nerve distribution. When the therapist evaluates the patient's work tasks, the therapist notes that the patient is required to key in the zip codes of about 58 letters/min/. An appropriate administrative control to decrease exposure would be to:

CHOICES:

1. Provide the worker with a resting splint to support the wrist.
2. Provide a height adjustable chair to position the wrists and hands in a neutral alignment.
3. Use job rotation during the workday.
4. Require the worker to attend a cumulative trauma disorder educational class.

TEACHING POINTS

CORRECT ANSWER: 3

Administrative controls reduce the duration, frequency, and severity of exposures to ergonomic stressors. Job rotation reduces fatigue and stress by rotating the worker to jobs that use different muscle-tendon groups during the workday.

INCORRECT CHOICES:

The other choices represent either clinical, engineering, or educational interventions and do not address the essential question of an administrative control.

TYPE OF REASONING: DEDUCTIVE

This question requires one to recall the parameters of an administrative control in ergonomic assessment. This is factual recall of ergonomic knowledge, which encourages the use of deductive reasoning skill. If this question was answered incorrectly, review administrative controls in ergonomic assessment.

C192 | Devices, Admin., etc. | Equipment, Modalities

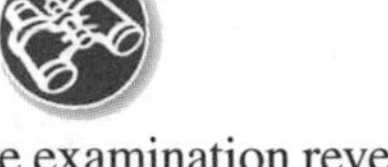

A patient with a traumatic brain injury presents with hemiparesis. The examination reveals slight cutaneous and proprioceptive impairment, fair (3/5) strength of the shoulder muscles and triceps, and slight spasticity of the biceps. Voluntary control of the patient's left arm has not progressed since admission. The therapist decides to use FES and place the active electrode on the triceps to facilitate active extension of the elbow. The timing sequence **BEST** to apply is:

CHOICES:

1. 2-sec ramp up, 5-sec stimulation, 2-sec ramp down.
2. 5-sec ramp up, 5-sec stimulation, 5-sec ramp down.
3. 2-sec ramp up, 10-sec stimulation, no ramp down.
4. No ramp up, 10-sec stimulation, 2-sec ramp down.

TEACHING POINTS

CORRECT ANSWER: 2

A relatively long ramp up time over a 5-sec period is used to minimize stimulating the muscle too quickly and increasing the spasticity. The ramp down time has no effect on spasticity.

INCORRECT CHOICES:

The other choices have too short or no ramp up time and this could increase the spasticity of the biceps.

TYPE OF REASONING: INDUCTIVE

This question requires one to predict the possible outcome of what will happen when each of the four possible approaches is applied. Via clinical judgment and the process of prediction, an inductive reasoning skill, one should determine that a 5-sec ramp up, 5-sec stimulation, and 5-sec ramp down will be **MOST** beneficial for this patient. If this question was answered incorrectly, refer to guidelines for FES for spastic upper extremities.

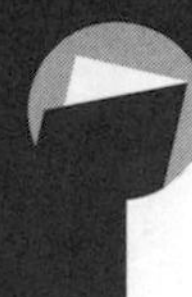

C193 | Devices, Admin., etc. | Teaching, Research, Roles

After a traumatic brain injury, a patient presents with significant difficulties in learning how to use a wheelchair. Memory for new learning is present but limited (Rancho Lelel of Cognitive Functioning, level VII). The patient is wheelchair-dependent and needs to learn how to transfer from the wheelchair to the mat (a skill never done before). The **BEST** strategy to enhance motor learning is to:

CHOICES:

1. Provide consistent feedback using a blocked practice schedule.
2. Use only guided movement to ensure correct performance.
3. Provide summed feedback after every few trials using a serial practice schedule.
4. Provide bandwidth feedback using a random practice schedule.

TEACHING POINTS

CORRECT ANSWER: 1

Early learning should focus on consistent feedback given after every trial to improve initial performance. A blocked practice schedule with repeated practice of the same skill will also reinforce early learning.

INCORRECT CHOICES:

Variable feedback schedules (summed or bandwidth) and variable practice schedules (serial and random) are indicated for later learning to improve retention. Using only guided movement is contraindicated in this case because it minimizes active participation and active learning.

TYPE OF REASONING: INFERENCE

One must infer the **BEST** strategy to enhance this patient's motor learning for transfer skills. Given the patient's current functional level, it is **BEST** to provide consistent feedback using a blocked practice schedule to reinforce early learning. Questions that require one to draw conclusions and infer strategies often utilize inferential reasoning skill. If this question was answered incorrectly, refer to strategies to enhance early learning after traumatic brain injury.

C194 | Neuromuscular | Evaluation, Diagnosis, Prognosis

A patient recovering from a CVA presents with predominant involvement of the contralateral lower extremity and lesser involvement of the contralateral upper extremity. The patient also demonstrates mild apraxia. These clinical manifestations are characteristic of:

CHOICES:

1. Middle cerebral artery syndrome.
2. Anterior cerebral artery syndrome.
3. Posterior cerebral artery syndrome.
4. Basilar artery syndrome.

TEACHING POINTS

CORRECT ANSWER: 2

These clinical manifestations are consistent with anterior cerebral artery syndrome (lower extremity is more involved than upper extremity).

INCORRECT CHOICES:

Patients with middle cerebral artery syndrome demonstrate the opposite findings, greater involvement of the upper than the lower extremity. Patients with posterior cerebral artery syndrome demonstrate primary involvement of the visual cortex (contralateral homonymous hemianopsia) along with dyslexia (difficulty reading), prosopagnosia (difficulty naming people on sight), and memory defect (temporal lobe lesion). Patients with basilar artery syndrome demonstrate a combination of brainstem syndromes along with signs of posterior cerebral artery syndrome.

TYPE OF REASONING: ANALYSIS

This question requires the test taker to determine the location of the patient's CVA based on symptoms presented, which is an analytical reasoning skill. Knowledge of neuroscience and the various arterial syndromes related to CVA are beneficial for arriving at the correct conclusion. If this question was answered incorrectly, refer to symptoms of cerebral artery syndromes.

C195 | Cardiovascular-Pulmonary | Evaluation, Diagnosis, Prognosis

A patient presents with significant intermittent claudication with onset after 2 minutes of walking. On further examination, the therapist would expect to find:

CHOICES:

1. Brownish color just above the ankle in both gravity-dependent and -independent positions.
2. Little or no changes in color with changes in extremity position.
3. Persistent local redness of the extremity in both gravity-dependent and -independent positions.
4. Elevation-induced pallor and dependent redness with the extremity in the gravity-dependent position.

TEACHING POINTS

CORRECT ANSWER: 4

Intermittent claudication (episodic muscular ischemia induced by exercise) is due to obstruction of large or middle-sized arteries by atherosclerosis. The rubor of dependency test is used to assess the adequacy of arterial circulation by evaluating the skin color changes that occur with first extremity elevation (pallor) and then lowering of the extremities (delayed color changes, redness).

INCORRECT CHOICES:

Color changes are expected with change of position. Brownish color just above the ankle suggests chronic venous insufficiency. Persistent local redness is indicative of a thrombosed vein in the area.

TYPE OF REASONING: INFERENCE

One must infer the likely findings for this patient, given that the patient's symptoms are in response to walking. It is beneficial to have prior knowledge of the rubor of dependency test in order to arrive at the correct conclusion. Through inferential reasoning, one should conclude that the patient would demonstrate elevation-induced pallor and dependent redness with the extremity in a gravity dependent position. If this question was answered incorrectly, review examination of the patient with PVD.

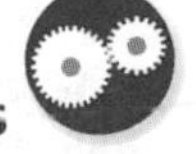

C196 | Other Systems | Evaluation, Diagnosis, Prognosis

After her cesarean section, a patient tells the therapist that she is anxious to return to her prepregnancy level of physical activity (working out at the gym 3 days/wk and running 5 miles every other day). The therapist's **BEST** advice is to tell her to resume activities with:

CHOICES:

1. Pelvic floor exercises and refrain from all other exercise and running for at least 12 weeks.
2. Pelvic floor and gentle abdominal exercises for the first 4–6 weeks.
3. Abdominal crunches with return to running after 5 weeks.
4. A walking program progressing to running after 4 weeks.

TEACHING POINTS

CORRECT ANSWER: 2

Postcesarean physical therapy can include postoperative TENS, assisted breathing and coughing techniques, and gentle abdominal exercises with incisional support provided by a pillow. Pelvic floor exercises are also important because hours of labor and pushing are typically present before surgery.

INCORRECT CHOICES:

Vigorous exercise (abdominal crunches, running) is contraindicated for at least 6 weeks. Without complications, 12 weeks is too long to refrain from exercises and running.

TYPE OF REASONING: EVALUATION

This question requires one to evaluate the merits of each of the four statements and then determine which response to the patient is **BEST** given her recent cesarean section. Evaluative reasoning skills are utilized whenever one must make value judgments and assess the worth of ideas presented. If this question was answered incorrectly, refer to guidelines on exercise for women postpartum.

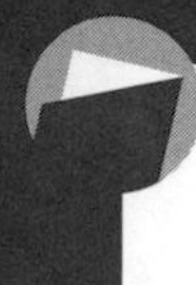

C197 | Other Systems | Evaluation, Diagnosis, Prognosis

A 26 year-old who was diagnosed with schizophrenia, disorganized type, at the age of 22 is referred for gait training after a compound fracture of the tibia. The individual recently experienced an exacerbation of the condition. The therapist recognizes this from the patient's demonstrated behaviors, which include:

CHOICES:

1. Sleep disturbances and flashbacks.
2. Increased fear of going out in public.
3. Frequent verbalizations of pervasive feelings of low self-esteem.
4. Poor ability to perform multistep tasks requiring abstract problem solving.

TEACHING POINTS

CORRECT ANSWER: 4

Schizophrenia is characterized by disordered thinking (fragmented thoughts, errors of logic or abstract reasoning, delusions, poor judgment, and so forth).

INCORRECT CHOICES:

Sleep disturbances and flashbacks are common with posttraumatic stress disorder. Increased fear of going out in public is agoraphobia. Pervasive feelings of low self-esteem can accompany depression or anxiety disorder.

TYPE OF REASONING: INFERENCE

This question requires one to infer or draw a conclusion about the likely symptoms of disorganized schizophrenia. This necessitates inferential reasoning skill. For this situation, the therapist should expect behaviors of poor ability to perform multistep tasks requiring abstract problem solving. If this question was answered incorrectly, review symptoms of schizophrenia, especially disorganized type.

C198 | Devices, Admin., etc. | Equipment, Modalities

The rehabilitation team is completing a home visit to recommend environmental modifications for a patient who is scheduled to be discharged next week. The patient is wheelchair-dependent. The home has not been adapted. Which of the following recommendations is correct?

CHOICES:

1. Installing a entry way ramp with a running slope of 1:10.
2. Widening the door entrance to 28 inches.
3. Adding horizontal grab bars in the bathroom positioned at 34 inches.
4. Raising the toilet seat to 25 inches.

TEACHING POINTS

CORRECT ANSWER: 3

Horizontal grab bars should be positioned at an optimal height of 33–36 inches.

INCORRECT CHOICES:

The minimum ramp grade (slope) is 1:12 (not 1:10, which would be too steep for functional use). The toilet seat should be raised to a height of 17–19 inches (not 25). Minimum clearance width for doorways is 32 inches (not 28); 36 inches is ideal.

TYPE OF REASONING: INFERENCE

This question requires one to determine appropriate recommendations for patients utilizing wheelchairs for mobility in the home. This necessitates recall of factual knowledge and clinical judgment, which is an inferential reasoning skill. If this question was answered incorrectly, review guidelines for environmental (home) modifications for patients utilizing wheelchairs for mobility.

C199 | Musculoskeletal | Patient Examination 

During an examination of gait, the therapist observes lateral pelvic tilt on the side of the swing leg during frontal plane analysis. The therapist recognizes this finding functions to:

CHOICES:

1. Control forward and backward rotations of the pelvis.
2. Reduce peak rise of the pelvis.
3. Reduce physiological valgum at the knee.
4. Reduce knee flexion at mid stance.

TEACHING POINTS

CORRECT ANSWER: 2

Lateral pelvic tilt in the frontal plane keeps the peak of the sinusoidal curve lower than it would have been if the pelvis did not drop. Lateral pelvic tilt to the right is controlled by the left hip abductors.

INCORRECT CHOICES:

Forward and backward rotations of the pelvis assist the swing leg. The normal physiologic valgum at the knee reduces the width of the base of support. Knee flexion at midstance is another adjustment in keeping the center of gravity from rising too much. All are termed determinants of gait.

TYPE OF REASONING: INFERENCE

One must infer the purpose of the lateral pelvic tilt on the side of the swing leg during gait in order to arrive at the correct conclusion. This necessitates inferential reasoning skill, where one must draw conclusions based on the evidence presented. If this question was answered incorrectly, review gait analysis guidelines.

C200 | Devices, Admin., etc. | Teaching, Research, Roles 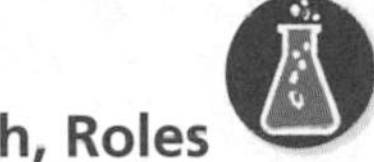

A group of researchers investigated the effect of tai chi on perceived health status in older, frail adults. The subjects were 269 women who were older than 70 years of age and recruited from five independent senior living facilites. Participants took part in a 48-week single-blind RCT. Perceived health status was measured by five pretrained testers using the Sickness Impact Profile (SIP). The researchers found significant perceived health benefits. Analysis of the design reveals:

CHOICES:

1. Limited generalizibility to a larger population.
2. Important findings on the effects of tai chi exercise in the frail elderly.
3. Errors in validity due to the selection of the outcome measure.
4. Errors in reliability due to the number of testers.

TEACHING POINTS

CORRECT ANSWER: 2

This study provides important findings on the effects ot tai chi in the elderly. It has a large number of subjects from multiple centers and thus has good generalizability (not limited). The SIP is a gold standard instrument with extensive testing and established validity and reliability.

INCORRECT CHOICES:

Errors in reliability are not automatically inherent with multiple testers. Pretrial training reduces the likelihood of errors in reliability. There is no error in validity because of the use of the SIP.

TYPE OF REASONING: ANALYSIS

This question requires the test taker to analyze the design of the research study and then draw a conclusion about this design. This necessitates analysis of many factors, which is an analytical reasoning skill. For this scenario, the test taker should reasonably conclude that the study had good generalizability due to the number of subjects in the study and multiple centers involved in the study and good validity and reliability. If this question was answered incorrectly, review research design guidelines.

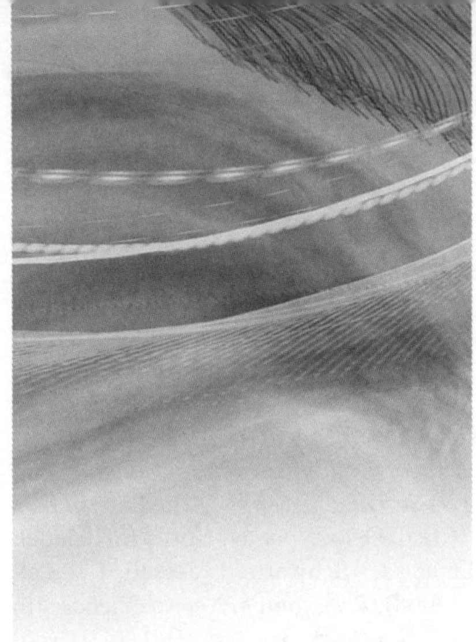

References

Adler S, Beckers D, Buck M (2008). *PNF in Practice*, 3rd ed. New York, Springer.

American College of Sports Medicine (2009). *ACSM's Exercise Management for Persons with Chronic Diseases and Disabilities*, 3rd ed. Resources for Clinical Exercise Physiology. Philadelphia, Lippincott Williams & Wilkins.

American College of Sports Medicine (2009). *ACSM's Guidelines for Exercise Testing and Prescription*, 8th ed. Philadelphia, Lippincott Williams & Wilkins.

American Physical Therapy Association (2001). *Guide to Physical Therapist Practice*, 2nd ed. Alexandria, VA, APTA.

American Physical Therapy Association. *Occupational Health Physical Therapy Guidelines: Prevention of Work-Related Injury/Illness*. Initial BOD11-99-25-71, APTA;

The Role of the Physical Therapist in Occupational Health. BOD 03-97-27-71, APTA;

Physical Therapist Management of the Acutely Injured Worker. BOD 03-01-17-56, APTA;

Evaluation Functional Capacity. BOD11-01-07-11, APTA;

Work Conditioning and Work Hardening Programs. BOD 03-01-17-58, APTA.

Andrews J, Wilk K, Harrelson G (2004). *Physical Rehabilitation of the Injured Athlete*, 3rd ed. Philadelphia, Elsevier Saunders.

Baranoski S, Ayello E (2007). *Wound Care Essentials: Practice & Principles*, 2nd ed. Philadelphia, Lippincott Williams & Wilkins.

Batavia M. (2000). *Clinical Research for Health Professionals: A User-Friendly Guide*. Boston, Butterworth-Heinemann.

Batavia M. (2006). *Contraindications in Physical Rehabilitation—Doing No Harm*. St Louis, Elsevier Saunders.

Bear M, Connors B, Paradiso M (2007). *Neuroscience—Exploring the Brain*, 3rd ed. Philadelphia, Lippincott Williams & Wilkins.

Behrens B, Michlovitz S (2005). *Physical Agents: Theory & Practice*, 2nd ed. Philadelphia, FA Davis.

Belanger AY (2002). *Evidence-Based Guide to Therapeutic Physical Agents*. Philadelphia, Lippincott Williams & Wilkins.

Bickley L (2009). *Bates' Guide to Physical Examination and History Taking*, 10th ed. Philadelphia, Lippincott Williams & Wilkins.

Bloom, B, Krathwohl, D et al. (1956). *Taxonomy of Educational Objectives: Handbook I, Cognitive Domain and Handbook II, Affective Domain.* New York, David McKay Co.

Boissonnault W (2010). *Primary Care for the Physical Therapist—Examination and Triage*, 2nd ed. St Louis, Elsevier Saunders.

Brotzman S (2007). *Handbook of Orthopaedic Rehabilitation*, 2nd ed. St Louis, Elsevier Mosby.

Brown S, Miller W, Eason J (2005). *Exercise Physiology Basis of Human Movement in Health and Disease*. Philadelphia, Lippincott Williams & Wilkins.

Cameron M (2008). *Physical Agents in Rehabilitation*, 3rd ed. St Louis, Elsevier Saunders.

Campbell S (2006). *Physical Therapy for Children*, 3rd ed. St Louis, Elsevier Saunders.

Carroll K, Edelstein J (2006). *Prosthetics and Patient Management: A Comprehensive Clinical Approach.* Thorofare NJ, Slack Inc.

Carter R, Lubinski J, Domholdt E (2010). *Rehabilitation Research: Principles and Applications,* 4th ed. St Louis, Elsevier Saunders.

Chaffin D, Andersson G, Martin B (2006). *Occupational Biomechanics*, 4th ed. New York, John Wiley & Sons.

Childs J, Cleland J, Elliott J, et al (2008). Neck Pain. Clinical Practice Guidelines Linked to International Classification of Functioning, Disability, and Health from the Orthopaedic Section of the American Physical Therapy Association. J Orthop Sports Phys Ther 38(9): A1–A31.

Cibulka M, White D, Woehrle J (2009). Hip Pain and Mobility Deficits – Hip Osteoarthritis. Clinical Practice Guidelines Linked to International Classification of Functioning, Disability, and Health from the Orthopaedic Section of the American Physical Therapy Association. J Orthop Sports Phys Ther 39(4): A1–A25.

Ciccone C (2007). *Pharmacology in Rehabilitation,* 4th ed. Philadelphia, FA Davis.

Cleland, J. (2007). *Orthopaedic Clinical Examination: An Evidence-Based Approach for Physical Therapists.* Philadelphia: Saunders, an Imprint of Elsevier.

Cook C (2006). *Orthopedic Manual Therapy: An Evidence-Based Approach.* Upper Saddle River, NJ, Pearson Education.

Davies P (2000). *Steps to Follow*, 3rd ed. New York, Springer.

Davis C (2006). *Patient Practitioner Interaction*, 4th ed. Thorofare, NJ, Slack.

DeDomenico G (2008). *Beard's Massage*, 5th ed. St Louis, Elsevier.

Deglin J, Vallerand A (2009). *FA Davis's Drug Guide for Nurses*, 11th ed. Philadelphia, FA Davis.

Denegar C, Saliba E, Saliba S (2006) *Therapeutic Modalities for Musculoskeletal Injuries*, 2nd ed. Champaign, IL, Human Kinetics.

DeTurk W, Cahalin L (2010). *Cardiovascular and Pulmonary Physical*

Therapy, 2nd ed. New York, McGraw-Hill.

Domholdt E (2005). *Rehabilitation Research: Principles and Applications*, 3rd ed. St Louis, Elsevier Saunders.

Donatelli R (2007) *Sports-Specific Rehabilitation*. St Louis, Elsevier.

Donatelli R, Wooden M (2009). *Orthopedic Physical Therapy*, 4th ed. New York, Churchill Livingstone.

Drake R, et al (2008) *Gray's Atlas of Anatomy*. Maryland Heights, MO, Elsevier.

Drench M, Noonan A, Sharby N, Ventura S (2012). *Psychosocial Aspects of Health Care*, 3rd ed. Upper Saddle River, NJ, Prentice Hall.

Durstine J, Moore, G, Durstine (2002). ACSM's Exercise Management for Persons with Chronic Diseases and Disabilities. Champaign, IL, Human Kinetics.

Dutton M (2008). *Orthopaedic Examination, Evaluation, and Intervention*, 2nd ed. New York, McGraw-Hill.

Edelstein J, Moroz A (2010). *Lower-Limb Prosthetics and Orthotics: Clinical Concepts. Thorofare NJ, Slack Inc.*

Effgen S (2005). *Meeting the Physical Therapy Needs of Children*. Philadelphia, FA Davis.

Erickson M, McKnight B, Utzman R (2008). *Physical Therapy Documentation: From Examination to Outcome*. Thorofare, NJ, Slack.

Erkonen, WE. (1998). Radiology 101: *The basics and fundamentals of imaging*. Philadelphia, Lippincott, Williams & Wilkins.

Field-Fote E (2009). *Spinal Cord Injury Rehabilitation*. Philadelphia, F A Davis.

Finch E, Brooks D, Stratford P, et al. (2002). *Physical Rehabilitation Outcome Measures: A Guide to Enhanced Clinical Decision Making*, 2nd ed. Toronto, Canadian Physiotherapy Association.

Frontera W, Slovik D, Dawson D (eds) (2006). *Exercise in Rehabilitation Medicine*, 2nd ed. Champaign, IL, Human Kinetics.

Frownfelter D, Dean E (2006). *Cardiovascular and Pulmonary Physical Therapy: Evidence and Practice*, 4th ed. St Louis, Elsevier Mosby.

Gabard D, Martin M (2003). *Physical Therapy Ethics*. Philadelphia, FA Davis.

Goodman C, Fuller K (2009). *Pathology: Implications for the Physical Therapist*, 3rd ed. St Louis, Elsevier Saunders.

Goodman C, Snyder T (2007). *Differential Diagnosis in Physical Therapy: Screening for Referral,* 4th ed. St Louis, Elsevier Saunders.

Griffin L (2005). *Essentials of Musculoskeletal Care*, 3rd ed. Rosemont, IL, American Academy of Orthopedic Surgeons.

Gutman S (2008). *Quick Reference Neuroscience for Rehabilitation Professionals: The Essential Neurological Principles Underlying Rehabilitation Professionals*, 2nd ed. Thorofare, NJ, Slack.

Guyton A, Hall J (2006). *Textbook of Medical Physiology*, 10th ed. St Louis, Elsevier Saunders.

Hall C, Brody L (2004). *Therapeutic Exercise: Moving Toward Function*, 2nd ed. Philadelphia, Lippincott Williams & Wilkins.

Hengveld E, Banks K (2005). *Maitland's Peripheral Manipulation*. 4th ed. Philadelphia: Elsevier.

Hertling D, Kessler R (2006). *Management of Common Musculoskeletal Disorders: Physical Therapy Principles and Methods*, 4th ed. Philadelphia, Lippincott Williams & Wilkins.

Hillegass E, Sadowsky H (2001). *Essentials of Cardiopulmonary Physical Therapy*, 2nd ed. St Louis, Elsevier Saunders.

Hislop H, Montgomery J (2007). *Daniels and Worthingham's Muscle Testing: Techniques of Manual Examination*, 8th ed. St Louis, Elsevier Saunders.

Hoppenfeld S (1982). *Physical Evaluation of the Spine and Extremities*. New York, Appleton-Century-Crofts.

Howle J (2002). *Neuro-Developmental Treatment Approach: Theoretical Foundations and Principles of Clinical Practice*. Laguna Beach, CA, Neuro-Developmental Treatment Association.

Huber F, Wells C (2006). *Therapeutic Exercise—Treatment Planning for Progression*. St Louis, Elsevier Saunders.

Irion G (2009). *Comprehensive Wound Management*, 2nd ed. Thorofare, NJ, Slack.

Irion J, Irion G (2009). *Women's Health in Physical Therapy*. Baltimore, Lippincott Williams & Wilkins, Wolters Kluwer.

Irwin S, Tecklin J (2004). *Cardiopulmonary Physical Therapy*, 4th ed. St Louis, Elsevier Mosby.

Jenkins D (2009). *Hollinshead's Functional Anatomy of the Limbs and Back*, 9th ed. Maryland Heights, MO, Elsevier.

Jewell D (2008). *Guide to Evidence-Based Physical Therapy Practice*. Sudbury, MA, Jones & Bartlett.

Kaltenborn F (2003). *Manual Mobilization of the Joints*. The Spine, 4th ed. Oslo, Norway,Olaf Norlis Bokhandel.

Kaltenborn F (2007). *Manual Mobilization of the Joints. Vol 1*. The Extremities, 6th ed. Oslo, Norway,Olaf Norlis Bokhandel.

Kaltenborn FM (2003). *Manual Mobilization of the Joints: The Kaltenborn Method of Joint Examination and Treatment, Vol 2*. The Spine. 4th ed. Oslo, Norway: Norlis Bokhandel.

Kaltenborn FM (2007). *Manual Mobilization of the Joints: Joint Examination and Basic Treatment. Vol 1,* The Extremities. 6th ed. Oslo, Norway: Norlis Bokhandel.

Kandel E, Schwartz J, Jessell T, et al. (2008). *Principles of Neural Science*, 4th ed. New York, McGraw-Hill.

Kauffman T, Barr J, Moran M (2007). *Geriatric Rehabilitation Manual*, 2nd ed. St Louis, Elsevier Health Sciences.

Kendall F, McCreary E, Provance P, et al (2005). *Muscle Testing and Function*, 5th ed. Philadelphia, Lippincott Williams & Wilkins.

Kiernan J (2006). *Barr's The Human Nervous System: An Anatomical Viewpoint*, 8th ed. Philadelphia, Lippincott Williams & Wilkins.

Kisner C, Colby L (2007). *Therapeutic Exercise Foundations and Techniques*, 5th ed. Philadelphia, FA Davis.

Kitchen S (2002). Electrotherapy: *Evidence-Based Practice*, 2nd ed. St Louis, Elsevier Mosby.

Kizior R, Hodgson B (2009). *Saunders Drug Handbook for Health Professionals*. St Louis, Elsevier Saunders.

Kloth L, McCulloch J (2002). *Wound Healing: Alternatives in Management*, 3rd ed. Philadelphia, FA Davis.

Kolt G, Snyder-Mackler L (2007). *Physical Therapies in Sport and Exercise*, 2nd ed. St Louis, Elsevier Churchill Livingstone.

Lacy C, Amstrong L, Goldman M, et al (2007). *Drug Information Handbook*, 15th ed. Hudson, OH, Lexi-Comp.

Law M, MacDermid J (2007). *Evidence-Based Rehabilitation: A Guide to Practice*, 2nd ed. Thorofare, NJ, Slack.

Leavitt R, ed. (1999). *Cross-cultural Rehabilitation: An International Perspective*. St Louis, Elsevier Saunders.

Levangie P, Norkin C (2011). *Joint Structure and Function: A Comprehensive Analysis*, 5th ed. Philadelphia, FA Davis.

LeVeau B (2010) *Biomechanics of Human Motion: Basics and Beyond for the Health Professions*. Thorofare NY, Slack Inc

Lewis C, Bottomley J, (2007). *Geriatric Rehabilitation—A Clinical Approach*, 3rd ed. Upper Saddle River, NJ, Pearson Education.

Logerstedt D, Snyder-Mackler L, Ritter R et al. (2010). Knee Pain and Mobility

Impairments: Meniscal and Articular Cartilage Lesions. Clinical Practice Guidelines Linked to International Classification of Functioning, Disability, and Health from the Orthopaedic Section of the American Physical Therapy Association. J Orthop Sports Phys Ther 40(6): A1–A35.

Long T, Toscanok (2001). *Handbook of Pediatric Physical Therapy*, 2nd ed. Baltimore, Lippincott Williams & Wilkins.

Lundy-Ekman L (2007). *Neuroscience Fundamentals for Rehabilitation*, 3rd ed. St Louis, Elsevier Saunders.

Lusardi MM, Nielsen CC (eds) (2006). *Orthotics and Prosthetics in Rehabilitation*, 2nd ed. St Louis, Elsevier Butterworth-Heinemann.

Magee D (2008). *Orthopedic Physical Assessment*, 5th ed. St Louis, Elsevier Saunders.

Magee D, Zachazewski J, Quillen W (2007). *Scientific Foundations and Principles of Practice in Musculoskeletal Rehabilitation*. St Louis, Elsevier Saunders.

Magee D, Zachazewski J, Quillen W (2009). *Pathology and Intervention in Musculoskeletal Rehabilitation*. St Louis, Elsevier Saunders.

Maitland GD (2005). *Maitland's Peripheral Manipulation*. 4th ed. Philadelphia: Elsevier.

Maitland GD (2005). *Maitland's Vertebral Manipulation*. 7th ed. Philadelphia: Elsevier.

Malone D, Lindsay K (2006). *Physical Therapy in Acute Care: A Clinician's Guide*. Thorofare, NJ, Slack.

Malone, TR, Hazle, C, and Grey, ML (2008). *Imaging in rehabilitation*. New York, McGraw-Hill.

Martin S, Kessler M (2006). *Neurologic Interventions for Physical Therapy*, 2nd ed. St Louis, Elsevier Saunders.

McArdle W, Katch F, Katch V (2006). *Exercise Physiology: Energy, Nutrition and Human Performance*, 5th ed. Philadelphia, Lippincott Williams & Wilkins.

McCulloch J, Kloth L (2010). *Wound Healing: Evidence-Based Management* (Contemporary Perspectives in Rehabilitation, 4th ed. Philadelphia, FA Davis.

McKinnis L (2010). *Fundamentals of Musculoskeletal Imaging*, 3rd ed. Philadelphia, FA Davis.

McPoil T, Martin R, RnWa, M (2008). Heel Pain – Plantar Fasciitis. Clinical Practice Guidelines Linked to International Classification of Functioning, Disability, and Health from the Orthopaedic Section of the American Physical Therapy Association. J Orthop Sports Phys Ther 38(4): A1–A18.

Michlovitz S (2011). *Modalities for Therapeutic Intervention*, 5th ed. Philadelphia, FA Davis.

Minor SM, Minor MS (2010). *Patient Care Skills*, 6th ed. Upper Saddle River, NJ, Prentice Hall Health.

Moore K (2006). *Clinically Oriented Anatomy*, 5th ed. Baltimore, Lippincott Williams & Wilkins.

Myers B (2012). *Wound Management: Principles and Practice*, 3rd ed. Upper Saddle River, NJ, Prentice Hall.

Netter FH (2010) *Atlas of Human Anatomy*, 5th ed. St Louis, Saunders Elsevier.

Neumann DA (2009). *Kinesiology of the Musculoskeletal System: Foundations for Physical Rehabilitation*, 2nd 3rd.. St Louis, Elsevier Mosby.

Nordin M, Frankel (2001). *Basic Biomechanics of the Musculoskeletal System*. Philadelphia, Lippincott Williams & Wilkins.

Norkin C, White J (2009). *Measurement of Joint Motion: A Guide to Goniometry*, 4th ed. Philadelphia, FA Davis.

Nosse L, Friberg D (2004). *Managerial and Supervisory Principles for Physical Therapists*, 2nd ed. Philadelphia, Lippincott Willliams & Wilkins.

Nyland J (2006). *Clinical Decisions in Therapeutic Exercise—Planning and Implementation*. Upper Saddle River NJ, Pearson Prentice Hall.

Oatis C (2008). *Kinesiology: The Mechanics & Pathomechanics of Human Movement*. Philadelphia, Lippincott Williams & Wilkins.

OConnell D, OConnell J, Hinman M (2011). *Special Tests of Cardiopulmonary, Vascular and Gastrointestinal Systems*. Thorofare NJ, Slack Inc.

Olson KA (2009). *Manual Physical Therapy of the Spine*. St. Louis: Saunders, an Imprint of Elsevier.

O'Sullivan S, Schmitz T (2007). *Physical Rehabilitation*, 5th ed. Philadelphia, F A Davis.

O'Sullivan S, Schmitz T (2010). *Improving Functional Outcomes in Physical Rehabilitation*. Philadelphia, FA Davis.

Pagliarulo M (2007). *Introduction to Physical Therapy*, 3rd ed. St Louis, Elsevier Mosby.

Paz J, West M (2008). *Acute Care Handbook for Physical Therapists*, 3rd ed. St Louis, Elsevier Butterworth-Heinneman.

Perry J, Burnfield J (2010) *Gait Analysis – Normal and Pathological Function*, 2nd ed. Thorofare NJ, Slack Inc.

Pierson F, Fairchild S (2008). *Principles and Techniques of Patient Care*, 4th ed. St Louis, Elsevier Saunders.

Porth C (2005). *Pathophysiology*, 7th ed. Philadelphia, Lippincott Williams & Wilkins.

Portney L, Watkins M (2008). *Foundations of Clinical Research*, 3rd ed. Upper Saddle River, NJ, Prentice Hall Health.

Prentice Q (2011). *Therapeutic Modalities for Allied Health Professionals*, 4th ed. New York, McGraw-Hill Medical.

Purtilo R (2005). *Ethical Dimensions in the Health Professions*, 4th ed. St Louis, Elsevier.

Purtilo R, Haddad A (2007). Health Professional and Patient Interaction, 7th ed. St Louis, Elsevier Saunders.

Quinn L, Gordon J (2009). *Documentation for Rehabilitation: A Framework for Clinical Decision-Making*, 2nd ed. Maryland Heights, MO, Elsevier.

Reese N (2011). *Muscle and Sensory Testing*, 3rd ed. St Louis, Elsevier Saunders.

Reese N B, Bandy WD (2009). *Joint Range of Motion and Muscle Length*, 2nd ed. St Louis, Elsevier Saunders.

Robertson V, Ward A, Law J, Reed A (2006). *Electrotherapy Explained: Principles and Practice*, 3rd ed. Philadelphia, Butterworth-Heinemann.

Robinson A, Snyder-Mackler L (2008). *Clinical Electrophysiology – Electrotherapy and Electrophysiologic Testing*, 3rd ed. Philadelphia, Lippincott Williams & Wilkins.

Rothstein J, Roy S, Wolf S (2005). *The Rehabilitation Specialist's Handbook*, 3rd ed. Philadelphia, FA Davis.

Rubin M, Safdieh J (2007). *Netter's Concise Neuroanatomy*. St Louis, Elsevier Health Sciences.

Sahrmann S (2010). *Diagnosis and Treatment of Movement System Impairment Syndromes of the Extremities, Cervical and Thoracic Spines*. St Louis, Elsevier. Mosby.

Saidoff D, McDonough A (2002). *Critical Pathways in Therapeutic Intervention—Extremities and Spine*. St Louis, Elsevier Mosby.

Salter R (1999). *Textbook of Disorders and Injuries of the Musculoskeletal System*, 3rd ed. Baltimore, Williams & Wilkins.

Saunders H, Saunders R (eds) (2004). *Evaluation, Treatment and Prevention of Musculoskeletal Disorders & Spine*, 4th ed. Chaska, MN, Saunders Group.

Schmidt R, Lee T (2005). *Motor Control and Learning*, 4th ed. Champaign, IL, Human Kinetics.

Scifers J (2008). *Special Tests for Neurologic Examination*. Thorofare, NJ, Slack.

Scott R (1998). *Professional Ethics: A Guide for Rehabilitation Professionals*. St. Louis, Elsevier Mosby.

Scott R (2006). *Legal Aspects of Documenting Patient Care for Rehabilitation Professionals*, 3rd ed. Boston, Jones & Barlett.

Scott R, Petrosinol L (2008). *Physical Therapy Management*. St Louis, Elsevier Mosby.

Scuderi G, McCann P, Bruno P (eds) (2005). *Sports Medicine*, 2nd ed. St. Louis, Elsevier Mosby.

Seymour R (2002). *Prosthetics and Orthotics: Lower Limb and Spinal*. Philadelphia, Lippincott Williams & Wilkins.

Shepard K, Jensen G (2002). *Handbook of Teaching for Physical Therapists*, 2nd ed. St Louis, Elsevier Butterworth-Heinemann.

Shumway-Cook A, Woollacott M (2012). *Motor Control—Theory and Practical Applications*, 4th ed. Philadelphia, Lippincott Williams & Wilkins.

Shurr D, Michael J (2001). *Prosthetics and Orthotics*, 2nd ed. Upper Saddle River, NJ, Prentice Hall.

Snell R (2005). *Clinical Neuroanatomy for Medical Students*, 6th ed. Philadelphia, Lippincott Williams & Wilkins.

Somers M (2009). *Spinal Cord Injury Rehabilitation*, 3rd ed. Upper Saddle River, NJ, Prentice Hall.

Standring S (2008). *Gray's Anatomy: The Anatomical Basis of Clinical Practice*. St Louis, Elsevier Churchill Livingstone.

Starkey C and Johnson G (2005). *Athletic Training and Sports Medicine*. American Academy of Orthopedic Medicine. Sudbury MA, Jones and Bartlett.

Starkey C, Ryan J (2009). *Evaluation of Orthopedic and Athletic Injuries*, 3rd ed. Philadelphia, FA Davis.

Stephenson R, O'Connor L (2000) *Obstetric and Gynecologic Care in Physical Therapy*, 2nd ed. Thorofare, NJ, Slack.

Straus S, Sackett, D, et al. (2011). *Evidence-Based Medicine*, 4th ed. Philadelphia, Churchill Livingstone.

Sussman C, Bates-Jenson B (2006). *Wound Care: A Collaborative Practice Manual for Physical Therapists and Nurses*, 3rd ed. Philadelphia, Lippincott Williams & Wilkins.

Swain J, Bush K, Brosing J (2009). *Diagnostic Imaging for Physical Therapists*. St Louis, Elsevier.

Tecklin J (2007). *Pediatric Physical Therapy*, 4th ed. Philadelphia, Lippincott Williams & Wilkins.

Thompson JC (2001). *Netter's Concise Atlas of Orthopedic Anatomy*. St Louis, Elsevier.

Umphred D (ed) (2007). *Neurological Rehabilitation*, 5th ed. St Louis, Elsevier Mosby.

Watchie J (2009). *Cardiovascular and Pulmonary Physical Therapy: A Clinical Manual*, 2nd ed. Maryland Heights, MO, Elsevier.

Watson T (ed) (2008). *Electrotherapy: Evidenced-Based Practice*, 12th ed. St Louis, Churchill Livingston Elsevier.

Waxman S (2002). *Correlative Neuroanatomy*, 25th ed. New York, McGraw-Hill.

Whittle M (2007). *Gait Analysis*, 4th ed. St Louis, Elsevier.

Wilmore J, Costill D, Kenney W (2007). *Physiology of Sport and Exercise*, 4th ed. Champaign, IL, Human Kinetics.

Wong M (2009). *Pocket Orthopaedics: Evidence-Based Survival Guide*. Sudbury MA, Jones and Bartlett Pub.

Young P, Young P, Tolbert D (2007). *Basic Clinical Neuroscience*. Philadelphia, Lippincott Williams & Wilkins.

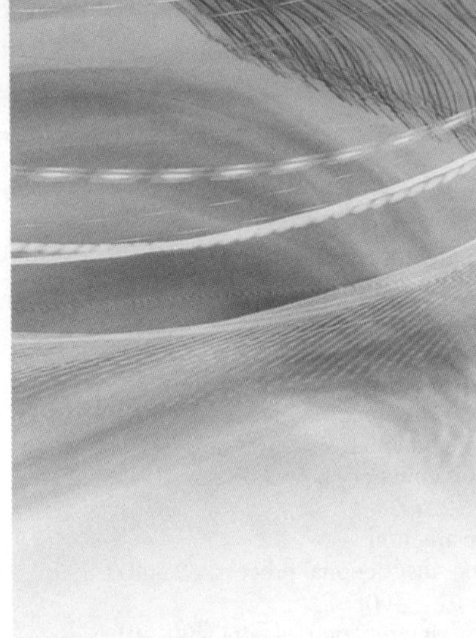

Index

Page numbers followed by f and t indicate figures and tables.